The Essential Guide to Prescription Drugs

THE ESSENTIAL GUIDE TO PRESCRIPTION DRUGS

1996 EDITION

James J. Rybacki, Pharm. D.
James W. Long, M.D.

HarperPerennial
A Division of HarperCollins *Publishers*

THE ESSENTIAL GUIDE TO PRESCRIPTION DRUGS 1996. Copyright © 1996 by James J. Rybacki and James W. Long. Copyright © 1994 by James W. Long and James J. Rybacki. Copyright © 1977, 1980, 1982, 1985, 1987, 1988, 1989, 1990, 1991, 1992, 1993 by James W. Long. All rights reserved. Printed in the United States of America. No part of this book may be used or reproduced in any manner whatsoever without written permission except in the case of brief quotations embodied in critical articles and reviews. For information address HarperCollins Publishers Inc., 10 East 53rd Street, New York, NY 10022.

HarperCollins books may be purchased for educational, business, or sales promotional use. For information please write: Special Markets Department, HarperCollins Publishers Inc., 10 East 53rd Street, New York, NY 10022.

Designed by C. Linda Dingler

ISSN 0894–7058
ISBN 0–06–271600-X

Contents

Author's Note for the 1996 Edition — vii
Points for Consideration by the Patient — xi
Points for Consideration by the Pharmacist — xv
Points for Consideration by the Physician — xix

SECTION ONE:

1. How to Use This Book — 3
2. Guidelines for Safe and Effective Drug Use — 14
   - Do Not — 14
   - Do — 15
   - Preventing Adverse Drug Reactions — 16
   - Drugs and the Elderly — 19
   - Therapeutic Drug Monitoring (Measuring Drug Levels in Blood) — 21

SECTION TWO:
Drug Profiles — 25

SECTION THREE:
The Leading Edge — 1057

SECTION FOUR:
Drug Classes — 1059

SECTION FIVE:
A Glossary of Drug-Related Terms   **1075**

SECTION SIX:
Tables of Drug Information   **1097**

1. Drugs That May Adversely Affect the Fetus and Newborn Infant   1099
2. Drugs That May Cause Photosensitivity on Exposure to Sun   1100
3. Drugs That May Adversely Affect Behavior   1100
4. Drugs That May Adversely Affect Vision   1103
5. Drugs That May Cause Blood Cell Dysfunction or Damage   1105
6. Drugs That May Cause Heart Dysfunction or Damage   1107
7. Drugs That May Cause Lung Dysfunction or Damage   1108
8. Drugs That May Cause Liver Dysfunction or Damage   1110
9. Drugs That May Cause Kidney Dysfunction or Damage   1112
10. Drugs That May Cause Nerve Dysfunction or Damage   1114
11. Drugs That May Adversely Affect Sexuality   1115
12. Drugs That May Interact With Alcohol   1120
13. High-Potassium Foods   1124
14. Your Personal Drug Profile   1125

Sources   **1127**

Index   **1131**

About the Authors   **1157**

Controlled Drug Classes   **1159**

Pregnancy Risk Categories   **1160**

Author's Note for the 1996 Edition

This edition marks a bold new direction for *The Essential Guide to Prescription Drugs*. So many loyal readers have asked for coverage of a greater and greater number of medicines that we had to make a decision. Dr. James Long and I have decided to expand the number of medicines and type of information that can be provided. We are accomplishing this goal by creating a separate book for information on chronic disorders. Dr. Long is at work on *The Essential Guide To Chronic Disorders* to provide broad and extensive information on chronic disorders. *The Essential Guide To Prescription Drugs* continues to use Dr. Long's excellent framework to provide expanded coverage of more drugs than possible before and adds a new section on promising new medicines.

In the United States, we continue to take medicines for granted. Many lives are lost each year because of the misuse of prescription and non-prescription medicines. The loss of life is senseless and preventable. The consumer and professional press all too often includes accounts of serious drug errors at outstanding hospitals where the culprit was human error. We can *not* continue to take medicines for granted. Readers are encouraged to study this book, to know the Points For Consideration by the Patient, and to become an advocate for their own safe and effective drug use. Always ask questions and do *not* assume that the correct medicine has been given.

Health care is constantly in transition. In the coming year, I believe that more Americans will have access to health care, but will *quality* health care be offered? Some organizations have established blind cost containment as a goal. There have been reports of cancer patients being denied potent medicines to stop vomiting because the prescribed medicines were deemed too expensive. I am personally appalled that an administrator is given the authority to make that decision. Yet we all need to become aware of the balance of outcome and expense: what medicine at what expense achieves the best result. I expect the thinking behind the way in which the health care system dispenses medicines will continue to evolve, and I have included new glossary terms and comments in the drug profiles to reflect this evolution. It is no longer enough to provide a medicine in the correct dose. The drug which offers the individual patient the best outcome for the money spent—as well as the best quality of life—must be our collective goal.

Many excellent hospitals and health care facilities have adopted an interdisciplinary team approach to providing care. These teams organize tests and therapy to make the most efficient use of the money available to fight disease. Their ultimate goal is to help the patient achieve the fullest potential possible with the most effective therapy. Some HMOs and hospital systems are taking a disease management approach to critical conditions and will begin to seek to prevent them. The hospital will become a staging ground for transition to home or out-patient therapy. The Agency for Health Care Policy and Research is bringing the awareness that effective and timely management of pain is a fundamental patient right. Consistent with this view is the concept that the outcomes from a particular therapy *must* be considered when a medicine is selected.

I have made a deliberate attempt to further simplify the language used in this book. This year I had the privilege to work with Dr. Stuart Grossman of Johns Hopkins and Dr. Edward Creagan of the Mayo Clinic on a physician education program. Once again, I've learned more about words as tools and have put this learning to work in this book.

The use of existing medicines, as well as the development of new medicines continues to evolve. The reader will find many new drugs in this edition of *The Essential Guide to Prescription Drugs.* Current FDA approved uses as well as cutting edge unlabeled uses for these drugs are now clearly defined in all profiles. Capital letters again define more important benefits and highlight critical risks in therapy.

Science moves forward, and new understanding is captured in each of the drug profiles in explaining how the medicines work. The latest publications and important research are included in updates of everything from dosing to effects in pregnancy. A new section called The Leading Edge aims to help the reader become aware of medicines which offer great promise and are waiting just over the next horizon. Genetic therapy is much closer to reality. Profiles will follow in subsequent editions of this book once fuller data is available.

What research shows us about chronic diseases of the kidney or liver continue to impact dosing of medicines. I have broadened last year's section in all of the profiles which details how medication dose or frequency should be adjusted for people with kidney or liver compromise. I believe that this will help us avoid dangerous and unnecessary toxic drug reactions.

Dr. James Long has continued his efforts to broaden my ability and skill, and I could not ask for a more capable, accomplished or effective mentor. It is with a heavy heart that I see him move into his new work on chronic disorders. I will be fortunate to retain his guidance and consultation as the years go by. It is rare in one's life to be privileged to know such a brilliant man, rarer still to be groomed to take a project such as this book further into the future.

Remember, the health care which you receive is **your** health care. Be an active participant. Your understanding can help make your medicines work their best in treating the condition which you are facing, and protect you from possible harmful effects. My opinions and profiles are unclouded by any pharmaceutical company support or research funding. I will be there to bring you the truth and the best possible information about your medicines. Welcome to the future of health care.

As noted in each previous edition, no claim is made that *all* known actions, uses, side-effects, adverse effects, precautions, interactions, etc., for a drug are included in the information provided in the sections that comprise this book. While diligent care has been taken to ensure the accuracy of the information provided during the preparation of this revision, the continued accuracy and currentness are ever subject to change relative to the dissemination of new information derived from drug research, development and general usage.

James Joseph Rybacki, Pharm. D.
July 1995

Points for Consideration by the Patient

A recent study by Dr. Lucian L. Leape of Harvard found 334 drug errors in six months at two major teaching hospitals in the United States. Fourteen of these errors were life-threatening. Studies of medication usage performed over the past 15 years have shown that more than 50% of patients take their prescription drugs incorrectly. There are a variety of reasons that contribute to this wasteful and sometimes hazardous practice. The following suggestions are offered to reduce confusion and misunderstanding and to increase the likelihood that you take the right drug for the right reason at the right time and in the right way.

General Recommendations

1. If you are being treated for a recurrent or chronic disorder (such as asthma or diabetes), **learn as much as you can** about the nature and medical management of your condition. Ask your physician and pharmacist for written information they may have available; visit your local libraries and book stores for pertinent publications; consult local chapters of national organizations that provide educational materials for specific disorders. The more you know about your disorder and its treatment, the more able you will be to use your prescribed medications safely and effectively.
2. Cooperate fully with your physician and pharmacist to ensure that the diagnosis of your disorder is as accurate as possible and that the treatment prescribed is the most appropriate for you. It is incumbent upon you to **share the responsibility** for obtaining safe and effective drug treatment.
3. Do not be unduly influenced by seductive advertising of prescription

drug products to the public through television commercials, magazine displays, celebrity endorsements, etc. Ask your physician and pharmacist for **printed information sheets** that provide unbiased, objective information regarding the drug's benefits and risks—and its appropriateness for you.

4. Some specific points to consider when your physician prescribes a drug for you:
- Inform your physician of any known drug allergies and of any prior drug-induced adverse effects.
- Inform your physician of **all other drugs** (prescription and nonprescription) that you are taking currently.
- Ask if there are any special precautions to observe: avoidance of certain foods, alcohol, exposure to sun, other drugs, hazardous activities.
- Ask how long you should take the drug; if applicable, determine an approximate time for discontinuation.
- Ask your physician to include on the prescription label both the **name of the drug** and the **disorder** for which the drug is taken. For example: Capoten for hypertension.
- Ask your physician to give you a **written summary** of appropriate information about the drug prescribed. (It is impossible for you to remember all of the information and instructions that you have been given verbally. A written summary will allow you to clarify and verify pertinent information as necessary.)
- Ask your doctor if the medicine prescribed offers the best balance of price and outcomes for you.
- Inform your physician if new symptoms develop after you start taking the drug(s) prescribed.
- Be certain to keep follow-up appointments with your physician; the performance of many drugs must be monitored closely.
- If you go to a second physician, or to a dentist, inform him or her of all medications you are taking currently—prescription and nonprescription.

5. Some specific points to consider when you obtain your prescription drug(s) from your pharmacist:
- Read your prescription carefully before submitting it to be filled. Verify that both the **name of the drug** and the **disorder** are specified. If these are not present, ask your pharmacist to contact your physician for permission to add them.
- If your prescription is a refill, verify that the drug issued is identical to the drug in your original supply. If it is not the same, ask your pharmacist to explain the difference. (Generic drug products from different manufacturers often vary in size, shape, color, etc.)
- Be aware that there are over 1000 drug names that "look alike" in print or "sound alike" in speech. Examples: acetazolamide—aceto-

hexamide, Acutrim—Accutane, Aralen—Arlidin, cyclosporine—cycloserine, Orinase—Ornade, Prilosec—Prozac, Xanax—Zantac. Mistaking one drug for the other can lead to serious dispensing errors. "Sound alike" drugs are easily confused when a prescription is given by telephone. Since each drug of the pair is used to treat a distinctively different condition, the statement of the **disorder** within the prescription will alert the pharmacist and the patient to the mistake. Use the Color Chart insert in this book to verify that you are taking the correct drug.
- Ask the pharmacist to give you **printed information sheets** that provide specific information about the drug(s) prescribed for you. A variety of such sources of information (written for the patient) is now available to physicians and pharmacists and intended for the patient's use. The information provided is similar to that presented in the Drug Profiles found in Section Two of this book. However, it is usually less comprehensive and less detailed.
- Read each warning label that the pharmacist attaches to the container—in addition to the main prescription label. These are important reminders regarding the proper use of the drug. They serve to distinguish between eye drops and ear drops; they identify dosage forms that should not be altered (opened, crushed or chewed); they provide numerous precautions that improve the effectiveness of your medication.
- If your pharmacist utilizes a computer system that records and analyzes each patient's drug history, take advantage of this excellent tool to prevent serious allergic reactions and significant drug interactions. Inform your pharmacist of all drugs you are taking currently.

6. Your responsibilities—to yourself—as a patient:
   - Know both the generic and brand name of all drugs prescribed for you.
   - If you are taking more than one drug, be sure that the label of each container includes the **name of the drug** and the **condition it treats**.
   - If you do not clearly understand the directions for using a drug, ask your physician or pharmacist before taking it.
   - Follow all dosing instructions carefully and completely. Comply fully to obtain the maximal benefit the drug can provide. If you have trouble remembering to take your medications "on time," ask your pharmacist for a dosing calendar or a weekly medication box.
   - If you are taking medications prescribed by more than one physician, check the **generic names** of all prescriptions to ensure that you are not taking duplicate drugs with different brand names. This could cause serious overdosage.
   - Nonprescription drugs can interact unfavorably with prescription

medications. Ask your physician or pharmacist **before** you begin taking any new over-the-counter preparations.
- Be certain all drugs you take are "in date"—have not expired according to the dating on the label.
- Consider the effective and timely control of pain a basic right to which you are entitled when you are in the hospital. The Agency for Health Care Policy and Research has released Clinical Practice Guidelines which clearly outline the management of cancer pain, but also broadly apply to the management of pain in general. It is reasonable to expect that your pain is responded to with as much care and attention as a high fever from an infection or a dangerously elevated blood pressure.

Suggestions for Containing the Costs of Drug Therapy

1. Cooperate fully with your physician to ensure accurate diagnosis so that the initial selection of drugs will be as safe and effective as possible.

2. Ask your physician to prescribe the drug that is most appropriate for you, selecting the product which offers the best balance of price and outcomes for you.

3. Ask your physician if the drug prescribed is available as an acceptable generic product that is less expensive than the brand name product.

4. Comply fully with your physician's instructions regarding how to take the drugs prescribed.

5. The outcomes of a given therapy or procedure have emerged as a critical factor in deciding how to approach a particular disease or medical management issue. If there appear to be several options to treat the condition which you are facing, ask your doctor what the expected outcomes of the various treatments will be. For example, if you are challenged by several chronic diseases at the same time, what appears to be a more expensive therapy may have a better outcome for you than a less costly one. In a patient facing a single infection, unchallenged by other chronic diseases, a less costly, very specific antibiotic may offer an equal outcome and decreased expense.

Points for Consideration by the Pharmacist

The pharmacist is in a unique position to enhance and reinforce communication between the patient and the physician relative to the optimal use of drugs. In a setting where the pressure of time is somewhat less restrictive, the pharmacist is able to focus more considerately on the identification, selection and utilization of prescription drugs.

Today's pharmacist endorses the FDA initiative to define his or her role and responsibility as counselor to consumers regarding the proper use of medicinal drugs. The FDA's position is that the patient has a right to demand and receive essential drug information, and that the pharmacist should voluntarily initiate the appropriate dialogue to accomplish this. The FDA recommends that **printed information** be dispensed with the prescribed drug to reinforce verbal consultation by the pharmacist. Studies have established that the combined use of verbal consultation and printed information is the most effective means of patient education in drug use.

Yet another study, this one by Dr. Lucian L. Leape of the Harvard School of Public Health, has said that serious medication errors are still occurring. Some of the errors were attributed to pharmacist dispensing. In the retail setting, you are the final check before the patient gets the medicine. Guard and value this role above any distraction or volume of prescriptions which must be filled.

General Recommendations

1. Some specific points to consider when you fill a prescription:
   - Clarify any prescription information that is illegible, uncertain, or a potential source for erroneous interpretation—by you or the patient.

- Be alert to the inherent hazard of "look alike" and "sound alike" drug names. This is an ongoing problem that increases with the proliferation of brand names; it is a significant cause of dispensing error. In accepting prescriptions by telephone, ask the caller to spell the name of the drug—as appropriate.
- As the situation warrants (multiple drugs taken concurrently, the older patient, etc.), include both the **name of the drug** and the respective **disorder** on the label. (Examples: Micronase for diabetes; Zantac for ulcer.) If required by jurisdictional regulation, consult the prescribing physician. The inclusion of the **disorder** on the label will serve to (1) reduce potential dispensing error caused by "look alike" and "sound alike" drug names; (2) prevent the confusion that often occurs during the concurrent use of multiple drugs: mistaken identity of drug and purpose, mistakenly altered dosing schedules, etc.
- As appropriate, use the full complement of instructional add-on labels designed to enhance compliance and drug performance.
- Check the stock bottle for accurate identification and appropriate dating. Be certain the appearance of the drug is uniform. If a technician fills the prescription, be certain you open the dispensing container and check the drug personally.

2. Some specific points to consider when you counsel the patient (as you dispense the filled prescription):
   - If it seems advisable, ask the patient to read all of the labeling on the container. Clarify any points of confusion or misunderstanding.
   - Verify that the patient recognizes the **name of the drug** and the **disorder being treated**. Explain what the drug is supposed to do.
   - Review with the patient the details of dosing instructions: How much to take, when to take it, and for how long.
   - Discuss the possibility of side-effects and adverse effects that may occur while taking the drug(s) dispensed. Advise the patient about what to do if any of these occur.
   - As appropriate, inform the patient of any precautions to observe while taking the drug. This includes the possibility of interactions with foods, beverages, and other drugs the patient may be taking. Specify any activities that should be avoided or modified.
   - Provide **written information** about the drug(s) dispensed and the patient's **disorder** (if available).
   - Be certain the patient knows how to store the medication properly. If the patient is elderly and requests a non-childproof lid, remind him/her to keep the drug out of reach whenever children are visiting.
   - Encourage the patient to call his/her physician if new symptoms develop while taking the medication.
   - Remind the patient that nonprescription (over-the-counter) drugs

can alter the effects of prescription drugs. Encourage the patient to call your pharmacy or his or her physician whenever guidance is needed in this regard.
- Offer medication calendars or daily/weekly dose holders if you feel that compliance may be a problem. Reinforce the importance of taking medications exactly as directed.
- If your pharmacy utilizes a computerized information system that includes patient profiles (drug histories), invite the patient to participate in this program. Explain the service it provides in detecting possible contraindications and adverse drug effects, notably allergic reactions and drug interactions. Some systems provide a "reminder" service to alert patients that they are due for a refill of certain drugs being used for long-term therapy.
- Encourage the patient to ask questions—at time of dispensing and later—whenever the need arises.

3. Get a copy of the Agency for Health Care Policy and Research Clinical Practice Guidelines Number 9 on the management of cancer pain, as well as copies of the patient guide on cancer pain. The Agency for Health Care Policy and Research is advocating effective and timely control of pain as a basic human right. This is a clear opportunity for you to help in offering effective therapeutic options and superb pharmaceutical care.

Suggestions for Containing the Costs of Drug Therapy

1. As judgment dictates, fill the prescription with the most reasonably priced drug available—within legally possible and appropriate guidelines. Consult with the prescribing physician regarding generic substitution when feasible.

2. If the patient is taking other drugs (prescribed by other physicians), explore the possibility of drug duplication—taking the same generic drug under more than one brand name.

3. In conjunction with verbal counseling, provide written information designed to enhance patient compliance with dosing instructions.

4. The outcomes of available therapeutic options will be the hallmark of the use of medicines for the future. Understand the concepts of outcomes research; the FDA will be applying them to patient-directed advertising, physicians will be facing questions about who gets better on what medicine, and you will have a role in retrospective and potentially concurrent drug use review.

Points for Consideration by the Physician

Way back in 1991 in his introduction to the *Yearbook of Drug Therapy*, Michael Weintraub, M.D., stated, "In looking for trends in the medical literature, it is apparent that the need for the physician to be an educator of patients and their families is becoming greater and greater." In addition, citing an increased need for patient education, he summarized with the following opinion: "Treatment principles correctly applied by patients educated about their condition and involved in its management seem to be the wave of the future."

More than ever before, the volume and characteristics of the drugs in use today require deliberate individualization of treatment. The overall effectiveness of any drug therapy is directly dependent upon how considerately the drug is selected, how carefully the drug is dispensed, and how accurately the drug is administered. Responsible communication between physician, pharmacist, nurse and patient must be achieved to the greatest extent possible. This process begins with the physician.

General Recommendations

1. Some specific points to consider when you evaluate a patient for drug therapy:
- Review the patient's drug history for known drug allergies and prior drug-induced adverse reactions.
- Determine if the patient is currently under treatment by other physicians or dentists.
- Ask about all drugs used currently—prescription and OTC.
- Establish the nature and severity of the disorder under consideration for drug treatment.

- Elicit significant coexisting disorders—possible absolute contraindications for certain drugs.
- Evaluate any suspected or obvious organ dysfunction—possible relative contraindications for certain drugs. When creatinine values are available, take the time to calculate creatinine clearance. Many drugs have break points for adjustment of dosage at various levels of renal impairment.
- Assess the patient's potential for compliance or noncompliance with drug therapy.

2. Some specific points to consider when selecting drugs for therapy.
    - Try to match the drug's power to the patient's problem. Avoid overprescribing—medicinal "over-kill." For example: mild to moderate stress reactions (situational anxiety-tension states) respond well to antianxiety drugs; they do not require antipsychotic medication. An uncomplicated urinary tract infection with a broadly sensitive single organism does not require a broad spectrum anti-infective drug.
    - Many new oral anti-infectives are effective against pathogens which historically required intravenous therapy. This fact may allow you to avoid hospitalization, but it also makes the patient's compliance more critical.
    - Choose the drug with the most favorable benefit/risk ratio: the best clinical effects with the least adverse reactions.
    - When you prescribe narrow-therapeutic-window drugs that require periodic blood level determinations, be certain that blood sampling is done after the drug has reached its steady state. Understand which level is preferable to measure: "peak" level (as for theophylline), or "trough" level (as for digoxin).
    - Give due consideration to the patient's prior experience with other drugs similar to the one you are considering.
    - When drug treatment fails after a reasonable trial with good compliance, change to a drug of another chemical class if one is available for the specific disorder.
    - The "most frequently prescribed" drug is not necessarily the best drug within its class. The large volume of a drug's use is frequently a reflection of its maker's marketing strategies and techniques and not an endorsement of any therapeutic advantage. Select the drugs you prescribe critically—utilizing independent, objective reviews of available information.
    - Even "drugs of choice" in objective reviews can be poor choices when you consider the characteristics of individual patients. A renally compromised patient may better tolerate an "alternate drug" with dual elimination (hepatic and renal) than a drug of choice that is limited to renal elimination.
    - Only 20% of newly approved drugs each year are classified by FDA as truly innovative or more advantageous than similar drugs in

current use. The remaining 80% are largely "me too" drugs with a limited history of use and a potential for "surprises" after a period of general use. Be objective and discerning as you review the claims made for a newly released drug within a sizable class of drugs already available. It is advisable to select drugs with established records that show them to be the best within their respective classes.

3. Some specific points to consider when you issue prescriptions in writing or by telephone:

- When prescribing for outpatient use, consider the value and advantage of including both the **name of the drug** and the **therapeutic indication** (the patient's disorder) on the prescription label. For example: Cafergot for migraine; Isordil for angina; Sinemet CR for Parkinson's. The inclusion of the **disorder** on the label will serve to (1) reduce potential dispensing error caused by "look alike" and "sound alike" drug names; (2) prevent the confusion that so often occurs during the concurrent use of multiple drugs, especially among the elderly: mistaken identity of drug and purpose, mistakenly altered dosing schedules, etc.
- If, in your judgment, there are valid reasons against public disclosure of certain **disorders**, suggest that the patient (or the family) add the name of the disorder to the respective label *after* the prescription is dispensed. The need for clear identity of both drug and purpose is paramount.
- Keep dosing instructions and schedules as simple as possible. When applicable, once-a-day dosing will do much to improve compliance.
- Alert the pharmacist to "look alike" and "sound alike" drug names. Print the drug name on written prescriptions. Spell the drug name when prescribing by telephone.

4. Some specific points to consider when counseling patients about drug therapy:

- Briefly explain the nature of the patient's disorder and its treatment. (Informed consent procedure.) Avoid the use of medical jargon; use language that is readily understood by the average person.
- Provide written information or references for educational material about the disorder. If the disorder is chronic in nature (diabetes, hypertension), explain the need to continue drug therapy indefinitely, possibly for life.
- Briefly explain the name and nature of the drugs you are prescribing. Stress the importance of strict compliance with the instructions given for each medication. (Informed consent procedure.) It is wise to alert the patient—in advance—to any potential adverse effects that may be characteristic of the drugs you are prescribing. The patient who experiences such an event is more likely to be understanding and forgiving.
- To supplement your verbal discussion, **provide a printed document**

that summarizes the essential information the patient needs to use the drug(s) safely and effectively. Be certain the patient knows what to do if a dose is missed. (Informed consent procedure.)
- Explain the need (as appropriate) for follow-up visits to monitor the effects of drug treatment and the course of the disorder. (Informed consent procedure.)
- Explain that quite often drugs do not work in practice exactly as expected. Inform the patient to be alert to the possibility that a new symptom or sign *may* be drug-related. Encourage the patient to call as needed regarding any aspect of drug treatment. Recognize the need to adjust drug selection and/or dosage regimens to accommodate individual variability. When altering medication schedules, be certain you adjust the size of the dose and/or the intervals of administration, as appropriate.
- As appropriate, give special attention to the older patient on drug therapy. Because the elderly (1) generally use multiple drugs concurrently, and (2) are more prone to experience adverse drug effects, it is advisable to conduct routine reviews of all drugs being taken each time a new drug is prescribed.
- Explore the feasibility of using an available computerized drug information program that will print out relevant information for the patient to take home. Such services can provide detailed descriptions of drugs, general guidelines for drug use, and personalized instructions.
- The point to remember: An informed patient can be your greatest ally in optimal therapeutics!

5. Obtain a copy of the Agency for Health Care Policy and Research Clinical Practice Guidelines Number 9. The AHCPR is advocating effective and timely pain control as a basic human right. Increase your awareness of the World Health Organization pain ladder and the use of the agents which are primary analgesics and adjuvants.

Suggestions for Containing the Costs of Drug Therapy

1. When you have selected the most appropriate drug, consider its cost. Which product of that drug is the most reasonably priced? If the patient requests an available generic product, direct the pharmacist to dispense one with certified bioequivalence. Because of generic product variability, caution the patient to have the prescription refilled with the identical generic (same manufacturer) each time.

2. Avoid polypharmacy whenever possible. Limit the number of drugs that the patient is taking concurrently to the fewest required. Medicate serious, significant disorders; discourage the use of drugs for minor, transient complaints.

3. Consider carefully any requests from patients for a prescription drug they have learned about through direct-to-consumer advertising, especially those with added inducements. Explain the profit motive of the producer. Assure your patients that you will prescribe the drug that, in your judgment, is the most appropriate for them.

4. In conjunction with verbal counseling, provide written information designed to enhance patient compliance with all aspects of using the drug prescribed.

5. When circumstances permit, utilize home intravenous drug therapy in preference to hospitalization.

6. The growing focus on managed care and health care reform will deliver a clear expectation and tracking of the outcomes of your therapeutic and clinical decisions. Become more familiar with the expense of various medicinal options, as well as the specific patient populations where the benefit-to-risk and cost-to-outcome ratios make the most sense.

SECTION ONE

1
HOW TO USE THIS BOOK

2
GUIDELINES FOR SAFE AND EFFECTIVE DRUG USE

1

How to Use This Book

Your physician has advised you to take a drug (or drugs), or you have been directed to administer a drug (or drugs) to someone under your care. The kind and amount of information you have been given about how to use these drugs, and what to expect from them, may vary tremendously. In many instances it will not be practical or possible for the physician to provide you with *all* the information that could be considered appropriate and useful, or it will be difficult for you to remember it. From time to time you will find it desirable—even necessary—to seek clarification and guidance about some aspect of drug action or drug use. The aim of this book is to give you the kind of information you may need to supplement the direction and guidance you receive from your physician.

The book consists of six sections. The first section will give you the orientation and insight necessary to appreciate the complexities of modern drug therapy and help you to make the best use of the information contained in Sections Two through Six.

Section Two is a compilation of Drug Profiles covering more than 300 generic prescription drugs, covering more than 2,000 brand names used widely in the United States and Canada. The selection of each drug is based upon three considerations: the extent of its use; the urgency of the conditions for which it is prescribed; the volume and complexity of the information essential to its proper utilization. The Drug Profiles are arranged alphabetically by generic name. (Some generic names have spellings similar to other generic names; be careful not to confuse one with another.)

The Profile of each drug is presented in a uniform sequence of information categories. (When you become familiar with the format, you will be able to find quickly specific items of information on any drug, without having to read the entire Profile.) Each Drug Profile contains 45 (or more) separate categories of information. The principal categories include the following.

Year Introduced

This tells you how long the drug has been in general use. The older the drug, the more likely its full spectrum of actions is known and the less likely its continued use will produce new surprises. The date given represents the year the drug was introduced for human use anywhere in the world.

Drug Class

This identifies the principal therapeutic class(es) to which the drug belongs. When appropriate, the chemical and/or pharmacological class designations are also given. You will find it helpful to recognize the class of the drug you are taking because many actions, reactions and interactions with other drugs are often shared by drugs of the same class. Throughout this book (and in most literature on drug information) you will find reference to drugs by their class designation. (Section Four provides alphabetically arranged listings of the classes of drugs referred to in this guide.)

Prescription Required

This indicates whether a drug is a prescription or a nonprescription (over-the-counter) purchase. Because there are significant differences in prescription requirements between the United States and Canada, the designation for each country is given when appropriate.

Controlled Drug

Drugs subject to regulation under the Controlled Substances Act of 1970 (those with potential for abuse) are so designated by the particular schedule that governs their dispensing in the United States. A corresponding schedule is also given for Canada when applicable. A description of the Schedules of Controlled Drugs is found at the back of this guide.

Available for Purchase by Generic Name

Increasing interest in the availability of prescription drugs for purchase by their generic names has been prompted by two issues of major significance. The first is concerned with the cost of prescription drugs. The comparison shopper realizes that in general the cost of prescription medication is significantly less when a generic equivalent of a brand name product is purchased. The second issue relates to what is termed "bioavailability and bioequivalence"—the comparative composition, quality and effectiveness of the generic versus the brand name drug product. Further discussion of bioavailability and bioequivalence of drug products will be found in the Glossary, Section Five.

Brand Names

These are provided to confirm that you are looking at the correct Drug Profile. They may also help you recognize a brand name that caused problems for you when you took it in the past. Brand names are listed for the United States and for Canada (♦). A combination drug (a drug product with more than one active ingredient) is identified by [CD] following the brand name.

In some cases a brand name in use in both the United States and Canada will represent entirely different generic drugs (in a single drug product), or a significantly different mixture of generic medicines (in a combination drug product). The generic composition of such brand name products is identified by country in the index. Travelers between the two countries who obtain their medications by brand name in either country must check to see that the drug contains the same generic medicine(s).

Benefits versus Risks

This section summarizes the "pros" and "cons" for each drug. The format adopted for this category utilizes capital letters to give weight (emphasis) to the drug's principal benefits and risks, while lower case letters are used for less critical benefits and risks. One look reveals the "comparative weights" of the two columns and gives an initial impression as to whether a drug's benefits exceed its risks, or vice versa, or whether its benefits and risks are about equal.

This presentation is not intended to be the principal basis for decision on whether or not to use the drug. Its purpose is to enjoin the reader to be more circumspect and discriminating in his or her use of drugs. The failure to give adequate attention to the individualization of drug selection and dosage is perhaps the greatest weakness seen in the current management of drug therapy.

Principal Uses

A drug may be available as a single drug product or in combination with other drugs. In this section of the Profile under the designation As a Single Drug Product, you will find the primary use(s) of the drug when used alone. Under the designation As a Combination Drug Product [CD], you will find the primary use(s) when combined with other active drugs within the same tablet, capsule, etc. The uses stated are those determined by consensus within the medical community and substantiated by current scientific study. Combination drugs have been developed because some conditions that warrant drug therapy have more than one cause, are characterized by a variety of symptoms or may be treated in more than one way. Where appropriate, in this guide, the logic for combining certain drugs to enhance their therapeutic value is explained. When you find the designation for Combination Drugs [CD] in the Brand Name list at the beginning of the Drug Profile, read under the Principal Uses section to learn more about the drug's use in combination products.

How This Drug Works

This simplified explanation is limited to consideration of how the drug acts to produce its principal (intended) therapeutic effect(s). If a specific method of action has not been established, the currently held theory is given.

Available Dosage Forms and Strengths

This represents a composite of available manufacturers' dosage forms (tablets, capsules, elixirs, etc.) and strengths, without company identification. Included are those dosage forms appropriate for use by outpatients and in extended care facilities and nursing homes. Dosage forms limited to hospital use are not included. Refer to Dosage Forms and Strengths in the Glossary for an explanation of those few abbreviations used to designate the strengths of each dosage form.

Usual Adult Dosage Range

The dosage information given represents a carefully derived consensus by appropriate authorities and is the currently recommended standard. It is provided as a guide that indicates the amount of the drug that is reasonably expected to be both effective and safe when properly used for its intended purpose. Under certain circumstances, your physician may elect to modify this "standard" dosage scheme. Adhere strictly to his or her prescribed dosages and schedules.

Conditions Requiring Dosing Adjustments

This section provides you with the latest information on conditions which require adjustments in the medicine dose or dosing. Problems in eliminating medicines from the body are suprisingly common causes of adverse drug effects. This is also a waste of money and may result in serious injury and hospitalization. It is critical to ask your doctor if the medicine dose has been adjusted for any compromise in kidney or liver function that you might have.

Dosing Instructions

Specific guidance is given here regarding the timing of oral medication with regard to food intake. In addition, there are occasions when an individual finds it difficult or impossible to swallow a tablet or a capsule, and the drug to be taken is not available in a liquid dosage form. On those occasions when the patient's condition urgently requires the medication, one may wish to crush the tablet or open the capsule and mix the contents with a palatable food or beverage for administration. Many of today's drugs are available in a bewildering array of solid dosage forms, some of which should *not* be altered to accommodate administration. This information category identifies those dosage forms of each drug that may be and those that should not be altered for administration. In addition, your pharmacist can provide appropriate guidance if you should need it.

Usual Duration of Use

Many factors influence the period of time required for any drug to exert beneficial effects. Among them are the nature and severity of the symptoms being treated, the formulation and strength of the drug, the presence or absence of food in the stomach, the ability of the patient to respond and the concurrent use of other drugs. The information in this category is helpful in preventing premature termination of medication in treatment situations where improvement may seem to you to be unreasonably delayed. Where appropriate, limitations in the duration of use are given.

This Drug Should Not Be Taken If

This category consists of the *absolute* contraindications to the use of the drug (see Contraindications in Glossary). It is most important that you alert your physician or dentist if any information in this category applies to you.

Inform Your Physician Before Taking This Drug If

This category lists the *relative* contraindications to the use of the drug. Here again, it is important that you communicate all relevant information to your physician or dentist.

Possible Side-Effects

This category describes the natural, expected and usually unavoidable actions of the drug—the normal and anticipated consequences of taking it. It is important that you maintain a realistic perspective that balances properly the occurrence of side-effects and the goals of treatment. Consult your physician for guidance whenever side-effects are troublesome or distressing, so that appropriate adjustments of your treatment program can be made.

Possible Adverse Effects

This category includes those unusual, unexpected and infrequent drug effects that are commonly referred to as adverse drug reactions. For the sake of evaluation, adverse effects are classified as mild or serious in nature. It is always wise to inform your physician as soon as you have reason to suspect you may be experiencing an adverse drug effect. Serious adverse reactions usually announce their development initially in the form of mild, unthreatening symptoms. It is important that you remain alert to significant changes in your well-being when you are taking a drug that is known to be capable of producing a serious adverse effect. It is also possible to experience an adverse reaction that has not yet been reported. Do not discount the possibility of an adverse effect just because it is not listed in this category. Following standard practice, some adverse reactions (and interactions) of certain drugs are listed, as a precaution, because these reactions are associated with the use of a particular class of drugs. Although the literature may not document such reactions in connection with the use of an individual drug within that class, the possibility of their occurrence must be considered.

A word of caution is appropriate here. You have consulted your physician for medical evaluation and management. He or she has advised you to take a drug (or administer it to someone else). It is important that you recognize and understand that *in the vast majority of instances a properly selected drug has a comparatively small chance of producing serious harm.* Most of the drugs included in this book produce serious adverse effects rarely. Knowledge that a drug is capable of causing a serious adverse reaction should not deter you from using it when it has been properly selected and its use will be carefully supervised.

Possible Effects on Sexual Function

The growing interest and concern of the medical community and the general public regarding the potential effects of many drugs on sexual function justify this designated category for the provision of relevant information. This aspect of drug performance has not received the professional scrutiny or public disclosure commensurate with its importance. Currently available information (often inadequate and vague) from all reliable sources is presented for consideration. In the interest of compliance and effective management, both physician and patient are well advised to discuss frankly the full significance of any potential effect that proposed drug therapy could have on all aspects of sexual expression.

Adverse Effects That May Appear Similar to Natural Diseases or Disorders

The failure to recognize that a given symptom or disorder is actually drug induced occurs with surprising frequency. Quite often this inadvertent error is compounded by the administration of yet another drug to relieve the "symptoms" (unrecognized manifestations) of a drug being taken on a regular basis. For milder symptoms (*e.g.*, the nasal congestion and diarrhea caused by reserpine), the oversight may not be too serious. But in the case of parkinsonlike effects of some drugs, the mistake can be devastating. This category can alert you to this common flaw in the management of drug therapy.

Natural Diseases or Disorders That May Be Activated by This Drug

Similar to the situation described in the previous category, many drugs in common use are capable of "activating" latent disorders that may not be recognized as drug induced. The development of a new and seemingly unrelated disorder during the course of any treatment program should arouse suspicion that it may be drug related.

Possible Effects on Laboratory Tests

Most of the drugs in current use have multiple and significant effects on body chemistry and organ system functions. Some of these effects are intended and beneficial (therapeutic); others are unintended, unavoidable and potentially harmful. Many of these effects can be detected and evaluated by a variety of specific laboratory tests. The timely use of appropriate tests enables the physician to monitor the performance of a drug and the course of the condition being treated. The tests included in this category are limited to those of practical importance for effective physician–patient communication and cooperation in managing the use of certain drugs. Knowledge of selected test results can greatly enhance the patient's understanding and skill in the proper use of medications.

Caution

This category provides information on certain aspects of drug action and/or drug use that require special emphasis. Occasionally these warnings may relate to information provided in other categories. When included here, such entries are of sufficient importance to warrant repetition.

Precautions for Use by Infants and Children

In addition to mandatory adjustments of drug dosage for infants and children under twelve years of age, some drugs and/or treatment situations call for special precautions. This category provides such information for selected drugs. When administering *any* drug (whether prescription or over-the-counter), it is advisable to ask the attending physician about precautions to observe or procedures to follow.

Precautions for Use by Those over 60 Years of Age

Changes in body composition and function occur naturally as part of normal aging. As would be expected, there is enormous individual variation in the speed with which such changes occur and the degree of these changes. With regard to medical management—and to drug therapy in particular—the assessment of one's "age" must be based upon the individual's mental and physical condition and never upon years alone. In general, however, it should be recognized that changes that accompany aging may affect the actions of the body on the drug, as well as the actions of the drug on the body. Appropriate precautions are outlined in this category.

Advisability of Use During Pregnancy: Pregnancy Category

Information regarding the safe use of a particular drug during pregnancy was one of the most forceful concerns that led to the formal petitioning of the Food and Drug Administration in 1975 for the provision of such guidance to the public. The FDA definitions of the five Pregnancy Categories are listed at the back of the book. It should be noted that the FDA does not make the initial category assignment; this is the responsibility of the manufacturer that markets the drug. The initial designation is then subject to review and modification by the FDA as deemed appropriate. The Pregnancy Category designations presented in each Profile were determined by the author after thorough review of pertinent literature and consultation with appropriate authorities. They are offered at this time for initial guidance only. They are in no sense "official" and do not have the endorsement of either the manufacturer or the FDA.

Advisability of Use If Breast-Feeding

Information presented here includes what could be ascertained regarding the effects of the drug on milk production, the presence of the drug in human milk and the possible effects of the drug on the nursing infant. Prudent recommendations are given where appropriate.

Suggested Periodic Examinations While Taking This Drug

This category lists those examinations your physician may recommend you undergo while taking the drug(s) he or she has prescribed, in order to monitor your reaction to them and the course of your condition. You should remember that the advisability of performing such examinations varies greatly from one situation to another, and is best left to the judgment of your physician. The selection and timing of examinations are based on many variables, including your past and present medical history, the nature of the condition under treatment, the dosage and anticipated duration of drug use and your physician's observations of your response to treatment. There may be many occasions when he or she will feel no examinations are necessary.

To assure optimal results from drug treatment, it is important that you keep your physician informed of all developments you think may be drug related.

While Taking This Drug, Observe the Following: Marijuana Smoking

The widespread "social" use of marijuana by virtually all age groups has led to inquiries regarding the possibility of interactions between the pharmacologically active chemicals in marijuana smoke and medicinal drugs in common use. Currently available literature on the health aspects of marijuana use contains very little practical information concerning the potential for drug interactions. The limited information presented in this category of selected Drug Profiles represents those *possible interactions* that are considered likely to occur in view of the known pharmacological effects of the principal components of marijuana and of the medicinal drug reviewed in the Profile. In most instances, the interaction statements are not based on documented evidence since very little is available. However, the conclusions stated—derived by logical inductive reasoning—represent the concurrence of authorities with expertise in this field.

While Taking This Drug, Observe the Following: Other Drugs

For clarification of this confusing and often controversial area of drug information, this category is divided into five subcategories of possible interactions between drugs. Observe carefully the wording of each subcategory heading (see also Interaction in Glossary). Some of the drugs listed as possible interactants do not have a representative Profile in Section Two. If you are using one of these drugs, consult your physician or pharmacist for guidance regarding potential interactions. A brand name (or names) that follows the generic name of an interacting drug is given for purposes of illustration only. It is not intended to mean that the particular brand(s) named have interactions that are different from other brands of the same generic drug. If you are taking the generic drug, *all* brand names under which it is marketed are to be considered as possible interactants.

Driving, Hazardous Activities

In addition to driving motor vehicles, the information in this category applies to any activity of a dangerous nature, such as operating machinery, working on ladders, using power tools and handling weapons.

Aviation Note

Until the publication of Dr. Stanley Mohler's *Medication and Flying: A Pilot's Drug Guide* in 1982, there was no authoritative source of current drug information written specifically to serve the needs of civil aviation. Military pilots enjoy the expert guidance and surveillance provided by the flight surgeon, but no tightly structured control system exists for their civilian counterparts. However, the need for practical information regarding the possible effects of medicinal drugs on flight performance is the same for pilots in all settings. This category is designed to inform the civilian pilot how a particular drug may affect his or her eligibility to fly and when it is advisable or necessary to consult a designated Aviation Medical Examiner or an FAA medical officer.

Occurrence of Unrelated Illness

This category relates to those drugs that require careful regulation of daily doses to maintain a constant drug effect within critical limits. Anticoagulants, antidiabetic medication and digitalis are examples of such drugs. Emphasis is given to those interim illnesses, separate from the condition for which the drug has been prescribed, that might affect the established schedule of drug use.

Discontinuation

This aspect of drug use is often overlooked when a plan of drug therapy is first discussed. However, for some drugs it is mandatory that the patient be fully informed on *when* to discontinue, when *not* to discontinue and precisely *how* to discontinue use of the drug.

Another consideration in discontinuation is the need to adjust the dosage schedules of other drugs being taken concurrently. The physician who is primarily responsible for your overall management must be kept informed of *all* the drugs you are taking at a given time.

The remaining information categories in the Drug Profile are self-explanatory.

Section Three is a new section which offers what are in the author's opinion those medicines which show great promise and are just over the horizon from FDA approval. Some of these medicines may not actually attain approval, but give significant hope that they are worth consideration. The information may actually allow patients facing serious diseases to request to be included in scientific studies and actually obtain the medicine prior to actual approval.

Section Four is a presentation of Drug Classes arranged alphabetically according to their chemical or therapeutic class designation. The drugs within each class are listed alphabetically by their generic names. Because of their chemical composition and biological activities some drugs appear in two or more classes. For example, the drug product with the brand name Diuril will be represented by its generic name, chlorothiazide, in three drug classes: the Thiazide Diuretics (a chemical classification), the Diuretics (a drug action classification) and the Antihypertensives (a disease-oriented classification).

Frequently in the Drug Profiles in Section Two you are advised to "See (a particular) Drug Class." This alerts you to a possible contraindication for drug use, or to possible interactions with certain foods, alcohol or other drugs. In each case, you can determine the more readily recognized brand names for each drug listed generically within a drug class by consulting the appropriate Drug Profile. Timely use of these references will enable you to avoid many possible hazards of medication.

Section Five is a glossary of drug-related terms used throughout the book. The preferred use of each term is explained. Frequent references to the Glossary are made in the Drug Profiles. Use of the Glossary will increase your understanding of how to recognize and interpret significant drug effects.

Section Six consists of tables of drug information. The title and introductory material explain the content and purpose of each table. The information in the tables is drawn from certain information categories in the Profiles and is rearranged to emphasize pertinent aspects of drug behavior. The tables are intended to provide another source of ready reference.

The index of Brand and Generic Names in the back of the book is a single alphabetical listing that provides page references to the appropriate Drug Profile(s) for all drugs found in this book. Its usefulness will be enhanced if you read first the introductory explanation of the special features of this combined index.

2

Guidelines for Safe and Effective Drug Use

DO NOT

- pressure your physician to prescribe drugs that, in his or her judgment, you do not need.
- take prescription drugs on your own or on the advice of friends and neighbors because your symptoms are "just like theirs."
- offer drugs prescribed for you to anyone else without a physician's guidance.
- change the dose or timing of any drug without the advice of your physician (except when the drug appears to be causing adverse effects).
- continue to take a drug that you feel is causing adverse effects, until you are able to reach your physician for clarification.
- take *any* drug (prescription or nonprescription) while pregnant or nursing an infant until you are assured by your physician that no harmful effects will occur to either mother or child.
- take any more medicines than are absolutely necessary. (The greater the number of drugs taken simultaneously, the greater the likelihood of adverse effects.)
- withhold from your physician important information about previous prescription or non-prescription drug experiences. He or she will want to know both beneficial and undesirable drug effects you have had.
- take any drug in the dark. Identify every dose of medicine carefully in adequate light to be certain you are taking the drug intended.
- keep drugs on a bedside table. Drugs for emergency use, such as nitroglycerin, are an exception. It is advisable to have only one such drug at the bedside for use during the night.

DO

- know the name (and correct spelling) of the drug(s) you are taking. It is advisable to know both the brand name and the generic name.
- read the package labels of all nonprescription drugs to become familiar with the contents of the product.
- follow your physician's instructions regarding dosage schedules as closely as possible. Notify him or her if it becomes necessary to make major changes in your treatment routine.
- thoroughly shake all liquid suspensions of drugs to ensure uniform distribution of ingredients.
- use a standardized measuring device for giving liquid medications by mouth. The household "teaspoon" varies greatly in size.
- follow your physician's instruction on dietary and other treatment measures designed to augment the actions of the drugs prescribed. This makes it possible to achieve desired drug effects with smaller doses. (A familiar example is to decrease or eliminate salt from the diet when medicine is being taken for drug treatment of high blood pressure.)
- keep your personal physician informed of all drugs prescribed for you by someone else. Consult him or her regarding nonprescription drugs you intend to take on your own initiative at the same time that you are taking drugs prescribed by him or her.
- inform your anesthesiologist, surgeon and dentist of *all* drugs you are taking, prior to any surgery.
- inform your physician if you become pregnant while you are taking any drugs from any source.
- keep a written record of *all* drugs (and vaccines) you take during your entire pregnancy—name, dose, dates taken and reasons for use.
- keep a written record of *all* drugs (and vaccines) to which you become allergic or experience an adverse reaction. This should be done for each member of the family, especially the elderly and infirm.
- keep a written record of *all* drugs (and vaccines) to which *your children* become allergic or experience an adverse reaction.
- inform your physician of all known or suspected allergies, especially allergies to drugs. Be certain that this information is included in your medical record. (Allergic individuals are four times more prone to drug reactions than those who are free of allergy).
- inform your physician promptly if you think you are experiencing an overdose, a side-effect or an adverse effect from a drug.
- determine if it is safe to drive a car, operate machinery or engage in other hazardous activities while taking the drug(s) prescribed.
- determine if it is safe to drink alcoholic beverages while taking the drug(s) prescribed.
- determine if any particular foods, beverages or other drugs should be avoided while taking the drug(s) prescribed.

- keep all appointments for follow-up examinations or laboratory tests to determine the effects of the drugs and the course of your illness.
- ask for clarification of any point that is confusing or difficult to understand, at the time the drug(s) are prescribed or later if you have forgotten. Request information in writing if circumstances justify it.
- discard all outdated prescription drugs. This will prevent the use of drugs that have deteriorated with time.
- store all drugs to be retained for intermittent use out of the reach of children to prevent accidental poisoning.

PREVENTING ADVERSE DRUG REACTIONS

Our knowledge of the mechanisms of adverse reactions is very limited. For the most part, we cannot identify with certainty the person who is at greater risk of experiencing a true adverse effect. Available tests for the early detection of toxicity are of definite value, but they do not provide as full a measure of protection as we could wish.

As our understanding of drug actions and reactions expands, it becomes more apparent that there *is* a sizable proportion of adverse effects that are, to some extent, predictable and preventable. The exact percentage of preventable reactions is yet to be determined, but several contributing factors are now well recognized, and specific recommendations are available to guide both physician and patient. These fall into eleven categories of consideration.

Previous Adverse Reaction to a Drug

There is evidence to indicate that an individual who has experienced an adverse drug reaction in the past is more likely to have adverse reactions to other drugs, even though the drugs are unrelated. This suggests that some individuals may have a genetic (inborn) predisposition to unusual and abnormal drug responses. *The patient should inform the physician of any history of prior adverse drug experiences.*

Allergies

Individuals who are allergic by nature (hayfever, asthma, eczema, hives) are more likely to develop allergies to drugs than are nonallergic individuals. The allergic patient must be observed very closely for the earliest indication of a developing hypersensitivity to any drug. Known drug allergies must be noted in the medical record. The patient must inform every physician and dentist consulted that he or she is allergic by nature and is allergic to specific drugs by name. *The patient should provide this information without waiting to be asked.* The physician will then be able to avoid those drugs that could provoke an allergic reaction, as well as those related drugs to which the patient may have developed a cross-sensitivity.

Contraindications

Both patient and physician must strictly observe all known contraindications to any drug under consideration. *Absolute contraindications* include those conditions and situations that prohibit the use of the drug for any reason. *Relative contraindications* include those conditions that, in the judgment of the physician, do not preclude the use of the drug altogether, but make it essential that special considerations be given to its use to prevent the intensification of preexisting disease or the development of new disease. Such conditions and situations usually require adjustment of dosage, additional supportive measures and close supervision.

Precautions in Use

The patient should know about any special precautions to observe while taking the drug. This includes the advisability of use during pregnancy or while nursing an infant; precautions regarding exposure to the sun (or ultraviolet lamps); the avoidance of extreme heat or cold, heavy physical exertion, etc.

Dosage

The patient must adhere to the prescribed dosage schedule as closely as possible. *This is most important with those drugs that have narrow margins of safety.* Even medications which are taken only once every 24 hours should be taken at the same time of day or night to ensure the most constant blood drug levels. Circumstances that interfere with taking the drug as prescribed (nausea, vomiting, diarrhea) must be reported to the physician so that appropriate adjustments can be made.

Interactions

Much is known today about how some drugs can interact unfavorably with certain foods, alcohol and other drugs to produce serious adverse effects. *The patient must be informed regarding all likely interactants* that could alter the action of the drug he or she is using. If, during the course of treatment, the patient has reason to feel he or she has discovered a new interaction of importance, the physician should be informed so that its full significance can be determined. (It is through such observations that much of our understanding of drug interactions has come.)

Warning Symptoms

Experience has shown that many drugs will produce symptoms that are actually early indications of a developing adverse effect. Examples include the appearance of severe headaches and visual disturbances *before* the onset of a stroke in a woman taking oral contraceptives; the development of acid indigestion and stomach distress *before* the activation of a bleeding peptic ulcer in a man taking phenylbutazone (Butazolidin) for shoulder bursitis. *It is imperative that the patient be familiar with those symptoms and signs that could be early indicators of impending adverse reactions.* With this knowledge he or she can act in his or her own behalf by discontinuing the drug and consulting the physician for additional guidance.

Examinations to Monitor Drug Effects

Certain drugs (less than half of those in common use) are capable of damaging vital body tissues (bone marrow, liver, kidney, eye structures, etc.)—especially when these drugs are used over an extended period or taken in high doses. Such adverse effects are relatively rare, and many of them are not discovered until the drug has been in wide use for a long time. As our knowledge of such effects accumulates, we learn which kinds of drugs (that is, which chemical structures) are most likely to produce such tissue reactions. Hence, we know those drugs that should be monitored periodically to detect as early as possible any evidence of tissue injury resulting from their use. *The patient should cooperate fully with the physician in the performance of periodic examinations for evidence of adverse drug effects.*

Advanced Age and Debility

The altered functional capacity of vital organs that accompanies advancing age and debilitating disease can greatly influence the body's response to drugs. Such patients tend not to tolerate drugs with inherent toxic potential well; it is usually necessary for them to use smaller doses at longer intervals. *The effects of drugs on the elderly and severely ill are often unpredictable.* The frequent need for dosage adjustments or change in drug selection requires continuous observation of these patients if adverse effects are to be prevented or minimized.

Appropriate Drug Choice

The drug(s) selected to treat any condition should be the most appropriate of those available. Many adverse reactions can be prevented if both physician and patient exercise good judgment and restraint. *The wise patient will not demand overtreatment.* He or she will cooperate with the physician's attempt to balance properly the seriousness of the illness and the hazard of the drug.

Polypharmacy

This term refers to the concurrent use by an individual of several drugs prescribed separately by two (or more) physicians for different disorders—often without appropriate communication between patient and prescriber. This frequent practice is conducive to potentially serious drug/drug interactions. *The patient should routinely inform each physician and dentist consulted of all the drugs—prescription and nonprescription—that he or she may be taking at the time.* It is mandatory that each physician and dentist has this information before prescribing additional drugs.

DRUGS AND THE ELDERLY

Advancing age brings changes in body structure and function that may alter significantly the action of drugs. An impaired digestive system may interfere with drug absorption. Reduced capacity of the liver and kidneys to metabolize and eliminate drugs may result in the accumulation of drugs in the body to toxic levels. By impairing the body's ability to maintain a "steady state" (homeostasis), the aging process may increase the sensitivity of many tissues to the actions of drugs, thereby altering greatly the responsiveness of the nervous and circulatory systems to standard drug doses. If aging should cause deterioration of understanding, memory, vision or physical coordination, people with such impairments may not always use drugs safely and effectively.

Adverse reactions to drugs occur three times more frequently in the older population. An unwanted drug response can render a functioning and independent older person whose health and reserves are at marginal levels, confused, incompetent or helpless. For these reasons, drug treatment in the elderly must always be accompanied by the most careful consideration of the individual's health and tolerances, the selection of drugs and dosage schedules and the possible need for assistance in treatment routines.

Guidelines for the Use of Drugs by the Elderly

- Be certain that drug treatment is necessary. Many health problems of the elderly can be managed without the use of drugs.
- Avoid if possible the use of many drugs at one time. It is advisable to use not more than three drugs concurrently.
- Dosage schedules should be as uncomplicated as possible. When feasible, a single daily dose of each drug is preferable.
- In order to establish individual tolerance, treatment with most drugs is usually best begun by using smaller than standard doses. Maintenance doses should also be determined carefully. A maintenance dose is often smaller for persons over 60 years of age than for younger persons.
- Avoid large tablets and capsules if other dosage forms are available. Liquid preparations are easier for the elderly or debilitated to swallow.

- Have all drug containers labeled with the drug name and directions for use in large, easy-to-read letters.
- Ask the pharmacist to package drugs in easy-to-open containers. Avoid "child-proof" caps and stoppers.
- Do not take any drug in the dark. Identify each dose of medicine carefully in adequate light to be certain you are taking the drug intended.
- To avoid taking the wrong drug or an extra dose, do not keep drugs on a bedside table. Drugs for emergency use, such as nitroglycerin, are an exception. It is advisable to have only one such drug at the bedside for use during the night.
- Drug use by older persons may require supervision. Observe drug effects continuously to ensure safe and effective use.
- Remember the adage: "Start low, go slow and (when appropriate) learn to say no."

Drugs Best Avoided by the Elderly Because of Increased Possibility of Adverse Reactions

antacids (high sodium)*
barbiturates*
benzodiazepines (long-acting)
cyclophosphamide
diethylstilbestrol
estrogens
indomethacin
monoamine oxidase (MAO) inhibitors*
oxyphenbutazone
phenacetin
phenylbutazone
tetracyclines*

Drugs That Should Be Used by the Elderly in Reduced Dosages Until Full Effect Has Been Determined

anticoagulants (oral)*
antidepressants*
antidiabetic drugs*
antihistamines*
antihypertensives*
anti-inflammatory drugs*
barbiturates*
beta-blockers*
colchicine
cortisonelike drugs*
digitalis preparations*
diuretics* (all types)
ephedrine
epinephrine
haloperidol
isoetharine
nalidixic acid
narcotic drugs
prazosin
pseudoephedrine
quinidine
sleep inducers (hypnotics)*
terbutaline
thyroid preparations

Drugs That May Cause Confusion and Behavioral Disturbances in the Elderly

acyclovir
albuterol
amantadine
antidepressants*
antidiabetic drugs*
antihistamines*
anti-inflammatory drugs*
asparaginase
atropine* (and drugs containing belladonna)
barbiturates*
benzodiazepines*
beta-blockers*
carbamazepine
cimetidine
digitalis preparations*
diuretics*

ergoloid mesylates
famotidine
levodopa
meprobamate
methocarbamol
methyldopa
narcotic drugs

nizatidine
pentazocine
phenytoin
primidone
reserpine
ranitidine
sedatives

sleep inducers
 (hypnotics)*
thiothixene
tranquilizers (mild)*
trihexyphenidyl

Drugs That May Cause Orthostatic Hypotension in the Elderly

antidepressants*
antihypertensives*
diuretics* (all types)

phenothiazines*
sedatives
selegiline

tranquilizers (mild)*
vasodilators*

Drugs That May Cause Sluggishness, Unsteadiness and Falling in the Elderly

barbiturates*
beta blockers*
chlordiazepoxide
clorazepate

diazepam
diphenhydramine
flurazepam
halazepam

methyldopa
prazepam
sleep inducers
 (hypnotics)*

Drugs That May Cause Constipation and/or Retention of Urine in the Elderly

acebutolol
amantadine
androgens
antidepressants*
antiparkinsonism drugs*

atropinelike drugs*
epinephrine
ergoloid mesylates
isoetharine
ketorolac

narcotic drugs
phenothiazines*
ranitidine
terbutaline

Drugs That May Cause Loss of Bladder Control (Urinary Incontinence) in the Elderly

diuretics* (all
 types)
sedatives

sleep inducers
 (hypnotics)*
tacrine

thioridazine
tranquilizers (mild)*

THERAPEUTIC DRUG MONITORING
(Measuring Drug Levels in Blood)

The routine use of measuring drug levels in blood as an aid in managing drug therapy has evolved gradually over the past 25 years. Because individuals vary so greatly in the nature and degree of their responses to drugs, it became apparent that greater precision in determining optimal dosage for the individual was needed. For many drugs, the responses observed by the physician (clinical changes) clearly indicate

*See Drug Class, Section Four.

that the drug is working as intended and that the dosage scheme is satisfactory. However, for some drugs—especially those with narrow safety margins—the toxic reactions closely resemble the symptoms of the disorder for which the drugs are prescribed. In many instances the patient's response is not in keeping with his or her clinical condition or program of drug therapy. By measuring the blood levels of certain drugs at appropriate times, the physician can adjust dosage schedules more accurately, predict drug response more precisely, reduce the risk of toxicity and achieve greater benefit.

The timing of the blood samples is an important consideration. As a general rule, the best time for sampling is just before the next scheduled dose of the drug to be measured (the "trough" level). Sampling should be avoided during the two hours following oral administration; during this absorption period, blood levels do not represent tissue levels of the drug. Some medications require both a peak and trough level to ensure best results.

The following drugs are those most suitable for therapeutic drug monitoring. If you are using any of these on a regular basis, consult your physician regarding the advisability or need for periodic measurement of drug levels in your blood. These numbers are ranges where effects are usually seen. Some people may have a therapeutic response with a level that is a little lower than the range. In this case, the level should be followed closely, and left alone. "Treat the patient, not the level."

Generic Name/Brand Name	Blood Level Range
acetaminophen/Tylenol, etc.	10–20 mcg/ml
amikacin/Amikin	12–25 mcg/ml (peak)
	5–10 mcg/ml (trough)
amitriptyline/Elavil, etc.	120–250 ng/ml
(combined with nortriptylline)	
amoxapine/Asendin	200–500 ng/ml
aspirin (other salicylates)	100–250 mcg/ml
carbamazepine/Tegretol	5–10 mcg/ml
chloramphenicol/Chloromycetin	10–25 mcg/ml
chlorpromazine/Thorazine	50–300 ng/ml
ciprofloxacin/Cipro	0.94–3.4 mcg/ml
clonazepam/Klonopin	10–50 ng/ml
cyclosporine/Sandimmune	100–150 ng/ml
desipramine/Norpramin, Pertofrane	150–300 ng/ml
digitoxin/Crystodigin	15–30 ng/ml
digoxin/Lanoxin	0.5–2.0 ng/ml
diltiazem/Cardizem	100–200 ng/ml
disopyramide/Norpace	2.0–4.5 mcg/ml
doxepin/Adapin, Sinequan	100–275 ng/ml
ethosuximide/Zarontin	40–100 mcg/ml
flecainide/Tambocor	0.2–1.0 mcg/ml
flucytosine/Ancobon	50–100 mcg/ml

Generic Name/Brand Name	Blood Level Range
gentamicin/Garamycin	4.0–10 mcg/ml (peak) less than 2 mcg/ml (trough)
gold salts/Auranofin, etc.	1.0–2.0 mcg/ml
imipramine/Janimine, Tofranil, etc.	150–300 ng/ml
kanamycin/Kantrex	25–35 mcg/ml
lidocaine/Xylocaine, etc.	2.0–5.0 mcg/ml
lithium/Lithobid, Lithotabs, etc.	0.3–1.3 mEq/L
mephobarbital/Mebaral	1–7 mcg/ml
methotrexate/Mexate	up to 0.1 mcmol/L
methsuximide/Celontin	up to 1.0 mcg/ml
metoprolol/Lopressor	20–200 ng/ml
mexiletine/Mexitil	0.75–2.0 mcg/ml
nifedipine/Procardia	25–100 ng/ml
nortriptyline/Aventyl, Pamelor	50–150 ng/ml
combined with amitriptyline	125–250 ng/ml
phenobarbital/Luminal, etc.	10–25 mcg/ml
phenytoin/Dilantin	10–20 mcg/ml
primidone/Mysoline	6–12 mcg/ml
procainamide/Pronestyl	4–10 mcg/ml
(napa metabolite)	4–10 mcg/ml
propranolol/Inderal	50–100 ng/ml
protriptyline/Vivactil	70–250 ng/ml
quinidine/Quinaglute, etc. (specific quinidine assay method)	1.0–4.0 mcg/ml
sulfadiazine/Microsulfon	100–120 mcg/ml
sulfamethoxazole/Gantanol	90–100 mcg/ml
theophylline/Aminophylline, etc.	10–20 mcg/ml
thioridazine/Mellaril	50–300 ng/ml
tobramycin/Nebcin	4.0–10 mcg/ml (peak) less than 2 mcg/ml (trough)
tocainide/Tonocard	5–12 mcg/ml
trimethadione/Tridione	10–30 mcg/ml
trimethoprim/Proloprim	1–3 mcg/ml
valproic acid/Depakene	50–100 mcg/ml
vancomycin/Vancocin	30–40 mcg/ml (peak) 5–10 mcg/ml (trough)
verapamil/Calan	50–200 ng/ml

SECTION TWO

DRUG PROFILES

Drugs Reviewed in This Section

Section Two consists of detailed Drug Profiles of more than 300 drugs of major importance. Drug selection was governed by consideration of the following criteria:

1. The drug is used to treat or prevent a relatively serious or significant disease or disorder.
2. The drug is recognized by experts to be among the "best choices" within its class.
3. The drug has a benefit-to-risk ratio that compares favorably with those available in its class.
4. The safe and effective use of the drug requires special information and guidance for both the health care practitioner (physician, dentist, pharmacist, nurse) and the health care consumer (patient and family).
5. The drug is suitable (safe and practical) for use in an outpatient setting (home, work site, school, etc.). It can be self-administered, or may require administration by trained medical personnel (as with home intravenous therapy, free-standing cancer, emergency or pain centers).

GENERIC NAMES

The generic names of the drugs included are listed below in alphabetic order.

acebutolol
acetazolamide
acetic acid NSAIDs
acyclovir
albuterol
allopurinol
alprazolam
amantadine
amiloride
aminophylline
amitriptyline
amlodipine
amoxapine
amoxicillin
amoxicillin/clavulanate
ampicillin
aspirin
astemizole
atenolol
auranofin
azathioprine
azithromycin
bacampicillin
beclomethasone
benazepril
benztropine
betaxolol
bitolterol
bromocriptine
bumetanide
bupropion
buspirone
calcitonin
captopril
carbamazepine
carteolol
cefaclor
cefadroxil
cefixime
cefprozil
ceftriaxone

cefuroxime
cephalexin
chlorambucil
chloramphenicol
chloroquine
chlorothiazide
chlorpromazine
chlorpropamide
chlorthalidone
cholestyramine
cimetidine
ciprofloxacin
cisapride
clarithromycin
clindamycin
clofazimine
clomipramine
clonazepam
clonidine
clotrimazole
cloxacillin
clozapine
codeine
colchicine
colestipol
cromolyn
cyclophosphamide
cyclosporine
dapsone
desipramine
dexamethasone
diazepam
diclofenac
didanosine
dideoxycytidine
  (see zalcitabine)
diflunisal
digitoxin
digoxin
diltiazem
diphenhydramine

dipyridamole
disopyramide
disulfiram
dornase alpha
doxazosin
doxepin
doxycycline
enalapril
epinephrine
ergotamine
erythromycin
estrogens
ethambutol
ethanol
ethosuximide
etidronate
etodolac
etretinate
famciclovir
famotidine
felbamate
felodipine
fenamate NSAIDs
fenoprofen
fentanyl transdermal
filgrastim
finasteride
fluconazole
flucytosine
flunisolide
fluoxetine
fluphenazine
flurazepam
flurbiprofen
flutamide
fluticasone
fluvoxamine
foscarnet
fosinopril
furosemide
ganciclovir

27

Generic Names

gemfibrozil
glipizide
glyburide
griseofulvin
guanfacine
haloperidol
histamine (H-2) blocking drugs
hydralazine
hydrochlorothiazide
hydrocodone
hydroxychloroquine
hydroxyurea
ibuprofen
imipramine
indapamide
indomethacin
influenza vaccine
insulin
iodoquinol
ipratropium
isoniazid
isosorbide dinitrate
isosorbide mononitrate
isotretinoin
isradipine
ketoconazole
ketoprofen
ketorolac
labetalol
lamotrigine
lansoprazole
levodopa/carbidopa
levothyroxine
lidocaine/prilocaine cream
liothyronine
lisinopril
lithium
lomefloxacin
loperamide
loratadine
lorazepan
losartan
lovastatin
maprotiline
meclofenamate
medroxyprogesterone
mefenamic acid
meperidine
mercaptopurine
mesalamine
metaproterenol
metformin
methadone
methotrexate
methyclothiazide
methylphenidate
methylprednisolone
methysergide
metoclopramide
metolazone
metoprolol
metronidazole
mexiletine
minoxidil
misoprostol
molindone
morphine
mupirocin
nabumetone
nadolol
nafarelin
naltrexone
naproxen
nedocromil
nefazodone
neostigmine
niacin
nicardipine
nicotine
nifedipine
nitrofurantoin
nitroglycerin
nizatidine
norfloxacin
nortriptyline
ofloxacin
olsalazine
omeprazole
ondansetron
oral contraceptives
oxaprozin
oxicam NSAIDs
oxtriphylline
oxycodone
paroxetine
penbutolol
penicillamine
penicillin V
pentamidine
pentazocine
pentoxifylline
pergolide
perphenazine
phenelzine
phenobarbital
phenytoin
pilocarpine
pindolol
pirbuterol
piroxicam
pravastatin
prazosin
prednisolone
prednisone
prilocaine cream (see lidocaine/prilocaine cream)
primaquine
primidone
probenecid
probucol
procainamide
prochlorperazine
propionic acid NSAIDs
propranolol
protriptyline
pyrazinamide
pyridostigmine
pyrimethamine
quazepam
quinacrine
quinapril
quinidine
ramipril
ranitidine
rifabutin
rifampin
risperidone
salmeterol
selegiline
sertraline
simvastatin
spironolactone
stavudine
strontium-89
sucralfate
sulfadiazine
sulfamethoxazole

sulfasalazine
sulfisoxazole
sulindac
sumatriptan
tacrine
tamoxifen
terazosin
terbutaline
terfenadine
tetracycline
theophylline
thiazide diuretics

thioridazine
thiothixene
ticlopidine
timolol
tolazamide
tolbutamide
tolmetin
trazodone
triamcinolone
triamterene
trichlormethiazide
trifluoperazine

trimethoprim
valproic acid
vancomycin
varicella virus vaccine
venlafaxine
verapamil
warfarin
zalcitabine
   (dideoxycytidine)
zidovudine
zolpidem

Author's note: It is now possible to report serious Adverse Drug Reactions by phone by calling 1-800-332-1088.

ACEBUTOLOL (a se BYU toh lohl)

Introduced: 1973 **Prescription:** USA: Yes **Available as Generic:** Yes **Class:** Antihypertensive, heart rhythm regulator, beta-adrenergic blocker **Controlled Drug:** USA: No
Brand Name: Sectral, ♦Monitan, ♦Rhotral

BENEFITS versus RISKS	
Possible Benefits	*Possible Risks*
EFFECTIVE ANTIHYPERTENSIVE in mild to moderate high blood pressure CAN DECREASE the number of deaths occuring after a heart attack	CONGESTIVE HEART FAILURE in advanced heart disease Worsening of angina in coronary heart disease (abrupt withdrawal) Masking of low blood sugar (hypoglycemia) in drug-treated diabetes Rare lupus erythematosus syndrome

▷ **Principal Uses**
  As a Single Drug Product: Uses currently included in FDA approved labeling: (1) Treatment of mild to moderately high blood pressure. Used alone or combined with other drugs. Also used to prevent premature ventricular heartbeats.
  Other (unlabeled) generally accepted uses: Treatment of stable angina pectoris, use after a heart attack to help prolong life, may have a role in easing the symptoms of panic attacks.
How This Drug Works: By blocking part of the sympathetic nervous system, this drug slows the rate and contraction force of the heart. This reduces the extent of blood vessel contraction, expanding the walls and lowering the blood pressure. It also slows the speed of nerve impulses through the heart, of benefit in management of some heart rhythm disorders.
Available Dosage Forms and Strengths
  Capsules — 100 mg (in Canada), 200 mg, 400 mg
▷ **Recommended Dosage Ranges: (Actual dosage and administration schedule must be determined by the physician or clinical pharmacist for each patient individually.)**
  Infants and Children: Not indicated.
  18 to 65 Years of Age: Initially 400 mg daily, either as a single dose in the morning or as 200 mg taken morning and evening (12 hours apart). The usual maintenance dose is 400 to 800 mg/24 hours. The total dose should not exceed 1200 mg/24 hours, given as 600 mg twice daily.
  Over 65 Years of Age: Bioavailability (amount taken into your body) doubles. Lower maintenance doses are needed. **Maximum** daily dose is 800 mg per day.
Conditions Requiring Dosing Adjustments
  Liver function: Acebutolol is extensively metabolized in the liver. Used with caution in compromised liver function.
  Kidney function: Dose must be decreased by up to 75% in kidney failure.

Acebutolol

▷ **Dosing Instructions:** May be taken without regard to eating. Capsule may be opened for administration. Do not stop this drug abruptly.

Usual Duration of Use: Use on a regular schedule for 5 to 11 days is needed to see this drug's peak effect in lowering blood pressure or stopping premature heartbeats. Long-term use of this drug is determined by sustained benefit and patient response to a combined program (weight reduction, salt restriction, smoking cessation, etc.). See your doctor regularly.

Possible Advantages of This Drug
Slows the heart less than most other beta blocker drugs, and is less likely to cause asthma (in susceptible individuals) when used in low doses.

▷ **This Drug Should Not Be Taken If**
- you have had an allergic reaction to it previously.
- you have congestive heart failure.
- you have an abnormally slow heart rate or a serious form of heart block.
- you are taking, or have taken within the past 14 days, any monoamine oxidase (MAO) type A inhibitor drug (see Drug Class, Section Four).

▷ **Inform Your Physician Before Taking This Drug If**
- you have had an adverse reaction to any beta blocker (see Drug Class, Section Four).
- you have serious heart disease, or episodes of heart failure.
- you have hay fever (allergic rhinitis), asthma, chronic bronchitis or emphysema. Some drugs in this class should not be taken if you have asthma.
- you have an overactive thyroid function (hyperthyroidism).
- you have a history of low blood sugar (hypoglycemia).
- you have impaired liver or kidney function.
- you have diabetes or myasthenia gravis.
- you currently take any form of digitalis, quinidine or reserpine, or any calcium blocker drug (see Drug Class, Section Four).
- you plan to have surgery under general anesthesia in the near future.
- you take other prescription or non-prescription medications which were not discussed when acebutolol was prescribed for you.
- you are unsure of how much to take or how often to take acebutolol.

Possible Side-Effects (natural, expected and unavoidable drug actions)
Lethargy and fatigability (11%), cold extremities (0.2%), slow heart rate, light-headedness in upright position (see Orthostatic Hypotension in Glossary).

▷ **Possible Adverse Effects** (unusual, unexpected and infrequent reactions)
If any of the following develop, consult your physician promptly for guidance.
Mild Adverse Effects
Allergic Reactions: Skin rash, itching.
Headache, dizziness, insomnia, fatigue or abnormal dreams.
Indigestion, nausea, constipation, diarrhea.
Joint and muscle discomfort, fluid retention (edema).
Serious Adverse Effects
Mental depression (2%), anxiety, low blood sugar.
Chest pain, shortness of breath, precipitation of congestive heart failure.

Acebutolol

Induction of bronchial asthma (in people with asthma).
Positive ANA and lupus erythematosus.

▷ **Possible Effects on Sexual Function:** Impotence (2%), decreased libido, Peyronie's disease (see Glossary).

Possible Effects on Laboratory Tests
Antinuclear Antibodies (ANA) and LE cells: often positive after 3 to 6 months. Free fatty acids (FFA): decreased.
Glucose tolerance test (GTT): decreased; abnormal tests at 60 and 120 minutes.

CAUTION
1. ***Do not stop this drug suddenly*** without the knowledge and guidance of your physician. Carry a note on your person that you take this drug.
2. Call your physician or pharmacist before using nasal decongestants. These can cause sudden increases in blood pressure if taken with beta blockers.
3. Report the development of any tendency to emotional depression.

Precautions for Use
By Infants and Children: Safety and effectiveness for use by those under 12 years of age have not been established. If this drug is used, watch for fainting as a sign of low blood sugar (hypoglycemia) if a meal is skipped.
By Those over 60 Years of Age: All antihypertensive drugs should be used *cautiously*. High blood pressure should be lowered slowly, avoiding the risks (such as stroke or heart attack) of excessively low blood pressure. Small doses and frequent blood pressure checks are indicated. Total daily dosage should not exceed 800 mg. Watch for dizziness, unsteadiness, tendency to fall, confusion, hallucinations, depression or urinary frequency.

▷ **Advisability of Use During Pregnancy**
Pregnancy Category: B. See Pregnancy Code at the back of this book.
Animal studies: No significant increase in birth defects in rats or rabbits.
Human studies: Adequate studies of pregnant women are not available.
Use this drug only if clearly needed. Ask physician for guidance.

Advisability of Use if Breast-Feeding
Presence of this drug in breast milk: Yes.
Avoid drug or refrain from nursing.

Habit-Forming Potential: None.

Effects of Overdosage: Weakness, slow pulse, low blood pressure, fainting, cold and sweaty skin, congestive heart failure, possible coma and convulsions.

Possible Effects of Long-Term Use: Decreased heart reserve and heart failure in some individuals with advanced heart disease.

Suggested Periodic Examinations While Taking This Drug (at physician's discretion)
Measurements of blood pressure, evaluation of heart function.

▷ **While Taking This Drug, Observe the Following**
Foods: No restrictions. Avoid excessive salt intake.
Beverages: No restrictions. May be taken with milk.

34 Acetazolamide

▷ *Alcohol:* Alcohol may exaggerate this drug's ability to lower the blood pressure and may increase its mild sedative effect.

Tobacco Smoking: Nicotine may reduce this drug's effectiveness in treating high blood pressure. May increase the closing of bronchial tubes seen in regular smokers.

▷ *Other Drugs*

Acebutolol may *increase* the effects of
- other antihypertensive drugs and excessively lower the blood pressure. Dosage adjustments may be necessary.
- reserpine (Ser-Ap-Es, etc.) and cause sedation, depression, slow heart rate and low blood pressure.

Acebutolol *taken concurrently* with
- clonidine (Catapres) may cause rebound high blood pressure if clonidine is withdrawn while acebutolol is still being taken.
- insulin may cause hypoglycemia (see Drug Class).
- oral hypoglycemic agents (see Drug Class) may result in slow recovery from low blood sugars.
- NSAIDS (see Glossary) may result in decreased lowering of blood pressure.

The following drugs may *decrease* the effects of acebutolol
- indomethacin (Indocin), and some other "aspirin substitutes,"(NSAIDS) can blunt acebutolol's antihypertensive effect.

▷ *Driving, Hazardous Activities:* Use caution until you see how drowsy and lethargic you may become.

Aviation Note: The use of this drug *is a disqualification* for piloting. Consult a designated Aviation Medical Examiner.

Exposure to Sun: No restrictions.

Exposure to Heat: Hot environments can exaggerate the effects of this drug.

Exposure to Cold: The elderly must be careful in preventing hypothermia (see Glossary).

Heavy Exercise or Exertion: This drug can intensify the hypertensive response to isometric exercise.

Avoid exertion causing dizziness, excessive fatigue or muscle cramps.

Occurrence of Unrelated Illness: Fevers can lower the blood pressure and require adjustment of dosage. Nausea or vomiting may interrupt the dosing schedule. Ask your doctor for help.

Discontinuation: Avoid stopping the drug suddenly. Slow reduction of dose over a period of 2 to 3 weeks is recommended. Ask your physician for guidance.

ACETAZOLAMIDE (a set a ZOHL a mide)

Introduced: 1953   **Prescription:** USA: Yes; Canada: Yes   **Available as Generic:** USA: Yes; Canada: No   **Class:** Anticonvulsant, antiglaucoma, diuretic, sulfonamides   **Controlled Drug:** USA: No; Canada: No

Brand Names: ✦Acetazolam, Ak-Zol, ✦Apo-Acetazolamide, Dazamide, Diamox, Diamox Sustained release, Diamox Seques, Storzolamide

Acetazolamide

BENEFITS versus RISKS	
Possible Benefits	*Possible Risks*
REDUCTION OF INTERNAL EYE PRESSURE in selected cases of glaucoma CONTROL OF ABSENCE (PETIT MAL) SEIZURES TREATMENT OF PERIODIC PARALYSIS REDUCTION OF FLUID IN CONGESTIVE HEART FAILURE OR DRUG-INDUCED EDEMA. PREVENTION OR LESSENING OF SYMPTOMS OF ACUTE MOUNTAIN CLIMBING SICKNESS.	Acidosis with long-term use Increased risk of kidney stone Rare bone marrow, liver or kidney injury Tingling in the arms and legs (paresthesias) Paralysis (rare) Bone weakening (with long term use)

▷ **Principal Uses**

As a Single Drug Product: Uses currently included in FDA approved labeling: (1) Treatment of certain types of glaucoma; (2) used with other drugs to manage petit mal epilepsy; (3) treats familial periodic paralysis and prevents altitude sickness.

Other (unlabeled) generally accepted uses: (1) Taken orally as a urine alkalinizing agent in patients who have had uric acid kidney stones; (2) Given intravenously to increase elimination of some drugs in overdoses; (3) May be used in patients in intensive care units on ventilators to correct chemical imbalances.

How This Drug Works: By blocking the effect of the enzyme carbonic anhydrase, it slows the formation of fluid (the aqueous humor) in the eye and increases the volume of urine. It causes fluid loss by lowering the hydrogen ion concentration in the the kidney and increasing elimination of bicarbonate (a basic chemical), potassium, sodium and water.

Available Dosage Forms and Strengths

Capsules, prolonged-action (sustained release) — 500 mg
Injection — 500 mg per vial
Tablets — 125 mg, 250 mg

▷ **Recommended Dosage Ranges (Actual dosage and administration schedule must be determined by the physician or clinical pharmacist for each patient individually.)**

Infants and Children: Not indicated in infants.

Acute glaucoma in children: Give 5–10 mg/kg intramuscularly (IM) or intravenously (IV) every 6 hours.

Children with glaucoma: Give 8–30 mg/kg per day in three divided doses.

Epilepsy in children: Give 8–30 mg/kg per day in 1–4 divided doses. Lower doses used if drug is combined with other medications. (250 mg per day).

Diuretic in children: Give 5 mg/kg IV or orally once daily in the morning.

18 to 65 Years of Age: For glaucoma: 250 to 1000 mg/24 hours, in 2 or 3 doses. For epilepsy: 250 to 1000 mg/24 hours. As a diuretic: 250 to 375 mg/24 hours, in one morning dose for one or two days.

36   Acetazolamide

Over 65 Years of Age: Most of a given dose is eliminated via the kidneys. Use with caution in this age group, and start with the lower end of the dosage range.

Conditions Requiring Dosing Adjustments
Liver function: Used with extreme caution in patients with cirrhosis.
Kidney function: Used with extreme caution and the kidney patient closely followed.

▷ **Dosing Instructions:** Best taken with food or milk to prevent stomach irritation. Tablet may be crushed. Diamox Sequels may be opened, but do not chew or crush contents.

Usual Duration of Use: Treatment of glaucoma and epilepsy require long-term use. If taken to control seizures, do not stop this drug abruptly. See your doctor regularly.

▷ **This Drug Should Not Be Taken If**
- you have had an allergic reaction to any form of it previously.
- you have serious liver or kidney disease.
- you have Addison's disease.
- you have electrolyte problems (low sodium or potassium).
- you have some types of glaucoma.

▷ **Inform Your Physician Before Taking This Drug If**
- you have had an allergic reaction to any "sulfa" drug.
- you have gout or lupus erythematosus.
- you have emphysema or blockages of your lungs.
- you have a history of low blood platelets.

Possible Side-Effects (natural, expected and unavoidable drug actions)
Drowsiness, temporary nearsightedness.

▷ **Possible Adverse Effects** (unusual, unexpected and infrequent reactions)
If any of the following develop, consult your physician promptly for guidance.
Mild Adverse Effects
Allergic Reactions: Skin rash, hives, drug fever.
Reduced appetite, indigestion, nausea.
Confusion, fatigue; weakness; dizziness; tingling of face, arms or legs.
Excessive growth of hair in females.

Serious Adverse Effects
Allergic Reactions: Hemolytic anemia (see Glossary), spontaneous bruising (reduced blood platelet count, see Glossary).
Bone marrow depression (see Glossary)—fatigue, weakness, fever, sore throat, abnormal bleeding or bruising.
Hepatitis with jaundice (see Glossary)—yellow eyes and skin, dark-colored urine, light-colored stools.
Severe muscle weakness leading to paralysis (rare).
Weakness of the bones with long-term use.

▷ **Possible Effects on Sexual Function:** Decreased libido (male and female), impotence (both infrequent). Effects may begin after 2 weeks of use and subside when drug is stopped.

▷ **Adverse Effects That May Mimic Natural Diseases or Disorders**
Toxic liver reaction may suggest viral hepatitis.
Lupus erythematosuslike syndrome.

Acetazolamide 37

Natural Diseases or Disorders That May Be Activated by This Drug
Gout, acidosis caused by chronic obstructive lung disease—asthma, bronchitis, emphysema.

Possible Effects on Laboratory Tests
Complete blood counts: decreased red cells, hemoglobin, white cells and platelets.
Blood chloride level: increased.
Blood glucose level: increased in prediabetics and with use of oral antidiabetic drugs (see Drug Class, Section Four).
Blood lupus erythematosus (LE) cells: positive.
Blood uric acid level: increased.

CAUTION
1. Watch for loss of diuretic (fluid) or seizure control effect.
2. Emotional depression can be an adverse effect of this drug.
3. May cause excessive loss of potassium. Ask your doctor about a high-potassium diet or potassium supplements.

Precautions for Use
By Infants and Children: Excess dose may cause drowsiness and numbness of the face and extremities. Not recommended for use as a diuretic in children.
By Those over 60 Years of Age: Do not exceed recommended doses. Increased dose may lead to weakness, confusion, numbness in the extremities and nausea. If taking a digitalis preparation (digitoxin, digoxin), you may need a high-potassium diet or potassium supplements. Ask your doctor for advice.

▷ **Advisability of Use During Pregnancy**
Pregnancy Category: C. See Pregnancy Code at the back of this book.
Animal studies: Limb and skeletal defects reported in mice and rats.
Human studies: Adequate studies of pregnant women not available.
Avoid completely during the first 3 months and during labor and delivery.

Advisability of Use if Breast-Feeding
Presence of this drug in breast milk: Yes.
Diuretic effect may temporarily impair milk production. Watch nursing infant closely and stop drug or nursing if adverse effects develop.

Habit-Forming Potential: None.

Effects of Overdosage: Drowsiness, numbness and tingling, thirst, nausea, vomiting, confusion, excitement, convulsions, coma.

Possible Effects of Long-Term Use: The development of low blood potassium and/or acidosis.

Suggested Periodic Examinations While Taking This Drug (at physician's discretion)
Complete blood cell counts, measurements of blood sodium, potassium and uric acid levels, liver and kidney function tests.

▷ **While Taking This Drug, Observe the Following**
Foods: Ask your doctor about the need for a high-potassium diet. See Section Six for the Table of High Potassium Foods.
Beverages: No restrictions. May be taken with milk.
▷ *Alcohol:* Alcohol can blunt the anticonvulsant effect of this drug and reduce seizure control.
Tobacco Smoking: No interactions expected.

▷ *Other Drugs*
  Acetazolamide may *increase* the effects of
  • quinidine.
  Acetazolamide may *decrease* the effects of
  • lithium.
▷ *Driving, Hazardous Activities:* Usually no restrictions. Drowsiness or dizziness may occur.
  Aviation Note: The use of this drug *may be a disqualification* for piloting. Consult a designated Aviation Medical Examiner.
  Exposure to Sun: No restrictions.

ACETIC ACIDS
(Nonsteroidal Antiinflammatory Drugs)

Indomethacin (in doh METH a sin) **Diclofenac** (di KLOH fen ak) **Etodolac** (E TOE do lak) **Ketorolac** (KEY tor o lak) **Nabumentone** (na BYU me tohn) **Sulindac** (sul IN dak) **Tolmetin** (TOHL met in)

Introduced: 1963, 1976, 1986, 1991, 1984, 1976, 1976 **Prescription:** USA: Yes; Canada: Yes **Available as Generic:** USA: Yes: indomethacin, sulindac, tolmetin.; Canada: No **Class:** NSAID, Mild analgesic **Controlled Drug:** USA: No; Canada: No

Brand Names: Indomethacin: ✦Apo-Indomethacin, Indameth, ✦Indocid, ✦Indocid-SR, ✦Indocid PDA, Indocin, Indocin-SR, ✦Novomethacin, ✦Nu-Indo, Zendole, Diclofenac:, ✦Apo-Diclo, Cataflam, ✦Novo-Difenac, ✦Nu-Diclo, Voltaren, Voltaren SR, Voltaren Ophthalmic, Etodolac: Lodine, Ketorolac: Toradol, Acular (ketorolac ophthalmic), Nabumetone: Relafen, Sulindac: ✦Apo-Sulin, Clinoril, ✦Novo-Sundac, Tolmetin: Tolectin, Tolectin DS, Tolectin 600

BENEFITS versus RISKS	
Possible Benefits	*Possible Risks*
EFFECTIVE RELIEF OF MILD TO MODERATE PAIN AND INFLAMMATION	Gastrointestinal pain, ulceration, bleeding (rare)
Easy change from the IM form to the oral form (ketorolac)	Rare liver or kidney damage
Decreased stomach (GI) problems (etodolac)	Rare fluid retention
	Rare bone marrow depression
	Mental depression, confusion
	Rare lung fibrosis (nabumetone)
	Rare pneumonitis (sulindac)
	Rare aseptic meningitis (diclofenac)
	Rare severe skin reaction (diclofenac, etodolac, ketorolac and sulindac)

▷ **Principal Uses**
  As a Single Drug Product: Uses currently included in FDA approved labeling:
  (1) All of the drugs in this class except ketorolac are approved to treat

osteoarthritis; (2) all of the drugs in this class except ketorolac and etodolac are approved to relieve rheumatoid arthritis; (3) etodolac and ketorolac are used to treat mild to moderate pain; (4) diclofenac is useful in ankylosing spondylitis; (5) the sustained release form of indomethacin as well as the immediate release form of sulindac help symptoms of tendonitis, bursitis and acute painful shoulder; (6) tolmetin eases symptoms of juvenile rheumatoid arthritis; (7) sulindac therapy is useful in acute gout; (8) ophthalmic form of diclofenac is useful after cataract surgery.

Other (unlabeled) generally accepted uses: (1) Diclofenac used intramuscularly is effective in acute migraine headache and kidney colic; (2) indomethacin has recently proven to be useful in reducing systemic reactions in kidney transplants, and addressing low grade neonatal intraventricular hemorrhage; (3) ketorolac has been helpful in reducing swelling after cataract surgery and in treating reflex sympathetic dystrophy by injection; (4) sulindac is effective in treating colon polyps (Gardner's syndrome) and easing diabetic neuropathic pain.

How These Drugs Work: It is thought that these drugs reduce tissue concentrations of prostaglandins (and related compounds), chemicals involved in the production of inflammation and pain.

Available Dosage Forms and Strengths

Indomethacin:
  Capsules — 25 mg, 50 mg, 75 mg
  Gelatin Capsule (Canada) — 25 mg, 50 mg
  Capsules, SR (prolonged action) — 75 mg
  Oral suspension — 25 mg per 5-ml teaspoonful
  Suppositories — 50 mg

Diclofenac potassium:
  Tablets — 50 mg

Diclofenac sodium:
  Suppositories — 50 mg, 100 mg (Canada)
  Enteric tablets — 25 mg, 50 mg
  Prolonged action tablets — 75 mg, 100 mg (Canada)
  Ophthalmic solution — 1 mg per ml

Etodolac:
  Capsules — 200 mg, 300 mg

Ketorolac:
  Tablets — 10 mg
  Ophthalmic solution — 0.5%
  Injection — 15 mg, 30 mg

Nabumetone:
  Tablets — 500 mg, 750 mg

Sulindac:
  Tablets — 150 mg, 200mg

Tolmetin:
  Capsules — 400 mg
  — 492 mg
  Gelatin Capsule — 400 mg (Canada)
  Tablets — 200 mg, 600 mg

▷ **Usual Adult Dosage Range:** Indomethacin: For arthritis and related conditions: 25 to 50 mg 2 to 4 times daily. If needed and tolerated, dose may be increased by 25 or 50 mg/day at intervals of 1 week. For acute gout: 100 mg initially; then 50 mg 3 times/day until pain is relieved. Maximum daily dose is 200 mg.

Diclofenac potassium: Maximum daily dose is 200 mg.

Diclofenac sodium: 100 to 200 mg daily to start in 2 to 5 divided doses. Reduction to the minimum efective dose is advisable. Maximum daily dose is 225 mg.

Etodolac: For osteoarthritis: A starting dose of 800 to 1200 mg is given in divided doses. The lowest effective dose is advisable, and effective treatment has been accomplished with 200 to 400 mg daily. Maximum dose is 1200 mg daily.

Ketorolac: 10 mg is used every 4 to 6 hours for short-term treatment of pain. Maximum daily dose is 40 mg orally.

Nabumentone: 1000 mg daily as a single dose is given. Dosage is increased as needed and tolerated to 1500 mg daily. The lowest effective daily dose is advisable. Maximum daily dose is 2000 mg.

Sulindac: Therapy is started with 150 to 200 mg twice daily taken 12 hours apart. Maximum daily dose is 400 mg.

Tolmetin: 400 mg 3 times daily is started, with usual ongoing doses of 600 to 1600 mg as needed and tolerated. Total daily dose should not exceed 1600 mg for osteoarthritis or 2000 mg for rheumatoid arthritis.

Children two years of age or older may be given 20 mg per kg orally, divided into three or four doses daily. The dose may be increased as needed and tolerated to a maximum daily dose of 30 mg per kg.

Note: Actual dose and dosing schedule must be determined by the physician for each patient individually.

Conditions Requiring Dosing Adjustments

Liver function: These drugs are extensively metabolized in the liver. They should be used with caution in patients with liver compromise.

Kidney function: All nonsteroidal anti-inflammatory drugs may inhibit prostaglandins and alter kidney blood flow in patients with kidney (renal) compromise. Used with caution in patients with kidney compromise.

▷ **Dosing Instructions:** Take with or following food to prevent stomach irritation. Take with a full glass of water and remain upright (do not lie down) for 30 minutes. Regular release tablets may be crushed, but not extended release forms. The regular capsules may be opened for administration, but not the prolonged-action capsules. Food actually increases absorption of nabumetone.

Usual Duration of Use: Continual use on a regular schedule for 1 to 2 weeks is usually necessary to determine drug effectiveness in relieving the discomfort of arthritis. The usual length of treatment for bursitis or tendinitis for indomethacin or sulindac is 7 to 14 days. Ketorolac is used for short-term pain treatment. Long-term use of the other agents in this class requires physician supervision and periodic evaluation.

▷ **These Drugs Should Not Be Taken If**
- you have had an allergic reaction to them previously.
- you are subject to asthma or nasal polyps caused by aspirin.

ACEBUTALOL
Sectral
capsules 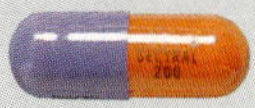
- 200 mg 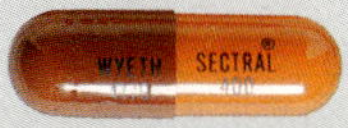
- 400 mg

ACETAZOLAMIDE
Diamox
tablets 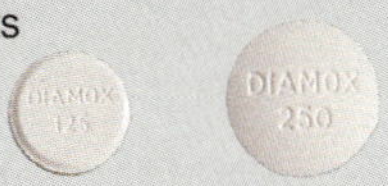
- 125 mg
- 250 mg

sequel 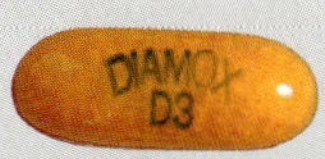
- 500 mg

ACYCLOVIR
Zovirax
capsule 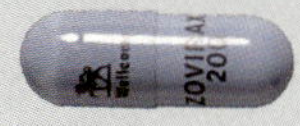
- 200 mg

tablet 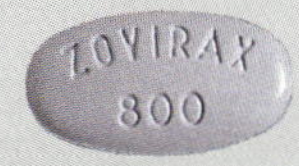
- 800 mg

ALBUTEROL
Ventolin
tablet 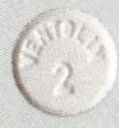
- 2 mg

Proventil
tablet 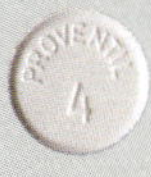
- 4 mg

tablet, extended-release 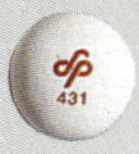
- 4 mg

ALLOPURINOL
Zyloprim
tablets 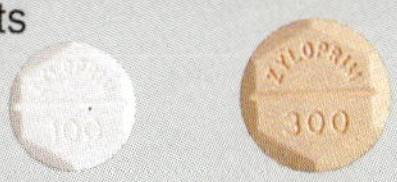
- 100 mg
- 300 mg

ALPRAZOLAM
Xanax
tablets
- 0.25 mg
- 0.5 mg 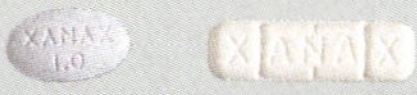
- 1 mg
- 2 mg

AMANTADINE
Symmetrel
capsule 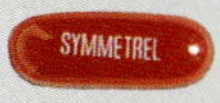
- 100 mg

AMILORIDE
Moduretic
tablet 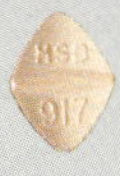
- 5/50 mg

AMINOPHYLLINE
Aminophylline Generic
tablet 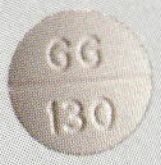
- 100 mg

Mudrane-2
tablet 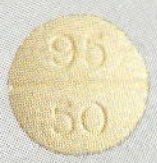
- 130 mg

AMITRIPTYLINE
Elavil
tablets
- 10 mg
- 25 mg 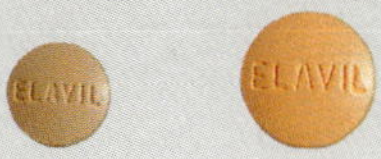
- 50 mg
- 75 mg

Elavil (cont.)
- 100 mg
- 150 mg

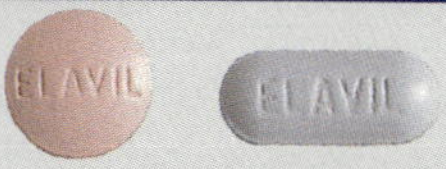

AMLODIPINE
Norvasc
tablet 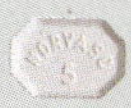
- 5 mg

AMOXAPINE
Asendin
tablets 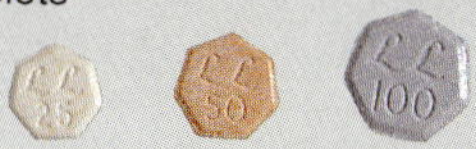
- 25 mg
- 50 mg
- 100 mg

AMOXICILLIN
Amoxil
capsules 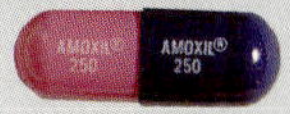
- 250 mg 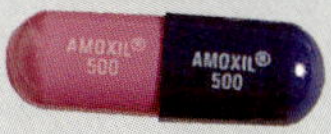
- 500 mg

tablets, chewable 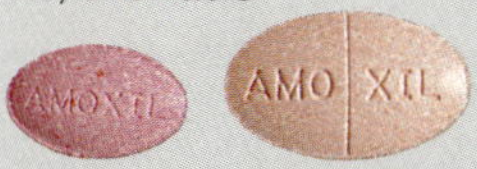
- 125 mg
- 250 mg

Polymox
capsules 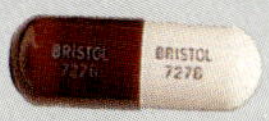
- 250 mg 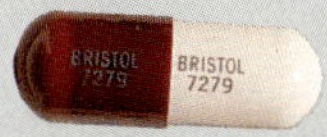
- 500 mg

AMOXICILLIN/CLAVULANATE
Augmentin
tablets 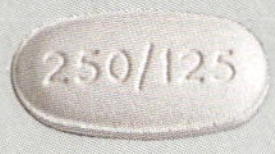
- 250/125 mg

AMOXICILLIN/CLAVULANATE
Augmentin
tablets (cont.)
500/125 mg

tablet, chewable
250/62.50 mg

AMPICILLIN
Omnipen
capsule
500 mg

Polycillin
capsules
250 mg
500 mg

Totacillin
capsule
250 mg

ASTEMIZOLE
Hismanal
tablet
10 mg

ATENOLOL
Tenormin
tablets
25 mg 50 mg 100 mg

AURANOFIN
Ridaura
capsule
3 mg

AZATHIOPRINE
Imuran
tablet
50 mg

AZITHROMYCIN
Zithromax
capsule
250 mg

BECLOMETHASONE
Beclovent
inhaler

Vanceril
inhaler

BENAZEPRIL
Lotensin
tablets
5 mg 10 mg 20 mg

BENZTROPINE
Cogentin
tablets
0.5 mg 1 mg 2 mg

BETAXOLOL
Kerlone
tablets
10 mg 20 mg

BITOLTEROL
Tornalate
inhaler

BROMOCRIPTINE
Parlodel
tablet
2.5 mg

BUMETANIDE
Bumex
tablets
0.5 mg 1 mg 2 mg

BUPROPION
Wellbutrin
tablets
75 mg 100 mg

BUSPIRONE
BuSpar
tablets
5 mg 10 mg

CAPTOPRIL
Capoten
tablets
12.5 mg 25 mg 50 mg

CARBAMAZEPINE
Tegretol

tablet — 200 mg

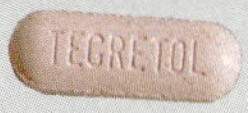

tablet, chewable — 100 mg

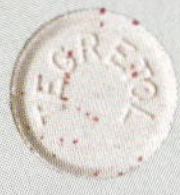

CARTEOLOL
Cartrol

tablet — 2.5 mg

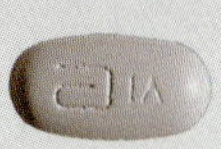

CEFACLOR
Ceclor

capsules — 250 mg, 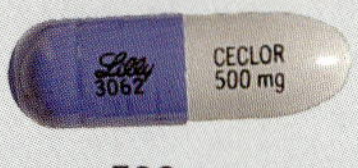 500 mg

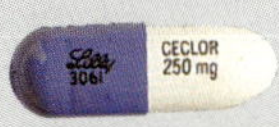

CEFADROXIL
Duricef

capsule — 500 mg

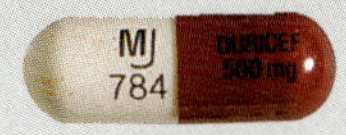

tablet — 1 gram

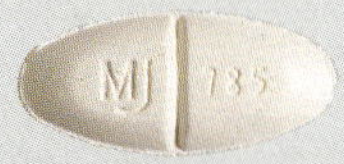

CEFIXIME
Suprax

tablet — 400 mg

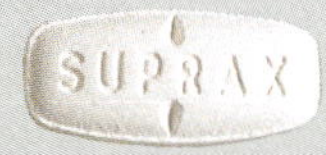

CEFPROZIL
Cefzil

tablets — 250 mg, 500 mg

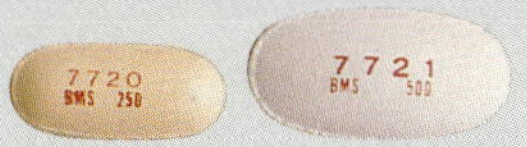

CEFUROXIME
Ceftin

tablets — 125 mg, 250 mg, 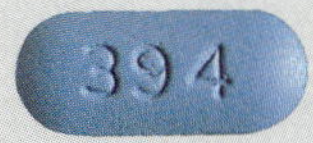 500 mg

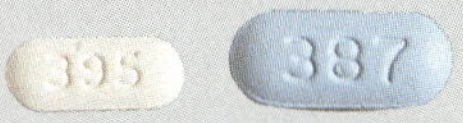

CEPHALEXIN
Keflex

capsules — 250 mg, 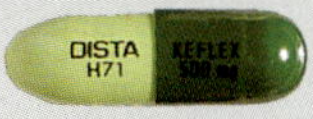 500 mg

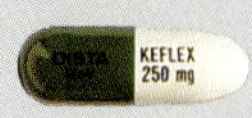

Keftab

tablet — 500 mg

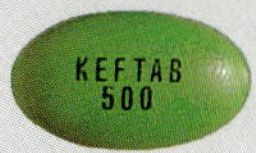

CHLORAMBUCIL
Leukeran

tablet — 2 mg

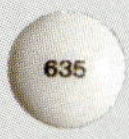

CHLORAMPHENICOL
Chloromycetin

capsule — 250 mg

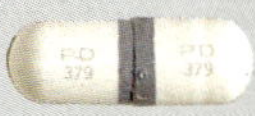

CHLOROQUINE
Aralen

tablet — 500 mg

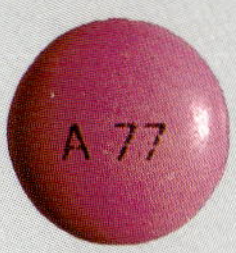

CHLOROTHIAZIDE
Diuril

tablets — 250 mg, 500 mg

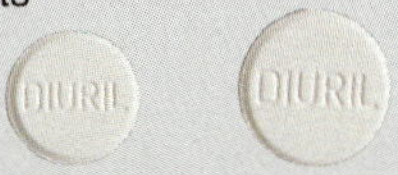

CHLORPROMAZINE
Thorazine

capsules, extended-release — 75 mg, 150 mg

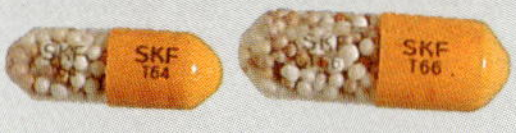

tablets — 100 mg, 200 mg

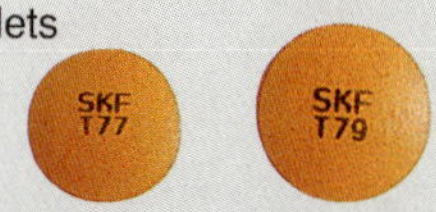

CHLORPROPAMIDE
Diabinese

tablet — 250 mg

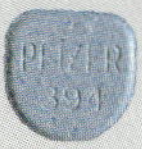

CHLORTHALIDONE
Hygroton

tablets — 25 mg, 50 mg

CHOLESTYRAMINE

Questran Light

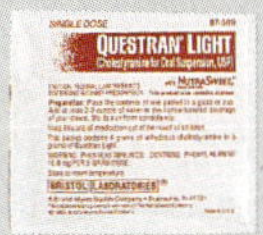

CHOLESTYRAMINE (cont.)
Questran Powder

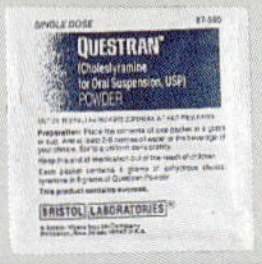

CIMETIDINE
Tagamet

tablets 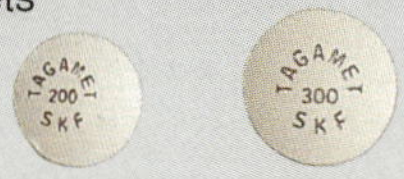
- 200 mg
- 300 mg 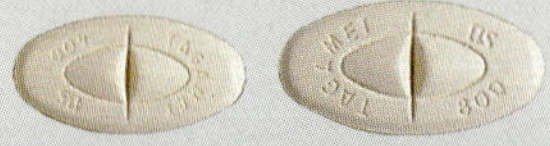
- 400 mg
- 800 mg

CIPROFLOXACIN
Cipro

tablets 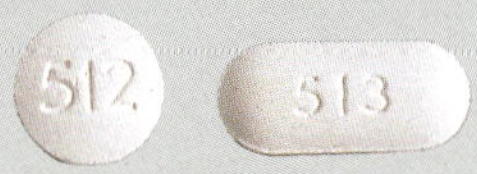
- 250 mg
- 500 mg 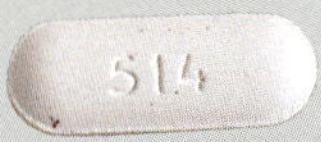
- 750 mg

CLARITHROMYCIN
Biaxin

tablets 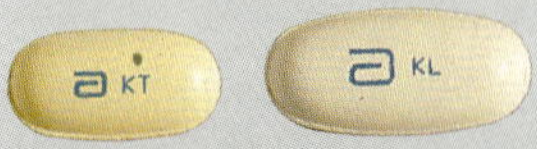
- 250 mg
- 500 mg

CISAPRIDE
Prospulsid

tablets
- 10 mg
- 20 mg

CLOFAZIMINE
Lamprene

capsule 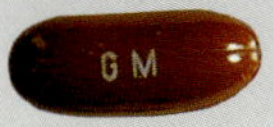
- 100 mg

CLOMIPRAMINE
Anafranil

capsules 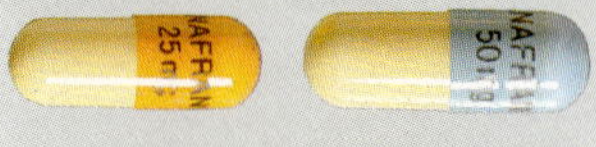
- 25 mg
- 50 mg 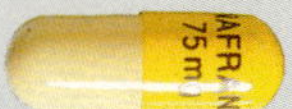
- 75 mg

CLONAZEPAM
Klonopin

tablets 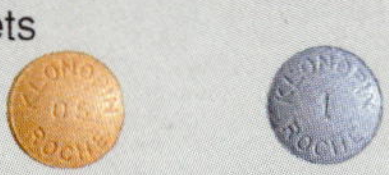
- 0.5 mg
- 1 mg

CLONIDINE
Catapres

tablets 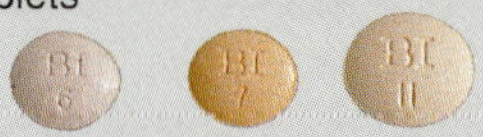
- 0.1 mg
- 0.2 mg
- 0.3 mg

CLOTRIMAZOLE
Mycelex

troche 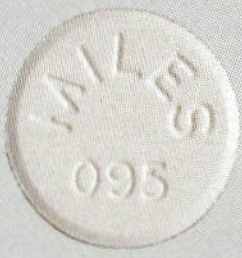
- 10 mg

CLOXACILLIN
Tegopen

capsules 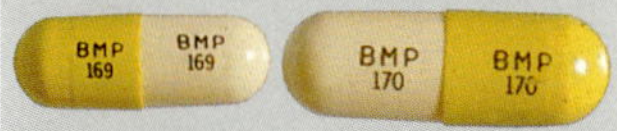
- 250 mg
- 500 mg

CLOZAPINE
Clozaril

tablets 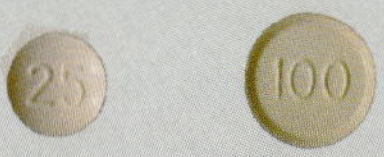
- 25 mg
- 100 mg

COLCHICINE
ColBENEMID

tablet

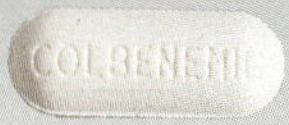

CROMOLYN
Intal

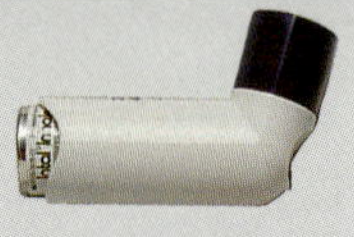

inhaler

CYCLOPHOSPHAMIDE
Cytoxan

tablets 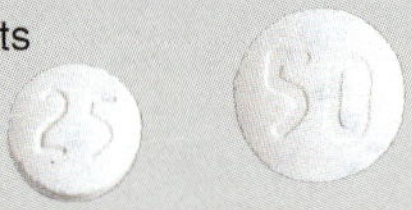
- 25 mg
- 50 mg

CYCLOSPORINE
Sandimmune

capsule 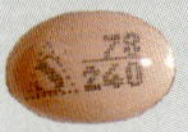
- 25 mg

DAPSONE
(Generic only)

tablets 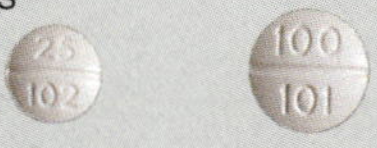
- 25 mg
- 100 mg

DESIPRAMINE
Norpramin

tablets 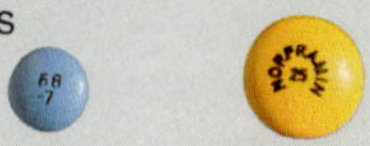
- 10 mg
- 25 mg 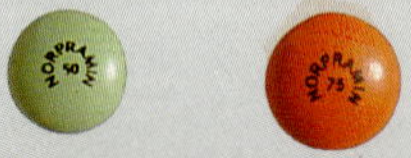
- 50 mg
- 75 mg

DEXAMETHASONE
Decadron (0.75mg) & Generic

tablets 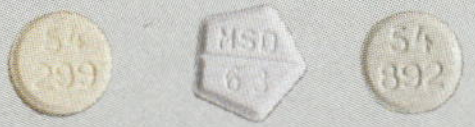
- 0.5 mg
- 0.75 mg
- 4 mg

DIAZEPAM
Valium

tablets 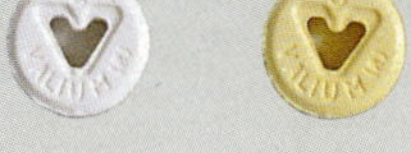
- 2 mg
- 5 mg

Valrelease
capsule, extended-release
15 mg

DICLOFENAC
Voltaren
tablets
- 25 mg
- 75 mg

DIDANOSINE
Videx
tablet
- 25 mg

DIFLUNISAL
Dolobid
tablets
- 250 mg
- 500 mg

DIGOXIN
Lanoxicaps
capsules
- 0.1 mg
- 0.2 mg

Lanoxin
tablets
- 0.125 mg
- 0.25 mg
- 0.5 mg

DILTIAZEM
Cardizem
tablets
- 30 mg
- 60 mg

Cardizem (cont.)
- 90 mg
- 120 mg

Cardizem CD
capsules
- 180 mg
- 240 mg
- 300 mg

Cardizem SR
capsules
- 60 mg
- 90 mg
- 120 mg

DIPHENHYDRAMINE
Benadryl
capsules
- 25 mg
- 50 mg

DIPYRIDAMOLE
Persantine
tablets
- 50 mg
- 75 mg

DISOPYRAMIDE
Norpace
capsules
- 100 mg

Norpace (cont.)
- 150 mg

Norpace CR
capsules, extended-release
- 100 mg
- 150 mg

DISULFIRAM
Antabuse
tablets
- 250 mg
- 500 mg

DOXAZOSIN
Cardura
tablets
- 1 mg
- 2 mg
- 4 mg
- 8 mg

DOXEPIN
Sinequan
capsules
- 10 mg
- 25 mg
- 50 mg

DOXYCYCLINE
Zenith generic
tablet
- 100 mg

ENALAPRIL
Vasotec
tablet
2.5 mg

ERGOTAMINE
Ergostat
tablet
2 mg

ERYTHROMYCIN
Ery-Tab
tablet, delayed-release
333 mg

E-Mycin
tablets, delayed-release
250 mg   333 mg

Eryc
capsule, delayed-release
250 mg

Erythrocin
tablets
250 mg   500 mg

ESTROGENS
Estrace
tablets
1 mg   2 mg

Ogen
tablets
0.625 mg   1.5 mg

Premarin
tablets
0.3 mg   0.625 mg
0.9 mg   1.25 mg
2.5 mg

ETHAMBUTOL
Myambutol
tablet
400 mg

ETHOSUXIMIDE
Zarontin
capsule
250 mg

ETIDRONATE
Didronel
tablets
200 mg   400 mg

ETRETINATE
Tegison
capsules
10 mg   25 mg

FAMOTIDINE
Pepcid
tablets
20 mg   40 mg

FELODIPINE
Plendil
tablets
5 mg   10 mg

FENOPROFEN
Nalfon
capsule
200 mg

FINASTERIDE
Proscar
tablet
5 mg

FLUCONAZOLE
Diflucan
tablets
50 mg   100 mg

FLUCYTOSINE
Ancobon
capsule
500 mg

FLUOXETINE
Prozac
capsule
20 mg

FLUPHENAZINE
Prolixin
tablets
- 1 mg
- 5 mg

FLURAZEPAM
Dalmane
capsules
- 15 mg
- 30 mg

FLURBIPROFEN
Ansaid
tablets
- 50 mg
- 100 mg

FLUTAMIDE
Eulexin
capsule
- 125 mg

FOSINOPRIL
Monopril
tablets
- 10 mg
- 20 mg

FUROSEMIDE
Lasix
tablets
- 20 mg
- 40 mg
- 80 mg

GEMFIBROZIL
Lopid
tablet
- 600 mg

GLIPIZIDE
Glucotrol
tablets
- 5 mg
- 10 mg

GLYBURIDE
DiaBeta
tablets
- 1.25 mg
- 2.5 mg
- 5 mg

Micronase
tablets
- 1.25 mg
- 2.5 mg
- 5 mg

GRISEOFULVIN
Fulvicin P/G
tablets
- 250 mg
- 330 mg

GUANFACINE
Tenex
tablets
- 1 mg
- 2 mg

HALOPERIDOL
Haldol
tablets
- 0.5 mg
- 1 mg
- 2 mg

Haldol (cont.)
- 5 mg
- 10 mg

HYDRALAZINE
Apresoline
tablet
- 100 mg

HYDROCHLOROTHIAZIDE
Esidrix
tablets
- 25 mg
- 50 mg

HYDROCODONE
(& acetaminophen)
Vicodin
tablet
- 5/500 mg

Vicodin ES
tablet
- 7.5/750 mg

HYDROXYCHLOROQUINE
Plaquenil
tablet
- 200 mg

IBUPROFEN
Motrin
tablets
- 400 mg
- 600 mg
- 800 mg

IMIPRAMINE
Tofranil

tablets 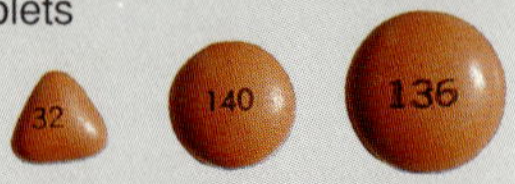
- 10 mg
- 25 mg
- 50 mg

Tofranil-PM

capsule 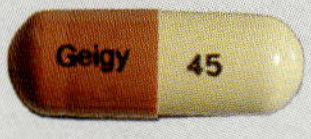
- 125 mg

INDAPAMIDE
Lozol

tablet 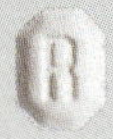
- 2.5 mg

INDOMETHACIN
Indocin

capsules 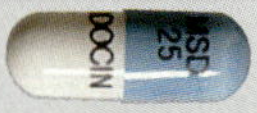
- 25 mg 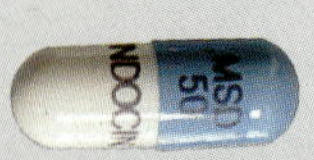
- 50 mg

Indocin SR

capsule 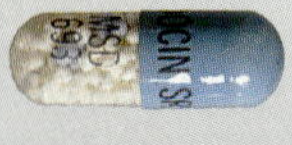
- 75 mg

IODOQUINOL
Yodoxin

tablet 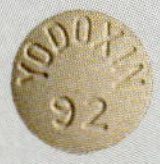
- 210 mg

ISONIAZID
INH

tablet 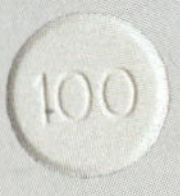
- 100 mg

ISOSORBIDE DINITRATE
Isordil

tablets 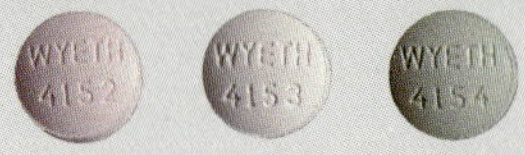
- 5 mg
- 10 mg
- 20 mg 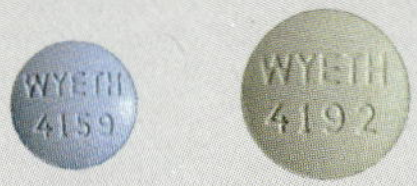
- 30 mg
- 40 mg

tablet, extended-release 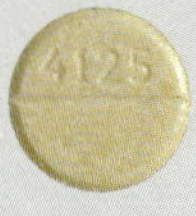
- 40 mg

tablet, sublingual
- 5 mg

ISOSORBIDE MONONITRATE
Ismo

tablet 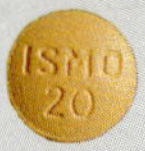
- 20 mg

ISOTRETINOIN
Accutane

capsules 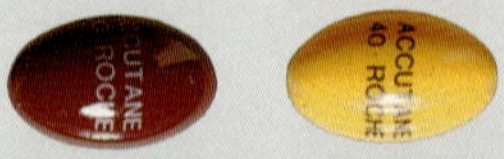
- 20 mg
- 40 mg

ISRADIPINE
DynaCirc

capsules 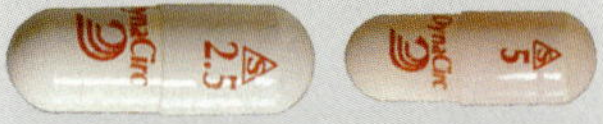
- 2.5 mg
- 5 mg

KETOCONAZOLE
Nizoral

tablet 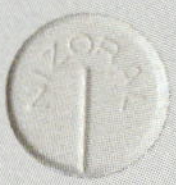
- 200 mg

KETOPROFEN
Orudis

capsules 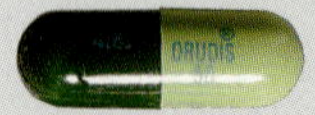
- 50 mg 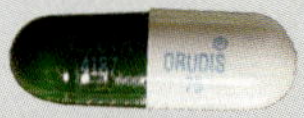
- 75 mg

KETOROLAC
Toradol oral

tablet 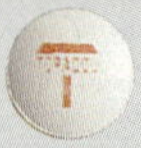
- 10 mg

LABETALOL
Normodyne

tablets 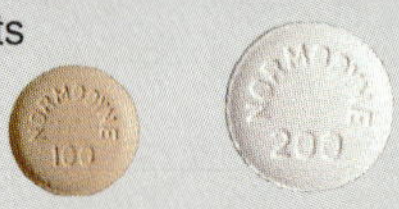
- 100 mg
- 200 mg 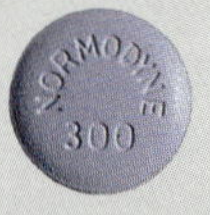
- 300 mg

Trandate

tablets 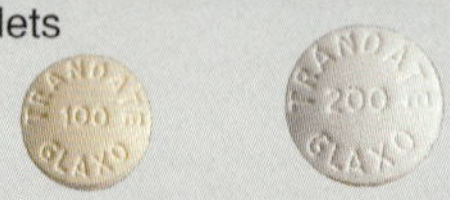
- 100 mg
- 200 mg 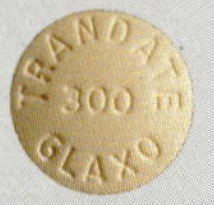
- 300 mg

LEVODOPA/CARBIDOPA
Sinemet

tablets 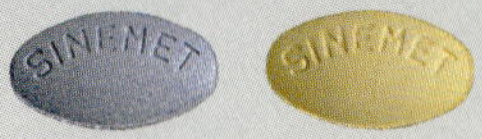
- 10/100 mg
- 25/100 mg 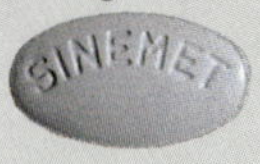
- 25/250 mg

Sinemet CR
tablet, sustained-release
50/200 mg

LEVOTHYROXINE
Synthroid
tablets
- 0.025 mg
- 0.05 mg
- 0.075 mg
- 0.1 mg
- 0.112 mg
- 0.125 mg
- 0.15 mg
- 0.175 mg

LIOTHYRONINE
Cytomel
tablets
- 5 mcg
- 25 mcg

LISINOPRIL
Prinivil
tablets
- 5 mg
- 10 mg
- 20 mg

Zestril
tablets
- 5 mg
- 10 mg
- 20 mg

LITHIUM
Eskalith CR
tablet, controlled-release
450 mg

Lithobid
tablet
300 mg

LOMEFLOXACIN
Maxaquin
tablet
400 mg

LOPERAMIDE
Imodium
capsule
2 mg

LOVASTATIN
Mevacor
tablets
- 20 mg
- 40 mg

MAPROTILINE
Ludiomil
tablets
- 25 mg
- 50 mg

MECLOFENAMATE
Meclomen
capsule
100 mg

MEDROXYPROGESTERONE
Provera
tablets
- 2.5 mg
- 5 mg
- 10 mg

MEPERIDINE
Demerol
tablets
- 50 mg
- 100 mg

MERCAPTOPURINE
Purinethol
tablet
50 mg

MESALAMINE
Asacol
tablet
400 mg

METAPROTERENOL
Alupent
tablet
20 mg

METHADONE
Dolophine
tablet
5 mg

METHOTREXATE
Lederle generic
tablet
2.5 mg

METHYLPHENIDATE
Ritalin
tablets
- 5 mg
- 10 mg
- 20 mg

METHYLPREDNISOLONE
Medrol

tablet — 4 mg

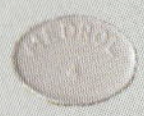

METHYSERGIDE
Sansert

tablet — 2 mg

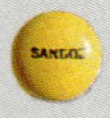

METOCLOPRAMIDE
Reglan

tablets — 5 mg, 10 mg

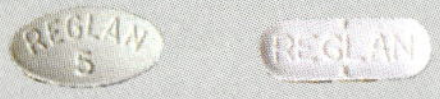

METOLAZONE
Zaroxolyn

tablets — 2.5 mg, 5 mg

METOPROLOL
Lopressor

tablets — 50 mg, 100 mg

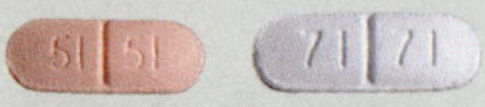

Toprol XL

tablets, extended-release — 50 mg, 100 mg

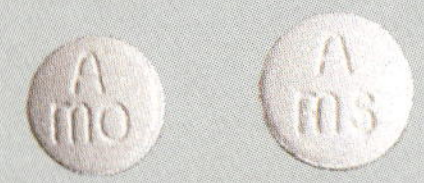

METRONIDAZOLE
Flagyl

tablets — 250 mg, 500 mg

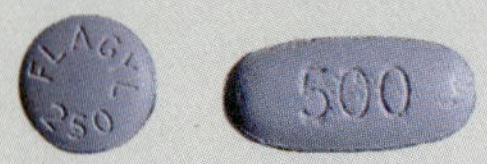

MEXILETINE
Mexitil

capsules — 150 mg, 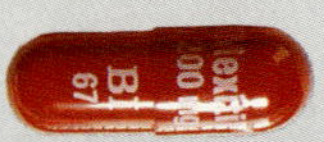 200 mg

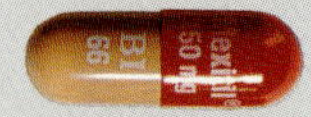

MINOXIDIL
Loniten

tablet — 2.5 mg

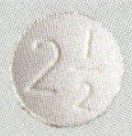

MISOPROSTOL
Cytotec

tablets — 0.1 mg, 0.2 mg

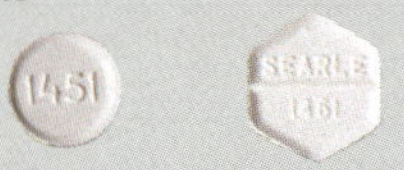

MOLINDONE
Moban

tablets — 10 mg, 25 mg, 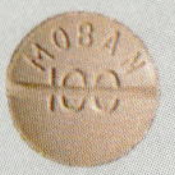 100 mg

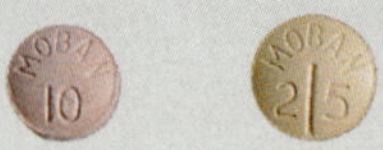

MORPHINE
MS Contin

tablets — 15 mg, 30 mg, 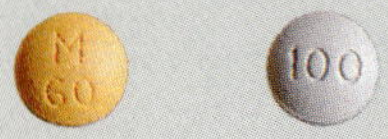 60 mg, 100 mg

NABUMETONE
Relafen

tablets — 500 mg, 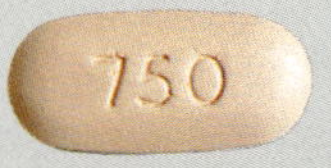 750 mg

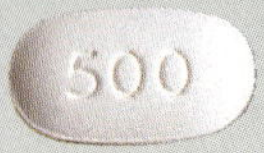

NADOLOL
Corgard

tablets — 20 mg, 40 mg, 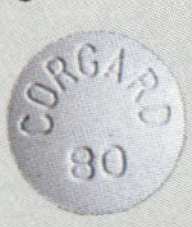 80 mg

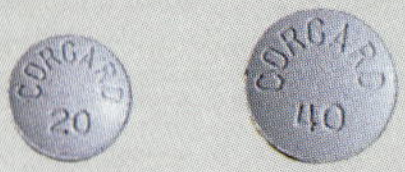

NAPROXEN
Anaprox

tablets — 275 mg, 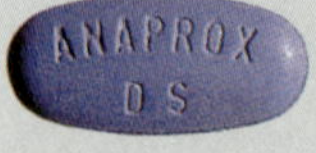 550 mg

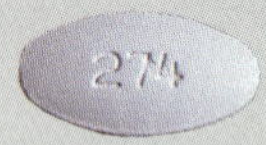

Naprosyn

tablets — 250 mg, 375 mg, 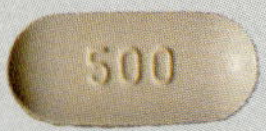 500 mg

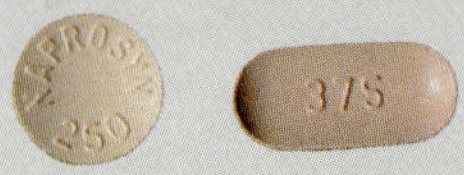

NEOSTIGMINE
Prostigmin

tablet — 15 mg

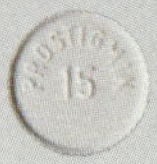

NIACIN
Nicobid
capsules, extended-release
- 250 mg

Slo-Niacin
tablets, extended-release
- 500 mg

NICARDIPINE
Cardene
capsules
- 20 mg
- 30 mg

NICOTINE
Nicorette chewing gum
- 2 mg
tablet
- 4 mg

NIFEDIPINE
Adalat
capsules
- 10 mg
- 20 mg

Procardia
capsules
- 10 mg
- 20 mg

Procardia XL
tablets, extended-release
- 30 mg
- 60 mg
- 90 mg

NITROFURANTOIN
Furadantin
tablets
- 50 mg

Macrodantin
capsules
- 50 mg
- 100 mg

NITROGLYCERIN
Nitrostat
tablets, sublingual
- 0.4 mg

NIZATIDINE
Axid
capsules
- 150 mg
- 300 mg

NORFLOXACIN
Noroxin
tablet
- 400 mg

NORTRIPTYLINE
Pamelor
capsules
- 10 mg
- 25 mg
- 50 mg
- 75 mg

OFLOXACIN
Floxin
tablets
- 200 mg
- 300 mg
- 400 mg

OLSALAZINE
Dipentum
capsule
- 250 mg

OMEPRAZOLE
Prilosec
capsule
- 20 mg

OXTRIPHYLLINE
Choledyl
tablet
- 200 mg

Choledyl SA
tablet, sustained-action
400 mg

OXYCODONE
Roxicodone
tablet
5 mg

OXYCODONE (& acetaminophen)
Percocet
tablet
5/325 mg

PAROXETINE
Paxil
tablet
20 mg • 30 mg

PENICILLAMINE
Cuprimine
capsules
125 mg • 250 mg

Depen
tablet
250 mg

PENICILLIN V
Beepen VK
tablets
250 mg • 500 mg

Pen-Vee-K
tablet
250 mg

V-Cillin K
tablets
250 mg
500 mg

PENTAZOCINE/NALOXONE
Talwin Nx
tablet
50/0.5 mg

PENTOXIFYLLINE
Trental
tablet
400 mg

PERGOLIDE
Permax
tablets
0.05 mg • 1 mg

PERPHENAZINE
Trilafon
tablets
2 mg • 4 mg

PHENELZINE
Nardil
tablet
15 mg

PHENOBARBITAL
Warner Chilcott generic
tablets
15 mg • 30 mg
60 mg • 100 mg

PHENYTOIN
Dilantin
capsule
100 mg

tablet, chewable
50 mg

PINDOLOL
Visken
tablets
5 mg • 10 mg

PIROXICAM
Feldene
capsules
10 mg
20 mg

PRAVASTATIN
Pravachol

tablets 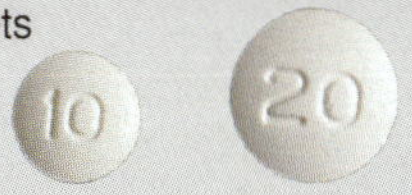
- 10 mg
- 20 mg

PRAZOSIN
Minipress

capsules 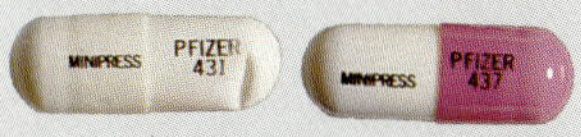
- 1 mg
- 2 mg 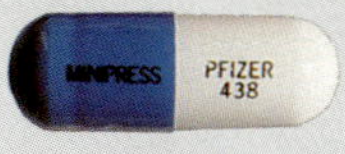
- 5 mg

PREDNISONE
Deltasone

tablets 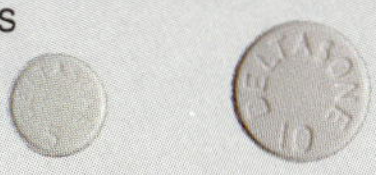
- 5 mg
- 10 mg 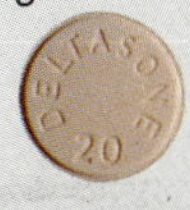
- 20 mg

PRIMIDONE
Mysoline

tablets 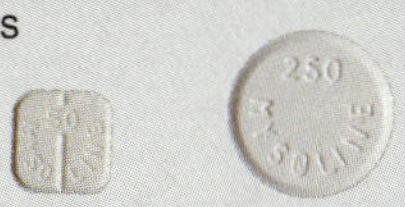
- 50 mg
- 250 mg

PROBENECID
Benemid

tablet 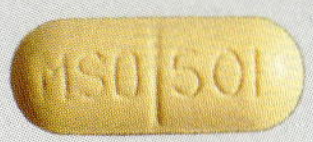
- 500 mg

PROBUCOL
Lorelco

tablets 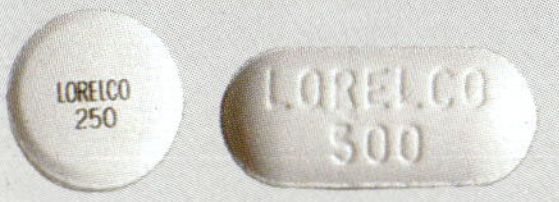
- 250 mg
- 500 mg

PROCAINAMIDE
Pronestyl

capsule 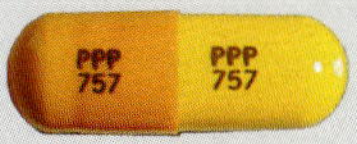
- 500 mg

Procan-SR
tablets, extended-release 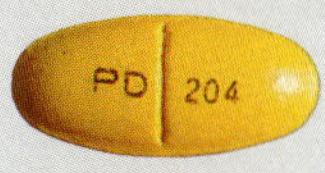
- 500 mg
- 750 mg

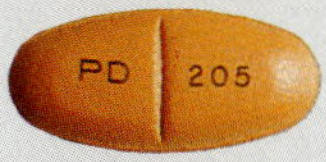

PROCHLORPERAZINE
Compazine

capsules 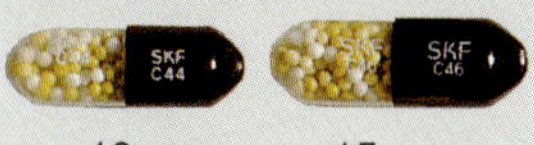
- 10 mg
- 15 mg

tablet 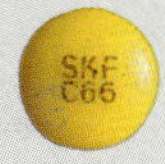
- 5 mg

PROPRANOLOL
Inderal

tablets 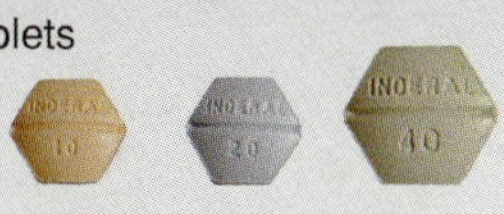
- 10 mg
- 20 mg
- 40 mg 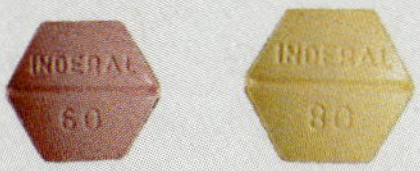
- 60 mg
- 80 mg

Inderal LA
capsules, extended-release 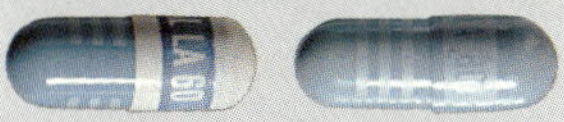
- 60 mg
- 80 mg 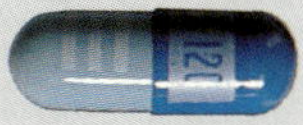
- 120 mg

Inderal LA (cont.)
- 160 mg

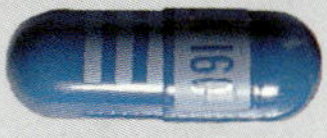

PROTRIPTYLINE
Vivactil

tablet 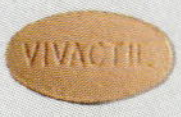
- 5 mg

PYRAZINAMIDE
Lederle generic

tablet 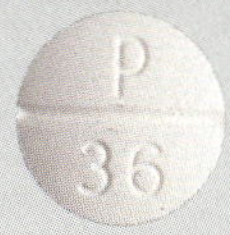
- 500 mg

PYRIDOSTIGMINE
Mestinon

tablet 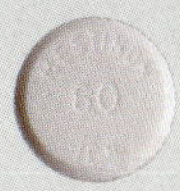
- 60 mg

PYRIMETHAMINE
Daraprim

tablet 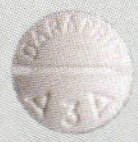
- 25 mg

QUAZEPAM
Doral

tablets 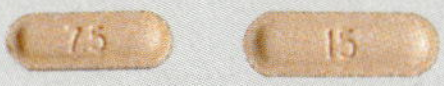
- 7.5 mg
- 15 mg

QUINAPRIL
Accupril

tablets 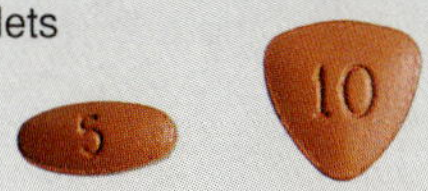
- 5 mg
- 10 mg 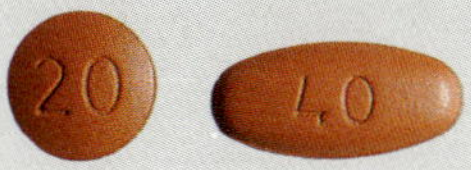
- 20 mg
- 40 mg

QUINIDINE
Quinaglute
tablet — 324 mg

Quinidex
tablet — 300 mg

RAMIPRIL
Altace
capsules — 2.5 mg, 5 mg, 10 mg

RANITIDINE
Zantac
tablets — 150 mg, 300 mg

RIFABUTIN
Mycobutin
tablet — 150 mg

RIFAMPIN
Rifadin
capsules — 150 mg

Rifadin (cont.)
300 mg

SELEGILINE
Eldepryl
tablet — 5 mg

SERTRALINE
Zoloft
tablets — 50 mg, 100 mg

SIMVASTATIN
Zocor
tablets — 5 mg, 10 mg

SPIRONOLACTONE
Aldactone
tablets — 25 mg, 50 mg, 100 mg

SUCRALFATE
Carafate
tablet — 1 gram

SULFAMETHOXAZOLE/TRIMETHOPRIM
Bactrim
tablets — 400/80 mg

Bactrim (cont.)
800/160 mg

Septra
tablets — 400/80 mg, 800/160 mg

SULFASALAZINE
Azulfidine
tablet — 500 mg

Azulfidine EN-Tab
tablet, enteric-coated — 500 mg

SULFISOXAZOLE
Gantrisin
tablet — 500 mg

SULINDAC
Clinoril
tablets — 150 mg, 200 mg

SUMATRIPTAN
Imitrex
auto-injector system

TAMOXIFEN
Nolvadex
tablet 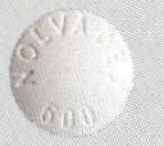
- 10 mg

TERAZOSIN
Hytrin
tablets 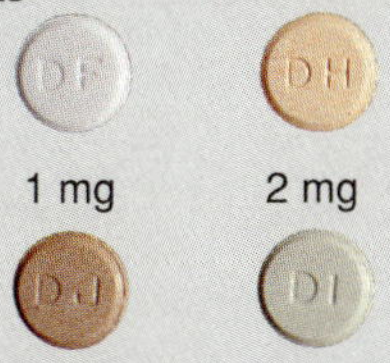
- 1 mg
- 2 mg
- 5 mg
- 10 mg

TERBUTALINE
Brethine
tablets 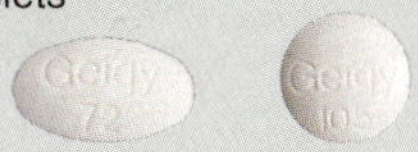
- 2.5 mg
- 5 mg

TERFENADINE
Seldane
tablet 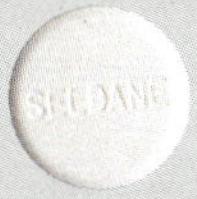
- 60 mg

TETRACYCLINE
Achromycin V
capsule 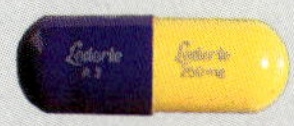
- 250 mg

Sumycin
capsules 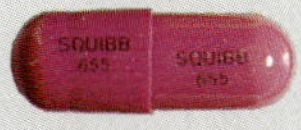
- 250 mg 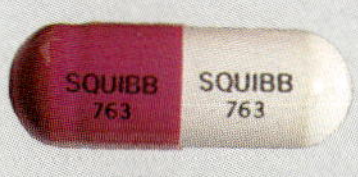
- 500 mg

THEOPHYLLINE
Quibron-T/SR Dividose
tablet 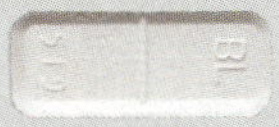
- 300 mg

Slo-bid
capsules 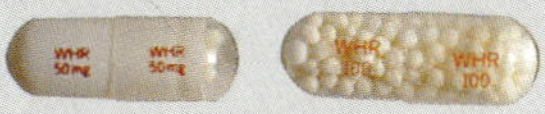
- 50 mg
- 100 mg 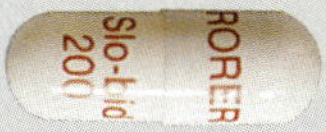
- 200 mg 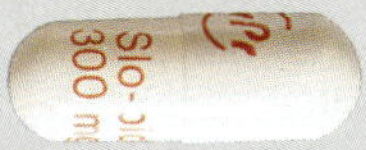
- 300 mg

Slo-Phyllin
capsules 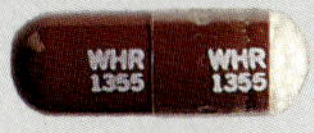
- 125 mg 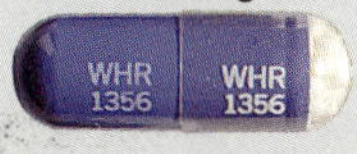
- 250 mg

tablet 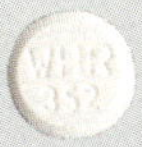
- 200 mg

Theo-Dur
capsules 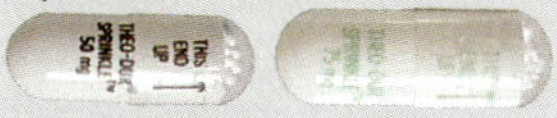
- 50 mg
- 75 mg 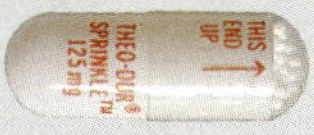
- 125 mg 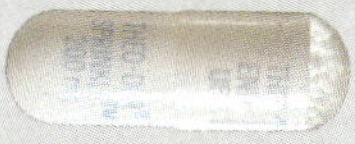
- 200 mg

tablets 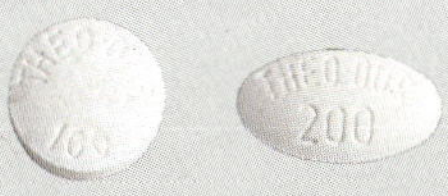
- 100 mg
- 200 mg

Theo-Dur (cont.)
- 300 mg
- 450 mg

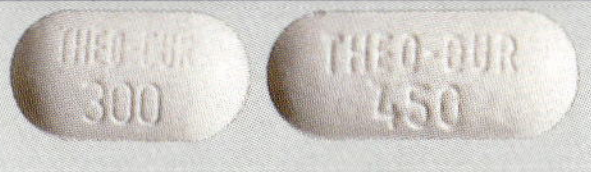

Theo-24
capsule 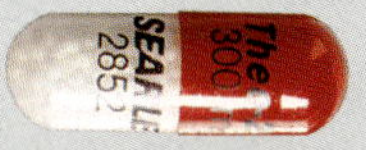
- 300 mg

THIORIDAZINE
Mellaril
tablets 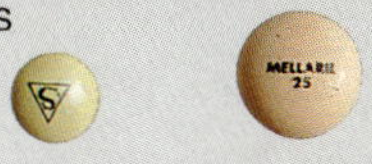
- 10 mg
- 25 mg 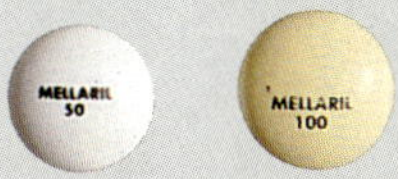
- 50 mg
- 100 mg

THIOTHIXENE
Navane
capsules 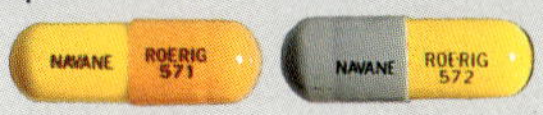
- 1 mg
- 2 mg 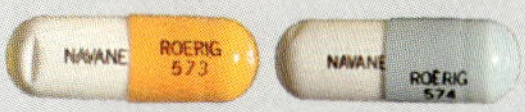
- 5 mg
- 10 mg 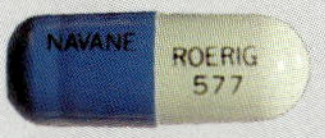
- 20 mg

TICLOPIDINE
Ticlid
tablet 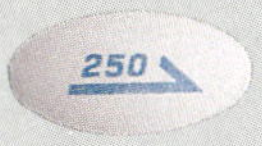
- 250 mg

TIMOLOL
Blocadren
tablets 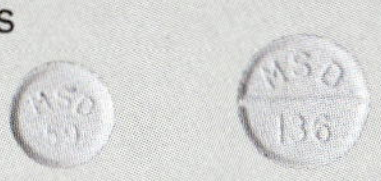
- 5 mg
- 10 mg 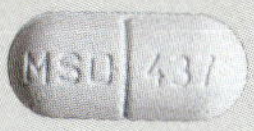
- 20 mg

TOLAZAMIDE
Tolinase
tablets
- 250 mg
- 500 mg

TOLBUTAMIDE
Orinase
tablet
- 500 mg

TOLMETIN
Tolectin
tablet
- 600 mg

Tolectin DS
capsule
- 400 mg

TRAZODONE
Desyrel
tablets
- 50 mg
- 100 mg
- 150 mg

TRIAMTERENE/HYDROCHLOROTHIAZIDE
Dyazide
capsule
- 50/25 mg

Maxzide
tablets
- 37.5/25 mg
- 75/50 mg

TRIFLUOPERAZINE
Stelazine
tablets
- 1 mg
- 2 mg
- 5 mg

TRIMETHOPRIM
Trimpex
tablet
- 100 mg

VALPROIC ACID
Depakote Sprinkle
capsule
- 125 mg

Depakote
tablets
- 125 mg
- 250 mg
- 500 mg

VANCOMYCIN
Vancocin
capsule
- 125 mg

VERAPAMIL
Calan
tablets
- 80 mg
- 120 mg

Calan SR
tablets, extended-release
- 120 mg
- 180 mg
- 240 mg

Verelan
capsules, extended-release
- 120 mg
- 180 mg
- 240 mg

WARFARIN
Coumadin
tablets
- 1 mg
- 2 mg
- 2.5 mg
- 5 mg
- 7.5 mg
- 10 mg

ZALCITABINE
Hivid
tablets
- 0.375 mg
- 0.750 mg

ZIDOVUDINE
Retrovir
capsule
- 100 mg

- you are pregnant (all NSAIDS during the last three months of pregnancy) or you are breast-feeding.
- you have active peptic ulcer disease or any form of gastrointestinal ulceration or bleeding.
- you have active liver disease.
- you have a bleeding disorder or a blood cell disorder.
- you have severe impairment of kidney function.
- you have porphyria (diclofenac, indomethacin).

▷ **Inform Your Physician Before Taking This Drug If**
- you are allergic to aspirin or to other aspirin substitutes.
- you have a history of peptic ulcer disease, Crohn's disease, ulcerative colitis or any type of bleeding disorder.
- you have a history of epilepsy, Parkinson's disease or mental illness (psychosis).
- you have impaired liver or kidney function.
- you have high blood pressure or a history of heart failure.
- you are taking any of the following: acetaminophen, aspirin or other aspirin substitutes or anticoagulants.

Possible Side-Effects (natural, expected and unavoidable drug actions)
Drowsiness, ringing in ears, fluid retention.

▷ **Possible Adverse Effects** (unusual, unexpected and infrequent reactions)
If any of the following develop, consult your physician promptly for guidance.

Mild Adverse Effects
Allergic Reactions: Skin rash, hives, itching, localized swellings of face and/or extremities.
Headache, dizziness, feelings of detachment.
Mouth sores, indigestion, nausea, vomiting, diarrhea.
Ringing in the ears.
Temporary loss of hair (indomethacin).

Serious Adverse Effects
Allergic Reactions: Asthma, difficult breathing, mouth irritation.
Blurred vision, confusion, depression.
Active peptic ulcer, with or without bleeding.
Liver damage with jaundice (see Glossary).
Kidney damage with painful urination, bloody urine, reduced urine formation.
Rare bone marrow depression (see Glossary)—fatigue, weakness, fever, sore throat, abnormal bleeding or bruising.
Severe skin rash (Stevens-Johnson syndrome-diclofenac, ketorolac, etodolac, sulindac).
Peripheral neuritis (see Glossary)—numbness, pain or weakness in extremities (indomethacin).
Rare lung fibrosis (nabumetone).
Rare pneumonitis (sulindac).
Rare aseptic meningitis (diclofenac).

▷ **Possible Effects on Sexual Function**
Enlargement and tenderness of both male and female breasts (indomethacin, sulindac).

Nonmenstrual vaginal bleeding (indomethacin).
Rare impotence (diclofenac, nabumetone).
Rare uterine bleeding (etodolac, sulindac).

Possible Delayed Adverse Effects: Mild anemia due to "silent" blood loss from the stomach (less than that caused by aspirin).

▷ **Adverse Effects That May Mimic Natural Diseases or Disorders**
Liver reactions may suggest viral hepatitis.

Natural Diseases or Disorders That May Be Activated by These Drugs
Peptic ulcer disease, ulcerative colitis.

Possible Effects on Laboratory Tests
Complete blood cell counts: decreased red cells, hemoglobin, white cells and platelets.
Prothrombin time: increased.
Blood lithium level: increased.
Liver function tests: increased liver enzymes (ALT/GPT, AST/GOT and alkaline phosphatase), increased bilirubin.
Kidney function tests: increased blood creatinine and urea nitrogen (BUN) levels (kidney damage).
Fecal occult blood test: positive.

CAUTION
1. Dosage should always be limited to the smallest amount that produces reasonable improvement.
2. These drugs may mask early indications of infection. Inform your physician if you think you are developing an infection of any kind.

Precautions for Use
By Infants and Children: Indomethacin: this drug frequently causes impairment of kidney function in infants. Fatal liver reactions have occurred in children between 6 and 12 years of age; avoid the use of this drug in this age group.
Diclofenac, etodolac, ketorolac, nabumetone, sulindac: Safety and efficacy for those under 12 years of age not established.
Tolmetin: Safety and efficacy for those under two years of age not established.
By Those over 60 Years of Age: Small doses are advisable until tolerance is determined. Watch for any indications of liver or kidney toxicity, fluid retention, dizziness, confusion, impaired memory, depression, peptic ulcer or diarrhea, often with rectal bleeding.

▷ **Advisability of Use During Pregnancy**
Pregnancy Category: Diclofenac, tolmetin: B. Ketorolac, nabumetone, sulindac and etodolac: C. Indomethacin, sulindac and tolmetin: (last three months): D. See Pregnancy Code at the back of this book.
Animal studies: Indomethacin: significant toxicity and birth defects reported in mice and rats.
Diclofenac: mouse, rat and rabbit studies reveal toxic effects on the embryo but no birth defects.
Ketorolac: rat and rabbit studies did not reveal teratogenicity, however, oral dosing after the 17th day of pregnancy caused increased pup mortality.
Nabumetone, tolmetin: rat and rabbit studies revealed no defects.

Human studies: Indomethacin: adequate studies of pregnant women are not available. However, birth defects have been attributed to the use of this drug during pregnancy.

The manufacturer recommends that this drug not be taken during pregnancy.

Diclofenac, nabumetone, sulindac, tolmetin: adequate studies of pregnant women are not available. Avoid this drug completely during the last 3 months of pregnancy. Use it during the first 6 months only if clearly needed. Ask your doctor for guidance.

Ketorolac: adequate studies of pregnant women are not available. Ask your doctor for guidance.

Etodolac: adequate studies of pregnant women not available. The manufacturer advises that this drug be avoided during pregnancy.

Advisability of Use if Breast-Feeding
Presence of this drug in breast milk: Yes: indomethacin, diclofenac, ketorolac.
Unknown: Etodolac, nabumetone, sulindac, tolmetin.
Avoid drug or refrain from nursing.

Habit-Forming Potential: None.

Effects of Overdosage: Drowsiness, agitation, confusion, nausea, vomiting, diarrhea, disorientation, seizures, coma.

Possible Effects of Long-Term Use: Indomethacin and tolmetin: eye changes: deposits in the cornea, alterations in the retina.

Suggested Periodic Examinations While Taking These Drugs (at physician's discretion)
Complete blood cell counts, liver and kidney function tests, complete eye examinations if vision is altered in any way.

▷ **While Taking These Drugs, Observe the Following**
Foods: No restrictions.
Nutritional Support: Indomethecin: take 50 mg of vitamin C (ascorbic acid) daily.
Beverages: No restrictions. May be taken with milk.

▷ *Alcohol:* Use with caution. The irritant action of alcohol on the stomach lining, added to the irritant action of this drug in sensitive individuals, can increase the risk of stomach ulceration and/or bleeding.
Tobacco Smoking: No interactions expected.

▷ *Other Drugs*
Medications in this class may *increase* the effects of
- acetaminophen (Tylenol, etc.), and increase the risk of kidney damage; avoid prolonged use of this combination.
- anticoagulants such as warfarin (Coumadin, etc.), and increase the risk of bleeding; monitor prothrombin time, adjust dose accordingly.
- lithium, and cause lithium toxicity.
- cyclosporine (Sandimmune) and cause toxicity.
- methotrexate (Mexate, others) and cause toxic levels.
- thrombolytics such as streptokinase or TPA.

Medications in this class may *decrease* the effects of
- beta blocker drugs (see Drug Class section), and reduce their antihypertensive effectiveness.

- bumetanide (Bumex).
- captopril (Capoten).
- ethacrynic acid (Edecrin).
- furosemide (Lasix).

Medications in this class *taken concurrently* with the following drugs may increase the risk of bleeding; avoid these combinations:
- aspirin.
- diflunisal (Dolobid).
- dipyridamole (Persantine).
- sulfinpyrazone (Anturane).
- valproic acid (Depakene).

▷ *Driving, Hazardous Activities:* This drug may cause drowsiness, dizziness or impaired vision. Restrict activities as necessary.

Aviation Note: The use of this drug *may be a disqualification* for piloting. Consult a designated Aviation Medical Examiner.

Exposure to Sun: Use caution. Several of the medicines in this class have caused increased sensitivity (photosensitivity—see Glossary) to the sun.

ACYCLOVIR (ay SI kloh ver)

Introduced: 1979 **Prescription:** USA: Yes; Canada: Yes **Available as Generic:** No **Class:** Antiviral **Controlled Drug:** USA: No; Canada: No
Brand Name: Zovirax

Author's note: This medication was recently rejected by the FDA for a change to non-prescription "over the counter" OTC status.

BENEFITS versus RISKS	
Possible Benefits	*Possible Risks*
Hastened recovery from initial episode of genital herpes	Nausea, vomiting, diarrhea (8% in long-term use)
Prevention of recurrence of genital herpes	Nervousness, depression (less than 3%)
Lessen the severity of chicken pox in some children	Joint and muscle pain (3%)
	Seizures or coma with IV use (1%)

▷ **Principal Uses**

As a Single Drug Product: Uses currently included in FDA approved labeling: (1) Treats or helps prevent genital herpes; (2) used to lessen the severity of chicken pox in children using inhaled steroids or who have a lung disease; (3) treats shingles (Herpes zoster) which has recurred; (4) treats skin and mucous infections (mucocutaneous) caused by Herpes simplex in patients with immune problems; (5) used to treat brain infections caused by Herpes simplex.

Other (unlabeled) generally accepted uses: Acyclovir is also beneficial in the treatment of herpes simplex infections of the eye and rectum and pneumonia caused by the chicken pox virus. Some data to support its use in non-malignant skin growths in the throat (laryngeal papillomatosis). It is a trial AIDS treatment.

How This Drug Works: By blocking genetic material formation of the herpes simplex virus, this drug stops viral multiplication and spread, reducing severity and duration of the herpes infection.

Available Dosage Forms and Strengths
 Capsules — 200 mg
 Intravenous — 500 mg, one gram
 Oral suspension — 200 mg/5 ml
 Tablets — 200 mg, 400 mg (Canada only) and 800 mg
 Ointment — 5%

▷ **Recommended Dosage Ranges (Actual dosage and administration schedule must be determined by the physician or clinical pharmacist for each patient individually.)**

Infants and Children: Safety and efficacy in children younger than 2 years of age has NOT been established.

Information about use of topical acyclovir in children is lacking.

18 to 65 Years of Age: For initial episode of genital herpes—200 mg/4 hours for a total of 5 capsules daily for 10 consecutive days (total dose of 50 capsules). For intermittent recurrence—200 mg/4 hours for a total of 5 capsules daily for 5 consecutive days (total dose of 25 capsules). Start treatment at the earliest sign of recurrence. For prevention of frequent recurrence—400 mg taken 2 times daily for up to 12 months. For the ointment form—cover all infected areas every 3 hours for a total of 6 times daily for 7 consecutive days. Start treatment at the earliest sign of infection.

Treatment of chicken pox: 20 mg/kg (do not exceed 800 mg) orally, four times a day for 5 days. Start treatment at the first symptom or sign.

Over 65 Years of Age: The dose must be adjusted if the kidneys are impaired.

Conditions Requiring Dosing Adjustments

Liver function: Specific adjustment in liver dysfunction is not defined.

Kidney function: The dose **must** be adjusted in people with compromised kidney function.

▷ **Dosing Instructions:** May be taken without regard to food. Capsule may be opened to take it. Take the full course of the exact dose prescribed. Use a finger cot or rubber glove to apply the ointment.

Usual Duration of Use: Use on a regular schedule for 10 days is usually needed to see this drug's effect in reducing the severity and duration of the initial infection. Continual use for 6 months to 3 years may be needed to prevent frequent recurrence of herpes eruptions.

▷ **This Drug Should Not Be Taken If**
- you have had an allergic reaction to it previously.

▷ **Inform Your Physician Before Taking This Drug If**
- you have impaired liver or kidney function.
- you are taking any other drugs at this time.
- you are unsure of how much or how often to take acyclovir.

Possible Side-Effects (natural, expected and unavoidable drug actions)
With use of capsules—none.
With use of ointment—mild pain, or stinging at site of application (28%).

Acyclovir

▷ **Possible Adverse Effects** (unusual, unexpected and infrequent reactions)
   If any of the following develop, consult your physician promptly for guidance.
   Mild Adverse Effects
     Allergic Reaction: Skin rash.
     Headache, dizziness, nervousness, insomnia, depression, fatigue.
     Nausea, vomiting, diarrhea.
     Joint pains, muscle cramps.
     Acne, hair loss.
   Serious Adverse Effects
     Superficial thrombophlebitis, enlarged lymph glands.
     Seizures or coma with IV use (1%).
     Kidney problems (rare).

▷ **Possible Effects on Sexual Function:** Altered timing and pattern of menstruation.

Possible Effects on Laboratory Tests
   Complete blood cell counts: decreased red cells and hemoglobin.
   Blood urea nitrogen (BUN): increased.
   Serum creatinine: increased.

CAUTION
   1. This drug does not eliminate all herpes virus and is not a cure. Recurrence is possible. Resume treatment at the earliest sign of infection.
   2. Avoid sexual intercourse if herpes blisters and swelling are present.
   3. Do not exceed the prescribed dosage.
   4. Tell your doctor if frequency or severity of infections don't improve.

Precautions for Use
   By Infants and Children: Safety and effectiveness for use by those under 12 not established.
   By Those over 60 Years of Age: Avoid dehydration. Drink 2 to 3 quarts of liquids daily.

▷ **Advisability of Use During Pregnancy**
   Pregnancy Category: C. See Pregnancy Code at the back of this book.
     Animal studies: No birth defects found in mouse, rat or rabbit studies.
     Human studies: Adequate studies of pregnant women are not available.
     Avoid use if possible. Use only if clearly needed.

Advisability of Use if Breast-Feeding
   Presence of this drug in breast milk: Yes.
   Ask your physician for guidance.

Habit-Forming Potential: None.

Effects of Overdosage: Possible impairment of kidney function.

Possible Effects of Long-Term Use: Development of acyclovir resistant strains of herpes virus.

Suggested Periodic Examinations While Taking This Drug (at physician's discretion)
   Kidney function tests.

▷ **While Taking This Drug, Observe the Following**
   Foods: No restrictions.
   Beverages: No restrictions. May be taken with milk. Drink 2 to 3 quarts of liquids daily.

▷ *Alcohol:* Use caution; dizziness or fatigue may be accentuated.
Tobacco Smoking: No interactions expected.
▷ *Other Drugs*
The following drugs may *increase* the effects of acyclovir
- cyclosporine use may result in increased risk of kidney toxicity.
- probenecid (Benemid) may delay its elimination.
▷ *Driving, Hazardous Activities:* Use caution if dizziness or fatigue occurs.
Aviation Note: The use of this drug *may be a disqualification* for piloting. Consult a designated Aviation Medical Examiner.
Exposure to Sun: No restrictions.

ALBUTEROL (al BYU ter ohl)

Other Name: Salbutamol

Introduced: 1968 **Prescription:** USA: Yes; Canada: Yes **Available as Generic:** Yes **Class:** Antiasthmatic, bronchodilator **Controlled Drug:** USA: No; Canada: No

Brand Names: ✦Apo-Salvent, ✦Novo-Salmol, Proventil Inhaler, Proventil Repetabs, Proventil Tablets, ✦Salbutamol, ✦Ventodisk, Ventolin Inhaler, Ventolin Rotacaps, Ventolin syrup, Ventolin tablets, Volmax extended release tablets, ✦Volmax controlled release tablets

BENEFITS versus RISKS	
Possible Benefits	*Possible Risks*
VERY EFFECTIVE RELIEF OF BRONCHOSPASM	Increased blood pressure Fine hand tremor Irregular heart rhythm and fatalities (with excessive use)

▷ **Principal Uses**
As a Single Drug Product: (1)Relieves acute bronchial asthma and reduces the frequency and severity of chronic, recurrent asthmatic attacks. Helps prevent exercise induced bronchospasm in children ages 4–11.

How This Drug Works: By increasing cyclic AMP, this drug relaxes constricted bronchial muscles to relieve asthmatic wheezing.

Available Dosage Forms and Strengths
Aerosol — 90 mcg per actuation
Capsules for inhalation — 200 mcg
Solution for inhalation — 0.83 mg per ml and 5 mg per ml
Syrup — 2 mg per 5-ml teaspoonful
Rotacaps — 200 mcg
Tablets — 2 mg, 4 mg
— 2.4 mg, 4.8 mg (Canada)
Tablets, controlled release (Canada) — 4 mg, 8 mg
Tablets, extended release — 4 mg, 8 mg, 9 mg
Ventodisk (Canada) — 200 mcg and 400 mcg per disk

48   Albuterol

▷ **Recommended Dosage Ranges (Actual dosage and administration schedule must be determined by the physician or clinical pharmacist for each patient individually.)**

Inhaler—Adults and children 12 or older: Two inhalations repeated every 4 to 6 hours. For some patients, one inhalation every 4 hours may be enough. Taking a larger number of inhalations is **not** recommended. If the dose which has worked for you before does not provide relief, call your physician immediately as the status of your asthma must be examined. Tablets—2 to 4 mg 3 to 4 times daily, every 4 to 6 hours. **Do not exceed 8 inhalations (720 mcg)/24 hours, or 32 mg (tablet form)/24 hours.**

Conditions Requiring Dosing Adjustments

Liver function: Use with caution and in low doses in people with liver compromise.

Kidney function: No specific changes in dosing are available.

Coronary artery disease: A maximum starting dose should be 1 mg in order to avoid chest pain (angina).

Thyroid disease

People with low (hypoactive) thyroid may require increased doses to attain a therapeutic effect.

▷ **Dosing Instructions:** May be taken on empty stomach or with food or milk. Tablet may be crushed. For inhaler, follow the written instructions carefully. Do not overuse.

Usual Duration of Use: Do not use beyond the time necessary to stop episodes of asthma.

▷ **This Drug Should Not Be Taken If**
- you have had an allergic reaction to any dosage form of it.
- you currently have an irregular heart rhythm.
- you are taking, or have taken within the past 2 weeks, any monoamine oxidase (MAO) type A inhibitor drug (see Drug Class, Section Four).

▷ **Inform Your Physician Before Taking This Drug If**
- you have a heart or circulatory disorder, especially high blood pressure or coronary heart disease.
- you have diabetes.
- you have an over active thyroid (hyperthyroid).
- you are taking any form of digitalis or any stimulant drug.
- you take other prescription or non-prescription medications which were not discussed when albuterol was prescribed for you.
- you are unsure of how much to take or how often to take albuterol.

Possible Side-Effects (natural, expected and unavoidable drug actions)

Aerosol—dryness or irritation of mouth or throat, altered taste.

Tablet—nervousness, palpitation.

▷ **Possible Adverse Effects** (unusual, unexpected and infrequent reactions)

If any of the following develop, consult your physician promptly for guidance.

Mild Adverse Effects

Headache (7%), dizziness (2%), restlessness, insomnia, fine hand tremor (20%).

Nausea (2%), heartburn, vomiting.
Leg cramps (3%), flushing of skin.
Serious Adverse Effects
A pattern of loss of response followed by increased dose and frequency have resulted in rapid or irregular heart rhythm and fatalities.
High blood sugar (hyperglycemia).

▷ **Possible Effects on Sexual Function:** None reported.

Natural Diseases or Disorders That May Be Activated By This Drug
Latent coronary artery disease, diabetes or high blood pressure.

Possible Effects on Laboratory Tests
Blood HDL Cholesterol level: increased.
Blood glucose level: increased.

CAUTION
1. Use of this drug by inhalation with beclomethasone aerosol (Beclovent, Vanceril) may increase the risk of fluorocarbon propellant toxicity. Use albuterol aerosol 20 to 30 minutes *before* beclomethasone aerosol to reduce toxicity and enhance the penetration of beclomethasone.
2. Serious heart rhythmn problems or cardiac arrest can result from excessive or prolonged inhalation.
3. Call your doctor if you begin to increase the number of times you use this drug on a daily basis.

Precautions for Use
By Infants and Children: Used to help prevent bronchospasm caused by exercise in children ages 4–11.
By Those over 60 Years of Age: Avoid excessive and continual use. If asthma is not relieved promptly, other drugs will have to be tried. Watch for nervousness, palpitations, irregular heart rhythm and muscle tremors.

▷ **Advisability of Use During Pregnancy**
Pregnancy Category: C. See Pregnancy Code at the back of this book.
Animal studies: Cleft palate reported in mice.
Human studies: Adequate studies of pregnant women are not available.
Avoid use during first 3 months if possible.

Advisability of Use if Breast-Feeding
Presence of this drug in breast milk: Unknown.
Avoid drug or refrain from nursing.

Habit-Forming Potential: None.

Effects of Overdosage: Nervousness, palpitation, rapid heart rate, sweating, headache, tremor, vomiting, chest pain.

Possible Effects of Long-Term Use: Loss of effectiveness.

Suggested Periodic Examinations While Taking This Drug (at physician's discretion)
Blood pressure measurements, evaluation of heart status.

▷ **While Taking This Drug, Observe the Following**
Foods: No restrictions.
Beverages: Avoid excessive caffeine as found in coffee, tea, cola, chocolate.
▷ *Alcohol:* No interactions expected.
Tobacco Smoking: No interactions expected.

Allopurinol

▷ **Other Drugs**
   Albuterol *taken concurrently* with
   - amphetamines may result in worsening of cardiovascular side effects.
   - beta blockers such as propranolol results in loss of effect of both medications.
   - monoamine oxidase (MAO) type A inhibitor drugs can cause very high blood pressure and undesirable heart stimulation.
   - theophylline may result in rapid removal of theophylline and loss of therapeutic theophylline effect.
   - tricyclic antidepressants (see Glossary) may cause a severe increase in blood pressure.

▷ *Driving, Hazardous Activities:* Use caution if excessive nervousness or dizziness occurs.
   Aviation Note: The use of this drug *is a disqualification* for piloting. Consult a designated Aviation Medical Examiner.
   Exposure to Sun: No restrictions.
   Heavy Exercise or Exertion: Use caution. Excessive exercise can induce asthma in sensitive people.

ALLOPURINOL (al oh PURE i nohl)

Introduced: 1963 **Prescription:** USA: Yes; Canada: Yes **Available as Generic:** USA: Yes; Canada: No **Class:** Antigout **Controlled Drug:** USA: No; Canada: No

Brand Names: ✦Alloprin, ✦Apo-Allopurinol, Lopurin, ✦Novopurol, ✦Purinol, Zurinol, Zyloprim

BENEFITS versus RISKS	
Possible Benefits	*Possible Risks*
EFFECTIVE CONTROL OF GOUT	Increased frequency of acute gout initially
CONTROL OF HIGH BLOOD URIC ACID due to polycythemia, leukemia, cancer and chemotherapy	Peripheral neuritis
	Allergic reactions in skin, lung, blood vessels and liver
	Bone marrow depression
	Kidney toxicity

▷ **Principal Uses**
   As a Single Drug Product: Uses currently included in FDA approved labeling: (1) Used in the long-term management of gout to *prevent* episodes of acute gout (It does not relieve the symptoms of acute gout attacks.); (2) helps prevent abnormally high blood levels of uric acid in people who have recurrent uric acid kidney stones, those who are receiving chemotherapy or radiation therapy for cancer or people taking thiazide diuretics (see Drug Classes).
   Other (unlabeled) generally accepted uses: (1) May be a great benefit in decreasing pain and occurance of mouth sores in people receiving 5-fluorouacil chemotherapy.

Allopurinol

How This Drug Works: By blocking the action of the enzyme xanthine oxidase, this drug decreases the formation of uric acid.

Available Dosage Forms and Strengths
Tablets — 100 mg, 300 mg (and 200 mg in Canada)

▷ **Usual Adult Dosage Range:** Initially 100 mg/24 hours. Increase by 100 mg/24 hours at intervals of 1 week until uric acid blood level is 6 mg/dl or less. Usual dose is 200 to 300 mg/24 hours for mild gout, and 400 to 600 mg/24 hours for moderate to severe gout. Daily doses of 300 mg or less may be taken as a single dose. Doses exceeding 300 mg daily should be divided into 2 or 3 equal portions; for the high uric acid levels associated with cancer, 600 to 800 mg/24 hours, divided into 3 equal portions. **Note: Actual dosage and administration schedule must be determined by the physician for each patient individually.**

Conditions Requiring Dosing Adjustments
Liver function: Dose adjustment in liver compromise is not documented.
Kidney function: Allopurinol dosing **must** be adjusted in renal compromise.
Malnutrition
Patients who are malnourished or who have been placed on low protein diets will not eliminate allopurinol normally and are at risk for toxicity. Doses must be decreased.

▷ **Dosing Instructions:** Best taken with food or milk to reduce stomach irritation. Tablet may be crushed. Drink 2 to 3 quarts of liquids daily.

Usual Duration of Use: Blood uric acid levels usually begin to decrease in 48 to 72 hours and may reach a normal range in 1 to 3 weeks. Regular use for several months may be needed to prevent attacks of acute gout. Continual use for many years may be necessary for adequate control. See your doctor regularly.

▷ **This Drug Should Not Be Taken If**
- you have had an allergic reaction to it previously.
- you are experiencing an acute attack of gout at the present time.

▷ **Inform Your Physician Before Taking This Drug If**
- you have a personal or family history of hemochromatosis.
- you have a history of liver or kidney disease.
- you have had a blood cell or bone marrow disorder.
- you have any type of convulsive disorder (epilepsy).
- you take other prescription or non-prescription medications which were not discussed when allopurinol was prescribed for you.
- you are unsure of how much to take or how often to take allopurinol.
- you are on a low protein diet.

Possible Side-Effects (natural, expected and unavoidable drug actions)
The frequency and severity of episodes of acute gout may occur during the first several weeks of drug use. Ask your doctor about the need for other drugs during this period.

▷ **Possible Adverse Effects** (unusual, unexpected and infrequent reactions)
If any of the following develop, consult your physician promptly for guidance.
Mild Adverse Effects
Allergic Reactions: Skin rash, hives, itching, drug fever.

Headache, dizziness, drowsiness.
Nausea, vomiting, diarrhea, stomach cramps.
Loss of scalp hair.

Serious Adverse Effects
Allergic Reactions: Severe skin reactions, high fever, chills, joint pains, swollen glands, kidney damage.
Hepatitis with or without jaundice (see Glossary)—yellow eyes and skin, dark-colored urine, light-colored stools.
Bone marrow depression (see Glossary).
Seizures, peripheral neuritis.
Bronchospasm (rare).
Eye damage (macular), cataract formation.

▷ **Possible Effects on Sexual Function:** Less than 1% and questionable cause: male infertility, male breast enlargement, impotence.

▷ **Adverse Effects That May Mimic Natural Diseases or Disorders**
Toxic liver reaction may suggest viral hepatitis.
Severe skin reactions may resemble the Stevens-Johnson syndrome (erythema multiforme).

Possible Effects on Laboratory Tests
Complete blood cell counts: decreased red cells, hemoglobin and platelets; increased eosinophils.
Liver function tests: increased ALT/GPT, AST/GOT, and alkaline phosphatase.

CAUTION
1. During the early weeks of treatment, the frequency of acute attacks of gout may increase. These subside with continuation of treatment.
2. This drug will not relieve the symptoms of acute gout. It should not be started during the presence of acute gout symptoms.
3. Vitamin C in doses of 2 grams or more daily can increase the risk of kidney stone formation during the use of allopurinol.
4. Allergic-type kidney damage can result from the concurrent use of thiazide diuretics (see Drug Class, Section Four). Avoid this combination.
5. Patients on low protein diets will not eliminate allopurinol normally and decreased doses are indicated.

Precautions for Use
By Infants and Children: Watch closely for allergic skin reactions and blood cell disorders. The toxicity of azathioprine (Imuran) or mercaptopurine (Purinethol) may be increased in children receiving chemotherapy for cancer.
By Those over 60 Years of Age: Smaller initial and maintenance doses of this drug must be used.

▷ **Advisability of Use During Pregnancy**
Pregnancy Category: C. See Pregnancy Code at the back of this book.
Animal studies: Results are conflicting and inconclusive.
Human studies: Adequate studies of pregnant women are not available.
Avoid use of drug during the first 3 months. Use during the last 6 months only if clearly needed.

Advisability of Use if Breast-Feeding
Presence of this drug in breast milk: Yes.
Avoid drug or refrain from nursing.

Habit-Forming Potential: None.

Effects of Overdosage: Nausea, vomiting or diarrhea may occur as a result of individual sensitivity. Hypersensitivity reactions, kidney and liver function decline.

Possible Effects of Long-Term Use: None identified.

Suggested Periodic Examinations While Taking This Drug (at physician's discretion)
Blood uric acid levels, complete blood cell counts, liver and kidney function tests. If appropriate, eye examinations for possible cataract formation or macular damage. Complete blood counts.

▷ **While Taking This Drug, Observe the Following**
Foods: Follow physician's advice regarding the need for a low-purine diet.
Beverages: No restrictions. May be taken with milk.

▷ *Alcohol:* No interactions expected.
Tobacco Smoking: No interactions expected.

▷ *Other Drugs*
Allopurinol may *increase* the effects of
- azathioprine (Imuran) and mercaptopurine (Purinethol), making it necessary to reduce their dosages.
- oral anticoagulants such as warfarin (see Drug Class Section).
- theophylline (aminophylline, Elixophyllin, Theo-Dur, etc.)

Allopurinol *taken concurrently* with
- ampicillin may increase the incidence of skin rash.
- antacids containing aluminum will decrease the therapeutic effect of allopurinol.
- captopril or other ACE inhibitors (see Drug Classes) can increase the likelihood of allergic reactions.
- cyclophosphamide may result in cyclophosphamide toxicity.
- cyclosporine can result in cyclosporine toxicity.
- tamoxifen may result in increased allopurinol levels and increased risk of liver toxicity.
- theophylline may increase theophylline to toxic levels.
- vidarabine may increase risk of neurotoxicity.

▷ *Driving, Hazardous Activities:* Drowsiness may occur in some people. Use caution.
Aviation Note: The use of this drug *may be a disqualification* for piloting. Consult a designated Aviation Medical Examiner.
Exposure to Sun: No restrictions.

ALPRAZOLAM (al PRAY zoh lam)

Introduced: 1973 **Prescription:** USA: Yes; Canada: Yes **Available as Generic:** Yes **Class:** Mild tranquilizer, benzodiazepines **Controlled Drug:** USA: C-IV*; Canada: No

Brand Name: Xanax, Alprazolam Intensol, ◆Apo-Alpraz, ◆Nu-Alpraz

Warning: The brand names Xanax and Zantac are similar and can be mistaken for each other; this can lead to serious medication errors. These names represent very different drugs. Xanax is the mild tranquilizer alprazolam. Zantac is the generic drug ranitidine, used to treat peptic ulcer disease. Verify that you are taking the correct drug.

BENEFITS versus RISKS	
Possible Benefits	*Possible Risks*
RELIEF OF ANXIETY AND NERVOUS TENSION	Habit-forming potential with prolonged use
EFFECTIVE TREATMENT OF PANIC DISORDER	Minor impairment of mental functions with therapeutic doses
Wide margin of safety with therapeutic doses	Tachycardia and palpitations

▷ **Principal Uses**

As a Single Drug Product: Uses currently included in FDA approved labeling: (1) Used as a mild tranquilizer for the short-term relief of mild to moderate anxiety and nervous tension; (2) helps relieve anxiety associated with neurosis; (3) works to end irritable bowel syndrome (se Glossary); (4) can help ease the frequency and severity of panic attacks.

Other (unlabeled) generally accepted uses: (1) May have a role in helping to control extreme PMS symptoms; (2) can help ease a variety of types of cancer pain when added on to various narcotic therapy.

How This Drug Works: Produces a calming effect by enhancing the action of the nerve transmitter gamma-aminobutyric acid (GABA), which in turn blocks higher brain centers.

Available Dosage Forms and Strengths
 Tablets — 0.25 mg, 0.5 mg, 1 mg, 2 mg
 Oral Solution — 0.25 mg, 0.5 mg, 1 mg/5ml

▷ **Usual Adult Dosage Range:** For anxiety and nervous tension: 0.25 mg to 0.5 mg 3 times daily. Maximum dose is 4 mg/24 hours, taken in divided doses. For panic disorder: Initially 0.5 mg 3 times daily; increase dose by 1 mg every 3 to 4 days as needed and tolerated. Maximum daily dose is 10 mg.

Note: Actual dosage and administration schedule must be determined by the physician for each patient individually.

Conditions Requiring Dosing Adjustments

Liver function: Manufacturer recommends a starting dose of 0.25 mg in patients with advanced liver disease, with slow increase in dose if needed.

Kidney function: Specific dosage reductions are not defined by the manufacturer.

---

*See Schedules of Controlled Drugs at the back of this book.

Obesity
: This drug takes a longer time to reach final concentrations in obese people. Doses should be calculated based on ideal rather than actual body weight.

Alcoholism
: Because of some of the physiological and liver changes that can occur in alcoholism, the removal of this drug from the body may be delayed. Lower doses or longer times (intervals) between doses are indicated.

▷ **Dosing Instructions:** May be taken on empty stomach or with food or milk. Tablet may be crushed. Do not stop this drug abruptly if taken for more than 4 weeks.

Usual Duration of Use: Several days to several weeks. Avoid prolonged and uninterrupted use. Continual use should not exceed 8 weeks without evaluation by your doctor.

▷ **This Drug Should Not Be Taken If**
- you have had an allergic reaction to it previously.
- you are pregnant (first 3 months).
- you have acute narrow-angle glaucoma.
- you have myasthenia gravis.

▷ **Inform Your Physician Before Taking This Drug If**
- you have a history of palpitations and tachycardis (this drug may worsen these problems).
- you are allergic to benzodiazepine drugs (see Drug Class, Section Four).
- you are pregnant (last 6 months) or planning pregnancy.
- you are breast-feeding.
- you have a history of depression or serious mental illness (psychosis).
- you have a history of alcoholism or drug abuse.
- you have impaired liver or kidney function.
- you have open-angle glaucoma.
- you have a seizure disorder (epilepsy).
- you have severe chronic lung disease.
- you take other prescription or non-prescription medications which were not discussed when alprazolam was prescribed for you.
- you are unsure of how much alprazolam to take or how often to take it.

Possible Side-Effects (natural, expected and unavoidable drug actions)
Drowsiness, light-headedness.

▷ **Possible Adverse Effects** (unusual, unexpected and infrequent reactions)
If any of the following develop, consult your physician promptly for guidance.

Mild Adverse Effects
Allergic Reactions: Skin rash, hives.
Headache, dizziness, fatigue, blurred vision, dry mouth.
Nausea, vomiting, constipation.

Serious Adverse Effects
Confusion, hallucinations, depression, unexpected excitement, agitation (paradoxical reaction).
Tachycardia and palpitations (8%).
Increased liver enzymes (rare).
Low blood pressure (hypotension).

56   Alprazolam

▷ **Possible Effects on Sexual Function:**   Rare but documented: inhibited female orgasm (5 mg/day); impaired ejaculation (3.5 mg/day); decreased libido, impaired erection (4.5 mg/day); altered timing and pattern of menstruation (0.75 to 4 mg/day).

Possible Effects on Laboratory Tests
Liver function tests: increased ALT/GPT, AST/GOT, rare and insignificant.
Urine screening tests for drug abuse: may be **positive**. (Test results depend upon amount of drug taken and testing method used.)

CAUTION
1. This drug should not be discontinued abruptly if it has been taken continually for more than 4 weeks.
2. Some over-the-counter drug products contain antihistamines (allergy and cold preparations, sleep aids) and can cause excessive sedation.

Precautions for Use
By Infants and Children: Safety and effectiveness for use by those under 18 not established.
By Those over 60 Years of Age: Starting dose should be 0.25 mg 2 or 3 times daily. Watch for excessive drowsiness, dizziness, unsteadiness and incoordination (possible low blood pressure).

▷ **Advisability of Use During Pregnancy**
Pregnancy Category: D. See Pregnancy Code see at the back of this book.
Animal studies: Diazepam (a closely related benzodiazepine) can cause cleft palate in mice and skeletal defects in rats. No data on alprazolam.
Human studies: Some studies suggest a possible association between the use of diazepam and defects such as cleft lip and heart deformities. Adequate studies on the use of alprazolam by pregnant women are not available.
Avoid use during entire pregnancy if possible.

Advisability of Use if Breast-Feeding
Presence of this drug in breast milk: Yes.
Avoid drug or refrain from nursing.

Habit-Forming Potential: This drug can cause psychological and/or physical dependence (see Glossary) if used in large doses for an extended period of time.

Effects of Overdosage: Marked drowsiness, weakness, feeling of drunkenness, staggering gait, tremor, stupor progressing to deep sleep or coma.

Possible Effects of Long-Term Use: Psychological and/or physical dependence.

Suggested Periodic Examinations While Taking This Drug (at physician's discretion)
None required for short-term use.

▷ **While Taking This Drug, Observe the Following**
Foods: No restrictions.
Beverages: Avoid excess intake of caffeine-containing beverages: coffee, tea, cola. This drug may be taken with milk.
▷ *Alcohol:* Use with extreme caution. Alcohol may increase the sedative effects of alprazolam. Alprazolam may increase the intoxicating effects of alcohol. Avoid alcohol completely—throughout the day and night—if you find it necessary to drive or to engage in *any* hazardous activity.

Tobacco Smoking: Heavy smoking may reduce the calming action of alprazolam.
Marijuana Smoking
 Occasional (once or twice weekly): Mild increase in the sedative effect.
 Daily: Marked increase in the sedative effect of this drug.
▷ *Other Drugs*
 Alprazolam may *increase* the effects of
 • digoxin (Lanoxin), and cause digoxin toxicity.
 Alprazolam may *decrease* the effects of
 • levodopa (Sinemet, etc.), and reduce its effect in treating Parkinson's disease.
 The following drugs may *increase* the effects of alprazolam
 • cimetidine (Tagamet).
 • disulfiram (Antabuse).
 • isoniazid (INH, Rifamate, etc.).
 • oral contraceptives.
 • valproic acid (Depakene).
 The following drugs may *decrease* the effects of alprazolam
 • carbamazepine (Tegretol).
 • rifampin (Rimactane, etc.).
 • theophylline (aminophylline, Theo-Dur, etc.).
 Alprazolam *taken concurrently* with
 • benzodiazepines (see Drug Class) may result in increased central nervous system (CNS) depression.
 • tricyclic antidepressants (see Drug Class Section) will result in additional (CNS) depression.
 • buspirone (Buspar) can result in additive CNS depression.
 • alcohol (ethanol) will worsen coordination and mental abilities.
▷ *Driving, Hazardous Activities:* This drug can impair mental alertness, judgment, physical coordination and reaction time. Avoid hazardous activities accordingly.
Aviation Note: The use of this drug *is a disqualification* for piloting. Consult a designated Aviation Medical Examiner.
Exposure to Sun: Use caution, rare photosensitivity reports (see Glossary).
Discontinuation: If this drug has been taken for an extended period of time, do not stop it abruptly. Slowly reduce dose by 1 mg per week until a total daily dose of 4 mg is reached; by 0.5 mg per week until a total daily dose of 2 mg is reached; then by 0.25 mg per week thereafter. Ask physician for guidance.

AMANTADINE (a MAN ta deen)

Introduced: 1966 **Prescription:** USA: Yes; Canada: Yes **Available as Generic:** USA: Yes; Canada: No **Class:** Antiparkinsonism, antiviral
Controlled Drug: USA: No; Canada: No

Brand Names: Symadine, Symmetrel

Amantadine

BENEFITS versus RISKS	
Possible Benefits	**Possible Risks**
Partial relief of rigidity, tremor and impaired motion in all forms of parkinsonism	Skin rashes, mild to severe
	Confusion, hallucinations
	Congestive heart failure
Prevention and treatment of respiratory tract infections caused by influenza type A viruses*	Increased prostatism (see Glossary)
	Abnormally low white blood cell counts

▷ **Principal Uses**

As a Single Drug Product: Uses currently included in FDA approved labeling: (1) Treatment of all forms of parkinsonism; (2) prevention or treatment of respiratory tract infections caused by influenza type A virus (although rimantidine is currently the drug of first choice because of amantidine's higher occurance of CNS side effects); (3) treatment of drug-induced extrapyramidal symptoms (see Glossary).

Other (unlabeled) generally accepted uses: (1) May have a small role in helping manage behavioral problems which can happen after some brain injuries; (2) has had some success in reversing symptoms of mild dementia; (3) can ease some resistant myoclonic or absence seizures.

How This Drug Works: By increasing the nerve impulse transmitter known as dopamine in some nerve centers, this drug reduces muscular rigidity, tremor and impaired movement associated with parkinsonism. By blocking penetration of infectious material from viruses into cells, this drug prevents development of influenza.

Available Dosage Forms and Strengths
Capsules — 100 mg
Syrup — 50 mg per 5-ml teaspoonful

▷ **Usual Adult Dosage Range:** Antiparkinsonism: 100 mg once or twice daily. The total daily dose should not exceed 400 mg. Antiviral: 200 mg once daily; or 100 mg/12 hours. **Note: Actual dosage and administration schedule must be determined by the physician for each patient individually.**

Conditions Requiring Dosing Adjustments
Liver function: The liver is not known to be involved in the elimination of amantadine.
Kidney function: Must be carefully adjusted to blood levels in patients with kidney problems.

▷ **Dosing Instructions:** May be taken with or following meals. Can open the capsule to take it.

Usual Duration of Use: Use on a regular schedule for up to 2 weeks is usually needed to see this drug's effectiveness in relieving the symptoms of parkinsonism. Long-term use (months to years) requires periodic check of response and dose changes. Consult your physician on a regular basis.

---

*NOT effective for the prevention or treatment of viral infections other than those caused by influenza type A viruses.

Following exposure to influenza type A, peak protection requires continual daily dosage for at least 10 days. During influenza epidemics, this drug may be given for 6 to 8 weeks.

▷ **This Drug Should Not Be Taken If**
- you have had an allergic reaction to it previously.

▷ **Inform Your Physician Before Taking This Drug If**
- you have any type of seizure disorder.
- you have a history of serious emotional or mental disorder.
- you have a history of heart disease, especially previous heart failure.
- you have impaired liver or kidney function.
- you have a history of peptic ulcer disease.
- you have eczema or recurring eczemalike skin rashes.
- you are taking any drugs for emotional or mental disorders.
- you take other prescription or non-prescription medications which were not discussed when amantadine was prescribed for you.
- you have a history of low white blood cell counts.
- you are unsure of how much amantadine to take or how often to take it.

Possible Side-Effects (natural, expected and unavoidable drug actions)
Light-headedness, dizziness, weakness, feeling of impending faint in upright position (see Orthostatic Hypotension in Glossary). Dry mouth, constipation. Reddish-blue network pattern or patchy discoloration of the skin of the legs and feet (livedo reticularis); this is transient and unimportant.

▷ **Possible Adverse Effects** (unusual, unexpected and infrequent reactions)
If any of the following develop, consult your physician promptly for guidance.

Mild Adverse Effects
Allergic Reaction: Skin rash.
Headache, nervousness, irritability, inability to concentrate, insomnia, nightmares.
Unsteadiness, visual disturbances, slurred speech.
Loss of appetite, nausea, vomiting.

Serious Adverse Effects
Allergic Reaction: Severe eczemalike skin rashes.
Idiosyncratic Reactions: Confusion, depression, hallucinations.
Increased seizure activity in presence of epilepsy.
Swelling (fluid retention) of the arms, feet or ankles.
Development of congestive heart failure (rare).
Aggravation of prostatism (see Glossary).
Difficulty breathing.
Elevated liver function tests.
Abnormally low white blood cell counts: fever, sore throat, infections.
Catatonia or seizures (if abruptly stopped).

▷ **Possible Effects on Sexual Function:** None reported.

▷ **Adverse Effects That May Mimic Natural Diseases or Disorders**
Mood changes, confusion or hallucinations may suggest a psychotic disorder.

Swelling of the legs and feet may suggest (but not necessarily be indicative of) heart, liver or kidney disorder.

Natural Diseases or Disorders That May Be Activated by This Drug
Latent epilepsy, incipient congestive heart failure.

Possible Effects on Laboratory Tests
Liver function tests: increased liver enzymes (AST/GOT, alkaline phosphatase).
Kidney function tests: Transient increase in blood urea nitrogen (BUN).

CAUTION
1. NARROW margin of safety. Do not exceed a total dose of 400 mg/24 hours. Watch closely for adverse effects with doses over 200 mg/24 hours.
2. After initial benefit lasting 3 to 6 months, this drug may lose its effectiveness in the treatment of parkinsonism. If this occurs, consult your physician regarding dosage adjustment or drug replacement.
3. May increase susceptibility to German measles. Avoid exposure to anyone with active German measles infection.
4. Watch for early signs of congestive heart failure: shortness of breath on exertion or during the night while sleeping, mild cough, swelling of the feet and ankles. Report these developments promptly to your doctor.

Precautions for Use
By Infants and Children: Safety and effectiveness for use by those under 1 not established.
By Those over 60 Years of Age: Confusion, delirium, hallucinations and disorderly conduct may develop. Prostatism may be aggravated by this drug.

▷ **Advisability of Use During Pregnancy**
Pregnancy Category: C. See Pregnancy Code at the back of this book.
Animal studies: Birth defects reported in rat studies; no defects reported in rabbit studies.
Human studies: Adequate studies of pregnant women are not available. Avoid this drug during the first 3 months if possible. Ask your doctor for help.

Advisability of Use if Breast-Feeding
Presence of this drug in breast milk: Yes.
Nursing infant may develop skin rash, vomiting or retention of urine. Avoid drug or refrain from nursing.

Habit-Forming Potential: This drug does have a potential for abuse because of its ability to cause euphoria, hallucinations and feelings of detachment.

Effects of Overdosage: Hyperactivity, disorientation, confusion, visual hallucinations, aggressive behavior, severe toxic psychosis, seizures, heart rhythm disturbances, drop in blood pressure.

Possible Effects of Long-Term Use: Livedo reticularis (see Possible Side-Effects above). Congestive heart failure in predisposed individuals.

Suggested Periodic Examinations While Taking This Drug (at physician's discretion)
White blood cell counts, liver and kidney function tests.
Evaluation of heart function.

▷ **While Taking This Drug, Observe the Following**
  Foods: No restrictions.
  Beverages: No restrictions. May be taken with milk.
▷ *Alcohol:* This combination may impair mental function and lower blood pressure excessively.
  Tobacco Smoking: No interactions expected.
  Marijuana Smoking: No interactions expected.
▷ *Other Drugs*
  Amantadine may *increase* the effects of
  • those atropinelike drugs that are used to treat parkinsonism, especially benztropine (Cogentin), orphenadrine (Disipal) and trihexyphenidyl (Artane). Amantadine can increase their therapeutic effectiveness, but if doses are too large, these drugs taken concurrently with amantadine may cause mental confusion, delirium, hallucinations and nightmares.
  • levodopa (Dopar, Larodopa, Sinemet, etc.), and enhance its therapeutic effectiveness. Combination may cause acute mental disturbances.
  The following drugs may *increase* the effects of amantadine
  • amphetamine and amphetaminelike stimulant drugs may cause excessive stimulation and adverse behavioral effects.
  • hydrochlorothiazide + triamterene may increase the blood level of amantadine and cause toxicity.
  Taken *concurrently* with
  • cotrimoxazole may increase risk of CNS stimulation or arrhythmias.
  • sulfamethoxazole may increase risk of CNS stimulation or arrhythmia.
  • trimethoprim may increase risk of CNS stimulation or arrhythmias.
▷ *Driving, Hazardous Activities:* This drug may cause drowsiness, dizziness, blurred vision or confusion. If these drug effects occur, avoid all hazardous activities.
  Aviation Note: The use of this drug **may be a disqualification** for piloting. Consult a designated Aviation Medical Examiner.
  Exposure to Sun: No restrictions.
  Exposure to Heat: No restrictions.
  Exposure to Cold: Use caution. Excessive chilling may enhance the development of livedo reticularis (see Possible Side-Effects above).
  Discontinuation: When used to treat parkinsonism, this drug should not be stopped abruptly. Sudden discontinuation may cause an acute parkinsonian crisis. When used to treat influenza A infections, this drug should be continued for 48 hours after the disappearance of all symptoms.

AMILORIDE (a MIL oh ride)

Introduced: 1967   **Prescription:** USA: Yes; Canada: Yes   **Available as Generic:** Yes   **Class:** Diuretic   **Controlled Drug:** USA: No; Canada: No

Brand Names: ✦Apo-Amilzide, Midamor, ✦Moduret [CD], Moduretic [CD], ✦Nu-Amilzide [CD]

Amiloride

BENEFITS versus RISKS	
Possible Benefits	*Possible Risks*
EFFECTIVE DIURETIC WITH DECREASED POTASSIUM LOSS	ABNORMALLY HIGH BLOOD POTASSIUM with excessive use Rare bone marrow depression Rare heart arrhythmias Rare kidney failure Rare liver toxicity

▷ **Principal Uses**
  As a Single Drug Product: Uses currently included in FDA approved labeling: (1) To eliminate excessive fluid retention (edema) seen in congestive heart failure; (2) Treats high blood pressure, especially good in those prone to low potassium; (3) trement of thiazide caused low blood potassium.
  As a Combination Drug Product [CD]: Combined with other thiazide diuretics to prevent excess potassium loss.
  Other (unlabeled) generally accepted uses: (1) May be able to help dissolve kidney stones in patients unable to tolerate surgery; (2) can help correct the increased urination which occurs in patients taking lithium.

How This Drug Works: This drug promotes the loss of sodium and water from the body and potassium retention by altering kidney enzymes that control urine formation.

Available Dosage Forms and Strengths
  Tablets — 5 mg

▷ **Usual Adult Dosage Range:** One 5 mg dose a day, preferably in the morning. May increase up to 15 mg daily as needed and tolerated. Should not exceed 20 mg/24 hours. **Note: Actual dosage and administration schedule must be determined by the physician for each patient individually.**

Conditions Requiring Dosing Adjustments
  Liver function: Used with extreme caution in patients with severe liver disease.
  Kidney function: NOT used in patients who can't make urine or acute or chronic kidney failures.

▷ **Dosing Instructions:** Best taken when you wake up, with the stomach empty. Withhold food for 4 hours. May be taken with food if necessary to reduce stomach irritation. Tablet may be crushed for administration.

Usual Duration of Use: As needed to loose abnormal fluid or to normalize normal blood pressure. Intermittent or alternate-day use is recommended to minimize imbalance of sodium and potassium. Consult your physician on a regular basis.

▷ **This Drug Should Not Be Taken If**
  • you have had an allergic reaction to any form of it previously.
  • your blood potassium level is above the normal range.
  • your kidneys are not producing urine.

▷ **Inform Your Physician Before Taking This Drug If**
  • you have diabetes or glaucoma.
  • you have a history of kidney disease or impaired kidney function.
  • you take any other diuretic, blood pressure drug, any form of digitalis or lithium.
  • you are unsure of how much amiloride to take or how often to take it.

Possible Side-Effects (natural, expected and unavoidable drug actions)
Abnormally high blood potassium level (10% of users), abnormally low blood sodium level, dehydration, constipation.

▷ **Possible Adverse Effects** (unusual, unexpected and infrequent reactions)
If any of the following develop, consult your physician promptly for guidance.
Mild Adverse Effects
Allergic Reactions: Skin rash, itching.
Headache, dizziness, weakness, fatigue, numbness and tingling.
Dry mouth, nausea, vomiting, stomach pains, diarrhea.
Loss of scalp hair.
Serious Adverse Effects
Idiosyncratic Reactions: Joint and muscle pains.
Abnormally high potassium level—marked fatigue and weakness, confusion, numbness and tingling of lips or extremities, slow and irregular heartbeats.
Rare liver or kidney toxicity.
Abnormally high sodium level.
Increased internal eye pressure (of concern in glaucoma).
Mental depression, visual disturbances, ringing in ears, tremors.
Aplastic anemia (see Glossary)—unusual fatigue or weakness, fever, sore throat, abnormal bleeding or bruising.
Palpitations and arrhythmias (rare).

▷ **Possible Effects on Sexual Function:** More than 1%: decreased libido and impotence (5 to 10 mg/day).

▷ **Adverse Effects That May Mimic Natural Diseases or Disorders**
Nervousness, confusion or depression may mimic spontaneous mental disorder.

Natural Diseases or Disorders That May Be Activated by This Drug
Preexisting peptic ulcer, latent glaucoma.

Possible Effects on Laboratory Tests
Blood cholesterol level: decreased.
Blood creatinine level: increased with long-term use.
Blood potassium level: increased.
Blood uric acid level: increased with long-term use, especially if taken with thiazide diuretics.
Blood sodium level: decreased

CAUTION
1. Do NOT take potassium supplements, or eat more high-potassium foods.
2. More frequent potassium levels needed if you take digitalis compounds.
3. Do not stop this drug abruptly unless your doctor says you must.

Precautions for Use
By Infants and Children: Safety and effectiveness for use by those under 12 not established.
By Those over 60 Years of Age: Declines in kidney function may predispose to retention of potassium. Limit use of this drug to periods of 2 to 3 weeks if possible. Extended use can cause excessive loss of water, increased

thickness of the blood and increased risk of abnormal blood clotting (thrombosis, heart attack, stroke).

▷ **Advisability of Use During Pregnancy**
Pregnancy Category: C. See Pregnancy Code at the back of this book.
Animal studies: No birth defects reported.
Human studies: Adequate studies of pregnant women are not available.
Use only if clearly needed.

Advisability of Use if Breast-Feeding
Presence of this drug in breast milk: Unknown, but probably present.
This drug may suppress milk production.
Avoid drug if possible. If use is necessary, monitor nursing infant closely and discontinue drug or nursing if adverse effects develop.

Habit-Forming Potential: None.

Effects of Overdosage: Thirst, drowsiness, fatigue, weakness, nausea, vomiting, confusion, numbness and tingling of face and extremities, irregular heart rhythm, shortness of breath.

Suggested Periodic Examinations While Taking This Drug (at physician's discretion)
Complete blood counts; blood levels of sodium, potassium and chloride; kidney function tests; and check of water balance (state of hydration).

▷ **While Taking This Drug, Observe the Following**
Foods: Avoid excessive salt restriction and high-potassium foods.
Beverages: No restrictions. May be taken with milk.
▷ *Alcohol:* Use caution. Alcohol can exaggerate the blood-pressure-lowering effect of this drug and cause orthostatic hypotension (see Glossary).
Tobacco Smoking: No interactions expected.
▷ *Other Drugs*
Amiloride may *increase* the effects of
- other blood-pressure-lowering drugs. Dosage decreases may be needed.

Amiloride may *decrease* the effects of
- digoxin (Lanoxin, etc.), and reduce its effect in treating heart failure.

Amiloride *taken concurrently* with
- spironolactone (Aldactone, Aldactazide) or triamterene (Dyrenium, Dyazide) may cause dangerous blood potassium levels. Avoid combination.
- lithium may cause lithium accumulation to toxic levels.
- ACE inhibitors (see Drug Classes) such as benazopril may result in abnormally high blood potassium.
- NSAIDs (see Drug Classes) may decrease the lowering of blood pressure.
- potassium supplements may result in extremely elevated blood potassium levels.

▷ *Driving, Hazardous Activities:* May cause drowsiness, dizziness and orthostatic hypotension. If these drug effects occur, avoid hazardous activities.
Aviation Note: The use of this drug *may be a disqualification* for piloting. Consult a designated Aviation Medical Examiner.
Exposure to Sun: No restrictions.
Exposure to Heat: Caution advised. Excessive sweating can cause water, sodium and potassium imbalance. Hot environments can cause lowering of blood pressure.

Occurrence of Unrelated Illness: Call your doctor if you contract an illness causing vomiting or diarrhea.

Discontinuation: With high dosage or prolonged use, withdraw this drug gradually. Sudden withdrawal can cause excessive loss of potassium from the body.

AMINOPHYLLINE (am in OFF i lin)

Other Name: theophylline ethylenediamine

Introduced: 1910 **Prescription:** USA: Yes; Canada: Yes **Available as Generic:** Yes **Class:** Antiasthmatic, bronchodilator, xanthines **Controlled Drug:** USA: No; Canada: No

Brand Names: Aminophyllin, Mudrane [CD], Mudrane GG [CD], ✦Palaron, Phyllocontin, Somophyllin, ✦Somophyllin-12, Truphylline

BENEFITS versus RISKS	
Possible Benefits	*Possible Risks*
EFFECTIVE PREVENTION AND RELIEF OF ACUTE BRONCHIAL ASTHMA	NARROW TREATMENT RANGE FREQUENT STOMACH DISTRESS Gastrointestinal bleeding
MODERATELY EFFECTIVE CONTROL OF CHRONIC, RECURRENT BRONCHIAL ASTHMA	Central nervous system toxicity, seizures Heart rhythm disturbances
Moderately effective symptomatic relief in chronic bronchitis and emphysema	

▷ **Principal Uses**

As a Single Drug Product: Uses currently included in FDA approved labeling: (1) Relieves shortness of breath and wheezing in acute bronchial asthma, and helps prevent recurrence of asthmatic episodes; (2) Also useful in chronic obstructive pulmonary disease (COPD) typically used in combination with beta agonists and anticholinergics.

Other (unlabeled) generally accepted uses: None at present.

As a Combination Drug Product [CD]: Available in combination with several other drugs that are beneficial in the management of bronchial asthma and related conditions. Ephedrine enhances the bronchodilator effects; guaifenesin provides an expectorant effect that thins mucus secretions; mild sedatives such as phenobarbital are added to allay the anxiety that is often seen in acute attacks of asthma.

How This Drug Works: This drug yields 79% theophylline, the active medicine. It inhibits the enzyme phosphodiesterase, and increases cyclic AMP. This causes relaxation of the muscles in the bronchial tubes and lung blood vessels, resulting in relief of bronchospasm, and improved lung circulation.

Available Dosage Forms and Strengths

Enema — 65.14 mg per ml

Injection — 25 mg per ml and 50 mg per ml (Canada)

Aminophylline

        Oral solution — 105 mg per 5-ml teaspoonful
        Suppositories — 250 mg, 500 mg
        Tablets — 100 mg, 200 mg
    Tablets, enteric-coated — 100 mg, 200 mg
Tablets, extended release — 225 mg, 350 mg (Canada)

▷ **Recommended Dosage Ranges** (Actual dosage and administration schedule must be determined by the physician for each patient individually.)

Note: All doses of aminophylline are to be calculated as theophylline-equivalents; all dosages cited below are for theophylline.

Infants and Children: For acute attack of asthma (not currently taking theophylline)—loading dose of 5 to 6 mg/kg of body weight.

For acute attack if taking theophylline—a single dose of 2.5 mg/kg of body weight, if no signs of theophylline toxicity. Check blood levels.

For maintenance during acute attack—dosage is based on age:

    Up to 6 months of age—0.07 for each week of age + 1.7 = the mg/kg of body weight, given every 8 hours.

    6 months to 1 year of age—0.05 for each week of age + 1.25 = the mg/kg of body weight, given every 6 hours.

    1 to 9 years of age—5 mg/kg of body weight, every 6 hours.

    9 to 12 years of age—4 mg/kg of body weight, every 6 hours.

    12 to 16 years of age—3 mg/kg of body weight, every 6 hours.

For chronic treatment to prevent recurrence of asthma—dosage is based on age:

    Initially 16 mg/kg of body weight, in 3 or 4 divided doses at 6 to 8 hour intervals, up to a maximum of 400 mg daily. Increase dose as needed and tolerated by increments of 25% every 2 to 3 days. Limit total daily dosage as follows:

    Up to 1 year of age—0.3 for each week of age + 8.0 = the mg/kg of body weight, per day.

    1 to 9 years of age—22 mg/kg of body weight, per day.

    9 to 12 years of age—20 mg/kg of body weight, per day.

    12 to 16 years of age—18 mg/kg of body weight, per day.

    16 years of age and over—13 mg/kg of body weight or 900 mg per day, whichever is less.

Note: Theophylline blood levels are needed periodically.

16 to 60 Years of Age: For acute attack of asthma (not currently taking theophylline)—loading dose of 5 to 6 mg/kg of body weight.

For acute attack while currently taking theophylline—a single dose of 2.5 mg/kg of body weight, if no signs of theophylline toxicity. Check blood levels of theophylline.

For maintenance during acute attack—for nonsmokers: 3 mg/kg of body weight, every 8 hours; for smokers: 4 mg/kg of body weight, every 6 hours.

For chronic treatment to prevent recurrence of asthma—Initially 6 to 8 mg/kg of body weight, in 3 or 4 divided doses at 6 to 8 hour intervals, up to a maximum of 400 mg daily. Increase dose as needed and tolerated by increments of 25% every 2 to 3 days. The total daily dosage should not exceed 13 mg/kg of body weight or 900 mg, whichever is less.

Over 60 Years of Age: For acute attack—same as 16 to 60 years of age.

For maintenance during acute attack—2 mg/kg of body weight, every 8 hours.

Conditions Requiring Dosing Adjustments
Liver function: Dose **must** be decreased in liver compromise, and blood levels checked.
Kidney function: Lower doses will be needed and accumulation may occur. Check blood levels.
Obesity: This drug does not enter fatty tissue. Doses **must** be calculated on lean body weight.
Pulmonary edema: When fluid accumulates in the lungs, particularly in acute situations, the dose needed should be decreased to half of the normal dose.
Fever: Extended periods of fever change the amount of space into which the drug distributes and also lowers the point at which seizures may occur. The dose of aminophylline may need to be decreased.
Congestive heart failure: Patients with this kind of heart failure should have their doses decreased by 50% in order to avoid toxicity.

▷ **Dosing Instructions:** May be taken with or following food to reduce stomach irritation. The regular tablets may be crushed before taking. Enteric-coated and prolonged-action tablets should be swallowed whole and not altered. Shake the oral solution gently before measuring each dose. Do not refrigerate any liquid dosage forms of this drug.

Usual Duration of Use: Use on a regular schedule for 48 to 72 hours is usually needed to see this drug's effectiveness in helping bronchial asthma and chronic lung disease. Long-term use (months to years) requires supervision and periodic evaluation by your physician. Consult your physician on a regular basis.

▷ **This Drug Should Not Be Taken If**
- you have had an allergic reaction to it, or to dyphylline, oxtriphylline or theophylline.
- you have active peptic ulcer disease.
- you have an uncontrolled seizure disorder.

▷ **Inform Your Physician Before Taking This Drug If**
- you have had an unfavorable reaction to any xanthine drug (see Drug Class, Section Four).
- you have a seizure disorder of any kind.
- you have a history of peptic ulcer disease.
- you have impaired liver or kidney function.
- you have had a temperature for a significant period of time.
- you have hypertension, heart disease or any heart rhythm disorder.
- you take other prescription or non-prescription medications which were not discussed when aminophylline was prescribed for you.
- you see a lung specialist for chronic pulmonary edema.
- you are unsure of how much aminophylline to take or how often to take it.

Possible Side-Effects (natural, expected and unavoidable drug actions)
Nervousness, insomnia, rapid heart rate, increased urine volume.

Aminophylline

▷ **Possible Adverse Effects** (unusual, unexpected and infrequent reactions)
   If any of the following develop, consult your physician promptly for guidance.
   Mild Adverse Effects
   Allergic Reactions: Skin rash, hives.
   Headache, dizziness, irritability, tremor, fatigue, weakness.
   Appetite loss, nausea, vomiting, abdominal pain, diarrhea, excessive thirst.
   Flushing of face.
   Serious Adverse Effects
   Idiosyncratic Reactions: Marked anxiety, confusion, behavioral disturbances.
   Central nervous system toxicity: muscle twitching, seizures.
   Heart rhythm abnormalities, rapid breathing, low blood pressure.
   Gastrointestinal bleeding.
   Worsening of migraines.
   Increased fluid loss via the kidneys.

▷ **Possible Effects on Sexual Function:** None reported.

Natural Diseases or Disorders That May Be Activated by This Drug
   Latent peptic ulcer disease.

Possible Effects on Laboratory Tests
   Blood uric acid level: increased.
   Fecal occult blood test: positive (large doses may cause stomach bleeding).
   Phenobarbital level: falsely decreased.

CAUTION
   1. Do not combine this drug with other antiasthmatic drugs unless you are directed to do so by your doctor. Serious overdose could result.
   2. Influenza vaccine may delay elimination and cause toxicity.

Precautions for Use
   By Infants and Children: Do not exceed recommended doses. Watch for toxicity: irritability, agitation, tremors, lethargy, fever, vomiting, rapid heart rate and breathing, seizures. Check blood levels of drug during long-term use.
   By Those over 60 Years of Age: Small starting doses are indicated. You may be more susceptible to stomach irritation, nausea, vomiting or diarrhea. This drug may cause a hyperactivity syndrome when used with coffee (caffeine) or nasal decongestants.

▷ **Advisability of Use During Pregnancy**
   Pregnancy Category: C. See Pregnancy Code at the back of this book.
   Animal studies: Significant birth defects due to this drug reported in mice.
   Human studies: Adequate studies of pregnant women are not available. No increase in birth defects reported in 394 exposures to theophylline.
   Avoid this drug during the first 3 months. Use it otherwise only if clearly needed. Ask your physician for guidance.

Advisability of Use if Breast-Feeding
   Presence of this drug in breast milk: Yes.
   Ask your doctor for help. It may be possible to take a typical dose after nursing and avoid the peak effect of the drug.

Habit-Forming Potential: None.

Effects of Overdosage: Nausea, vomiting, restlessness, irritability, confusion, delirium, seizures, high fever, weak pulse, coma.

Possible Effects of Long-Term Use: Gastrointestinal irritation.

Suggested Periodic Examinations While Taking This Drug (at physician's discretion)
Check of blood theophylline levels, especially with high dosage or long-term use. (See Therapeutic Drug Monitoring in Section One.)

▷ **While Taking This Drug, Observe the Following**
Foods: High carbohydrate meals may decrease absorption. High fat meals may decrease absorption.

Beverages: Avoid excess use of caffeine-containing beverages: coffee, tea, or cola.

▷ *Alcohol:* No interactions expected. May increase stomach irritation.

Tobacco Smoking: Can increase drug elimination and reduce effectiveness. Higher doses may be needed to maintain a therapeutic blood level.

▷ *Other Drugs*
Aminophylline may *decrease* the effects of
- adenosine (Adenocard).
- lithium (Lithane, Lithobid, etc.), and reduce its effectiveness.
- midazolam (Versed).

Aminophylline *taken concurrently* with
- amiodarone (Codarone) may cause a large increase in theophylline blood level.
- halothane (anesthesia) may cause heart rhythm abnormalities.
- imipenam-cilastatin (Primaxin) may result in large increases in theophylline levels and toxicity.
- phenytoin (Dilantin) may cause decreased effects of both drugs. Check blood levels and adjust dosages as appropriate.

The following drugs may *increase* the effects of aminophylline
- allopurinol (Lopurin, Zyloprim).
- caffeine (greater than 6 cups or IV form).
- cimetidine (Tagamet).
- ciprofloxacin (Cipro), and other Quinolones to various degrees.
- clarithromycin (Biaxin).
- disulfiram (Antabuse).
- erythromycin (E-Mycin, Erythrocin, etc.).
- ilsoniazid (INH).
- interferon alfa (Roferon).
- mexiletine (Mexitil).
- norfloxacin (Noroxin).
- oral contraceptives.
- pentoxyfylline (Trental).
- ranitidine (Zantac).
- tacrine (Cognex).
- thiabendazole (Mintezol)
- ticlopidine (Ticlid).
- troleandomycin (TAO).
- verapamil (Calan, Verelan, etc.)

The following drugs may *decrease* the effects of aminophylline
- albuterol.
- barbiturates (phenobarbital, etc.).
- beta blocker drugs (see Drug Class).
- carbamazepine (Tegretol).
- primidone (Mysoline).
- rifampin (Rifadin, Rimactane, etc.).
- rifabutin (Mycobutin).
- tobacco smoke.

▷ *Driving, Hazardous Activities:* This drug may cause dizziness. Restrict activities as necessary.

Aviation Note: The use of this drug *may be a disqualification* for piloting. Consult a designated Aviation Medical Examiner.

Exposure to Sun: No restrictions.

Occurrence of Unrelated Illness: Acute viral respiratory infections can delay drug elimination. Watch closely for toxicity and the need to reduce dose or lengthen the dosing interval.

Discontinuation: Avoid prolonged and unnecessary use of this drug. When you have achieved an asthma-free state, slowly withdraw this drug over several days.

AMITRIPTYLINE (a mee TRIP ti leen)

Introduced: 1961 **Prescription:** USA: Yes; Canada: Yes **Available as Generic:** Yes **Class:** Antidepressant **Controlled Drug:** USA: No; Canada: No

Brand Names: Amitril, ✦Apo-Amitriptyline, Elavil, ✦Elavil Plus [CD], Emitrip, Endep, Enovil, Etrafon [CD], Etrafon-A [CD], Etrafon-Forte [CD], ✦Levate, Limbitrol [CD], ✦Novotriptyn, PMS-Levazine [CD], SK-amitriptyline, Triavil [CD]

BENEFITS versus RISKS	
Possible Benefits	*Possible Risks*
EFFECTIVE RELIEF OF ENDOGENOUS DEPRESSION Additive therapy in some pain syndromes	ADVERSE BEHAVIORAL EFFECTS: Confusion, disorientation, hallucinations CONVERSION OF DEPRESSION TO MANIA in manic-depressive disorders Irregular heart rhythms Rare blood cell abnormalities

▷ **Principal Uses**

As a Single Drug Product: Uses currently included in FDA approved labeling: (1) Relieves symptoms seen in spontaneous (endogenous) depression, and helps restore normal mood. This drug should be used only when a diagnosis of a true, primary depression of significant degree has been made.

Other (unlabeled) generally accepted uses: (1) Additive (adjuvant) therapy in chronic pain and other pain syndromes; (2) helps ease agitation; (3) may have a role in diabetic neuropathic pain; is an alternative treatment in intractable hiccups; (4) used in combination with other medicines to ease the pain of postherpetic neuralagia; (5) may be of some benefit in easing the pain of chronic vulvar burning (vulvodynia).

As a Combination Drug Product [CD]: Combined with chlordiazepoxide, a mild benzodiazepine tranquilizer, to relieve anxiety that may accompany depression. Also available in combination with perphenazine, a strong phenothiazine tranquilizer, to relieve severe agitation that may accompany depression.

How This Drug Works: This drug relieves depression by slowly restoring normal levels of norepinephrine and serotonin, chemicals that transmit nerve impulses.

Available Dosage Forms and Strengths
    Tablets — 10 mg, 25 mg, 50 mg, 75 mg, 100 mg, 150 mg
Oral suspension — 10 mg/5 ml

▷ **Usual Adult Dosage Range:** Initially 25 mg 2 to 4 times daily. Dose may be increased cautiously as needed and tolerated by 10 to 25 mg daily at intervals of 1 week. Usual maintenance dose is 50 to 100 mg/24 hours. Total dose should not exceed 150 mg/24 hours. When the optimal requirement is determined, it may be taken at bedtime as one dose. **Note: Actual dosage and administration schedule must be determined by the physician for each patient individually.**

Conditions Requiring Dosing Adjustments
Liver function: Specific guidelines not available, however, low doses and a check of blood levels is prudent.
Kidney function: Low doses and blood level checks are needed with kidney failure.

▷ **Dosing Instructions:** May be taken without regard to meals. Tablet may be crushed to take it.

Usual Duration of Use: Some benefit may occur in 1 to 2 weeks, but adequate response may require continual use for 4 to 6 weeks or longer. Long-term use should not exceed 6 months without follow up evaluation.

▷ **This Drug Should Not Be Taken If**
- you are allergic to any of the brand names listed above.
- you are taking or have taken within the past 14 days any monoamine oxidase (MAO) type A inhibitor drug (see Drug Class, Section Four).
- you are recovering from a recent heart attack.
- you have narrow-angle glaucoma.
- you are pregnant.
- you have congestive heart failure.

▷ **Inform Your Physician Before Taking This Drug If**
- you are allergic to any tricyclic antidepressant (see Drug Class, Section Four).
- you have a history of: diabetes, epilepsy, glaucoma, heart disease, prostate gland enlargement or overactive thyroid function.
- you plan to have surgery under general anesthesia in the near future.
- you take other prescription or non-prescription medications which were not discussed when amitriptyline was prescribed for you.
- you are unsure of how much amitriptyline to take or how often to take it.

Amitriptyline

- you have a history of schizophrenia—this drug may worsen any paranoia.
- you have a history of prostate problems.
- you have a liver or kidney disorder.
- you have a blood cell disorder.
- you have a history of intestinal ileus.
- you have a history of sexual dysfunction.

Possible Side-Effects (natural, expected and unavoidable drug actions)
Drowsiness, blurred vision, dry mouth, constipation, impaired urination.

▷ **Possible Adverse Effects** (unusual, unexpected and infrequent reactions)
If any of the following develop, consult your physician promptly for guidance.

Mild Adverse Effects
Allergic Reactions: Skin rash, hives, swelling of face or tongue, drug fever (see Glossary).
Headache, dizziness, weakness, fainting, unsteady gait, tremors.
Peculiar taste, irritation of tongue or mouth, nausea, indigestion.
Fluctuation of blood sugar levels.
Change in the ability to perceive tones.

Serious Adverse Effects
Allergic Reactions: Hepatitis, with or without jaundice (see Glossary).
Idiosyncratic Reactions: Neuroleptic malignant syndrome (see Glossary).
Confusion, hallucinations, agitation, restlessness, nightmares.
Heart palpitation and irregular rhythm.
Bone marrow depression (see Glossary)—fatigue, weakness, fever, sore throat, abnormal bleeding or bruising.
Peripheral neuritis (see Glossary)—numbness, tingling, pain, loss of arm or leg strength.
Parkinson-like disorders (see Glossary)—usually mild and infrequent; more likely to occur in the elderly.
Liver toxicity.

▷ **Possible Effects on Sexual Function:** Decreased libido (8%), increased libido (antidepressant effect), impotence (19%), inhibited female orgasm, inhibited ejaculation, male and female breast enlargement, milk production, swelling of testicles. These effects usually disappear within 2 to 10 days after discontinuation of the drug.

▷ **Adverse Effects That May Mimic Natural Diseases or Disorders**
Liver toxicity may suggest viral hepatitis.

Natural Diseases or Disorders That May Be Activated by This Drug
Latent diabetes, epilepsy, glaucoma, impaired urination due to prostate.

Possible Effects on Laboratory Tests
Complete blood counts: decreased white cells and platelets; increased eosinophils.
Liver function tests: increased ALT/GPT, AST/GOT, alkaline phosphatase, increased bilirubin.
Blood glucose levels: increased and decreased (fluctuations).

CAUTION
1. Dosage must be individualized. Report for follow-up evaluation and laboratory tests as directed by your physician.

2. It is advisable to withhold this drug if electroconvulsive therapy (ECT, "shock" treatment) is to be used to treat your depression.

Precautions for Use
By Infants and Children: Safety and effectiveness for those under 12 years old not established.

By Those over 60 Years of Age: During the first 2 weeks of treatment, watch for the development of confusion, agitation, forgetfulness, disorientation, delusions and hallucinations. Decreased dose or discontinuation may be needed. Unsteadiness may predispose to falling and injury. May worsen impaired urination associated with prostate gland enlargement (prostatism).

▷ **Advisability of Use During Pregnancy**
Pregnancy Category: D. See Pregnancy Code at the back of this book.
Animal studies: Skull deformities reported in rabbits.
Human studies: No defects reported in 21 exposures. Adequate studies of pregnant women are not available.
Avoid use of drug during first 3 months. Use during last 6 months only if clearly needed.

Advisability of Use if Breast-Feeding
Presence of this drug in breast milk: Yes, in small amounts.
Watch nursing infant closely and stop drug or nursing if adverse effects start.

Habit-Forming Potential: Psychological or physical dependence is rare and unexpected.

Effects of Overdosage: Confusion, hallucinations, marked drowsiness, heart palpitations, dilated pupils, tremors, stupor, deep sleep, coma, convulsions.

Suggested Periodic Examinations While Taking This Drug (at physician's discretion)
Complete blood cell counts, liver function tests, serial blood pressure readings and electrocardiograms.

▷ **While Taking This Drug, Observe the Following**
Foods: No restrictions. May increase appetite and cause excessive weight gain.
Beverages: No restrictions. May be taken with milk.
▷ *Alcohol:* Avoid completely. Can markedly increase the intoxicating effects of alcohol and brain function depression.
Tobacco Smoking: May hasten the elimination of this drug. Higher doses may be necessary.

▷ *Other Drugs*
Amitriptyline may *increase* the effects of
- atropinelike drugs (see Drug Class).
- cimetadine (Tagamet)
- phenytoin.

Amitriptyline may *decrease* the effects of
- clonidine (Catapres).
- guanethidine (Ismelin).
- guanfacine (Hytrin).

Amitriptyline *taken concurrently* with
- anticoagulants such as warfarin may cause an increased risk of bleeding.
- carbamazepine (Tegretol) may decrease the blood level of amitriptyline.
- epinephrine may cause an increased risk of rapid heart rate and high blood pressure.
- estrogens (see Drug Classes) may result in abnormal body movements.
- ethanol (alcohol) may result in additive toxicity to the central nervous system.
- fluvoxetine (Prozac) can result in very high levels of anitriptyline.
- monoamine oxidase (MAO) type A inhibitor drugs may cause high fever, delirium and convulsions (see Drug Class).
- quinidine (Quinaglute, etc.) can result in increased antidepressant blood levels.
- thyroid preparations may impair heart rhythm and function. Ask physician for guidance regarding adjustment of thyroid dose.

▷ *Driving, Hazardous Activities:* This drug may impair mental alertness, judgment, physical coordination and reaction time. Avoid hazardous activities.
Aviation Note: The use of this drug *is a disqualification* for piloting. Consult a designated Aviation Medical Examiner.
Exposure to Sun: This drug may cause photosensitivity (see Glossary).
Exposure to Heat: This drug can inhibit sweating and impair the body's adaptation to hot environments, increasing the risk of heat stroke. Avoid saunas.
Exposure to Cold: Elderly should avoid conditions conducive to hypothermia (see Glossary).
Discontinuation: It is advisable to stop this drug gradually. Abrupt withdrawal after long-term use can cause headache, malaise and nausea.

AMLODIPINE (am LOH di peen)

Introduced: 1986 **Prescription:** USA: Yes **Available as Generic:** No **Class:** Antianginal, antihypertensive, calcium channel blocker
Controlled Drug: USA: No
Brand Name: Norvasc

Warning: **Controversies In Medicine:** New study data indicates that medicines in this class should NOT be used in some patients with extremely compromised hearts. Be certain to ask your doctor about your cardiac output and if the benefits of this medicine outweigh the risks of its use.

BENEFITS versus RISKS	
Possible Benefits	*Possible Risks*
EFFECTIVE PREVENTION OF BOTH MAJOR TYPES OF ANGINA EFFECTIVE TREATMENT OF HYPERTENSION	Peripheral edema (fluid retention in feet and ankles) 9.8%

▷ **Principal Uses**
As a Single Drug Product: Uses currently included in FDA approved labeling: Treatment of (1) angina pectoris due to coronary artery spasm (Prinzmetal's variant angina) that happens spontaneously and is not associated

Amlodipine

with exertion; (2) classical angina-of-effort (due to atherosclerotic disease of the coronary arteries) in people who have not responded to or can't tolerate nitrates or beta blocker drugs; (3) mild to moderate hypertension.
Other (unlabeled) generally accepted uses: (1) Research has continued to accumulate which says medicines in this class can reverse the build up of fat and calcium on the inside of blood vessels (atherosclerosis); (2) can help stop premature labor; (3) may help prevent migraine headaches.

How This Drug Works: By blocking the normal passage of calcium through cell walls, this drug inhibits the contraction of coronary arteries and peripheral arterioles. As a result of these combined effects, this drug
- prevents spontaneous spasm of the coronary arteries (Prinzmetal's type of angina).
- decreases the rate and contraction force of the heart during exertion, reducing the frequency of effort-induced angina.
- reduces contraction of peripheral arterial walls, resulting in lower blood pressure. This decreases the work of the heart during exertion and helps prevent angina.

Available Dosage Forms and Strengths
Tablets — 2.5 mg, 5 mg, 10 mg

▷ **Recommended Dosage Ranges** (Actual dosage and administration schedule must be determined by the physician for each patient individually.)
Infants and Children: Dosage not established.
12 to 60 Years of Age: 2.5 to 10 mg daily, in a single dose for high blood pressure.
5 to 10 mg daily in treating chronic angina.
Over 60 Years of Age: Same as 12 to 60 years of age.

Conditions Requiring Dosing Adjustments
Liver function: Patients with damaged livers should be started on a daily 2.5 mg dose, and have the medicine slowly increased as needed or tolerated.
Kidney function: No adjustment in dosing is needed.
Low protein or starvation
This drug is transported about the body by a protein called albumin. If protein is low as in liver failure or starvation, an increased effect may be seen with "normal" doses. Therapy should be started with low doses and increased only if needed or tolerated.

▷ **Dosing Instructions:** May be taken with or following food to reduce stomach irritation. The tablet may be crushed for administration.

Usual Duration of Use: Use on a regular schedule for 2 to 4 weeks is usually needed to see this drug's effectiveness in reducing the frequency and severity of angina and in controlling hypertension. For long-term use (months to years), determine the smallest effective dose. Periodic evaluation by your doctor is needed.

Possible Advantages of This Drug
Slow onset and prolonged effect, allowing effective once-a-day treatment for both angina and hypertension.
No adverse effects on heart function.

▷ **This Drug Should Not Be Taken If**
- you have had an allergic reaction to it previously.
- you have active liver disease.

- you have low blood pressure—systolic pressure below 90.
- you have a seriously contracted or narrowed (stenosed) aorta.

▷ **Inform Your Physician Before Taking This Drug If**
- you have had an unfavorable response to any calcium blocker drug.
- you are currently taking any form of digitalis or a beta blocker drug (see Drug Class, Section Four).
- you are taking any drugs that lower blood pressure.
- you have had congestive heart failure, heart attack or stroke.
- you are subject to disturbances of heart rhythm.
- you have a history of drug-induced liver damage.
- you are unsure of how much amlodipine to take or how often to take it.
- you have circulation problems in your hands.
- you have muscular dystrophy.

Possible Side-Effects (natural, expected and unavoidable drug actions)
Swelling of feet and ankles (9.8%), flushing and sensation of warmth (2.4%).

▷ **Possible Adverse Effects** (unusual, unexpected and infrequent reactions)
If any of the following develop, consult your physician promptly for guidance.

Mild Adverse Effects
Allergic Reactions: Skin rash.
Headache (8%), dizziness (3%), fatigue (4%).
Nausea (2%).
Overgrowth of the gums (gingival hyperplasia) (up to 10% with drugs in the same class).
Increased urge to urinate at night.

Serious Adverse Effects
Allergic Reactions: None reported.
Idiosyncratic Reactions: None reported.
Palpitations (up to 4.5% with the 10 mg dose).

▷ **Possible Effects on Sexual Function:** Sexual dysfunction has been reported in both men and women as frequently as 1–2%.

▷ **Adverse Effects That May Mimic Natural Diseases or Disorders**
An allergic rash and swelling of the legs may resemble erysipelas.

Possible Effects on Laboratory Tests
None reported.

CAUTION
1. Tell all doctors and dentists you see that you are taking this drug. Note the use of this drug on your card of personal identification.
2. You may use nitroglycerin and other nitrate drugs as needed to relieve acute episodes of angina pain. If you notice that your angina attacks are becoming more frequent or intense, call your doctor promptly.

Precautions for Use
By Infants and Children: Safety and effectiveness for use by those under 12 not established.
By Those over 60 Years of Age: May be more susceptible to the development of weakness, dizziness, fainting and falling. Take necessary precautions to prevent injury.

Amlodipine

▷ **Advisability of Use During Pregnancy**
Pregnancy Category: C. See Pregnancy Code at the back of this book.
Animal studies: No information available.
Human studies: Adequate studies of pregnant women are not available.
Avoid this drug during the first 3 months. Use during the last 6 months only if clearly needed. Ask physician for guidance.

Advisability of Use if Breast-Feeding
Presence of this drug in breast milk: Unknown.
Avoid drug or refrain from nursing.

Habit-Forming Potential: None.

Effects of Overdosage: Weakness, light-headedness, fainting, fast pulse, low blood pressure, slow heart beat, sinus arrest, heart attack, shortness of breath, flushed and warm skin, seizures, metabolic acidosis, low potassium and calcium.

Possible Effects of Long-Term Use: Overgrowth of the gums.

Suggested Periodic Examinations While Taking This Drug (at physician's discretion)
Evaluations of heart function, including electrocardiograms; measurements of blood pressure in supine, sitting and standing positions.

▷ **While Taking This Drug, Observe the Following**
Foods: No restrictions. Avoid excessive salt intake.
Beverages: No restrictions. May be taken with milk.
▷ *Alcohol:* Use caution. Alcohol may exaggerate the drop in blood pressure.
Tobacco Smoking: Nicotine may reduce the effectiveness of this drug. Ask your doctor to help.
Marijuana Smoking: Possible reduced effectiveness of this drug; mild to moderate increase in angina; possible changes in electrocardiogram, confusing interpretation.

▷ *Other Drugs*
Amlodipine ***taken concurrently*** with
- adenosine (Adenocard) may cause extended problems with slow heart rate.
- beta blocker drugs or digitalis preparations (see Drug Classes) may cause heart rate and rhythm problems.
- cyclosporine (Sandimmune) causes increased cyclosporine blood levels and increased risk of toxicity.

The following drug may ***increase*** the effects of amlodipine
- cimetidine (Tagamet).

▷ *Driving, Hazardous Activities:* This drug may cause dizziness. Restrict activities as necessary.
Aviation Note: Coronary artery disease ***is a disqualification*** for piloting. Consult a designated Aviation Medical Examiner.
Exposure to Sun: No restrictions.
Exposure to Heat: Caution advised. Hot environments can exaggerate the blood-pressure-lowering effects of this drug. Observe for light-headedness or weakness.
Heavy Exercise or Exertion: This drug may improve your ability to be more active without resulting angina pain. Use caution.

Discontinuation: Do not stop this drug abruptly. Ask your doctor about gradual withdrawal. Observe for the possible development of rebound angina.

AMOXAPINE (a MOX a peen)

Introduced: 1970 **Prescription:** USA: Yes; Canada: Yes **Available as Generic:** Yes **Class:** Antidepressant **Controlled Drug:** USA: No; Canada: No
Brand Name: Asendin

BENEFITS versus RISKS	
Possible Benefits	*Possible Risks*
EFFECTIVE RELIEF OF PRIMARY DEPRESSIONS: Endogenous, neurotic, reactive	ADVERSE BEHAVIORAL EFFECTS: Confusion, delusions, disorientation, hallucinations
	CONVERSION OF DEPRESSION TO MANIA in manic-depressive disorders
	Rare blood cell abnormalities
	Rare movement disorders
	Rare seizures
	Rare liver toxicity

▷ **Principal Uses**
As a Single Drug Product: Uses currently included in FDA approved labeling: (1) Provides symptomatic relief in all depressive neurosis, psychotic depression, psychotic depressive reaction and depression.
Other (unlabeled) generally accepted uses: (1) May be a second line agent in panic attacks.

How This Drug Works: By increasing some nerve impulse transmitters (norepinephrine and serotonin) in brain tissue, this drug relieves symptoms of depression.

Available Dosage Forms and Strengths
Tablets — 25 mg, 50 mg, 100 mg, 150 mg

▷ **Usual Adult Dosage Range:** Initially 50 mg 2 or 3 times daily. Dose may be increased cautiously on the fifth or sixth day as needed and tolerated to 100 mg 3 times daily. Usual maintenance dose is 200 to 300 mg/24 hours. Total dosage should not exceed 600 mg/24 hours. When determined, the optimal requirement may be taken at bedtime as one dose, not to exceed 300 mg. If the dose is greater than 300 mg per day it should be separated into several smaller doses that are taken two or three times a day. **Note: Actual dosage and administration schedule must be determined by the physician for each patient individually.**

Conditions Requiring Dosing Adjustments
Liver function: Lower doses, careful watch for adverse effects and blood levels are needed.
Kidney function: The steps taken for liver compromise are prudent with compromised kidneys.

▷ **Dosing Instructions:** May be taken without regard to meals. May crush tablet to take it.

Usual Duration of Use: Benefit may be apparent within 4 to 7 days in some individuals, but continual use on a regular schedule for 2 to 3 weeks is usually needed to see the peak effect. Long-term use should not exceed 6 months without evaluation regarding the need for continuation. Ask your doctor.

▷ **This Drug Should Not Be Taken If**
- you have had an allergic reaction to it previously.
- you are taking or have taken within the past 14 days any monoamine oxidase (MAO) type A inhibitor drug (see Drug Class, Section Four).
- you are recovering from a recent heart attack.

▷ **Inform Your Physician Before Taking This Drug If**
- you are allergic or overly sensitive to other antidepressant drugs.
- you have a history of: diabetes, epilepsy, glaucoma, heart disease, paranoia, prostate gland enlargement, schizophrenia or overactive thyroid.
- you plan to have surgery under general anesthesia in the near future.
- you are unsure of how much amoxapine to take or how often to take it.
- you are pregnant or breast-feeding.
- you have asthma.
- you have liver or kidney disease.
- you have a history of a blood cell disorder.

Possible Side-Effects (natural, expected and unavoidable drug actions)
Drowsiness, blurred vision, dry mouth, constipation, impaired urination.

▷ **Possible Adverse Effects** (unusual, unexpected and infrequent reactions)
If any of the following develop, consult your physician promptly for guidance.
Mild Adverse Effects
Allergic Reactions: Skin rash, hives, swellings, drug fever (see Glossary).
Insomnia, nervousness, palpitations, dizziness, unsteadiness, tremors, fainting.
Constipation.
Blurred vision.
Lowered blood pressure.
Peculiar taste, indigestion, nausea, vomiting.
Serious Adverse Effects
Idiosyncratic Reactions: Neuroleptic malignant syndrome (see Glossary).
Behavioral effects: anxiety, confusion, excitement, disorientation, hallucinations, delusions.
Rapid heart rate (tachycardia).
Aggravation of paranoid psychosis and schizophrenia.
Aggravation of epilepsy (seizures).
Seizures in those without a history of epilepsy.
Parkinson-like disorders (see Glossary).
Peripheral neuritis (see Glossary)—numbness, tingling, pain, loss of strength in arms and legs.
Reduced white blood cell count—fever, sore throat.
Movement disorders (akathisia and antipyramidal effects).
Hepatitis (rare).

▷ **Possible Effects on Sexual Function:** Decreased libido (150 mg/day), increased libido (antidepressant effect), inhibited ejaculation (75 to 150 mg/day), painful ejaculation (75 mg/day), inhibited female orgasm (100 mg/day), female breast enlargement/milk production (300 mg/day), altered menstrual timing and pattern (300 mg/day), swelling of testicles. These effects usually disappear within 2 to 10 days after discontinuation of the drug.

Natural Diseases or Disorders That May Be Activated by This Drug
Latent epilepsy, glaucoma, prostatism.

Possible Effects on Laboratory Tests
White blood cell counts: decreased.

CAUTION
1. Drug dose must be individualized. Blood levels may be needed.
2. Watch for toxicity: confusion, agitation, rapid heartbeat.
3. It is advisable to withhold this drug if electroconvulsive therapy (ECT, "shock" treatment) is to be used.

Precautions for Use
By Infants and Children: Safety and effectiveness for use by those under 16 not established.
By Those over 60 Years of Age: During the first 2 weeks of treatment, watch for development of confusion, restlessness, agitation, forgetfulness, disorientation, delusions and hallucinations. Reduced dose or discontinuation may be necessary. Unsteadiness may predispose to falling and injury. This drug can increase the degree of impaired urination associated with prostate gland enlargement (prostatism). Taking the total dose at bedtime can reduce the risk of postural hypotension (see Glossary).

▷ **Advisability of Use During Pregnancy**
Pregnancy Category: C. See Pregnancy Code at the back of this book.
Animal studies: Reveal toxic effects on the embryo in rats and rabbits but no birth defects in the newborn.
Human studies: Adequate studies of pregnant women are not available.
Avoid drug during first 3 months. Use during the last 6 months only if clearly needed.

Advisability of Use if Breast-Feeding
Presence of this drug in breast milk: Yes, in small amounts.
Watch infant closely and stop drug or nursing if adverse effects start.

Habit-Forming Potential: None.

Effects of Overdosage: Confusion, hallucinations, marked drowsiness, tremors, dilated pupils, cold skin, stupor, coma, convulsions, rapid heartbeat, low blood pressure.

Suggested Periodic Examinations While Taking This Drug (at physician's discretion)
Complete blood cell counts, serial blood pressure readings and electrocardiograms.

▷ **While Taking This Drug, Observe the Following**
Foods: No restrictions. Drug may increase appetite and cause excessive weight gain.
Beverages: No restrictions. May be taken with milk.

▷ *Alcohol:* Avoid completely. This drug can markedly increase the intoxicating effects of alcohol and accentuate its depressant action on brain function.
　Tobacco Smoking: May hasten the elimination of this drug. Higher doses may be necessary.
▷ *Other Drugs*
　Amoxapine may *increase* the effects of
　• atropinelike drugs (see Drug Class).
　Amoxapine may *decrease* the effects of
　• clonidine (Catapres).
　• guanethidine (Ismelin).
　Amoxapine *taken concurrently* with
　• antihistamines may increase urinary retention and dry mouth.
　• monoamine oxidase (MAO) type A inhibitor drugs may cause high fever, delirium and convulsions (see Drug Class).
　• carbamazepine (Tegretol) may result in decreased antidepressant action.
　• cimetidine (Tagamet) may increase amoxapine levels and result in toxicity.
　• phenytoin (Dilantin) may result in increased phenytoin levels.
　• quinidine (Quinaglute) may result in amoxapine toxicity.
　• thyroid preparations may impair heart rhythm and function. Ask physician for guidance regarding adjustment of thyroid dose.
▷ *Driving, Hazardous Activities:* This drug may impair mental alertness, judgment, physical coordination and reaction time. Avoid hazardous activities.
　Aviation Note: The use of this drug *is a disqualification* for piloting. Consult a designated Aviation Medical Examiner.
　Exposure to Sun: Caution, this drug may cause photosensitivity (see Glossary).
　Exposure to Heat: This drug can inhibit sweating and impair the body's adaptation to hot environments, increasing the risk of heat stroke. Avoid saunas.
　Exposure to Cold: The elderly should use caution. Avoid conditions conducive to hypothermia (see Glossary).
　Discontinuation: Slowly stop this drug. Abrupt withdrawal after long-term use can cause headache, malaise and nausea.

AMOXICILLIN (a mox i SIL in)

Introduced: 1969　　**Prescription:** USA: Yes; Canada: Yes　　**Available as Generic:** USA: Yes; Canada: No　　**Class:** Anti-infective, penicillins
Controlled Drug: USA: No; Canada: No
Brand Names: Amoxil, ✦Apo-Amoxi, ✦Clavulin, Larotid, ✦Novamoxin, ✦Nu-Amoxi, Polymox, Trimox, Utimox, Wymox

BENEFITS versus RISKS	
Possible Benefits	*Possible Risks*
EFFECTIVE TREATMENT OF INFECTIONS due to susceptible microorganisms	ALLERGIC REACTIONS, mild to severe, in 3% of the general population and 15% of allergic individuals
	Superinfections (yeast)
	Drug-induced colitis

Amoxicillin

▷ **Principal Uses**

As a Single Drug Product: Uses currently included in FDA approved labeling: Treatment of the following infections: (1) Some genitourinary tract infections; (2) Acute uncomplicated gonorrhea, male and female; (3) A Drug of Choice for acute otitis media (middle ear infection); (4) Some acute bacterial infections of the sinuses and throat; (5) Some acute bacterial infections of the skin and soft tissues; (6) Haemophilus influenzae infections.

Other (unlabeled) generally accepted uses: Treatment of the following infections: (1) Bronchitis; (2) biliary tract infections; (3) Lyme disease; (4) typhoid fever; (5) gonorrheal infection of the urethra; (6) combination antibiotic treatment of duodenal ulcer caused by H. pylori; (7) prevention of bacterial endocarditis.

As a Combination Drug Product [CD]: See the following Drug Profile of Amoxicillin and Clavulanate.

How This Drug Works: This drug destroys susceptible infecting bacteria by interfering with their ability to produce new protective cell walls as they multiply and grow.

Available Dosage Forms and Strengths

    Capsules — 250 mg, 500 mg
Chewable tablets — 125 mg, 250 mg
Oral liquid — 3 gram
Oral suspension — 50 mg per ml; 125 mg, 250 mg per 5 ml teaspoonful
Pediatric drops — 50 mg/ml

▷ **Recommended Dosage Ranges** (Actual dosage and administration schedule must be determined by the physician for each patient individually.)

Infants and Children: Up to 6 kg of body weight—25 to 50 mg every 8 hours. 6 to 8 kg of body weight—50 to 100 mg every 8 hours. 8 to 20 kg of body weight—6.7 to 13.3 mg/kg of body weight every 8 hours. 20 kg of body weight and over—same as 12 to 60 years of age.

12 to 60 Years of Age: Usual dose—250 to 500 mg every 8 hours. The total daily dose should not exceed 4.5 grams.

For gonorrhea—3 grams, together with 1 gram of probenecid, taken as a single dose.

For Lyme disease—250 to 500 mg, 3 or 4 times a day, for 10 to 30 days; dose and duration of treatment depends on severity of infection and response to treatment.

Over 60 Years of Age: Same as 12 to 60 years of age.

Conditions Requiring Dosing Adjustments

Liver function: Adjustments in dosing in liver compromise are not needed.
Kidney function: Dosing interval **must** be adjusted in renal compromise.

▷ **Dosing Instructions:** May be taken on an empty stomach or with food, milk, fruit juice, ginger ale or other cold drinks. The capsule may be opened for administration. Shake the oral suspension well before measuring each dose. The tablets should be chewed or crushed.

Usual Duration of Use: For all streptococcal infections—not less than 10 consecutive days (without interruption) to reduce the possibility of rheumatic fever or glomerulonephritis. For all other infections—as long as needed to treat the infection.

▷ **This Drug Should Not Be Taken If**
- you have had an allergic reaction to any dosage form of it previously.
- you are certain you are allergic to *any* form of penicillin.

▷ **Inform Your Physician Before Taking This Drug If**
- you suspect you are allergic to penicillin or have had a previous "reaction" to penicillin.
- you are allergic to any cephalosporin drugs (Ancef, Ceporan, Ceporex, Kafocin, Keflex, Keflin, Kefzol, Loridine, others).
- you are allergic by nature (hay fever, asthma, hives, eczema).
- you are unsure of how much amoxicillin to take or how often to take it.
- you have a history of liver or kidney disease.

Possible Side-Effects (natural, expected and unavoidable drug actions)
Superinfections (see Glossary), often due to yeast organisms.

▷ **Possible Adverse Effects** (unusual, unexpected and infrequent reactions)
If any of the following develop, consult your physician promptly for guidance.

Mild Adverse Effects
Allergic Reactions: Skin rashes, hives, itching.
Irritations of mouth and tongue, "black tongue," nausea, vomiting, mild diarrhea, dizziness (rare).

Serious Adverse Effects
Allergic Reactions: Anaphylactic reaction (see Glossary), severe skin reactions, drug fever, swollen painful joints, sore throat, abnormal bleeding or bruising.
Drug-induced pseudomembranous colitis: severe abdominal pain and cramping, marked diarrhea, bloody stools, fever.
Rare liver toxicity.

▷ **Possible Effects on Sexual Function:** None reported.

Possible Effects on Laboratory Tests
White blood cell counts: decreased.

CAUTION
1. Take the exact dose and the full course prescribed.
2. Should not be used with antibiotics such as erythromycin or tetracycline.

Precautions for Use
By Infants and Children: A rash occurs in approximately 90% of people who take this drug during an episode of infectious mononucleosis. The drug commonly causes diarrhea.
By Those over 60 Years of Age: Natural changes in the skin may predispose to prolonged itching reactions in the genital and anal regions. Report such reactions promptly.

▷ **Advisability of Use During Pregnancy**
Pregnancy Category: B. See Pregnancy Code at the back of this book.
Animal studies: No information available.
Human studies: Information from adequate studies of pregnant women indicates no increased risk of birth defects in 3546 pregnancies exposed to penicillin derivatives.
Ask physician for guidance.

Amoxicillin/Clavulanate

Advisability of Use if Breast-Feeding
Presence of this drug in breast milk: Yes.
The nursing infant may be sensitized to penicillin and may be at risk for developing diarrhea or yeast infections.
Avoid drug if possible or refrain from nursing.

Habit-Forming Potential: None.

Effects of Overdosage: Possible nausea, vomiting and/or diarrhea.

Possible Effects of Long-Term Use: Superinfections, often due to yeast organisms.

Suggested Periodic Examinations While Taking This Drug (at physician's discretion)
Complete blood cell counts.

▷ **While Taking This Drug, Observe the Following**
Foods: No restrictions, minor decrease in absorption.
Beverages: No restrictions. May be taken with milk, fruit juices or carbonated drinks.
▷ *Alcohol:* No interactions expected.
Tobacco Smoking: No interactions expected.
▷ *Other Drugs*
Amoxicillin may *decrease* the effects of
- oral contraceptives—PREGNANCY risk.

The following drugs may *decrease* the effects of amoxicillin
- antacids reduce the absorption of amoxicillin.
- chloramphenicol (Chloromycetin).
- erythromycin (Erythrocin, E-Mycin, etc.).
- tetracyclines (Achromycin, Declomycin, Minocin, etc.). (See Drug Class.)

▷ *Driving, Hazardous Activities:* Be alert to the rare occurrence of dizziness and/or nausea, and restrict activities accordingly.
Aviation Note: The use of this drug **may be a disqualification** for piloting. Consult a designated Aviation Medical Examiner.
Exposure to Sun: No restrictions.
Special Storage Instructions: Oral suspension and pediatric drops should be refrigerated.
Observe the Following Expiration Times: Do not take the oral suspension or drops of this drug if older than 7 days when kept at room temperature or 14 days when kept refrigerated.

AMOXICILLIN/CLAVULANATE (a mox i SIL in/ KLAV yu lan ayt)

Introduced: 1982 **Prescription:** USA: Yes; Canada: Yes **Available as Generic:** USA: No; Canada: No **Class:** Anti-infective, penicillins, beta-lactamase inhibitor **Controlled Drug:** USA: No; Canada: No

Brand Names: Augmentin, ✦Clavulin

BENEFITS versus RISKS	
Possible Benefits	*Possible Risks*
EFFECTIVE TREATMENT OF INFECTIONS due to susceptible microorganisms	ALLERGIC REACTIONS, mild to severe, in 3% of the general population and 15% of allergic individuals Superinfections (yeast) Drug-induced colitis Low white blood cells (rare)

▷ **Principal Uses**

As a Combination Drug Product [CD]: Uses currently included in FDA approved labeling: Treatment of the following infections: (1) Some genitourinary tract infections; (2) Some bacterial pneumonias; (3) Acute otitis media (middle ear infection) and sinusitis caused by certain bacteria; (4) Some acute bacterial infections of the skin and soft tissues.

Other (unlabeled) generally accepted uses: Treatment of the following infections: (1) Bronchitis; (2) biliary tract infections; (3) chancroid; (4) cat bite infections.

How This Drug Works: Amoxicillin destroys susceptible infecting bacteria by interfering with their ability to produce new protective cell walls as they multiply and grow.

Clavulanate inhibits beta-lactamase enzymes produced by resistant bacteria. Clavulanate enhances the action of amoxicillin against resistant bacteria.

Available Dosage Forms and Strengths

Oral suspension — 125 mg (amoxicillin) and 31.25 mg (clavulanate) per 5 ml teaspoonful
— 250 mg (amoxicillin) and 62.5 mg (clavulanate) per 5 ml teaspoonful
Tablets — 250 mg (amoxicillin) and 125 mg (clavulanate)
— 500 mg (amoxicillin) and 125 mg (clavulanate)
Tablets, chewable — 125 mg (amoxicillin) and 31.25 mg (clavulanate)
— 250 mg (amoxicillin) and 62.5 mg (clavulanate)

▷ **Recommended Dosage Ranges** (Actual dosage and administration schedule must be determined by the physician for each patient individually.)

Infants and Children: Up to 40 kg of body weight—6.7 to 13.3 mg (amoxicillin)/kg of body weight every 8 hours.

40 kg of body weight and over—same as 12 to 60 years of age.

12 to 60 Years of Age: Usual dose—250 to 500 mg (amoxicillin) every 8 hours. The total daily dose (of amoxicillin) should not exceed 4.5 grams.

Over 60 Years of Age: Same as 12 to 60 years of age.

Note: The above dosages refer to the amoxicillin component of this combination drug. The 250 mg regular tablet and the 250 mg chewable tablet contain different amounts of clavulanate and are not interchangeable. See **Dosage Forms** above.

Conditions Requiring Dosing Adjustments

Liver function: Specific guidelines do not exist regarding adjustment in liver failure.

Kidney function: Dose **must** be decreased in kidney compromise.

Amoxicillin/Clavulanate

▷ **Dosing Instructions:** May be taken on an empty stomach or with food, milk, fruit juice, ginger ale or other cold drinks. The oral suspension should be shaken well before measuring each dose. The regular tablets may be crushed for administration. The chewable tablets should be chewed or crushed.

Usual Duration of Use: For all streptococcal infections—not less than 10 consecutive days (without interruption) to reduce the possibility of developing rheumatic fever or glomerulonephritis. For all other infections—as long as necessary to eradicate the infection.

▷ **This Drug Should Not Be Taken If**
- you have had an allergic reaction to any dosage form of it previously.
- you are certain you are allergic to *any* form of penicillin.

▷ **Inform Your Physician Before Taking This Drug If**
- you suspect you are allergic to penicillin or have had a previous "reaction" to penicillin.
- you are allergic to cephalosporin drugs (Ancef, Ceporan, Ceporex, Kafocin, Keflex, Keflin, Kefzol, Loridine, others).
- you are allergic by nature (hay fever, asthma, hives, eczema).
- you are unsure of how much amoxicillin/clavulanate to take or how often to take it.
- you have a history of low blood counts.
- you have a history of liver or kidney disease.

Possible Side-Effects (natural, expected and unavoidable drug actions)
Superinfections (see Glossary), often due to yeast organisms.

▷ **Possible Adverse Effects** (unusual, unexpected and infrequent reactions)
If any of the following develop, consult your physician promptly for guidance.
Mild Adverse Effects
Allergic Reactions: Skin rashes, hives, itching.
Irritations of mouth and tongue, "black tongue," nausea, vomiting, mild diarrhea, dizziness (rare).
Serious Adverse Effects
Allergic Reactions: Anaphylactic reaction (see Glossary), severe skin reactions, drug fever, swollen painful joints, sore throat, abnormal bleeding or bruising.
Drug-induced pseudomembranous colitis: severe abdominal pain and cramping, marked diarrhea, bloody stools, fever.
Low white blood cells (rare).
Hepatitis (rare).
Candidal vaginitis.

▷ **Possible Effects on Sexual Function:** None reported.

Possible Effects on Laboratory Tests
White blood cell counts: decreased.

CAUTION
1. Take the exact dose and the full course prescribed.
2. Should not be used with erythromycin or tetracycline.

Precautions for Use
By Infants and Children: A generalized rash occurs in approximately 90% of individuals who take this drug during an episode of infectious mononucleosis. This drug may cause diarrhea, which sometimes necessitates discontinuation.
By Those over 60 Years of Age: Natural changes in the skin may predispose to prolonged itching reactions in the genital and anal regions. Report such reactions promptly.

▷ **Advisability of Use During Pregnancy**
Pregnancy Category: B. See Pregnancy Code at the back of this book.
Animal studies: No information available.
Human studies: Information from adequate studies of pregnant women indicates no increased risk of birth defects in 3546 pregnancies exposed to penicillin derivatives.
Ask physician for guidance.

Advisability of Use if Breast-Feeding
Presence of this drug in breast milk: Yes.
The nursing infant may be sensitized to penicillin and may be at risk for developing diarrhea or yeast infections.
Avoid drug if possible or refrain from nursing.

Habit-Forming Potential: None.

Effects of Overdosage: Possible nausea, vomiting and/or diarrhea.

Possible Effects of Long-Term Use: Superinfections, often due to yeast organisms.

Suggested Periodic Examinations While Taking This Drug (at physician's discretion)
Complete blood cell counts.

▷ **While Taking This Drug, Observe the Following**
Foods: No restrictions.
Beverages: No restrictions. May be taken with milk, fruit juices or carbonated drinks.
▷ *Alcohol:* No interactions expected.
Tobacco Smoking: No interactions expected.
▷ *Other Drugs*
Amoxicillin may *decrease* the effects of
• oral contraceptives in some women, and impair their effectiveness.
The following drugs may *decrease* the effects of amoxicillin
• antacids reduce the absorption of amoxicillin.
• chloramphenicol (Chloromycetin).
• erythromycin (Erythrocin, E-Mycin, etc.).
• tetracyclines (Achromycin, Declomycin, Minocin, etc.). (See Drug Class.)
▷ *Driving, Hazardous Activities:* Be alert to the rare occurrence of dizziness and/or nausea, and restrict activities accordingly.
Aviation Note: The use of this drug **may be a disqualification** for piloting. Consult a designated Aviation Medical Examiner.
Exposure to Sun: No restrictions.
Special Storage Instructions: Oral suspension and pediatric drops should be refrigerated.

Observe the Following Expiration Times: Do not take the oral suspension or drops of this drug if older than 7 days when kept at room temperature or 14 days when kept refrigerated.

AMPICILLIN (am pi SIL in)

Introduced: 1961 **Prescription:** USA: Yes; Canada: Yes **Available as Generic:** Yes **Class:** Antibiotic, penicillins **Controlled Drug:** USA: No; Canada: No

Brand Names: Amcill, ✦Ampicin, ✦Ampicin PRB [CD], ✦Ampilean, ✦Apo-Ampi, D-Amp, 500 Kit [CD], Nu-Ampi, ✦Novo-Ampicillin, Omnipen, Omnipen Pediatric Drops, ✦Penbritin, Polycillin, Polycillin Pediatric Drops, Polycillin-PRB [CD], ✦Pondocillin, Principen, Probampacin [CD], ✦Pro-Biosan, SK-Ampicillin, Totacillin

BENEFITS versus RISKS	
Possible Benefits	*Possible Risks*
EFFECTIVE TREATMENT OF INFECTIONS due to susceptible microorganisms	ALLERGIC REACTIONS, mild to severe Superinfections (yeast) Drug-induced colitis Rare blood cell disorders Rare kidney problems

▷ **Principal Uses**

As a Single Drug Product: Treats some infections of the skin and soft tissues, of the respiratory tract, of the gastrointestinal tract, and of the genitourinary tract (including gonorrhea in females). Also used to treat certain types of septicemia and meningitis.

As a Combination Drug Product [CD]: May be combined with probenecid (Benemid) to keep a therapeutic blood level.

How This Drug Works: This drug destroys susceptible infecting bacteria by interfering with their ability to produce new protective cell walls as they multiply and grow.

Available Dosage Forms and Strengths
 Capsules — 250 mg, 500 mg
 Oral suspension — 100 mg per ml, 125 mg, 250 mg, 500 mg per 5 ml teaspoonful
 Pediatric drops — 100 mg per ml

▷ **Usual Adult Dosage Range:** 500 to 1000 mg/6 hours. The usual maximal dose is 6000 mg/24 hours. **Note: Actual dosage and administration schedule must be determined by the physician for each patient individually.**

Conditions Requiring Dosing Adjustments

Liver function: The liver is not significantly involved in the elimination of ampicillin.

Kidney function: Dose must be decreased in people with kidney damage.

▷ **Dosing Instructions:** Best taken on an empty stomach, 1 hour before or 2 hours after eating. Capsule may be opened for administration.

Usual Duration of Use: For all streptococcal infections—not less than 10 consecutive days (without interruption) to reduce the possibility of developing rheumatic fever or glomerulonephritis. For all other infections—as long as necessary to eradicate the infection.

▷ **This Drug Should Not Be Taken If**
- you have had an allergic reaction to any dosage form of it previously.
- you are certain you are allergic to *any* form of penicillin.

▷ **Inform Your Physician Before Taking This Drug If**
- you suspect you are allergic to penicillin or you have a previous "reaction" to penicillin.
- you are allergic to cephalosporin antibiotics (Ancef, Ceporan, Ceporex, Kafocin, Keflex, Keflin, Kefzol, Loridine).
- you are allergic by nature (hay fever, asthma, hives, eczema).
- you are unsure of how much ampicillin to take or how often to take it.
- you have mono (mononucleosis) as you are more likely to get a rash.
- you have a history of blood disorders.
- you have a history of kidney problems.

Possible Side-Effects (natural, expected and unavoidable drug actions)
Superinfections (see Glossary), often due to yeast organisms.

▷ **Possible Adverse Effects** (unusual, unexpected and infrequent reactions)
If any of the following develop, consult your physician promptly for guidance.

Mild Adverse Effects
Allergic Reactions: Skin rashes, hives, itching.
Irritations of mouth and tongue, "black tongue," nausea, vomiting, mild diarrhea, dizziness (rare).

Serious Adverse Effects
Allergic Reactions: Anaphylactic reaction (see Glossary), severe skin reactions, drug fever, swollen painful joints.
Blood cell problems: sore throat, abnormal bleeding or bruising.
Rare kidney problems (interstitial nephritis).
Rare seizures (high blood levels).
Rare severe colon inflammation (pseudomembranous colitis).

▷ **Possible Effects on Sexual Function:** May have a small effect in decreasing sperm counts in men.

Possible Effects on Laboratory Tests
Complete blood cell counts: decreased red cells, white cells and platelets; increased eosinophils.
Bleeding time: may be prolonged, related to dose of drug.
Coombs' antiglobulin test: may be positive.
Urine analysis: positive for red blood cells and casts.
Urine sugar tests: using Tes-Tape—no drug effect; using Clinistix or Diastix—false low or negative; using Clinitest—false positive.

CAUTION
1. Take the exact dose and the full course prescribed.
2. Should not be used with erythromycin or tetracycline.

Precautions for Use
By Infants and Children: A generalized rash occurs in approximately 90% of individuals who take this drug during an episode of infectious mononu-

cleosis. This drug may cause diarrhea, which sometimes necessitates discontinuation.

By Those over 60 Years of Age: Natural changes in the skin may predispose to prolonged itching reactions in the genital and anal regions. Report such reactions promptly.

▷ **Advisability of Use During Pregnancy**
Pregnancy Category: B. See Pregnancy Code at the back of this book.
Animal studies: No birth defects due to this drug found in mice or rats.
Human studies: Information from adequate studies of pregnant women indicates no increased risk of birth defects in 3546 pregnancies exposed to penicillin derivatives.
Ask physician for guidance.

Advisability of Use if Breast-Feeding
Presence of this drug in breast milk: Yes, in small amounts.
The nursing infant may be sensitized to penicillin and may be at risk for developing diarrhea or yeast infections.
Avoid drug if possible or refrain from nursing.

Habit-Forming Potential: None.

Effects of Overdosage: Possible nausea, vomiting and/or diarrhea, seizures.

Possible Effects of Long-Term Use: Superinfections, often due to yeast organisms.

Suggested Periodic Examinations While Taking This Drug (at physician's discretion)
Complete blood cell counts.

▷ **While Taking This Drug, Observe the Following**
Foods: No restrictions.
Beverages: No restrictions. May be taken with milk.
▷ *Alcohol:* No interactions expected, however alcohol may blunt the immune response and lessen your ability to fight infection.
Tobacco Smoking: No interactions expected.
▷ *Other Drugs*
Ampicillin may *decrease* the effects of
- oral contraceptives in some women, and impair their effectiveness in preventing pregnancy.

The following drugs may *decrease* the effects of ampicillin
- antacids reduce the absorption of amoxicillin.
- chloramphenicol (Chloromycetin).
- erythromycin (Erythrocin, E-Mycin, etc.).
- tetracyclines (Achromycin, Declomycin, Minocin, etc.). (See Drug Class.)

▷ *Driving, Hazardous Activities:* Be alert to the rare occurrence of dizziness and/or nausea, and restrict activities accordingly.
Aviation Note: The use of this drug **may be a disqualification** for piloting. Consult a designated Aviation Medical Examiner.
Exposure to Sun: No restrictions.
Special Storage Instructions: Oral suspension and pediatric drops should be refrigerated.
Observe the Following Expiration Times: Do not take the oral suspension or drops of this drug if older than 7 days when kept at room temperature or 14 days when kept refrigerated.

ASPIRIN* (AS pir in)

Other Names: ASA, acetylsalicylic acid
Introduced: 1899   **Prescription:** USA: No; Canada: No   **Available as Generic:** Yes   **Class:** Mild analgesic, anti-inflammatory, antiplatelet, antipyretic, salicylates   **Controlled Drug:** USA: No; Canada: No
Brand Names: Alka-Seltzer Effervescent Pain Reliever & Antacid [CD], Alka-Seltzer Plus Cold, Alka-Seltzer Night Time [CD], Alka-Seltzer Plus [CD], Anacin [CD], Anacin Maximum Strength [CD], ◆Anacin w/Codeine [CD], ◆Ancasal, APC [CD], Arthritis Pain Formula [CD], A.S.A. Enseals, ◆Asasantine [CD], Ascriptin [CD], Ascriptin A/D [CD], Aspergum, ◆Aspirin*, ◆Astrin, Axotal [CD], Azdone [CD], Bayer Aspirin, Bayer Children's Chewable Aspirin, Bayer Enteric Aspirin, Bufferin [CD], Bufferin Arthritis Strength [CD], Bufferin Extra Strength [CD], Bufferin w/Codeine [CD], Cama Arthritis Pain Reliever [CD], Carisoprodol Compound [CD], ◆C2 buffered [CD], Cope [CD], Coricidin [CD], ◆Coryphen, ◆Coryphen-Codeine [CD], Darvon Compound [CD], ◆Dristan [CD], Easprin, Ecotrin Preparations, 8-Hour Bayer, Empirin, Empirin w/Codeine No. 2, 4 [CD], ◆Entrophen, Excedrin [CD], Fiorinal [CD], Fiorinal w/Codeine [CD], ◆Fiorinal-C 1/4, -C 1/2 [CD], Genprin, Halprin, Hepto [CD], Lortab ASA [CD], Marnal [CD], Maximum Bayer Aspirin, Measurin, Midol Caplets [CD], Momentum [CD], Norgesic [CD], Norgesic Forte [CD], ◆Novasen, Orphenadrine [CD], PAP with codeine [CD], Percodan [CD], Percodan-Demi [CD], ◆Phenaphen [CD], ◆Phenaphen No. 2, 3, 4 [CD], Propoxyphene compound [CD], ◆Riphen-10, Robaxisal [CD], ◆Robaxisal-C [CD], Roxiprin [CD], ◆Sal-Adult, ◆Sal-Infant, SK-65 Compound [CD], St. Joseph Children's Aspirin, ◆Supasa, Synalgos [CD], Synalgos-DC [CD], Talwin Compound [CD], Talwin Compound-50 [CD], ◆Tecnal tablet [CD], ◆Triaphen-10, ◆217 [CD], ◆217 Strong [CD], Vanquish [CD], Verin, Wesprin, Zorprin

BENEFITS versus RISKS	
Possible Benefits	*Possible Risks*
EFFECTIVE RELIEF OF MILD TO MODERATE PAIN and INFLAMMATION REDUCTION OF FEVER PREVENTION OF BLOOD CLOTS (as in heart attack, phlebitis and stroke)	Stomach irritation, bleeding, and/or ulceration Hearing loss Decreased numbers of white blood cells and platelets Hemolytic anemia Rare liver toxicity Bronchospasm in asthmatics

▷ **Principal Uses**
As a Single Drug Product: Uses currently included in FDA approved labeling: (1) Relieves mild to moderate pain, and provides symptomatic relief in conditions causing inflammation or high fever. Treats musculoskeletal disorders, especially acute and chronic arthritis. Used selectively in low dosage to (2) reduce the risk of recurrent heart attack; (3) prevent platelet

---

*In the United States *aspirin* is an official generic designation. In Canada *Aspirin* is the Registered Trade Mark of the Bayer Company Division of Sterling Drug Limited.

embolism to the brain (in men); (4) reduce the risk of clots (thromboembolism) in patients who have had a heart attack, in people with artificial heart valves and after hip surgery; (See Blood Platelets in the Glossary.) (5) helps prevent recurrance of stroke in people who have suffered a stroke; (6) helps prevent stroke in patients who have had a transient ischemic attack (TIA).

Other (unlabeled) generally accepted uses: (1) Can help prevent toxemia of pregnancy when used in low doses, (2) may decrease the risk of colon polyps or colon cancer.

As a Combination Drug Product [CD]: Frequently combined with other mild or strong analgesic drugs to enhance pain relief. Also combined with antihistamines and decongestants in many cold preparations to relieve headache and general discomfort.

How This Drug Works: Reduces prostaglandins, chemicals involved in the production of inflammation and pain. By modifying the temperature-regulating center in the brain, dilating blood vessels, and increasing sweating, aspirin reduces fever. By preventing the production of thromboxane in blood platelets, aspirin inhibits formation of blood clots.

Available Dosage Forms and Strengths

Capsules, enteric-coated — 500 mg
Capsules, enteric-coated granules — 325 mg
Gum tablets — 227.5 mg
Suppositories — 60 mg, 120 mg, 125 mg, 130 mg, 195 mg, 200 mg, 300 mg, 325 mg, 600 mg, 650 mg, 1.2 grams
Tablets — 65 mg, 81 mg, 325 mg, 500 mg
Tablets, chewable — 81 mg
Tablets, enteric-coated — 81 mg, 165 mg, 325 mg, 500 mg, 650 mg, 975 mg
Tablets, prolonged-action — 650 mg, 800 mg

▷ **Usual Adult Dosage Range:** For pain or fever—325 to 650 mg/4 hours as needed. For arthritis (and related conditions)—3600 to 5400 mg daily in divided doses. For the prevention of blood clots—80 to 150 mg/24 to 48 hours. **Note: For long-term use, actual dosage and administration schedule must be determined by the physician for each patient individually.**

Conditions Requiring Dosing Adjustments

Liver function: This medication should be avoided in severe liver disease.
Kidney function: It should be avoided or used with caution in patients with kidney problems.
Glucose-6-Phosphate Dehydrogenase Deficiency
May cause destruction of red blood cells in patients with G-6-PD deficiency.

▷ **Dosing Instructions:** Take with food, milk, or a full glass of water to reduce stomach upset. Regular tablets may be crushed and capsules opened for administration. Enteric-coated tablets, prolonged-action tablets, A.S.A. Enseals, Cama tablets and Ecotrin tablets should not be crushed.

Usual Duration of Use: Short-term use is recommended—3 to 5 days. Daily use should not exceed 10 days without physician supervision. Use on a regular schedule for 1 week is usually needed to determine this drug's effectiveness in relieving the symptoms of chronic arthritis. Must evaluate response and adjust dose in long-term use. Consult your physician on a regular basis.

▷ **This Drug Should Not Be Taken If**
- you have had an allergic reaction to any form of aspirin.
- you have any type of bleeding disorder (such as hemophilia).
- you have active peptic ulcer disease.
- you are in the last 3 months of pregnancy.
- it smells like vinegar. This indicates decomposition of aspirin.

▷ **Inform Your Physician Before Taking This Drug If**
- you are taking any anticoagulant drug.
- you are taking oral antidiabetic drugs.
- you have a history of peptic ulcer disease or gout.
- you have lupus erythematosus.
- you are pregnant or planning pregnancy.
- you have asthma, carditis or nasal polyps.
- you plan to have surgery of any kind in the near future.
- you take other prescription or non-prescription medications which were not discussed when aspirin was prescribed for you.
- you are unsure of how much aspirin to take or how often to take it.
- you have a history of liver or kidney problems.
- you have a deficiency of G-6-PD.
- you have a history of angina (may be worsened by this drug).

Possible Side-Effects (natural, expected and unavoidable drug actions)
Mild drowsiness in sensitive individuals.

▷ **Possible Adverse Effects** (unusual, unexpected and infrequent reactions)
If any of the following develop, consult your physician promptly for guidance.
Mild Adverse Effects
Allergic Reactions: Skin rash, hives, nasal discharge (resembling hay fever), nasal polyps.
Stomach irritation, heartburn, nausea, vomiting, constipation.
Serious Adverse Effects
Allergic Reactions: Acute anaphylactic reaction (see Glossary), allergic destruction of blood platelets (see Glossary) and bruising.
Idiosyncratic Reactions: Hemolytic anemia (see Glossary).
Erosion of stomach lining, with silent bleeding.
Activation of peptic ulcer, with or without hemorrhage.
Bone marrow depression (see Glossary)—fatigue, weakness, fever, sore throat, abnormal bleeding or bruising.
Hepatitis with jaundice (see Glossary)—yellow skin and eyes, dark-colored urine, light-colored stool (very rare).
Kidney damage, if used in large doses or for a prolonged period of time.
Bronchospasm when used in patients with nasal polyps, asthma.
May worsen angina attacks and increase their frequency.
Reye's syndrome if used during viral illness.

▷ **Possible Effects on Sexual Function:** None reported.

▷ **Adverse Effects That May Mimic Natural Diseases or Disorders**
Liver damage may suggest viral hepatitis.

Possible Effects on Laboratory Tests
Complete blood counts: decreased red cells, hemoglobin, white cells and platelets.
Bleeding time: prolonged.
Prothrombin time: increased by large doses; decreased by small doses.
Blood glucose level: decreased in diabetics.
Blood uric acid level: increased by small doses; decreased by large doses.
Liver function tests: increased ALT/GPT, AST/GOT, alkaline phosphatase.
Kidney function tests: increased blood creatinine and urea nitrogen levels with long-term use; increased protein and kidney cells in urine.
Thyroid function tests: increased T_3 uptake, free T_3 and free T_4; decreased TSH, T_3, T_4, and free thyroxine index (FTI).
Urine sugar tests: false positive with Clinitest or Benedict's solution.
Fecal occult blood test: positive with large doses of aspirin.

CAUTION

1. It must be remembered that aspirin is a drug. While it is one of our most useful drugs, we have an unrealistic sense of safety and its potential for adverse effects.
2. Make it a point to learn the contents of all drugs you take—those prescribed by your physician and over-the-counter (OTC) medicines.
3. Do NOT take more than 3 tablets (975 mg) at one time, allow at least 4 hours between doses and take no more than 10 tablets (3250 mg) in 24 hours without physician supervision.
4. Remember that aspirin can
   - cause new illnesses.
   - complicate existing illnesses.
   - complicate pregnancy.
   - complicate surgery.
   - interact unfavorably with other drugs.
5. When your physician asks "Are you taking any drugs?" the answer is yes if you are taking aspirin. This also applies to *any* nonprescription drug you may be taking. (See OTC Drugs in the Glossary.)

Precautions for Use

By Infants and Children: Reye's syndrome (brain and liver damage in children, often fatal) can follow flu or chicken pox in children and teenagers. Some reports suggest that the use of aspirin by children with flu or chicken pox can increase the risk of developing this complication. Consult your physician before giving aspirin to a child or teenager with chicken pox, flu or similar infection.

Usual dosage schedule for children:
  Up to 2 years of age—consult physician.
  2 to 4 years of age—160 mg/4 hours, up to 5 doses/24 hours.
  4 to 6 years of age—240 mg/4 hours, up to 5 doses/24 hours.
  6 to 9 years of age—320 mg/4 hours, up to 5 doses/24 hours.
  9 to 11 years of age—400 mg/4 hours, up to 5 doses/24 hours.
  11 to 12 years of age—480 mg/4 hours, up to 5 doses/24 hours.

Do not exceed 5 days of continual use without consulting your physician.
Give all doses with food, milk or a full glass of water.

By Those over 60 Years of Age: Watch for signs of excessive dosage: nervous irritabilty, confusion, ringing in the ears, deafness, loss of appetite, nausea and stomach upset. Aspirin can cause serious bleeding from the stomach. This can occur as "silent" bleeding of small amounts over a long time, resulting in anemia. Sudden hemorrhage can occur, even without a history of stomach ulcer. Watch for gray to black colored stools—an indication of stomach bleeding.

▷ **Advisability of Use During Pregnancy**

Pregnancy Category: C. See Pregnancy Code at the back of this book.

Animal studies: Significant birth defects due to this drug have been reported.

Human studies: Information from studies of pregnant women indicates no increased risk of birth defects in 32,164 pregnancies exposed to aspirin. However, studies show that the regular use of aspirin during pregnancy is often detrimental to the health of the mother and to the welfare of the fetus. Anemia, hemorrhage before and after delivery and an increased incidence of stillbirths and newborn deaths have been reported. It is advisable to limit aspirin use during pregnancy to small doses and for brief periods of time. There are data which support use of aspirin in low doses to prevent toxemia of pregnancy in some women with a history of this problem. Ask your doctor for help. Avoid aspirin altogether during the last 3 months.

Advisability of Use if Breast-Feeding

Presence of this drug in breast milk: Yes.
Avoid drug or refrain from nursing.

Habit-Forming Potential: Extended high dose use may cause a psychological dependence (see Glossary).

Effects of Overdosage: Stomach distress, nausea, vomiting, ringing in the ears, dizziness, impaired hearing, blood chemistry imbalance, sweating, stupor, fever, deep and rapid breathing, muscular twitching, delirium, shock, hallucinations, convulsions.

Possible Effects of Long-Term Use

A form of psychological dependence (see Glossary).
Anemia due to chronic blood loss from erosion of stomach lining.
The development of stomach ulcer.
The development of "aspirin allergy"—nasal discharge, nasal polyps, asthma.
Kidney damage.
Prolonged bleeding time, critical in the event of injury or surgery.

Suggested Periodic Examinations While Taking This Drug (at physician's discretion)

Complete blood cell counts.
Kidney function tests and urine analyses.
Liver function tests.

Aspirin

▷ **While Taking This Drug, Observe the Following**
  Foods: No restrictions.
  Nutritional Support: Do not take large doses of vitamin C while taking aspirin regularly.
  Beverages: No restrictions. May be taken with milk.
▷ *Alcohol:* Concurrent use of alcohol and aspirin may significantly increase the risk of stomach damage and may prolong bleeding time.
  Tobacco Smoking: No interactions expected.
▷ *Other Drugs*
  Aspirin may *increase* the effects of
  - oral anticoagulants (see Drug Classes), and cause abnormal bleeding.
  - insulin and require dosage adjustment.
  - oral antidiabetic drugs and insulin, and cause hypoglycemia (see Drug Classes). Dosage decrease is often necessary.
  - heparin, and cause abnormal bleeding.
  - methotrexate, and increase its toxic effects.
  - valproic acid (Depakene).

  Aspirin may *decrease* the effects of
  - beta-adrenergic-blocking drugs (see Drug Class).
  - captopril (Capoten).
  - furosemide (Lasix).
  - spironolactone.
  - other NSAIDS (see Drug Classes).
  - probenecid (Benemid), and reduce its effectiveness in the treatment of gout—with aspirin doses of less than 2 grams/24 hours.
  - spironolactone (Aldactone), and reduce its diuretic effect.
  - sulfinpyrazone (Anturane), and reduce its effectiveness in the treatment of gout—with aspirin doses of less than 2 grams/24 hours.

  Aspirin *taken concurrently* with
  - diltiazem (Cardizem) may result in increased risk of bleeding.
  - methotrexate (Mexate) and cause toxicity.
  - valproic acid and cause toxic blood levels.
  - verapamil and cause increased bleeding risk.

  The following drugs may *increase* the effects of aspirin
  - acetazolamide (Diamox).
  - para-aminobenzoic acid (Pabalate).
  - cimetidine (Tagamet)

  The following drugs may *decrease* the effects of aspirin
  - antacids, in regular continual use.
  - cortisonelike drugs (see Drug Class).
  - urinary alkalizers (sodium bicarbonate, sodium citrate).
▷ *Driving, Hazardous Activities:* No restrictions or precautions.
  Aviation Note: It is advisable to watch for mild drowsiness and restrict activities accordingly.
  Exposure to Sun: Use caution, may cause photosensitivity.
  Discontinuation: Aspirin should be stopped at least 1 week before surgery of any kind.

ASTEMIZOLE (a STEM i zohl)

Introduced: 1982   **Prescription:** USA: Yes; Canada: No   **Available as Generic:** No   **Class:** Antihistamines   **Controlled Drug:** USA: No; Canada: No
Brand Name: Hismanal

BENEFITS versus RISKS	
Possible Benefits	*Possible Risks*
EFFECTIVE, LONG-LASTING RELIEF OF ALLERGIC RHINITIS AND ALLERGIC SKIN DISORDERS	RARE HEART RHYTHM DISTURBANCES Mild fatigue (infrequent)

▷ **Principal Uses**
   As a Single Drug Product: Uses currently included in FDA approved labeling: (1) Provides symptomatic relief in allergic and related disorders: seasonal and perennial allergic rhinitis (hay fever), allergic conjunctivitis and vasomotor rhinitis; and hives or localized allergic swellings (angioedema); (2) helps relieve vertigo; (3) of use in chronic urticaria.
   Other (unlabeled) generally accepted uses: (1) May have a role in relieving Lichen nitidus lesions.

How This Drug Works: Antihistamines block the action of histamine, and the development of swelling and itch in the eyes, nose and skin.

Available Dosage Forms and Strengths
   Suspension — 10 mg per 5 ml teaspoonful (Canada)
   Tablets — 10 mg

▷ **Usual Adult Dosage Range:** 10 mg once daily. The total daily dosage should not exceed 10 mg. **Note: Actual dosage and administration schedule must be determined by the physician for each patient individually.**

Conditions Requiring Dosing Adjustments
   Liver function: This drug should be used with caution in hepatic disease.
   Kidney function: Routine adjustment in kidney problems is not expected to be needed.

▷ **Dosing Instructions:** Take on an empty stomach, 1 hour before eating or 2 hours after eating. The tablet may be crushed for administration.

Usual Duration of Use: Regular use for 3 days is usually needed to see this drug's effectiveness in helping symptoms of allergic rhinitis and dermatosis. Some people may need to take this drug during the entire pollen season. However, antihistamines should not be taken continually (without interruption). Limit use to relieve symptoms. Consult your physician on a regular basis.

Possible Advantages of This Drug
   Effective relief with once-a-day dosage.
   No loss of effectiveness with continual use.
   Minimal drowsiness or decreased alertness characteristic of many other antihistamines.
   No or very slight atropinelike effects.

Astemizole

▷ **This Drug Should Not Be Taken If**
- you have had an allergic reaction to any form of it.
- you are currently undergoing allergy skin tests.
- you take: erythromycin, itraconazole, fluconazole or ketoconazole.

▷ **Inform Your Physician Before Taking This Drug If**
- you have had allergic reactions to antihistamines.
- you have a history of heart rhythm disorders.
- you have impaired liver or kidney function.
- you take other prescription or non-prescription medications which were not discussed when astemizole was prescribed for you.
- you are unsure of how much astemizole to take or how often to take it.

Possible Side-Effects (natural, expected and unavoidable drug actions)
Dry nose, mouth or throat.

▷ **Possible Adverse Effects** (unusual, unexpected and infrequent reactions)
If any of the following develop, consult your physician promptly for guidance.
Mild Adverse Effects
Allergic Reactions: Skin rash, itching.
Headache, nervousness, fatigue.
Increased appetite and weight (3.6%), dry mouth, indigestion, nausea, diarrhea.
Rare muscle aches.
Serious Adverse Effects
Significant heart rhythm disorders (from excess dose or drug interactions).
Rare paresthesias.
Rare convulsions.
Rare bronchospasm.

▷ **Possible Effects on Sexual Function**
None reported.

Possible Effects on Laboratory Tests
None reported.

CAUTION
1. Do not take more than prescribed; excess levels may cause serious heart rhythm disturbances.
2. Do not take this drug with any form of erythromycin, itraconazole fluconazole, ketoconazole or sotolol.
3. Report faintness, dizziness, heart palpitation or chest pain promptly.
4. Stop this drug 4 days before diagnostic skin test. This drug can hide true allergy to the substances being skin tested (false negative).
5. Do not use this drug if you have active bronchial asthma, bronchitis or pneumonia. It can thicken mucus, making it more difficult to remove.

Precautions for Use
By Infants and Children: Safety and effectiveness for those under 12 years of age not established.
By Those over 60 Years of Age: Increased risk of headache or fatigue. Use smaller doses at longer intervals.

▷ **Advisability of Use During Pregnancy**
   Pregnancy Category: C. See Pregnancy Code at the back of this book.
   Animal studies: No birth defects due to this drug reported.
   Human studies: Adequate studies of pregnant women are not available.
   Use this drug only if clearly needed. Ask your physician for guidance.

Advisability of Use if Breast-Feeding
   Presence of this drug in breast milk: Unknown.
   Avoid drug or refrain from nursing.

Habit-Forming Potential: None.

Effects of Overdosage: Serious heart rhythm abnormalities.

Possible Effects of Long-Term Use: None reported.

Suggested Periodic Examinations While Taking This Drug (at physician's discretion)
   Electrocardiograms for those with heart disorders.

▷ **While Taking This Drug, Observe the Following**
   Foods: No restrictions.
   Beverages: No restrictions. May be taken with milk.
▷ *Alcohol:* No interactions expected.
   Tobacco Smoking: No interactions expected.
▷ *Other Drugs:* Astemizole **taken concurrently** with the following drugs may cause increased blood levels of astemizole and resulting heart rhythm disturbances
   • azithromycin (Zithromax)
   • clarithromycin (Biaxin)
   • erythromycin
   • itraconazole
   • ketoconazole
   • fluconazole
   • sotolol can cause heart arrhythmias by prolonging the QTC interval additively with astemizole.
   Hazardous Activities: No restrictions.
   Aviation Note: The use of this drug *is probably not a disqualification* for piloting. Consult a designated Aviation Medical Examiner.
   Exposure to Sun: Rare cases of photosensitivity have been reported (see Glossary).

ATENOLOL (a TEN oh lohl)

Introduced: 1973   **Prescription:** USA: Yes; Canada: Yes   **Available as Generic:** Yes   **Class:** Antianginal, antihypertensive, beta-adrenergic blocker   **Controlled Drug:** USA: No; Canada: No

Brand Names: ♣Apo-Atenolol, ♣Novo-Atenolol, ♣Nu-Atenolol, Tenoretic [CD], Tenormin

Atenolol

BENEFITS versus RISKS	
Possible Benefits	**Possible Risks**
EFFECTIVE ANTIANGINAL DRUG in the management of effort-induced angina	CONGESTIVE HEART FAILURE in advanced heart disease
EFFECTIVE, WELL-TOLERATED ANTIHYPERTENSIVE in mild to moderate high blood pressure	Worsening of angina in coronary heart disease (abrupt withdrawal)
	Masking of low blood sugar (hypoglycemia) in drug-treated diabetes
	Provocation of bronchial asthma (with high doses)

▷ **Principal Uses**

As a Single Drug Product: Uses currently included in FDA approved labeling: (1) Treats classical, effort-induced angina pectoris; (2) mild to moderately severe high blood pressure. May be used alone or in combination with other antihypertensive drugs, such as diuretics; (3) used following heart attacks to help decrease risk of a second heart attack, decrease the size of the heart attack and reduce risk of abnormal heart beats.

Other (unlabeled) generally accepted uses: (1) Can help people with stage fright; (2) may have a role in preventing migraine headaches.

How This Drug Works: By blocking certain actions of the sympathetic nervous system, this drug
- reduces the rate and contraction force of the heart, reducing the oxygen requirement for the heart as it works.
- reduces blood vessel wall contraction, resulting in their relaxation and expansion and consequent lowering of blood pressure.

Available Dosage Forms and Strengths
Tablets — 25 mg, 50 mg, 100 mg

▷ **Usual Adult Dosage Range:** Initially 50 mg once daily. Dose may be increased gradually at intervals of 7 to 10 days as needed and tolerated up to 100 mg/24 hours. The usual maintenance dose is 50 to 100 mg/24 hours. The total dose should not exceed 100 mg/24 hours. **Note: Actual dosage and administration schedule must be determined by the physician for each patient individually.**

Conditions Requiring Dosing Adjustments

Liver function: No decreases needed as the liver has a small role in eliminating atenolol.

Kidney function: The dose must be decreased with 25 mg a day as a maximum dose in some people.

▷ **Dosing Instructions:** May be taken without regard to eating. Tablet may be crushed to take it. **Do not** stop this drug abruptly.

Usual Duration of Use: Use on a regular schedule for 3 to 7 days is usually needed to see this drug's effectiveness in lowering blood pressure. Long-term use of this drug will be decided by how much your blood pressure decreases over time in response to an overall treatment program (weight reduction, salt restriction, smoking cessation, etc.). See your physician on a regular basis.

Possible Advantages of This Drug: Least likely of all beta blocker drugs to cause central nervous system adverse effects: confusion, hallucinations, nervousness, nightmares.

Currently a "Drug of Choice"
for starting treatment of hypertension with a single drug, especially for those subject to diabetes.

▷ **This Drug Should Not Be Taken If**
- you have had an allergic reaction to it previously.
- you have congestive heart failure.
- you have an abnormally slow heart rate or a serious form of heart block.
- you are taking, or have taken within the past 14 days, any monoamine oxidase (MAO) type A inhibitor drug (see Drug Class, Section Four).
- you have recently had a heart attack.

▷ **Inform Your Physician Before Taking This Drug If**
- you have had an adverse reaction to any beta blocker drug (see Drug Class, Section Four).
- you have a history of serious heart disease, with or without episodes of heart failure.
- you have a history of hay fever (allergic rhinitis), asthma, chronic bronchitis or emphysema.
- you have been taking clonidine.
- you have a history of overactive thyroid function (hyperthyroidism).
- you have a history of low blood sugar (hypoglycemia)—this drug may hide some of the symptoms occurring with hypoglycemia.
- you have impaired liver or kidney function.
- you have diabetes or myasthenia gravis.
- you are currently taking any form of digitalis, quinidine or reserpine, or any calcium blocker drug (see Drug Class, Section Four).
- you plan to have surgery under general anesthesia in the near future.
- you take other prescription or non-prescription medications which were not discussed when atenolol was prescribed for you.
- you are unsure of how much atenolol to take or how often to take it.

Possible Side-Effects (natural, expected and unavoidable drug actions)
Lethargy, fatigability, cold extremities, slow heart rate, light-headedness in upright position (see Orthostatic Hypotension in Glossary).

▷ **Possible Adverse Effects** (unusual, unexpected and infrequent reactions)
If any of the following develop, consult your physician promptly for guidance.

Mild Adverse Effects
Allergic Reactions: Skin rash, itching.
Headache, dizziness, drowsiness, abnormal dreams.
Indigestion, nausea, diarrhea.
Joint and muscle discomfort, fluid retention (edema).

Serious Adverse Effects
Mental depression, anxiety.
Chest pain, shortness of breath, can lead to congestive heart failure.
Induction of bronchial asthma (in asthmatic individuals).
Angina (if abruptly stopped).
Rebound hypertension (if abruptly stopped).

Psychosis (very rare).
Systemic lupus erythematosus (rare).

▷ **Possible Effects on Sexual Function:** Decreased libido and impaired potency (50 to 100 mg/day). This drug is less likely to cause reduced erectile capacity than most drugs of its class.

Possible Effects on Laboratory Tests
Blood cholesterol levels: no effect with doses of 50 mg/day; increased with doses of 100 mg/day.
Blood HDL cholesterol levels: no effect with doses of 50 mg/day; decreased with doses of 100 mg/day.
Blood LDL cholesterol levels: no effect with doses of 50 mg/day; increased with doses of 100 mg/day.
Blood VLDL cholesterol levels: no effect with doses of 50 mg/day; increased with doses of 100 mg/day.
Blood triglyceride levels: no effect with doses of 50 mg/day; increased with doses of 100 mg/day.

CAUTION
1. ***DO NOT stop this drug suddenly*** without the knowledge and guidance of your physician. Carry a note on your person that take this drug.
2. Consult your physician or pharmacist before using nasal decongestants. These can cause sudden increases in blood pressure when combined with beta blocker drugs.
3. Report the development of any tendency to emotional depression.

Precautions for Use
By Infants and Children: Safety and effectiveness by those under 12 years of age not established. However, if this drug is used, watch for development of low blood sugar (hypoglycemia) especially if meals are skipped.
By Those over 60 Years of Age: Proceed ***cautiously*** with all antihypertensive drugs. High blood pressure should be reduced slowly, avoiding excessively low blood pressure. Small doses, and frequent blood pressure checks are needed. Sudden and excessive decrease in blood pressure can predispose to stroke or heart attack. Maximum daily dosage is 100 mg. Watch for dizziness, unsteadiness, tendency to fall, confusion, hallucinations, depression or urinary frequency.

▷ **Advisability of Use During Pregnancy**
Pregnancy Category: D. See Pregnancy Code at the back of this book.
Animal studies: Increased resorptions of embryo and fetus reported in rats, but no birth defects.
Human studies: Adequate studies of pregnant women are not available.
This drug has been used during the last three months of pregnancy, however fetal growth may be slowed and the child may be born with low blood pressure and temperature. Ask your doctor for guidance.

Advisability of Use if Breast-Feeding
Presence of this drug in breast milk: Yes.
Avoid drug if possible. If drug is necessary, observe nursing infant for slow heart rate and indications of low blood sugar.

Habit-Forming Potential: None.

Effects of Overdosage: Weakness, slow pulse, low blood pressure, fainting, cold and sweaty skin, congestive heart failure, possible coma and convulsions.

Possible Effects of Long-Term Use: Reduced heart reserve and eventual heart failure in some people with advanced heart disease.

Suggested Periodic Examinations While Taking This Drug (at physician's discretion)
Measurements of blood pressure, evaluation of heart function.

▷ **While Taking This Drug, Observe the Following**
Foods: No restrictions. Avoid excessive salt intake.
Beverages: No restrictions. May be taken with milk.

▷ *Alcohol:* Use caution. Alcohol may exaggerate this drug's ability to lower blood pressure and may increase its mild sedative effect.
Tobacco Smoking: Nicotine may reduce this drug's effectiveness in treating high blood pressure. High doses may worsen bronchial tightening caused by regular smoking.

▷ *Other Drugs*
Atenolol may *increase* the effects of
- other antihypertensive drugs and cause excessive lowering of blood pressure. Dosage adjustments may be necessary.
- reserpine (Ser-Ap-Es, etc.) and cause sedation, depression, slowing of heart rate and lowering of blood pressure.

Atenolol *taken concurrently* with
- amiodarone (Codarone) may result in cardiac arrest.
- calcium carbonate may result in large increases in atenolol blood levels and toxic effects.
- clonidine (Catapres) requires close monitoring for rebound high blood pressure if clonidine is stopped while atenolol is still being taken.
- insulin requires close monitoring to avoid undetected hypoglycemia (see Glossary).
- phenothiazines (see Drug Classes) may increase the effects of both agents and result in phenothiazine toxicity or excessively low blood pressure.
- quinidine (Quinaglute) may cause additive lowering of the blood pressure.
- oral hypoglycemics (see Drug Classes) may result in prolonged low blood sugar.

The following drugs may *decrease* the effects of atenolol
- indomethacin (Indocin), and possibly other "aspirin substitutes," or NSAIDs may impair atenolol's antihypertensive effect.

▷ *Driving, Hazardous Activities:* Use caution until the full extent of drowsiness, lethargy, and blood pressure change has been determined.
Aviation Note: The use of this drug *is a disqualification* for piloting. Consult a designated Aviation Medical Examiner.
Exposure to Sun: No restrictions.
Exposure to Heat: Caution advised. Hot environments can lower blood pressure and exaggerate the effects of this drug.
Exposure to Cold: Caution advised. Can enhance the circulatory deficiency that may occur with this drug. Elderly should be careful to prevent hypothermia (see Glossary).

Heavy Exercise or Exertion: Avoid exertion that causes light-headedness, excessive fatigue, or muscle cramping. This drug may worsen the blood pressure response to isometric exercise.

Occurrence of Unrelated Illness: Fever can lower blood pressure and require decreased dose. Nausea or vomiting may interrupt the dosing schedule. Ask your physician for help.

Discontinuation: Avoid stopping this drug suddenly. If possible, gradual reduction of dose over a period of 2 to 3 weeks is recommended. Ask your physician for help.

AURANOFIN (aw RAY noh fin)

Introduced: 1976   **Prescription:** USA: Yes; Canada: Yes   **Available as Generic:** No   **Class:** Antiarthritic, gold compounds   **Controlled Drug:** USA: No; Canada: No

Brand Name: Ridaura

BENEFITS versus RISKS

Possible Benefits	*Possible Risks*
REDUCTION OF JOINT PAIN, TENDERNESS AND SWELLING in active, severe RHEUMATOID ARTHRITIS Medication effective when taken by mouth	SIGNIFICANTLY REDUCED LEVELS OF RED AND WHITE BLOOD CELLS AND BLOOD PLATELETS (1% to 3%) LIVER DAMAGE WITH JAUNDICE (less than 0.1%) Diarrhea (47%), ulcerative colitis (less than 0.1%) Skin rash (24%) Mouth sores (13%) Kidney toxicity Rare lung damage

▷ **Principal Uses**

As a Single Drug Product: Uses currently included in FDA approved labeling: Used *only* for severe rheumatoid arthritis in adults who have had an inadequate response to aspirin, aspirin substitutes or other antiarthritic drugs and treatment programs. Usually added to a well-established program of antiarthritic drugs of the aspirin-substitute (NSAID) class.

Other (unlabeled) generally accepted uses: (1) May have a role in helping decrease the need for steroid use in people with asthma; (2) can ease the symptoms of nodular vasculitis.

How This Drug Works: Unknown. It suppresses but does not cure arthritis and associated synovitis. It has an effect on specific cells (macrophages) and stops them from engulfing cell debris and also inhibits lysosomes.

Available Dosage Forms and Strengths
Capsules — 3 mg

▷ **Usual Adult Dosage Range:** 6 mg daily, taken either as one dose every 24 hours or as two doses of 3 mg each every 12 hours. If response is inadequate after 6 months of regular continual use, the dose may be increased to 9 mg daily, taken as 3 doses of 3 mg each. If response remains inadequate after 3 months of 9 mg daily, this drug should be stopped. **Note: Actual dosage and administration schedule must be determined by the physician for each patient individually.**

Conditions Requiring Dosing Adjustments
Liver function: The liver is not involved in auranofin elimination. No dose decreases needed.

Kidney function: Blood levels are recommended, and decreased doses may be needed.

▷ **Dosing Instructions:** Take with or following food to reduce stomach irritation. Take the capsule whole with milk or a full glass of water.

Usual Duration of Use: Use on a regular schedule for 3 to 4 months is usually needed to see this drug's effectiveness in reducing joint pain, tenderness and swelling associated with rheumatoid arthritis. Long-term use will depend on how much benefit or the pattern of adverse effects experienced. Consult your physician on a regular basis.

▷ **This Drug Should Not Be Taken If**
- you have had an allergic reaction from previous use of gold.
- you have active ulcerative colitis.
- you have a current blood cell or bone marrow disorder.
- you have active liver or kidney disease.
- you are pregnant or breast-feeding.
- you have exfoliative dermatitis (ask your doctor).
- you are taking penicillamine or antimalarial drugs for arthritis.
- you have fibrous replacement of lung tissue (pulmonary fibrosis).

▷ **Inform Your Physician Before Taking This Drug If**
- you have a history of allergic reactions to drugs.
- you have diabetes.
- you have a history of heart disease, high blood pressure, circulatory disorders, liver or kidney disease, or ulcerative colitis.
- you are taking any other drugs at this time.
- you are planning pregnancy in the near future.
- you take other prescription or non-prescription medications which were not discussed when auranofin was prescribed for you.
- you are unsure of how much auranofin to take or how often to take it.

Possible Side-Effects (natural, expected and unavoidable drug actions)
Metallic taste.

▷ **Possible Adverse Effects** (unusual, unexpected and infrequent reactions)
If any of the following develop, consult your physician promptly for guidance.

Mild Adverse Effects
Allergic Reactions: Itching, skin rash.
Sores in mouth and throat and on tongue, loss of appetite, nausea, vomiting, stomach cramps, diarrhea (47%).
Taste problems.
Headache, partial or complete hair loss.
Conjunctivitis (3–9%).

Serious Adverse Effects
   Allergic Reactions: Severe skin reactions, exfoliative dermatitis.
   Fever, cough, shortness of breath, drug-induced pneumonia and lung damage.
   Liver damage with jaundice, ulcerative colitis.
   Kidney damage.
   Blood cell and bone marrow toxicity—fatigue, weakness, sore throat, abnormal bleeding or bruising.
   Peripheral neuritis—pain, numbness, weakness of arms and legs.
   Pancreatitis (less than 1%).

▷ **Possible Effects on Sexual Function:** Breast tenderness and swelling of male breast tissue (gynecomastia).

Possible Delayed Adverse Effects: Adverse effects may occur many months after treatment is stopped. This is due to accumulation of gold in body tissues and its slow elimination. Report any signs of toxicity to your physician promptly.

▷ **Adverse Effects That May Mimic Natural Diseases or Disorders**
   Fever, cough and chest discomfort may suggest respiratory tract infections such as bronchitis or pneumonia.
   Liver damage may suggest viral hepatitis.

Possible Effects on Laboratory Tests
   Complete blood counts: decreased red cells, hemoglobin and white cells; increased eosinophils and platelets; these occur in about 13% of users.

CAUTION
   1. Periodic examinations (blood and urine tests) are mandatory. Keep all appointments as directed by your physician.
   2. Promptly tell your doctor if any signs of toxic reactions occur. If there is a delay in reaching your doctor, stop this drug until you obtain medical guidance.

Precautions for Use
   By Infants and Children: Safety and effectiveness for those under 12 years of age not established.
   By Those over 60 Years of Age: Use small doses initially and watch closely for indications of adverse effects.

▷ **Advisability of Use During Pregnancy**
   Pregnancy Category: C. See Pregnancy Code at the back of this book.
      Animal studies: Rabbit studies revealed an increase in resorptions, abortions and birth defects.
      Human studies: Adequate studies of pregnant women are not available.
      The manufacturer does not recommend the use of this drug during pregnancy.

Advisability of Use if Breast-Feeding
   Presence of this drug in breast milk: Yes.
   Avoid drug or refrain from nursing.

Habit-Forming Potential: None.

Effects of Overdosage: Nausea, vomiting, diarrhea, confusion, low blood platelets, kidney dysfunction, delirium, peripheral neuritis, lung damage, encephalopathy, necrosis of the liver.

Suggested Periodic Examinations While Taking This Drug (at physician's discretion)
Complete blood cell counts, urine analyses, liver and kidney function tests.

▷ **While Taking This Drug, Observe the Following**
Foods: No restrictions.
Beverages: No restrictions. May be taken with milk.

▷ *Alcohol:* Use caution. Alcohol may intensify the irritant effect of this drug on the Stomach and intestines (gastrointestinal tract).
Tobacco Smoking: No interactions expected.

▷ *Other Drugs*
Auranofin may *increase* the effects of
- phenytoin (Dilantin), by increasing its blood level. Watch closely for indications of phenytoin toxicity.

Auranofin *taken concurrently* with
- Penicillamine may result in increased bone marrow depression.

▷ *Driving, Hazardous Activities:* Usually no restrictions.
Aviation Note: The use of this drug *may be a disqualification* for piloting. Consult a designated Aviation Medical Examiner.
Exposure to Sun: This drug may cause photosensitivity (see Glossary). Avoid sun and sun lamps.

AZATHIOPRINE (ay za THI oh preen)

Introduced: 1965 **Prescription:** USA: Yes; Canada: Yes **Available as Generic:** Yes **Class:** Antiarthritic, immunosuppressive **Controlled Drug:** USA: No; Canada: No
Brand Name: Imuran

BENEFITS versus RISKS	
Possible Benefits	*Possible Risks*
REDUCTION OF JOINT PAIN, TENDERNESS AND SWELLING in active, severe RHEUMATOID ARTHRITIS (66% of users) PREVENTION OF REJECTION IN ORGAN TRANSPLANTATION	UNACCEPTABLE ADVERSE EFFECTS IN 15% OF USERS REDUCED LEVELS OF WHITE BLOOD CELLS (28% in rheumatoid arthritis, 50% in kidney transplants) REDUCED LEVELS OF RED BLOOD CELLS AND PLATELETS LIVER DAMAGE WITH JAUNDICE (less than 1%) POSSIBLE INCREASED RISK OF MALIGNANCY (3%)

▷ **Principal Uses**
As a Single Drug Product: Uses currently included in FDA approved labeling: (1) Used to prevent rejection of transplanted organs (mainly kidney transplants); (2) also used in active, severe rheumatoid arthritis (in adults) that has failed conventional treatment.
Other (unlabeled) generally accepted uses: (1) Used to treat lupus ery-

thematosus, ulcerative colitis, chronic active hepatitis and other "autoimmune" disorders.

How This Drug Works: It is thought that by impairing purine metabolism, DNA and RNA, and inhibiting cell multiplication, this drug decreases the immune reaction that is responsible for rheumatoid arthritis, lupus erythematosus, etc.

Available Dosage Forms and Strengths
 Injection — 100 mg per 20-ml vial
 Tablets — 50 mg

▷ **Usual Adult Dosage Range:** As immunosuppressant—3 to 5 mg/kilogram of body weight daily, 1 to 3 days before transplantation surgery; for postoperative maintenance—1 to 2 mg/kilogram of body weight daily. As antiarthritic—1 mg/kilogram of body weight daily for 6 to 8 weeks; increase dose by 0.5 mg/kilogram of body weight every 4 weeks as needed and tolerated. Maximal daily dose is 2.5 mg/kilogram of body weight. Total dose may be taken once daily or divided into 2 equal doses taken 12 hours apart. **Note: Actual dosage and administration schedule must be determined by the physician for each patient individually.**

Conditions requiring dosing adjustments
 Liver function: No specific dosing guidelines are available, however, the drug may need to be stopped if jaundice occurs. Liver function must be closely watched.
 Kidney function: The dose must be decreased by up to 50% in kidney failure.

▷ **Dosing Instructions:** Take with or following food to reduce stomach upset. Tablet may be crushed.

Usual Duration of Use: Use on a regular schedule for 12 weeks is usually needed to determine this drug's effectiveness in helping rheumatoid arthritis. Successful use for up to 11 years has been reported. See your physician on a regular basis.

▷ **This Drug Should Not Be Taken If**
- you have had an allergic reaction to it previously.
- you are pregnant, and this drug is prescribed to treat rheumatoid arthritis.
- you have an active blood cell or bone marrow disorder.
- you are taking, or have recently taken, any form of chlorambucil (Leukeran), cyclophosphamide (Cytoxan) or melphalan (Alkeran).

▷ **Inform Your Physician Before Taking This Drug If**
- you have any kind of active infection.
- you have any form of cancer.
- you have gout or are taking allopurinol (Zyloprim).
- you have a history of blood cell or bone marrow disorders.
- you have impaired liver or kidney function.
- you are taking any form of gold, penicillamine or an antimalarial drug for arthritis.
- you plan pregnancy in the near future.
- you take other prescription or non-prescription medications which were not discussed when azathioprine was prescribed for you.
- you are unsure of how much azathioprine to take or how often to take it.

Possible Side-Effects (natural, expected and unavoidable drug actions)
Development of infection (2.4%).

▷ **Possible Adverse Effects** (unusual, unexpected and infrequent reactions)
If any of the following develop, consult your physician promptly for guidance.
Mild Adverse Effects
Allergic Reaction: Skin rash (2%).
Loss of appetite, nausea, vomiting, diarrhea (19%).
Sores on lips and in mouth.
Muscle aches.
Serious Adverse Effects
Allergic Reactions: Drug fever (see Glossary), joint and muscle pain.
Pancreatitis—severe stomach pain with nausea and vomiting (0.18%).
Bone marrow depression (see Glossary)—fatigue, weakness, fever, sore throat, abnormal bleeding or bruising.
Liver damage—yellow eyes and skin, dark-colored urine, light-colored stools (0.37%). (See Hepatitis and Jaundice in Glossary.)
Rare liver (hepatic) veno-occlusive disease.
Drug-induced pneumonia—cough, shortness of breath.
Development of cancer—skin cancer, reticulum-cell sarcoma, lymphoma, leukemia (3.3%).

▷ **Possible Effects on Sexual Function:** Reversal of male infertility due to sperm antibodies; this drug suppresses autoantibodies and permits the normal accumulation of sperm.

Possible Delayed Adverse Effects: Bone marrow depression may occur many weeks after stopping this drug.

▷ **Adverse Effects That May Mimic Natural Diseases or Disorders**
Liver damage may suggest viral hepatitis.

Possible Effects on Laboratory Tests
Complete blood cell counts: decreased red cells, hemoglobin, white cells and platelets.
Blood amylase and lipase levels: increased—possible pancreatitis.
Blood uric acid levels: increased with rapid tissue destruction; decreased in patients with gout.
Liver function tests: increased liver enzymes (ALT/GPT, AST/GOT and alkaline phosphatase); increased bilirubin.
Sperm counts: decreased.

CAUTION
1. Promptly report any indications of a developing infection—fever, chills, lip or mouth sores, etc.
2. Inform your physician promptly if you become pregnant.
3. Periodic blood counts are mandatory for the safe use of this drug.

Precautions for Use
By Infants and Children: Safety and effectiveness in those under 12 years of age not established.
By Those over 60 Years of Age: The smallest effective dose should be used as this reduces the risk of toxic reactions.

▷ **Advisability of Use During Pregnancy**
Pregnancy Category: D. See Pregnancy Code at the back of this book.
Animal studies: Birth defects reported in rodent studies.
Human studies: Two incidents of birth defects reported.
Adequate studies of pregnant women are not available.
Avoid completely during entire pregnancy if possible.

Advisability of Use if Breast-Feeding
Presence of this drug in breast milk: Yes.
Avoid drug or refrain from nursing.

Habit-Forming Potential: None.

Effects of Overdosage: Immediate—nausea, vomiting, diarrhea. Delayed—lowered white blood cell and platelet counts, liver and kidney toxicity.

Possible Effects of Long-Term Use: Susceptibility to infection, bone marrow depression, development of malignancies.

Suggested Periodic Examinations While Taking This Drug (at physician's discretion)
Complete blood cell counts, liver function tests.

▷ **While Taking This Drug, Observe the Following**
Foods: No restrictions.
Beverages: No restrictions. May be taken with milk.
▷ *Alcohol:* No interactions expected.
Tobacco Smoking: No interactions expected.
▷ *Other Drugs*
Azathioprine may **decrease** the effects of
- oral anticoagulants (warfarin, etc.), and require increased doses.
- certain muscle relaxants (gallamine, pancuronium, tubocurarine), and make it necessary to increase their dosage.

The following drugs may **increase** the effects of azathioprine
- allopurinol (Zyloprim) may increase its activity and toxicity and make it necessary to reduce its dosage.

Azathioprine *taken concurrently* with
- ACE inhibitors (see Drug Classes) such as captopril or enalapril may cause severe anemias.

▷ *Driving, Hazardous Activities:* No restrictions.
Aviation Note: The use of this drug **may be a disqualification** for piloting. Consult a designated Aviation Medical Examiner.
Exposure to Sun: No restrictions.
Discontinuation: A gradual reduction in dosage is preferable. Consult your physician for a withdrawal schedule.

AZITHROMYCIN (a zith roh MY sin)

Introduced: 1991 **Prescription:** USA: Yes **Available as Generic:** USA: No **Class:** Anti-infective, macrolides **Controlled Drug:** USA: No
Brand Name: Zithromax

BENEFITS versus RISKS

Possible Benefits	Possible Risks
Effective treatment of upper and lower respiratory tract infections due to susceptible microorganisms	Mild gastrointestinal symptoms
	Drug-induced colitis (rare)
	Superinfections (rare)
Effective treatment of skin infections due to susceptible microorganisms	
Effective treatment of urethral and cervical infections due to chlamydia trachomatis	

▷ **Principal Uses**
   As a Single Drug Product: Uses currently included in FDA approved labeling: (1) Treatment of some upper respiratory tract infections—streptococcal pharyngitis and tonsillitis; (2) Treatment of certain lower respiratory tract infections—acute bronchitis and pneumonia; (3) Treatment of some skin (and skin structure) infections; (4) Treatment of non-gonococcal urethritis and cervicitis due to chlamydia trachomatis. Cultures and sensitivity testing needed.
   Other (unlabeled) generally accepted uses: (1) This drug may be useful in treatment of AIDS-related infection due to Mycobacterium avium-intracellulare; (2) may have a role in toxoplasmosis AIDS patients.

How This Drug Works: This drug prevents the growth of susceptible organisms by blocking the formation of life-sustaining proteins.

Available Dosage Forms and Strengths
   Capsules — 250 mg

▷ **Recommended Dosage Ranges** (Actual dosage and administration schedule must be determined by the physician for each patient individually.)
   Infants and Children: Dosage not established.
   16 to 60 Years of Age: For pharyngitis/tonsillitis, bronchitis, pneumonia, and skin infections—500 mg as a single dose on the first day; then 250 mg once daily on days 2 through 5 for a total dose of 1.5 grams.
   For non-gonococcal urethritis and cervicitis—a single 1 gram dose.
   Over 60 Years of Age: Same as 16 to 60 years of age. If liver or kidney function is limited, the dose must be reduced.

Conditions Requiring Dosing Adjustments
   Liver function: Caution must be used in patients with impaired livers or bile tract disease.
   Kidney function: No data available about use of azithromycin in renal (kidney) compromise.

▷ **Dosing Instructions:** Do not take with food. Take at least 1 hour before eating or 2 hours after eating. Do not take antacids containing aluminum or magnesium with this drug. The capsule may be opened for administration.

Usual Duration of Use: Use on a regular schedule for 3 to 5 days is usually needed to see this drug's effectiveness in controlling infections. For streptococcal throat infections: the drug must be taken for at least 5 consecu-

Azithromycin

tive days (without interruption) to reduce the risk of rheumatic fever or glomerulonephritis.

Possible Advantages of This Drug
Broader spectrum of infectious microorganism ceverage; equivalent to erythromycin, some penicillins and some cephalosporins.
Effective with only 1 dose daily.
Very well tolerated; infrequent and minor adverse effects.

▷ **This Drug Should Not Be Taken If**
- you have had an allergic reaction to it previously.
- you are taking astemizole.

▷ **Inform Your Physician Before Taking This Drug If**
- you are allergic to related drugs: clarithromycin, erythromycin, or troleandomycin.
- you have impaired liver or kidney function.
- you have a history of drug-induced colitis.
- you take other prescription or non-prescription medications which were not discussed when azithromycin was prescribed for you.
- you are unsure of how much azithromycin to take or how often to take it.

Possible Side-Effects (natural, expected and unavoidable drug actions)
Superinfections (see Glossary), usually due to yeast.

▷ **Possible Adverse Effects** (unusual, unexpected and infrequent reactions)
If any of the following develop, consult your physician promptly for guidance.

Mild Adverse Effects
Allergic Reactions: Skin rash (1%).
Headache, dizziness, drowsiness, fatigue (all 1%).
Palpitation, chest pain (1%).
Nausea, stomach pain, indigestion (3%), diarrhea (5%).

Serious Adverse Effects
Allergic Reactions: Rare angioedema (swelling of soft tissues).
Rare drug-induced jaundice (see Glossary).
Rare drug-induced colitis.

▷ **Possible Effects on Sexual Function:** None reported.

Possible Effects on Laboratory Tests
Complete blood cell counts: decreased white cells and platelets (1%).
Liver function tests: increased enzymes (ALT/GPT, AST/GOT and alkaline phosphatase), increased bilirubin (all 1–2%).
Kidney function tests: increased blood urea nitrogen (1%).

CAUTION
1. If diarrhea starts and continues for more than 24 hours, call your doctor promptly. This could be drug-induced colitis.
2. Take the full dosage and amount prescribed to prevent resistance.

Precautions for Use
By Infants and Children: Safety and effectiveness for use by those under 16 years of age have not been established.
By Those over 60 Years of Age: Consider dosage adjustment if liver or kidney function is severely impaired.

▷ **Advisability of Use During Pregnancy**
  Pregnancy Category: B. See Pregnancy Code at the back of this book.
    Animal studies: No drug-induced birth defects reported.
    Human studies: Adequate studies of pregnant women are not available.
    Use this drug only if clearly needed. Ask your physician for guidance.
  Advisability of Use if Breast-Feeding
    Presence of this drug in breast milk: Unknown.
    Watch nursing infant closely and stop drug or nursing if adverse effects develop.
  Habit-Forming Potential: None.
  Effects of Overdosage: Possible nausea, vomiting, abdominal discomfort and diarrhea.
  Possible Effects of Long-Term Use: Superinfections, drug-induced colitis.
  Suggested Periodic Examinations While Taking This Drug (at physician's discretion)
    None.
▷ **While Taking This Drug, Observe the Following**
  Foods: No restrictions.
  Beverages: No restrictions.
▷ *Alcohol:* No interactions expected.
  Tobacco Smoking: No interactions expected.
▷ *Other Drugs*
    Azithromycin may *increase* the effects of
    • carbamazepine (Tegretol) may result in increased levels.
    • cyclosporine (Sandimmune) may result in increased cyclosporine levels and toxicity.
    • digoxin may result in increased blood levels of digoxin.
    • phenytoin (Dilantin) may result in increased phenytoin levels.
    • terfenadine may result in heart (cardiac) toxicity.
    • theophylline (Theo-Dur, Theolair, etc.); monitor blood levels of theophylline if appropriate.
    • warfarin (Coumadin); monitor prothrombin times if appropriate.
    The following drugs may *decrease* the effects of azithromycin
    • antacids containing aluminum or magnesium.
    Azithromycin *taken concurrently* with
    • astemizole (and perhaps other non-sedating antihistamines) may lead to severe adverse heart (cardiac) effects.
▷ *Driving, Hazardous Activities:* May cause dizziness, nausea and/or diarrhea. Restrict activities as needed.
  Aviation Note: The use of this drug ***may be a disqualification*** for piloting. Consult a designated Aviation Medical Examiner.
  Exposure to Sun: Use caution. This drug can cause photosensitivity (see Glossary).

BACAMPICILLIN (bak am pi SIL in)

Introduced: 1979 **Prescription:** USA: Yes; Canada: Yes **Available as Generic:** No **Class:** Antibiotic, penicillins **Controlled Drug:** USA: No; Canada: No

Brand Names: ◆Penglobe, Spectrobid

BENEFITS versus RISKS	
Possible Benefits	*Possible Risks*
EFFECTIVE TREATMENT OF INFECTIONS due to susceptible microorganisms	ALLERGIC REACTIONS, mild to severe, in 3% of the general population and 15% of allergic individuals
	Superinfections (yeast)
	Drug-induced colitis

▷ **Principal Uses**

As a Single Drug Product: To treat some infections of the skin and skin structures, the upper and lower respiratory tract, and the genitourinary tract, including gonorrhea.

How This Drug Works: When it is absorbed from the gastrointestinal tract, bacampicillin is changed to ampicillin. When given in equivalent doses, bacampicillin provides peak blood levels that are 3 times higher than provided by ampicillin. This lets bacampicillin be effective when given every 12 hours; while ampicillin requires a dosing every 6 hours. (See ampicillin Drug Profile.)

Available Dosage Forms and Strengths

Oral suspension — 125 mg per 5-ml teaspoonful

Tablets — 400 mg

▷ **Usual Adult Dosage Range:** 400 to 800 mg/12 hours. **Note: Actual dosage and administration schedule must be determined by the physician for each patient individually.**

Conditions Requiring Dosing Adjustments

Liver function: Caution is advised with use in moderate to severe liver compromise.

Kidney function: The dose must be decreased to 400 mg per day in moderate kidney failure. In severe kidney failure a dose of 400 mg every 36 hours is used.

▷ **Dosing Instructions:** Tablets may be taken without regard to eating. Oral suspensions should be taken on an empty stomach, 1 hour before or 2 hours after eating. The tablet may be crushed to take it.

Usual Duration of Use: Use on a regular schedule for 5 to 7 days is usually needed to see the effectiveness in eliminating the infection. Therapy is usually continued for 2 to 3 days after all indications of infection are gone. All streptococcal infections should be treated for at least 10 consecutive days (without interruption) to reduce risk of rheumatic fever or glomerulonephritis.

▷ **While Taking This Drug, Observe the Following**

▷ *Other Drugs*

Bacampicillin *taken concurrently* with

- allopurinol (Zyloprim) substantially increases skin rash occurence.
- disulfiram (Antabuse) can cause a disulfiramlike reaction (see Glossary). Avoid the combination of these 2 drugs.
- birth control pills (oral contraceptives) may result in loss of contraceptive effectiveness and pregnancy.

The following drugs may *decrease* the effects of bacampicillin
- chloramphenicol (Chloromycetin).
- erythromycins (E-Mycin, Erythrocin, etc.).
- sulfonamides ("Sulfa" drugs, see Drug Classes).
- tetracyclines (see Drug Class).

Note: The information categories provided in this Profile are appropriate for bacampicillin. For specific information that is normally found in those categories that have been omitted from this Profile, see the Drug Profile of ampicillin.

BECLOMETHASONE (be kloh METH a sohn)

Introduced: 1976 **Prescription:** USA: Yes; Canada: Yes **Available as Generic:** No **Class:** Antiallergic, antiasthmatic, cortisonelike drugs
Controlled Drug: USA: No; Canada: No

Brand Names: ✦Beclodisk, Becloforte, Beclovent, ✦Beclovent Rotacaps, ✦Beclovent Rotahaler, Beconase AQ Nasal Spray, Beconase Nasal Inhaler, ✦Propaderm, ✦Propaderm-C, Vancenase AQ Nasal Spray, Vancenase Nasal Inhaler, Vanceril

BENEFITS versus RISKS	
Possible Benefits	*Possible Risks*
EFFECTIVE RELIEF OF ALLERGIC RHINITIS	FUNGUS INFECTIONS OF THE MOUTH AND THROAT
EFFECTIVE CONTROL OF SEVERE, CHRONIC ASTHMA	Localized areas of "allergic" pneumonia
	Changes in nasal mucosa

▷ **Principal Uses**

As a Single Drug Product: Uses currently included in FDA approved labeling: (1) Used to treat bronchial asthma in people who do not respond to bronchodilators and who need cortisonelike drugs for asthma control. This inhalation dosage form is much more advantageous than cortisone taken by mouth (swallowed) or by injection in that it works directly on the respiratory tract and does not require absorption and systemic distribution. This prevents the more serious adverse effects of long-term use of systemic cortisone; (2) prevention of nasal polyps once they have been surgically removed; (3) treats seasonal and perennial rhinitis in children and adults.

Other (unlabeled) generally accepted uses: None.

How This Drug Works: By increasing the amount of cyclic AMP, this drug may increase epinephrine, which opens the bronchial tubes and fights asthma. The drug can also reduce local inflammation in the lining of the respiratory tract.

Beclomethasone

Available Dosage Forms and Strengths
  Nasal inhaler — 16.8 grams (200 doses of 42 mcg each)
  Nasal spray — 0.042%
  Oral inhaler — 16.8 grams (200 doses of 42 mcg each)

▷ **Usual Adult Dosage Range:** Nasal inhaler—1 inhalation (42 mcg) 2 to 4 times daily. Oral inhaler—2 inhalations (84 mcg) 3 or 4 times daily. For severe asthma—12 to 16 inhalations daily. The maximal daily dose should not exceed 20 inhalations. **Note: Actual dosage and administration schedule must be determined by the physician for each patient individually.**

Conditions Requiring Dosing Adjustments
  Liver function: Use with caution in patients with liver compromise.
  Kidney function: No adjustments in dosing expected to be needed.

▷ **Dosing Instructions:** May be used without regard to eating. Rinse the mouth and throat (gargle) with water thoroughly after each inhalation.

Usual Duration of Use: Use on a regular schedule for 1 to 4 weeks is usually needed to see this drug's effectiveness in relieving severe, chronic allergic rhinitis and in controlling severe, chronic asthma. Long-term use must be physician supervised. See your doctor on a regular basis.

▷ **This Drug Should Not Be Taken If**
- you have had an allergic reaction to any of the brand names listed above.
- you are experiencing severe acute asthma or status asthmaticus that requires more intense treatment for prompt relief.
- your asthma can be controlled by other antiasthmatic drugs that are not related to cortisone.
- your asthma requires cortisonelike drugs infrequently for control.
- you have a form of nonallergic bronchitis with asthmatic features.

▷ **Inform Your Physician Before Taking This Drug If**
- you are now taking or have recently taken any cortisone-related drug (including ACTH by injection) for any reason (see Drug Class, Section Four).
- you have a history of tuberculosis of the lungs.
- you have chronic bronchitis or bronchiectasis.
- you think you have an active infection of any kind, especially a respiratory infection.
- you have recently been exposed to chicken pox.
- you are prone to nose bleeds (epistaxis).
- you are unsure of how much or how often to take beclomethasone.

Possible Side-Effects (natural, expected and unavoidable drug actions)
  Fungus infections (thrush) of the mouth and throat.

▷ **Possible Adverse Effects** (unusual, unexpected and infrequent reactions)
  If any of the following develop, consult your physician promptly for guidance.
  Mild Adverse Effects
  Allergic Reaction: Skin rash (rare).
  Dryness of mouth, hoarseness, sore throat.
  Nose bleeds (epistaxis).
  Serious Adverse Effects
  Allergic Reaction: Localized areas of "allergic" pneumonitis (lung inflammation).

Bronchospasm, asthmatic wheezing (rare).
Yeast infections (up to 41%).

▷ **Possible Effects on Sexual Function:** None reported.

Natural Diseases or Disorders That May Be Activated by This Drug
Cortisone-related drugs having systemic effects impair immunity and lead to reactivation of "healed" or dormant tuberculosis. People with a history of tuberculosis must be watched closely while using this drug.

Possible Effects on Laboratory Tests
Blood cortisol levels: decreased.

CAUTION
1. This drug should not be relied upon for immediate relief of acute asthma.
2. If you were using cortisone-related drugs for your asthma *before* starting this inhaler, it may be necessary to resume the former cortisone-related drug if you experience injury or infection of any kind, or if you require surgery. Tell your doctor of your prior use of cortisone-related drugs taken either by mouth or by injection.
3. If severe asthma returns while using this drug, notify your doctor immediately so that supportive treatment with cortisone-related drugs by mouth or injection can be provided as needed.
4. Carry a personal identification card with a notation (if applicable) that you have used cortisone-related drugs within the past year. During periods of stress it may be necessary to resume cortisone treatment.
5. Wait 5 to 10 minutes after using a bronchodilator inhaler like epinephrine, isoetharine, or isoproterenol (which should be used first) and inhalation of this drug. This will permit greater penetration of beclomethasone into the bronchial tubes. The delay between inhalations will also reduce the possibility of adverse propellant effects.
6. This drug does NOT replace systemic steroids.

Precautions for Use
By Infants and Children: Safety and effectiveness for use of the nasal inhaler by those under 12 years of age have not been established. Safety and effectiveness for use of the oral inhaler by those under 6 years of age have not been established. The maximal daily dose in children 6 to 12 years of age should not exceed 10 inhalations.

By Those over 60 Years of Age: People with bronchiectasis should be watched closely for the development of lung infections.

▷ **Advisability of Use During Pregnancy**
Pregnancy Category: C. See Pregnancy Code at the back of this book.
Animal studies: Mouse, rat and rabbit studies reveal significant birth defects due to this drug.
Human studies: Adequate studies of pregnant women are not available.
Avoid drug during the first 3 months. Use infrequently and only as clearly needed during the last 6 months.

Advisability of Use if Breast-Feeding
Presence of this drug in breast milk: Probably yes.
Avoid drug or refrain from nursing.

Habit-Forming Potential: With recommended dosage, a state of functional dependence (see Glossary) is not likely to develop.

Effects of Overdosage: Indications of cortisone excess (due to systemic absorption)—fluid retention, flushing of the face, stomach irritation, nervousness.

Suggested Periodic Examinations While Taking This Drug (at physician's discretion)
Inspection of nose, mouth and throat for evidence of fungus infection.
Assessment of adrenal function status in people who have used cortisone-related drugs over an extended period of time prior to using this drug.
Lung X-ray of people with a prior history of tuberculosis.

▷ **While Taking This Drug, Observe the Following**
Foods: No specific restrictions beyond those advised by your physician.
Beverages: No specific restrictions.
▷ *Alcohol:* No interactions expected.
Tobacco Smoking: No interactions expected. However, smoking can reduce the effectiveness of this drug. Follow your physician's advice.
▷ *Other Drugs*
The following drugs may *increase* the effects of beclomethasone
- inhalant bronchodilators—epinephrine, isoetharine, isoproterenol.
- oral bronchodilators—aminophylline, ephedrine, terbutaline, theophylline, etc.

▷ *Driving, Hazardous Activities:* No restrictions.
Aviation Note: The use of this drug and the disorder for which this drug is prescribed *may be disqualifications* for piloting. Consult a designated Aviation Medical Examiner.
Exposure to Sun: No restrictions.
Occurrence of Unrelated Illness: Acute infections, serious injuries, and surgical procedures can create an urgent need for additional supportive cortisone-related drugs given by mouth and/or injection. Notify your physician immediately in the event of new illness or injury of any kind.
Discontinuation: If the regular use of this drug has made it possible to reduce or discontinue maintenance doses of cortisonelike drugs by mouth, *do not* stop this drug abruptly. If you must stop this drug, call your doctor. It may be necessary to resume cortisone preparations and to institute other measures for satisfactory management.
Special Storage Instructions
Store at room temperature. Avoid exposure to temperatures above 120 degrees F (49 degrees C). Do not store or use this inhaler near heat or open flame. Protect from light.

BENAZEPRIL (ben AY ze pril)

Introduced: 1985 **Prescription:** USA: Yes **Available as Generic:** No **Class:** Antihypertensive, ACE inhibitor **Controlled Drug:** USA: No
Brand Name: Lotensin

BENEFITS versus RISKS	
Possible Benefits	*Possible Risks*
EFFECTIVE CONTROL OF MILD TO MODERATE HIGH BLOOD PRESSURE	Headache (6.2%), dizziness (3.6%), fatigue (2.4%) Low blood pressure (0.3%) Allergic swelling of face, tongue, throat, vocal cords (0.5%) Rare decreased hemoglobin

▷ **Principal Uses**
  As a Single Drug Product: Uses currently included in FDA approved labeling: Treatment of mild to moderate high blood pressure, alone or in combination with a thiazide diuretic.
  Other (unlabeled) generally accepted uses: (1) Helps relieve symptoms of congestive heart failure.

How This Drug Works: It is thought that by blocking certain enzyme systems (angiotensin-converting enzyme, ACE) that effect arteries, benazepril helps relax arterial walls throughout the body and lowers the blood pressure. This, in turn, reduces the workload of the heart and improves its performance.

Available Dosage Forms and Strengths
  Tablets — 5 mg, 10 mg, 20 mg, 40 mg

▷ **Recommended Dosage Ranges** (Actual dosage and administration schedule must be determined by the physician for each patient individually.)
  Infants and Children: Dosage not established.
  12 to 60 Years of Age: Initially 10 mg once daily for those not taking a diuretic; 5 mg once daily for those taking a diuretic. Usual maintenance dose is 20 to 40 mg/day taken in a single dose. If once-a-day dosing does not give stable control of blood pressure over a 24 hour period, divide the dose equally into morning and evening doses. The total daily dosage should not exceed 80 mg.
  Over 60 Years of Age: Same as 12 to 60 years of age, if kidney function is normal. If kidney function is significantly impaired, reduce dose by 50%. The total daily dose should not exceed 40 mg.

Conditions Requiring Dosing Adjustments
  Liver function: Dosage adjustment in cirrhosis is not currently considered necessary.
  Kidney function: Some of this medicine is removed by the kidneys. People with creatinine clearances of less than 30 ml/min, or serum creatinine concentrations of greater than 3 mg/dl, the initial dose should be 5 mg once daily.

▷ **Dosing Instructions:** Take on an empty stomach or with food, at same time each day. The tablet may be crushed for administration.

Usual Duration of Use: Use on a regular schedule for 2 to 3 weeks is usually needed to see this drug's peak effect in controlling high blood pressure. Therapy may be long-term. See your physician on a regular basis.

Benazepril

Possible Advantages of This Drug
   Usually controls blood pressure effectively with one daily dose.
   Relatively low incidence of adverse effects.
   No adverse influence on asthma, cholesterol blood levels or diabetes.
   Sudden withdrawal does not result in a rapid increase in blood pressure.

▷ **This Drug Should Not Be Taken If**
   - you have had an allergic reaction to it previously.
   - you are pregnant (last 6 months).
   - you currently have a blood cell or bone marrow disorder.
   - you have an abnormally high level of blood potassium.

▷ **Inform Your Physician Before Taking This Drug If**
   - you have had an allergic reaction to other ACE inhibitor drugs (see Drug Class, Section Four).
   - you are planning pregnancy.
   - you have a history of kidney disease or impaired kidney function.
   - you have scleroderma or systemic lupus erythematosus.
   - you have cerebral artery disease.
   - you have any form of heart disease.
   - you are taking: other antihypertensives, diuretics, nitrates or potassium supplements.
   - you plan to have surgery under general anesthesia in the near future.
   - you are unsure of how much benazepril to take or how often to take it.
   - you have renal artery stenosis (ask your doctor).
   - you have liver disease.
   - you have any history of autoimmune disease.

Possible Side-Effects (natural, expected and unavoidable drug actions)
   Dizziness (3.6%), orthostatic hypotension (0.4%) (see Glossary), fainting (0.1%), increased blood potassium level (1%).

▷ **Possible Adverse Effects** (unusual, unexpected and infrequent reactions)
   If any of the following develop, consult your physician promptly for guidance.
   Mild Adverse Effects
   Allergic Reactions: Skin rash, itching (less than 1%).
   Headache (6.2%), fatigue (2.4%), drowsiness (1.6%), numbness and tingling (less than 1%), weakness (less than 1%).
   Cough (up to 39%), chest pain, palpitation (less than 1.0%).
   Indigestion, nausea (1.3%), vomiting, constipation (less than 1%).
   Back pain (2%).
   Serious Adverse Effects
   Allergic Reactions: Swelling (angioedema) of face, tongue and/or vocal chords (0.5%); can be life-threatening.
   Impairment of kidney function (2.0%).
   Decreased hemoglobin (rare).
   Angina and palpitations.
   First dose low blood pressure.
   Elevated blod potassium.
   Psoriasis (rare).

▷ **Possible Effects on Sexual Function:** Decreased libido, impotence (less than 1%).

Possible Effects on Laboratory Tests
  Blood potassium level: increased.
  Kidney function tests: blood urea nitrogen (BUN) and creatinine increased.

CAUTION
  1. Ask your doctor if you should stop other antihypertensive drugs (especially diuretics) for 1 week before starting this drug.
  2. **Inform your physician immediately if you become pregnant.** This drug should not be taken beyond the first 3 months of pregnancy.
  3. **Report promptly** any signs of infection (fever, sore throat), and any weight gain, puffiness, swollen feet or ankles.
  4. Do not use a salt substitute without your physician's knowledge and approval. (Many salt substitutes contain potassium.)
  5. It is advisable to obtain blood cell counts and urine analyses **before** starting this drug.

Precautions for Use
  By Infants and Children: Safety and effectiveness for use by those in this age group not established.
  By Those over 60 Years of Age: Small starting doses are advisable. Sudden or excessive lowering of blood pressure can cause stroke or heart attack in people with impaired brain circulation or coronary artery heart disease.

▷ **Advisability of Use During Pregnancy**
  Pregnancy Category: D. See Pregnancy Code at the back of this book.
  Animal studies: No birth defects found in mouse, rat or rabbit studies.
  Human studies: The use of ACE inhibitor drugs during the last 6 months of pregnancy is known to possibly cause very serious injury and possible death to the fetus; skull and limb malformations, lung defects, and kidney failure have been reported in over 50 cases worldwide.
  Avoid this drug completely during the last 6 months. During the first 3 months of pregnancy, use this drug only if clearly needed. Ask your physician for guidance.

Advisability of Use if Breast-Feeding
  Presence of this drug in breast milk: Yes, in small amounts.
  Ask your doctor for guidance.

Habit-Forming Potential: None.

Effects of Overdosage: Excessive drop in blood pressure, light-headedness, dizziness, fainting.

Possible Effects of Long-Term Use: Gradual increase in blood potassium level.

Suggested Periodic Examinations While Taking This Drug (at physician's discretion)
  Before starting drug: Complete blood cell counts; urine analysis with measurement of protein content; blood potassium level.
  During use of drug: Blood cell counts; measurements of blood potassium.

▷ **While Taking This Drug, Observe the Following**
  Foods: Consult physician regarding salt intake.
  Nutritional Support: **Do not take** potassium supplements unless directed by your physician.
  Beverages: No restrictions. May be taken with milk.

▷ *Alcohol:* Use caution. Alcohol may enhance the blood-pressure-lowering effect of this drug.
Tobacco Smoking: No interactions expected.
▷ *Other Drugs*
Benazepril *taken concurrently* with
- aspirin may decrease the benefit of benazepril on heart function.
- bumetanide or furosemide may cause severe lowering of blood pressure if patients suddenly stand.
- cyclosporine (Sandimune) may cause increased kidney toxicity.
- lithium may triple blood levels of lithium and result in lithium toxicity.
- phenothiazines (see Drug CLasses) may cause sudden lowering of the blood pressure to undesirable levels.
- potassium preparations (K-Lyte, Slow-K, etc.) may cause increased blood levels of potassium with risk of serious heart rhythm disturbances.
- potassium-sparing diuretics: amiloride (Moduretic), spironolactone (Aldactazide), triamterene (Dyazide) may cause increased blood levels of potassium with risk of serious heart rhythm disturbances.

▷ *Driving, Hazardous Activities:* Be aware of possible drops in blood pressure with resultant dizziness or faintness.
Aviation Note: The use of this drug **may be a disqualification** for piloting. Consult a designated Aviation Medical Examiner.
Exposure to Sun: Caution advised. A similar drug of this class can cause photosensitivity.
Exposure to Heat: Caution advised. Excessive perspiring with resultant loss of body water may drop blood pressure.
Occurrence of Unrelated Illness: Promptly report vomiting or diarrhea. Fluid and chemical imbalances must be corrected as soon as possible.
Discontinuation: Consult your physician regarding withdrawal of this drug for any reason.

BENZTROPINE (BENZ troh peen)

Introduced: 1954 **Prescription:** USA: Yes; Canada: No **Available as Generic:** USA: Yes; Canada: Yes **Class:** Antiparkinsonism, atropinelike drugs **Controlled Drug:** USA: No; Canada: No
Brand Names: ◆Apo-Benztropine, ◆Bensylate, Cogentin, ◆PMS Benztropine

BENEFITS versus RISKS	
Possible Benefits	*Possible Risks*
PARTIAL RELIEF OF SYMPTOMS OF PARKINSON'S DISEASE	Atropinelike side-effects: blurred vision, dry mouth, constipation, impaired urination
	Rare toxic psychosis
	Rare movement problems (tardive dyskenesia)

▷ **Principal Uses**
As a Single Drug Product: Uses currently included in FDA approved labeling: (1) Used in combination with other therapy in of all types of parkinsonism

Benztropine

to relieve the characteristic rigidity, tremor and sluggish movement. If relief is inadequate, it may be supplemented with more potent drugs such as levodopa and bromocriptine; (2) also used to control parkinsonian reactions that can result from some antipsychotic drugs, such as phenothiazines and related medicines.

Other (unlabeled) generally accepted uses: (1) Combined with psychotherapy, this drug can help excessively sweaty palms; (2) can help drooling in developmentally disabled patients; (3) can relieve painful erections (priapism).

How This Drug Works: It decreases the symptoms of parkinsonism by restoring a more normal balance of chemicals responsible for nerve impulses in the brain (basal ganglia).

Available Dosage Forms and Strengths
Injection — 1 mg per ml
Tablets — 0.5 mg, 1 mg, 2 mg

▷ **Usual Adult Dosage Range:** For Parkinson's disease—0.5 to 2 mg daily, taken in a single dose at bedtime. For drug-induced parkinsonian reactions—1 to 4 mg daily, either in a single dose or in 2 to 3 divided doses. The total daily dose should not exceed 6 mg. **Note: Actual dosage and administration schedule must be determined by the physician for each patient individually.**

Conditions Requiring Dosing Adjustments
Liver function: Use with caution in patients with impaired liver function.
Kidney function: Caution. Decreased kidney function may lead to an increased blood level and an increased risk of adverse effects.

▷ **Dosing Instructions:** May be taken with or following food to reduce stomach irritation. Tablet may be crushed for administration.

Usual Duration of Use: Use on a regular schedule for 2 to 4 weeks is usually necessary to see this drug's peak benefit in relieving symptoms of parkinsonism and to determine the best dosage schedule. Long-term use (months to years) requires physician supervision. See your doctor regularly.

▷ **This Drug Should Not Be Taken If**
- you have had an allergic reaction to any dosage form of it previously.
- it is prescribed for a child under 3 years of age.
- you have tardive dyskenesia.
- you have narrow angle glaucoma.

▷ **Inform Your Physician Before Taking This Drug If**
- you have had an unfavorable reaction to atropine or atropinelike drugs.
- you have glaucoma or myasthenia gravis.
- you have heart disease or high blood pressure.
- you have a history of liver or kidney disease.
- you have difficulty emptying the urinary bladder, especially if due to an enlarged prostate gland.
- you are taking, or have taken within the past 2 weeks, any monoamine oxidase (MAO) type A inhibitor drug (see Drug Class, Section Four).
- you take other prescription or non-prescription medications which were not discussed when benztropine was prescribed for you.

- you are unsure of how much benztropine to take or how often to take it.
- you will be exposed to extreme heat for extended periods such as some iron smelters or travelers to tropical climates.
- you have a history of bowel obstructions.

Possible Side-Effects (natural, expected and unavoidable drug actions)
Nervousness, blurring of vision, dryness of mouth, constipation, impaired urination. (These often subside as drug use continues.)

▷ **Possible Adverse Effects** (unusual, unexpected and infrequent reactions)
If any of the following develop, consult your physician promptly for guidance.

Mild Adverse Effects
Allergic Reaction: Skin rashes.
Headache, dizziness, drowsiness, muscle cramps.
Indigestion, nausea, vomiting.
Memory problems.

Serious Adverse Effects
Idiosyncratic Reactions: Abnormal behavior, confusion, delusions, hallucinations, agitation.
Tardive dyskinesia (rare).
Dystonia (rare).
Bowel obstruction (rare).
Abnormal elevations of temperature (hyperthermia)

▷ **Possible Effects on Sexual Function**
Reversal of male impotence due to the use of fluphenazine (a phenothiazine antipsychotic drug).
Male infertility (0.5 to 6 mg/day).
May help treat priapism.

Natural Diseases or Disorders That May Be Activated by This Drug
Latent glaucoma, latent myasthenia gravis.

Possible Effects on Laboratory Tests
None reported.

CAUTION
1. Many over-the-counter (OTC) medications for allergies, colds and coughs contain drugs that should NOT be combined with benztropine. Ask your physician or pharmacist for help.
2. This drug may aggravate tardive dyskinesia (see Glossary). Ask physician for guidance.

Precautions for Use
By Infants and Children: Safety and effectiveness for those under 3 years of age not established. Children are especially susceptible to the atropinelike effects.
By Those over 60 Years of Age: Small starting doses are advisable. Increased susceptibility to impaired thinking, confusion, nightmares, hallucinations, increased internal eye pressure (glaucoma) and impaired urination associated with prostate gland enlargement (prostatism).

▷ **Advisability of Use During Pregnancy**
Pregnancy Category: C. See Pregnancy Code at the back of this book.
Animal studies: No data available.

Human studies: Adequate studies of pregnant women are not available. Avoid use if possible, especially close to delivery. This drug can impair the infant's intestinal tract following birth.

Advisability of Use if Breast-Feeding
Presence of this drug in breast milk: Unknown.
Ask your doctor for guidance.

Habit-Forming Potential: None with recommended doses. At higher doses it may cause euphoria and hallucinations, creating a potential for abuse.

Effects of Overdosage: Weakness; drowsiness; stupor; impaired vision; rapid pulse; excitement; confusion; hallucinations; dry, hot skin; skin rash; dilated pupils.

Possible Effects of Long-Term Use: Increased internal eye pressure—possible glaucoma, especially in the elderly.

Suggested Periodic Examinations While Taking This Drug (at physician's discretion)
Measurement of internal eye pressure at regular intervals.

▷ **While Taking This Drug, Observe the Following**
Foods: No restrictions.
Beverages: No restrictions.
▷ *Alcohol:* Use caution. Alcohol may increase the sedative effects of this drug.
Tobacco Smoking: No interactions expected.
▷ *Other Drugs*
Benztropine may *decrease* the effects of
- haloperidol (Haldol), and reduce its effectiveness.
- phenothiazines (Thorazine, etc.), and reduce their effectiveness.

The following drugs may *increase* the effects of benztropine
- antihistamines may add to the dryness of mouth and throat.
- tricyclic antidepressants (Elavil, etc.) may add to eye effects and further increase internal eye pressure (dangerous in glaucoma).
- monoamine oxidase (MAO) type A inhibitor drugs may intensify all effects of this drug (see Drug Class, Section Four).

Benztropine *taken concurrently* with
- amantadine (Symmetrel) may cause increased confusion and possible hallucinations.

▷ *Driving, Hazardous Activities:* Drowsiness and dizziness may occur in sensitive individuals. Avoid hazardous activities until full effects and tolerance have been determined.
Aviation Note: The use of this drug *is a disqualification* for piloting. Consult a designated Aviation Medical Examiner.
Exposure to Sun: No restrictions.
Exposure to Heat: Use caution. This drug may reduce sweating, cause an increase in body temperature, and increase risk of heat stroke.
Heavy Exercise or Exertion: Use caution. Avoid in hot environments.
Discontinuation: Do not stop this drug abruptly. Ask your doctor how to reduce the dose gradually.

BETAXOLOL (be TAX oh lohl)

Introduced: 1983   **Prescription:** USA: Yes   **Available as Generic:** No   **Class:** Antihypertensive, beta-adrenergic blocker   **Controlled Drug:** USA: No

Brand Names: Betoptic, Betoptic-S, Kerlone

BENEFITS versus RISKS	
Possible Benefits	*Possible Risks*
EFFECTIVE, WELL-TOLERATED ANTIHYPERTENSIVE in mild to moderate high blood pressure EFFECTIVE TREATMENT OF CHRONIC, OPEN-ANGLE GLAUCOMA Treatment of ocular hypertension	CONGESTIVE HEART FAILURE in advanced heart disease Worsening of angina in coronary heart disease (abrupt withdrawal) Masking of low blood sugar (hypoglycemia) in drug-treated diabetes Provocation of bronchial asthma (with high doses) Rare anemia and low blood platelets

▷ **Principal Uses**

As a Single Drug Product: Uses currently included in FDA approved labeling: Used to treat: (1) mild to moderately severe high blood pressure; (2) chronic open-angle glaucoma (eye drops). May be used alone or combined with other antihypertensive drugs, such as diuretics; (3) ocular hypertension.

Other (unlabeled) generally accepted uses: (1) The oral form may help decrease mortality by reducing damage from a heart attack and making abnormal heart beats less likely; (2) helps decrease the occurrence and severity of chest pain (angina); (3) can be of help in easing aggressive behavior in selected psychiatric patients; (4) may help panic attacks; (5) can treat selected cases of stuttering.

How This Drug Works: By blocking certain actions of the sympathetic nervous system, this drug
- reduces the rate and contraction force of the heart, thus lowering the ejection pressure of the blood and reducing the oxygen needed by the heart to work.
- relaxes contracted blood vessel walls, resulting in expansion and consequent lowering of blood pressure.
- reduces the internal pressure of the eye.

Available Dosage Forms and Strengths
Eye drops — 2.8 mg/ml
— 5.6 mg/ml
Tablets — 10 mg, 20 mg

▷ **Usual Adult Dosage Range:** Initially 10 mg once daily. Dose may be increased gradually at intervals of 7 to 14 days as needed and tolerated up to 20 mg/24 hours. The usual maintenance dose is 10 to 15 mg/24 hours. The total dose should not exceed 20 mg/24 hours.

For use in glaucoma: One or two drops of the 2.8 mg/ml solution or one drop of the 5.6 mg/ml. **Note: Actual dosage and administration schedule must be determined by the physician for each patient individually.**

Conditions Requiring Dosing Adjustments
Liver function: Use with caution, this drug is metabolized in the liver.
Kidney function: Up to 12% of a dose is removed by the kidney. Reduced doses are needed in severe kidney (renal) compromise.

▷ **Dosing Instructions:** May be taken without regard to eating. The tablet may be crushed for administration. Do not stop this drug abruptly.

Usual Duration of Use: Use on a regular schedule for 10 to 14 days is usually needed to see this drug's effectiveness in lowering blood pressure. Long-term use will be determined by the success in lowering your blood pressure over time and your response to an overall treatment program of weight reduction, salt restriction, smoking cessation, etc. See your doctor regularly.

Possible Advantages of This Drug: Usually effective and well tolerated with a single dose daily.

▷ **This Drug Should Not Be Taken If**
- you have had an allergic reaction to it previously.
- you have congestive heart failure.
- you have an abnormally slow heart rate or a serious heart block.
- you are taking, or have taken within the past 14 days, any monoamine oxidase (MAO) type A inhibitor drug (see Drug Class, Section Four).

▷ **Inform Your Physician Before Taking This Drug If**
- you have had an adverse reaction to any beta blocker drug (see Drug Class, Section Four).
- you have a history of serious heart disease or episodes of heart failure.
- you have a history of hay fever (allergic rhinitis), asthma, chronic bronchitis or emphysema. Some drugs in this class are contraindicated in asthmatics.
- you have a history of overactive thyroid function (hyperthyroidism).
- you have a history of low blood sugar (hypoglycemia).
- you have impaired liver or kidney function.
- you have diabetes or myasthenia gravis.
- you currently take: digitalis, quinidine or reserpine, or any calcium blocker drug (see Drug Class, Section Four).
- you plan to have surgery under general anesthesia in the near future.
- you take other prescription or non-prescription medications which were not discussed when betaxolol was prescribed for you.
- you are unsure of how much betaxolol to take or how often to take it.

Possible Side-Effects (natural, expected and unavoidable drug actions)
Lethargy (2.8%), fatigue (up to 10%), cold extremities (1.9%), slow heart rate (8.1%), light-headedness in upright position (see Orthostatic Hypotension in Glossary).

▷ **Possible Adverse Effects** (unusual, unexpected and infrequent reactions)
If any of the following develop, consult your physician promptly for guidance.
Mild Adverse Effects
Allergic Reactions: Skin rash (1.2%), itching.

Headache (up to 15%), dizziness (4.5%), drowsiness, insomnia (1.2%), abnormal dreams (1.0%).
Indigestion (4.7%), nausea (1.6%), diarrhea (2.0%).
Joint and muscle discomfort (3.1%), fluid retention (edema) (1.8%).
Difficulty breathing (< 2%).

Serious Adverse Effects
Mental depression (0.8%), anxiety (0.8%).
Chest pain (2.4%), shortness of breath (2.4%), congestive heart failure.
Induction of bronchial asthma (in asthmatic individuals).
Low blood platelets and anemia (< 2%).
Congestive heart failure (< 2%).
Angina (if drug abruptly stopped).
Very rare myocardial infarction.

▷ **Possible Effects on Sexual Function:** Decreased libido, impotence (1.2%). Altered menstrual patterns.

▷ **Adverse Effects That May Mimic Natural Diseases or Disorders**
Reduced blood flow to extremities may mimic Raynaud's disease (see Glossary).

Possible Effects on Laboratory Tests
Glaucoma-screening test (measurement of internal eye pressure): pressure is decreased (false low or normal value).
Antinuclear antibodies (ANA) test: positive in 5.3% of users.
Blood platelet counts and hemoglobin: decreased (rarely).

CAUTION
1. ***Do not stop this drug suddenly*** without the knowledge of your doctor. Always carry a note with you that says you are taking this drug.
2. Ask your physician or pharmacist before using nasal decongestants. These can cause sudden increases in blood pressure when combined with beta blocker drugs.
3. Report the development of any tendency to emotional depression.

Precautions for Use
By Infants and Children: Safety and effectiveness for those under 12 years of age not established. However, if this drug is used, watch for the development of low blood sugar (hypoglycemia), especially if a meal is missed.
By Those over 60 Years of Age: Caution: High blood pressure should be slowly reduced, avoiding the risks associated with excessively low blood pressure. Treatment should be started with 5 mg daily and blood pressure checked often. Sudden, rapid and excessive reduction of blood pressure can cause stroke or heart attack. Total daily dosage should not exceed 10 to 15 mg. Watch for dizziness, unsteadiness, tendency to fall, confusion, hallucinations, depression or urinary frequency. This age group is more prone to develop excessively slow heart rates and hypothermia.

▷ **Advisability of Use During Pregnancy**
Pregnancy Category: C. See Pregnancy Code at the back of this book.
Animal studies: Rat studies reveal increased resorptions of embryo and fetus, retarded growth and development of newborn and mild skeletal defects.
Human studies: Adequate studies of pregnant women are not available.

Avoid use of drug during the first 3 months if possible. Avoid use during labor and delivery because of the possible effects on the newborn infant.

Advisability of Use if Breast-Feeding
Presence of this drug in breast milk: Yes.
Avoid drug if possible. If drug is necessary, observe nursing infant for slow heart rate and indications of low blood sugar.

Habit-Forming Potential: None.

Effects of Overdosage: Weakness, slow pulse, low blood pressure, fainting, cold and sweaty skin, congestive heart failure, possible coma and convulsions.

Possible Effects of Long-Term Use: Reduced heart reserve and eventual heart failure in susceptible individuals with advanced heart disease.

Suggested Periodic Examinations While Taking This Drug (at physician's discretion)
Measurements of blood pressure, evaluation of heart function.

▷ **While Taking This Drug, Observe the Following**
Foods: No restrictions. Avoid excessive salt intake.
Beverages: No restrictions. May be taken with milk.

▷ *Alcohol:* Use with caution. Alcohol may exaggerate this drug's ability to lower blood pressure and may increase its mild sedative effect.
Tobacco Smoking: Nicotine may reduce this drug's effectiveness in treating high blood pressure. In addition, high drug doses worsen the constriction of bronchial tubes caused by regular smoking.

▷ *Other Drugs*
Betaxolol may *increase* the effects of
- other antihypertensive drugs and cause excessive lowering of blood pressure. Dosage decreases may be necessary.
- reserpine (Ser-Ap-Es, etc.) and cause sedation, depression, slowing of heart rate and lowering of blood pressure (light-headedness, fainting).

Betaxolol *taken concurrently* with
- clonidine (Catapres) requires close monitoring for rebound high blood pressure if clonidine is stopped while betaxolol is still taken.
- insulin requires close following to avoid hypoglycemia (see Glossary).
- oral hypoglycemic drugs (see Drug Classes) may prolong recovery from low blood sugars.
- calcium channel blockers may cause severe lowering of blood pressure.
- phenothiazines (see Drug Classes) may result in additive blood pressure lowering effects.

The following drugs may *decrease* the effects of betaxolol
- indomethacin (Indocin), and possibly other "aspirin substitutes," or NSAIDs may impair betaxolol's antihypertensive effect.

▷ *Driving, Hazardous Activities:* Use caution until the full extent of drowsiness, lethargy, and blood pressure change has been determined.
Aviation Note: The use of this drug *is a disqualification* for piloting. Consult a designated Aviation Medical Examiner.
Exposure to Sun: No restrictions.
Exposure to Heat: Caution advised. Hot environments can lower blood pressure and exaggerate the effects of this drug.

Exposure to Cold: Caution advised. Cold environments can enhance the circulatory deficiency in the extremities that may occur with this drug. The elderly should be careful to prevent hypothermia (see Glossary).

Heavy Exercise or Exertion: It is advisable to avoid exertion that produces light-headedness, excessive fatigue, or muscle cramping. The use of this drug may intensify the hypertensive response to isometric exercise.

Occurrence of Unrelated Illness: Fever can lower blood pressure and require adjustment of dosage. Nausea or vomiting may interrupt the dosing schedule. Ask your physician for help.

Discontinuation: Avoid sudden discontinuation of this drug in all situations. If possible, gradual reduction of dose over a period of 2 to 3 weeks is recommended. Ask your physician for specific guidance.

BITOLTEROL (bi TOHL ter ohl)

Introduced: 1985   **Prescription:** Yes   **Available as Generic:** No
Class: Antiasthmatic, bronchodilator   **Controlled Drug:** No
Brand Name: Tornalate

BENEFITS versus RISKS	
Possible Benefits	*Possible Risks*
EFFECTIVE PREVENTION AND RELIEF OF ASTHMA for 5 to 8 hours	Fine hand tremor (14%) Nervousness (5%) Throat irritation (5%) Irregular heart rhythm (with excessive use)

▷ **Principal Uses**

As a Single Drug Product: Uses currently included in FDA approved labeling: (1) To relieve acute bronchial asthma and to reduce the frequency and severity of chronic, recurrent asthmatic attacks; (2) used to prevent asthma triggered by exercise.

Other (unlabeled) generally accepted uses: (1) may be more useful than other agents in helping open the bronchi in patients with chronic obstructive pulmonary disease (COPD).

How This Drug Works: By increasing cyclic AMP, this drug relaxes bronchial muscles and relieves asthmatic wheezing.

Available Dosage Forms and Strengths
Aerosol inhaler — 15 ml (300 inhalations of 0.37 mg each)

▷ **Usual Adult Dosage Range:** For acute bronchospasm—2 inhalations at intervals of 1 to 3 minutes, followed by a third inhalation in 3 to 4 minutes if needed. For prevention of bronchospasm—2 inhalations/8 hours.

For children over 12: same as adult bronchospasm dose. **Note: Actual dosage and administration schedule must be determined by the physician for each patient individually.**

Conditions Requiring Dosing Adjustments
Liver function: Use with caution in severe liver compromise.
Kidney function: Significant kidney removal, however, specific dosage guidelines are unavailable.

▷ **Dosing Instructions:** May be used without regard to eating. Follow the written directions for use carefully. Do not overuse.

Usual Duration of Use: Do not use beyond the time needed to stop episodes of acute asthma. Ask physician for help regarding use in preventing asthma attacks.

▷ **This Drug Should Not Be Taken If**
- you have had an allergic reaction to it previously.
- you currently have an irregular heart rhythm.
- you are taking, or have taken within the past 2 weeks, any monoamine oxidase (MAO) type A inhibitor drug (see Drug Class, Section Four).

▷ **Inform Your Physician Before Taking This Drug If**
- you have any type of heart or circulatory disorder, especially high blood pressure or coronary heart disease.
- you have diabetes, epilepsy or an overactive thyroid gland.
- you are taking any form of digitalis or any stimulant drug.
- you are unsure of how much bitolterol to take or how often to take it.

Possible Side-Effects (natural, expected and unavoidable drug actions)
Dryness or irritation of mouth or throat (5%).

▷ **Possible Adverse Effects** (unusual, unexpected and infrequent reactions)
If any of the following develop, consult your physician promptly for guidance.
Mild Adverse Effects
Headache (4%), dizziness (3%), nervousness (5%), insomnia (less than 1%), fine tremor of hands (14%).
Nausea (3%), indigestion.
Coughing (4%).
Serious Adverse Effects
Excess use can cause irregular heart rate, rhythm or increased blood pressure.
Paradoxical bronchospasm (rare).

▷ **Possible Effects on Sexual Function:** None reported.

Natural Diseases or Disorders That May Be Activated by This Drug
Latent coronary artery disease, diabetes or high blood pressure.

Possible Effects on Laboratory Tests
None reported.

CAUTION
1. Combination use of this drug by inhalation with beclomethasone aerosol (Beclovent, Vanceril) may increase the risk of toxicity due to fluorocarbon propellants. Use bitolterol aerosol 20 to 30 minutes *before* beclomethasone aerosol. This will reduce toxicity risk and enhances penetration of beclomethasone.
2. Excessive or prolonged use of this drug by inhalation can reduce effectiveness and cause serious heart rhythm disturbances.

Precautions for Use
By Infants and Children: Safety and effectiveness for children under 12 years of age not established.

132   Bromocriptine

By Those over 60 Years of Age: Avoid excessive and continual use. If acute asthma is not relieved promptly, other drugs will be needed. Watch for development of nervousness, palpitations, irregular heart rhythm and muscle tremors.

▷ **Advisability of Use During Pregnancy**
Pregnancy Category: C. See Pregnancy Code at the back of this book.
Animal studies: Cleft palate reported in mice.
Human studies: Adequate studies of pregnant women are not available.
Avoid use during first 3 months if possible.

Advisability of Use if Breast-Feeding
Presence of this drug in breast milk: Unknown.
Avoid drug or refrain from nursing.

Habit-Forming Potential: None.

Effects of Overdosage: Nervousness, palpitation, rapid heart rate, sweating, headache, tremor, vomiting, abnormal heart rhythms, chest pain.

Possible Effects of Long-Term Use: Loss of effectiveness.

Suggested Periodic Examinations While Taking This Drug (at physician's discretion)
Blood pressure measurements, evaluation of heart status.

▷ **While Taking This Drug, Observe the Following**
Foods: No restrictions.
Beverages: Avoid excessive caffeine—coffee, tea, cola, chocolate.
▷ *Alcohol:* No interactions expected.
Tobacco Smoking: No interactions expected.
▷ *Other Drugs*
Bitolterol **taken concurrently** with
- monoamine oxidase (MAO) type A inhibitor drugs (see Drug Class, Section Four) may cause large increases in blood pressure and undesirable heart stimulation.

▷ *Driving, Hazardous Activities:* Use caution if excessive nervousness or dizziness occurs.
Aviation Note: The use of this drug **is a disqualification** for piloting. Consult a designated Aviation Medical Examiner.
Exposure to Sun: No restrictions.
Heavy Exercise or Exertion: Use caution. Excessive exercise can induce asthma in some people.

BROMOCRIPTINE (broh moh KRIP teen)

Introduced: 1975   **Prescription:** USA: Yes; Canada: Yes   **Available as Generic:** No   **Class:** Antiparkinsonism, dopamine agonist, ergot derivative
Controlled Drug: USA: No; Canada: No

Brand Name: Parlodel, Normatine

BENEFITS versus RISKS	
Possible Benefits	*Possible Risks*
PARTIAL RELIEF OF SYMPTOMS OF PARKINSON'S DISEASE	ABNORMAL INVOLUNTARY MOVEMENTS AND ALTERED BEHAVIOR IN 20% to 35% of users taking high doses
CORRECTION OF INFERTILITY AND ABSENT MENSTRUATION in women with high prolactin levels	Raynaud's phenomenon (see Glossary) in 30% to 60% of users taking high doses
	Low blood pressure

▷ **Principal Uses**

As a Single Drug Product: Uses currently included in FDA approved labeling: (1) Treats Parkinson's disease. Can be used to treat early-stage symptoms. Often it is used in conjunction with levodopa when levodopa starts to lose its effectiveness, or the patient cannot tolerate the adverse effects of levodopa and dosage adjustment or withdrawal is necessary; (2) treat disorders due to excessive production of prolactin by the pituitary gland: absence of menstruation, infertility, and inappropriate production of milk; (3) helps as an adjunct to surgery in acromegaly; (4) eases breast engorgement and galactorrhea in stress induced hyperprolactinemia, (5) can help in functional infertility in females; (6) reduces the size of pituitary tumors.

Other (unlabeled) generally accepted uses: (1) Can help in patients who have had a stroke and have problems in speaking; (2) may have a small role in helping cocaine withdrawal; (3) can have selected use in patients with weak bones (osteopenia); (4) may help return growth to normal in children experiencing abnormal skeletal growth.

Author's note: Bromocriptine is no longer FDA approved for the treatment of physiological lactation. This indication was withdrawn because the risks of the use of the drug outweigh the benefits for this indication.

How This Drug Works: By stimulating receptor sites (dopamine) in the brain (corpus striatum), this drug helps increase dopamine and relieve rigidity, tremor, and sluggish movement characteristic of Parkinson's disease. By inhibiting the production of the hormone prolactin by the anterior pituitary gland, this drug
- reduces the amount of prolactin in the blood and blocks breast milk production.
- reduces abnormally high levels of prolactin in the blood, restoring it to normal levels that permit menstrual regularity and fertility.

Available Dosage Forms and Strengths
Capsules — 5 mg
Tablets — 2.5 mg
Elixir — 4 mg/5ml

▷ **Usual Adult Dosage Range:** For Parkinson's disease—initially 1.25 to 2.5 mg once daily; for maintenance, 2.5 to 100 mg daily in divided doses. Increase dose by no more than 2.5 to 5 mg on alternate days. The usual dosage range is 10 to 40 mg daily. Do not exceed 300 mg daily. For suppression of lactation—2.5 mg 2 times a day for 14 days; may extend to 21 days if needed. For absent menstruation and infertility—initially 1.25 to 2.5 mg daily; for maintenance, 2.5 mg 2 or 3 times a day. **Note: Actual dosage and administration schedule must be determined by the physician for each patient individually.**

Conditions Requiring Dosing Adjustments
Liver function: The dose should be decreased or the dosing interval lengthened, however, specific guidelines are not available.
Kidney function: Used with caution in severe renal failure only.

▷ **Dosing Instructions:** Take with food or milk to reduce stomach irritation. Capsule may be opened and tablet may be crushed for administration.

Usual Duration of Use: Use on a regular schedule for 3 to 4 months is usually neesded to determine this drug's effectiveness in controlling the symptoms of Parkinson's disease. Treatment for 4 to 12 weeks restores fertility and normal menstruation in most women; however, treatment may be necessary for 6 to 12 months. Long-term use (up to 3 years or more) must be under physician supervision and guidance. Consult your physician on a regular basis.

▷ **This Drug Should Not Be Taken If**
- you have had an allergic reaction to it previously.
- you have had a serious adverse effect from any ergot preparation.
- you have severe coronary artery disease or peripheral vascular disease.
- you are pregnant.

▷ **Inform Your Physician Before Taking This Drug If**
- you have constitutionally low blood pressure.
- you are taking any antihypertensive drugs or phenothiazines (see Drug Classes).
- you have coronary artery disease, especially with a history of heart attack (myocardial infarction).
- you have a history of heart rhythm abnormalities.
- you have impaired liver function.
- you have a seizure disorder (epilepsy).
- you take other prescription or non-prescription medications which were not discussed when bromocriptine was prescribed for you.
- you have an ulcer.
- you have a history of mental illness.
- you take other medicines that can lower blood pressure.
- you are unsure of how much bromocriptine to take or how often to take it.

Possible Side-Effects (natural, expected and unavoidable drug actions)
Fatigue, lethargy, light-headedness in upright position (see Orthostatic Hypotension in Glossary).

▷ **Possible Adverse Effects** (unusual, unexpected and infrequent reactions)
If any of the following develop, consult your physician promptly for guidance.
Mild Adverse Effects
Allergic Reaction: Skin rash.
Headache, drowsiness, dizziness, fainting, nervousness, nightmares.

Nasal congestion, dry mouth, loss of appetite, nausea, vomiting, stomach cramps, constipation, diarrhea.

Serious Adverse Effects

Abnormal involuntary movements, confusion, hallucinations, incoordination, visual disturbances, depression, seizures.

Swelling of feet and ankles (edema).

Loss of urinary bladder control, inability to empty bladder.

Indications of "ergotism": numbness and tingling of fingers, cold hands and feet, muscle cramps of legs and feet.

Vomiting blood, bloody or black stools (gastrointestinal bleeding).

Retroperitoneal fibrosis.

May worsen existing ulcers.

Excessive lowering of blood pressure.

Worsening of mania in manic patients.

Vasospasms and potential for heart attack (very rare).

Lung changes (pulmonary fibrosis) with long-term use.

▷ **Possible Effects on Sexual Function:** Rare occurrence of impotence. However, this drug can correct impotence and reduced libido when the problem is due to high blood levels of prolactin (a pituitary hormone).

▷ **Adverse Effects That May Mimic Natural Diseases or Disorders**

Effects on mental function and behavior may resemble psychotic disorders.

Natural Diseases or Disorders That May Be Activated by This Drug

Coronary artery disease with anginal syndrome, Raynaud's syndrome.

Possible Effects on Laboratory Tests

Blood alkaline phosphatase level: increased.

CAUTION

1. During treatment of parkinsonism, avoid excessive and hurried activity as improvement occurs; this will reduce the risk of falls and injury.
2. The neurological and psychiatric disturbances due to this drug may last for 2 to 6 weeks after stopping it.
3. During treatment to reduce the blood level of prolactin and restore normal menstruation and fertility, it is mandatory that you use a barrier method of contraception to prevent pregnancy. Oral contraceptives should not be used while taking bromocriptine.
4. If pregnancy occurs, notify your physician immediately.

Precautions for Use

By Infants and Children: Safety and effectiveness for those under 15 years of age not established.

By Those over 60 Years of Age: Your initial test dose should be 1.25 mg. Watch closely for light-headedness or faintness on attempting to stand after this first dose. You may be more susceptible to the development of impaired thinking, confusion, agitation, nightmares, hallucinations, nausea or vomiting. Close monitoring and careful dosage adjustments are mandatory.

▷ **Advisability of Use During Pregnancy**

Pregnancy Category: C. See Pregnancy Code at the back of this book.

Animal studies: Rabbit studies reveal an increase in cleft lip.

Human studies: Serious birth defects have been reported in infants whose mothers took this drug during early pregnancy. Because the incidence of these defects (3.3%) does not exceed that reported for the general population, a cause-and-effect relationship is uncertain. Information from adequate studies of pregnant women is not available.

Ask your doctor for advice on stopping therapy.

Advisability of Use if Breast-Feeding
This drug prevents the production of milk and makes nursing impossible.

Habit-Forming Potential: Use to treat cocaine craving may result in a chemical dependence on bromocriptine.

Effects of Overdosage: Weakness, low blood pressure, nausea, vomiting, diarrhea, confusion, agitation, hallucinations, loss of consciousness.

Possible Effects of Long-Term Use: Changes in lung tissue, thickening of the pleura and pleural effusion (fluid formation within the chest cage). These changes appear reversible after stopping the drug. Fibrosis (scar tissue formation) in the back wall of the abdominal cavity and contractures of the extremities have been reported.

Suggested Periodic Examinations While Taking This Drug (at physician's discretion)

Blood pressure measurements; CAT scan of the pituitary gland for enlargement due to tumor; pregnancy test; blood tests for anemia; evaluation of heart, lung and liver functions.

▷ **While Taking This Drug, Observe the Following**
Foods: No restrictions.
Beverages: No restrictions. May be taken with milk.
▷ *Alcohol:* Caution—alcohol can exaggerate the blood-pressure-lowering effects and sedative effects of this drug and also worsen nausea and abdominal side effects.
▷ *Other Drugs*
Bromocriptine *taken concurrently* with
- antihypertensive drugs (and other drugs that can lower blood pressure) requires careful monitoring for excessive drops in pressure. Dosage adjustments may be necessary.
- erythromycins (see Drug Classes) may result in increased bromocriptine levels and toxicity.
- phenylpropanolamine can result in bromocritpine toxicity.

The following drugs may *decrease* the effects of bromocriptine
- phenothiazines (see Drug Classes). It is probably best to avoid the concurrent use of these drugs until the results of further studies are available.

▷ *Driving, Hazardous Activities:* Be alert to the possible occurrence of orthostatic hypotension, dizziness, drowsiness or impaired coordination.

Aviation Note: Parkinsonism *is a disqualification* for piloting. The use of this drug otherwise *may be a disqualification* for piloting. Consult a designated Aviation Medical Examiner.

Exposure to Sun: No restrictions.

Discontinuation
Once this medicine is stopped, pituitary tumor regrowth and symptoms of hyperprolactinemia may occur again.

BUMETANIDE (byu MET a nide)

Introduced: 1983 **Prescription:** USA: Yes **Available as Generic:** No **Class:** Diuretic **Controlled Drug:** USA: No
Brand Name: Bumex

BENEFITS versus RISKS	
Possible Benefits	*Possible Risks*
POTENT, EFFECTIVE DIURETIC BY MOUTH OR INJECTION	ABNORMALLY LOW BLOOD POTASSIUM with excessive use Impaired sexual function Blood disorders (rare)

▷ **Principal Uses**

As a Single Drug Product: Uses currently included in FDA approved labeling: (1) Relieves retained fluid associated with congestive heart failure, liver disease or kidney disease; (2) helps edema in patients who don't respond or can't tolerate furosemide.

Other (unlabeled) generally accepted uses: (1) Used as an adjunct to other therapy in high blood pressure (hypertension); (2) can help older people decrease the number of times they must get up at night to urinate (nocturia); (3) eases the amount of fluid which can build up in the lungs (pulmonary edema).

How This Drug Works: Increases removal of salt and water from the body (through increased urine production), and reduces sodium and the volume of fluid in the blood.

Available Dosage Forms and Strengths
Injection — 0.25 mg per ml (2-ml ampules)
Tablets — 0.5 mg, 1 mg, 2 mg

▷ **Usual Adult Dosage Range:** 0.5 to 2 mg daily, usually taken in the morning as a single dose. If needed, an additional second or third dose may be taken later in the day at 4- to 5-hour intervals. The total daily dose should not exceed 10 mg. Alternate-day dosage (taken every other day) may be adequate for some individuals. **Note: Actual dosage and administration schedule must be determined by the physician for each patient individually.**

Conditions Requiring Dosing Adjustments
Liver function: Rapid body fluid removal can cause a coma in liver failure patients.
Kidney function: **Not** recommended for use in progressive renal failure.

▷ **Dosing Instructions:** May be crushed when taken and given with or following food to reduce stomach irritation.

Usual Duration of Use: Two to three days of use on a regular schedule is usually needed to see peak effect in relieving fluid buildup (edema). Once peak benefit is realized, intermittent use reduces the risk of sodium, potassium and water imbalance. Long-term use requires physician supervision.

Bumetanide

Possible Advantages of This Drug
Diuretic effect is usually complete in 4 hours; diuretic effect of furosemide usually lasts from 6 to 8 hours.

▷ **This Drug Should Not Be Taken If**
- you have had an allergic reaction to either dosage form previously.
- coma caused by liver failure is present.
- your kidneys are unable to produce urine.
- severe electrolyte or fluid imbalance.

▷ **Inform Your Physician Before Taking This Drug If**
- you are allergic to any form of "sulfa" drug.
- you are pregnant or planning pregnancy.
- you have a blood disorder.
- you have impaired liver or kidney function.
- you have diabetes, a diabetic tendency or a history of gout.
- you have impaired hearing, or develop hearing loss during therapy.
- you are taking: cortisone, digitalis, oral antidiabetic drugs, insulin, probenecid (Benemid), indomethacin (Indocin), lithium or drugs for high blood pressure.
- you plan to have surgery under general anesthesia in the near future.
- you are unsure of how much to take or how often to take bumetanide.

Possible Side-Effects (natural, expected and unavoidable drug actions)
Light-headedness on arising from sitting or lying position (see Orthostatic Hypotension in Glossary).
Increase in level of blood sugar, affecting control of diabetes.
Increase in level of blood uric acid, affecting control of gout.
Decreased blood potassium and sodium with muscle weakness and cramping.

▷ **Possible Adverse Effects** (unusual, unexpected and infrequent reactions)
If any of the following develop, consult your physician promptly for guidance.

Mild Adverse Effects
Allergic Reactions: Skin rashes, hives, itching.
Headache, dizziness, vertigo, fatigue, weakness, sweating, earache.
Nausea, vomiting, stomach pain, diarrhea.
Breast nipple tenderness, joint and muscle pains.

Serious Adverse Effects
Impaired hearing, development of liver coma (in preexisting liver disease).
Abnormally low magnesium, potassium and sodium (electrolytes).
Low white blood cells and platelets (leukopenia and thrombocytopenia).
Kidney failure (rare).
Pancreatitis (rare).
Eye defects (rare).
Lung fibrosis (rare).
Hearing toxicity (ototoxicity) (rare).

▷ **Possible Effects on Sexual Function:** Difficulty maintaining an erection; premature ejaculation (0.5 to 2 mg/day).
Male breast enlargement and tenderness (gynecomastia) (rare).

Natural Diseases or Disorders That May Be Activated by This Drug
Latent diabetes, gout.
Possible Effects on Laboratory Tests
White blood cell counts: increased (usual); decreased (rare).
Blood platelets: decreased.
Blood lithium levels: increased.
Blood uric acid levels: increased.
CAUTION
1. High doses can cause excessive excretion of water, sodium and potassium, with loss of appetite, nausea, weakness, confusion and profound drop in blood pressure (circulatory collapse).
2. May cause digitalis toxicity by depleting potassium. If you are taking a digitalis preparation (digitoxin, digoxin), ensure an adequate intake of high-potassium foods.
3. People with cirrhosis of the liver must not increase their dose unless told to do so by their doctor. Excess dosing can cause liver coma.
4. People who take lithium may experience lithium toxicity.

Precautions for Use
By Infants and Children: Safety and effectiveness for those under 18 years of age not established.
By Those over 60 Years of Age: Small starting doses are advisable. You may be more susceptible to the development of impaired thinking, orthostatic hypotension, potassium loss and elevation of blood sugar. Overdosage and prolonged use can cause excessive loss of body water, thickening of the blood, and an increased risk of blood clots, stroke, heart attack or thrombophlebitis.

▷ **Advisability of Use During Pregnancy**
Pregnancy Category: C. See Pregnancy Code at the back of this book.
Animal studies: Ten times the maximum therapeutic human dose caused bone defects in rabbits.
Human studies: Adequate studies of pregnant women are not available.
Only used in pregnancy if a very serious complication of pregnancy occurs for which this drug is significantly beneficial.

Advisability of Use if Breast-Feeding
Presence of this drug in breast milk: Unknown.
Avoid drug or refrain from nursing.

Habit-Forming Potential: None.

Effects of Overdosage: Weakness, lethargy, dizziness, confusion, nausea, vomiting, muscle cramps, thirst, electrolyte disturbances, drowsiness progressing to deep sleep or coma, weak and rapid pulse.

Possible Effects of Long-Term Use: Impaired balance of water, salt, and potassium in blood and body tissues. Dehydration with resultant increase in blood viscosity and potential for abnormal clotting. Development of diabetes in some patients.

Suggested Periodic Examinations While Taking This Drug (at physician's discretion)
Complete blood counts; blood levels of sodium, potassium, chloride, sugar, uric acid; liver and kidney function tests.

While Taking This Drug, Observe the Following

Foods: Salt restriction and a high-potassium diet may be needed. Ask your doctor. See Section Six for the Table of High Potassium Foods.

Beverages: No restrictions unless directed by your doctor. May be taken with milk.

▷ *Alcohol:* Alcohol can exaggerate the blood-pressure-lowering effect of this drug and cause orthostatic hypotension (see Glossary).

Tobacco Smoking: No interactions expected. Follow your physician's advice regarding smoking.

▷ **Other Drugs**

Bumetanide may *increase* the effects of
- antihypertensive drugs. Careful decreases in dose are needed to prevent excessive lowering of the blood pressure.

Bumetanide *taken concurrently* with
- aminoglycoside antibiotics (amikacin, gentamicin, kanamycin, neomycin, streptomycin, tobramycin, viomycin) increase the risk of hearing loss.
- cortisone-related drugs may cause excessive potassium loss.
- digitalis-related drugs require very careful monitoring and dose adjustments to prevent serious disturbances of heart rhythm.
- lithium may increase the risk of lithium toxicity.

The following drugs may *decrease* the effects of bumetanide
- indomethacin (Indocin) or other NSAIDs may reduce its diuretic effect.

▷ *Driving, Hazardous Activities:* **Caution:** Varying degrees of dizziness, weakness or orthostatic hypotension (see Glossary) may occur.

Aviation Note: The use of this drug **may be a disqualification** for piloting. Consult a designated Aviation Medical Examiner.

Exposure to Sun: No restrictions.

Occurrence of Unrelated Illness: Report vomiting or diarrhea promptly to your doctor.

Discontinuation: It may be advisable to stop this drug 5 to 7 days before major surgery. Consult your physician, surgeon, or anesthesiologist for help.

BUPROPION (byu PROH pee on)

Other Name: Amfebutamone
Introduced: 1986 **Prescription:** USA: Yes **Available as Generic:** USA: No **Class:** Antidepressant **Controlled Drug:** USA: No
Brand Name: Wellbutrin

BENEFITS versus RISKS	
Possible Benefits	*Possible Risks*
EFFECTIVE TREATMENT OF MAJOR DEPRESSIVE DISORDERS	DRUG-INDUCED SEIZURES (0.4%) Excessive mental stimulation: excitement, anxiety, confusion, hallucinations, insomnia Conversion of depression to mania in manic-depressive disorders

Bupropion

▷ **Principal Uses**
As a Single Drug Product: Uses currently included in FDA approved labeling: Treatment of major depressive disorders.
Other (unlabeled) generally accepted uses: (1) Chronic fatigue syndrome symptoms may be relieved by this medicine; (2) can significantly reduce cocaine craving when combined with psychotherapy; (3) is the agent of choice in patients who have had significant weight gain while taking tricyclic antidepressants.

How This Drug Works: Bupropion increases the levels of two nerve transmitters (norepinephrine and dopamine.) Animal studies demonstrate that this drug is primarily a brain stimulant.

Available Dosage Forms and Strengths
Tablets — 75 mg, 100 mg

▷ **Recommended Dosage Ranges** (Actual dosage and administration schedule must be determined by the physician for each patient individually.)
Infants and Children: Dosage not established for those under 18 years of age.
18 to 60 Years of Age: Initially (first 3 days), 100 mg in the morning, 100 mg in the evening; total daily dose of 200 mg.
On the fourth day, if needed and tolerated, increase dose to 100 mg in the morning, at noon, and in the evening; total daily dose of 300 mg.
This schedule of 100 mg, 3 times daily, 6 hours apart, is now continued for 3 to 4 weeks.
If tolerated and improvement continues, the dose may be slowly increased if needed up to a maximum of 450 mg daily. Increases should not exceed 100 mg per day within a period of 3 days. No single dose should exceed 150 mg. If a daily dose of 450 mg is reached, take 150 mg in the morning, then 100 mg every 4 hours for 3 more doses.
The lowest dose that maintains remission of depression should be used.
This drug should be stopped if significant improvement is not seen after an adequate trial of 450 mg daily.
Over 60 Years of Age: Same as 18 to 60 years of age.

Conditions Requiring Dosing Adjustments
Liver function: In liver cirrhosis, lower dosages and caution in monitoring should be used.
Kidney function: The dose must be decreased in patients with compromised kidneys.

▷ **Dosing Instructions:** May be taken with food to reduce stomach upset. Best to swallow the tablet whole, not chewing or crushing it; this drug has a bitter taste and a local numbing effect on the lining of the mouth.

Usual Duration of Use: Use on a regular schedule for 4 to 6 weeks is usually needed to realize this drug's effectiveness in decreasing the symptoms of depression. Long-term use (months to years) requires periodic evaluation of response and dosage adjustment. Consult your physician on a regular basis.

Possible Advantages of This Drug
Causes less atropinelike side-effects: Blurred vision, dry mouth, constipation, impaired urination.
Does not cause sedation or orthostatic hypotension (see Glossary).

Bupropion

▷ **This Drug Should Not Be Taken If**
- you have had an allergic reaction to it previously.
- you have a history of anorexia nervosa or bulimia.
- you have a seizure disorder of any kind.
- you are taking, or have taken within the past 14 days, any monoamine oxidase (MAO) type A inhibitor drug (see Drug Class, Section Four).

▷ **Inform Your Physician Before Taking This Drug If**
- you have had any adverse effects from antidepressant drugs.
- you are pregnant or planning pregnancy.
- you are breast-feeding currently.
- you have a history of mental illness, head injury, or brain tumor.
- you have a history of alcoholism or drug abuse.
- you have any kind of heart disease, especially a recent heart attack.
- you have impaired liver or kidney function.
- you take other prescription or non-prescription medications which were not discussed when bupropion was prescribed for you.
- you are unsure of how much to take or how often to take bupropion.
- you have a history of mental illness.

Possible Side-Effects (natural, expected and unavoidable drug actions)
Nervousness (31%), anxiety (3%), confusion (8%), insomnia (18%).
Weight loss of more than 5 pounds (28%).

▷ **Possible Adverse Effects** (unusual, unexpected and infrequent reactions)
If any of the following develop, consult your physician promptly for guidance.

Mild Adverse Effects
Allergic Reactions: Skin rash (8%), itching (2%).
Headache (25%), dizziness (22%), blurred vision (4%), tremor (21%).
Indigestion (3%), nausea and vomiting (22%), constipation (26%).
Dry mouth (13%).
Excessive sweating (diaphoresis) (up to 22%).

Serious Adverse Effects
Drug-induced seizures (0.4%), more common with high doses.
Change of depression to mania in manic-depressive (bipolar) disorders.
Psychosis in patients with psychotic predisposition (up to 33%).
Liver toxicity (rare).
Ringing in the ears (tinitis).

▷ **Possible Effects on Sexual Function:** Impotence (3%), altered menstruation (4%).

Possible Delayed Adverse Effects: None reported.

Natural Diseases or Disorders That May Be Activated by This Drug
Latent epilepsy, latent psychosis, manic phase of bipolar affective disorder.

Possible Effects on Laboratory Tests
White blood cell count: decreased.

CAUTION
1. Take exactly the amount prescribed; rapid dose increases can cause seizures. Watch closely for excessive stimulation.
2. Ask your physician or pharmacist before taking any other prescription or over-the-counter drug while taking this drug.

3. Do not take any monoamine oxidase (MAO) type A inhibitor drug while taking this drug (see Drug Class, Section Four). If you have taken an MAO inhibitor, then stopped it, wait 2 weeks before starting bupropion.

Precautions for Use
By Infants and Children: Safety and effectiveness for those under 18 years of age not established.
By Those over 60 Years of Age: Age-related liver or kidney function decline may require dose decreases.

▷ **Advisability of Use During Pregnancy**
Pregnancy Category: B. See Pregnancy Code at the back of this book.
Animal studies: Rat and rabbit studies reveal no significant birth defects.
Human studies: Adequate studies of pregnant women are not available.
Use this drug only if clearly needed. Ask your physician for guidance.

Advisability of Use if Breast-Feeding
Presence of this drug in breast milk: Yes.
Avoid drug or refrain from nursing.

Habit-Forming Potential: Remote with use of recommended doses. Slight potential for abuse by those who abuse stimulant drugs.

Effects of Overdosage: Headache, agitation, confusion, hallucinations, seizures, loss of consciousness.

Possible Effects of Long-Term Use: Electrocardiographic (ECG) changes: Premature beats, nonspecific ST-T wave changes.

Suggested Periodic Examinations While Taking This Drug (at physician's discretion)
Liver and/or kidney function tests as appropriate.

▷ **While Taking This Drug, Observe the Following**
Foods: No restrictions.
Beverages: No restrictions. May be taken with milk.
▷ *Alcohol:* Avoid completely. Alcohol may predispose to the development of seizures.
Tobacco Smoking: No interactions expected.
Marijuana Smoking: Avoid completely; it may induce psychotic behavior.
▷ *Other Drugs*
The following drugs **taken concurrently** with bupropion may increase the risk of major seizures
- antidepressants (tricyclic).
- clozapine.
- fluoxetine.
- haloperidol.
- lithium.
- loxapine.
- maprotiline.
- molindone.
- phenothiazines.
- thioxanthenes.
- trazodone.

Bupropion *taken concurrently* with
- carbamazepine (Tegretol) may result in lowered carbamazepine levels.
- levodopa results in increased nausea, restlessness and tremor.
- phenytoin (Dilantin) may result in decreased phynytoin levels.

▷ *Driving, Hazardous Activities:* This drug may cause dizziness, drowsiness or seizures. Restrict activities as necessary.

Aviation Note: The use of this drug *is a disqualification* for piloting. Consult a designated Aviation Medical Examiner.

Exposure to Sun: No restrictions.

Discontinuation: Do not stop this drug abruptly. Ask your physician for help.

BUSPIRONE (byu SPI rohn)

Introduced: 1979 **Prescription:** USA: Yes **Available as Generic:** No **Class:** Mild tranquilizer **Controlled Drug:** USA: No
Brand Name: Buspar

BENEFITS versus RISKS	
Possible Benefits	*Possible Risks*
EFFECTIVE RELIEF OF MILD TO MODERATE ANXIETY without significant sedation or risk of dependence	Mild dizziness, faintness or headache (uncommon) Rapid heart rate (tachycardia—2%) Rare restlessness, depression, tremor or rigidity (with high doses)

▷ **Principal Uses**

As a Single Drug Product: Uses currently included in FDA approved labeling: (1) Relieves mild to moderate anxiety and nervous tension. Particularly useful in the elderly, alcoholics and addiction-prone people because of its lack of significant sedative effects or abuse potential; (2) beneficial in decreasing self-injurious behaviors or aggression in developmentally disabled adults.

Other (unlabeled) generally accepted uses: (1) May have a benefit in reducing alcohol craving in alcoholics; (2) can help aggression or hyperactivity in autistics; (3) may decrease symptoms in obsessive-compulsive disorder; (4) can be of help in sexual dysfunction in people with generalized anxiety disorder.

How This Drug Works: This drug is thought to be a "mid-brain modulator" which causes changes in brain chemicals (dopamine, norepinephrine and serotonin) resulting in a calming effect. It is also a partial agonist at serotonin reuptake sites.

Available Dosage Forms and Strengths
Tablets — 5 mg, 10 mg

▷ **Usual Adult Dosage Range:** 20 to 30 mg/day, in divided doses. Initially, 5 mg three times/day; if needed, increase dose by 5 to 10 mg/day every 2 to 3 days, with individual doses every 6 to 8 hours. The total daily dose should not exceed 60 mg. **Note: Actual dosage and administration schedule must be determined by the physician for each patient individually.**

Conditions Requiring Dosing Adjustments
Liver function: Used with caution in severe liver failure. Doses must be decreased.
Kidney function: Used with caution in severe kidney problems. Dose should be decreased to 25–50% of normal dose.

▷ **Dosing Instructions:** The tablet may be crushed to take it and given without regard to food.

Usual Duration of Use: Use on a regular schedule for 7 to 10 days is usually needed to see this drug's benefit in relieving anxiety and nervous tension. Avoid uninterrupted use. Use intermittently and only as needed.

Possible Advantages of This Drug
Relieves anxiety or tension without severe sedation or impaired thinking. Does not cause withdrawal when it is stopped.

▷ **This Drug Should Not Be Taken If**
- you have had an allergic reaction to it previously.
- you take or have taken in the last two weeks, one of the MAO inhibitor drugs (see Drug Classes Section). May increase blood pressure.

▷ **Inform Your Physician Before Taking This Drug If**
- you take other drugs that affect the brain or nervous system: Tranquilizers, sedatives, hypnotics, analgesics, narcotics, antidepressants, antipsychotic drugs, anticonvulsants or antiparkinsonians.
- you have impaired liver or kidney function.
- you take fluoxetine (Prozac) for depression.

Possible Side-Effects (natural, expected and unavoidable drug actions)
Mild drowsiness (less than with benzodiazepines), lethargy, fatigue.

▷ **Possible Adverse Effects** (unusual, unexpected and infrequent reactions)
If any of the following develop, consult your physician promptly for guidance.
Mild Adverse Effects
Headache, dizziness, faintness, excitement, nausea.
Insomnia and dream disturbances.
Serious Adverse Effects
Depression (3%).
Tachycardia (2%).
With high doses: dysphoria, restlessness, rigidity, tremors.
Movement disorders (rare).

▷ **Possible Effects on Sexual Function:** Increased or decreased libido, difficult or absent orgasm, inhibited ejaculation, impotence, breast milk production, altered timing or pattern of menstruation (10 to 40 mg/day).
May increase prolactin; however no reports of male breast tenderness or enlargement have been reported.

Possible Effects on Laboratory Tests
Conflicting increases or lack of effect on growth hormone levels.

CAUTION
This drug is reported to have very mild sedative effects and no abuse potential, however, it should be used with caution and only when clearly needed. Most use has been short-term. Some unexpected side-effects or

adverse effects may still be reported. Actual dysphoria has been reported with higher doses and may preclude its recreational use.

Precautions for Use

By Infants and Children: Safety and effectiveness by those under 18 years of age not established.

By Those over 60 Years of Age: Expected to be tolerated much better than benzodiazepines and barbiturates. Watch for increased dizziness or weakness and avoid falls.

▷ **Advisability of Use During Pregnancy**

Pregnancy Category: B. See Pregnancy Code at the back of this book.
Animal studies: No birth defects found in rat and rabbit studies.
Human studies: Adequate studies of pregnant women are not available.
Use this drug during pregnancy only when clearly needed. Advisable to avoid this drug during the first 3 months of pregnancy.

Advisability of Use if Breast-Feeding

Presence of this drug in breast milk: Unknown; probably yes.
Avoid drug or refrain from nursing.

Habit-Forming Potential: Does not appear to cause addiction, however, more studies are needed. Higher doses result in a dysphoric reaction which may keep it from becoming a drug involved in recreational use.

Effects of Overdosage: Drowsiness, fatigue, nausea, dysphoria, tingling sensations) paresthesias, and a rare chance of seizures.

Possible Effects of Long-Term Use: None reported.

Suggested Periodic Examinations While Taking This Drug (at physician's discretion)
Periodic check of heart rate.

▷ **While Taking This Drug, Observe the Following**

Foods: No restrictions.
Beverages: No restrictions.

▷ *Alcohol:* Milder problems than diazepam (Valium), however, avoid the combination.

Tobacco Smoking: No interactions expected.
Marijuana Smoking: Additive increase in drowsiness.

▷ *Other Drugs:* Buspirone **taken concurrently** with
- MAO inhibitors (see Drug Class Section) such as phenylzine (Parnate) may result in large blood pressure increases. Do not combine.
- Fluoxetine (Prozac) may increase underlying anxiety or mental disorder such as obsessive compulsive disorder. Do not combine.
- narcotics such as oxycodone (Percodan) may result in additive sedation and potential decreases in breathing (respiratory depression).

▷ *Driving, Hazardous Activities:* This drug may cause dizziness, faintness or fatigue. Restrict activities as necessary.

Aviation Note: The use of this drug **may be a disqualification** for piloting. Consult a designated Aviation Medical Examiner.

Exposure to Sun: No restrictions.

CALCITONIN (kal si TOH nin)

Other Names: Salcatonin, thyrocalcitonin
Introduced: 1977 **Prescription:** USA: Yes; Canada: Yes **Available as Generic:** USA: No; Canada: No **Class:** Calcium regulator, hormones
Controlled Drug: USA: No; Canada: No
Brand Names: Calcimar, Cibacalcin, Miacalcin

BENEFITS versus RISKS	
Possible Benefits	*Possible Risks*
PARTIAL RELIEF OF SYMPTOMS OF PAGET'S DISEASE OF BONE	Nausea (with or without vomiting)
Effective adjunctive treatment of postmenopausal osteoporosis	Allergic reactions
Effective adjunctive treatment of abnormally high blood calcium levels (associated with malignant disease)	

▷ **Principal Uses**

As a Single Drug Product: Uses currently included in FDA approved labeling: (1) Treatment of symptomatic Paget's disease of bone (excessive bone growth of skull, spine and long bones); (2) combination treatment of postmenopausal osteoporosis, taken with calcium and vitamin D; (3) adjunctive treatment of high blood calcium levels seen in bone cancer; (4) relieves symptoms of neurologic compression in Paget's disease.

Other (unlabeled) generally accepted uses: (1) Combination treatment of osteoporosis due to medicinal drugs, hormonal disorders, or immobilization taken with calcium and vitamin D; (2) may help aneurysmal bone cysts when directly injected into the cyst; (3) preliminary study indicates that this drug may be of benefit in preventing migraine headaches and reduce or eliminate the need for prophylatic medicines; (4) useful adjunct in cancer pain; (5) very beneficial in treating pain which occurs when an arm or leg has been amputated (phantom limb).

How This Drug Works: This natural hormone slows the abnormally accelerated processes of "bone turnover" that occur in Paget's disease. The excessive replacement of bone loss is gradually reduced and a more normal balance is restored. In cancer of the bone, this drug slows bone destruction and decreases the transfer of calcium from bone to blood stream.

Available Dosage Forms and Strengths
Calcitonin-Human Injection — 500 mcg (0.5 mg)
Calcitonin-Salmon Injection — 200 IU per ml

▷ **Recommended Dosage Ranges** (Actual dosage and administration schedule must be determined by the physician for each patient individually.)

Skin Testing: Skin testing is accomplished by diluting 10 IU to one ml with 0.9% sodium chloride. One tenth ml of this dilution is injected onto the inner forearm (about one IU). A positive reaction occurs if more than mild skin reddening or weal is seen within 15 minutes. The drug should NOT be used if this positive reaction is seen.

Infants and Children: Dosage not established.

12 to 60 Years of Age: Calcitonin-Human

For Paget's disease—Initially 500 mcg (0.5 mg) daily, injected subcutaneously; after adequate response, dose may be decreased to 250 mcg (0.25 mg) daily, or 500 mcg (0.5 mg) 2 or 3 times per week. Severe cases may require 1 mg per day.

Calcitonin-Salmon

For Paget's disease—50 to 100 IU daily or every other day, injected subcutaneouly or intramuscularly; after adequate response, dose may be decreased to 50 IU daily, every other day, or 3 times per week.

For postmenopausal osteoporosis—100 IU daily, every other day, or 3 times per week, injected under the skin. If adverse effects are marked, reduce dose to 50 IU daily; then increase dose gradually over a period of 2 weeks. Calcium and vitamin D replacement is strongly recommended.

For high blood calcium levels—Initially 4 IU/kg of body weight every 12 hours, injected subcutaneously or intramuscularly; as needed and tolerated, increase dose to 8 IU/kg of body weight every 12 hours; if necessary, the dose may be increased to a maximum of 8 IU/kg of body weight every 6 hours.

For adjunctive pain treatment: 100 to 200 IU daily, given intramuscularly or subcutaneously.

Over 60 Years of Age: Same as 12 to 60 years of age.

Conditions Requiring Dosing Adjustments

Liver function: No changes indicated.

Kidney function: Should be used with caution in blocked kidneys, as the attempt to lose water via the kidney (diuresis) will put added pressure on an overloaded system.

▷ **Dosing Instructions:** Subcutaneous (under the skin) injection is preferred for self-administration. Your doctor will teach you about proper injection technique. The daily dose may be given at bedtime with the stomach empty if you become nauseated.

Usual Duration of Use: Peak effect in treating Paget's disease is usually seen after 1–3 months of use on a regular schedule. If effective, the usual treatment is 6 months; and if response continues, the dose may be reduced during the next 6 months. Peak response may require treatment for up to 24 months. Long-term use (months to years) requires periodic physician evaluation.

Possible Advantages of This Drug

Calcitonin-human is less likely to induce allergic reactions than calcitonin-salmon, permitting treatment for longer periods of time.

▷ **This Drug Should Not Be Taken If**
- you have had an allergic reaction to it previously.
- you recently fractured a bone that has not healed completely.

Calcitonin

▷ **Inform Your Physician Before Taking This Drug If**
- you are allergic by nature (history of eczema, hives, hay fever, asthma).
- you have known allergies to foreign proteins.
- you are unsure of how much to take or how often to take.
- you will be unable to have follow up laboratory testing of calcium.

Possible Side-Effects (natural, expected and unavoidable drug actions)
Salty or metallic taste in mouth.

▷ **Possible Adverse Effects** (unusual, unexpected and infrequent reactions)
If any of the following develop, consult your physician promptly for guidance.

Mild Adverse Effects
Allergic Reactions: Skin rash, hives, itching.
Headache, dizziness, weakness.
Loss of appetite, nausea, vomiting, stomach pain, diarrhea.
Increased frequency of urination.
Pedal edema.
Shivering.
Metallic taste (rare).
Urination at night (nocturia).

Serious Adverse Effects
Allergic Reactions: Flushing, redness, tingling of face or extremities.
Glucose intolerance.
Increased urination.
Excessive lowering of calcium and rigidity (tetany) of muscles due to lack of calcium.
Anaphylactic reactions.

▷ **Possible Effects on Sexual Function:** None reported.

Possible Effects on Laboratory Tests
Blood alkaline phosphatase levels: decreased.
Blood calcium levels: decreased.
Urine hydroxyproline values: decreased.

CAUTION
1. It is advisable to perform a skin test before beginning treatment with calcitonin-salmon.
2. Eat a well-balanced diet with adequate calcium and vitamin D.
3. Tell your doctor if bone pain persists while taking this drug.

Precautions for Use
By Infants and Children: No specific information.
By Those over 60 Years of Age: Watch fluid balance closely if this drug is given to lower blood calcium.

▷ **Advisability of Use During Pregnancy**
Pregnancy Category:
C. See Pregnancy Code at the back of this book.
Animal studies: No drug-induced birth defects reported.

Human studies: Adequate studies of pregnant women are not available. Use this drug only if clearly needed. Ask your physician for help.

Advisability of Use if Breast-Feeding
Presence of this drug in breast milk: Yes.
Calcitonin taken in with breast milk is typically destroyed by infant stomach acids before it has any effect. Ask your doctor for guidance.

Habit-Forming Potential: None.

Effects of Overdosage: Nausea, vomiting.

Possible Effects of Long-Term Use: Antibodies may cause resistance and loss of effect. This occurs in approximately 50% of people after 2 to 18 months of treatment.

Suggested Periodic Examinations While Taking This Drug (at physician's discretion)
Measurements of blood calcium, phosphate, and alkaline phosphatase levels.
Measurement of urine hydroxyproline content.
Measurement of bone density by DEXA densitometry scanning.

▷ **While Taking This Drug, Observe the Following**
Foods: No restrictions.
Nutritional Support: Ensure adequate intake of calcium and vitamin D.
Beverages: No restrictions.
▷ *Alcohol:* No interactions expected.
Tobacco Smoking: No interactions expected.
▷ *Other Drugs:*
Calcitonin *taken concurrently* with
• Plicamycin will cause additive loss of calcium.
▷ *Driving, Hazardous Activities:* No restrictions.
Aviation Note: The use of this drug **may be a disqualification** for piloting. Consult a designated Aviation Medical Examiner.
Exposure to Sun: No restrictions.
Discontinuation:
Your doctor should decide when to stop this drug.
Special Storage Instructions:
Calcitonin-human—Store at a temperature below 25 degrees C (77 degrees F). Do not refrigerate. Protect from light.
Calcitonin-salmon—Store in refrigerator, between 2 and 8 degrees C (36 and 46 degrees F). Do not freeze.

CAPTOPRIL (KAP toh pril)

Introduced: 1979   **Prescription:** USA: Yes; Canada: Yes   **Available as Generic:** No   **Class:** Antihypertensive, ACE inhibitor   **Controlled Drug:** USA: No; Canada: No

Brand Names: ✦Apo-Capto, Capoten, Capozide [CD], ✦Novo-Captopril, ✦Nu-Capto, ✦Syn-Captopril

BENEFITS versus RISKS	
Possible Benefits	*Possible Risks*
EFFECTIVE CONTROL OF MILD TO SEVERE HIGH BLOOD PRESSURE	Rash, itching, fever (10%)
	Lost or altered taste (7%)
USEFUL ADJUNCTIVE TREATMENT FOR CONGESTIVE HEART FAILURE	Impaired white blood cell production (0.3%)
	Bone marrow depression (rare)
	Kidney damage (rare)
MAY DECREASE RISK OF KIDNEY PROBLEMS IN DIABETICS TAKING INSULIN	Liver damage (rare)
	Profound decreases in blood pressure
MAY REDUCE RISK OF DEATH AFTER A HEART ATTACK	(in some patients who have taken diuretics)

▷ **Principal Uses**
  As a Single Drug Product: Uses currently included in FDA approved labeling: (1) Treats all degrees of high blood pressure; (2) may help prevent death after heart attacks; (3) used in advanced heart failure; (4) used in type one insulin dependent diabetics who have kidney problems and damage to the retina of the eye.
  Other (unlabeled) generally accepted uses: (1) Helps relieve symptoms of cystinuria.

  How This Drug Works: It is thought that by blocking an enzyme system, this drug relaxes arterial walls and lowers the blood pressure. This, in turn, decreases the heart's work load and improves its performance.

  Available Dosage Forms and Strengths
  Tablets — 12.5 mg, 25 mg, 50 mg, 100 mg

▷ **Usual Adult Dosage Range:** Initially 12.5 to 25 mg 2 or 3 times daily for 2 weeks. If necessary, dose may be increased to 50 mg 3 times daily. Usual maintenance dose is 50 to 100 mg 3 times daily. Total daily dose should not exceed 450 mg. **Note: Actual dosage and administration schedule must be determined by the physician for each patient individually.**

  Conditions Requiring Dosing Adjustments
  Liver function: Must used with extreme caution, and started at a lower dose in liver failure.
  Kidney function: Increased blood level and risk of adverse effects (low blood counts and protein in the urine) if used in kidney failure. Must decrease dose.

▷ **Dosing Instructions:** Take on empty stomach, 1 hour before meals, at same time each day. Tablet may be crushed for administration.

  Usual Duration of Use: Several weeks of use on a regular schedule is usually needed to see high blood pressure control. Use may be continued for life.

▷ **This Drug Should Not Be Taken If**
  - you have had an allergic reaction to it previously.
  - you are pregnant (last 6 months).
  - you currently have a blood cell or bone marrow disorder.
  - you have an abnormally high level of blood potassium.

Captopril

▷ **Inform Your Physician Before Taking This Drug If**
- you are allergic to ACE inhibitors (see Drug Class).
- you are planning pregnancy.
- you have a history of kidney disease or impaired kidney function.
- you have scleroderma or systemic lupus erythematosus.
- you have any form of heart or liver disease.
- you have diabetes.
- you have an elevated potassium level.
- you have a blood cell disorder.
- you take: Other antihypertensives, diuretics, nitrates, allopurinol (Zyloprim), Indocin or potassium supplements.
- you plan to have surgery under general anesthesia in the near future.
- you have renal artery stenosis (ask your doctor).
- you are unsure of how much to take or how often to take captopril.

Possible Side-Effects (natural, expected and unavoidable drug actions)
Dizziness, light-headedness, fainting (excessive drop in blood pressure).

▷ **Possible Adverse Effects** (unusual, unexpected and infrequent reactions)
If any of the following develop, consult your physician promptly for guidance.

Mild Adverse Effects
Allergic Reactions: Skin rash; swelling of face, hands or feet; fever.
Lost or altered taste, mouth or tongue sores.
Rapid heart rate, palpitation.

Serious Adverse Effects
Bone marrow depression—weakness, fever, sore throat, bleeding or bruising.
Kidney damage—water retention (edema).
Liver damage—with or without jaundice.

▷ **Possible Effects on Sexual Function:** Decreased male libido (20% to 30%) with recommended dosage.

Possible Effects on Laboratory Tests
Complete blood counts: decreased red cells, hemoglobin, white cells and platelets; increased eosinophils.
Blood antinuclear antibodies (ANA): increased.
Blood cholesterol and triglycerides: no effects.
Blood sodium level: decreased.
Blood urea nitrogen level (BUN): increased.
Liver function tests: increased liver enzymes (alkaline phosphatase, AST/GOT, LDH), increased bilirubin.
Urine ketone tests: false positive results with Keto-diastix and Chemstrip-6.

CAUTION
1. If possible, advisable to stop all other antihypertensive drugs (especially diuretics) for 1 week before starting captopril.
2. **Inform your physician immediately if you become pregnant.** This drug should not be taken beyond the first 3 months of pregnancy.
3. **Report promptly** any signs of infection (fever, sore throat), and any indications of water retention (weight gain, swollen feet or ankles).
4. Many salt substitutes contain potassium, ask your doctor before using.
5. Blood counts and urine analyses are needed **before** taking captopril.

Precautions for Use
  By Infants and Children: Safety and effectiveness have not been established.
  By Those over 60 Years of Age: Small starting doses are advisable. Sudden and excessive lowering of blood pressure can cause stroke or heart attack.

▷ **Advisability of Use During Pregnancy**
  Pregnancy Category: D. See Pregnancy Code at the back of this book.
  Animal studies: No birth defects found in rat, rabbit or hamster studies. However, this drug was found to be toxic to the embryo and newborn.
  Human studies: The use of ACE inhibitor drugs during the last 6 months of pregnancy is known to possibly cause very serious injury and possible death to the fetus; skull and limb malformations, lung defects, and kidney failure have been reported in over 50 cases worldwide.
  Avoid this drug completely during the last 6 months. During the first 3 months of pregnancy, use this drug only if clearly needed. Ask your physician for guidance.

Advisability of Use if Breast-Feeding
  Presence of this drug in breast milk: Yes, in small amounts.
  Monitor nursing infant closely and discontinue drug or nursing if adverse effects develop.

Habit-Forming Potential: None.

Effects of Overdosage: Excessive drop in blood pressure—light-headedness, dizziness, fainting.

Possible Effects of Long-Term Use: Gradual increase in blood potassium level.

Suggested Periodic Examinations While Taking This Drug (at physician's discretion)
  Complete blood cell count, urine analysis and blood potassium level before drug started. Once started: Blood counts every 2 weeks during the first 3 months, then periodically for duration of use. Urine protein every month for the first 9 months of treatment, then periodically for duration of use. Periodic measurements of blood potassium.

▷ **While Taking This Drug, Observe the Following**
  Foods: Consult physician regarding salt intake.
  Nutritional Support: **Do not take** potassium supplements unless directed by your physician.
  Beverages: No restrictions. May be taken with milk.
▷ *Alcohol:* Alcohol can further lower blood pressure. Use with caution.
  Tobacco Smoking: No interactions expected.
▷ *Other Drugs*
  Captopril *taken concurrently* with
  - allopurinol (Zyloprim) may increase risk of serious skin reactions.
  - azathioprine may result in severe anemia.
  - cyclosporine (Sandimune) may result in kidney failure that takes a while to appear (delayed acute renal dysfunction).
  - lithium may result in three times the expected lithium levels and toxicity.
  - loop diuretics (see Drug Classes) may result in excessively low blood pressure on standing (postural hypotension).
  - phenothiazines (see Drug Classes) may result in postural hypotension.

- potassium preparations (K-Lyte, Slow-K, etc.) will increase blood potassium with risk of serious heart rhythm disturbances.
- potassium-sparing diuretics: amiloride (Moduretic), spironolactone (Aldactazide), triamterene (Dyazide) may increase blood levels of potassium with risk of serious heart rhythm disturbances.

The following drugs may *decrease* the effects of captopril
- indomethacin (Indocin) or other NSAIDS (see Drug Classes).
- salicylates (aspirin, etc.).

▷ *Driving, Hazardous Activities:* Usually no restrictions. Be aware of possible drops in blood pressure with resultant dizziness or faintness.

Aviation Note: The use of this drug **may be a disqualification** for piloting. Consult a designated Aviation Medical Examiner.

Exposure to Sun: Caution advised. This drug can cause photosensitivity.

Exposure to Heat: Caution advised. Excessive perspiring may drop blood pressure.

Occurrence of Unrelated Illness: Report promptly any disorder that causes nausea, vomiting or diarrhea. Fluid and chemical imbalances must be corrected as soon as possible.

CARBAMAZEPINE (kar ba MAZ e peen)

Introduced: 1962 **Prescription:** USA: Yes; Canada: Yes **Available as Generic:** Yes **Class:** Anticonvulsant, antineuralgic **Controlled Drug:** USA: No; Canada: No

Brand Names: ◆Apo-Carbamazepine, Epitol, ◆Mazepine, ◆Novo-Carbamaz, ◆PMS Carbamazepine, Tegretol, Tegretol Chewable tablet

BENEFITS versus RISKS	
Possible Benefits	*Possible Risks*
RELIEF OF PAIN IN TRIGEMINAL NEURALGIA	RARE BONE MARROW DEPRESSION (reduced formation of all blood cells)
EFFECTIVE CONTROL OF CERTAIN TYPES OF EPILEPTIC SEIZURES	Liver damage with jaundice
Relief of pain in some rare forms of nerve pain (neuralgia)	

▷ **Principal Uses**

As a Single Drug Product: Uses currently included in FDA approved labeling: Management of two uncommon but serious disorders: (1) for relief of pain in true trigeminal neuralgia (tic douloureux) and glossopharyngeal neuralgia; (2) for control of several types of epilepsy, namely grand mal, tonic-clonic, psychomotor or temporal lobe, complex partial and mixed seizure patterns. Precise diagnosis and careful management are mandatory for its proper use.

Other (unlabeled) generally accepted uses: (1) Beneficial in bipolar affective disorders; (2) schizoaffective disorders; (3) resistant schizophrenia; (4) posttraumatic stress disorder; (5) tabes dorsalis; (6) diabetic neuropathy; (7) hemifacial spasm; (8) cocaine withdrawal; (9) helps aggression in some Alzheimer's patients; (10) hiccups and belching associated with flutter of the diaphragm; (11) treats nerve problems resulting from thiamine deficiency; (12) may have a role in treating pain that occurs when an arm or leg is amputated (phantom limb pain).

How This Drug Works: By reducing impulses at certain nerve terminals, this drug relieves or reduces pain (of trigeminal neuralgia) and also reduces the excitability of nerve fibers in the brain decreasing the likelihood of seizures or reducing their frequency and severity.

Available Dosage Forms and Strengths
  Oral suspension — 100 mg per 5-ml teaspoonful
  Tablets — 200 mg
  Tablets, chewable — 100 mg

▷ **Usual Adult Dosage Range:** Initially 200 mg/12 hours. Dose may be increased at weekly intervals by 200 mg/24 hours as needed and tolerated. Total daily dosage should not exceed 1200 mg. **Note: Actual dosage and administration schedule must be determined by the physician for each patient individually.**

Conditions Requiring Dosing Adjustments
  Liver function: Used with extreme caution, in lower doses and watched closely in liver failure patients.
  Kidney function: Capable of being toxic to the kidneys. Used with extreme caution and in decreased dose in patients with kidneys that already do not work well.

▷ **Dosing Instructions:** Take at same time each day, with or following food to reduce stomach irritation. Tablet may be crushed for administration.

Usual Duration of Use: Use on a regular schedule for 3 months is usually needed to see this drug's effect in relieving the pain of trigeminal neuralgia. Longer periods, with dosage adjustment, may be required to determine its ability to control epileptic seizures. Careful evaluation of individual tolerance and response should be made every 3 months during long-term treatment.

▷ **This Drug Should Not Be Taken If**
  - you have had an allergic reaction to it previously.
  - you have active liver disease.
  - you currently have a blood cell or bone marrow disorder.
  - you currently take, or have taken within the past 14 days, a monoamine oxidase (MAO) type A inhibitor (see Drug Class, Section Four).

▷ **Inform Your Physician Before Taking This Drug If**
  - you have had an allergic reaction to any tricyclic antidepressant drug (see Drug Class).
  - you have taken this drug in the past.
  - you have had any blood or bone marrow disorder, especially drug induced.
  - you have a history of liver or kidney disease.
  - you have had serious mental depression or other mental disorder.
  - you have had thrombophlebitis.
  - you have high blood pressure, heart disease or glaucoma.

156   Carbamazepine

- you take more than 2 alcoholic drinks a day.
- you take other prescription or non-prescription medications which were not discussed when carbamazepine was prescribed for you.
- you are unsure of how much to take or how often to take carbamazepine.

Possible Side-Effects (natural, expected and unavoidable drug actions)
Dry mouth and throat, constipation, impaired urination.

▷ **Possible Adverse Effects** (unusual, unexpected and infrequent reactions)
If any of the following develop, consult your physician promptly for guidance.

Mild Adverse Effects
Allergic Reactions: Skin rash, hives, itching, drug fever.
Headache, dizziness, drowsiness, unsteadiness, fatigue, blurred vision, confusion.
Exaggerated hearing, ringing in ears.
Loss of appetite, nausea, vomiting, indigestion, diarrhea.
Water retention (edema), frequent urination.
Changes in skin pigmentation, hair loss.
Aching of muscles and joints, leg cramps.

Serious Adverse Effects
Allergic Reactions: Severe dermatitis with peeling of skin, irritation of mouth and tongue, swelling of lymph glands.
Idiosyncratic Reactions: Lung inflammation (pneumonitis): cough, shortness of breath.
Abnormal heart beats (bradyarrhythmias).
Bone marrow depression (see Glossary)—fatigue, weakness, fever, sore throat, abnormal bleeding or bruising.
Liver damage with jaundice (see Glossary)—yellow eyes and skin, dark-colored urine, light-colored stools.
Kidney damage—reduced urine volume, uremic poisoning.
Mental depression and agitation/psychosis.
Paradoxical increase in seizures.
Drug induced meningitis (aseptic meningitis).
Low thyroid hormones.
Abnormally elevated urine output (SIADH).
Neuroleptic malignant syndrome (rare).
Rare abnormal movement and muscle contractions.
Double vision, visual hallucinations, speech disturbances, peripheral neuritis (see Glossary).
Thrombophlebitis.

▷ **Possible Effects on Sexual Function**
Decreased libido and/or impotence (13%), male infertility.
This drug is used to control hypersexuality (exaggerated sexual behavior) that can result from injury to the temporal lobe of the brain.

▷ **Adverse Effects That May Mimic Natural Diseases or Disorders**
Liver reactions may suggest viral hepatitis.
Rare lung reactions may suggest interstitial pneumonitis.

Natural Diseases or Disorders That May Be Activated by This Drug
Latent psychosis, systemic lupus erythematosus.

Carbamazepine

Possible Effects on Laboratory Tests
    Complete blood cell: decreased red cells, hemoglobin, white cells and platelets; increased eosinophils, increased white cells.
    Blood calcium level: decreased.
    Blood prothrombin time: decreased.
    Blood urea nitrogen level (BUN): increased.
    Liver function tests: increased liver enzymes (ALT/GPT, AST/GOT and alkaline phosphatase), increased bilirubin.
    Urine pregnancy tests: false negative or inconclusive results with Prepurex, Predictor, Gonavislide, Pregnosticon.

CAUTION
1. Should be used only after less toxic drugs have failed.
2. *Before* the first dose is taken, blood cell counts, liver function tests and kidney function tests should be obtained.
3. Careful periodic testing for blood cell or bone marrow toxicity is **mandatory**.
4. *Should not be used* to prevent recurrence of trigeminal neuralgia when it is in remission.
5. *Do not stop this drug suddenly* if it is being used to control seizures.
6. If exposed to humidity, the tablet form hardens; this results in poor absorption from the gastrointestinal tract and erratic control of seizures. Store this drug in a cool, dry place; avoid bathrooms or other humid areas.

Precautions for Use
    By Infants and Children: Safety and effectiveness by those under 6 years of age not established. Careful testing of blood production, liver and kidney function must be performed regularly. This drug can reduce the effectiveness of other anticonvulsant drugs. Blood levels of all anticonvulsant drugs should be checked if this drug is added to the treatment program.
    By Those over 60 Years of Age: Can cause confusion and agitation. Watch for aggravation of glaucoma, coronary artery disease (angina) or prostatism (see Glossary).

▷ **Advisability of Use During Pregnancy**
    Pregnancy Category: C. See Pregnancy Code at the back of this book.
    Animal studies: Rat studies reveal significant birth defects.
    Human studies: Adequate studies of pregnant women are not available.
    Avoid completely during the first 3 months. Use during the last 6 months only if clearly needed.

Advisability of Use if Breast-Feeding
    Presence of this drug in breast milk: Yes.
    Avoid drug or refrain from nursing.

Habit-Forming Potential: None.

Effects of Overdosage: Dizziness, drowsiness, disorientation, tremor, involuntary movements, nausea, vomiting, flushed skin, dilated pupils, stupor progressing to coma.

Possible Effects of Long-Term Use: Water retention (edema), impaired liver function, possible jaundice.

158   Carbamazepine

Suggested Periodic Examinations While Taking This Drug (at physician's discretion)
   Complete blood counts weekly during the first 3 months of treatment, and then monthly until the drug is stopped. Liver and kidney function tests. Complete eye examinations.

▷ **While Taking This Drug, Observe the Following**
   Foods: No restrictions.
   Beverages: No restrictions. May be taken with milk.
▷ *Alcohol:* Avoid alcohol use, unless your doctor approves alcohol use.
   Tobacco Smoking: No interactions expected.
▷ *Other Drugs*
   Carbamazepine may *increase* the effects of
   - sedatives, tranquilizers, hypnotics, narcotics, and enhance their sedative effects.

   Carbamazepine may *decrease* the effects of
   - antidepressants (see Drug Classes).
   - corticosteroids (see Drug Classes).
   - cyclosporine (Sandimmune).
   - doxycycline (Doxy-II, Vibramycin, etc.).
   - haloperidol (Haldol) or other phenothiazines.
   - itraconazole (Sporanox).
   - birth control pills (oral contraceptives).
   - tetracyclines (see Drug Classes).
   - valproic acid (Depakene, etc.).
   - warfarin (Coumadin).

   Carbamazepine *taken concurrently* with
   - clozapine (Clozaril) may result in serious bone marrow suppression.
   - felbamate (Felbatol) may result in decreased carbamazepine levels and seizures.
   - lithium may cause serious neurological problems: Confusion, drowsiness, weakness, unsteadiness, tremors, and twitching.
   - monoamine oxidase (MAO) type A inhibitor drugs (see Drug Class) may cause severe toxic reactions.
   - phenytoin (Dilantin, etc.) may cause unpredictable fluctuations of blood levels of both drugs and impair seizure control.
   - terfenadine (Seldane) may result in carbamazepine toxicity.
   - theophylline (Theo-Dur, etc.) may reduce the effects of both drugs.

   The following drugs may *increase* the effects of carbamazepine
   - cimetidine (Tagamet).
   - danazol (Danocrine).
   - diltiazem (Cardizem)—and perhaps other calcium channel blockers.
   - macrolide antibiotics—erythromycin, clarithramycin and azithromycin.
   - isoniazid (INH).
   - nicotinamide (nicotinic acid amide).
   - propoxyphene (Darvon, Darvocet, etc.).
   - troleandomycin (Tao).
   - verapamil (Calan, Isoptin).

▷ *Driving, Hazardous Activities:* Can cause dizziness, drowsiness or blurred vision. Adjust activities.

Aviation Note: The use of this drug *is a disqualification* for piloting. Consult a designated Aviation Medical Examiner.

Exposure to Sun: This drug can cause photosensitivity (see Glossary). Use caution until sensitivity to sun is known.

Heavy Exercise or Exertion: Use caution if you have coronary artery disease. Can intensify angina and reduce tolerance for physical activity.

Occurrence of Unrelated Illness: Because of potential for serious adverse effects, you **must** tell each physician and dentist you see that you take carbamazepine.

Discontinuation: If treating trigeminal neuralgia, every 3 months attempts to reduce the maintenance dose or to stop this drug are needed. If used to control epilepsy, this drug *must not be stopped abruptly.*

Special Storage Instructions

Store the tablet form of this drug in a cool, dry place. Protect it from exposure to humid conditions.

CARTEOLOL (KAR tee oh lohl)

Introduced: 1983 **Prescription:** USA: Yes **Available as Generic:** No **Class:** Antihypertensive, beta-adrenergic blocker **Controlled Drug:** USA: No

Brand Name: Cartrol, Ocupress, Optipress

BENEFITS versus RISKS	
Possible Benefits	*Possible Risks*
EFFECTIVE, WELL-TOLERATED ANTIHYPERTENSIVE EFFECTIVE GLAUCOMA TREATMENT	CONGESTIVE HEART FAILURE in advanced heart disease Worsening of angina in coronary heart disease (abrupt withdrawal) Masking of low blood sugar (hypoglycemia) in drug-treated diabetics Provocation of asthma in asthmatics

▷ **Principal Uses**

As a Single Drug Product: Uses currently included in FDA approved labeling: (1) Treatment of mild to moderate high blood pressure. May be used alone or in combination with other drugs, such as diuretics; (2) helps lower eye (intraocular) pressure in people with glaucoma.

Other (unlabeled) generally accepted uses: (1) Effective in helping increase the amount of exercise which can be performed before angina occurs; (2) can have a role in helping decrease aggressive behavior.

How This Drug Works: By blocking certain actions of the sympathetic nervous system, this drug

- reduces the rate and contraction force of the heart, lowering the ejection pressure of blood leaving the heart.
- reduces the extent of blood vessel wall contraction, resulting in relaxation and expansion and lowering of blood pressure.
- reduces elevated eye pressure (intraocular) and relieves glaucoma symptoms.

Carteolol

Available Dosage Forms and Strengths
    Tablets — 2.5 mg, 5 mg
Ophthalmic solution — 1 %

▷ **Usual Adult Dosage Range:** For high blood pressure (hypertension): Initially 2.5 mg once daily. The dose may be increased gradually by 2.5 mg/day at intervals of 2 weeks as needed and tolerated up to 10 mg/day. For maintenance, 2.5 to 7.5 mg once daily is usually adequate. The total daily dose should not exceed 10 mg.

For glaucoma: One drop in the affected eye or eyes two times a day. **Note: Actual dosage and administration schedule must be determined by the physician for each patient individually.**

Conditions Requiring Dosing Adjustments
Liver function: Decreased doses needed in severe liver failure.
Kidney function: The kidney is the main route of elimination for this drug. Dosing interval **must** be decreased in kidney failure. In severe compromise, the drug is given every 48 to 72 hours.

▷ **Dosing Instructions:** Tablet may be crushed and taken without regard to eating. Do not stop this drug abruptly.

Usual Duration of Use: Use on a regular schedule for up to 3 weeks may be needed to see this drug's effectiveness in lowering blood pressure. Long-term use of this drug (months to years) will be determined by the benefit in lowering your blood pressure over time and your response to a treatment program of weight reduction, salt restriction, smoking cessation, etc. See your doctor on a regular basis.

Possible Advantages of This Drug
Adequate control of blood pressure with a single daily dose.
Causes less slowing of the heart rate than most other beta blocker drugs.

▷ **This Drug Should Not Be Taken If**
- you have bronchial asthma
- you have had an allergic reaction to it previously.
- you have congestive heart failure.
- you have an abnormally slow heart rate or a serious heart block.
- you are subject to bronchial asthma.
- you have a dissecting aortic aneurysm (ask your doctor).

▷ **Inform Your Physician Before Taking This Drug If**
- you have had an adverse reaction to any beta blocker (see Drug Class).
- you have serious heart disease or episodes of heart failure.
- you have had hay fever (allergic rhinitis), asthma, chronic bronchitis or emphysema.
- you have a history of overactive thyroid function (hyperthyroidism).
- you have a history of low blood sugar (hypoglycemia).
- you have a history of diabetes.
- you have impaired liver or kidney function.
- you have diabetes or myasthenia gravis.
- you have a circulation problem (Raynaud's disorder, claudication pains in legs).
- you take any form of digitalis, quinidine or reserpine, or any calcium blocker drug (see Drug Class).
- you plan to have surgery under general anesthesia in the near future.

Possible Side-Effects (natural, expected and unavoidable drug actions)
Lethargy and fatigability, cold extremities, slow heart rate, light-headedness in upright position (see Orthostatic Hypotension in Glossary).

▷ **Possible Adverse Effects** (unusual, unexpected and infrequent reactions)
If any of the following develop, consult your physician promptly for guidance.
Mild Adverse Effects
Allergic Reactions: Skin rash.
Dizziness, nervousness, drowsiness, insomnia, abnormal dreams.
Indigestion, nausea, vomiting, constipation, diarrhea.
Joint and muscle discomfort, numbness of fingers or toes.
Tearing and irritation with use in the eye (25%).
Serious Adverse Effects
Mental depression, anxiety.
Chest pain, irregular heartbeat, shortness of breath, can cause congestive heart failure.
Induction of bronchial asthma (in asthmatic individuals).
Aggravation of myasthenia gravis.
May hide symptoms of low blood sugar.

▷ **Possible Effects on Sexual Function:** Decreased libido, impotence.

▷ **Adverse Effects That May Mimic Natural Diseases or Disorders**
Decreased extremity blood flow may mimic Raynaud's phenomenon (see Glossary).

Natural Diseases or Disorders That May Be Activated by This Drug
Raynaud's disease, intermittent claudication, myasthenia gravis.

Possible Effects on Laboratory Tests
Blood creatine kinase level: increased.

CAUTION
1. *Do not stop this drug suddenly* without the knowledge of your doctor. Carry a note that says you are taking this drug.
2. Ask your physician or pharmacist before using nasal decongestants. These can cause sudden increases in blood pressure when combined with beta blocker drugs.
3. Report any new tendency to emotional depression.

Precautions for Use
By Infants and Children: Safety and effectiveness by those under 12 years of age not established. However, if this drug is used, watch for the development of low blood sugar (hypoglycemia) especially if meals are skipped.
By Those over 60 Years of Age: **Caution:** Unacceptably high blood pressure should be reduced without creating excessively low blood pressure. Treatment should begin with small doses, and blood pressure should be checked often. Sudden and excessive reduction of blood pressure can lead to stroke or heart attack. Watch for dizziness, tendency to fall, confusion, hallucinations, depression or urinary frequency.

▷ **Advisability of Use During Pregnancy**
Pregnancy Category: C. See Pregnancy Code at the back of this book.
Animal studies: No birth defects due to this drug found in rat or rabbit studies.

Human studies: Adequate studies of pregnant women are not available. Use this drug only if clearly needed. Ask physician for guidance.

Advisability of Use if Breast-Feeding
Presence of this drug in breast milk: Unknown.
Avoid drug or refrain from nursing.

Habit-Forming Potential: None.

Effects of Overdosage: Weakness, slow pulse, low blood pressure, fainting, cold and sweaty skin, congestive heart failure, possible coma and convulsions.

Possible Effects of Long-Term Use: Reduced heart reserve and eventual heart failure in susceptible individuals with advanced heart disease.

Suggested Periodic Examinations While Taking This Drug (at physician's discretion)
Measurements of blood pressure, evaluation of heart function.

▷ **While Taking This Drug, Observe the Following**
Foods: No restrictions. Avoid excessive salt intake.
Beverages: No restrictions. May be taken with milk.

▷ *Alcohol:* Use caution. Alcohol may exaggerate this drug's ability to lower the blood pressure and may increase its mild sedative effect.
Tobacco Smoking: Nicotine may reduce this drug's effectiveness in treating high blood pressure. In addition, high doses may worsen constriction of the bronchial tubes caused by regular smoking.

▷ *Other Drugs*
Carteolol may *increase* the effects of
- other antihypertensive drugs, and cause excessive lowering of the blood pressure. Dosage adjustments may be necessary.
- reserpine (Ser-Ap-Es, etc.), and cause sedation, depression, slowing of the heart rate and low blood pressure. This combination is best avoided.
- theophyllines (aminophylline, dyphylline, oxtriphylline, etc.).
- verapamil (Calan, Isoptin), and cause excessive depression of heart function; monitor this combination closely.

Carteolol *taken concurrently* with
- amiodarone (Codarone) may cause severe slowing of the heart and sinus arrest. Do not combine these agents.
- clonidine (Catapres) requires close monitoring for rebound high blood pressure if clonidine is stopped while carteolol is still being taken. Severe rebound hypertension may occur.
- epinephrine (Adrenalin, etc.) may cause sudden rise in blood pressure followed by slowing of the heart rate. Avoid the combination.
- ergot preparations (ergotamine, methysergide, etc.) may enhance serious ergot-induced constriction of peripheral circulation.
- insulin requires close monitoring to avoid hypoglycemia (see Glossary).
- oral hypoglycemic agents (see Drug Classes) may cause prolonged recovery from hypoglycemia should it occur.
- phenothiazines (see Drug Class) can cause increased effects of both drugs.

The following drugs may *decrease* the effects of carteolol
- indomethacin (Indocin), and possibly other "aspirin substitutes," or NSAIDs may impair carteolol's antihypertensive effect.

▷ *Driving, Hazardous Activities:* Use caution until the full extent of fatigue, dizziness and blood pressure change have been determined.
Aviation Note: The use of this drug ***is a disqualification*** for piloting. Consult a designated Aviation Medical Examiner.
Exposure to Sun: No restrictions.
Exposure to Heat: Caution advised. Hot environments can lower the blood pressure and exaggerate the effects of this drug.
Exposure to Cold: Caution advised. The elderly should take precautions to prevent hypothermia (see Glossary).
Heavy Exercise or Exertion: Avoid exertion that produces light-headedness, excessive fatigue or muscle cramping. The use of this drug can cause dangerously increased blood pressure with isometric exercise.
Occurrence of Unrelated Illness: Fever can lower the blood pressure and require decreased doses. Illnesses that cause nausea or vomiting may interrupt the regular dosage schedule. Ask your physician for guidance.
Discontinuation: Avoid sudden discontinuation of this drug in all situations. If possible, gradual reduction of dose over a period of 2 to 3 weeks is recommended. Ask your physician for specific guidance.

CEFACLOR (SEF a klor)

Introduced: 1979   **Prescription:** USA: Yes; Canada: Yes   **Available as Generic:** No   **Class:** Antibiotic, cephalosporins   **Controlled Drug:** USA: No; Canada: No
Brand Name: Ceclor

BENEFITS versus RISKS	
Possible Benefits	*Possible Risks*
EFFECTIVE TREATMENT OF INFECTIONS due to susceptible microorganisms	ALLERGIC REACTIONS mild to severe (may also be seen in those allergic to penicillin)
	Drug-induced colitis (rare)
	Superinfections (see Glossary)

▷ **Principal Uses**
As a Single Drug Product: Uses currently included in FDA approved labeling: (1) To treat certain infections of the skin and skin structures, the upper and lower respiratory tract (including middle ear infections and "strep" throat), certain infections of the urinary tract and postoperative wounds.
Other unlabeled, generally accepted uses: (1) may have an alternative role in helping prevent rheumatic fever if the bacteria are resistant to erythromycin.

How This Drug Works: This drug destroys susceptible infecting bacteria by interfering with their ability to produce new protective cell walls as they multiply and grow.

Available Dosage Forms and Strengths
Capsules — 250 mg, 500 mg
Oral suspension — 125 mg, 187mg, 250 mg, 375 mg per 5-ml teaspoonful

Cefaclor

▷ **Usual Adult Dosage Range:** 250 to 500 mg/8 hours. Total daily dose should not exceed 4 grams.
   In children: 20 to 40 mg per kg of body weight per day is given in divided doses every 8 hours. Maximum dose is 1 gram (1,000 mg) daily. **Note: Actual dosage and administration schedule must be determined by the physician for each patient individually.**

Conditions Requiring Dosing Adjustments
   Liver function: Elmination by the liver has not been identified as yet.
   Kidney function: Cefaclor is 40–80% eliminated by the kidney. For creatinine clearances (CrCl) of 10–50 ml/min, use 50–100% of the usual dose at the normal interval. For CrCl of less than 10 ml/min, use 50% of the usual dose at the usual interval.

▷ **Dosing Instructions:** May be taken on an empty stomach or with food if stomach irritation occurs. Capsule may be opened for administration. Shake suspension well before measuring (use a measured dose cup or other calibrated dose measure) dose. Take the full course prescribed.

Usual Duration of Use: Continual use on a regular schedule for 3 to 5 days is usually necessary to determine this drug's effectiveness in controlling the infection under treatment. Response varies with the nature of the infection. Total treatment time will vary from 1 to 4 weeks. Certain infections require that this drug be taken for 10 consecutive days to prevent the development of rheumatic fever. Follow your doctor's instructions about how long to take this medicine.

▷ **This Drug Should Not Be Taken If**
   • you are allergic to any cephalosporin antibiotic (see Drug Class).

▷ **Inform Your Physician Before Taking This Drug If**
   • you have a history of allergy to any penicillin (see Drug Class).
   • you have a history of regional enteritis or ulcerative colitis.
   • you have impaired kidney function.

Possible Side-Effects (natural, expected and unavoidable drug actions)
   Superinfections (see Glossary).

▷ **Possible Adverse Effects** (unusual, unexpected and infrequent reactions)
   If any of the following develop, consult your physician promptly for guidance.
   Mild Adverse Effects
   Allergic Reactions: Skin rash, itching, hives.
   Nausea and vomiting (1 in 90), mild diarrhea (1 in 70), sore mouth or tongue.
   Mild and reversable decrease in white blood cells (neutrophils).
   Confusion, nervousness, insomnia, dizziness (rare).
   Serious Adverse Effects
   Allergic Reactions: Drug fever (see Glossary), joint aches and pains, anaphylactic reaction (see Glossary).
   Idiosyncratic Reactions: Minor and temporary changes in white blood cell counts and liver function tests (infrequent).
   Genital itching (may represent a fungus superinfection).
   Severe diarrhea, possibly indicating a drug-induced form of colitis (rare).
   Increases in liver enzymes and jaundice (cholestatic) (rare).

Cefaclor 165

▷ **Possible Effects on Sexual Function:** None reported.
▷ **Adverse Effects That May Mimic Natural Diseases or Disorders**
  Skin rash and fever may resemble measles.

Possible Effects on Laboratory Tests
  Blood platelet counts: decreased (rare).
  Liver enzymes: increased.
  BUN and creatinine: increased.

CAUTION
  In the management of diabetes it should be noted that this drug can cause a false positive test result for urine sugar when using Clinitest tablets, Benedict's solution or Fehling's solution, but not with Tes-Tape.

Precautions for Use
  By Infants and Children: Not recommended for use in infants less than 1 month old. The maximal dose in children should not exceed 1 gram/24 hours.
  By Those over 60 Years of Age: Dosage must be carefully individualized and based upon evaluation of kidney function. Natural changes in the skin may predispose to severe and prolonged itching reactions in the genital and anal regions. Such reactions should be reported promptly. The natural decline in kidney function often requires a decrease in dose and achieves the same effect as a larger dose.

▷ **Advisability of Use During Pregnancy**
  Pregnancy Category: B. See Pregnancy Code at the back of this book.
  Animal studies: No birth defects reported.
  Human studies: Information from adequate studies of pregnant women is not available.
  Generally considered to be safe. Ask physician for guidance.

Advisability of Use if Breast-Feeding
  Presence of this drug in breast milk: Yes, in small amounts.
  Ask your doctor for advice.

Habit-Forming Potential: None.

Effects of Overdosage: Nausea, vomiting, stomach cramps and/or diarrhea.

Possible Effects of Long-Term Use: Superinfections (see Glossary).

Suggested Periodic Examinations While Taking This Drug (at physician's discretion)
  Complete blood cell counts.
  Liver enzymes.
  BUN and creatinine with long-term therapy.

▷ **While Taking This Drug, Observe the Following**
  Foods: Delays the absorption of this drug and may result in decreased antibiotic effect.
  Beverages: No restrictions. May be taken with milk.
▷ *Alcohol:* No interactions expected.
  Tobacco Smoking: No interactions expected.
▷ *Other Drugs*
    Cefaclor **taken concurrently** with
    • use of this drug with any aminoglycoside (see Drug Classes) may result in increased kidney toxicity.

- birth control pills (oral contraceptives) may result in decreased effectiveness in preventing conception and pregnancy.
- probenecid (Benemid) will slow the elimination of cefaclor, resulting in higher blood levels and prolonged effect.

▷ *Driving, Hazardous Activities:* Usually no restrictions.
Aviation Note: The use of this drug **may be a disqualification** for piloting. Consult a designated Aviation Medical Examiner.
Exposure to Sun: No restrictions.
Special Storage Instructions: Oral suspension should be refrigerated.
Observe the Following Expiration Times: Do not take the oral suspension of this drug if it is older than 14 days.

CEFADROXIL (sef a DROX il)

Introduced: 1977 **Prescription:** USA: Yes; Canada: Yes **Available as Generic:** Yes **Class:** Antibiotic, cephalosporins **Controlled Drug:** USA: No; Canada: No
Brand Names: Duricef, Ultracef

BENEFITS versus RISKS	
Possible Benefits	*Possible Risks*
EFFECTIVE TREATMENT OF INFECTIONS due to susceptible microorganisms	ALLERGIC REACTIONS mild to severe Drug-induced colitis (rare) Superinfections (see Glossary)

▷ **Principal Uses**
As a Single Drug Product: Uses currently included in FDA approved labeling: (1) To treat certain infections of the skin and skin structures, the upper respiratory tract (including tonsillitis and "strep" throat) and certain infections of the urinary tract.
Other (unlabeled) generally accepted uses: None.

How This Drug Works: This drug destroys susceptible infecting bacteria by interfering with their ability to produce new protective cell walls as they multiply and grow.

Available Dosage Forms and Strengths
Capsules — 500 mg
Gelatin capsules (Canada) — 500 mg
Oral suspension — 125 mg, 250 mg, 500 mg per 5-ml teaspoonful
Tablets — 1000 mg (1 gram)

▷ **Usual Adult Dosage Range:** Skin infections—500 mg/12 hours, or 1 gram daily. "Strep" throat—500 mg/12 hours for 10 days. Urinary tract infections—500 mg to 1 gram/12 hours, or 1 to 2 grams daily. Total daily dosage should not exceed 6 grams.
For children: 30 mg per kg per day, given in divided doses every 12 hours.
Note: Actual dosage and administration schedule must be determined by the physician for each patient individually.

Conditions Requiring Dosing Adjustments
  Liver function: The liver is involved to a minimal degree, and no dosing changes are anticipated in liver compromise.
  Kidney function: With creatinine clearances of 10–50 ml/min, use the usual doses every 12 to 24 hours. For creatinine clearances less than 10 ml/min, use the usual doses given every 24–48 hours.

▷ **Dosing Instructions:** May be taken on an empty stomach or with food if stomach irritation occurs. Capsule may be opened for administration. Shake suspension well before measuring dose. Take the full course prescribed.

Usual Duration of Use: Continual use on a regular schedule for 3 to 5 days is usually necessary to determine this drug's effectiveness in controlling the infection under treatment. Response varies with the nature of the infection. Total treatment time will vary from 1 to 4 weeks. Certain infections require that this drug be taken for 10 consecutive days to prevent the development of rheumatic fever. Follow your physician's instructions about how long to take this medicine.

Possible Advantages of This Drug
  Higher cure rate (90%) than penicillin V (76%) in treating streptococcal infections of the throat; also, lower recurrence rate (7%) than penicillin V (15%).

▷ **This Drug Should Not Be Taken If**
  • you are allergic to any cephalosporin antibiotic (see Drug Class).

▷ **Inform Your Physician Before Taking This Drug If**
  • you have a history of allergy to any form of penicillin (see Drug Class).
  • you have a history of regional enteritis or ulcerative colitis.
  • you have impaired kidney function.

Possible Side-Effects (natural, expected and unavoidable drug actions)
  Superinfections (see Glossary).

▷ **Possible Adverse Effects** (unusual, unexpected and infrequent reactions)
  If any of the following develop, consult your physician promptly for guidance.
  Mild Adverse Effects
  Allergic Reactions: Skin rash, itching, hives, localized swellings.
  Headache, drowsiness, dizziness.
  Indigestion, stomach cramping, nausea, vomiting, mild diarrhea, sore mouth or tongue.
  Serious Adverse Effects
  Allergic Reactions: Drug fever (see Glossary), joint aches and pains, anaphylactic reaction (see Glossary).
  Idiosyncratic Reactions: Minor and temporary changes in white blood cell counts and liver function tests (infrequent).
  Genital itching (may represent a fungus superinfection).
  Severe diarrhea, possibly indicating a drug-induced form of colitis (rare).

▷ **Possible Effects on Sexual Function:** None reported.

▷ **Adverse Effects That May Mimic Natural Diseases or Disorders**
  Skin rash and fever may resemble measles.

Possible Effects on Laboratory Tests
  No significant effects reported.

Cefadroxil

CAUTION
> In the management of diabetes it should be noted that this drug can cause a false positive test result for urine sugar when using Clinitest tablets, Benedict's solution or Fehling's solution, but not with Tes-Tape.

Precautions for Use
By Infants and Children: Dosage is based upon weight, and must be determined by the physician for each individual. Follow your physician's instructions exactly.

By Those over 60 Years of Age: Dosage must be carefully individualized and based upon evaluation of kidney function. Natural changes in the skin may predispose to severe and prolonged itching reactions in the genital and anal regions. Such reactions should be reported promptly.

▷ **Advisability of Use During Pregnancy**
Pregnancy Category: B. See Pregnancy Code at the back of this book.
Animal studies: No birth defects reported.
Human studies: Information from adequate studies of pregnant women is not available.
Generally considered to be safe. Ask physician for guidance.

Advisability of Use if Breast-Feeding
Presence of this drug in breast milk: Yes, in small amounts.
Ask your doctor for guidance.

Habit-Forming Potential: None.

Effects of Overdosage: Nausea, vomiting, stomach cramps and/or diarrhea.

Possible Effects of Long-Term Use: Superinfections (see Glossary).

Suggested Periodic Examinations While Taking This Drug (at physician's discretion)
Complete blood cell counts. Liver and kidney function tests.

▷ **While Taking This Drug, Observe the Following**
Foods: No restrictions.
Beverages: No restrictions. May be taken with milk.
▷ *Alcohol:* No interactions expected.
Tobacco Smoking: No interactions expected.
▷ *Other Drugs*
Cefadroxil **taken concurrently** with
- aminoglycoside antibiotics (see Drug Class) may cause an increased risk of kidney toxicity.
- birth control pills (oral contraceptives) may result in inhibition of the contraceptive and pregnancy.
- probenecid (Benemid) will slow the elimination of cefadroxil, resulting in higher blood levels and prolonged effect.

▷ *Driving, Hazardous Activities:* Usually no restrictions. If drowsiness or dizziness occurs, restrict activities accordingly.

Aviation Note: The use of this drug **may be a disqualification** for piloting. Consult a designated Aviation Medical Examiner.

Exposure to Sun: No restrictions.
Special Storage Instructions: Oral suspension should be refrigerated.
Observe the Following Expiration Times: Do not take the oral suspension of this drug if it is older than 14 days.

CEFIXIME (sef IX eem)

Introduced: 1986 **Prescription:** USA: Yes **Available as Generic:** No **Class:** Antibiotic, cephalosporin **Controlled Drug:** USA: No
Brand Name: Suprax

BENEFITS versus RISKS

Possible Benefits	Possible Risks
EFFECTIVE TREATMENT OF INFECTIONS due to susceptible microorganisms	ALLERGIC REACTIONS Drug-induced colitis (rare) Superinfections (see Glossary) Low white blood cells ($<2\%$) Low blood platelets ($<2\%$)

▷ **Principal Uses**
  As a Single Drug Product: Uses currently included in FDA approved labeling: (1) Treats some infections of the middle ear, tonsils, throat, bronchial tubes and urinary tract.
  Other (unlabeled) generally accepted uses: (1) Effective in uncomplicated cervical or urethral gonorrhea, (2) may have a role in treating resistant Salmonella infections.

How This Drug Works: Destroys susceptible infecting bacteria by interfering with their ability to produce new protective cell walls as they multiply and grow.

Available Dosage Forms and Strengths
  Oral suspension — 100 mg per 5 ml teaspoonful
  Tablets — 200 mg, 400 mg

▷ **Usual Adult Dosage Range:** 400 mg daily, taken as a single dose or as 200 mg every 12 hours.
  For children over 6 months of age: 8 mg per kg/day, all in one dose or divided into 2 doses.
  For treatment of multi-drug resistant Salmonella: 20 mg per kg per day in divided doses every 12 hours for at least 12 days. **Note: Actual dosage and administration schedule must be determined by the physician for each patient individually.**

Conditions Requiring Dosing Adjustments
  Liver function: Dose changes not needed.
  Kidney function: Dose must be decreased in mild to moderate kidney problems. In severe failure, a single dose every 48 hours is needed.

▷ **Dosing Instructions:** May take on an empty stomach or with food if stomach irritation occurs. The tablet may be crushed and mixed with food (such as applesauce or ice cream) to help swallowing. Take the full course prescribed.

Usual Duration of Use: Continual use on a regular schedule for 3 to 5 days is needed to see this drug's effectiveness in controlling infections. Some infections require that the drug be taken for 10 consecutive days to prevent rheumatic fever. Follow your physician's instructions regarding duration of use.

Cefixime

▷ **This Drug Should Not Be Taken If**
- you are allergic to cephalosporin antibiotics (see Drug Class).
- you have active colitis of any type.

▷ **Inform Your Physician Before Taking This Drug If**
- you are allergic to penicillin (see Drug Class).
- you have a history of regional enteritis or ulcerative colitis.
- you have impaired kidney function.
- you have a history of low platelets or white blood cells.

Possible Side-Effects (natural, expected and unavoidable drug actions)
Superinfections (see Glossary): vaginitis (yeast infection).

▷ **Possible Adverse Effects** (unusual, unexpected and infrequent reactions)
If any of the following develop, consult your physician promptly for guidance.

Mild Adverse Effects
Allergic Reactions: Skin rash, hives, itching, drug fever (see Glossary).
Nausea (7%), indigestion (3%), loose stools (6%), diarrhea (16%), abdominal pain (3%).
Headache, dizziness.

Serious Adverse Effects
Severe diarrhea, possibly indicating a drug-induced form of colitis (rare). This can occur during use of the drug or months after it was stopped.
Low blood platelets ($<2\%$).
Low white blood cells ($<2\%$).
Kidney toxicity ($<2\%$).
Superinfections (see Glossary).

▷ **Possible Effects on Sexual Function:** None reported.

▷ **Adverse Effects That May Mimic Natural Diseases or Disorders**
Skin rash may resemble measles.

Possible Effects on Laboratory Tests
Complete blood cell counts: transient decreases in white blood cells and platelets; no serious consequences reported.

CAUTION
1. Otitis media (middle ear infection) should be treated with the oral suspension. Tablets should not be substituted for the suspension.
2. This drug can cause a false positive test result for urine sugar with using Clinitest tablets, Benedict's solution or Fehling's solution. Also causes a false positive reaction for urine ketones (nitroprusside tests).

Precautions for Use
By Infants and Children: Safety and effectiveness for use by those under 6 months of age have not been established.
By Those over 60 Years of Age: Must be individualized based on kidney function. Natural skin changes may make severe and prolonged itching reactions in genitals and anus likely. Such reactions should be reported promptly.

▷ **Advisability of Use During Pregnancy**
Pregnancy Category: B. See Pregnancy Code at the back of this book.
Animal studies: No birth defects reported in mouse and rat studies.
Human studies: Adequate studies of pregnant women are not available.
Generally considered to be safe. Ask physician for guidance.

Advisability of Use if Breast-Feeding
  Presence of this drug in breast milk: Unknown.
  Ask your doctor for help.

Habit-Forming Potential: None.

Effects of Overdosage: Nausea, vomiting, stomach cramps and/or diarrhea.

Possible Effects of Long-Term Use: Superinfections (see Glossary).

Suggested Periodic Examinations While Taking This Drug (at physician's discretion)
  Complete blood cell counts.

▷ **While Taking This Drug, Observe the Following**
  Foods: No restrictions.
  Beverages: No restrictions. May be taken with milk.
▷ *Alcohol:* No interactions expected.
  Tobacco Smoking: No interactions expected.
▷ *Other Drugs*
  Cefixime *taken concurrently* with
  • aminoglycoside antibiotics (see Drug Class) may pose an increased risk of kidney toxicity.
▷ *Driving, Hazardous Activities:* Usually no restrictions. Observe for the rare occurrence of dizziness.
  Aviation Note: The use of this drug **may be a disqualification** for piloting. Consult a designated Aviation Medical Examiner.
  Exposure to Sun: No restrictions.
  Special Storage Instructions: Keep oral suspension at room temperature. Do not refrigerate. Shake well before measuring dose.
  Observe the Following Expiration Time: Do not take the oral suspension of this drug if older than 14 days.

CEFPROZIL (SEF pro zil)

Introduced: 1991   **Prescription:** USA: Yes   **Available as Generic:** No   **Class:** Anti-infective, cephalosporins   **Controlled Drug:** USA: No
Brand Name: Cefzil

BENEFITS versus RISKS	
Possible Benefits	*Possible Risks*
EFFECTIVE TREATMENT OF INFECTIONS due to susceptible microorganisms	ALLERGIC REACTIONS mild to severe Drug-induced colitis (rare) Superinfections (see Glossary)

▷ **Principal Uses**
  As a Single Drug Product: Uses currently included in FDA approved labeling (when caused by susceptible organisms): (1) Treatment of upper respiratory tract infections: Pharyngitis, tonsillitis, otitis media; (2) Treatment of lower respiratory tract infections: Acute bronchitis and exacerbation of chronic bronchitis; (3) Treatment of skin and skin structure infections.
  Other (unlabeled) generally accepted uses: None.

Cefprozil

How This Drug Works: This drug destroys susceptible infecting bacteria by interfering with their ability to produce new protective cell walls as they multiply and grow.

Available Dosage Forms and Strengths
Oral suspension — 125 mg, 250 mg per 5-ml teaspoonful
Tablets — 250 mg, 500 mg

▷ **Recommended Dosage Ranges** (Actual dosage and administration schedule must be determined by the physician for each patient individually.)

Infants and Children: For otitis media (6 months to 12 years of age)—15 mg/kg of body weight every 12 hours, for 10 days.

13 to 60 Years of Age: Pharyngitis or tonsillitis—500 mg every 24 hours, for 10 days.
Acute or chronic bronchitis—500 mg every 12 hours, for 10 days.
Skin or skin structure infections—250 to 500 mg every 12 to 24 hours, for 10 days.

Over 60 Years of Age: Same as 13 to 60 years of age. Decreased dose in kidney failure.

Conditions Requiring Dosing Adjustments

Liver function: The liver is not known to be involved in elimination of this drug.

Kidney function: With severe kidney failure, half the dose can be given at the usual time.

Phenylketonuria (PKU): The suspension has 28 mg of phenylalanine in every 5 ml. This may preclude use of the drug in these patients.

▷ **Dosing Instructions:** Can take on an empty stomach or with food if stomach irritation occurs. The tablet may be crushed and mixed with food (such as applesauce or ice cream) if needed to help swallowing. Shake the oral suspension well before measuring each dose. Take the full course prescribed.

Usual Duration of Use: Continual use on a regular schedule for 3 to 5 days is needed to see how effective treatment will be. Some infections require 10 consecutive days to prevent the development of rheumatic fever. Follow your physician's instructions regarding how long it should be taken.

▷ **This Drug Should Not Be Taken If**
- you are allergic to cephalosporins (see Drug Class).

▷ **Inform Your Physician Before Taking This Drug If**
- you are allergic to penicillin (see Drug Class).
- you have a history of regional enteritis or ulcerative colitis.
- you have impaired kidney function.
- you have a history of blood clotting disorders.
- you have a history of low white blood cell count.

Possible Side-Effects (natural, expected and unavoidable drug actions)
Superinfections (see Glossary) 1.5%; vaginitis 1.6%.

▷ **Possible Adverse Effects** (unusual, unexpected and infrequent reactions)
If any of the following develop, consult your physician promptly for guidance.

Mild Adverse Effects
Allergic Reactions: Skin rash (0.9%), hives (0.1%).
Nausea (3.5%), vomiting (1.0%), mild diarrhea (2.9%).

Headache (1%), dizziness (1%).
Increased liver enzymes.
Serious Adverse Effects
Low white blood cell count.
Increased time for clotting to occur.

▷ **Possible Effects on Sexual Function:** None reported.

▷ **Adverse Effects That May Mimic Natural Diseases or Disorders**
Skin rash may resemble measles.

Possible Effects on Laboratory Tests
White blood cell counts: decreased (very rare).
Liver function tests: increased liver enzymes (ALT/GPT, AST/GOT).
Extended PTT tests.

CAUTION
This drug may cause a false positive test result for urine sugar when using Clinitest tablets, Benedict's solution or Fehling's solution.

Precautions for Use
By Infants and Children: Safety and effectiveness for those under 6 months of age not established.
By Those over 60 Years of Age: Dose must be individualized based on kidney function. Natural changes in the skin may predispose to severe and prolonged itching in the genital and anal regions. Such reactions should be reported promptly.

▷ **Advisability of Use During Pregnancy**
Pregnancy Category: B. See Pregnancy Code at the back of this book.
Animal studies: No birth defects reported in mouse, rat and rabbit studies.
Human studies: Adequate studies of pregnant women are not available.
Generally considered to be safe. Ask physician for guidance.

Advisability of Use if Breast-Feeding
Presence of this drug in breast milk: Unknown.
Ask your doctor for guidance.

Habit-Forming Potential: None.

Effects of Overdosage: Nausea, vomiting, stomach cramps and/or diarrhea.

Possible Effects of Long-Term Use: Superinfections (see Glossary).

Suggested Periodic Examinations While Taking This Drug (at physician's discretion)
Complete blood counts.

▷ **While Taking This Drug, Observe the Following**
Foods: No restrictions.
Beverages: No restrictions. May be taken with milk.

▷ *Alcohol:* No interactions expected.
Tobacco Smoking: No interactions expected.

▷ *Other Drugs*
Cefprozil ***taken concurrently*** with
- aminoglycosides (see Drug Class) may result in increased kidney toxicity.
- probenecid (Benemid) may cause higher blood levels and prolonged effect.

▷ *Driving, Hazardous Activities:* Usually no restrictions. Observe for the rare occurrence of dizziness.

Aviation Note: The use of this drug **may be a disqualification** for piloting. Consult a designated Aviation Medical Examiner.
Exposure to Sun: No restrictions.
Special Storage Instructions: Oral suspensions should be refrigerated.
Observe the Following Expiration Times: Discard unused portion after 14 days.

CEFTRIAXONE (SEF try ax own)

Introduced: 1984 **Prescription:** USA: Yes; Canada: Yes **Available as Generic:** USA: No; Canada: No **Class:** Antibiotic, cephalosporin **Controlled Drug:** USA: No; Canada: No
Brand Name: Rocephin

BENEFITS versus RISKS	
Possible Benefits	*Possible Risks*
HOME IV TREATMENT OF ADVANCED LYME DISEASE (STAGE TWO OR THREE) AFTER HOSPITAL INDUCTION (INITIATION OF INTRAVENOUS THERAPY IN THE HOSPITAL). HOME IV TREATMENT OF OSTEOMYELITIS (BONE INFECTIONS) AFTER HOSPITAL INDUCTION. Home IV treatment of other serious infections.	PALPITATIONS Hematologic effects: Thrombocytosis, Leukopenia and anemia Pseudomembranous colitis (a serious colon inflammation)

▷ **Principal Uses**
  As a Single Drug Product: Uses currently included in FDA approved labeling: (1) Treatment of: Lower respiratory infections, skin and skin structure infections, urinary tract infections, uncomplicated gonorrhea, pelvic inflammatory disease, bacterial septicemia, bone and joint infections, intra-abdominal infections, diabetic foot infections, gonorrhea, prosthetic joint infections, meningitis and surgical prophylaxis.
  Other (unlabeled) generally accepted uses: (1) Intravenous treatment of late (stage two or three) Lyme disease; (2) treatment of chancroid; (3) Initial treatment of epididymitis; (4) Shigella infection.
How This Drug Works: Ceftriaxone inhibits the ability of bacteria to make protective cell walls. Ceftriaxone usually causes the death of the bacteria.
Available Dosage Forms and Strengths
  250 mg of Rocephin—Boxes of one vial (NDC #0004-1962-02) and boxes of ten vials (NDC #0004-1962-01)
  500 mg of rocephin—Boxes of one and ten vials (NDC #0004-1963-02 and 0004-1963-01)
  1 gm of Rocephin—Boxes of one and ten vials (NDC #0004-1964-04 and 0004-1964-01), also piggyback bottles of ten (NDC #0004-1964-03)
  2 gm of Rocephin—Boxes of ten vials (NDC #0004-1965-01), also piggyback bottles of ten (NDC #0004-1965-03)
  10 gm of Rocephin—Box of one (NDC #0004-1971-01)

1 gm (NDC #0004-1964-05) and 2 gm (NDC #0004-1965-05) ADD-Vantage packaging

How To Store
Following reconstitution with 0.9% sodium chloride, 5% dextrose or sterile water for injection—ceftriaxone solutions having 100 mg per ml are stable for three (3) days at room temperature or ten (10) days in the refrigerator. Consult guidelines and outdates from your provider regarding frozen ceftriaxone.

▷ **Recommended Dosage Ranges (Actual dosage and administration schedule must be determined by the physician for each patient individually.)**
Infants and Children: For neonates and children less than 12 for treatment of serious infections caused by suceptible organisms (other than CNS infections such as meningitis) is 50 to 75 mg per kg (mg/kg) per day given in two equally divided doses twelve hours apart. (Not to exceed 2 grams daily). Some doctors suggest that neonates one week old or younger be given 50 mg/kg per day, and that neonates older than one week and weighing 2 kg or less also receive 50 mg/kg per day, and 50–75 mg/kg per day be given to neonates older than one week and weighing more than 2 kg.

For meningitis (caused by susceptible organisms) the dose for neonates and children 12 or younger is 100 mg/kg daily, divided into two equal doses given every 12 hours. The American Academy of Pediatrics suggests 80–100 mg/kg be given once daily or in two equally divided doses every 12 hours for children older than one month. Because the once daily regimen is relatively new, we suggest that the 12 hour regimen be used.

12 to 60 Years of Age: The dosing of ceftriaxone for treatment of most infections (caused by susceptible organisms) is: 1–2 grams daily or in equally divided doses two times a day depending on the type and severity of the infection. Children older than 12 can be given the adult dose. Some physicians recommend that CNS infections in adults may require 4 grams daily. This is the maximum adult dosage recommended by the manufacturer.

Uncomplicated gonorrhea caused by penicillinase producing strains of Neisseria gonorrhea (PPNG) or nonpenicillinase producing strains may be treated by a single IM 250 mg dose of ceftriaxone. Disseminated gonococcal infection should be treated by 1 (one) gram of ceftriaxone IV or IM once a day for seven days. Acute sexually transmitted epididymitis in adults may be treated with a single 250 mg IM dose of ceftriaxone followed by seven days of oral tetracycline or erythromycin. For treatment of acute pelvic inflammatory disease (PID), a single 250 mg IM dose of ceftriaxone should be given and then followed by 100 mg of oral doxycycline two times a day for 10–14 days.

Treatment of serious arthritis, cardiac or neurologic complications of early or late (stage two or three) Lyme disease:

Arthritis—Ceftriaxone at a dose of 2 grams IV daily for adults. Children should be given 75–100mg/kg/day IV.

Serious CNS Disease—Ceftriaxone at a dose of 2 grams IV daily for 21 days in adults. Children can be treated with 75–100 mg/kg IV daily for 21 days.

Cardiac Disease—Ceftriaxone 2 grams IV per day for 21 days in adults. Children can be given 75–100 mg/kg/day IV.

Surgical prophylaxis—Although ceftriaxone is FDA approved for surgical prophylaxis, we do not recommend its routine use. Other readily available

Ceftriaxone

agents are equally as effective, and much less expensive. Ceftriaxone use for surgical prophylaxis also increases the potential for resistance to this drug, and could decrease its usefulness in treating later infections.

Over 60 Years of Age: Same as 12 to 60 years of age.

Conditions Requiring Dosing Adjustments

Liver function: Patients with both liver and kidney problems should have drug levels checked, and a maximum total daily dose of 2 grams.

Kidney function: Compromise of the kidneys alone (see above) is cause for careful monitoring.

▷ **Dosing Instructions:** Bring refrigerated IV solutions to room temperature before using them. Do not use any IV solutions which contain particles or precipitates (are cloudy). Do not use outdated solutions—they will not treat your infection as effectively as IVs that have not expired.

Usual Duration of Use: In general, therapy should be continued (except gonorrhea) for at least 48 hours after the infection is gone and you are asymptomatic. For invasive infections, antibiotic therapy is usually continued for 5–7 days after negative bacteriologic cultures are obtained.

Gram negative bacillary meningitis should be treated for at least 21 days.

Osteomyelitis (bone infection) may require six weeks (42 days) of intravenous therapy with reassessment when the course of antibiotics is completed.

Continual use on a regular schedule for three weeks is usually needed to see this drug's effectiveness in Lyme disease. Lyme tests may remain positive for a significant amount of time even though the infection has been cured.

Possible Advantages of This Drug

Once or twice a day dosing is especially convenient for home IV therapy. Can be used with other antibiotics for a synergistic (much larger effect than either drug alone) effect against bacteria.

Currently a "Drug of Choice"

For second and third stage Lyme disease, for treatment of chancroid, for treatment of meningitis and epiglotitis caused by Hemophilus influenzae, meningitis caused by Neisseria meningitidis, Neisseria gonorrhoeae, and Salmonella typhi.

▷ **This Drug Should Not Be Taken If**
- you have had an allergic reaction to any dosage form of it previously or to any other cephalosporin (see Drug Class).
- you have active colitis of any type.

▷ **Inform Your Physician Before Taking This Drug If**
- you have a hematologic (blood) disorder such as anemia.
- you have liver or kidney problems.
- you have a history of regional enteritis or ulcerative colitis.
- you have an allergy to any prescription or non-prescription medicines.
- you have an allergy to penicillin.
- you have a history of gall bladder disease.
- you have a clotting disorder of the blood.
- you are pregnant or plan to become pregnant.
- you take other prescription or non-prescription medicines which were not discussed with your doctor when this medicine was prescribed.

Possible Side-Effects (natural, expected and unavoidable drug actions)
Superinfections (see glossary) such as vaginitis (a vaginal yeast infection), oral yeast infections, and overgrowth of organisms with long term use.

▷ **Possible Adverse Effects** (unusual, unexpected and infrequent reactions)
If any of the following develop, consult your physician promptly for guidance.
Mild Adverse Effects
Allergic Reactions: Skin rash (erythemetous and urticarial) (2%), pruritis (itching) fever and chills ($<1\%$).
Headache, flushing, dizziness and sweating (1%), palpitations ($<0.1\%$), transient diarrhea (42–44%) of children and (28%) of adults, asymptomatic gall bladder concretions (43%) of children receiving 60–100 mg/kg/day in one study, diarrhea (2–4%), nausea and vomiting ($<1\%$), pain and induration at the injection site (intramuscular use) (1–2%), increased liver enzymes (SGOT and SGPT) (3%), increased BUN and the occurance of urinary casts (1%), hematuria and glycosuria (blood and sugar in the urine) ($<0.1\%$), epistaxis (nose bleeds) ($<0.1\%$).
Serious Adverse Effects
Allergic Reactions: Bronchospasm, anaphylaxis and serum sickness.
Palpitations (rare), leukopenia (2%), jaundice ($<1\%$), hypoprothrombinemia ($<0.1\%$), neutropenia, anemia, lymphopenia, and thrombocytopenia (1%), leukocytosis, lymphocytosis, monocytosis and basophilia ($<0.1\%$), rare gallbladder concretions, rare pseudomembranous colitis, rare reversible symptomatic biliary symptoms, very rare urolithiasis (kidney stone) with renal colic, decreased kidney function and cholelithiasis.

▷ **Possible Effects on Sexual Function:** None reported.

Possible Delayed Adverse Effects: Biliary symptoms can be more likely with longer term high-dose therapy.

▷ **Adverse Effects That May Mimic Natural Diseases or Disorders**
Has been associated with the formation of biliary sludge in the gallbladder which mimics cholecystitis (gallbladder inflammation).
May result in jaudice as seen in hepatitis.
Markedly alters bacterial flora in the colon and may lead to hypoprothrombinemia as seen in malnutrition and chronic liver disease.

Natural Diseases or Disorders That May Be Activated by This Drug
Additive hypoprothrombinemia in malnutrition or chronic liver disease.

Possible Effects on Laboratory Tests
Complete blood cell counts: Eosinophilia, basophilia, monocytosis, leukocytosis, thrombocytosis, leukopenia, neutropenia, lymphopenias and thrombocytopenia have all occurred.
Prolongation of prothrombin times and hypoprothrombinemia has been reported.
Increased SGOT, SGPT, alkaline phosphatase and bilirubin.
Increased BUN, serum creatinine, urinary casts, glycosuria and hematuria.
Interferes with cupric sulfate (a specific chemical indicator) based tests for urine sugar such as Clinitest.
Manual tests for creatinine may be falsely elevated by ceftriaxone.

Ceftriaxone

CAUTION
1. Ceftriaxone should be used with caution in people who are allergic to penicillin, whatever the symptoms were.
2. Jaundiced neonates are at risk of bilirubin encephalopathy.
3. Ceftriaxone made with bacteriostatic water containing benzyl alcohol should not be used for IM (intramuscular) use in neonates.

Precautions for Use
By Infants and Children:
Specific dosing schedules have been developed for children less than 12.
By Those over 60 Years of Age: No changes indicated.

▷ **Advisability of Use During Pregnancy**
Pregnancy Category: B. See Pregnancy Code at the back of this book.
Animal studies: High dose studies in primates have not revealed teratogenicity or embryotoxicity. Mouse and rat studies using up to twenty (20) times the usual human dose have not shown any toxicity to the embryo or fetus.
Human studies: Adequate studies of pregnant women are not available.
Ask your physician for guidance.

Advisability of Use if Breast-Feeding
Presence of this drug in breast milk: Ceftriaxone is distributed into the milk of nursing mothers.
This drug should be used with caution in nursing mothers.

Habit-Forming Potential:
None.

Effects of Overdosage: This drug is safe over a wide dosage range, however, severe overdoses may increase the likelihood of listed adverse effects.

Possible Effects of Long-Term Use: Symptoms consistant with cholelithiasis (gallstones), Clostridium difficile mediated colitis, overgrowth of nonsusceptible organisms, prolongation of the prothrombin time.

Suggested Periodic Examinations While Taking This Drug (at physician's discretion)
Prothrombin time, CBC (complete blood count), SGOT and SGPT, BUN, creatinine and routine urinalysis.

▷ **While Taking This Drug, Observe the Following**
Foods: No restrictions as this is an IM or IV medication.
Nutritional Support: Some studies have been performed with nutritional support compatibility—we recommend calling the manufacturer's scientific services division for TPN formulation combinations and percent decomposition over time.
Beverages: No restrictions.
▷ *Alcohol:* Severe nausea and vomiting reported rarely. Alcohol also blunts the immune response. Avoid alcohol while taking this drug.
Tobacco Smoking: No interactions expected.
Marijuana Smoking: No interactions expected.
▷ *Other Drugs*
Ceftriaxone may *increase* the effects of
- anticoagulants such as coumadin or heparin.

Ceftriaxone *taken concurrently* with
- alcohol may cause severe nausea and vomiting.
- aminoglycosides may increase the effectiveness of both drugs against certain bacteria. Can be a great therapeutic benefit.
- aminoglycosides may increase the likelihood of kidney damage.
- colistimethate may increase the renal toxicity of colistin.
- cyclosporine may increase the cyclosporin level and toxicity risk.
- ethacrynic acid may increase the risk of kidney damage.
- furosemide may increase renal toxicity.
- methotrexate may decrease the antibiotic effect.

The following drugs may *decrease* the effects of ceftriaxone
- methotrexate.
- probenecid in high dose (1–2 grams).

▷ *Driving, Hazardous Activities:* Rarely cause of dizziness. Restrict activities as necessary.

Aviation Note: The use of this drug may be a disqualification for piloting. Consult a designated Aviation Medical Examiner.

Exposure to Sun: No restrictions.

Special Storage Instructions: Refrigeration is preferred once the medicine is reconstituted as the time until expiration is greatly prolonged. Storage at room temperature is possible, but the medicine does not keep as long.

Observe the Following Expiration Times: Because of the complexity of the situation, contact the home IV service or hospital who provided the IV solutions to you.

CEFUROXIME (sef yur OX eem)

Introduced: 1976   **Prescription:** USA: Yes   **Available as Generic:** Yes   **Class:** Antibiotic, cephalosporins   **Controlled Drug:** USA: No
Brand Name: Ceftin, Kefurox, Zinacef

BENEFITS versus RISKS	
Possible Benefits	*Possible Risks*
EFFECTIVE TREATMENT OF INFECTIONS due to susceptible microorganisms	ALLERGIC REACTIONS mild to severe Drug-induced colitis (rare) Superinfections (see Glossary)

▷ **Principal Uses**

As a Single Drug Product: Uses currently included in FDA approved labeling: (1) Used to treat some infections of the middle ear, bone, joints, wounds, tonsils, throat, bronchial tubes, urinary tract and skin, open fractures and gonorrhea.

Other (unlabeled) generally accepted uses: (1) Transition to an agent taken by mouth (oral) from the intravenous form.

How This Drug Works: This drug destroys susceptible infecting bacteria by interfering with their ability to produce new protective cell walls as they multiply and grow.

Cefuroxime

Available Dosage Forms and Strengths
    Tablets — 125 mg, 250 mg, 500 mg
    Intravenous — 750 mg/10 ml
        — 750 mg/50 ml
        — 750 mg/100 ml
        — 1.5 g/100 ml
        — 1.5 g/50 ml
        — 1.5 g/20 ml

▷ **Usual Adult Dosage Range:** Oral: 250 to 500 mg/12 hrs. Total daily dosage should not exceed 4 grams.
Intravenous: 750 mg to 1.5 grams every 8 hours.
For children:
Oral: 125 mg twice a day, 250 mg twice daily for treatment of otitis media.
Intravenous: Those over 3 months should be given 50 to 100 mg/kg per day divided every 6 to 8 hours. Maximum dose is 4 grams. **Note: Actual dosage and administration schedule must be determined by the physician for each patient individually.**

Conditions Requiring Dosing Adjustments
Liver function: Changes in dose or dosing interval are not anticipated.
Kidney function: Dosage changes needed in severe kidney compromise with a dose of 750 mg once daily in the most compromised kidneys. Dose must be repeated after dialysis as the drug is dialyzable.

▷ **Dosing Instructions:** May be taken on an empty stomach or with food if stomach irritation occurs. The tablet may be crushed and mixed with food (such as applesauce or ice cream) if necessary to facilitate swallowing. (Note: The crushed tablet has a persistent, bitter taste.) Take the full course prescribed.

Usual Duration of Use: Continual use on a regular schedule for 3 to 5 days is needed to see this drug's effectiveness in controlling infections. Response varies with the nature of the infection. Some infections require 10 consecutive days to prevent the development of rheumatic fever. Follow your doctor's advice.

▷ **This Drug Should Not Be Taken If**
- you are allergic to cephalosporins (see Drug Class).

▷ **Inform Your Physician Before Taking This Drug If**
- you are allergic to penicillins (see Drug Class).
- you have a history of regional enteritis or ulcerative colitis.
- you have a history of low white blood cell counts.
- you have impaired kidney function.

Possible Side-Effects (natural, expected and unavoidable drug actions)
Superinfections (see Glossary): vaginitis (1.9%).

▷ **Possible Adverse Effects** (unusual, unexpected and infrequent reactions)
If any of the following develop, consult your physician promptly for guidance.
Mild Adverse Effects
Allergic Reactions: Skin rash (0.6%), hives (0.2%), itching (0.3%).
Nausea (2.4%), vomiting (2.0%), loose stools (1.3%), mild diarrhea (3.5%).
Headache (0.7%), dizziness (0.2%).

Cefuroxime

Serious Adverse Effects
Severe diarrhea, possibly a sign of colitis caused by the drug (rare).
Low white blood cell counts.
Thrombophlebitis with the intravenous form (rare).

▷ **Possible Effects on Sexual Function:** None reported.

▷ **Adverse Effects That May Mimic Natural Diseases or Disorders**
Skin rash may resemble measles.

Possible Effects on Laboratory Tests
White blood cell counts: decreased (very rare).
Liver function tests: increased liver enzymes (ALT/GPT, AST/GOT) in people with impaired liver function.

CAUTION
This drug can cause a false positive test result for urine sugar when using Clinitest tablets, Benedict's solution or Fehling's solution.

Precautions for Use
By Infants and Children: The usual dose is 125 mg/12 hours. For middle ear infection, the recommended dose for those under 2 years of age is 125 mg/12 hours, and 250 mg/12 hours for those over 2 years of age.
By Those over 60 Years of Age: Must be individualized based on kidney function. Skin changes may predispose to severe and prolonged itching in the genital and anal regions. Such reactions should be reported promptly.

▷ **Advisability of Use During Pregnancy**
Pregnancy Category: B. See Pregnancy Code at the back of this book.
Animal studies: No birth defects reported in mouse and rat studies.
Human studies: Adequate studies of pregnant women are not available.
Generally considered to be safe. Ask physician for guidance.

Advisability of Use if Breast-Feeding
Presence of this drug in breast milk: Yes, in small amounts.
Ask your doctor for help.

Habit-Forming Potential: None.

Effects of Overdosage: Nausea, vomiting, stomach cramps and/or diarrhea.

Possible Effects of Long-Term Use: Superinfections (see Glossary).

Suggested Periodic Examinations While Taking This Drug (at physician's discretion)
None.

▷ **While Taking This Drug, Observe the Following**
Foods: No restrictions. Food enhances the absorption of this drug.
Beverages: No restrictions. May be taken with milk.

▷ *Alcohol:* No interactions expected.
Tobacco Smoking: No interactions expected.

▷ *Other Drugs*
Cefuroxime ***taken concurrently*** with
- aminoglycoside antibiotics (see Drug Class) may result in increased risk of kidney toxicity.
- birth control pills (oral contraceptives) may result in loss of contraception and pregnancy.
- probenecid (Benemid) will cause higher blood levels and prolonged effect.

▷ *Driving, Hazardous Activities:* Usually no restrictions. Observe for the rare occurrence of dizziness.
Aviation Note: The use of this drug **may be a disqualification** for piloting. Consult a designated Aviation Medical Examiner.
Exposure to Sun: No restrictions.

CEPHALEXIN (sef a LEX in)

Introduced: 1969   **Prescription:** USA: Yes; Canada: Yes   **Available as Generic:** Yes   **Class:** Antibiotic, cephalosporins   **Controlled Drug:** USA: No; Canada: No
Brand Names: ✦Apo-Cephalex, Cefanex, ✦Ceporex, Keflet, Keflex, Keftab, ✦Novo-lexin, ✦Nu-Cephalex

BENEFITS versus RISKS	
Possible Benefits	*Possible Risks*
EFFECTIVE TREATMENT OF INFECTIONS due to susceptible microorganisms	ALLERGIC REACTIONS mild to severe Drug-induced colitis (rare) Hemolytic anemia (rare) Superinfections (see Glossary)

▷ **Principal Uses**
As a Single Drug Product: Uses currently included in FDA approved labeling: (1) To treat certain infections of the skin and skin structures, the upper respiratory tract (including middle ear infections and "strep" throat), the genitourinary tract, prostate infections and certain infections involving bones and joints.
Other (unlabeled) generally accepted uses: (1) May have a role in preventing infections from animal bites; (2) can have a role in treating Streptococcal infections in patients who are penicillin allergic.

How This Drug Works: This drug destroys susceptible infecting bacteria by interfering with their ability to produce new protective cell walls as they multiply and grow.

Available Dosage Forms and Strengths
Capsules — 250 mg, 500 mg
Oral suspension — 125 mg, 250 mg per 5-ml teaspoonful
Pediatric oral suspension — 100 mg per ml
Tablets — 250 mg, 500 mg, 1000 mg (1 gram)

▷ **Usual Adult Dosage Range:** 250 to 500 mg/6 hours. Total daily dose should not exceed 4 grams.
Use in children: 25 to 50 mg/kg per day in 2 to 4 divided doses. Maximum dose is 4 grams (4,000 mg).
For otitis media: 75–100 mg/kg per day in 4 divided doses. **Note: Actual dosage and administration schedule must be determined by the physician for each patient individually.**

Conditions Requiring Dosing Adjustments
Liver function: The liver is not significantly involved in the elimination of this drug.

Kidney function: For creatinine clearances (CrCl) of 10–50 ml/min, give the usual dose every 6 hours. For CrCl less than 10 ml/min, give the usual dose every 8–12 hours.

▷ **Dosing Instructions:** May be taken on an empty stomach or with food if stomach irritation occurs. Capsule may be opened and tablet may be crushed for administration. Shake suspension well before measuring dose. Take the full course prescribed.

Usual Duration of Use: Continual use on a regular schedule for 3 to 5 days is usually necessary to determine this drug's effectiveness in controlling the infection under treatment. Response varies with the nature of the infection. Total treatment time will vary from 1 to 4 weeks. Certain infections require that this drug be taken for 10 consecutive days to prevent the development of rheumatic fever. Follow your physician's instructions regarding duration of use.

▷ **This Drug Should Not Be Taken If**
- you are allergic to any cephalosporin antibiotic (see Drug Class).

▷ **Inform Your Physician Before Taking This Drug If**
- you have a history of allergy to any form of penicillin (see Drug Class).
- you have a history of regional enteritis or ulcerative colitis.
- you have impaired kidney function.
- you have a history of a blood cell disorder, especially hemolytic anemia.
- you have a seizure disorder.
- you have a hearing disorder.

Possible Side-Effects (natural, expected and unavoidable drug actions)
Superinfections (see Glossary).

▷ **Possible Adverse Effects** (unusual, unexpected and infrequent reactions)
If any of the following develop, consult your physician promptly for guidance.

Mild Adverse Effects
Allergic Reactions: Skin rash (0.8%), itching, hives (0.3%).
Headache, drowsiness, dizziness.
Irritation of mouth or tongue, indigestion, stomach cramping, nausea, vomiting (1.8%), diarrhea (1.1%).

Serious Adverse Effects
Allergic Reactions: Drug fever (see Glossary), joint aches and pains, anaphylactic reaction (see Glossary).
Idiosyncratic Reactions: Minor and temporary changes in white blood cell counts and liver function tests (infrequent).
Genital itching (may represent a fungus superinfection).
Severe diarrhea, possibly indicating a drug-induced form of colitis (rare).
Low white blood cells.
Hemolytic anemia (rare).

▷ **Possible Effects on Sexual Function:** None reported.

▷ **Adverse Effects That May Mimic Natural Diseases or Disorders**
Skin rash and fever may resemble measles.

Possible Effects on Laboratory Tests
Complete blood cell counts: decreased white blood cells, increased eosinophils.

184 Cephalexin

Urine sugar tests: false positive results with Benedict's solution, Fehling's solution and Clinitest.

CAUTION
1. In the management of diabetes it should be noted that this drug can cause a false positive test result for urine sugar when using Clinitest tablets, Benedict's solution or Fehling's solution, but not with Tes-Tape.
2. Do not use this drug concurrently with other antibiotics such as erythromycin or tetracyclines.

Precautions for Use

By Infants and Children: Not recommended for use in infants less than 1 year old. Monitor allergic children closely for evidence of developing allergy to this drug.

By Those over 60 Years of Age: Dosage must be carefully individualized and based upon evaluation of kidney function. Natural changes in the skin may predispose to severe and prolonged itching reactions in the genital and anal regions. Such reactions should be reported promptly.

▷ **Advisability of Use During Pregnancy**

Pregnancy Category: B. See Pregnancy Code at the back of this book.
Animal studies: No birth defects reported.
Human studies: Information from adequate studies of pregnant women is not available.
Generally considered to be safe. Ask physician for guidance.

Advisability of Use if Breast-Feeding
Presence of this drug in breast milk: Yes, in small amounts.
Ask your doctor for guidance.

Habit-Forming Potential: None.

Effects of Overdosage: Nausea, vomiting, stomach cramps and/or diarrhea, seizures.

Possible Effects of Long-Term Use: Superinfections (see Glossary).

Suggested Periodic Examinations While Taking This Drug (at physician's discretion)
Complete blood cell counts. Liver and kidney function tests.

▷ **While Taking This Drug, Observe the Following**
Foods: No restrictions.
Beverages: No restrictions. May be taken with milk.
▷ *Alcohol:* No interactions expected.
Tobacco Smoking: No interactions expected.
▷ *Other Drugs*
Cephalexin *taken concurrently* with
- aminoglycoside antibiotics (see Drug Classes) as there is an increased risk of kidney toxicity.
- birth control pills (oral contraceptives) may cause loss of contraception and pregnancy.
- cholestyramine as it will result in decreased cephalexin absorption and lower benefit as an antibiotic.
- probenecid (Benemid) will slow the elimination of cephalexin, resulting in higher blood levels and prolonged effect.

▷ *Driving, Hazardous Activities:* Usually no restrictions. Use caution if drowsiness or dizziness occurs.

Aviation Note: The use of this drug *may be a disqualification* for piloting. Consult a designated Aviation Medical Examiner.
Exposure to Sun: No restrictions.
Special Storage Instructions: Oral suspension should be refrigerated.
Observe the Following Expiration Times: Do not take the oral suspension of this drug if it is older than 14 days.

CHLORAMBUCIL (klor AM byu sil)

Introduced: 1974   **Prescription:** USA: Yes; Canada: Yes   **Available as Generic:** USA: No; Canada: No   **Class:** Anticancer, immunosuppressant
Controlled Drug: USA: No; Canada: No
Brand Name: Leukeran

BENEFITS versus RISKS	
Possible Benefits	*Possible Risks*
EFFECTIVE PALLIATIVE TREATMENT FOR CHRONIC LYMPHOCYTIC LEUKEMIA	BONE MARROW DEPRESSION (see Glossary)
EFFECTIVE PALLIATIVE TREATMENT FOR HODGKIN'S DISEASE AND OTHER LYMPHOMAS	INCREASED SUSCEPTIBILITY TO INFECTIONS
	CENTRAL NERVOUS SYSTEM TOXICITY
	Male and female sterility
Immunosuppression of nephrotic syndrome	Drug-induced liver damage
	Drug-induced lung damage
Immunosuppression of rheumatoid arthritis	Development of secondary cancers

▷ **Principal Uses**
  As a Single Drug Product: Uses currently included in FDA approved labeling: Treats (1) chronic lymphocytic leukemia; (2) Hodgkin's lymphoma and other malignant lymphomas.
  Other (unlabeled) generally accepted uses: (1) Hairy cell leukemia; (2) multiple myeloma; (3) Letterer-Siwe disease; (4) nephrotic syndrome; (5) ovarian cancer; (6) may have a role in rheumatoid arthritis; (7) can have a short-term role in treating systemic lupus erythematosus.
How This Drug Works: This drug blocks genetic activity (impairs DNA and RNA), and inhibits production of essential proteins. This kills cancerous cells.
Available Dosage Forms and Strengths
  Tablets — 2 mg
▷ **Usual Adult Dosage Range:** For leukemia and lymphoma: Initially (induction phase of 3–6 weeks) 0.1 to 0.2 mg per kilogram of body weight daily, or 3 to 6 mg per square meter of body surface daily (usually 4 to 10 mg daily) as a single dose or in divided doses. Maintenance dose: 2–4 mg per day or a maximum of 0.1 mg/kg daily.
  For immunosuppression: 0.1 to 0.2 mg per kilogram of body weight daily, in a single dose, for 8 to 12 weeks.
Note: Actual dosage and administration schedule must be determined by the physician for each patient individually.

Chlorambucil

Conditions Requiring Dosing Adjustments
  Liver function: Can cause liver damage. Used with extreme caution in liver compromise.
  Kidney function: Can cause bladder inflammation; caution advised in compromised urine outflow.

▷ **Dosing Instructions:** Tablet may be crushed, however food may decrease absorption by up to 20%. Avoid this combination. See your doctor if vomiting prevents you from taking chlorambucil.

Usual Duration of Use: Use on a regular schedule for 3 to 4 weeks is usually required to see this drug's effectiveness in controlling leukemia or lymphoma; several months are needed to assess immunosuppression. Long-term use requires periodic evaluation of response and dose changes.

▷ **This Drug Should Not Be Taken If**
- you have had an allergic reaction to it previously.
- you have a significant degree of bone marrow depression.
- you currently have an uncontrolled infection.

▷ **Inform Your Physician Before Taking This Drug If**
- you are allergic to melphalan (Alkeran).
- you are pregnant, planning pregnancy, or breast-feeding.
- you have a history of bone marrow depression or a blood cell disorder.
- you have a history of gout or urate kidney stones.
- you have a seizure disorder of any kind.
- you have a history of porphyria.
- you have impaired liver or kidney function.
- you have had cancer chemotherapy or radiation therapy previously.
- you are taking drugs than can impair your immunity.
- you have recently had or been exposed to chicken pox or herpes zoster.

Possible Side-Effects (natural, expected and unavoidable drug actions)
  Decreased white blood cell and platelet counts.
  Decreased immunity, susceptibility to infections.
  Increased blood levels of uric acid, formation of kidney stones.

▷ **Possible Adverse Effects** (unusual, unexpected and infrequent reactions)
  If any of the following develop, consult your physician promptly for guidance.

Mild Adverse Effects
  Allergic Reactions: Skin rash, itching, drug fever (see Glossary).
  Mouth and lip sores, nausea, vomiting.

Serious Adverse Effects
  Allergic Reactions: Drug-induced hepatitis with jaundice.
  Cataract formation with high-dose usage.
  Central nervous system toxicity: agitation, confusion, hallucinations, seizures, tremors, paralysis.
  Peripheral neuritis (see Glossary).
  Lung damage: Cough, shortness of breath.
  Bone marrow damage, aplastic anemia (see Glossary).
  Leukemia (may depend on dose and length of treatment).
  Liver damage (hepatotoxicity and jaundice).
  Severe skin damage (toxic epidermal necrolysis).

Chlorambucil

▷ **Possible Effects on Sexual Function:** Can inhibit reproduction: Stops sperm production (male sterility); altered menstrual patterns, blocks ovulation and menstruation (female sterility).

Possible Delayed Adverse Effects: Severe bone marrow depression can happen after the drug has been stopped.
Secondary cancers (especially leukemia) have been reported.
Lung damage (pulmonary fibrosis).

▷ **Adverse Effects That May Mimic Natural Diseases or Disorders**
Drug-induced seizures may suggest epilepsy.
Drug-induced jaundice may suggest viral hepatitis.

Natural Diseases or Disorders That May Be Activated by This Drug
Gout, urate kidney stones, porphyria, latent epilepsy.

Possible Effects on Laboratory Tests
Complete blood counts: decreased red cells, hemoglobin, white cells and platelets.
Blood uric acid level: increased.
Liver function tests: increased liver enzymes (ALT/GPT, AST/GOT), increased bilirubin, increased icterus index.
Sperm counts: decreased or absent.

CAUTION

1. Long-term use of this drug in noncancerous conditions requires extreme caution. Risks include permanent sterility, lung damage, and the development of secondary cancers. It should only be used where less toxic medicines have failed.
2. It is advisable to have any needed dental work done prior to using this drug. The bone marrow depression could lead to gum infection, excessive bleeding and delayed healing.
3. If gout develops, allopurinol is the drug of choice for chlorambucil-caused gout symptoms.
4. This drug impairs the body's ability to produce protective antibodies. Both killed virus vaccines and live virus vaccines will not work. There is an increased risk that live virus vaccines may actually cause infection.

Three months to 1 year is needed for the immune system to recover after stopping this and similar drugs. Family members or people in close contact with chlorambucil patients should not receive the oral poliovirus vaccine. This eliminates risk of accidental exposure.

5. Immediately report: Onset of infection, unusual bruising or bleeding, excessive fatigue, tremors or muscle twitching, difficulty walking, loss of appetite with nausea or vomiting.
6. It is advisable to avoid pregnancy while taking this drug. A nonhormonal method of contraception is recommended. Call your doctor promptly if you think pregnancy has occurred.

Precautions for Use
By Infants and Children: Dosage schedules and treatment monitoring should be supervised by a qualified pediatrician.
Children with nephrotic syndrome can be more prone to drug-induced seizures.

188 Chloroambucil

By Those over 60 Years of Age: Watch closely for central nervous system toxicity.

▷ **Advisability of Use During Pregnancy**
Pregnancy Category:
D. See Pregnancy Code at the back of this book.
Animal studies: Rat studies reveal drug associated defects of the nervous system, palate, skeleton and urogenital system.
Human studies: Adequate studies of pregnant women are not available. There are two known cases of an infant born with an absent kidney and ureter following exposure to this drug during early pregnancy.
If possible, this drug should be avoided during pregnancy, especially the first 3 months.
A nonhormonal contraceptive is generally advisable during treatment with this and similar drugs.

Advisability of Use if Breast-Feeding
Presence of this drug in breast milk: Unknown.
Avoid drug or refrain from nursing.

Habit-Forming Potential: None.

Effects of Overdosage: Fatigue, weakness, fever, sore throat, bruising, agitation, unstable gait, seizures.

Possible Effects of Long-Term Use: Permanent sterility; secondary cancers (leukemia); lung damage (pulmonary fibrosis).

Suggested Periodic Examinations While Taking This Drug (at physician's discretion)
Before drug treatment and *periodically* during drug use: Complete blood counts, uric acid levels, liver function tests, sperm counts.

▷ **While Taking This Drug, Observe the Following**
Foods: No restrictions.
Beverages: No restrictions. May be taken with milk. It is advisable to drink 2 to 3 quarts of liquids daily to reduce the risk of kidney stone formation.
▷ *Alcohol:* Use with caution. Avoid if platelet counts are low and there is a risk of stomach bleeding.
Tobacco Smoking: No interactions expected.
Marijuana Smoking: Best avoided. This could increase the risk of central nervous system toxicity.
▷ *Other Drugs*
Chlorambucil **taken concurrently** with
- aspirin may increase the risk of bruising or bleeding; the platelet-reduction effects of chlorambucil and the antiplatelet action of aspirin are additive; avoid aspirin while taking chlorambucil.
- antidepressant or antipsychotic (neuroleptic) drugs require careful monitoring; these drugs lower the seizure threshold and increase the risk of chlorambucil-induced seizures.
- other immunosuppressant drugs can increase the risk of infection and the development of secondary cancers.

▷ *Driving, Hazardous Activities:*
This drug may cause nervous agitation, confusion, hallucinations or seizures. Restrict activities as necessary.

Aviation Note:
   The use of this drug **may be a disqualification** for piloting. Consult a designated Aviation Medical Examiner.
Exposure to Sun: No restrictions.
Discontinuation: Whether used as an anticancer drug or as an immunosuppressant, many factors will determine when and how this drug should be stopped. In order to get the greatest benefit, follow your doctor's advice.

CHLORAMPHENICOL (klor am FEN i kohl)

Introduced: 1947 **Prescription:** USA: Yes; Canada: Yes **Available as Generic:** USA: Yes; Canada: No **Class:** Antibiotic **Controlled Drug:** USA: No; Canada: No

Brand Names: Ak-Chlor, Chloracol, Chloromycetin, Chlorofair, Chloroptic, Chloroptic SOP, Econochlor, ✦Elase-Chloromycetin, ✦Fenicol, I-Chlor, ✦Isopto Fenicol, ✦Minims, ✦Nova-Phenicol, ✦Novochlorocap, ✦Ocu-Chlor, Ophthochlor, ✦Ophtho-Chloram, Ophthocort, ✦Pentamycetin, ✦PMS-Chloramphenicol, ✦Sopamycetin, ✦Sopamycetin/HC

BENEFITS versus RISKS

Possible Benefits	*Possible Risks*
VERY EFFECTIVE TREATMENT OF INFECTIONS due to susceptible microorganisms	BONE MARROW DEPRESSION APLASTIC ANEMIA (see Glossary) Peripheral neuritis (see Glossary) Liver damage, jaundice

---

▷ **Principal Uses**
   As a Single Drug Product: Uses currently included in FDA approved labeling: (1) Very effective in a broad spectrum of serious infections. However, because of serious toxicity (fatal aplastic anemia), its is now reserved for life-threatening (such as meningitis) infections caused by resistant organisms, and for infections in people who cannot tolerate other appropriate anti-infective drugs; (2) used in eye (intraocular) infections.
   Other (unlabeled) generally accepted uses: (1) May have a role in prevention of plague, (2) can help when applied topically to pressure sores.

How This Drug Works: This drug prevents the growth and multiplication of susceptible microorganisms by interfering with their formation of essential proteins.

Available Dosage Forms and Strengths
   Capsules — 250 mg, 500 mg
   Cream — 1%
   Eye/ear solutions — 0.5%
   Eye ointment — 1%
   Injection — 100 mg per ml
   Oral suspension — 150 mg per 5-ml teaspoonful

▷ **Usual Adult Dosage Range:** Total daily dose is 250 mg for each 10 pounds of body weight, given in 4 equally divided doses, 6 hours apart. Total daily dose should not exceed 500 mg for each 10 pounds of body weight. **Note:**

Chloramphenicol

Actual dosage and administration schedule must be determined by the physician for each patient individually.

Conditions Requiring Dosing Adjustments
Liver function: Must be adjusted in liver failure based on blood levels.
Kidney function: Adjustments in dose or dosing interval are suggested based on blood levels.

▷ **Dosing Instructions:** Capsule may be opened to take it, and should be taken with a full glass of water on an empty stomach, 1 hour before or 2 hours after eating. Shake oral suspension well before measuring dose.

Usual Duration of Use: Use on a regular schedule for 3 to 5 days is needed to see this drug's effectiveness in controlling the infection. Limit use to the time required to treat the infection. Avoid repeated courses if possible.

▷ **This Drug Should Not Be Taken If**
- you have had an allergic reaction to it previously.
- you have an active blood cell or bone marrow disorder.
- for mild or trivial infections such as a sore throat.
- you are pregnant.
- the ophthalmic suspension has been prescribed in a patient with a viral disease of the cornea such as Herpes simplex or mycobacterial or fungal eye disease.
- prescribed for a premature or newborn infant (under 2 weeks of age).

▷ **Inform Your Physician Before Taking This Drug If**
- you have a history of a blood cell or bone marrow disorder.
- you have impaired liver or kidney function.
- you are taking anticoagulants.
- you have a G-6-PD deficiency (ask your doctor).
- you are planning pregnancy.

Possible Side-Effects (natural, expected and unavoidable drug actions)
Superinfections (see Glossary).

▷ **Possible Adverse Effects** (unusual, unexpected and infrequent reactions)
If any of the following develop, consult your physician promptly for guidance.

Mild Adverse Effects
Allergic Reactions: Skin rashes, hives, swelling of face or extremities, fever.
Headache, confusion, peripheral neuritis (see Glossary)—numbness, pain, weakness in hands and/or feet.
Sore mouth or tongue, "black tongue," nausea, vomiting, diarrhea.

Serious Adverse Effects
Allergic Reactions: Anaphylactic reaction (see Glossary), liver damage with jaundice (rare).
Bone marrow depression (see Glossary)—fatigue, weakness, fever, sore throat, abnormal bleeding or bruising.
Gray baby syndrome—heart and lung failure (cardiovascular-respiratory collapse).
Peripheral neuritis (with prolonged therapy).
Porphyria (rare).
Acidosis (metabolic).

Pseudomembranous colitis (rare).
Liver toxicity (rare).
Severe skin syndrome (Stevens-Johnson).
Optic neuritis (often dose related).

▷ **Possible Effects on Sexual Function:** None reported.

▷ **Adverse Effects That May Mimic Natural Diseases or Disorders**
Liver reaction with jaundice may suggest viral hepatitis.

Possible Effects on Laboratory Tests
Complete blood counts: decreased red cells, hemoglobin, white cells and platelets; increased white cells; increased eosinophils.
Prothrombin time: increased.
Blood glucose level: decreased.
Liver function tests: increased liver enzymes (ALT/GPT, AST/GOT, alkaline phosphatase), increased bilirubin.
Fecal occult blood: positive (intestinal bleeding or drug-induced colitis).

CAUTION
1. This drug can cause serious bone marrow depression and aplastic anemia (see Glossary). Must not be used to treat trivial infections or as a preventive medication. Restricted to serious or life-threatening infections not responding to other anti-infective drugs.
2. Troublesome and persistent diarrhea can develop. If diarrhea persists for more than 24 hours, stop this drug and call your doctor.

Precautions for Use
By Infants and Children: Follow prescribed dosage exactly. Blood cell counts should be checked twice a week. Long-term use of this drug can cause optic neuritis; however, this may be prevented by taking vitamin B complex. Idiosyncratic aplastic anemia is rare (1 in 40,000 users), but may occur long after (weeks or months) this drug is stopped.

By Those over 60 Years of Age: The natural decline in kidney function after 60 may require decreased doses. Skin changes after 60 may predispose to severe itching reactions in the genital and anal regions. Report such reactions promptly.

▷ **Advisability of Use During Pregnancy**
Pregnancy Category: C. See Pregnancy Code at the back of this book.
Animal studies: Results are inconclusive.
Human studies: Adequate studies of pregnant women are not available. Limited data (348 exposures) indicate that this drug does not cause birth defects. However, it has been shown to be potentially toxic for the fetus and newborn. Ask your physician for help.

Advisability of Use if Breast-Feeding
Presence of this drug in breast milk: Yes.
Avoid drug or refrain from nursing.

Habit-Forming Potential: None.

Effects of Overdosage: Possible nausea, vomiting, diarrhea.

Possible Effects of Long-Term Use: Superinfections, impaired vision, peripheral neuritis and bone marrow depression.

Suggested Periodic Examinations While Taking This Drug (at physician's discretion)
Complete blood counts—before treatment is started and every 2 to 3 days during administration of drug.
Liver and kidney function tests.

▷ **While Taking This Drug, Observe the Following**
Foods: No restrictions.
Nutritional Support: Supplemental vitamins B-2, B-6 and B-12 are recommended.
Beverages: No restrictions. May be taken with milk.

▷ *Alcohol:* Avoid completely if you have liver disease. Use caution: Some people may develop a disulfiramlike reaction (see Glossary).
Tobacco Smoking: No interactions expected.

▷ *Other Drugs*
Chloramphenicol may *increase* the effects of
- oral anticoagulants (Coumadin, dicumarol, etc.), and increase the risk of bleeding.
- barbiturates (phenobarbital, etc.), and cause excessive sedation.
- phenytoin (Dilantin), and cause phenytoin toxicity.
- sulfonylureas (Diabinese, Dymelor, Orinase, Tolinase), and cause hypoglycemia (see Glossary).

Chloramphenicol may *decrease* the effects of
- some cephalosporins, especially ceftazidime.
- cyclophosphamide.
- iron preparations, used to treat anemia.
- penicillins.
- vitamin B-12.

The following drugs may *decrease* the effects of chloramphenicol
- barbiturates (phenobarbital, etc.).
- rifibutin (Mycobutin).
- rifampin (Rifadin, Rimactane, etc.).

▷ *Driving, Hazardous Activities:* Usually no restrictions. Watch for rare occurrence of confusion, and restrict activities accordingly.
Aviation Note: The use of this drug *may be a disqualification* for piloting. Consult a designated Aviation Medical Examiner.
Exposure to Sun: No restrictions.

CHLOROQUINE (KLOR oh kwin)

Introduced: 1964   **Prescription:** USA: Yes; Canada: Yes   **Available as Generic:** USA: Yes; Canada: No   **Class:** Antiamebic, antimalarial, lupus suppressant, rheumatoid arthritis suppressant   **Controlled Drug:** USA: No; Canada: No

Brand Name: Aralen

Warning:
The brand names Aralen and Arlidin are similar and can be mistaken for each other; this can lead to serious medication errors. These names represent very different drugs. Verify that you are taking the correct drug.

Chloroquine

BENEFITS versus RISKS	
Possible Benefits	*Possible Risks*
EFFECTIVE PREVENTION AND TREATMENT OF CERTAIN FORMS OF MALARIA	INFREQUENT BUT SERIOUS DAMAGE OF CORNEAL AND RETINAL EYE TISSUES
EFFECTIVE COMBINATION TREATMENT OF SOME FORMS OF AMEBIC INFECTION	RARE BUT SERIOUS BONE MARROW DEPRESSION; aplastic anemia, deficient white blood cells and platelets
Possibly effective in acute and chronic rheumatoid arthritis and juvenile arthritis	Rare heart muscle damage
	Rare ear damage; hearing loss, ringing in ears
Possibly effective in the management of chronic discoid and systemic lupus erythematosus	Rare eye damage

▷ **Principal Uses**
As a Single Drug Product: Uses currently included in FDA approved labeling: (1) treatment of acute attacks of certain types of malarial infection; (2) treatment for certain forms of amebic infection.
Other (unlabeled) generally accepted uses: (1) reduce disease activity in rheumatoid and juvenile arthritis; (2) suppress disease activity in certain types of lupus erythematosus; (3) treatment of sarcoidosis, polymorphous light eruption and porphyria; (4) prevention of malaria in travelers.

How This Drug Works: In treating malaria and amebiasis, this drug impairs the function of DNA in the protozoa that cause these diseases.
As an antiarthritic and antilupus drug, it acts as a mild immunosuppressant. It accumulates in white blood cells and blocks many enzymes involved in tissue destruction.

Available Dosage Forms and Strengths
Injection — 50 mg per ml
Tablets — 250 mg, 500 mg

▷ **Usual Adult Dosage Range:** For malaria suppression: 500 mg once every 7 days.
For malaria treatment: Initially 1 gram, followed by 500 mg in 6 to 8 hours; then 500 mg once a day on the second and third days.
For amebiasis (other than intestinal): Initially 250 mg 4 times daily for 2 days; then 250 mg 2 times daily for 2 to 3 weeks.
For rheumatoid arthritis: Up to 4 mg per kilogram of lean body weight daily.
For lupus erythematosus: Up to 4 mg per kilogram of lean body weight daily.
Note: Actual dosage and administration schedule must be determined by the physician for each patient individually.

Conditions Requiring Dosing Adjustments
Liver function: Blood levels are needed, and the dose should be adjusted (probably decreased) appropriately.
Kidney function: In severe kidney failure 50% of the normal dose should be used. If therapy is extended, 50 to 100 mg of chloroquine base should be given daily.

▷ **Dosing Instructions:** Tablet may be crushed and taken with food or milk to reduce stomach irritation. Take full course of treatment as prescribed.

Chloroquine

Note: For malaria prevention, begin medication 2 weeks before entering malarious area; continue medication while in the area and for 4 weeks after leaving the area.

For treating arthritis and lupus, take medication on a regular schedule daily; use for 6 months may be needed to see peak effect.

Usual Duration of Use: Use on a regular schedule for 2 weeks before exposure, during period of exposure, and 4 weeks after exposure is needed to realize effectiveness in preventing malaria. Use on a regular schedule for up to 6 months may be required to evaluate benefits in treating rheumatoid arthritis and lupus erythematosus. If improvement is not achieved within this time, this drug should be stopped. Long-term use (months to years) requires periodic physician evaluation of response and dose adjustments.

Possible Advantages of This Drug
May be more effective than hydroxychloroquine in some cases of lupus erythematosus.

▷ **This Drug Should Not Be Taken If**
- you have an allergy to chloroquine or hydroxychloroquine.
- you have an active bone marrow or blood cell disorder.
- you have significant cardiomyopathy.

▷ **Inform Your Physician Before Taking This Drug If**
- you are pregnant or planning pregnancy.
- you have bone marrow depression or a blood cell disorder.
- you have a deficiency of glucose-6-phosphate dehydrogenase.
- you have any eye disorder, especially disease of the cornea or retina, or visual field changes.
- you have a history of movement disorders.
- you have a history of mental illness.
- you have impaired hearing or ringing in the ears.
- you have a seizure disorder.
- you have a history of peripheral neuritis.
- you have low blood pressure or a heart rhythm disorder.
- you have a history of peptic ulcer disease, Crohn's disease or ulcerative colitis.
- you have impaired liver or kidney function or porphyria.
- you have any form of psoriasis.
- you are taking antacids, cimetidine or penicillamine.

Possible Side-Effects (natural, expected and unavoidable drug actions)
Light-headedness (low blood pressure); blue-black discoloration of skin, fingernails, or mouth lining with long-term use.

▷ **Possible Adverse Effects** (unusual, unexpected and infrequent reactions)
If any of the following develop, consult your physician promptly for guidance.

Mild Adverse Effects
Allergic Reactions: Skin rash, itching (more common in African-Americans).
Loss of hair color, loss of hair.
Headache, blurring of near vision (reading), ringing in ears.
Loss of appetite, nausea, vomiting, stomach cramps, diarrhea.

Serious Adverse Effects
    Allergic Reactions: Severe skin rash (erythema multiforme).
    Idiosyncratic Reactions: Hemolytic anemia in those with glucose-6-phosphate dehydrogenase deficiency in red blood cells.
    Emotional or psychotic mental changes; seizures.
    Movement disorders (ataxia, dyskinesias).
    Loss of hearing.
    Excessive muscle weakness.
    Eye damage, (cornea and retina), with significant impairment of vision.
    Heart rhythm abnormalities.
    Aplastic anemia (see Glossary): abnormally low red cells (fatigue and weakness), low white blood cell counts (fever, sore throat, infections), abnormally low platelets (abnormal bruising or bleeding).

▷ **Possible Effects on Sexual Function:** None reported.

Possible Delayed Adverse Effects: Retinal damage (reports of development 7 years after stopping) is more likely to occur following high-dose and/or long-term use.

▷ **Adverse Effects That May Mimic Natural Diseases or Disorders**
    Central nervous system toxicity mimics unrelated neuropsychiatric disorder. Seizures may suggest the onset of epilepsy.

Natural Diseases or Disorders That May Be Activated by This Drug
    Porphyria, psoriasis.

Possible Effects on Laboratory Tests
    Complete blood counts: decreased red cells, hemoglobin, white cells and platelets.
    Liver function tests: increased liver enzymes (AST/GOT) and bilirubin.
    Urine tests for drug abuse: *initial* test result may be falsely **positive**; *confirmatory* test will be **negative**. (Test results depend upon amount of drug taken and testing method used.)
    Electrocardiogram: conduction abnormalities, prolonged QRS interval, T wave changes, heart block.

CAUTION
    1. Will not prevent relapses in certain types of malaria. Ask your doctor for advice.
    2. Not effective in treating acute amebic dysentery (intestinal infection) or asymptomatic carriers.
    3. High-dose and/or long-term use of this drug may cause irreversible retinal damage; such use may also cause hearing loss due to nerve damage. Promptly report any vision or hearing changes.

Precautions for Use
    By Infants and Children: This age group is very sensitive to the effects of this drug. Dosages should be chosen and therapy monitored by a qualified pediatrician.
    By Those over 60 Years of Age: Reduced tolerance for high-dose and/or long-term use. Watch for behavioral changes, low blood pressure, heart rhythm disturbances, muscle weakness and changes in vision or hearing.

▷ **Advisability of Use During Pregnancy**
    Pregnancy Category:
    C. See Pregnancy Code at the back of this book.

196 Chloroquine

Animal studies: 47% of rat fetuses revealed undeveloped or partially developed eyes.

Human studies: Adequate studies of pregnant women are not available. A 1964 report includes drug-induced congenital deafness, retinal damage, gait instability and asymmetric body growth. A 1991 study of use in systemic lupus erythematosus concluded that the benefit outweighed the fetal risk.

Avoid use during pregnancy except for the suppression or treatment of malaria or amebic infection of the liver. Seek your doctor's advice.

Advisability of Use if Breast-Feeding
Presence of this drug in breast milk: Yes.
Avoid drug or refrain from nursing.

Habit-Forming Potential: None.

Effects of Overdosage: Drowsiness, headache, blurred vision, excitability, low blood pressure, seizures, coma.

Possible Effects of Long-Term Use: Irreversible eye damage (cornea and retina), hearing loss, myocarditis, muscle weakness, aplastic anemia.

Suggested Periodic Examinations While Taking This Drug (at physician's discretion)

Complete blood counts; liver and kidney function tests.
Serial blood pressure readings and electrocardiograms.
Neurological examinations for significant muscle weakness.
Complete eye examinations before starting high-dose or long-term treatment, then every 3 to 6 months during drug use.
Hearing tests as indicated.

▷ **While Taking This Drug, Observe the Following**
Foods: No restrictions.
Beverages: No restrictions. May be taken with milk.
▷ *Alcohol:* Use sparingly to minimize stomach irritation.
Tobacco Smoking: No interactions expected.
▷ *Other Drugs*
Chloroquine may *increase* the effects of
• cyclosporine and increase risk of kidney toxicity.
• penicillamine (Cuprimine, Depen), and increase its toxic potential.
Chloroquine may *decrease* the effects of
• Rabies vaccine.
The following drug may *increase* the effects of chloroquine
• cimetidine (Tagamet).
The following drugs may *decrease* the effects of chloroquine
• magnesium salts and antacids.
▷ *Driving, Hazardous Activities:*
This drug may cause light-headedness, blurred vision or impaired hearing. Restrict activities as necessary.
Aviation Note:
The use of this drug **may be a disqualification** for piloting. Consult a designated Aviation Medical Examiner.
Exposure to Sun: This drug may cause photosensitivity (see Glossary).

Discontinuation: This drug should be stopped and prompt evaluation made if: any changes in vision or hearing, seizures, unusual muscle weakness, infection (fever, sore throat, etc.), abnormal bruising or bleeding occurs.

CHLOROTHIAZIDE (klor oh THI a zide)

Introduced: 1957 **Prescription:** USA: Yes **Available as Generic:** USA: Yes **Class:** Antihypertensive, diuretic, thiazides **Controlled Drug:** USA: No
Brand Names: Aldoclor [CD], Diachlor, Diupres [CD], Diurigen, Diuril, SK-Chlorothiazide, ✦Supres [CD]

BENEFITS versus RISKS	
Possible Benefits	*Possible Risks*
EFFECTIVE, WELL-TOLERATED DIURETIC	Loss of body potassium
POSSIBLY EFFECTIVE IN MILD HYPERTENSION	Increased blood sugar
	Increased blood uric acid
ENHANCES EFFECTIVENESS OF OTHER ANTIHYPERTENSIVES	Increased blood calcium
	Rare blood cell disorders
Beneficial in treatment of diabetes insipidus	

Please see the thiazide diuretic profile for further information.

CHLORPROMAZINE (klor PROH ma zeen)

Introduced: 1952 **Prescription:** USA: Yes; Canada: Yes **Available as Generic:** Yes **Class:** Strong tranquilizer, phenothiazines **Controlled Drug:** USA: No; Canada: No
Brand Names: ✦Chlorpromanyl, ✦Largactil, ✦Novochlorpromazine, Ormazine, Promapar, Sonazine, Thorazine, Thorazine SR

BENEFITS versus RISKS	
Possible Benefits	*Possible Risks*
EFFECTIVE CONTROL OF ACUTE MENTAL DISORDERS in the majority of patients	SERIOUS TOXIC EFFECTS ON BRAIN with long-term use
Beneficial effects on thinking, mood and behavior	Liver damage with jaundice (less than 0.5%)
Moderately effective control of nausea and vomiting	Rare blood disorders: hemolytic anemia, abnormally low white blood count
	Eye toxicity

▷ **Principal Uses**

As a Single Drug Product: Uses currently included in FDA-approved labeling: (1) Treats acute and chronic psychotic disorders such as agitated depression, schizophrenia and mania; (2) it can be used for presurgical anxiety; (3) helps reduce symptoms in porphyrias and tetanus; (4) is used to stop

Chlorpromazine

prolonged hiccups; (5) lessens or stops vomiting caused by toxic chemotherapy or a potent drug used to treat fungal infections (amphotericin B). Other (unlabeled) generally accepted uses: (1) Can be of help in complicated drug withdrawal cases; (2) lessens the symptoms of Tourette's syndrome; (3) may be of help in combination therapy of tuberculosis; (4) can be used intravenously after some heart surgery.

How This Drug Works: By inhibiting the action of dopamine, this drug acts to correct an imbalance of nerve impulses found in some mental disorders.

Available Dosage Forms and Strengths
- Capsules, prolonged-action — 30 mg, 75 mg, 150 mg, 200 mg, 300 mg
- Concentrate — 30 mg per ml and 100 mg per ml
- Injection — 25 mg per ml
- Suppositories — 25 mg, 100 mg
- Syrup — 10 mg per 5-ml teaspoonful
- Tablets — 10 mg, 25 mg, 50 mg, 100 mg, 200 mg

▷ **Usual Adult Dosage Range:** Initially 10 to 25 mg 3 or 4 times daily. Dose may be increased by 20 to 50 mg at 3- to 4-day intervals as needed and tolerated. Usual dosage range is 300 to 800 mg daily. Extreme range is 25 to 2000 mg daily. Total daily dosage should not exceed 2000 mg. **Note: Actual dosage and administration schedule must be determined by the physician for each patient individually.**

Conditions Requiring Dosing Adjustments
Liver function: Used with caution and in decreased dose in patients with compromised livers. Can also be a cause of a specific kind of (cholestatic) jaundice.
Kidney function: Blood levels are recommended if used in severe kidney compromise.

▷ **Dosing Instructions:** Tablets may be crushed and taken with or after meals to reduce stomach irritation. Prolonged-action capsules may be opened, but not crushed or chewed.

Usual Duration of Use: Use on a regular schedule for several weeks is usually needed to see this drug's effectiveness in controlling psychotic disorders. If benefits are not seen in 6 weeks, it should be stopped. Long-term use (months to years) requires periodic physician evaluation.

▷ **This Drug Should Not Be Taken If**
- you are allergic to any form of this drug.
- you have active liver disease.
- you have taken a large amount of alcohol or narcotics.
- you have cancer of the breast.
- you have a current blood cell or bone marrow disorder.

▷ **Inform Your Physician Before Taking This Drug If**
- you are allergic or very sensitive to any phenothiazine drug (see Drug Class).
- you have impaired liver or kidney function.
- you have any type of seizure disorder.
- you have diabetes, glaucoma or heart disease.
- you have a history of lupus erythematosus.

- you are taking any drug with sedative effects.
- you plan to have surgery with anesthesia (general or spinal) soon.

Possible Side-Effects (natural, expected and unavoidable drug actions)
Drowsiness (usually during the first 2 weeks), orthostatic hypotension (see Glossary), blurred vision, dry mouth, nasal congestion, constipation, impaired urination.
Pink or purple coloration of urine, of no clinical significance.

▷ **Possible Adverse Effects** (unusual, unexpected and infrequent reactions)
If any of the following develop, consult your physician promptly for guidance.
Mild Adverse Effects
Allergic Reactions: Skin rash, hives, low-grade fever.
Lowering of body temperature, especially in the elderly.
Increased appetite and weight gain.
Weakness, agitation, insomnia, impaired day and night vision.
Chronic constipation, fecal impaction.

Serious Adverse Effects
Allergic Reactions: Hepatitis with jaundice (see Glossary), usually between second and fourth week; high fever; asthma; anaphylactic reaction (see Glossary).
Idiosyncratic Reactions: Neuroleptic malignant syndrome (see Glossary).
Depression, disorientation, seizures.
Disturbances of heart rhythm, rapid heart rate.
Hemolytic anemia (see Glossary).
Low blood platelets (rare).
Low white blood cells—fever, sore throat, infections.
Parkinson-like disorders (see Glossary); muscle spasms of face, jaw, neck, back, extremities.
Prolonged drop in blood pressure with weakness, perspiration and fainting.
Drop in blood pressure on standing (orthostatic hypotension).

▷ **Possible Effects on Sexual Function**
Decreased libido and impotence (1200 mg/day); inhibited ejaculation (400 mg/day); priapism (see Glossary) (250 mg/day); male infertility (30 to 800 mg/day); enlargement of male breasts, enlargement of female breasts with milk production, cessation of menstruation (30 to 800 mg/day).

▷ **Adverse Effects That May Mimic Natural Diseases or Disorders**
Nervous system reactions may suggest Parkinson's disease.
Liver reactions may suggest viral hepatitis.
Reactions resembling systemic lupus erythematosus can occur.

Natural Diseases or Disorders That May Be Activated by This Drug
Latent epilepsy, glaucoma, diabetes mellitus (25%), prostatism (see Glossary).

Possible Effects on Laboratory Tests
Complete blood counts: decreased red cells, hemoglobin, white cells and platelets; increased eosinophils (often warns of jaundice).
Antinuclear antibodies (ANA): positive in 63% of long-term users.
Blood cholesterol level: increased (with liver damage).
Blood glucose level: increased with long-term use.

Chlorpromazine

Glucose tolerance test (GTT): decreased; 40% abnormal with chronic use.
Prothrombin time: increased.
Blood uric acid level: decreased.
Liver function tests: increased liver enzymes (ALT/GPT, AST/GOT and alkaline phosphatase); increased bilirubin.
Urine pregnancy tests: false positive results with frog, rabbit and immunological tests.

CAUTION
1. Many over-the-counter medications (see OTC Drugs in Glossary) for allergies, colds and coughs should not be combined with this drug. Ask your physician or pharmacist for help.
2. Antacids that contain aluminum and/or magnesium can lower absorption of this drug and reduce its effect.
3. Obtain prompt evaluation of any change or disturbance of vision.
4. This drug can cause false positive pregnancy tests.

Precautions for Use
By Infants and Children: Do not use this drug in infants under 6 months of age, or in children of any age with symptoms suggestive of Reye syndrome (see Glossary). Watch carefully for blood cell changes.

By Those over 60 Years of Age: You may be more susceptible to the development of drowsiness, lethargy, constipation, lowering of body temperature (hypothermia) and orthostatic hypotension (see Glossary). Can worsen existing prostatism (see Glossary). Parkinson-like reactions and/or tardive dyskinesia (see discussion of these terms in Glossary) are more likely. Symptoms must be recognized early since they may become irreversible.

▷ **Advisability of Use During Pregnancy**
Pregnancy Category: C. See Pregnancy Code at the back of this book.
Animal studies: No birth defects reported in rodent studies. However, rodent studies suggest possible permanent neurological damage to the fetus.
Human studies: No increase in birth defects reported in 284 exposures. Adequate studies of pregnant women are not available.
Limit use to small and infrequent doses only when clearly needed. Avoid drug during the last month of pregnancy.

Advisability of Use if Breast-Feeding
Presence of this drug in breast milk: Yes, in small amounts.
Ask your doctor for advice.

Habit-Forming Potential: None.

Effects of Overdosage: Marked drowsiness, weakness, tremor, agitation, unsteadiness, deep sleep, coma, convulsions.

Possible Effects of Long-Term Use: Tardive dyskinesia in 10% to 20% (see Glossary); eye changes—cataracts and pigmentation of retina; gray to violet pigmentation of skin in exposed areas, more common in women; severe ulcerative colitis.

Suggested Periodic Examinations While Taking This Drug (at physician's discretion)
Complete blood counts, especially between four to ten weeks of treatment.
Liver function tests, electrocardiograms.
Complete eye examinations—eye structures and vision.

Careful tongue inspection for fine, involuntary, wavelike movements that could be the beginning of tardive dyskinesia.

▷ **While Taking This Drug, Observe the Following**

Foods: No restrictions.

Nutritional Support: A riboflavin (vitamin B-2) supplement should be taken with long-term use.

Beverages: No restrictions. May be taken with milk.

▷ *Alcohol:* Avoid completely. Increases phenothiazine sedative action and accentuates their depressant effects on brain function and blood pressure. Phenothiazines can increase the intoxicating effects of alcohol.

Tobacco Smoking: Possible reduction of drowsiness from drug.

Marijuana Smoking: Moderate increase in drowsiness; worsened orthostatic hypotension; increased risk of precipitating latent psychoses.

▷ *Other Drugs*

Chlorpromazine may *increase* the effects of
- all sedatives or narcotics, especially meperidine (Demerol).
- all atropinelike drugs, and cause nervous system toxicity.

Chlorpromazine may *decrease* the effects of
- guanethidine (Ismelin, Esimil), and reduce its effectiveness in lowering blood pressure.

Chlorpromazine *taken concurrently* with
- amphetamine will cause decreased effect of both drugs.
- ACE inhibitors (see Drug Classes) and cause excessive lowering of blood pressure.
- beta blockers (see Drug Classes) can intensify the effects of both drugs.
- lithium may result in a decrease in lithium or chlorpromazine effectiveness.
- propranolol (Inderal) may cause increased effects of both drugs; watch drug effects closely—doses may have to be decreased.
- valproic acid can result in elevated valproic acid blood levels and toxicity.

The following drugs may *decrease* the effects of chlorpromazine
- antacids containing aluminum and/or magnesium.
- benztropine (Cogentin).
- trihexyphenidyl (Artane).

▷ *Driving, Hazardous Activities:* This drug can impair mental alertness, judgment and physical coordination. Avoid hazardous activities.

Aviation Note: The use of this drug *is a disqualification* for piloting. Consult a designated Aviation Medical Examiner.

Exposure to Sun: Use caution. Some phenothiazines cause photosensitivity (see Glossary).

Exposure to Heat: Use caution and avoid excessive heat. This drug can impair body temperature regulation and increase the risk of heat stroke.

Exposure to Cold: Use caution and dress warmly. Increased risk of hypothermia in the elderly.

Discontinuation: After long-term use, do not stop this drug suddenly. Gradual withdrawal over 2 to 3 weeks. Do not stop this drug without your physician's knowledge and approval. Schizophrenia relapse rate after discontinuation is 50% to 60%.

CHLORPROPAMIDE (klor PROH pa mide)

Introduced: 1958 **Prescription:** USA: Yes; Canada: Yes **Available as Generic:** Yes **Class:** Antidiabetic, sulfonylureas **Controlled Drug:** USA: No; Canada: No
Brand Names: ✣Apo-Chlorpropamide, ✣Chloronase, Diabinese, Glucamide, ✣Novopropamide

BENEFITS versus RISKS	
Possible Benefits	*Possible Risks*
Help in regulating blood sugar in noninsulin-dependent diabetes (adjunctive to appropriate diet and weight control)	HYPOGLYCEMIA, severe and prolonged Allergic skin reactions (some severe) Water retention Liver damage Rare blood cell and bone marrow disorders

▷ **Principal Uses**
As a Single Drug Product: Uses currently included in FDA approved labeling: Helps control mild to moderate type II diabetes mellitus (adult, maturity-onset) that does not require insulin, but is not adequately controlled by diet alone.
Other (unlabeled) generally accepted uses: (1) May be of help in easing abnormal urine output (SIADH); (2) can be used as a test to define some genetic characteristics of diabetes (CPAF test); can be of benefit in some people who have an excessive reaction to sugar (reactive hypoglycemia).

How This Drug Works: This drug (1) stimulates the secretion of insulin if the pancreas is capable of responding to stimulation, and (2) enhances the utilization of insulin by appropriate tissues.

Available Dosage Forms and Strengths
Tablets — 100 mg, 250 mg

▷ **Usual Adult Dosage Range:** Initially 250 mg daily with breakfast. After 5 to 7 days, dose may be increased to 500 mg daily if needed and tolerated. Total daily dosage should not exceed 750 mg. A "loading" or priming dose is not necessary and should not be given. **Note: Actual dosage and administration schedule must be determined by the physician for each patient individually.**

Conditions Requiring Dosing Adjustments
Liver function: The dose **must** be decreased in patients with liver compromise.
Kidney function: Prudent to change to a drug such as tolbutamide in kidney failure.

▷ **Dosing Instructions:** Tablet may be crushed when taken. Taking with food reduces stomach irritation.

Usual Duration of Use: Use on a regular schedule for 1 to 2 weeks is usually needed to see peak effect in controlling diabetes. Failure to respond to maximum doses in 1 month is a primary failure. Up to 15% of those who respond initially may develop secondary failure of the drug within a year. Periodic measurement of blood sugar is needed. See your physician on a regular basis.

▷ **This Drug Should Not Be Taken If**
- you have had an allergic reaction to it previously.
- you have severe impairment of liver or kidney function.
- you are pregnant.
- you make ketone bodies (ketosis). Ask your doctor.
- you are a brittle, juvenile or unstable diabetic.

▷ **Inform Your Physician Before Taking This Drug If**
- you are allergic to other sulfonylurea drugs or to "sulfa" drugs.
- your diabetes has been unstable or "brittle" in the past.
- you have a history of blood disorders.
- you do not know how to recognize or treat hypoglycemia (see Glossary).
- you have a history of congestive heart failure, peptic ulcer disease, cirrhosis of the liver, hypothyroidism or porphyria.
- you have G6PD deficiency.

Possible Side-Effects (natural, expected and unavoidable drug actions)
If drug dose is excessive or food intake is delayed or inadequate, low blood sugar (hypoglycemia) will occur as a drug effect.

▷ **Possible Adverse Effects** (unusual, unexpected and infrequent reactions)
If any of the following develop, consult your physician promptly for guidance.

Mild Adverse Effects
Allergic Reactions: Skin rash, hives, itching, drug fever.
Headache, ringing in ears, weakness, numbness and tingling.
Indigestion, nausea, vomiting, diarrhea (may be severe).

Serious Adverse Effects
Allergic Reactions: Hepatitis with jaundice (see Glossary), severe skin reactions.
Idiosyncratic Reaction: Hemolytic anemia (see Glossary).
Disulfiramlike reaction with concurrent use of alcohol (see Glossary).
Water retention (edema), weight gain.
Lowered thyroid function (hypothyroidism).
Bone marrow depression (see Glossary)—fatigue, weakness, fever, sore throat, abnormal bleeding or bruising.
Abnormal heart beats (very rare).
Persistent diarrhea (pseudomembranous colitis) (rare).
Severe skin reactions (Stevens-Johnson syndrome) (rare).

▷ **Possible Effects on Sexual Function:** None reported.

▷ **Adverse Effects That May Mimic Natural Diseases or Disorders**
Liver reactions may suggest viral hepatitis.

Natural Diseases or Disorders That May Be Activated by This Drug
Acute intermittent porphyria, congestive heart failure (in predisposed individuals), peptic ulcer disease.

Possible Effects on Laboratory Tests
Complete blood cell counts: decreased red cells, hemoglobin, white cells and platelets; increased eosinophils (allergic reaction).
Prothrombin time: increased (with liver damage).
Blood thyroxine (T_4) level: decreased.

Chlorpropamide

Liver function tests: increased liver enzymes (ALT/GPT, AST/GOT and alkaline phosphatase), increased bilirubin.

CAUTION
1. Must be only one part of a total diabetes management program. It is not a substitute for a prescribed diet and regular exercise.
2. Over time (usually several months), this drug may lose its effectiveness in controlling blood sugar levels. Periodic follow-up examinations are necessary.
3. This drug has a long duration of action (up to 60 hours). It can produce severe and prolonged hypoglycemia, especially in the elderly.

Precautions for Use

By Infants and Children: This drug does not work in type I (juvenile, growth-onset) insulin-dependent diabetes.

By Those over 60 Years of Age: Should be avoided in this age group. Because its effect lasts such a long time, it can accumulate and cause marked and prolonged hypoglycemia. Repeated hypoglycemia in the elderly can cause brain damage.

▷ **Advisability of Use During Pregnancy**

Pregnancy Category: C by manufacturer, D by some researchers. See Pregnancy Code at the back of this book.

Animal studies: Specific studies have not been conducted in animals.

Human studies: Adequate studies of pregnant women are not available.

Ask your doctor for guidance. Insulin is clearly the drug of choice during pregnancy to control glucose levels.

Advisability of Use if Breast-Feeding

Presence of this drug in breast milk: Yes.

Avoid drug or refrain from nursing.

Habit-Forming Potential: None.

Effects of Overdosage: Symptoms of mild to severe hypoglycemia: headache, light-headedness, faintness, nervousness, confusion, tremor, sweating, heart palpitation, weakness, hunger, nausea, vomiting, stupor progressing to coma.

Possible Effects of Long-Term Use: Reduced function of the thyroid gland (hypothyroidism). Reports of increased frequency and severity of heart and blood vessel diseases associated with long-term use of this class of drugs was based on study of tolbutamide, but may apply to any drug in this class. A direct cause-and-effect relationship (see Glossary) is tenuous. Ask your physician for guidance.

Suggested Periodic Examinations While Taking This Drug (at physician's discretion)

Complete blood cell counts, liver function tests, thyroid function tests, periodic evaluation of heart and circulatory system.

▷ **While Taking This Drug, Observe the Following**

Foods: Follow the diabetic diet prescribed by your physician.

Beverages: As directed in the diabetic diet. May be taken with milk.

▷ *Alcohol:* Avoid this combination. Alcohol can exaggerate this drug's hypoglycemic effect. This drug can cause also cause a disulfiramlike reaction (see Glossary): facial flushing, sweating, palpitation.

Tobacco Smoking: No interactions expected.
▷ *Other Drugs*
The following drugs may *increase* the effects of chlorpropamide
- ammonium chloride.
- aspirin, aspirin containing combination drugs (see Aspirin profile) and other salicylates.
- beta blockers (see Drug Class) and cause slowed recovery from any low blood sugars which may occur.
- calcium channel blockers (see Drug Class).
- chloramphenicol (Chloromycetin).
- clofibrate (Atromid S).
- dicumarol.
- fenfluramine (Pondimin).
- monoamine oxidase (MAO) type A inhibitor drugs (see Drug Class).
- NSAIDs (see Drug Class).
- some "sulfa" drugs: sulfamethoxazole (Gantanol), sulfisoxazole (Gantrisin), Septra, Bactrim.

The following drugs may *decrease* the effects of chlorpropamide
- diazoxide (Proglycem).
- phenothiazines (see Drug Class).
- rifampin (Rifidin, Rimactane).
- sodium bicarbonate.
- thiazide diuretics (see Drug Class).

▷ *Driving, Hazardous Activities:* Dosing, eating schedule and physical activities must be carefully regulated to prevent hypoglycemia. Know the early symptoms of hypoglycemia so you can avoid hazardous activities and take corrective measures.
Aviation Note: Diabetes *is a disqualification* for piloting. Consult a designated Aviation Medical Examiner.
Exposure to Sun: Use caution. Drugs of this class can cause photosensitivity (see Glossary).
Occurrence of Unrelated Illness: Acute infections, illnesses causing vomiting or diarrhea, serious injuries and surgical procedures can change diabetic control and may require insulin use. Consult your physician promptly.
Discontinuation: Only about 12% of patients remain well controlled by this drug for more than 6 to 7 years. It is advisable to evaluate the continued benefit of this drug every 6 months.

CHLORTHALIDONE (klor THAL i dohn)

Introduced: 1960 **Prescription:** USA: Yes; Canada: Yes **Available as Generic:** USA: Yes; Canada: Yes **Class:** Antihypertensive, diuretic
Controlled Drug: USA: No; Canada: No

Brand Names: ✦Apo-Chlorthalidone, Combipres [CD], Demi-Regroton [CD], Hygroton, ✦Hygroton-Reserpine [CD], Hylidone, ✦Novothalidone, Regroton [CD], Tenoretic [CD], Thalitone, ✦Uridon

BENEFITS versus RISKS

Possible Benefits	*Possible Risks*
EFFECTIVE, WELL-TOLERATED DIURETIC	Loss of body potassium
POSSIBLY EFFECTIVE IN MILD HYPERTENSION	Increased blood sugar
ENHANCES EFFECTIVENESS OF OTHER ANTIHYPERTENSIVES	Increased blood uric acid
Beneficial in treatment of diabetes insipidus	Increased blood calcium
	Rare blood cell disorders

Please see the thiazide diuretic profile for further information.

CHOLESTYRAMINE (koh LES tir a meen)

Introduced: 1959 **Prescription:** USA: Yes; Canada: No **Available as Generic:** USA: No; Canada: No **Class:** Anticholesterol **Controlled Drug:** USA: No; Canada: No
Brand Names: Cholybar, Questran, Questran Light

BENEFITS versus RISKS

Possible Benefits	*Possible Risks*
EFFECTIVE REDUCTION OF TOTAL CHOLESTEROL AND LOW DENSITY CHOLESTEROL IN TYPE IIa CHOLESTEROL DISORDERS (15% to 25% reduction of total cholesterol, 25% to 35% reduction of LDL cholesterol)	Constipation (may be severe)
	Reduced absorption of fat, fat-soluble vitamins (A, D, E and K) and folic acid
EFFECTIVE RELIEF OF ITCHING associated with biliary obstruction	Reduced formation of prothrombin with resultant bleeding
Effective binding of medicines in drug overdoses	

▷ **Principal Uses**

As a Single Drug Product: Uses currently included in FDA approved labeling: Used to (1) treat a new condition called arteriohepatic dysplasia which results in liver and heart problems; (2) reduces abnormally high blood levels of total cholesterol and low density (LDL) cholesterol in Type IIa cholesterol disorders; (3) relieves itching due to the deposit of bile acids in the skin associated with partial biliary obstruction; (4) reduces risk of heart disease in men with type II hyperlipoproteinemia.

Other (unlabeled) generally accepted uses: (1) May be of help in biliary fistulas and skin irritations seen in colostomy; (2) can help lower thyroid hormone levels if too much thyroid hormone has been given in error; (3) may help treat cholesterol ester storage disease (CESD); (4) helps relapses of resistant diarrhea (pseudomembranous colitis).

Cholestyramine

How This Drug Works: It combines with bile acids and bile salts in the intestinal tract, and forms insoluble complexes that are excreted in the feces. This process stimulates conversion of cholesterol to bile acids to replace the loss; and reduces cholesterol levels. By reducing the blood levels of bile acids, this drug reduces bile acids deposited in the skin and relieves itching.

Available Dosage Forms and Strengths
    Bars — 4 grams
    Cans — 378 grams
    Packets — 4 grams and 9 grams

▷ **Usual Adult Dosage Range:** 9 grams of powder (equivalent to 4 grams of cholestyramine) 1 to 6 times daily. Dose may be increased slowly as needed and tolerated. The total daily dosage should not exceed 72 grams of powder (32 grams of cholestyramine). **Note: Actual dosage and administration schedule must be determined by the physician for each patient individually.**

Conditions Requiring Dosing Adjustments
Liver function: Cholestyramine is eliminated via the feces—no liver involvement.
Kidney function: This medication is **not** absorbed, and the kidney is not involved.

▷ **Dosing Instructions:** Always take just before or with a meal; this drug is ineffective when taken without food. Mix the powder thoroughly in 4 to 6 ounces of water, fruit juice, milk, thin soup or a soft food like applesauce; do not use carbonated beverages. **Do not take it in its dry form.**

Usual Duration of Use: Use on a regular schedule for up to 3 weeks may be needed to see this drug's benefit in lowering excessively high cholesterol. Duration of use should not exceed 3 months if an adequate response does not occur. Long-term use (months to years) requires periodic evaluation of response.

▷ **This Drug Should Not Be Taken If**
- you have had an allergic reaction to it previously.
- you have complete biliary obstruction.

▷ **Inform Your Physician Before Taking This Drug If**
- you are prone to constipation.
- you have peptic ulcer disease.
- you have a bleeding disorder of any kind.
- you have impaired kidney function.
- you have phenylketonuria (PKU).
- you have a bleeding disorder.

Possible Side-Effects (natural, expected and unavoidable drug actions)
Constipation (25%); interference with normal fat digestion and absorption; reduced absorption of vitamins A, D, E and K and folic acid.

▷ **Possible Adverse Effects** (unusual, unexpected and infrequent reactions)
    If any of the following develop, consult your physician promptly for guidance.
Mild Adverse Effects
Allergic Reactions: Skin rash, hives, tongue irritation, anal itching.

Loss of appetite, indigestion, heartburn, abdominal discomfort, excessive gas, nausea, vomiting, diarrhea.

Serious Adverse Effects
Allergic Reaction: Asthma-like wheezing.
Vitamin K deficiency and increased bleeding tendency.
Impaired absorption of calcium; predisposition to osteoporosis.
Gallbladder colic.
Disruption of acid/base balance (Acidosis).

▷ **Possible Effects on Sexual Function:** Increased libido (questionable).

Natural Diseases or Disorders That May Be Activated by This Drug
Peptic ulcer disease; steatorrhea (excessive fat in stools) with large doses.

Possible Effects on Laboratory Tests
Blood cholesterol and triglyceride levels: decreased (therapeutic effect).
Blood hemoglobin and iron levels: decreased (drug impairs absorption of iron).
Prothrombin time: increased (drug impairs absorption of vitamin K).
Liver function tests: increased liver enzymes (ALT/GPT, AST/GOT) in a few cases; not thought to be liver damage.
Urine calcium: increased (drug impairs absorption of calcium from intestine).

CAUTION
1. The powder should never be taken in its dry form; always mix it thoroughly with a suitable liquid before swallowing.
2. Use stool softeners and laxatives as needed if constipation develops.
3. This drug may bind other drugs and impair their absorption. It is advisable to take *all other drugs* 1 to 2 hours before or 4 to 6 hours after taking this drug.

Precautions for Use
By Infants and Children: Safety and effectiveness for those under 6 years of age not established. Watch carefully for development of acidosis and vitamin A or folic acid deficiency. (Ask your doctor for help.)
By Those over 60 Years of Age: Increased risk of developing severe constipation. Impaired kidney function may predispose to the development of acidosis.

▷ **Advisability of Use During Pregnancy**
Pregnancy Category: C. See Pregnancy Code at the back of this book.
Animal studies: No information available.
Human studies: Adequate studies of pregnant women are not available.
Use this drug only if clearly needed. Ensure adequate intake of vitamins and minerals. Ask physician for guidance.

Advisability of Use if Breast-Feeding
Presence of this drug in breast milk: No.
Breast-feeding is permitted.

Habit-Forming Potential: None.

Effects of Overdosage: Progressive constipation.

Possible Effects of Long-Term Use
Deficiencies of vitamins A, D, E and K and folic acid.
Calcium deficiency, osteoporosis.
Acidosis due to excessive retention of chloride.

Suggested Periodic Examinations While Taking This Drug (at physician's discretion)
Measurements of blood levels of total cholesterol, low density (LDL) cholesterol and high density (HDL) cholesterol.
Hemoglobin and red blood cell studies for possible anemia.

▷ **While Taking This Drug, Observe the Following**
Foods: Avoid foods that tend to constipate (cheeses, etc.).
Nutritional Support: Ask your doctor about the need for supplements of vitamins A, D, E and K, folic acid and calcium.
Beverages: Avoid carbonated beverages. Ensure adequate liquid intake (up to 2 quarts daily). This drug may be taken with milk.

▷ *Alcohol:* No interactions expected.
Tobacco Smoking: No interactions expected.

▷ *Other Drugs*
Cholestyramine may *decrease* the effects of
- acetaminophen; give 2 hours before cholestyramine.
- digitoxin and digoxin; give 2 hours before.
- furosemide (lasix).
- iron preparations; give 2 to 3 hours before.
- methotrexate; give 3 hours before cholestyramine.
- metronidazole (Flagyl).
- NSAIDS (some acidic ones such as piroxicam and sulindac).
- oral hypoglycemic agents (see Drug Classes).
- penicillin G.
- phenobarbital; give 2 hours before.
- thiazide diuretics (see Drug Class); give 2 hours before.
- thyroxin; give 5 hours before.
- warfarin; give 6 hours after.

Cholestyramine *taken concurrently* with
- amiodarone (Codarone) can result in lowered amiodarone blood levels and decreased effectiveness.

▷ *Driving, Hazardous Activities:* No restrictions.
Aviation Note: The use of this drug *is usually not a disqualification* for piloting. Consult a designated Aviation Medical Examiner.
Exposure to Sun: No restrictions.
Discontinuation: The dose of any potentially toxic drug taken concurrently must be reduced appropriately when this drug is discontinued.

CIMETIDINE (si MET i deen)

Introduced: 1976 **Prescription:** USA: Yes; Canada: Yes
Author's note: This drug is pending FDA approval as Tagamet HB, a nonprescription form.
Please see histamine (H-2) blocking drug for further information.

CIPROFLOXACIN (sip roh FLOX a sin)

Introduced: 1984   **Prescription:** USA: Yes   **Available as Generic:** USA: No   **Class:** Anti-infective   **Controlled Drug:** USA: No
Brand Name: Ciloxan, Cipro

Warning: Reports are being made for some drugs in this class which find tendon rupture as a rare adverse effect. Ask your doctor about limits on strenuous exercise while you are taking this medicine. A rare idiosyncratic reaction has also been reported which presents as mental confusion and disorientation. Use of this medicine after head trauma may be a risk factor. If you have suffered a fall, ask your doctor if a medicine in a different antibiotic class should be substituted. If you are taking this drug and notice a change in your thinking, call your doctor.

BENEFITS versus RISKS

Possible Benefits	*Possible Risks*
HIGHLY EFFECTIVE TREATMENT FOR INFECTIONS OF THE LOWER RESPIRATORY TRACT, URINARY TRACT, BONES, JOINTS AND SKIN TISSUES due to susceptible organisms	Nausea (1.6%), diarrhea (1.5%), very rare drug-induced colitis
	Mild allergic reactions (1.4%)
	Very rare hallucination or seizure
Effective treatment for some forms of bacterial gastroenteritis (diarrhea)	Tendon rupture (rare)

▷ **Principal Uses**

As a Single Drug Product: Uses currently included in FDA approved labeling: Treats responsive infections (in adults) of: (1) the lower respiratory tract (lungs and bronchial tubes); (2) the urinary tract (kidneys, bladder, urethra and prostate gland); (3) the digestive tract (small intestine and colon); (4) bones and joints; (5) skin and related tissues.

Other (unlabeled) generally accepted uses: (1) Can have a role in treating cholera where the organisms are resistant to doxycycline; (2) has a role in treatment of prostatitis; (3) lessens symptoms or prevents traveler's diarrhea; (4) can be of use in treating gonorrhea.

How This Drug Works: It blocks the bacterial enzyme DNA gyrase (required for DNA synthesis and cell reproduction), and arrests bacterial growth (in low concentrations) and kills bacteria (in high concentrations).

Available Dosage Forms and Strengths
Tablets — 250 mg, 500 mg, 750 mg
Ophthalmic solution — 0.3%

▷ **Usual Adult Dosage Range:** 250 mg to 750 mg/12 hours, depending upon the nature and severity of the infection. The total daily dosage should not exceed 1500 mg.

Ophthalmic: 1 or 2 drops instilled in the eye every 2 hours while awake for 2 days, then 1 or 2 drops for 5 more days which is given every 4 hours while awake. **Note: Actual dosage and administration schedule must be determined by the physician for each patient individually.**

Conditions Requiring Dosing Adjustments
Liver function: Used with caution in severe liver failure.
Kidney function: Dose **must** be decreased (or interval lengthened) in kidney compromise.
Cystic Fibrosis
A loading dose as well as ongoing doses of 750 mg every 8 hours is given in cystic fibrosis patients. This dosing gives blood levels which are more aggressive versus the bacteria which usually cause infections in these patients.

▷ **Dosing Instructions:** May be taken with or without food and may be crushed. Best taken 2 hours after eating. Drink large amounts of fluids during treatment. Avoid aluminum or magnesium antacids for 2 hours before and after taking.

Usual Duration of Use: Use on a regular schedule for 7 to 14 days is needed to see this drug's effectiveness in eradicating infection. The drug should be continued for at least 2 days after all indications of infection have disappeared. Bone and joint infections may be treated for 6 weeks or longer. Long-term use requires periodic evaluation of response.

Possible Advantages of This Drug
One of the broadest spectrums of antibacterial activity of all currently available oral antimicrobial drugs.
Among the most potent anti-infective actions of quinolones.
Highly effective in treating numerous types of infection caused by a wide spectrum of bacteria.
Provides effective drug levels in the prostate gland.

▷ **This Drug Should Not Be Taken If**
- you have had an allergic reaction to it previously.
- you are pregnant or breast-feeding.
- you have a seizure disorder that is not adequately controlled.
- it is prescribed for a person under 18 years of age.

▷ **Inform Your Physician Before Taking This Drug If**
- you are allergic to cinoxacin (Cinobac), nalidixic acid (NegGram), norfloxacin (Noroxin), or other quinolone drugs.
- you have a seizure disorder or a circulatory disorder of the brain.
- you have impaired liver or kidney function.
- you have a history of mental disorders (psychosis).
- you are taking any form of probenecid or theophylline.

Possible Side-Effects (natural, expected and unavoidable drug actions)
Superinfections (5%). (See Superinfection in the Glossary.)

▷ **Possible Adverse Effects** (unusual, unexpected and infrequent reactions)
If any of the following develop, consult your physician promptly for guidance.
Mild Adverse Effects
Allergic Reactions: Rash (0.83%), itching (0.47%), localized swelling (0.12%).
Dizziness (0.53%), headache (0.30%), weakness (0.36%), migraine (0.06%), anxiety (0.06%), abnormal vision (0.06%).
Nausea (1.6%), diarrhea (1.5%), vomiting (0.7%), indigestion (0.36%).

Ciprofloxacin

Muscle aches.
Burning feeling in the eye when the ophthalmic solution is used.
Serious Adverse Effects
Allergic Reactions: Anaphylaxis.
Idiosyncratic Reactions: Mental confusion and incapacitation.
Central nervous system stimulation: restlessness, tremor, confusion, hallucinations, seizures (all very rare).
Tendon rupture (rare).

▷ **Possible Effects on Sexual Function:** None reported.

▷ **Natural Diseases or Disorders That May Be Activated by This Drug**
Latent epilepsy, latent gout.

Possible Effects on Laboratory Tests
Kidney function: increased blood creatinine and urea nitrogen (BUN) (rare).

CAUTION
1. With high doses or prolonged use, crystal formation in the kidney may occur. This can be prevented by drinking large amounts of water, up to 2 quarts/24 hours.
2. May decrease saliva formation; make dental cavities or gum disease more likely. Consult your dentist if dry mouth persists.
3. Strenuous exercise is NOT recommended while this medicine is being taken.

Precautions for Use
By Infants and Children: Avoid the use of this drug completely. Impairs normal bone growth and development.
By Those over 60 Years of Age: Impaired kidney function may require dosage reduction.
If taking theophylline with this drug, the theophylline dose must be decreased.

▷ **Advisability of Use During Pregnancy**
Pregnancy Category: C. See Pregnancy Code at the back of this book.
Animal studies: No birth defects due to this drug found in mouse or rat studies. Rabbit studies showed maternal weight loss and increased abortions. This drug can impair normal bone development in immature dogs.
Human studies: Adequate studies of pregnant women are not available. However, the potential for adverse effects on fetal bone development contraindicates the use of this drug during entire pregnancy.

Advisability of Use if Breast-Feeding
Presence of this drug in breast milk: Probably yes.
Avoid drug or refrain from nursing.

Habit-Forming Potential: None.

Effects of Overdosage: Confusion, headache, abdominal pain, diarrhea, liver toxicity, seizures, kidney toxicity and hallucinations.

Possible Effects of Long-Term Use: Superinfections (see Glossary); crystal formation in kidneys.

Suggested Periodic Examinations While Taking This Drug (at physician's discretion)
Liver function tests, urine analysis.
▷ **While Taking This Drug, Observe the Following**
Foods: Caffeine will remain in your system longer than usual.
Dairy foods will decrease the effectiveness of ciprofloxacin by decreasing the amount absorbed.
Beverages: No restrictions. May be taken with milk.
▷ *Alcohol:* No interactions expected.
Tobacco Smoking: No interactions expected.
▷ *Other Drugs*
Ciprofloxacin may *increase* the effects of
- theophylline, and cause theophylline toxicity.

The following drug may *increase* the effects of ciprofloxacin
- probenecid (Benemid).

Ciprofloxacin *taken concurrently* with
- azlocillin may result in ciprofloxacin toxicity.
- caffeine will result in increased caffeine levels.
- cyclosporine (Sandimmune) may result in increased risk of kidney toxicity.
- foscarnet may result in an increased risk of seizures.
- phenytoin (Dilantin) may result in increased or decreased dilantin levels.
- warfarin can result in increased risk of bleeding.

The following drugs may *decrease* the effects of ciprofloxacin
- antacids containing aluminum or magnesium can reduce the absorption of ciprofloxacin and lessen its effectiveness.
- didanosine.
- iron salts.
- sucralfate.

▷ *Driving, Hazardous Activities:* May cause dizziness and impair vision. Restrict activities as necessary.
Aviation Note: The use of this drug *may be a disqualification* for piloting. Consult a designated Aviation Medical Examiner.
Exposure to Sun: May rarely cause photosensitivity (see Glossary). Sunglasses are advised if eyes are overly sensitive to bright light.
Heavy Exercise or Exertion: Several reports have surfaced regarding tendon rupture in patients on this medication. It is prudent to avoid heavy exercise or exertion while you are taking this medicine.
Discontinuation: If you experience no adverse effects from this drug, take the full course prescribed for best results. Ask your doctor when to stop treatment.

CISAPRIDE (SIS a pryde)

Introduced: July 1993   **Prescription:** USA: Yes; Canada: Yes   **Available as Generic:** USA: No; Canada: No   **Class:** GI Stimulant   **Controlled Drug:** USA: No; Canada: No
Brand Names: Propulsid, ✦Prepulsid

Cisapride

BENEFITS versus RISKS	
Possible Benefits	*Possible Risks*
EFFECTIVE TREATMENT OF NOCTURNAL HEARBURN	diarrhea (4%)
	sleep disturbances
FEW CENTRAL NERVOUS SIDE EFFECTS	

▷ **Principal Uses**

As a Single Drug Product: Uses currently included in FDA approved labeling: (1) Used to relieve symptoms of reflux esophagitis; (2) helps decrease nocturnal heartburn caused by gastroesophageal reflux disease.

Other (unlabeled) generally accepted uses: (1) May have a role in helping improve delayed stomach emptying which may lead to anorexia nervosa; (2) can help children with chronic constipation; (3) helps relieve slow emptying of the stomach (diabetic gastroparsis) often seen in diabetes; (4) relieves slowed stomach emptying caused by morphine; (5) decreases pain and flatulence in irritable bowel syndrome; (6) helps the gallbladder work better in patients with myotonic muscular dystrophy; (7) can be of help in promoting defecation in patients with spinal cord injury.

How This Drug Works: Increases the movement of the esophagus (by activating a specific muscarinic receptor) and increases contractions in the stomach and helps it to empty.

Available Dosage Forms and Strengths
Tablets — 10 mg, 20 mg

▷ **Recommended Dosage Ranges (Actual dosage and administration schedule must be determined by the physician for each patient individually.)**

Infants and Children: Safety and efficacy not established in children or infants.

12 to 60 Years of Age: For relief of nocturnal heartburn: 10 to 20 mg four times a day given 15 minutes before meals and at bedtime.

For reflux esophagitis: 10 mg four times a day combined with cimetidine one gram a day.

For diabetic gastroparesis: 10 mg four times a day given 15 minutes before meals and at bedtime.

Over 60 Years of Age: Same as 12 to 60 years of age.

Conditions Requiring Dosing Adjustments

Liver function: Patients with liver failure should be given 50% of the usual dose.

Kidney function: Dose changes are not needed in kidney failure.

▷ **Dosing Instructions:** This medicine should be taken 15 minutes before meals and at bedtime for best effect.

Usual Duration of Use: Use on a regular schedule for 8 to 12 weeks may be needed to see the peak benefit in treating chronic functional constipation. Up to 12 weeks may be needed to realize the full therapeutic effect when used in therapy of reflux esophagitis. Long-term use (months to years) requires periodic physician evaluation of response and dosage adjustment.

Possible Advantages of This Drug
Significant decrease in central nervous side effects compared to metoclopramide.

Currently a "Drug of Choice"
for patients who are unable to tolerate metoclopramide and are using it for a condition which cisapride effectively treats.

▷ **This Drug Should Not Be Taken If**
- you have had an allergic reaction to any dosage form of it previously.
- you have gastrointestinal obstruction, hemorrhage or perforation.

▷ **Inform Your Physician Before Taking This Drug If**
- you currently take a benzodiazepine drug (see Drug Classes Section).
- you have an abnormally fast heartbeat.
- you take other prescription or non-prescription medicines which were not discussed with your doctor when cisapride was prescribed.

Possible Side-Effects (natural, expected and unavoidable drug actions)
Sleepiness and fatigue (1.6%).

▷ **Possible Adverse Effects** (unusual, unexpected and infrequent reactions)
If any of the following develop, consult your physician promptly for guidance.

Mild Adverse Effects
Allergic Reactions: Skin rash and itching.
Somnolence and fatigue (1.6%).
Occasional headache, dizziness and sleep disturbances.
Rhinitis (7.3%).
Diarrhea (4%).

Serious Adverse Effects
Allergic Reactions: Anaphylactoid reaction (see Glossary).
Rare increases in heart rate.
Very rare bone marrow depression (see Glossary).

▷ **Possible Effects on Sexual Function:** None reported.

Possible Delayed Adverse Effects: None defined.

Possible Effects on Laboratory Tests
Complete blood count: decreased white cells, platelets and hemoglobin.
Liver function tests: increased liver enzymes (SGOT, SGPT and CPK).

CAUTION
1. May cause increased heart rate. Notify physician if this occurs.
2. Report promptly any increased tendency to infection.

Precautions for Use
By Infants and Children:
Safety and effectiveness for children not established.
By Those over 60 Years of Age: Specific changes not required.

▷ **Advisability of Use During Pregnancy**
Pregnancy Category: C. See Pregnancy Code at the back of this book.
Animal studies: Has caused prolongation of breeding interval in female rats.
Embryotoxic and fetotoxic in high dose studies in rats.
Human studies: Adequate studies of pregnant women are not available.
Used as a benefit to risk decision in pregnancy. Ask your doctor for help.

Advisability of Use if Breast-Feeding
Presence of this drug in breast milk: Yes.
Monitor nursing infant closely and discontinue drug or nursing if adverse effects develop.

Habit-Forming Potential: None.
Effects of Overdosage: Nausea, vomiting, flatulence, increased urination and diarrhea
Possible Effects of Long-Term Use: None defined.
Suggested Periodic Examinations While Taking This Drug (at physician's discretion)
   Complete blood counts: Periodically.
▷ **While Taking This Drug, Observe the Following**
   Foods: No restrictions.
   Beverages: No restrictions.
▷ *Alcohol:* Sedative effects of alcohol will be increased.
   Tobacco Smoking: No interactions expected.
   Marijuana Smoking: May cause additive drowsiness.
▷ *Other Drugs*
   Cisapride may *decrease* the effects of
   • warfarin (Coumadin) and decrease benefits. More frequent prothrombin times are indicated, and dosing should be adjusted if needed.
   Cisapride *taken concurrently* with
   • cimetidine (Tagamet) results in increased cisapride levels and potential cisapride toxicity. Cisapride dose may need to be decreased.
▷ *Driving, Hazardous Activities:* This drug may cause some drowsiness. Restrict activities as necessary.
   Aviation Note: The use of this drug **may be a disqualification** for piloting. Consult a designated Aviation Medical Examiner.
   Exposure to Sun: No restrictions.
   Discontinuation: If this medication is stopped and you have been taking an anticoagulant, prothrombin time testing will be needed.

CLARITHROMYCIN (klar ith roh MY sin)

Introduced: 1991   **Prescription:** USA: Yes   **Available as Generic:** USA: No   **Class:** Anti-infective, macrolides   **Controlled Drug:** USA: No
Brand Name: Biaxin

BENEFITS versus RISKS	
Possible Benefits	*Possible Risks*
EFFECTIVE TREATMENT OF UPPER AND LOWER RESPIRATORY TRACT INFECTIONS DUE TO SUSCEPTIBLE MICROORGANISMS	Mild gastrointestinal symptoms Drug-induced colitis (rare) Superinfections (rare)
EFFECTIVE TREATMENT OF SKIN INFECTIONS DUE TO SUSCEPTIBLE MICROORGANISMS	

▷ **Principal Uses**
   As a Single Drug Product: Uses currently included in FDA approved labeling:
      (1) Treatment of certain upper respiratory tract infections—maxillary

sinusitis, pharyngitis, tonsillitis; (2) treatment of certain lower respiratory tract infections—acute bronchitis and pneumonia; (3) treatment of certain skin (and skin structure) infections. As necessary, bacterial cultures and sensitivity testing should be performed; (4) treatment of mycobacterium avium complex (MAI) infections.

Other (unlabeled) generally accepted uses: (1) Combination antibiotic treatment of duodenal ulcer disease caused by H. pylori; (2) can have a role in combination therapy of some toxoplasmosis infections.

How This Drug Works: This drug prevents the growth and multiplication of susceptible organisms by interfering with their formation of essential proteins.

Available Dosage Forms and Strengths
Tablets — 250 mg, 500 mg

▷ **Recommended Dosage Ranges** (Actual dosage and administration schedule must be determined by the physician for each patient individually.)

Infants and Children: Dosage not established.

12 to 60 Years of Age: For pharyngitis/tonsillitis—250 mg/12 hours for 10 days.
For maxillary sinusitis—500 mg/12 hours for 14 days.
For acute bronchitis—250–500 mg/12 hours for 7 to 14 days.
For pneumonia—250 mg/12 hours for 7 to 14 days.
For skin infections—250 mg/12 hours for 7 to 14 days.

Over 60 Years of Age: Same as 12 to 60 years of age. Dose must be reduced in kidney compromise.

Conditions Requiring Dosing Adjustments
Liver function: If kidney function is normal, dose decrease not needed with liver problems.
Kidney function: The dose must be decreased in patients with compromised kidneys.

▷ **Dosing Instructions:** May be taken with or without food. The tablet may be crushed when taken.

Usual Duration of Use: Use on a regular schedule for 4 to 6 days is usually needed to see this drug's benefit in controlling responsive infections. For streptococcal throat infections; not less than 10 consecutive days (without interruption) will reduce the risk of rheumatic fever or glomerulonephritis. Use should stop when the infection is eliminated.

Possible Advantages of This Drug
Single drug effectiveness against a broader spectrum of bacteria; equivalent to erythromycin, some penicillins and some cephalosporins.
Effective with only 2 doses daily.
Can be taken without regard to eating.
Very well tolerated; infrequent and minor adverse effects.

▷ **This Drug Should Not Be Taken If**
- you have had an allergic reaction to it previously.

▷ **Inform Your Physician Before Taking This Drug If**
- you are allergic to: Azithromycin, erythromycin, or troleandomycin.
- you have impaired liver or kidney function.
- you have a history of drug-induced colitis.
- you have a history of low blood platelets.
- you are pregnant or planning pregnancy.

Clarithromycin

Possible Side-Effects (natural, expected and unavoidable drug actions)
Superinfections (see Glossary).

▷ **Possible Adverse Effects** (unusual, unexpected and infrequent reactions)
If any of the following develop, consult your physician promptly for guidance.
Mild Adverse Effects
Allergic Reactions: None reported.
Headache (2%).
Abnormal taste, nausea, stomach pain, indigestion, diarrhea (3%).
Serious Adverse Effects
Drug-induced colitis (rare).
Low blood platelets (rare).
Kidney toxicity (rare).
Acute psychosis (two recent case reports) (very rare).

▷ **Possible Effects on Sexual Function:** None reported.

Possible Effects on Laboratory Tests
Prothrombin time: increased (1%).
Liver function tests: increased liver enzymes (ALT/GPT, AST/GOT and alkaline phosphatase), increased bilirubin (all less than 1%).
Kidney function tests: increased blood urea nitrogen (4%).

CAUTION
1. If diarrhea starts and continues for more than 24 hours, call your doctor promptly. This could be the onset of drug-induced colitis.
2. Take the full amount prescribed to prevent resistant bacteria.

Precautions for Use
By Infants and Children: Safety and effectiveness for those under 12 years of age not established.
By Those over 60 Years of Age: Consider dosage adjustment if kidney function is severely impaired.

▷ **Advisability of Use During Pregnancy**
Pregnancy Category:
C. See Pregnancy Code at the back of this book.
Animal studies: Monkey, rabbit, rat and mouse studies have demonstrated adverse effects on fetal development and pregnancy outcome.
Human studies: Adequate studies of pregnant women are not available.
This drug should not be used during pregnancy except where no alternative treatment is appropriate. Ask your doctor for help.

Advisability of Use if Breast-Feeding
Presence of this drug in breast milk: Probably yes.
Watch nursing infant closely and stop the drug or nursing if adverse effects develop.

Habit-Forming Potential: None.

Effects of Overdosage: Possible nausea, vomiting, abdominal discomfort and diarrhea.

Possible Effects of Long-Term Use: Superinfections, drug-induced colitis.

Suggested Periodic Examinations While Taking This Drug (at physician's discretion)
None.

▷ **While Taking This Drug, Observe the Following**
   Foods: No restrictions.
   Beverages: No restrictions. May be taken with milk.
▷ *Alcohol:* No interactions expected.
   Tobacco Smoking: No interactions expected.
▷ *Other Drugs*
   Clarithromycin may *increase* the effects of
   • astemizole and cause life-threatening heart rhythms.
   • carbamazepine (Tegretol); check blood levels of carbamazepine.
   • terfenadine and cause life-threatening heart rhythms.
   • theophylline (Theo-Dur, Theolair, etc.); monitor blood levels of theophylline if appropriate.
   • warfarin and cause bleeding.
   Clarithromycin *taken concurrently* with
   • cyclosporine may lead to cyclosporine toxicity.
   • dihydroergotamine can lead to increased levels and dihydroergotamine toxicity.
   • ergotamine can cause toxicity.
   • zidovudine may lead to decreased levels and lack of zidovudine effectiveness.
▷ *Driving, Hazardous Activities:* This drug may cause nausea and/or diarrhea. Restrict activities as necessary.
   Aviation Note: The use of this drug *may be a disqualification* for piloting. Consult a designated Aviation Medical Examiner.
   Exposure to Sun: No restrictions.

CLINDAMYCIN (klin da MI sin)

Introduced: 1973 **Prescription:** USA: Yes; Canada: Yes **Available as Generic:** USA: Yes; Canada: No **Class:** Antibiotic **Controlled Drug:** USA: No; Canada: No

Brand Names: Cleocin, Cleocin T, ✦Dalacin C, ✦Dalacin T

BENEFITS versus RISKS	
Possible Benefits	*Possible Risks*
EFFECTIVE TREATMENT FOR SERIOUS INFECTIONS OF THE LOWER RESPIRATORY TRACT, ABDOMINAL CAVITY, GENITAL TRACT IN WOMEN, BLOOD STREAM (SEPTICEMIA), SKIN AND RELATED TISSUES caused by susceptible organisms	SEVERE DRUG-INDUCED COLITIS (fatalities reported) Rare liver injury with jaundice Rare reduction in white blood cell and platelet counts
Specific prevention and treatment of Pneumocystis carinii pneumonia	
Effective for the local treatment of acne	

Clindamycin

▷ **Principal Uses**
 As a Single Drug Product
   Uses currently included in FDA approved labeling: (1) Treats serious and unusual infections of the lungs and bronchial tubes, organs and tissues within the abdominal cavity, the genital tract and pelvic organs in women, the skin and soft tissue structures and generalized infections involving the bloodstream.
   Other (unlabeled) generally accepted uses: (1) Treatment of resistant gum disease, and malaria; (2) prevention of infection of the heart; (3) prevention and treatment of pneumocystis carinii pneumonia, an infection associated with AIDS; (4) may have a role in combination therapy of Toxoplasmosis infections of the brain in AIDS patients.

How This Drug Works: By blocking the formation of critical growth and reproductive proteins, this drug (in low concentrations) stops multiplication of bacteria and (in high concentrations) kills bacteria.

Available Dosage Forms and Strengths
   Capsules — 75 mg, 150 mg, 300 mg
   Injection — 150 mg per ml
   Oral solution — 75 mg per 5-ml teaspoonful
   Topical solution — 10 mg per ml

▷ **Usual Adult Dosage Range:** For infections of average severity: 150 to 300 mg/6 hours; for more severe infections: 300 to 450 mg/6 hours. The total daily dosage should not exceed 1800 mg. **Note: Actual dosage and administration schedule must be determined by the physician for each patient individually.**

Conditions Requiring Dosing Adjustments
 Liver function: The dose must be decreased with liver compromise.
 Kidney function: Serum levels should be checked in patients with renal compromise.

▷ **Dosing Instructions:** Take the capsule with a full glass of water or with food to prevent irritation. The capsule may be opened and the contents mixed with food for administration. Shake the oral solution well before measuring the dose. Do not refrigerate the oral solution; chilling can cause it to thicken, making it difficult to take.

Usual Duration of Use: Use on a regular schedule for 3 to 5 days is usually needed to see this drug's effect in controlling infections.

Possible Advantages of This Drug: Bacterial sensitivity testing may show this drug to be more effective than other antibiotics in treating some severe infections.

▷ **This Drug Should Not Be Taken If**
   • you are allergic to either clindamycin or lincomycin.
   • it is prescribed for a mild or trivial infection.
   • you have a history of Crohn's disease or ulcerative colitis.

▷ **Inform Your Physician Before Taking This Drug If**
   • you have a history of allergy to any drug.
   • you have a history of drug-induced colitis.
   • you are allergic by nature: Hay fever, asthma, hives, eczema.

- you have a history of previous yeast infections.
- you have a blood disorder.
- you have myasthenia gravis.
- you have impaired liver or kidney function.
- you plan to have surgery under general anesthesia in the near future.

Possible Side-Effects (natural, expected and unavoidable drug actions)
Superinfections (see Glossary).

▷ **Possible Adverse Effects** (unusual, unexpected and infrequent reactions)
If any of the following develop, consult your physician promptly for guidance.
Mild Adverse Effects
Allergic Reactions: Skin rashes (3% to 5%), hives.
Nausea, vomiting, mild diarrhea (3% to 30%), stomach pain.
Multiple joint pains (rare).
Serious Adverse Effects
Allergic Reactions: Severe skin reactions: erythema multiforme (Stevens-Johnson syndrome).
Toxic liver reaction with jaundice (see Glossary).
Severe colitis with persistent diarrhea (0.01% to 10%); stools may contain blood and/or mucus.
Rare reduction of white blood cell and platelet counts.

▷ **Possible Effects on Sexual Function:** None reported.

Possible Delayed Adverse Effects: Severe colitis with diarrhea (pseudomembranous colitis) may start several weeks after stopping this drug.

▷ **Adverse Effects That May Mimic Natural Diseases or Disorders**
Liver reactions may suggest viral hepatitis.
Multiple joint pains may suggest the onset of arthritis.

▷ **Natural Diseases or Disorders That May Be Activated by This Drug**
Crohn's disease, ulcerative colitis, myasthenia gravis.

Possible Effects on Laboratory Tests
Complete blood counts: decreased white cells and platelets; increased eosinophils (allergic reaction).
Liver function tests: uncommon, mild and transient increases in liver enzymes (ALT/GPT, AST/GOT, alkaline phosphatase).

CAUTION
1. Persistent diarrhea can develop in some patients. If diarrhea persists longer than 24 hours, stop the drug and call your doctor.
2. If surgery under general anesthesia is planned, the anesthetic must be carefully chosen to prevent clindamycin induced excessive muscle relaxation and breathing problems.

Precautions for Use
By Infants and Children: Safety and effectiveness for those under 1 month of age not established. Use with caution.
By Those over 60 Years of Age: Diarrhea will be more common in this age group. Watch for development of yeast infection of the skin in the genital and anal regions, a form of superinfection (see Glossary). Report such developments promptly to your physician.

Clindamycin

▷ **Advisability of Use During Pregnancy**
Pregnancy Category: B. See Pregnancy Code at the back of this book.
  Animal studies: No birth defects due to this drug found in mouse or rat studies.
  Human studies: Adequate studies of pregnant women are not available. Use this drug only if clearly needed. Ask your physician for guidance.

Advisability of Use if Breast-Feeding
  Presence of this drug in breast milk: Yes.
  Avoid drug or refrain from nursing.

Habit-Forming Potential: None.

Effects of Overdosage: Nausea, vomiting, cramping, diarrhea.

Possible Effects of Long-Term Use
  Superinfections, especially from yeast organisms.
  Severe colitis with persistent diarrhea.

Suggested Periodic Examinations While Taking This Drug (at physician's discretion)
  Complete blood cell counts, liver function tests.

▷ **While Taking This Drug, Observe the Following**
Foods: No restrictions.
Beverages: No restrictions. May be taken with milk.

▷ *Alcohol:* No interactions expected.
Tobacco Smoking: No interactions expected.

▷ *Other Drugs*
  Clindamycin *taken concurrently* with
  - antidiarrheal drugs (diphenoxylate, loperamide, paregoric) may result in worsening of the underlying colitis. Avoid the combination.
  - antimyasthenic drugs (ambenonium, neostigmine, pyridostigmine) may reduce their benefit in relieving muscle weakness of myasthenia gravis.

  The following drugs may *decrease* the effects of clindamycin
  - chloramphenicol (Chloromycetin).
  - erythromycin (E.E.S., E-Mycin, etc.).

▷ *Driving, Hazardous Activities:* This drug may cause nausea and diarrhea. Restrict activities as necessary.

Aviation Note: The use of this drug *may be a disqualification* for piloting. Consult a designated Aviation Medical Examiner.

Exposure to Sun: Use caution until sensitivity is determined.

Discontinuation: If tolerated, take the full course prescribed. When used to treat infections that may predispose to rheumatic fever or nephritis, take continually in full dosage for no less than 10 days.

Special Storage Instructions: Oral solution should be kept at room temperature; do not refrigerate.

Observe the Following Expiration Times: Do not take the oral solution if it is older than 14 days.

CLOFAZIMINE (kloh FA zi meen)

Introduced: 1973 **Prescription:** USA: Yes **Available as Generic:** USA: No **Class:** Anti-infective **Controlled Drug:** USA: No
Brand Name: Lamprene

BENEFITS versus RISKS	
Possible Benefits	*Possible Risks*
EFFECTIVE ADJUNCTIVE TREATMENT OF LEPROSY	RARE BOWEL OBSTRUCTION, GASTROINTESTINAL BLEEDING
Possibly effective adjunctive treatment of AIDS-related infection with M. avium-intracellulare (MAI)	Rare liver damage Skin pigmentation (red to brownish-black) in large majority of users, lasting up to 5 years

▷ **Principal Uses**
   As a Single Drug Product: Uses currently included in FDA approved labeling: Treatment of leprosy, in combination with other antileprosy drugs.
   Other (unlabeled) generally accepted uses: Treatment of AIDS-related infections with Mycobacterium avium-intracellulare; used in combination with other antimycobacterial drugs.

How This Drug Works: This drug binds to mycobacterial DNA and slowly kills the microorganism.

Available Dosage Forms and Strengths
   Capsules — 50 mg, 100 mg

▷ **Recommended Dosage Ranges** (Actual dosage and administration schedule must be determined by the physician for each patient individually.)
   Infants and Children: Dosage not established.
   12 to 60 Years of Age: For leprosy—50–100 mg once daily.
      For AIDS-related MAI infections—100 mg/8 hours.
      Total daily dosage should not exceed 300 mg.
   Over 60 Years of Age: Same as 12 to 60 years of age.

Conditions Requiring Dosing Adjustments
   Liver function: The dose **must** be decreased in liver compromise.
   Kidney function: Medication adjustments are not usually needed.

▷ **Dosing Instructions:** Take with food. Swallow capsule whole; do not alter or chew. Should be taken with one or more other antileprosy drugs to prevent the emergence of drug-resistance.

Usual Duration of Use: Use on a regular schedule for 1 to 3 months is usually needed to see this drug's effectiveness in controlling leprosy or MAI infection. Long-term use (months to years) requires periodic evaluation of response.

▷ **This Drug Should Not Be Taken If**
   • you have had an allergic reaction to it previously.
   • you have active peptic ulcer disease.
   • you have active inflammatory bowel disease—Crohn's disease or ulcerative colitis.
   • you have active liver disease.

Clofazimine

▷ **Inform Your Physician Before Taking This Drug If**
- you have a history of serious gastrointestinal disorders: peptic ulcer, Crohn's disease, ulcerative colitis, hepatitis.
- you have impaired liver function.
- you are pregnant or planning pregnancy.
- you have a history of blood disorders such as anemia or low blood platelets.

Possible Side-Effects (natural, expected and unavoidable drug actions)
Red to brownish-black coloration of the skin, hair, conjunctiva, tears, saliva, sweat, breast milk, urine and feces usually starting a few weeks after taking the drug. Depending upon the length of use, the skin may require 1 to 5 years to clear once the drug is stopped.

▷ **Possible Adverse Effects** (unusual, unexpected and infrequent reactions)
If any of the following develop, consult your physician promptly for guidance.

Mild Adverse Effects
Allergic Reactions: Skin rash, itching (5%).
Dry, rough or scaly skin changes (35%).
Headache, dizziness, drowsiness, fatigue (all less than 1%).
Irritation and burning of eyes (24%), impaired vision (12%).
Altered taste, loss of appetite (14%), nausea or vomiting (9%), diarrhea (9%).

Serious Adverse Effects
Severe abdominal symptoms: pain, burning, gastrointestinal bleeding (bloody or black stools), intestinal obstruction.
Drug-induced hepatitis with jaundice (see Glossary)(rare).
Vision changes (corneal deposits).

▷ **Possible Effects on Sexual Function:** None reported.

Possible Delayed Adverse Effects: Drug crystals may accumulate in the intestine, eye and abdominal lymph glands, causing abdominal pain, vision problems and digestive disorders for months after discontinuation of treatment.

▷ **Adverse Effects That May Mimic Natural Diseases or Disorders**
Liver reactions may suggest viral hepatitis.
Abdominal pain and digestive tract symptoms have caused exploratory surgery.

Possible Effects on Laboratory Tests
Erythrocyte sedimentation rate (ESR): increased.
Blood glucose level: increased.
Blood potassium level: decreased.
Liver function tests: increased liver enzymes and bilirubin.

CAUTION
1. Call your doctor if skin discoloration causes undue stress.
2. If you experience digestive symptoms or abdominal pain, watch for bloody or black stools that could indicate intestinal bleeding. Report this promptly.

Precautions for Use
  By Infants and Children: Safety and effectiveness for those under 12 years of age not established.
  By Those over 60 Years of Age: No information available.

▷ **Advisability of Use During Pregnancy**
  Pregnancy Category:
    C. See Pregnancy Code at the back of this book.
    Animal studies: Mouse studies reveal fetal toxicity but no drug-induced birth defects.
    Human studies: Adequate studies of pregnant women are not available.
    Use this drug only if clearly needed. Ask your physician for guidance.

Advisability of Use if Breast-Feeding
  Presence of this drug in breast milk: Yes.
  Avoid drug or refrain from nursing.

Habit-Forming Potential: None.

Effects of Overdosage: Nausea, vomiting, diarrhea.

Possible Effects of Long-Term Use: Intense discoloration of skin, cornea and conjunctiva. Visual disturbances.

Suggested Periodic Examinations While Taking This Drug (at physician's discretion)
  Liver function tests, as appropriate.

▷ **While Taking This Drug, Observe the Following**
  Foods: No restrictions.
  Beverages: No restrictions. May be taken with milk.
▷ *Alcohol:* No interactions expected. Avoid in the presence of liver dysfunction.
  Tobacco Smoking: No interactions expected.
▷ *Other Drugs*: No significant drug interactions reported.
▷ *Driving, Hazardous Activities:* This drug may cause dizziness or nausea. Restrict activities as necessary.
  Aviation Note: The use of this drug **may be a disqualification** for piloting. Consult a designated Aviation Medical Examiner.
  Exposure to Sun: Use caution. This drug can cause photosensitivity (see Glossary). If sensitive to sun, avoid use of sun lamps, tanning beds and booths.
  Discontinuation: Because of the nature of mycobacterial infections, long-term drug therapy is needed for control or cure. Discuss the probable length of treatment with your physician. Do not stop this drug without your doctor's help.

CLOMIPRAMINE (kloh MI pra meen)

Introduced: 1970 **Prescription:** USA: Yes; Canada: Yes **Available as Generic:** USA: No; Canada: No **Class:** Antiobsessive-compulsive, Antidepressant **Controlled Drug:** USA: No; Canada: No
Brand Name: Anafranil

Clomipramine

BENEFITS versus RISKS	
Possible Benefits	*Possible Risks*
EFFECTIVE TREATMENT OF SEVERE OBSESSIVE-COMPULSIVE NEUROSIS Effective relief of symptoms of some types of endogenous depression	DRUG-INDUCED SEIZURES (appoximately 1%) ADVERSE BEHAVIORAL EFFECTS: confusion, delirium, disorientation, hallucinations, delusions, paranoia Conversion of depression to mania in manic-depressive disorders Aggravation of schizophrenia Rare liver toxicity Rare bone marrow depression and blood cell disorders

▷ **Principal Uses**
  As a Single Drug Product: Uses currently included in FDA approved labeling: (1) Relieves manifestations of severe, disabling obsessive-compulsive disorder.
  Other (unlabeled) generally accepted uses: (1) Relieves symptoms of panic attacks; (2) helps some phobias; (3) may help repetitive symptoms in autistics; (4) could have a role in diabetic neuropathy; (5) can help premature ejaculation; (6) may relieve severity of hair pulling syndromes, severe nail biting and arm burning in obsessive-compulsive patients; (7) can help relieve symptoms in severe premenstrual syndrome.

How This Drug Works: By increasing brain levels of some nerve transmitters, principally serotonin, this drug reduces the frequency and intensity of obsessive and compulsive behavior patterns.

Available Dosage Forms and Strengths
  Capsules — 10 mg, 25 mg, 50 mg, 75 mg

▷ **Usual Adult Dosage Range:** Initially 25 mg daily, taken in the evening. Dose may be increased cautiously as needed and tolerated by 25 mg daily at intervals of 3 to 4 days until a dose of 100 mg daily is reached in 2 weeks. This larger dose should be divided and taken after meals. The usual maintenance dose is 50 mg to 150 mg/24 hours. The total daily dosage should not exceed 250 mg. (When determined, the optimal daily requirement may be given at bedtime as a single dose.) **Note: Actual dosage and administration schedule must be determined by the physician for each patient individually.**

Conditions Requiring Dosing Adjustments
  Liver function: The dose should be decreased in patients with liver compromise.
  Kidney function: Changes in dose are not usually needed.

▷ **Dosing Instructions:** May be taken without regard to meals. If needed, the capsule may be opened and may be taken taken with or following food to reduce stomach upset.

Usual Duration of Use: Use on a regular schedule for 3 to 4 weeks is usually needed to see this drug's benefit in controlling obsessive-compulsive behavior; peak response may require 3 or more months of use. Long-term use (months to years) requires periodic evaluation.

Currently a "Drug of Choice"
for the management of obsessive-compulsive disorder.

▷ **This Drug Should Not Be Taken If**
- you have had an allergic reaction to it previously.
- you are taking, or have taken within the past 14 days, any monoamine oxidase (MAO) type A inhibitor drug (see Drug Classes).
- you have active bone marrow depression or a current blood cell disorder.
- you have had a recent heart attack (myocardial infarction).
- you have narrow-angle glaucoma.

▷ **Inform Your Physician Before Taking This Drug If**
- you have had an adverse reaction to an antidepressant drug, especially one of the tricyclic class.
- you have a history of bone marrow or blood cell disorder.
- you have any type of seizure disorder.
- you have increased internal eye pressure.
- you have any type of heart disease, especially coronary artery disease or a heart rhythm disorder.
- you are subject to bronchial asthma.
- you have impaired liver or kidney function.
- you have any type of thyroid disorder or are taking thyroid medication.
- you have a history of suicide attempts.
- you have an adrenalin-producing tumor.
- you have prostatism (see Glossary).
- you have a history of alcoholism.
- you plan to have surgery under general anesthesia in the near future.

Possible Side-Effects (natural, expected and unavoidable drug actions)
Drowsiness (54%), increased sweating (29%), light-headedness (6%), blurred vision (18%), dry mouth (84%), constipation (47%), impaired urination (14%).

▷ **Possible Adverse Effects** (unusual, unexpected and infrequent reactions)
If any of the following develop, consult your physician promptly for guidance.

Mild Adverse Effects
Allergic Reactions: Skin rash (8%), itching (6%), drug fever (4%), (see Glossary).
Headache (52%), dizziness (54%), nervousness (18%), impaired memory (9%), weakness (39%), tremors (54%), insomnia (25%), muscle cramps (13%), flushing (8%).
Increased appetite (32%), weight gain (18%).
Altered taste (8%), indigestion (22%), nausea (33%), vomiting (7%), diarrhea (13%).

Serious Adverse Effects
Allergic Reactions: Drug-induced hepatitis, with or without jaundice.
Idiosyncratic Reactions: Neuroleptic malignant syndrome (see Glossary).
Adverse behavioral effects: confusion (3%), delirium, disorientation, delusions, hallucinations, paranoia.
Seizures; reduced control of epilepsy.

228   Clomipramine

Aggravation of paranoid psychoses and schizophrenia.
Heart rhythm disturbances.
Bone marrow depression (see Glossary): fatigue, weakness, fever, sore throat, infections, abnormal bleeding or bruising.
Liver toxicity.
Serotonin syndrome.

▷ **Possible Effects on Sexual Function**
Altered libido (21%), impaired ejaculation (42%), impotence (20%), inhibited male orgasm, inhibited female orgasm, female breast enlargement with milk production (4%).

▷ **Adverse Effects That May Mimic Natural Diseases or Disorders**
Liver toxicity may suggest viral hepatitis.

Natural Diseases or Disorders That May Be Activated by This Drug
Latent epilepsy, glaucoma, prostatism, schizophrenia.

Possible Effects on Laboratory Tests
Complete blood cell counts: decreased red cells, hemoglobin, white cells and platelets.
Liver function tests: increased liver enzymes (ALT/GPT, AST/GOT)—liver damage.
Thyroid function tests: decreased TT3 and FT3.

CAUTION
1. Watch for toxicity: Confusion, agitation, rapid heart rate, heart irregularity. Blood levels will clarify the situation.
2. Use with caution in schizophrenia. Observe closely for any deterioration of thinking or behavior.
3. Use with caution in epilepsy. Watch for any change in the frequency or severity of seizures.

Precautions for Use
By Infants and Children: Safety and effectiveness for those under 10 years of age not established. Dose and management should be supervised by a properly trained pediatrician. Total daily dosage should not exceed 200 mg.
By Those over 60 Years of Age: Start treatment with 10 mg at bedtime. Dose may be increased gradually as needed and tolerated to 75 mg daily in divided doses. During the first 2 weeks of treatment, watch for behavioral reactions: Restlessness, agitation, forgetfulness, disorientation, delusions or hallucinations. Also observe for unsteadiness and instability that may predispose to falling. This drug may aggravate prostatism.

▷ **Advisability of Use During Pregnancy**
Pregnancy Category:
C. See Pregnancy Code at the back of this book.
Animal studies: No drug-induced birth defects reported in mouse or rat studies.
Human studies: Adequate studies of pregnant women are not available.
Use only if clearly needed. Avoid use during the last 3 months, if possible, to prevent withdrawal symptoms in the newborn infant: irritability, tremors, seizures.

Advisability of Use if Breast-Feeding
   Presence of this drug in breast milk: Yes.
   Avoid drug or refrain from nursing.
Habit-Forming Potential: Psychological or physical dependence is rare and unexpected. This drug is not liable to abuse.
Effects of Overdosage: Confusion, delirium, hallucinations, drowsiness, tremors, unsteadiness, heart irregularity, seizures, stupor, sweating, fever.
Possible Effects of Long-Term Use: Neuroleptic malignant syndrome (see Glossary): Fever, fast or irregular heartbeat, fast breathing, sweating, weakness, muscle stiffness, seizures, loss of bladder control.
Suggested Periodic Examinations While Taking This Drug (at physician's discretion)
   Monitoring of blood drug levels as appropriate.
   Complete blood cell counts; liver and kidney function tests.
   Serial blood pressure readings and electrocardiograms.
   Measurement of internal eye pressure.

▷ **While Taking This Drug, Observe the Following**
   Foods: No specific restrictions. May need to limit food intake to avoid excessive weight gain.
   Beverages: No restrictions. May be taken with milk.
▷ *Alcohol:* Avoid completely. This drug can markedly increase the intoxicating effects of alcohol; the combination can depress brain function significantly.
   Tobacco Smoking: May delay the elimination of this drug and require dosage adjustment.
   Marijuana Smoking: Increased drowsiness and mouth dryness; and reduced effectiveness.
▷ *Other Drugs*
   Clomipramine may *increase* the effects of
   • all drugs with sedative effects; observe for excessive sedation.
   • all drugs with atropinelike effects (see Drug Classes).
   Clomipramine may *decrease* the effects of
   • clonidine (Catapres).
   • guanadrel (Hylorel).
   • guanethidine (Ismelin, Esimil).
   Clomipramine *taken concurrently* with
   • anticonvulsants requires careful monitoring for changes in seizure patterns and need to adjust anticonvulsant dosage.
   • monoamine oxidase (MAO) type A inhibitor drugs (see Drug Class) may cause high fever, seizures and excessive rise in blood pressure; avoid combining these drugs and provide periods of 14 days between administration of either.
   • stimulant drugs (amphetamine, cocaine, epinephrine, phenylpropanolamine, etc.) may cause severe high blood pressure and/or high fever.
   • thyroid preparations may increase the risk of heart rhythm disorders.
   • warfarin may cause an increased warfarin effect and bleeding.
   The following drugs may *increase* the effects of clomipramine
   • ACE inhibitors (see Drug Class).
   • cimetidine (Tagamet).

- estrogens.
- fluoxetine (Prozac).
- haloperidol (Haldol).
- methylphenidate (Ritalin).
- oral contraceptives.
- phenothiazines (see Drug Class).
- quinidine.
- ranitidine (Zantac).

The following drugs may *decrease* the effects of clomipramine
- barbiturates (see Drug Class).
- carbamazepine (Tegretol).
- chloral hydrate (Noctec, Somnos, etc.).
- lithium (Lithobid, Lithotab, etc.).
- reserpine (Serpasil, Ser-Ap-Es, etc.).

▷ *Driving, Hazardous Activities:*
This drug may cause seizures and impair alertness, judgment, physical coordination and reaction time. Restrict activities as necessary.

Aviation Note:
The use of this drug **is a disqualification** for piloting. Consult a designated Aviation Medical Examiner.

Exposure to Sun: No restrictions.

Exposure to Heat: Use caution. This drug may impair the body's adaptation to hot environments, increasing the risk of heat stroke. Avoid saunas.

Exposure to Environmental Chemicals: This drug may mask the symptoms of poisoning due to handling certain insecticides (organophosphorus types). Read their labels carefully.

Discontinuation: It is advisable to stop this drug gradually over a period of 3 to 4 weeks. Abrupt withdrawal after prolonged use may cause nausea, vomiting, diarrhea, headache, dizziness, malaise, disturbed sleep and irritability. Obsessive-compulsive behavior may worsen when this drug is stopped. It may be necessary to adjust the dosages of other drugs taken concurrently when this drug is discontinued.

CLONAZEPAM (kloh NA ze pam)

Introduced: 1977 **Prescription:** USA: Yes; Canada: Yes **Available as Generic:** No **Class:** Anticonvulsant, benzodiazepines **Controlled Drug:** USA: C-IV*; Canada: No

Brand Names: Klonopin, ✦Rivotril

Warning: The brand name Klonopin and the generic name clonidine are similar and can be mistaken for each other; this can lead to serious medication errors. These names represent very different drugs. Verify that you are taking the correct drug.

*See Schedules of Controlled Drugs at the back of this book.

Clonazepam

BENEFITS versus RISKS	
Possible Benefits	**Possible Risks**
EFFECTIVE CONTROL OF SOME TYPES OF PETIT MAL, AKINETIC AND MYOCLONIC SEIZURES	Paradoxical reactions: excitement, agitation, hallucinations
	Minor impairment of mental functions
Possibly effective in the management of panic disorders	Rare blood cell disorders: anemia, abnormally low white blood cell and platelet counts
	Increased salivation (of concern for those with chronic lung disease)

▷ **Principal Uses**

As a Single Drug Product: Uses currently included in FDA approved labeling: (1) Treats several types of epilepsy: petit mal variations, akinetic, myoclonic and absence seizure patterns

Other (unlabeled) generally accepted uses: (1) control panic disorders; (2) Helps control Tourette's syndrome; (3) Relieves pain in trigeminal neuralgia; (4) Can ease symptoms in resistant depression; (5) can ease drug-induced mania.

How This Drug Works: This drug produces an anticonvulsant effect by increasing the action of a nerve transmitter (gamma-aminobutyric acid), which then blocks seizures.

Available Dosage Forms and Strengths
Tablets — 0.5 mg, 1 mg, 2 mg

▷ **Usual Adult Dosage Range:** Initially 0.5 mg three times daily. The dose may be increased by 0.5 mg to 1.0 mg every three days, as needed and tolerated, until seizures are controlled. Total daily dose should not exceed 20 mg.
Note: Actual dosage and administration schedule must be determined by the physician for each patient individually.

Conditions Requiring Dosing Adjustments
Liver function: The dose must be decreased in liver compromise.
Kidney function: Watch for signs and symptoms of accumulation (see overdosage).

▷ **Dosing Instructions:** May be taken on empty stomach or with food or milk. The tablet may be crushed for administration. Do not stop this drug abruptly if taken for control of seizures, or if taken for more than 4 weeks to control panic attacks.

Usual Duration of Use: Use on a regular schedule for 2 to 3 weeks may be needed to see this drug's benefit in reducing the frequency and severity of seizures. Peak control will require careful dosage adjustments over a period of several months. Long-term use (months to years) requires ongoing supervision and periodic evaluation by your physician.

▷ **This Drug Should Not Be Taken If**
- you have had an allergic reaction to it previously.
- you have acute narrow-angle glaucoma.
- you have active liver disease.

Clonazepam

▷ **Inform Your Physician Before Taking This Drug If**
- you are allergic to any benzodiazepine (see Drug Class).
- you have a history of alcoholism or drug abuse.
- you are pregnant or planning pregnancy.
- you have impaired liver or kidney function.
- you have a history of serious depression or mental disorder.
- you have any of the following: asthma, emphysema, chronic bronchitis, myasthenia gravis.
- you have acute intermittant porphyria.

Possible Side-Effects (natural, expected and unavoidable drug actions)
Drowsiness (50%), lethargy, unsteadiness (30%), increased salivation (7%).

▷ **Possible Adverse Effects** (unusual, unexpected and infrequent reactions)
If any of the following develop, consult your physician promptly for guidance.
Mild Adverse Effects
Allergic Reactions: Skin rash, hives, itching.
Headache, dizziness, blurred vision, double vision, slurred speech, impaired memory, confusion, mental depression.
Muscle weakness, trembling, uncontrolled body movements.
Nausea, vomiting, constipation, diarrhea, impaired urination.
Serious Adverse Effects
Idiosyncratic Reactions: Paradoxical responses of excitement, hyperactivity, agitation, anger, hostility.
Hallucinations, seizures.
Rare blood disorders: Abnormally low red blood cell, white blood cell and platelet counts.
Porphyria.
Abnormal eye movements.
Increased secretions and breathing problems, especially in those with chronic lung disease.

▷ **Possible Effects on Sexual Function:** Increased libido, enlargement of male breasts. May cause abnormally early (precocious) secondary sex characteristics in children.

Possible Effects on Laboratory Tests
Complete blood cell counts: decreased red cells, hemoglobin, white cells and platelets.
Urine screening tests for drug abuse; may be **positive**. (Test results depend upon amount of drug taken and testing method used.)

CAUTION
1. This drug should not be stopped abruptly if used to control seizures.
2. Some over-the-counter drug products that contain antihistamines (allergy and cold preparations, sleep aids) can cause excessive sedation if combined with clonazepam.
3. Adverse behavioral reactions are more common in people with brain damage, mental retardation or psychiatric disorders.
4. A decreased response to this drug occurs in approximately 30% of users within 3 months after initiating treatment. Dosage adjustment may be necessary to restore seizure control.

Precautions for Use

By Infants and Children: This drug is used to treat infants and children of all ages. Careful dosage adjustment based on weight and age is mandatory. Abnormal behavioral responses are more common in children.

By Those over 60 Years of Age: Smaller doses and longer intervals are suggested. Watch for development of lethargy, indifference, fatigue, weakness, unsteadiness, disturbing dreams, nightmares and paradoxical reactions of excitement, agitation, anger, hostility and rage.

▷ **Advisability of Use During Pregnancy**

Pregnancy Category: C. See Pregnancy Code at the back of this book.

Animal studies: This drug causes cleft palates, open eyelids, fused rib structures and limb defects in rabbits.

Human studies: Adequate studies of pregnant women are not available.

It is advisable to avoid this drug during the first 3 months if possible. Frequent use in late pregnancy may cause the "floppy infant" syndrome in the newborn: weakness, lethargy, unresponsiveness, depressed breathing, low body temperature.

Advisability of Use if Breast-Feeding

Presence of this drug in breast milk: Probably yes.

Avoid drug or refrain from nursing.

Habit-Forming Potential: This drug can produce psychological and/or physical dependence (see Glossary) if used in large doses for an extended period of time.

Effects of Overdosage: Marked drowsiness, weakness, confusion, slurred speech, staggering gait, tremor, stupor progressing to deep sleep or coma.

Possible Effects of Long-Term Use: Benefits versus risks must be considered carefully during the extended use of this drug in children. Possible adverse effects on physical or mental development may not be apparent for many years.

Suggested Periodic Examinations While Taking This Drug (at physician's discretion)

During long-term use: Complete blood cell counts; liver function tests.

▷ **While Taking This Drug, Observe the Following**

Foods: No restrictions.

Beverages: No restrictions. May be taken with milk.

▷ *Alcohol:* Use with extreme caution. Alcohol may increase the depressant effects of this drug on the brain. It is advisable to avoid alcohol completely—throughout the day and night—if it is necessary to drive or to engage in any hazardous activity.

Tobacco Smoking: No interactions expected.

Marijuana Smoking: Increased sedation and significant impairment of intellectual and physical performance.

▷ **Other Drugs**

Clonazepam *taken concurrently* with

- amiodarone (Codarone) may decrease elimination of clonazepam and also worsen toxicity by causing low thyroid function.
- carbamazepine (Tegretol) may decrease blood levels and hence benefits of both medications.

- desipramine, imipramine and other tricyclic antidepressants (see Drug Class Section) can decrease the tricyclic antidepressant blood level and lessen its therapeutic benefit.
- valproic acid (Depakene, etc.) may cause continuous absence seizures.

The following drugs may *increase* the effects of clonazepam
- cimetidine (Tagamet).
- disulfiram (Antabuse).
- omeprazole (Losec).
- oral contraceptives.

The following drugs may *decrease* the effects of clonazepam
- theophylline (aminophylline, Theo-Dur, etc.).

▷ *Driving, Hazardous Activities:* This drug can impair mental alertness, judgment, physical coordination and reaction time. Avoid hazardous activities accordingly.

Aviation Note:
The use of this drug **is a disqualification** for piloting. Consult a designated Aviation Medical Examiner.

Exposure to Sun: No restrictions.

Discontinuation: Do not stop clonazepam suddenly if it is being used to control any type of seizure, or if it has been taken for more than 4 weeks to treat other conditions. Dosage should be tapered gradually to prevent a withdrawal syndrome that could include depression, confusion, hallucinations, tremor, seizures, muscle cramping, sweating and vomiting.

CLONIDINE (KLOH ni deen)

Introduced: 1969 **Prescription:** USA: Yes; Canada: Yes **Available as Generic:** USA: Yes; Canada: No **Class:** Antihypertensive **Controlled Drug:** USA: No; Canada: No

Brand Names: ◆Apo-Clonidine, Catapres, Catapres-TTS, Combipres [CD], ◆Dixarit, ◆Nu-Clonidine

BENEFITS versus RISKS	
Possible Benefits	*Possible Risks*
EFFECTIVE ANTIHYPERTENSIVE in mild to moderate high blood pressure	ACUTE WITHDRAWAL SYNDROME (rebound hypertension) with abrupt discontinuation
Effective control of menopausal hot flashes (in selected cases)	Raynaud's phenomenon (cold fingers or toes)
Effective help in narcotic withdrawal	

▷ **Principal Uses**

As a Single Drug Product: Uses currently included in FDA approved labeling: Used as a "step 2" drug in the treatment of mild to moderate high blood pressure. Generally not used to start therapy, but is added when a "step 1" drug doesn't work. It may be added as a "step 3 or 4" drug, replacing drugs that cause marked orthostatic hypotension (see Glossary).

Other (unlabeled) generally accepted uses: (1) Helps prevent migraine headache; (2) may help improve outcomes in patients with head injuries; (3)

can aid menopausal hot flashes and treat severe menstrual cramps; (4) helps to lessen symptoms of alcohol or narcotic drug withdrawal.

As a Combination Drug Product [CD]: This "step 2" antihypertensive is available in combination with the "step 1" antihypertensive drug chlorthalidone, a diuretic. The different ways in which these drugs work complement each other, making the combination a more effective antihypertensive.

How This Drug Works: By decreasing the activity of part of the brain (vasomotor center), this drug limits the ability of the sympathetic nervous system to constrict blood vessels and increase blood pressure.

Available Dosage Forms and Strengths
Patches — 2.5 mg, 5.0 mg, 7.5 mg
Tablets — 0.1 mg, 0.2 mg, 0.3 mg

▷ **Usual Adult Dosage Range:** Tablets—initially 0.1 mg twice daily. Increase by 0.1 to 0.2 mg daily as needed and tolerated. Usual range is 0.2 to 0.8 mg daily, taken in 2 doses. Total daily dosage should not exceed 2.4 mg. Medicated patches are applied once a week. **Note: Actual dosage and administration schedule must be determined by the physician for each patient individually.**

Conditions Requiring Dosing Adjustments
Liver function: This drug is changed into 6 active forms. The dose must be decreased in liver compromise.
Kidney function: The dose must be decreased by up to 75% in severe kidney failure.

▷ **Dosing Instructions:** Tablets may be taken without regard to eating. The tablet may be crushed for administration.

Usual Duration of Use: Use on a regular schedule for 2 to 3 weeks is usually needed to see this drug's benefit in lowering high blood pressure. Long-term use (months to years) requires physician supervision and guidance.

▷ **This Drug Should Not Be Taken If**
- you have had an allergic reaction to it previously.
- you have a problem in your heart that impacts the timing of the heartbeat or transmission of electrical impulses through the heart.

▷ **Inform Your Physician Before Taking This Drug If**
- you have a circulatory disorder of the brain.
- you have angina or coronary artery disease.
- you have or have had serious emotional depression.
- you have a very slow heart rate.
- you have Buerger's disease or Raynaud's phenomenon.
- you are taking a tricyclic antidepressant (see Drug Classes).
- you are taking any sedative or hypnotic drugs or an antidepressant.
- you plan to have surgery under general anesthesia in the near future.

Possible Side-Effects (natural, expected and unavoidable drug actions)
Drowsiness (35%), dry nose and mouth (40%), constipation (common), decreased heart rate, mild orthostatic hypotension (see Glossary).

▷ **Possible Adverse Effects** (unusual, unexpected and infrequent reactions)
If any of the following develop, consult your physician promptly for guidance.

Clonidine

Mild Adverse Effects
  Allergic Reactions: Skin rash, hives, localized swellings, itching.
  Headache, dizziness, fatigue, anxiety, nervousness, dryness and burning eyes.
  Painful parotid (salivary) gland, nausea, vomiting.
  Weight gain, urinary retention.
  Dry mouth.
  Urination at night (1%).
  Thinning of hair (rare).

Serious Adverse Effects
  Idiosyncratic Reaction: Raynaud's phenomenon (see Glossary).
  Aggravation of congestive heart failure, heart rhythm disorders, vivid dreaming, nightmares, depression, hallucinations.
  Sleep disorders.
  Corneal ulcers (rare).
  Acute pancreatitis (rare).
  Slow heart beat (bradycardia).

▷ **Possible Effects on Sexual Function:** Decreased libido in 10% (0.2 to 0.8 mg/day); impotence in 8% to 24% (0.5 to 3.6 mg/day); impaired ejaculation (rare); enlargement of male breasts (0.2 to 0.8 mg/day). Precocious puberty in females.

Possible Effects on Laboratory Tests
  Blood cholesterol or triglyceride levels: no consistent or significant effects.
  Blood sodium level: increased.
  Liver function: Rare increases of enzymes (ALT/GPT, AST/GOT, alkaline phosphatase).

CAUTION
  1. ***Do not stop this drug suddenly.*** Sudden withdrawal can cause a severe and possibly fatal reaction.
  2. Hot weather or fever can reduce blood pressure significantly. Dose adjustments may be necessary.
  3. Report the development of any tendency to emotional depression.

Precautions for Use
  By Infants and Children: Safety and effectiveness for those under 12 years of age not established.
  By Those over 60 Years of Age: ***Proceed cautiously*** with this drug. High blood pressure should be reduced slowly without the risks associated with excessively low blood pressure. Low initial doses and frequent blood pressure checks are needed. Watch for development of light-headedness, dizziness, unsteadiness, fainting and falling. Sedation and dry mouth occur in 50% of elderly users. Promptly report any changes in mood or behavior: Depression, delusions, hallucinations.

▷ **Advisability of Use During Pregnancy**
  Pregnancy Category: C. See Pregnancy Code at the back of this book.
    Animal studies: No birth defects reported. However, this drug is toxic to the embryo in low dosage.
    Human studies: Adequate studies of pregnant women are not available.
    The manufacturer recommends that this drug be avoided by women who are or who may become pregnant. Ask physician for guidance.

Advisability of Use if Breast-Feeding
   Presence of this drug in breast milk: Yes.
   This drug may impair milk production. Monitor nursing infant closely and discontinue drug or nursing if adverse effects begin.
Habit-Forming Potential: A small number of reports regarding abuse of this drug have surfaced. It may give extreme grogginess and lethargy when combined with diazepam (valium).
Effects of Overdosage: Marked drowsiness, weakness, dry mouth, slow pulse, low blood pressure, vomiting, stupor progressing to coma.
Possible Effects of Long-Term Use: Development of tolerance (see Glossary) with loss of drug effect; weight gain due to salt and water retention; temporary sexual impotence.
Suggested Periodic Examinations While Taking This Drug (at physician's discretion)
   Blood pressure measurements, monitoring of body weight.

▷ **While Taking This Drug, Observe the Following**
   Foods: Avoid excessive salt. Ask physician for help with degree of salt restriction.
   Beverages: No restrictions. May be taken with milk.
▷ *Alcohol:* Use with extreme caution. Combined effects can cause marked drowsiness and exaggerated reduction of blood pressure.
   Tobacco Smoking: No expected interactions. Heed your doctor's advice about stopping tobacco use.
▷ *Other Drugs*
   Clonidine may *decrease* the effects of
   • levodopa (Larodopa, Sinemet, etc.), causing an increase in parkinsonism symptoms.
   Clonidine *taken concurrently* with
   • beta-adrenergic-blocking drugs (Inderal, Lopressor, etc.) may increase the risk of rebound hypertension if clonidine is stopped first. Best to stop the beta blocker first and then withdraw clonidine gradually.
   • naloxone (Revia) may blunt the therapeutic effect of clonidine and result in a hypertensive response.
   The following drugs may *decrease* the effects of clonidine
   • tricyclic antidepressants (Elavil, Sinequan, etc.) may reduce its effectiveness in lowering blood pressure.
▷ *Driving, Hazardous Activities:* Use caution. This drug can cause drowsiness and can impair mental alertness, judgment and coordination.
   Aviation Note: Hypertension (high blood pressure) *is a disqualification* for piloting. Consult a designated Aviation Medical Examiner.
   Exposure to Sun: No restrictions.
   Exposure to Heat: Use caution. Hot environments may reduce the blood pressure; be alert to the possibility of orthostatic hypotension (see Glossary).
   Exposure to Cold: Use caution. May cause painful blanching and numbness of the hands and feet on exposure to cold air or water (Raynaud's phenomenon).
   Heavy Exercise or Exertion: Use caution. Isometric exercises—the "overload" technique for strengthening individual muscles—can raise blood pressure significantly. This drug may intensify the hypertensive response to isometric exercise. Ask physician for guidance.

238   Clotrimazole

Occurrence of Unrelated Illness: Fever may lower the blood pressure. Repeated vomiting may prevent the regular use of this drug and cause an acute withdrawal reaction. Consult your physician.

Discontinuation: **Do not stop this drug suddenly.** A severe withdrawal reaction can occur within 12 to 48 hours after the last dose. Best to gradually decrease the dose over 3 to 4 days, and check blood pressure often.

CLOTRIMAZOLE (kloh TRIM a zohl)

Introduced: 1976   **Prescription:** USA: Yes; Canada: Yes   **Available as Generic:** USA: No; Canada: No   **Class:** Antifungal   **Controlled Drug:** USA: No; Canada: No

Brand Names: ✦Canesten, Clotrimaderm, Gyne-Lotrimin, Lotrimin, Lotrimin AF, Lotrisone, Mycelex, Mycelex-7, Mycelex-G, ✦Myclo, ✦Neo-Zol

Warning: The brand names Mycelex and Myoflex are similar and can be mistaken for each other; this can lead to serious medication errors. These names represent very different drugs. Verify that you are using the correct drug.

BENEFITS versus RISKS	
Possible Benefits	*Possible Risks*
EFFECTIVE TREATMENT AND PREVENTION OF CANDIDA (YEAST) INFECTIONS OF THE MOUTH AND THROAT (THRUSH)	Skin and mucous membrane irritation due to sensitization (drug-induced allergy)
EFFECTIVE TREATMENT OF CANDIDA (YEAST) INFECTIONS OF THE SKIN	Nausea, vomiting, stomach cramping, diarrhea (when swallowed)
EFFECTIVE TREATMENT OF CANDIDA (YEAST) INFECTIONS OF THE VULVA AND VAGINA	
EFFECTIVE TREATMENT OF TINEA (RINGWORM) INFECTIONS OF THE SKIN	

▷ **Principal Uses**

As a Single Drug Product: Uses currently included in FDA approved labeling: (1) Treatment of candida (yeast) infections of the skin, mouth, throat, vulva and vagina; (2) Treatment of tinea and related infections: ringworm of the body, groin (jock itch), and feet (athlete's foot), due to susceptible fungal organisms.

Other (unlabeled) generally accepted uses: Prevention of candida (yeast) infections of the mouth and throat in the management of AIDS.

How This Drug Works: By damaging cell walls and blocking essential enzymes, this drug inhibits fungal cell growth and reproduction (with low drug concentrations) and kills fungus (with high drug concentrations).

Available Dosage Forms and Strengths
        Cream — 1% (10 mg per gram)
        Lotion — 1% (10 mg per gram)

Topical Solution — 1% (10 mg per ml)
Mouth lozenges — 10 mg
Vaginal Cream — 1% (10 mg per gram)
Vaginal Tablets — 100 mg, 500 mg

▷ **Recommended Dosage Ranges** (Actual dosage and administration schedule must be determined by the physician for each patient individually.)

Infants and Children: Use of lozenges not recommended for children under 5 years of age; for 5 years and older—dissolve 1 lozenge slowly and completely in mouth 5 times a day for 14 days, longer if necessary.

12 to 60 Years of Age: For Candida infections of mouth and throat—Dissolve 1 lozenge slowly and completely in mouth 5 times a day for 14 days; extended treatment may be necessary for people with AIDS.

For Candida and Tinea infections of skin—apply cream, lotion or solution to infected areas twice a day, morning and evening.

For Candida infections of vulva and vagina—1 applicatorful (5 grams) of cream intravaginally at bedtime for 7 to 14 consecutive days; or 1 100 mg tablet intravaginally at bedtime for 7 days, or 2 100 mg tablets intravaginally at bedtime for 3 days; one-dose treatment: 1 500 mg tablet intravaginally at bedtime, one time only.

Over 60 Years of Age: Same as 12 to 60 years of age.

Conditions Requiring Dosing Adjustments

Liver function: The drug goes out via the bile—dose decreased if bile duct is blocked.

Kidney function: Dosing changes are not needed.

▷ **Dosing Instructions:** Dissolve lozenge in mouth completely, swallowing saliva as it accumulates. Do not chew the lozenge or swallow it whole. Take full course prescribed.

Usual Duration of Use: Use on a regular schedule for 1 to 2 weeks is usually needed to see this drug's benefit in controlling yeast or tinea infection. Long-term use (as in management of AIDS) requires periodic evaluation of response and dosage adjustment.

Possible Advantages of This Drug
Reasonably effective with minimal toxicity.
More palatable than nystatin.

▷ **This Drug Should Not Be Taken If**
• you have had an allergic reaction to it previously.

▷ **Inform Your Physician Before Taking This Drug If**
• you are allergic to related antifungal drugs: fluconazole, itraconazole, ketoconazole, miconazole.

Possible Side-Effects (natural, expected and unavoidable drug actions)
None.

▷ **Possible Adverse Effects** (unusual, unexpected and infrequent reactions)
If any of the following develop, consult your physician promptly for guidance.

Mild Adverse Effects
Allergic Reactions: Skin rash, hives, itching, burning, swelling, blistering (not present prior to treatment).
Nausea, vomiting, stomach cramping, diarrhea (when swallowed).

Cloxacillin

Serious Adverse Effects
Allergic Reactions: Sensitization of tissues (where applied locally) that will react allergically with future drug application.

▷ **Possible Effects on Sexual Function:** None.

Possible Delayed Adverse Effects: Local tissue sensitization to this drug.

Possible Effects on Laboratory Tests
Liver function tests: Increased liver enzyme AST/GOT in 15% of users.

CAUTION
1. Avoid contact of cream, lotion and solution with the eyes.
2. Do not cover applied cream or lotion with an occlusive dressing.

Precautions for Use
By Infants and Children: Use of lozenges by those under 5 years of age is not recommended.
By Those over 60 Years of Age: No problems reported.

▷ **Advisability of Use During Pregnancy**
Pregnancy Category: B. See Pregnancy Code at the back of this book.
Animal studies: No drug-induced birth defects were found in mouse, rat or rabbit studies.
Human studies: Adequate studies of pregnant women are not available.
Use this drug only if clearly needed. Ask your physician for guidance.

Advisability of Use if Breast-Feeding
Presence of this drug in breast milk: Unknown.
Watch infant closely and stop drug or nursing if adverse effects start.

Habit-Forming Potential: None.

Effects of Overdosage: Excessive use of lozenges may cause nausea, vomiting or diarrhea.

Possible Effects of Long-Term Use: None reported.

Suggested Periodic Examinations While Taking This Drug (at physician's discretion)
None.

▷ **While Taking This Drug, Observe the Following**
Foods: No restrictions.
Beverages: No restrictions.
▷ *Alcohol:* No interactions expected.
Tobacco Smoking: No interactions expected.
▷ *Other Drugs:* Clotrimazole **taken concurrently** with
• cyclosporine may result in cyclosporine toxicity.
▷ *Driving, Hazardous Activities:* No restrictions.
Aviation Note: No restrictions.
Exposure to Sun: No restrictions.
Discontinuation: As directed by your physician.

CLOXACILLIN (klox a SIL in)

Introduced: 1962 **Prescription:** USA: Yes; Canada: Yes **Available as Generic:** USA: Yes; Canada: No **Class:** Antibiotic, penicillins **Controlled Drug:** USA: No; Canada: No

Brand Names: ✦Apo-Cloxi, ✦Bactopen, Cloxapen, ✦Novo-Cloxin, ✦Nu-Cloxi, ✦Orbenin, Tegopen

BENEFITS versus RISKS	
Possible Benefits	*Possible Risks*
EFFECTIVE TREATMENT OF INFECTIONS due to susceptible microorganisms	ALLERGIC REACTIONS, mild to severe Superinfections (yeast) Drug-induced colitis Rare blood cell disorders

▷ **Principal Uses**
 As a Single Drug Product: Uses currently included in FDA approved labeling: Used to (1) treat infections that are caused by bacteria (principally staphylococcus) that have developed resistance to the original types of penicillin. It is of value in treating infections of the skin and skin structures, the upper and lower respiratory tract (including strep throat) and infections that are widely scattered throughout the body.
 Other (unlabeled) generally accepted uses: (1) May have a limited role in treatment of bone infections where intravenous medicines are not tolerated.
How This Drug Works: This drug destroys susceptible infecting bacteria by interfering with their ability to produce new protective cell walls as they multiply and grow.
Available Dosage Forms and Strengths
 Capsules — 250 mg, 500 mg
 Oral solution — 125 mg per 5-ml teaspoonful
▷ **Usual Adult Dosage Range:** 250 to 500 mg/6 hours (4 doses/24 hours). The maximal dose is 6000 mg/24 hours. **Note: Actual dosage and administration schedule must be determined by the physician for each patient individually.**
Conditions Requiring Dosing Adjustments
 Liver function: Significantly metabolized to both active and inactive metabolites. This medication is also highly protein bound. Decrease the dose or interval in liver disease.
 Kidney function: This drug is eliminated through the bile and the urine. Monitor the patient closely if there is severe kidney compromise.
▷ **Dosing Instructions:** Take on empty stomach, 1 hour before or 2 hours after eating, at same times each day. Capsule may be opened for administration.
Usual Duration of Use: As long as necessary to eradicate the infection. For all streptococcal infections: not less than 10 consecutive days (without interruption) to reduce the possibility of developing rheumatic fever or glomerulonephritis.
▷ **This Drug Should Not Be Taken If**
 • you have had an allergic reaction to any dosage form of it previously.
 • you are certain you are allergic to *any* form of penicillin.
▷ **Inform Your Physician Before Taking This Drug If**
 • you suspect you may be allergic to penicillin or you have a history of a previous "reaction" to penicillin.
 • you are allergic to cephalosporin antibiotics (Ancef, Ceporan, Ceporex, Duricef, Kafocin, Keflex, Keflin, Kefzol, Loridine).

Cloxacillin

- you are allergic by nature—hay fever, asthma, hives, eczema.
- you have a history of kidney disease, regional enteritis or ulcerative colitis.
- you have a history of liver or kidney failure.

Possible Side-Effects (natural, expected and unavoidable drug actions)
Superinfections (see Glossary), often due to yeast organisms.

▷ **Possible Adverse Effects** (unusual, unexpected and infrequent reactions)
If any of the following develop, consult your physician promptly for guidance.
Mild Adverse Effects
Allergic Reactions: Skin rashes, hives, itching.
Irritations of mouth and tongue, unpleasant taste, nausea, vomiting, mild diarrhea.
Serious Adverse Effects
Allergic Reactions: Anaphylactic reaction (see Glossary), severe skin reactions, drug fever, swollen painful joints, sore throat.
Pseudomembranous colitis—severe diarrhea.
Kidney problems (interstitial nephritis).
Liver problems (cholestatic jaundice)(rare).

▷ **Possible Effects on Sexual Function:** None reported.

Possible Effects on Laboratory Tests
Complete blood cell counts: decreased white cells; increased eosinophils (allergic reaction).

CAUTION
1. Take the exact dose and the full course prescribed.
2. This drug should not be used concurrently with antibiotics like erythromycin or tetracycline.

Precautions for Use
By Infants and Children: Dosage is based on age and weight. Consult your physician for precise dosage schedule.
By Those over 60 Years of Age: It is advisable to evaluate kidney function before and during use of this drug to determine the need for dosage adjustment. Natural changes in the skin may predispose to prolonged itching reactions in the genital and anal regions. Report such reactions promptly.

▷ **Advisability of Use During Pregnancy**
Pregnancy Category: B. See Pregnancy Code at the back of this book.
Animal studies: No birth defects reported in rabbit studies.
Human studies: Information from adequate studies of pregnant women indicates no increased risk of birth defects in 3546 pregnancies exposed to penicillin derivatives.
Use only if clearly needed. Ask physician for guidance.

Advisability of Use if Breast-Feeding
Presence of this drug in breast milk: Probably, yes.
The nursing infant may be sensitized to penicillin and may be at risk for diarrhea or yeast infections. Avoid drug if possible or refrain from nursing.

Habit-Forming Potential: None.

Effects of Overdosage: Possible nausea, vomiting and/or diarrhea.

Possible Effects of Long-Term Use: Superinfections, often due to yeast organisms.

Suggested Periodic Examinations While Taking This Drug (at physician's discretion)
Complete blood cell counts. Liver and kidney function tests with long-term use.

▷ **While Taking This Drug, Observe the Following**
Foods: No restrictions.
Beverages: No restrictions.
▷ *Alcohol:* No interactions expected.
Tobacco Smoking: No interactions expected.
▷ *Other Drugs*
Cloxacillin may *decrease* the effects of
- Birth control pills (oral contraceptives) in some women, and impair their effectiveness in preventing pregnancy.

The following drugs may *decrease* the effects of cloxacillin
- antacids may reduce the absorption of cloxacillin.
- chloramphenicol (Chloromycetin).
- erythromycin (Erythrocin, E-Mycin, etc.).
- tetracyclines (Achromycin, Declomycin, Minocin, etc.). (See Drug Class.)

Cloxacillin *taken concurrently* with
- warfarin (Coumadin) may intensify the anticoagulant effect and increase risk of bleeding.

▷ *Driving, Hazardous Activities:* Usually no restrictions.
Aviation Note: The use of this drug *may be a disqualification* for piloting. Consult a designated Aviation Medical Examiner.
Exposure to Sun: No restrictions.
Special Storage Instructions: Keep capsules in a tightly closed container at room temperature. Keep oral solution in the refrigerator.
Observe the Following Expiration Times: Oral solution kept refrigerated is good for 14 days; when kept at room temperature, it is good for only 3 days.

CLOZAPINE (KLOH za peen)

Introduced: 1975   **Prescription:** USA: Yes   **Available as Generic:** USA: No   **Class:** Strong tranquilizer (Antipsychotic)   **Controlled Drug:** USA: No

Brand Name: Clozaril

Note: In the United States, this drug is available only by special arrangement through the Clozaril Patient Management System, administered by Caremark Homecare Corporation. Currently, this system is owned by HMI in New York. The toll free number is: 800-237-2767. Ask your doctor for help.

Clozapine

BENEFITS versus RISKS	
Possible Benefits	*Possible Risks*
EFFECTIVE CONTROL OF SEVERE SCHIZOPHRENIA that has failed to respond adequately to other appropriate drugs	SERIOUS BLOOD CELL DISORDERS: abnormally low white blood cell and platelet counts (3%)
Improvement in 30% of refractory cases	DRUG-INDUCED SEIZURES (1% to 5%, depending upon size of dose)

▷ **Principal Uses**
   As a Single Drug Product: Uses currently included in FDA approved labeling: Used solely in the management of severe schizophrenia that has failed to respond to adequate trials of at least two standard antipsychotic medications. Because of its potential for causing serious blood cell disorders and seizures, its use is reserved for the severely ill schizophrenic patient.
   Other (unlabeled) generally accepted uses: (1) Severe and refractory bipolar disorder; (2) severe tardive dyskinesia (dystonic subtype)—a syndrome which can happen after some medicines are used to treat psychosis; (3) Psychosis occurring after labor with lactation.

How This Drug Works: By blocking the place (receptor) where dopamine works in some parts of the brain, this drug helps correct an imbalance of nerve impulses that causes schizophrenic thought disorders.

Available Dosage Forms and Strengths
   Tablets — 25 mg, 100 mg

▷ **Usual Adult Dosage Range:** Initially 25 mg one or two times a day; the dose is gradually increased by 25 mg to 50 mg daily, as tolerated, to reach a dose of 300 mg to 450 mg daily by the end of two weeks. Later increases should be limited to 100 mg one or two times a week. Average dosage requirements are 600 mg daily. Total daily dosage should not exceed 900 mg. **Note: Actual dosage and administration schedule must be determined by the physician for each patient individually.**

Conditions Requiring Dosing Adjustments
   Liver function: Eliminated in the liver, however no specific dosing guidelines are available.
   Kidney function: Patients with kidney failure should be watched closely for adverse effects.

▷ **Dosing Instructions:** May be taken without regard to meals or with food if necessary to reduce stomach irritation. The tablet may be crushed for administration.

Usual Duration of Use: This drug's benefits may be seen after 2–4 weeks of regular use. Peak effect usually requires three months. If no significant benefit is seen within 6 to 8 weeks, the drug should be stopped. Long-term use requires periodic evaluation of response and dosage adjustment.

Possible Advantages of This Drug
   Rarely causes significant sexual dysfunction.
   Low incidence of Parkinson-like reactions (see Glossary).
   Does not cause tardive dyskinesia (see Glossary).

Currently a "Drug of Choice"
for treatment of severe schizophrenia in patients who have not responded to other standard antipsychotic drugs.

▷ **This Drug Should Not Be Taken If**
- you have had an allergic reaction to it previously.
- you have experienced severe bone marrow depression (impaired white blood cell production) with previous use of this drug.
- you presently have any type of bone marrow or blood cell disorder.
- you are currently taking any other drug that can cause bone marrow depression (see Glossary).

▷ **Inform Your Physician Before Taking This Drug If**
- you have a history of any type of seizure disorder.
- you have a history of narrow-angle glaucoma.
- you have any type of heart or circulatory disorder, especially heart rhythm abnormalities or hypertension.
- you have impaired liver or kidney function.
- you have prostatism (see Glossary).

Possible Side-Effects (natural, expected and unavoidable drug actions)
Drowsiness (39%), dizziness (19%), light-headedness, orthostatic hypotension (9%) (see Glossary).
Blurred vision (5%), salivation (31%), dry mouth (6%), impaired urination (2%), constipation (14%).

▷ **Possible Adverse Effects** (unusual, unexpected and infrequent reactions)
If any of the following develop, consult your physician promptly for guidance.
Mild Adverse Effects
Allergic Reactions: Skin rash (2%); drug fever (see Glossary) which usually occurs within the first 3 weeks of treatment and is self-limiting (5%).
Headache (7%), tremor (6%), fainting (6%), nightmares (4%), restlessness (4%), confusion (3%), depression (1%).
Weight gain.
Rapid heartbeat (25%), hypertension (4%), chest pain (1%).
Nausea (5%), indigestion (4%), vomiting (3%), diarrhea (2%).
Serious Adverse Effects
Allergic Reactions: Asthmatic type respiratory reaction (rare).
Bone marrow depression: specific impairment of white blood cell production with potential for serious infection (3%).
Drug-induced seizures, dose-related (1% to 5%).
Tardive dyskinesia (possible, not reported).
Abnormaly low blood pressure.
Anticholinergic syndrome (rare).
Sleep disorders.
Neuroleptic malignant syndrome (rare).

▷ **Possible Effects on Sexual Function**
Decreased libido and impotence (infrequent and dose related—over 150 mg), abnormal ejaculation (1%), priapism (see Glossary).

Clozapine

▷ **Adverse Effects That May Mimic Natural Diseases or Disorders**
Drug-induced fever may suggest systemic infection. Because of the risk of bone marrow depression and secondary infection, any occurrence of fever must be carefully evaluated.
Drug-induced seizures may suggest the possibility of epilepsy.

Natural Diseases or Disorders That May Be Activated by This Drug
Latent glaucoma, prostatism.

Possible Effects on Laboratory Tests
White blood cell counts: decreased.

CAUTION
1. Baseline white blood cell counts must be checked before clozapine treatment is started; follow-up counts must be made every week during the entire course of treatment and for 4 weeks after discontinuation of clozapine.
2. Promptly report any signs of infection: fever, sore throat, flulike symptoms, skin infections, painful urination, etc.
3. Report promptly light-headedness or dizziness on rising from a sitting or lying position; this could be orthostatic hypotension (see Glossary).
4. Call your doctor before taking any other medication. This includes all prescription and over-the-counter drugs.

Precautions for Use
By Infants and Children: Safety and effectiveness for those under 16 years of age not established.
By Those over 60 Years of Age: Increased risk of orthostatic hypotension, confusion, blood problems and prostatism. Report related symptoms promptly.

▷ **Advisability of Use During Pregnancy**
Pregnancy Category: B. See Pregnancy Code at the back of this book.
Animal studies: No birth defects due to this drug reported.
Human studies: Adequate studies of pregnant women are not available.
Use this drug only if clearly needed.

Advisability of Use if Breast-Feeding
Presence of this drug in breast milk: Unknown.
Avoid drug or refrain from nursing.

Habit-Forming Potential: None.

Effects of Overdosage: Marked drowsiness, delirium, hallucinations, rapid and irregular heartbeat, irregular breathing, fainting.

Possible Effects of Long-Term Use: None reported to date.

Suggested Periodic Examinations While Taking This Drug (at physician's discretion)
White blood and differential counts prior to starting therapy, every week during therapy and for 4 weeks after stopping therapy.
Serial blood pressure measurements and electrocardiograms.

▷ **While Taking This Drug, Observe the Following**
Foods: No restrictions.
Beverages: No restrictions. May be taken with milk.
▷ *Alcohol:* Avoid completely. Alcohol increases sedation and accentuates its brain function and blood pressure depression. This drug can increase the intoxicating effects of alcohol.

Tobacco Smoking: May accelerate the elimination of this drug and require increased dosage.

Marijuana Smoking: Moderate increase in drowsiness; accentuation of orthostatic hypotension; increased risk of aggravating psychosis.

▷ *Other Drugs*

Clozapine may *increase* the effects of
- drugs with sedative actions; observe for excessive sedation.
- drugs with atropinelike actions (see Drug Class).
- antihypertensive drugs; observe for excessive lowering of blood pressure.

Clozapine *taken concurrently* with
- other bone marrow depressant drugs such as carbamazepine (Tegretol) may increase the risk of impaired white blood cell production.
- cimetidine (Zantac) can result in a toxic level of clozapine.
- lithium (Lithobid, Lithotab, etc.) may increase the risk of confusional states, seizures and neuroleptic malignant syndrome (see Glossary).
- Monoamine Oxidase Inhibitors (MAO inhibitors—see Drug Class) may cause abnormally low blood pressure and exaggerated central nervous system response.
- phenytoin (Dilantin) can cause a decreased clozapine level and result in breakthrough schizophrenia.
- warfarin (Coumadin) and cause an increased risk of bleeding.

▷ *Driving, Hazardous Activities:*
This drug may cause drowsiness, dizziness, blurred vision, confusion and seizures. Restrict activities as necessary.

Aviation Note:
The use of this drug **is a disqualification** for piloting. Consult a designated Aviation Medical Examiner.

Exposure to Sun: No restrictions.

Exposure to Heat: Use caution. This drug can cause fever and can impair the body's adaptation to heat.

Occurrence of Unrelated Illness: Infections must be vigorously treated. White blood cell response to infection must be followed closely.

Discontinuation: If possible, this drug should be discontinued gradually over a period of 1 to 2 weeks. If abrupt withdrawal is necessary, observe carefully for recurrence of psychotic symptoms.

CODEINE (KOH deen)

Introduced: 1886   **Prescription:** USA: Yes; Canada: Yes   **Available as Generic:** Yes   **Class:** Analgesic, narcotic   **Controlled Drug:** USA: C-II*; Canada: N

Brand Names: A.B.C. compound with codeine [CD], AC & C [CD], Accopain, Actagen-C [CD], Actifed w/Codeine [CD], Afed-C [CD], Alamine-C [CD], Alamine Expectorant [CD], Ambenyl Expectorant [CD], Ambenyl Syrup [CD], Anacin 3 with Codeine #2–4, Anacin w/Codeine [CD], APC with Codeine [CD], Atasol-8, -15, -30 [CD], Ban-Tuiss C [CD], Benylin Syrup w/Codeine [CD], Bromanyl Cough Syrup [CD], Bromotuss, Bromphen DC

*See Schedules of Controlled Drugs at the back of this book.

Codeine

[CD], Bufferin w/Codeine [CD], Butalbital compound [CD], ◆C2 buffered, ◆C2 with codeine, Chemdal Expectorant [CD], Chem-Tuss NE [CD], Chlor-Trimeton Expectorant [CD], Coactifed [CD], Codehist Elixir, Codehist DH, ◆Coricidin with Codeine [CD], ◆Coryphen-Codeine [CD], Deproist [CD], Dimetane Cough Syrup-DC [CD], Dimetane Expectorant-C [CD], Dimetapp-C [CD], Dimetapp w/Codeine [CD], Empirin w/Codeine No. 2, 4 [CD], Empracet w/Codeine No. 3, 4 [CD], ◆Empracet-30, -60 [CD], ◆Emtec-30 [CD], ◆Exdol-8, -15, -30 [CD], ◆Extra Strength Acetaminophen, ◆Fiorinal-C 1/4, -C 1/2 [CD], Fiorinal w/Codeine No. 1, 2, 3 [CD], Gecil [CD], Glydeine, Isoclor Expectorant [CD], ◆Lenoltec w/Codeine No. 1, 2, 3, 4 [CD], ◆Mersyndol, Naldecon-CX [CD], Normatane [CD], Novadyne DH [CD], ◆Novahistex C [CD], ◆Novo-Gesic, Nucochem [CD], Nucofed [CD], ◆Omni-Tuss [CD], Oridol-C [CD], Panadol with codeine [CD], ◆Paveral, Pediacof [CD], Penntuss [CD], ◆Phenaphen No. 2, 3, 4 [CD], Phenaphen w/Codeine No. 2, 3, 4 [CD], Phenergan w/Codeine [CD], Poly-Histine [CD], Promethazine CS [CD], Pyra-Phed [CD], ◆Robaxacet-8, Robaxisal-C [CD], ◆Rounox w/Codeine [CD], SK-Apap [CD], Tamine Expectorant DC [CD], ◆Tecnal C [CD], Terpin Hydrate and Codeine [CD], Triafed with codeine [CD], Triaminic Expectorant w/Codeine [CD], ◆Triatec-8, 30 [CD], ◆Tussaminic C Forte [CD], ◆Tussaminic C Ped [CD], ◆Tussi-Organidin [CD], ◆Tylenol w/Codeine [CD], Tylenol w/Codeine No. 1, 2, 3, 4 [CD], Tylenol w/Codeine Elixir [CD], ◆222 [CD], ◆282 [CD], ◆292 [CD], ◆318 A.C. & C. [CD], ◆VC Expectorant with Codeine, ◆Veganin [CD]

BENEFITS versus RISKS

Possible Benefits	Possible Risks
EFFECTIVE RELIEF OF MODERATE TO SEVERE PAIN	Low potential for habit formation (dependence)
EFFECTIVE CONTROL OF COUGH	Mild allergic reactions (infrequent)
	Nausea, constipation

▷ **Principal Uses**
As a Single Drug Product: Uses currently included in FDA approved labeling: (1) relieves moderate to severe pain; (2) controls cough. Its widest use is as an ingredient in analgesic preparations and cough remedies.
Other (unlabeled) generally accepted uses: None.
As a Combination Drug Product [CD]: Codeine is combined with other analgesics (aspirin and acetaminophen) on the World Health Organization Pain Ladder to increase overall pain control. It is also added to cough mixtures containing antihistamines, decongestants and expectorants.

How This Drug Works: By depressing some brain functions, this drug decreases pain perception, calms emotional responses to pain and reduces cough reflex sensitivity.

Available Dosage Forms and Strengths
Injection — 30 mg per ml and 60 mg per ml
Tablets — 15 mg, 30 mg, 60 mg
Tablets, soluble — 15 mg, 30 mg, 60 mg

▷ **Usual Adult Dosage Range:** As analgesic—15 to 60 mg/3 to 6 hours. Current pain theory says that the drug should be scheduled, not taken in response to pain as in the past. For cough—10 to 20 mg/4 to 6 hours as needed.

Total daily dosage should not exceed 200 mg for pain or 120 mg for cough.
Note: Actual dosage and administration schedule must be determined by the physician for each patient individually.

Conditions Requiring Dosing Adjustments
Liver function: The dose must be decreased in liver compromise.
Kidney function: In moderate to severe kidney failure, the dose is decreased by up to 75%.

▷ **Dosing Instructions:** Tablet may be crushed, then taken with or following food to reduce stomach irritation or nausea.

Usual Duration of Use: As required to control pain or cough. Continual use should not exceed 5 to 7 days without reassessment of need.

▷ **This Drug Should Not Be Taken If**
- you have had an allergic reaction to any dosage form of it previously.
- you are having an acute attack of asthma.
- your breathing is depressed (respiratory depression).

▷ **Inform Your Physician Before Taking This Drug If**
- you have a history of drug abuse or alcoholism.
- you have impaired liver or kidney function.
- you have gallbladder disease, a seizure disorder or an underactive thyroid gland.
- you have chronic lung disease (COPD)
- you have low blood calcium (increased sensitivity to this medicine).
- you have a history of porphyria.
- you tend to be constipated.
- you are taking any other drugs that have a sedative effect.
- you plan to have surgery under general anesthesia in the near future.

Possible Side-Effects (natural, expected and unavoidable drug actions)
Drowsiness, light-headedness, dry mouth, urinary retention, constipation.

▷ **Possible Adverse Effects** (unusual, unexpected and infrequent reactions)
If any of the following develop, consult your physician promptly for guidance.
Mild Adverse Effects
Allergic Reactions: Skin rash, hives, itching.
Dizziness, impaired concentration, sensation of drunkenness, confusion, depression, blurred or double vision.
Nausea, vomiting.
Serious Adverse Effects
Allergic Reactions: Anaphylaxis (rare), severe skin reactions.
Idiosyncratic Reactions: Delirium, hallucinations, excitement, increased sensitivity to pain after the analgesic effect has worn off.
Seizures (rare), impaired breathing.
Porphyria (rare).

▷ **Possible Effects on Sexual Function:** None reported.

▷ **Adverse Effects That May Mimic Natural Diseases or Disorders**
Paradoxical behavioral disturbances may suggest psychotic disorder.

Possible Effects on Laboratory Tests
Blood platelet counts: decreased.
Blood amylase and lipase levels: increased (natural side-effect).

Urine screening tests for drug abuse: may be **positive**. (Test results depend upon amount of drug taken and testing method used.)

CAUTION
1. If you have asthma, chronic bronchitis or emphysema, excessive use of this drug may cause respiratory difficulty, thickening of bronchial secretions and decrease of needed cough reflex.
2. Combining this drug with atropinelike drugs can increase the risk of urinary retention and reduced intestinal function.
3. Do not take this drug following acute head injury.

Precautions for Use

By Infants and Children: Do not use this drug in children under 2 years of age because of their vulnerability to life-threatening respiratory depression.

By Those over 60 Years of Age: Small starting doses and short-term use is indicated. Expect increased risk of drowsiness, dizziness, unsteadiness, falling, urinary retention and constipation (often leading to fecal impaction).

▷ **Advisability of Use During Pregnancy**

Pregnancy Category: C. See Pregnancy Code at the back of this book.

Animal studies: Skull defects reported in hamster studies.

Human studies: Adequate studies of pregnant women are not available. Some studies suggest an increase in significant birth defects when this drug is taken during the first 6 months of pregnancy. Codeine taken during the last few weeks before delivery can cause withdrawal symptoms in the newborn.

Use this drug only if clearly needed and in small, infrequent doses.

Advisability of Use if Breast-Feeding

Presence of this drug in breast milk: Yes, in small amounts.

Avoid drug or refrain from nursing.

Habit-Forming Potential: Psychological and/or physical dependence can develop with use of large doses for an extended period of time. However, true dependence is infrequent and unlikely with prudent use.

Effects of Overdosage: Drowsiness, restlessness, agitation, nausea, vomiting, dry mouth, vertigo, weakness, lethargy, stupor, coma, seizures.

Possible Effects of Long-Term Use: Psychological and physical dependence, chronic constipation.

Suggested Periodic Examinations While Taking This Drug (at physician's discretion)

None.

▷ **While Taking This Drug, Observe the Following**

Foods: No restrictions.

Beverages: No restrictions. May be taken with milk.

▷ *Alcohol:* Use extreme caution. Codeine intensifies the intoxicating effects of alcohol, and alcohol intensifies the depressant effects of codeine on brain function, breathing and circulation.

Tobacco Smoking: No interactions expected.

Marijuana Smoking: Increased drowsiness and pain relief; mental and physical performance will be impaired.

▷ *Other Drugs*
  Codeine may *increase* the effects of
  • other drugs with sedative effects.
  • atropinelike drugs, and increase the risk of constipation and urinary retention.
  • monoamine oxidase inhibitors (MAO) and also increase central nervous symptoms and depression.
▷ *Driving, Hazardous Activities:* This drug can impair mental alertness, judgment, reaction time and physical coordination. Avoid hazardous activities accordingly.
  Aviation Note: The use of this drug *is a disqualification* for piloting. Consult a designated Aviation Medical Examiner.
  Exposure to Sun: No restrictions.
  Discontinuation: Best to limit this drug to short-term use. If extended use occurs, discontinuation should be gradual to minimize possible effects of withdrawal (usually mild with codeine).

COLCHICINE (KOL chi seen)

Introduced: 1763 **Prescription:** USA: Yes; Canada: No **Available as Generic:** Yes **Class:** Antigout **Controlled Drug:** USA: No; Canada: No
Brand Names: Colabid [CD], ColBenemid [CD], Cosalide, Proben-C [CD], ✦Verban [CD]

BENEFITS versus RISKS	
Possible Benefits	*Possible Risks*
EFFECTIVE RELIEF OF ACUTE GOUT SYMPTOMS	Loss of hair
Prevention of recurrent gout attacks	Rare bone marrow depression (see Glossary)
Prevention of attacks of Mediterranean fever	Rare peripheral neuritis (see Glossary)
	Rare liver damage

▷ **Principal Uses**
  As a Single Drug Product: Uses Currently included in FDA approved labeling: (1) Reduces the pain, swelling and inflammation associated with acute attacks of gout; (2) It is also used in smaller doses to prevent recurrent gout attacks.
    Other (unlabeled) generally accepted uses: (1) Prevention and control of attacks of familial Mediterranean fever; (2) may have a role in easing symptoms of Behcet's disease; (3) limited use in cirrhosis of the liver; (4) damaged disk syndrome may be helped in some patients; (5) may have a role in recurrent pericarditis; (6) can be of help in pseudogout; (7) appears to be of benefit in some lung disease (idiopathic pulmonary fibrosis); (8) has a role in treatment of some cases of refractory immune thrombocytopenic purpura.
  As a Combination Drug Product [CD]: Colchicine combined with probenecid enhances its ability to prevent recurrent attacks of gout. Colchicine is most effective in relieving acute gout, it has some effect in preventing

recurrent and chronic discomfort. Probenecid increases removal of uric acid by the kidneys and reduces risk of acute gout. This dual action is more effective than either drug used alone in the long-term management of gout.

How This Drug Works: By decreasing joint tissue acid, this drug decreases painful deposit of uric acid crystals and acute inflammation and pain. (Colchicine does not lower uric acid in the blood or increase urine removal.)

Available Dosage Forms and Strengths
Injection — 1 mg per 2 ml
Tablets — 0.5 mg, 0.6 mg

▷ **Usual Adult Dosage Range:** For acute attack—0.5 to 1.3 mg initially, followed by 0.5 to 0.65 mg/1 to 2 hours until pain is relieved or nausea, vomiting or diarrhea occurs. Maximum total dose is 10 mg. For prevention of recurrent attacks—0.5 to 0.65 mg, 1 to 3 times/day. **Note: Actual dosage and administration schedule must be determined by the physician for each patient individually.**

Conditions Requiring Dosing Adjustments
Liver function: Caution must be used, and the dose decreased if there is a bile obstruction.
This drug should **not** be used in people with both liver and kidney compromise.
Kidney function: For severe kidney failure, 50% of the usual dose should be given. Ongoing prophylactic use should be avoided in moderate (CCl < 50) kidney problems.

▷ **Dosing Instructions:** The tablet may be crushed, then either taken on an empty stomach or with food to reduce nausea or stomach irritation. Start treatment at the first sign of an acute attack. Take the exact dose prescribed.

Usual Duration of Use: For acute attack—stop the drug when pain is relieved or when nausea, vomiting or diarrhea occurs; do not start this drug for 3 days without asking your doctor. For prevention—use the smallest dose that works; consult your doctor about dosage schedule and duration.

▷ **This Drug Should Not Be Taken If**
- you have had an allergic reaction to it previously.
- you have an active stomach or duodenal ulcer.
- you have active ulcerative colitis.
- you have a serious heart disorder.
- you have a history of blood cell disorders.

▷ **Inform Your Physician Before Taking This Drug If**
- you have a history of peptic ulcer disease or ulcerative colitis.
- you develop diarrhea and vomiting while taking this drug.
- you have any type of heart disease.
- you have impaired liver or kidney function.
- you plan to have surgery in the near future.

Possible Side-Effects (natural, expected and unavoidable drug actions)
Nausea, vomiting, abdominal cramping, diarrhea.

▷ **Possible Adverse Effects** (unusual, unexpected and infrequent reactions)
If any of the following develop, consult your physician promptly for guidance.

Mild Adverse Effects
  Allergic Reactions: Skin rash, hives, fever.
Serious Adverse Effects
  Allergic Reaction: Anaphylactic reaction (see Glossary).
  Loss of hair.
  Bone marrow depression (see Glossary)—fatigue, weakness, fever, sore throat, abnormal bleeding or bruising.
  Peripheral neuritis (see Glossary)—numbness, tingling, pain, weakness in hands and/or feet.
  Myopathy with nerve symptoms (facial palsy and weakness) (especially with long-term use).
  Porphyria.
  Drooping of the eyes (ptosis).
  Inflammation of colon with bloody diarrhea.
  Thrombophlebitis with intravenous use.
  Liver damage.
▷ **Possible Effects on Sexual Function:** Reversable absence of sperm (azoospermia).
Possible Delayed Adverse Effects: Impaired production of sperm, possibly resulting in birth defects of child that was conceived while father was taking this drug.

Natural Diseases or Disorders That May Be Activated by This Drug
  Peptic ulcer disease, ulcerative colitis.

Possible Effects on Laboratory Tests
  Complete blood cell counts: decreased red cells, hemoglobin, white cells and platelets; increased white cells (follows initial decrease).
  Prothrombin time: decreased (with concurrent use of warfarin).
  Blood vitamin B_{12} level: decreased.
  Liver function tests: increased liver enzymes (ALT/GPT, AST/GOT and alkaline phosphatase), increased bilirubin.
  Fecal occult blood test: positive.
  Sperm counts: decreased (may be marked).

CAUTION
  1. If this drug causes vomiting and/or diarrhea before relief of joint pain, discontinue it and inform your physician.
  2. Try to limit each course of treatment for acute gout to 4 to 8 mg. Do not exceed 3 mg/24 hours or a total of 10 mg/course.
  3. Omit drug for 3 days between courses to avoid toxicity.
  4. Carry this drug with you while traveling if you are subject to attacks of acute gout.
  5. The stress of surgery can cause an acute attack of gout. Ask your doctor how much colchicine should be taken before and after surgery to prevent gout.

Precautions for Use
  By Infants and Children: Dosage has not been established. Ask physician for guidance.
  By Those over 60 Years of Age: Because the dosage needed to relieve acute gout often causes vomiting and/or diarrhea, extreme caution is advised if you have heart or circulatory disorders, reduced liver or kidney function or general debility.

▷ **Advisability of Use During Pregnancy**
  Pregnancy Category: C by one manufacturer, and D by another. See Pregnancy Code at the back of this book.
  Animal studies: This drug causes significant birth defects in hamsters and rabbits.
  Human studies: Adequate studies of pregnant women are not available. However, it is reported that colchicine can cause harm to the fetus.
  Avoid during entire pregnancy if possible. Ask physician for guidance.

Advisability of Use if Breast-Feeding
  Presence of this drug in breast milk: Yes.
  Ask your doctor for help.

Habit-Forming Potential: None.

Effects of Overdosage: Nausea, vomiting, abdominal cramping, diarrhea (may be bloody), burning sensation in throat and skin, weak and rapid pulse, progressive paralysis, inability to breathe.

Possible Effects of Long-Term Use: Hair loss, aplastic anemia (see Glossary), peripheral neuritis (see Glossary).

Suggested Periodic Examinations While Taking This Drug (at physician's discretion)
  Complete blood cell counts, uric acid blood levels to monitor status of gout, sperm analysis for quantity and condition, liver function tests.

▷ **While Taking This Drug, Observe the Following**
  Foods: Follow physician's advice regarding the need for a low-purine diet.
  Beverages: Drink at least 3 quarts of liquids/24 hours. This drug may be taken with milk. Some "herbal teas" (promoted as being beneficial for arthritis) contain phenylbutazone and other potentially toxic ingredients. Avoid herbal teas if you are not certain of their source, content and medicinal effects.

▷ *Alcohol:* No interactions expected. Combination may increase the risk of gastrointestinal irritation or bleeding and raise uric acid blood levels.
  Tobacco Smoking: No interactions expected.

▷ *Other Drugs*
  Colchicine **taken concurrently** with
  • allopurinol (Zyloprim), probenecid (Benemid) or sulfinpyrazone (Anturane) can prevent attacks of acute gout that often occur when treatment with these drugs is first started.
  • cyanocobalamin will decrease absorption of the vitamin B12.
  • cyclosporine may increase cyclosporine levels and result in toxicity.
  • erythromycins (EES, azithromycin, clarithromycin) and result in toxic colchicine blood levels.

▷ *Driving, Hazardous Activities:* Usually no restrictions when taken continually in small (preventive) doses. May cause nausea, vomiting and/or diarrhea when taken in larger (treatment) doses.
  Aviation Note: The use of this drug **may be a disqualification** for piloting. Consult a designated Aviation Medical Examiner.
  Exposure to Sun: No restrictions.
  Exposure to Cold: This drug can lower body temperature. Use caution to prevent excessive lowering (hypothermia), especially in those over 60 years of age.

Occurrence of Unrelated Illness: Acute attacks of gout may result from injury or illness. Call your doctor for dosing adjustment if injury or new illness occurs.

COLESTIPOL (koh LES ti pohl)

Introduced: 1974 **Prescription:** USA: Yes; Canada: Yes **Available as Generic:** USA: No; Canada: No **Class:** Anticholesterol **Controlled Drug:** USA: No; Canada: No
Brand Name: Colestid

BENIFITS versus RISKS	
Possible Benefits	*Possible Risks*
EFFECTIVE REDUCTION OF TOTAL CHOLESTEROL AND LOW DENSITY CHOLESTEROL IN TYPE IIa CHOLESTEROL DISORDERS (15% to 25% reduction of total cholesterol, 25% to 35% reduction of LDL cholesterol)	Constipation (may be severe)
	Reduced absorption of fat, fat-soluble vitamins (A, D, E and K) and folic acid
	Reduced formation of prothrombin with resultant bleeding
EFFECTIVE RELIEF OF ITCHING associated with biliary obstruction	

▷ **Principal Uses**

As a Single Drug Product: Uses currently included in FDA approved labeling: (1) Reduces abnormally high blood levels of total cholesterol and low density (LDL) cholesterol in Type IIa cholesterol disorders; (2) relieve the itching due to the deposit of bile acids in the skin associated with partial biliary obstruction; (3) helps remove buildup on interior of blood vessels (atherosclerosis).

Other (unlabeled) generally accepted uses: (1) Data from one study showed that colestipol in combination with lovastatin actually caused regression of plaque buildup (atherosclerosis) inside blood vessels.

How This Drug Works: This drug combines with bile acids and salts and is excreted in the feces. This removal of bile acids stimulates conversion of cholesterol to bile acids to replace the loss; this in turn reduces the blood levels of cholesterol. By reducing the blood levels of bile acids, this drug hastens clearance of bile acids in the skin and relieves itching.

Available Dosage Forms and Strengths
Bottles — 250 grams and 500 grams
Packets — 5 grams
Flavored Colestid Granules — 5 grams per dose

▷ **Usual Adult Dosage Range:** Initially 5 grams of powder 3 times daily. Dose may be increased slowly as needed and tolerated to 30 grams daily in 2 to 4 divided doses. **Note: Actual dosage and administration schedule must be determined by the physician for each patient individually.**

Conditions Requiring Dosing Adjustments

Liver function: This medication is eliminated via the feces, and the liver is not involved.

Kidney function: No changes are needed in renal compromise as the drug is not absorbed.

▷ **Dosing Instructions:** Always take just before or with a meal; this drug is ineffective when taken without food. Mix the powder thoroughly in 4 to 6 ounces of water, fruit juice, tomato juice, milk, thin soup or a soft food like applesauce. **Do not take it in its dry form.**

Usual Duration of Use: Use on a regular schedule for 4 to 6 weeks is usually needed to see this drug's effectiveness in lowering high blood levels of cholesterol. The drug should be stopped if an acceptable response is not seen after 3 months. Long-term use (months to years) requires periodic physician evaluation of response and dosage adjustment.

Currently a "Drug of Choice"
for initiating treatment of elevated LDL cholesterol. See Cholesterol Disorders in Section Two. Other medications are suggested as first line agents if you have had a heart attack or have severely increased cholesterol.

▷ **This Drug Should Not Be Taken If**
- you have had an allergic reaction to it previously.
- you have complete biliary obstruction.

▷ **Inform Your Physician Before Taking This Drug If**
- you are prone to constipation.
- you have low thyroid function (hypothyroidism).
- you have peptic ulcer disease.
- you have a bleeding disorder of any kind.
- you have impaired kidney function.

Possible Side-Effects (natural, expected and unavoidable drug actions)
Constipation (10%); interference with normal fat digestion and absorption; reduced absorption of vitamins A, D, E and K and folic acid.

▷ **Possible Adverse Effects** (unusual, unexpected and infrequent reactions)
If any of the following develop, consult your physician promptly for guidance.

Mild Adverse Effects
Allergic Reactions: Skin rash (0.1%), hives, tongue irritation, anal itching.
Headache, dizziness, weakness, muscle and joint pains.
Constipation, loss of appetite, indigestion, heartburn, abdominal discomfort, excessive gas, nausea, vomiting, diarrhea.

Serious Adverse Effects
Vitamin K deficiency with resultant deficiency of prothrombin and increased bleeding tendency.
Impaired absorption of calcium; predisposition to osteoporosis.
Gallbladder colic (questionable).
Hypothyroidism.
Disruption of normal acid base balance of the body (metabolic acidosis).

▷ **Possible Effects on Sexual Function:** None reported.

Natural Diseases or Disorders That May Be Activated by This Drug
Peptic ulcer disease; steatorrhea (excessive fat in stools) with large doses.

Possible Effects on Laboratory Tests
Blood cholesterol and triglyceride levels: decreased (therapeutic effect).
Blood thyroxine (T_4) level: decreased when colestipol and niacin are taken concurrently (in presence of normal thyroid function).

CAUTION
1. Never take the powder in its dry form; always mix it thoroughly with a suitable liquid before swallowing.
2. Watch carefully for constipation; use stool softeners and laxatives as needed.
3. This drug may bind other drugs taken concurrently and impair their absorption. It is advisable to take *all other drugs* 1 to 2 hours before or 4 to 6 hours after taking this drug.

Precautions for Use
By Infants and Children: Safety and effectiveness for those under 12 years of age not established. Watch carefully for the possible development of acidosis and vitamin A or folic acid deficiency. (Ask your physician for guidance.)
By Those over 60 Years of Age: Increased risk of severe constipation. Impaired kidney function may predispose to the development of acidosis.

▷ **Advisability of Use During Pregnancy**
Pregnancy Category: C. See Pregnancy Code at the back of this book.
Animal studies: No information available.
Human studies: Adequate studies of pregnant women are not available.
Use this drug only if clearly needed. Ensure adequate intake of vitamins and minerals to satisfy needs of mother and fetus.

Advisability of Use if Breast-Feeding
Presence of this drug in breast milk: No.
Breast-feeding is permitted.

Habit-Forming Potential: None.

Effects of Overdosage: Progressive constipation.

Possible Effects of Long-Term Use: Deficiencies of vitamins A, D, E and K and folic acid. Calcium deficiency, osteoporosis. Acidosis due to excessive retention of chloride.

Suggested Periodic Examinations While Taking This Drug (at physician's discretion)
Measurements of blood levels of total cholesterol, low density (LDL) cholesterol and high density (HDL) cholesterol.
Hemoglobin and red blood cell studies for possible anemia.
Thyroid function tests.

▷ **While Taking This Drug, Observe the Following**
Foods: Avoid foods that tend to constipate (cheeses, etc.).
Nutritional Support: Ask your doctor if you need supplements of vitamins A, D, E and K, folic acid and calcium.
Beverages: Ensure adequate liquid intake (up to 2 quarts daily). This drug may be taken with milk.

▷ *Alcohol:* No interactions expected.
Tobacco Smoking: No interactions expected.

▷ **Other Drugs**
Colestipol may *decrease* the effects of
- acetaminophen; give 2 hours before colestipol.
- aspirin; give 2 hours before.
- digitoxin and digoxin; give 2 hours before.
- furosemide; give 4 hours before.

- hydrocortisone; 2 hours before.
- iron preparations; give 2 to 3 hours before.
- penicillin G; give 2 hours before.
- phenobarbital; give 2 hours before.
- tetracycline; give 2 hours before.
- thiazide diuretics (see Drug Class Section); give 2 hours before.
- thyroxine; give 5 hours before.
- vitamin B12.
- warfarin; give 6 hours after.

▷ *Driving, Hazardous Activities:* No restrictions.

Aviation Note: The use of this drug *is usually not a disqualification* for piloting. Consult a designated Aviation Medical Examiner.

Exposure to Sun: No restrictions.

Discontinuation: The dose of any toxic drug combined with colestipol must be reduced when this drug is stopped. Once colestipol is stopped, cholesterol levels usually return to pretreatment levels in 1 month.

CROMOLYN (KROH moh lin)

Other Names: Cromolyn sodium, sodium cromoglycate
Introduced: 1968 **Prescription:** USA: Yes; Canada: Yes **Available as Generic:** USA: No; Canada: No **Class:** Asthma preventive, rhinitis preventive **Controlled Drug:** USA: No; Canada: No
Brand Names: ✦Fivent, Gastrocrom, Intal, ✦Intal Spincaps, ✦Intal Syncroner, ✦Nalcrom, Nasalcrom, Opticrom, ✦Rynacrom, ✦Vistacrom

BENEFITS versus RISKS	
Possible Benefits	*Possible Risks*
LONG-TERM PREVENTION OF RECURRENT ASTHMA ATTACKS	Rare anaphylactic reaction (see Glossary)
Prevention of acute asthma due to allergens or exercise	Rare spasm of bronchial tubes, increased wheezing
Prevention and treatment of allergic rhinitis	Rare allergic pneumonitis (allergic reaction in lung tissue)
Relief of allergic conjunctivitis	
Treatment of giant papillary conjunctivitis	

▷ **Principal Uses**

As a Single Drug Product: Uses currently included in FDA approved labeling: (1) *Prevents* allergic reactions in the nose (allergic rhinitis, hay fever) and the bronchial tubes (bronchial asthma). Does not relieve asthma once an attack has begun. It is also used to treat allergic rhinitis (70% effective) and conjunctivitis; (2) helps prevent exercise- or environmentally-induced asthma; (3) treatment of mastocytosis and management of several allergy-related skin disorders.

Other (unlabeled) generally accepted uses: (1) Helps modify the reactions in food allergies; (2) May have a small place in the therapy of Bell's palsy and ulcerative colitis.

How This Drug Works: It blocks the release of histamine (and other chemicals) that worsen allergic reactions, this drug prevents the sequence of events that lead to swelling and itching and to constriction of bronchial tubes (asthma).

Available Dosage Forms and Strengths
- Capsules, oral — 100 mg
- Eye drops — 2% and 4%
- Inhalation aerosol — 0.8 mg per metered spray
- Inhalation capsules (powder) — 20 mg
- Inhalation solution — 20 mg per ampul
- Nasal insufflation (powder) — 10 mg per cartridge
- Nasal solution — 40 mg per ml

▷ **Usual Adult Dosage Range**

Eye drops: 1 drop 4 to 6 times daily at regular intervals.

Inhalation aerosol: 1.6 mg (2 inhalations) 4 times daily at regular intervals for prevention of asthma, or as a single dose 10 to 15 minutes **before** exposure to prevent acute allergen-induced or exercise-induced asthma.

Inhalation powder: 20 mg (1 capsule) 4 times daily at regular intervals for long-term prevention of asthma; 20 mg (1 capsule) as a single dose 10 to 15 minutes before exposure to prevent acute allergen-induced or exercise-induced asthma. Total daily maximum dosage is 160 mg (8 capsules).

Inhalation solution: Same as inhalation powder.

Nasal insufflation: Initially 10 mg in each nostril every 4 to 6 hours as needed; reduce to every 8 to 12 hours for maintenance.

Nasal solution: 2.6 mg to 5.2 mg in each nostril 3 to 6 times daily as needed.

Note: Actual dosage and administration schedule must be determined by the physician for each patient individually.

Conditions Requiring Dosing Adjustments

Liver function: If the bile duct is damaged by liver disease, the dose must be decreased.

Kidney function: The dose should be decreased in kidney failure.

▷ **Dosing Instructions:** Follow instructions provided with all of the dosage forms, especially the inhalers. Do not swallow the capsules; the powder is intended for inhalation. (If the capsule is accidently swallowed, the drug will cause no beneficial or adverse effects.)

Usual Duration of Use: Use on a regular schedule for 4 to 6 weeks is usually needed to see this drug's benefit in preventing asthma attacks or allergic rhinitis. Long-term use (months to years) requires periodic physician evaluation.

Possible Advantages of This Drug

May be quite effective in the young asthmatic.

Usually well tolerated.

Serious adverse effects are very rare.

▷ **This Drug Should Not Be Taken If**
- you have had an allergic reaction to any dosage form of it previously.

▷ **Inform Your Physician Before Taking This Drug If**
- you are allergic to milk, milk products or lactose. (The inhalation powder contains lactose.)

Cromolyn

- you have impaired liver or kidney function.
- you have angina or a heart rhythm disorder. (The inhalation aerosol contains propellants that could be hazardous.)

Possible Side-Effects (natural, expected and unavoidable drug actions)
Unpleasant taste with use of inhalation aerosol.
Mild throat irritation, hoarseness, cough. (These can be minimized by a few swallows of water after each inhalation of powder.)

▷ **Possible Adverse Effects** (unusual, unexpected and infrequent reactions)
If any of the following develop, consult your physician promptly for guidance.
Mild Adverse Effects
Allergic Reactions: Skin rash, hives, itching.
Headache, dizziness.
Nausea, vomiting, urinary urgency and pain, joint and muscle pain.
Stinging or burning of the eyes with ophthalmic use.
Cough and bronchial irritation.
Nosebleed with nasal solution use.
Serious Adverse Effects
Allergic Reactions: Rare anaphylactic reaction (see Glossary). Allergic pneumonitis (allergic reaction in lung tissue).
Propellants in the metered dose inhaler may cause problems in patients with disease of the heart arteries or a history of abnormal heart rhythms.

▷ **Possible Effects on Sexual Function:** None reported.

Possible Effects on Laboratory Tests
None reported.

CAUTION

1. This drug only helps *prevent* bronchial asthma—used *before* the start of acute bronchial constriction (asthmatic wheezing).
2. ***Do not*** use this drug during an acute attack of asthma; it could worsen and prolong asthmatic wheezing.
3. This drug does ***not*** block the benefits of drugs which relieve acute asthma attacks after they start. Cromolyn is used ***before and between*** acute attacks to help keep them from starting; bronchodilators are used ***during*** acute attacks.
4. If you are using a bronchodilator drug by inhalation, it is best to take it about 5 minutes before inhaling cromolyn.
5. If this drug has allowed you to decrease or eliminate steroids, and you are unable to tolerate it, ask your doctor about the need to start steroids once again.

Precautions for Use
By Infants and Children: Safety and effectiveness for those under 5 years of age not established. Young children may find a nebulized solution easier than the powder.
By Those over 60 Years of Age: This drug does not work in the management of chronic bronchitis or emphysema.

▷ **Advisability of Use During Pregnancy**
Pregnancy Category: B. See Pregnancy Code at the back of this book.
Animal studies: Mouse, rat and rabbit studies revealed no birth defects due to this drug.

Human studies: Adequate studies of pregnant women are not available. Use this drug only if clearly needed.

Advisability of Use if Breast-Feeding
Presence of this drug in breast milk: Unknown.
Avoid drug or refrain from nursing.

Habit-Forming Potential: None.

Effects of Overdosage: No significant effects reported.

Possible Effects of Long-Term Use: Allergic reaction of lung tissue (allergic pneumonitis, very rare).

Suggested Periodic Examinations While Taking This Drug (at physician's discretion)
Sputum analysis and X-ray if symptoms suggest allergic pneumonitis.

▷ **While Taking This Drug, Observe the Following**
Foods: Follow physician prescribed diet. Avoid all foods to which you are allergic.
Beverages: Avoid all beverages to which you may be allergic.
▷ *Alcohol:* No interactions expected.
Tobacco Smoking: Follow your physician's advice regarding smoking.
▷ *Other Drugs:* Cromolyn may allow reduced dosage of cortisonelike drugs in the management of chronic asthma. Ask your doctor about dosage adjustment.
▷ *Driving, Hazardous Activities:* This drug may cause dizziness. Restrict activities as necessary.
Aviation Note: The use of this drug **may be a disqualification** for piloting. Consult a designated Aviation Medical Examiner.
Exposure to Sun: No restrictions.
Heavy Exercise or Exertion: This drug may prevent exercise-induced asthma if taken 10 to 15 minutes before exertion. It is most effective in young people.
Discontinuation: If cromolyn has made it possible to reduce or stop maintenance doses of cortisonelike drugs, and you find it necessary to discontinue cromolyn, watch closely for a sudden return of asthma. You may have to start a cortisonelike drug as well as other measures to control asthma.
Special Storage Instructions: Keep the powder cartridges in a dry, tightly closed container. Store in a cool place but not in the refrigerator. Do not handle the cartridges or the inhaler when hands are wet.

CYCLOPHOSPHAMIDE (si kloh FOSS fa mide)

Introduced: 1959 **Prescription:** USA: Yes; Canada: Yes **Available as Generic:** No **Class:** Anticancer, immunosuppressive **Controlled Drug:** USA: No; Canada: No

Brand Names: Cytoxan, Neosar, ✦Procytox

Cyclophosphamide

BENEFITS versus RISKS	
Possible Benefits	*Possible Risks*
CURE OR CONTROL OF CERTAIN TYPES OF CANCER	REDUCED WHITE BLOOD CELL COUNT
PREVENTION OF REJECTION IN ORGAN TRANSPLANTATION	SECONDARY INFECTION URINARY BLADDER BLEEDING
Possibly beneficial in the treatment of rheumatoid arthritis and lupus erythematosus	HEART, LUNG, LIVER OR KIDNEY DAMAGE Loss of hair
Possibly beneficial in selected cases of nephrotic syndrome in children	

▷ **Principal Uses**

As a Single Drug Product: Uses currently included in FDA approved labeling: (1) Treatment of various forms of cancer, notably malignant lymphomas, multiple myeloma, sarcomas, retinoblastomas, leukemias and cancers of the breast and ovary; (2) because this drug exerts a suppressant effect on the immune system, it is also used to prevent rejection in organ transplantation and to treat certain autoimmune disorders; (3) also used to treat some resistant forms of nephrotic syndrome.

Other (unlabeled) generally accepted uses: (1) Used to prepare patients for autologous bone marrow transplants; (2) part of several combination chemotherapy regmens; (3) improves survival in cancer of the cervix, lung and endometrium; (4) can be part of combination therapy for Ewing's sarcoma; (5) may be of help in helping patients with lupus erythematosus who have interstitial lung disease or nephritis; (6) secondary role in prostate cancer; (7) has a secondary role in treating the serious anemia (aplastic anemia) that can be seen in lupus erythematosus.

How This Drug Works: Because of its ability to kill cancer cells during all phases of their development and reproduction, this drug suppresses the primary growth and secondary spread (metastasis) of certain types of cancer.

Available Dosage Forms and Strengths
  Injection — vials of 100 mg, 200 mg, 500 mg, 1 gram and 2 grams
  Tablets — 25 mg, 50 mg

▷ **Usual Adult Dosage Range:** Oral form: 60 to 120 mg per square meter of body surface area daily or 400 mg per square meter of body surface area on days 1–5 every 3–4 weeks.
  Intravenous: 1000 to 1500 mg per square meter every 3 to 4 weeks. **Note: Actual dosage and administration schedule must be determined by the physician for each patient individually.**

Conditions Requiring Dosing Adjustments
  Liver function: If the bilirubin (a specific measure of liver function) is from 3.1–5.0, 75% of the dose is given at the typical interval. If the bilirubin is greater than 5.0, the dose is omitted.
  Kidney function: In moderate to severe kidney problems, the dose is decreased by 75–50%.

Cyclophosphamide

▷ **Dosing Instructions:** Tablets may be crushed, and are best taken on an empty stomach. However, if nausea or indigestion occurs, this drug may be taken with or following food. Total liquid intake should be no less than 3 quarts/24 hours to reduce the risk of bladder irritation.

Usual Duration of Use: Use on a regular schedule is required to achieve and maintain a significant remission of the cancer. Duration of use depends on the response of the cancer and patient tolerance of the drug.

▷ **This Drug Should Not Be Taken If**
- you have had an allergic reaction to any dosage form of it previously.
- you have an active infection of any kind.
- you have bloody urine for any reason.
- you have renal failure.
- you are pregnant.

▷ **Inform Your Physician Before Taking This Drug If**
- you have impaired liver or kidney function.
- you have a blood cell or bone marrow disorder.
- you have had previous chemotherapy or X-ray therapy for any type of cancer.
- you take, or have taken within the past year, any cortisonelike drug (adrenal corticosteroids).
- you have diabetes.
- you plan to have surgery under general anesthesia in the near future.

Possible Side-Effects (natural, expected and unavoidable drug actions)
Bone marrow depression (see Glossary)—low production of white blood cells and, to a lesser degree, red blood cells and blood platelets (see Glossary). Possible effects include fever, chills, sore throat, fatigue, weakness, abnormal bleeding or bruising.
Leukemia has been reported following cyclophosphamide therapy.
Impairment of natural resistance (immunity) to infection.
Weakening of the heart muscle (cardiomyopathy).
Excessive urination (SIADH).
Cystitis or hemorrhagic cystitis.

▷ **Possible Adverse Effects** (unusual, unexpected and infrequent reactions)
If any of the following develop, consult your physician promptly for guidance.

Mild Adverse Effects
Allergic Reaction: Skin rash (rare).
Headache, dizziness.
Loss of scalp hair (50% of users), darkening of skin and fingernails, transverse ridging of nails.
Loss of appetite, nausea (30%), vomiting (25%), ulceration of mouth, diarrhea (may be bloody).

Serious Adverse Effects
Idiosyncratic Reaction: Hemolytic anemia (see Glossary).
Liver damage with jaundice—yellow eyes and skin, dark-colored urine, light-colored stools.
Kidney damage—impaired kidney function, reduced urine volume, bloody urine.
Severe inflammation of bladder (10%)—painful urination, bloody urine.

264   Cyclophosphamide

Drug-induced damage of heart and lung tissue.
Blurred vision.
Severe lung damage (intersittial pneumonitis).

▷ **Possible Effects on Sexual Function**
Suppression of ovarian function—irregular menstrual pattern or cessation of menstruation (18% to 57% depending upon dose and duration of use).
Testicular suppression—reduced or no sperm production (100% of users).

Possible Delayed Adverse Effects
Development of other types of cancer (secondary malignancies).
Development of severe cystitis with bleeding from the bladder wall. (May occur many months after the last dose.)

Possible Effects on Laboratory Tests
Complete blood cell counts: decreased red cells, hemoglobin, white cells and platelets.
Prothrombin time: increased.
Liver function tests: increased liver enzymes (ALT/GPT, AST/GOT and alkaline phosphatase), increased bilirubin.

CAUTION
1. This drug may interfere with the normal healing of wounds.
2. This drug can cause significant changes in genetic material in both men and women (sperm and eggs or ova). Patients taking this drug **must** understand the potential for serious defects in children that are conceived during or following the course of medication.
3. This drug can suppress natural resistance (immunity) to infection, resulting in life-threatening illness.
4. Avoid live-virus vaccines while taking this drug.

Precautions for Use
By Infants and Children: This drug should not be given if the child is dehydrated. Adequate fluid intake to ensure a copious urine volume for 4 hours following each dose is needed. Prevent exposure of child to anyone with active chicken pox or shingles. This drug may cause ovarian or testicular sterility.
By Those over 60 Years of Age: Increased risk of serious chemical cystitis, and absolute need to maintain a copious volume of urine. This may increase the risk of urinary retention in men with prostatism (see Glossary).

▷ **Advisability of Use During Pregnancy**
Pregnancy Category: D. See Pregnancy Code at the back of this book.
Animal studies: Significant birth defects reported in mice, rat and rabbit studies.
Human studies: Information from studies of pregnant women indicates that this drug can cause serious birth defects or fetal death.
Avoid completely during the first 3 months. Use of this drug during the last 6 months must be carefully individualized.

Advisability of Use if Breast-Feeding
Presence of this drug in breast milk: Yes.
Avoid drug or refrain from nursing.

Habit-Forming Potential: None.

Effects of Overdosage: Nausea, vomiting, diarrhea, bloody urine, water retention, weight gain, severe bone marrow depression, severe infections.

Possible Effects of Long-Term Use: Development of fibrous tissue in lungs; secondary malignancies.

Suggested Periodic Examinations While Taking This Drug (at physician's discretion)
> Complete blood cell counts, every 2 to 4 days during initial treatment; then every 3 to 4 weeks during maintenance treatment.
> Liver and kidney function tests.
> Thyroid function tests (if symptoms warrant).

▷ **While Taking This Drug, Observe the Following**
> *Foods:* No restrictions.
> *Beverages:* No restrictions. May be taken with milk.

▷ *Alcohol:* No interactions expected.
> *Tobacco Smoking:* No interactions expected.

▷ *Other Drugs*
> Cyclophosphamide *taken concurrently* with
> - allopurinol (Zyloprim) may increase the extent of bone marrow depression.
> - chloramphenicol can decrease cyclophosphamide effectiveness.
> - digoxin may decrease digoxin absorption and impair digoxin effectiveness.
> - hydrochlorothiazide and other thiazide diuretics (see Drug Class) may worsen the lowering of white blood cells (myelosuppression) caused by cyclophosphamide.
> - influenza vaccine (and perhaps other vaccines) may have decreased ability to confer imunity.
> - pentostatin may cause fatal heart damage.

▷ *Driving, Hazardous Activities:* Use caution if dizziness occurs.
> *Aviation Note:* The use of this drug **may be a disqualification** for piloting. Consult a designated Aviation Medical Examiner.
> *Exposure to Sun:* No restrictions.
> *Occurrence of Unrelated Illness:* Any signs of infection—fever, chills, sore throat, cough or flulike symptoms must be promptly reported. This drug may have to be stopped until the infection is controlled. Consult your physician.

CYCLOSPORINE (SI kloh spor een)

Other Names: Ciclosporin, cyclosporin A

Introduced: 1983 **Prescription:** USA: Yes; Canada: Yes **Available as Generic:** USA: No; Canada: No **Class:** Immunosuppressant **Controlled Drug:** USA: No; Canada: No

Brand Name: Sandimmune

Cyclosporine

BENEFITS versus RISKS	
Possible Benefits	*Possible Risks*
EFFECTIVE PREVENTION AND TREATMENT OF REJECTION IN ORGAN TRANSPLANTATION Limited effectiveness in the treatment of Crohn's disease, myasthenia gravis, severe psoriasis, rheumatoid arthritis	MARKED KIDNEY TOXICITY (25% to 38%) DEVELOPMENT OF HYPERTENSION (13% TO 53%) Excessive hair growth (21% to 45%) Overgrowth of gums (5% to 16%) Liver toxicity (4% to 7%) Low white blood cell count Development of lymphoma (0.2%)

▷ **Principal Uses**

As a Single Drug Product: Uses included in FDA approved labeling: (1) helps prevent (in conjunction with cortisonelike drugs) organ rejection in kidney, liver and heart transplantation; (2) helps treat rejection crisis.

Other (unlabeled) generally accepted uses: (1) Used in transplantation of the bone marrow; (2) used investigationally in a variety of diseases involving the immune system such as: Sjogren's, Crohn's and Grave's disease, psoriasis, myasthenia gravis, bullous pemphigoid, pulmonary fibrosis associated with rheumatoid arthritis, rheumatoid arthritis, Sweet's syndrome, insulin-dependent diabetes, and aplastic anemia; (3) may have a role in treating male pattern baldness; (4) can help canker sores (apthous stomatitis); (5) used to help severe, steroid-dependent asthma.

How This Drug Works: By inhibiting some lymphocytes (white blood cells) and their growth factors, this drug suppresses the rejection of transplanted organs.

Available Dosage Forms and Strengths
   Capsules, soft gelatin — 25 mg, 100 mg
   Injection, intravenous — 50 mg per ml
   Oral solution — 100 mg per ml

▷ **Usual Adult Dosage Range:** Initially 15 mg/kg/day taken 4 to 12 hours prior to transplantation surgery. This dose is continued following surgery for 1 to 2 weeks; then gradually reduce the dose by 5% per week to a maintenance dose of 5 to 10 mg/kg/day. **Note: Actual dosage and administration schedule must be determined by the physician for each patient individually.**

Conditions Requiring Dosing Adjustments

Liver function: The dose must be adjusted (based on blood levels) in liver compromise.

Kidney function: This drug is capable of causing marked kidney toxicity. Caution is critical.

Diabetes
   People who are diabetic and subsequently have kidney or pancreatic transplants will need larger than usual doses.

Hypercholesterolemia: If the blood cholesterol is 50% above normal, the dose must be decreased by 50% in order to avoid toxicity.

Obesity: Because of the way the drug is distributed in the body, the dosing of this medication **must** be based on ideal (a calculation which helps eliminate the weight which is fat) body weight.

Cystic fibrosis: It is very difficult to appropriately dose this medication in patients who have this disease. Some patients will require as much as two times the usual dose. The dose should be adjusted to drug levels.

Multiple organ transplants:
Patients with multiple transplants (such as pancreas and kidney) often need an increased dose of cyclosporin in order to achieve the desired effect. The dose should be determined based on blood levels.

▷ **Dosing Instructions:** Preferably taken with or immediately following food to reduce stomach irritation. The capsule should be swallowed whole; do not open, crush or chew. The oral solution should be mixed with milk, chocolate milk or orange juice (at room temperature) in a glass or ceramic cup; do not use a wax-lined or plastic container. Stir well and drink immediately. It is advisable to take this drug at the same time each day to maintain steady blood levels.

Usual Duration of Use: Use on a regular schedule for several weeks is usually needed to see this drug's effectiveness in preventing organ rejection or stopping rejection that is already underway. Long-term use (months to years) requires periodic evaluation of response, blood tests and dosage adjustment.

▷ **This Drug Should Not Be Taken If**
- you have had an allergic reaction to it previously.
- you are taking any immunosuppressant drug other than cortisonelike preparations.
- you have an active lymphoma of any type.
- you have an active, uncontrolled infection, especially chicken pox or shingles.

▷ **Inform Your Physician Before Taking This Drug If**
- you are pregnant or breast-feeding.
- you have a history of liver or kidney disease, or impaired liver or kidney function.
- you have a history of hypertension or gout.
- you have a chronic gastrointestinal disorder.
- you are taking a potassium supplement or drugs that can raise the blood level of potassium.
- you have a seizure disorder.
- you have a history of a blood cell disorder.
- you are taking other medicines which may be toxic to the kidney.

Possible Side-Effects (natural, expected and unavoidable drug actions)
Predisposition to infections (74%).

▷ **Possible Adverse Effects** (unusual, unexpected and infrequent reactions)
If any of the following develop, consult your physician promptly for guidance.
Mild Adverse Effects
Allergic Reactions: Skin rash (15%), itching (3%).
Excessive hair growth (21 to 45%), acne (1 to 2%).
Headache (2 to 15%), confusion (2%), tremors (21 to 55%).
Mouth sores (2%), gum overgrowth (5 to 16%), nausea/vomiting (4 to 10%), diarrhea (3 to 8%).

Cyclosporine

Serious Adverse Effects
Allergic Reactions: Anaphylactoid reaction (see Glossary) to intravenous solution (0.1%).
Severe kidney injury (25 to 38%).
Hypertension, mild to severe (13 to 53%).
Seizures (1 to 5%).
Cortical blindness.
Liver injury (4 to 7%).
Changes in facial features.
Pancreatitis (rare).
Low white blood cell count (leukopenia)(1–6%).
Low blood platelets ($<2\%$).
High blood potassium levels.
High blood glucose.
High uric acid levels and gout.
Low blood magnesium.
Lymphoma (0.2 to 0.7%), possibly drug induced.
Elevation of blood potassium and uric acid levels.
Depressed ability to fight infections.

▷ **Possible Effects on Sexual Function**
Enlargement and tenderness of male breast (1 to 4%).

▷ **Adverse Effects That May Mimic Natural Diseases or Disorders**
Liver toxicity may suggest viral hepatitis.

Natural Diseases or Disorders That May Be Activated by This Drug
Latent infections, hypertension, gout.

Possible Effects on Laboratory Tests
Complete blood cell counts: decreased red cells, hemoglobin and white cells.
Blood potassium level: increased.
Blood uric acid level: increased.
Blood platelets, white cells, magnesium: decreased.
Liver function tests: increased liver enzymes (ALT/GPT, AST/GOT and alkaline phosphatase), increased bilirubin.
Kidney function tests: blood creatinine and urea nitrogen levels (BUN) increased; urine casts present.

CAUTION
1. Report promptly any indications of infection of any kind.
2. Promptly report swollen glands, sores or lumps in the skin, abnormal bleeding or bruising.
3. Inform your physician promptly if you become pregnant.
4. Periodic laboratory tests are mandatory.
5. Best to avoid immunizations and contact with people who have recently taken oral poliovirus vaccine.

Precautions for Use
By Infants and Children: This drug has been used successfully and safely in children of all ages.
By Those over 60 Years of Age: The dose must be adjusted to any decline in kidney function.

▷ **Advisability of Use During Pregnancy**
Pregnancy Category: C. See Pregnancy Code at the back of this book.
Animal studies: Rat and rabbit studies reveal that this drug is toxic to the embryo and fetus. No drug-induced birth defects were found.
Human studies: Adequate studies of pregnant women are not available.
Avoid this drug during entire pregnancy unless it is clearly needed.

Advisability of Use if Breast-Feeding
Presence of this drug in breast milk: Yes.
Avoid drug or refrain from nursing.

Habit-Forming Potential: None.

Effects of Overdosage: Headache, painful sensations in hands and feet, flushing of the face, gum soreness and bleeding, high blood pressure, atrial fibrillation, respiratory distress syndrome, seizures, coma, hallucinations, neurotoxicity, electrolyte disturbances, liver toxicity.

Possible Effects of Long-Term Use: Irreversible kidney damage, severe hypertension, abnormal growth of gums.

Suggested Periodic Examinations While Taking This Drug (at physician's discretion)
Measurement of cyclosporine blood levels.
Complete blood cell counts.
Liver and kidney function tests.
Measurement of magnesium, potassium and uric acid blood levels.
Serial blood pressure measurements.

▷ **While Taking This Drug, Observe the Following**
Foods: Avoid excessive intake of high-potassium foods. See Table section. Food may also increase the peak blood level of cyclosporine.
Beverages: No restrictions. May be taken with milk.
▷ *Alcohol:* No interactions expected.
Tobacco Smoking: No interactions expected.
▷ *Other Drugs*
Cyclosporine *taken concurrently* with
- ACE (see Drug Classes) inhibitors may increase the risk of kidney problems.
- amphotericin B can cause serious kidney toxicity.
- aspirin substitutes (nonsteroidal anti-inflammatory drugs or NSAIDs) may increase kidney toxicity.
- aminoglycoside antibiotics (see Drug Class) may increase kidney toxicity.
- calcium channel blockers (see Drug Class) may result in cyclosporine toxicity.
- ciprofloxacin (and other fluoroquinolones—see Drug Class) may increase risk of kidney toxicity.
- cotrimoxazole may result in decreased cyclosporine effectiveness as well as kidney toxicity.
- digoxin may result in serious digoxin toxicity.
- furosemide may result in increased risk of gout.
- histamine H2 inhibitors (see Drug Class) and ketoconazole may experience decreased cyclosporine blood levels.
- imipenem/cilastatin may result in neurotoxicity.

- metronidazole may result in increased cyclosporine levels and toxicity.
- simvastatin may cause myopathy.
- sulfamethoxazole and/or trimethoprim may increase kidney toxicity.
- methylprednisolone may cause seizures.
- nifedipine may worsen abnormal gum growth (gingival hyperplasia) and also cause nefedipine toxicity (low blood pressure and abnormal heart beats).
- pravastatin can cause myopathy.
- azathioprine may increase immunosuppression.
- cyclophosphamide may increase immunosuppression.
- tacrolimus can cause kidney toxicity.
- verapamil may increase immunosuppression.
- vaccines may blunt the benefit of the vaccine.
- lovastatin may cause muscle destruction and acute kidney failure.

The following drugs may *increase* the effects of cyclosporine
- acetazolamide.
- allopurinol.
- amiodarone.
- ceftriaxone.
- colchicine.
- danazol or other anabolic steroids.
- diltiazem.
- erythromycin.
- clarithramycin.
- azithramycin.
- ketoconazole.
- itraconazole.
- fluconazole.
- miconazole.
- methyltestosterone.
- metoclopramide.
- oral contraceptives.

The following drugs may *decrease* the effects of cyclosporine
- carbamazepine.
- isoniazid.
- nafcillin.
- octreotide.
- phenobarbital.
- phenytoin.
- quinine.
- rifabutin.
- rifampin.
- sulfadimidine, sulfadiazine and/or trimethoprim.
- ticlopidine.

▷ *Driving, Hazardous Activities:*
This drug may cause confusion or seizures. Restrict activities as necessary.

Aviation Note: The use of this drug **may be a disqualification** for piloting. Consult a designated Aviation Medical Examiner.

Exposure to Sun: No restrictions.

Discontinuation: Do not discontinue this drug without your physician's guidance.

Special Storage Instructions: Keep the gelatin capsules in the blister packets until ready for use. Store below 77 degrees F (25 degrees C).

Keep the oral solution in a tightly closed container. Store below 86 degrees F (30 degrees C). Do not refrigerate.

Observe the Following Expiration Times: The oral solution must be used within 2 months after opening.

DAPSONE (DAP sohn)

Other Name: DDS
Introduced: 1963 **Prescription:** USA: Yes; Canada: Yes **Available as Generic:** USA: Yes; Canada: No **Class:** Anti-infective **Controlled Drug:** USA: No; Canada: No
Brand Name: ♦Avlosulfon

BENEFITS versus RISKS	
Possible Benefits	*Possible Risks*
EFFECTIVE ADJUNCTIVE TREATMENT OF ALL TYPES OF LEPROSY	HEMOLYTIC ANEMIA (see Glossary)
	Rare aplastic anemia (see Glossary)
EFFECTIVE TREATMENT OF DERMATITIS HERPETIFORMIS	Rare but serious skin reactions
	Rare liver damage
Effective adjunctive prevention and treatment of Pneumocystis carinii pneumonia (AIDS related)	Rare peripheral neuritis (see Glossary)
	Rare kidney damage
Moderately effective adjunctive prevention of malaria (some types)	Rare severe skin reaction

▷ **Principal Uses**

As a Single Drug Product: Uses currently included in FDA approved labeling: (1) Treatment (in combination with other antileprosy drugs) of all types of leprosy; (2) Treatment of dermatitis herpetiformis.

Other (unlabeled) generally accepted uses: (1) Prevention and treatment (in combination with trimethoprim) of Pneumocystis carinii pneumonia; (2) prevention (in combination with pyrimethamine) of chloroquine-resistant P. falciparum malaria; (3) prevention (in combination with pyrimethamine and chloroquine) of P. vivax malaria; (4) treatment of certain skin disorders of systemic lupus erythematosus; (5) treatment of brown recluse spider bite; (6) may have a role in helping decrease steroid use in asthmatics; (7) offers some treatment option in Kaposi's sarcoma; can have a role in superficial pemphigus; (8) can help in rheumatoid arthritis; (9) offers temporal arteritis patients an augmentation to steroids; (10) can have a role in resistant idiopathic thrombocytopenic purpura.

How This Drug Works: By interfering with vitamin (folate) synthesis, this drug inhibits the growth of and kills M. leprae, the cause of leprosy. Its mechanism of action in dermatitis herpetiformis is not known.

Dapsone

Available Dosage Forms and Strengths
Tablets — 25 mg, 100 mg

▷ **Recommended Dosage Ranges** (Actual dosage and administration schedule must be determined by the physician for each patient individually.)

Infants and Children: For leprosy—1.4 mg/kg of body weight, once daily.

To suppress dermatitis herpetiformis—Initially 2 mg/kg of body weight daily. Increase if needed and tolerated. As soon as possible, reduce to lowest effective maintenance dose.

To prevent Pneumocystis carinii pneumonia in children over 1 month old—1 mg/kg of body weight, up to 100 mg daily.

12 to 60 Years of Age: For leprosy—50 to 100 mg, once daily; or 1.4 mg/kg of body weight, once daily.

To suppress dermatitis herpetiformis—Initially 50 mg daily; as needed and tolerated, increase up to 300 mg daily. As soon as possible, reduce to lowest effective maintenance dose.

To prevent Pneumocystis carinii pneumonia—50 to 100 mg, once daily.

To treat Pneumocystis carinii pneumonia—100 mg, once daily, in combination with trimethoprim 20 mg/kg of body weight daily, for 21 days.

To prevent malaria—100 mg, in combination with pyrimethamine 12.5 mg, once every 7 days.

Over 60 Years of Age: Same as 12 to 60 years of age.

Conditions Requiring Dosing Adjustments
Liver function: This drug should be used with caution in liver compromise.
Kidney function: The dose must be decreased in kidney compromise.

▷ **Dosing Instructions:** May be taken with or following food to reduce stomach irritation. Do not use antacids for 4 hours before and after taking this drug. The tablet may be crushed and mixed with jelly for administration to children.

Usual Duration of Use: Use on a regular schedule for 2 to 3 months is usually needed to see this drug's effectiveness in treating leprosy. Treatment for 1 week will determine its effectiveness in treating dermatitis herpetiformis; for 2 to 3 weeks in treating P. carinii pneumonia. Leprosy requires treatment for 2 to 10 years or longer. Long-term use requires periodic physician evaluation of response and dosage adjustment.

Currently a "Drug of Choice"
for the suppression of dermatitis herpetiformis.

▷ **This Drug Should Not Be Taken If**
- you have had an allergic reaction to it previously.
- you currently have a serious blood cell or bone marrow disorder.
- you have active liver disease.

▷ **Inform Your Physician Before Taking This Drug If**
- you are allergic to "sulfa" drugs.
- you have glucose-6-phosphate dehydrogenase (G6PD) deficiency.
- you have methemoglobin reductase deficiency.
- you have had a drug-induced adverse effect on blood cells or bone marrow.
- you have a history of liver disease or impaired liver function.

- you have a history of mental illness.
- you are currently taking any other drugs.

Possible Side-Effects (natural, expected and unavoidable drug actions)
Mild hemolytic anemia and mild methemoglobinemia occur in all users.

▷ **Possible Adverse Effects** (unusual, unexpected and infrequent reactions)
If any of the following develop, consult your physician promptly for guidance.

Mild Adverse Effects
Allergic Reactions: Mild skin rashes.
Headache, nervousness, insomnia, mood changes.
Blurred vision, ringing in ears.
Loss of appetite, nausea, vomiting.

Serious Adverse Effects
Allergic Reactions: After 6 to 8 weeks of use, a "sulfone syndrome" may develop: fever, fatigue, peeling skin rash, swollen lymph glands, and jaundice (see Glossary).
Other forms of severe and extensive dermatitis.
Idiosyncratic Reactions: Serious blood cell disorders, including aplastic anemia (see Glossary): fatigue, weakness, fever, sore throat, abnormal bruising or bleeding.
Hallucinations and psychosis (rare).
Severe skin rash (Toxic Epidermal Necrolysis).
Low blood albumin.
Drug-induced liver damage with jaundice (see Glossary).
Drug-induced kidney damage.
Peripheral neuritis (see Glossary): numbness, tingling, burning, weakness in hands and/or feet.

▷ **Possible Effects on Sexual Function:** Reversible male infertility.

Possible Delayed Adverse Effects: None reported.

▷ **Adverse Effects That May Mimic Natural Diseases or Disorders**
Drug-induced liver reaction may suggest viral hepatitis.
A syndrome resembling infectious mononucleosis.
Skin reactions resembling cutaneous lupus erythematosus.

Possible Effects on Laboratory Tests
Complete blood cell counts: decreased red cells, hemoglobin, white cells and platelets; increased eosinophils (allergic reaction).
Blood total cholesterol: increased.
Liver function tests: increased liver enzymes (ALT/GPT, AST/GOT and alkaline phosphatase), increased bilirubin.

CAUTION
1. Periodic blood counts are mandatory. This drug can cause serious (sometimes fatal) bone marrow depression (see Glossary). Complete blood cell counts should be performed before treatment, weekly for the first month, monthly for 6 months, and every 6 months thereafter.
2. High doses of this drug increase risk of peripheral neuropathy. Watch for weakness of the extremities.
3. Stop drug and call your doctor if new or severe skin reactions start.

Dapsone

Precautions for Use
By Infants and Children: Safety and effectiveness for those under 1 month of age not established.
By Those over 60 Years of Age: Reduced kidney function will require dosage adjustment.

▷ **Advisability of Use During Pregnancy**
Pregnancy Category: C. See Pregnancy Code at the back of this book.
Animal studies: None reported.
Human studies: Adequate studies of pregnant women are not available.
However, there are no reports of drug-induced birth defects when this drug has been used throughout pregnancy for the long-term treatment of leprosy and dermatitis herpetiformis.
Use this drug only if clearly needed. Ask your physician for guidance.

Advisability of Use if Breast-Feeding
Presence of this drug in breast milk: Yes.
Avoid drug or refrain from nursing.

Habit-Forming Potential: None.

Effects of Overdosage: Nausea, vomiting, excitability, headache, seizures, irreversible damage to retina and optic nerve.

Possible Effects of Long-Term Use: Increased risk of kidney damage and peripheral neuropathy.

Suggested Periodic Examinations While Taking This Drug (at physician's discretion)
Complete blood cell counts, including reticulocyte counts.
Liver and kidney function tests.
Complete eye examination if blurred vision develops.

▷ **While Taking This Drug, Observe the Following**
Foods: No restrictions. During treatment of dermatitis herpetiformis, a gluten-free diet may be advantageous.
Beverages: No restrictions.
▷ *Alcohol:* No interactions expected.
Tobacco Smoking: No interactions expected.
▷ *Other Drugs*
Dapsone *taken concurrently* with
- birth control pills (oral contraceptives) may decrease the effectiveness of the contraceptives and result in pregnancy.
- trimethoprim (Proloprim, Trimpex) may increase the blood levels of both drugs. Adjust dosage if necessary to prevent dapsone toxicity.

The following drug may *increase* the effects of dapsone
- cimetidine (Tagamet).
- probenecid (Benemid).

The following drugs may *decrease* the effects of dapsone
- didanosine (DDI). Dapsone should be taken at least 2 hours before or 2 hours after didanosine.
- rifampin (Rifadin, Rimactane, others).
- rifabutin.

▷ *Driving, Hazardous Activities:* This drug may cause dizziness. Restrict activities as necessary.

Aviation Note: The use of this drug *may be a disqualification* for piloting. Consult a designated Aviation Medical Examiner.

Exposure to Sun: Caution—this drug may cause photosensitivity (see Glossary).

Discontinuation: Consult your physician before deciding to alter your dosing schedule or discontinue this medication.

DESIPRAMINE (des IP ra meen)

Introduced: 1964 **Prescription:** USA: Yes; Canada: Yes **Available as Generic:** USA: Yes; Canada: Yes **Class:** Antidepressant **Controlled Drug:** USA: No; Canada: No

Brand Names: Norpramin, Pertofrane

BENEFITS versus RISKS	
Possible Benefits	*Possible Risks*
EFFECTIVE RELIEF OF ENDOGENOUS DEPRESSION Possibly beneficial in other depressive disorders	ADVERSE BEHAVIORAL EFFECTS: confusion, disorientation, delusions, hallucinations CONVERSION OF DEPRESSION TO MANIA in bipolar affective disorders Aggravation of paranoia and schizophrenia Drug-induced heart rhythm disorders Abnormally low white blood cell and platelet counts

▷ **Principal Uses**

As a Single Drug Product: Uses currently included in FDA approved labeling: (1) Relieves severe depression. This drug is more likely to work in primary (endogenous) depression than in secondary, reactive (exogenous) depression.

Other (unlabeled) generally accepted uses: (1) Chronic pain syndromes, including diabetic neuropathy; (2) treatment of attention deficit disorder in children over 6 years of age and in adolescents; (3) decreases the symptoms of panic disorder; (4) helps treat resistant malaria; (5) may help reduce binge eating in bulimia.

How This Drug Works: By increasing brain concentrations of some nerve impulse transmitters (norepinephrine and serotonin), this drug relieves the symptoms associated with depression.

Available Dosage Forms and Strengths
Capsules — 25 mg, 50 mg
Tablets — 10 mg, 25 mg, 50 mg, 75 mg, 100 mg, 150 mg

▷ **Usual Adult Dosage Range:** Initially 25 mg 2 to 4 times daily. Dose may be increased cautiously as needed and tolerated by 25 mg daily at intervals of 1 week. The usual maintenance dose is 100 mg to 200 mg/24 hours. The

total daily dosage should not exceed 300 mg. (When determined, the optimal daily requirement may be given at bedtime as a single dose.)
Note: Actual dosage and administration schedule must be determined by the physician for each patient individually.

Conditions Requiring Dosing Adjustments
Liver function: The dose should be decreased in patients with compromised livers.
Kidney function: Can cause urine retention—used with caution in kidney compromise with urine outflow problems.

▷ **Dosing Instructions:** May be taken without regard to meals. The capsule may be opened and the tablet may be crushed for administration.

Usual Duration of Use: Use on a regular schedule for 3 to 4 weeks is usually needed to see this drug's effectiveness in relieving depression; peak response may require 3 months of use. Delusional patients may require seven weeks to benefit. Long-term use (months to years) requires periodic evaluation of response and dosage adjustment.

▷ **This Drug Should Not Be Taken If**
- you have had an allergic reaction to it previously.
- you are taking, or have taken within the past 14 days, any monoamine oxidase (MAO) type A inhibitor drug (see Drug Class Section).
- you have had a recent heart attack (myocardial infarction).
- you have narrow-angle glaucoma.

▷ **Inform Your Physician Before Taking This Drug If**
- you have had an adverse reaction to any other antidepressant drug.
- you have any type of seizure disorder.
- you have increased internal eye pressure.
- you have any type of heart disease, especially a heart rhythm disorder.
- you have any type of thyroid disorder or are taking thyroid medication.
- you have thought about or attempted suicide.
- you have diabetes or sugar intolerance.
- you have prostatism (see Glossary).
- you plan to have surgery under general anesthesia in the near future.

Possible Side-Effects (natural, expected and unavoidable drug actions)
Mild drowsiness, light-headedness (low blood pressure), blurred vision, dry mouth, constipation, impaired urination.

▷ **Possible Adverse Effects** (unusual, unexpected and infrequent reactions)
If any of the following develop, consult your physician promptly for guidance.
Mild Adverse Effects
Allergic Reactions: Skin rash, hives, swelling of face or tongue, drug fever (see Glossary).
Headache, dizziness, weakness, unsteadiness, tremors, fainting.
Irritation of tongue or mouth, altered taste, indigestion, nausea.
Fluctuations of blood sugar.
Serious Adverse Effects
Allergic Reactions: Drug-induced hepatitis, with or without jaundice; anaphylactoid reaction (see terms in Glossary).

Adverse behavioral effects: confusion, disorientation, delusions, hallucinations.
Seizures; reduced control of epilepsy.
Aggravation of paranoid psychoses and schizophrenia.
Heart rhythm disturbances.
Parkinsonlike disorders, peripheral neuritis (see both terms in Glossary).
Abnormally low white blood cell and platelet counts: fever, sore throat, infections, abnormal bleeding or bruising.
Neuroleptic malignant syndrome.

▷ **Possible Effects on Sexual Function:** Decreased libido, increased libido (antidepressant effect), impotence, painful male orgasm, male breast enlargement, female breast enlargement with milk production, swelling of testicles, decreased sperm viability.

▷ **Adverse Effects That May Mimic Natural Diseases or Disorders**
Liver toxicity may suggest viral hepatitis.

Natural Diseases or Disorders That May Be Activated by This Drug
Latent diabetes, epilepsy, glaucoma, prostatism.

Possible Effects on Laboratory Tests
Complete blood cell counts: decreased red cells, hemoglobin, white cells and platelets; increased eosinophils (allergic reaction).
Blood glucose levels: unexplained fluctuations.
Liver function tests: increased liver enzymes (ALT/GPT, AST/GOT and alkaline phosphatase), increased bilirubin (all rare).
Thyroid function tests: decreased TSH and mean free thyroxin.

CAUTION
1. Should only be used when a true, primary, endogenous depression (not reactive) has been diagnosed.
2. Watch for indications of toxicity: confusion, agitation, rapid heart rate, heart irregularity. Blood levels will be needed.
3. It is advisable to withhold this drug if electroconvulsive therapy (ECT) is to be used to treat the depression.

Precautions for Use
By Infants and Children: Safety and effectiveness for those under 6 years of age not established. This drug is being used experimentally to treat children who have attention deficit syndrome, with or without hyperactivity. Dosage and management must be supervised by a properly trained pediatrician.
By Those over 60 Years of Age: Initiate treatment with 25 mg 1 or 2 times daily to evaluate tolerance. During the first 2 weeks of treatment, watch for confusion, restlessness, agitation, forgetfulness, disorientation, delusions or hallucinations. Also observe for unsteadiness and instability that may predispose to falling. This drug may aggravate prostatism.

▷ **Advisability of Use During Pregnancy**
Pregnancy Category: C. See Pregnancy Code at the back of this book.
Animal studies: Birth defects reported in rat and rabbit studies.
Human studies: Adequate studies of pregnant women are not available. Use only if clearly needed. Avoid during the first 3 months if possible.

Advisability of Use if Breast-Feeding
 Presence of this drug in breast milk: Yes, in small amounts.
 Monitor nursing infant closely and discontinue drug or nursing if adverse effects develop.

Habit-Forming Potential: Psychological or physical dependence is rare and unexpected. Some patients may seek to abuse this medicine for its ability to create anticholinergic delirium.

Effects of Overdosage: Confusion, hallucinations, drowsiness, tremors, heart irregularity, seizures, stupor, hypothermia (see Glossary).

Possible Effects of Long-Term Use: None reported.

Suggested Periodic Examinations While Taking This Drug (at physician's discretion)
 Complete blood cell counts, liver function tests.
 Serial blood pressure readings and electrocardiograms.

▷ **While Taking This Drug, Observe the Following**
 Foods: No specific restrictions. Limiting food intake may avoid excess weight gain.
 Beverages: No restrictions. May be taken with milk.
▷ *Alcohol:* Avoid completely. This drug can markedly increase the intoxicating effects of alcohol; the combination can depress brain function.
 Tobacco Smoking: May accelerate the elimination of this drug and require increased dosage.
 Marijuana Smoking
  Occasional (once or twice weekly): Transient increase in drowsiness and mouth dryness.
  Daily: Persistent drowsiness and mouth dryness; possible reduced effectiveness of this drug.

▷ *Other Drugs*
 Desipramine may *increase* the effects of
 • all drugs with sedative effects; observe for excessive sedation.
 • all drugs with atropinelike effects (see Drug Class Section).
 Desipramine may *decrease* the effects of
 • clonidine (Catapres).
 • guanfacine (Tenex).
 • guanethidine (Ismelin, Esimil).
 Desipramine *taken concurrently* with
 • anticonvulsants requires careful monitoring for changes in seizure patterns and need to adjust anticonvulsant dosage (carbamazepine or phenytoin are examples).
 • ethchlorvynol (Placidyl) may cause delirium; avoid concurrent use.
 • monoamine oxidase (MAO) type A inhibitor drugs (see Drug Class) may cause high fever, seizures and excessive rise in blood pressure; avoid concurrent use of these drugs and provide periods of 14 days between administration of either.
 • quinidine may cause desipramine toxicity.
 • stimulant drugs (amphetamine, cocaine, epinephrine, phenylpropanolamine, etc.) may cause severe high blood pressure and/or high fever.
 • thyroid preparations may increase the risk of heart rhythm disorders.

- warfarin may cause an increased risk of bleeding. Increased testing of INR is indicated.

The following drugs may *increase* the effects of desipramine
- cimetidine (Tagamet).
- fluoxetine (Prozac).
- methylphenidate (Ritalin).
- phenothiazines (see Drug Class).

The following drugs may *decrease* the effects of desipramine
- barbiturates (see Drug Class Section).
- chloral hydrate (Noctec, Somnos, etc.).
- clonazepam.
- estrogen (see Drug Profile for brand names).
- lithium (Lithobid, Lithotab, etc.).
- oral contraceptives (see Drug Profile for brand names).
- reserpine (Serpasil, Ser-Ap-Es, etc.).

▷ *Driving, Hazardous Activities:* This drug may impair mental alertness, judgment, physical coordination and reaction time. Restrict activities as necessary.

Aviation Note: The use of this drug *is a disqualification* for piloting. Consult a designated Aviation Medical Examiner.

Exposure to Sun: Use caution. This drug may cause photosensitivity (see Glossary) and changes in iris and skin pigment color with sun exposure.

Exposure to Heat: Use caution. This drug can inhibit sweating and impair adaptation to hot environments, increasing the risk of heat stroke. Avoid saunas.

Exposure to Cold: The elderly should use caution and avoid conditions conducive to hypothermia (see Glossary).

Exposure to Environmental Chemicals: This drug may mask the symptoms of poisoning due to handling certain insecticides (organophosphorus types). Read labels carefully.

Discontinuation: It is advisable to stop this drug gradually. Abrupt withdrawal after prolonged use may cause headache, malaise and nausea. When this drug is stopped, it may be necessary to adjust the dosages of other drugs taken concurrently.

DEXAMETHASONE (dex a METH a sohn)

Introduced: 1958   **Prescription:** USA: Yes; Canada: Yes   **Available as Generic:** USA: Yes; Canada: Yes   **Class:** Cortisonelike drugs   **Controlled Drug:** USA: No; Canada: No

Brand Names: Acroseb-Dex, ✦Ak-Dex, Dalalone, Dalalone DP, Dalalone LA, Decaderm, Decadron, Decadron Nasal Spray, Decadron-LA, Decadron Phosphate Ophthalmic, Decadron Phosphate Respihaler, Decadron Phosphate Turbinaire, Decadron w/Xylocaine [CD], Decaject, Decaject LA, Decaspray, Deenar [CD], ✦Deronil, Dex-4, Dexacen-4, Dexacen LA-8, Dexameth, Dexasone, Dexasone-LA, Dexo-LA, Dexone, Dexone-E, Dexone-LA, Hexadrol, Maxidex, Mymethasone, ✦Neodecadron Eye-Ear, Neomycin-Dex, ✦Oradexon, ✦PMS-Dexamethasone, ✦SK-Dexamethasone, ✦Sofracort, Solurex, Solurex-LA, ✦Spersadex, Tobradex

Dexamethasone

BENEFITS versus RISKS	
Possible Benefits	*Possible Risks*
EFFECTIVE RELIEF OF SYMPTOMS IN A WIDE VARIETY OF INFLAMMATORY AND ALLERGIC DISORDERS EFFECTIVE IMMUNOSUPPRESSION in selected benign and malignant disorders	Short-term use (up to 10 days) is usually well tolerated Long-term use (exceeding 2 weeks) is associated with many possible adverse effects: ALTERED MOOD AND PERSONALITY CATARACTS, GLAUCOMA HYPERTENSION ARRHYTHMIAS PEPTIC ULCERS PANCREATITIS OSTEOPOROSIS ASEPTIC BONE NECROSIS INCREASED SUSCEPTIBILITY TO INFECTIONS (See Possible Adverse Effects and Possible Effects of Long-Term Use below)

▷ **Principal Uses**

As a Single Drug Product: Uses currently included in FDA approved labeling: (1) Used in the management of serious skin disorders, asthma, lymphoma, brain edema, shock, systemic lupus erythematosus and all types of major rheumatic disorders including bursitis, systemic lupus erythematosus, tendonitis and most forms of arthritis; (2) topical cream is used to treat eczema, psoriasis, dermatitis and lichen planus.

Other (unlabeled) generally accepted uses: (1) Adrenal insufficiency; (2) acute airway obstruction; (3) mountain sickness; (4) vomiting caused by chemotherapy; (5) cardiopulmonary bypass; (6) refractory depression; (7) relief of symptoms of cancer which has spread to the brain (metastasis); (8) used in combination regimens to control multiple myeloma; (9) may have a role in extreme cases of pneumocystis carinii pneumonia.

How This Drug Works: Inhibits defensive functions of certain white blood cells. It reduces the production of lymphpocytes and some antibodies and acts as an immunosuppressant.

Available Dosage Forms and Strengths

Aerosol — 0.01% and 0.04%
Aerosol inhaler — 84 mcg per spray
Cream — 0.1%
Elixir — 0.5 mg per 5-ml teaspoonful
Eye ointment — 0.05%
Gel — 0.1%
Injection — 4 mg per ml, 8 mg per ml, 10 mg per ml, 16 mg per ml, 20 mg per ml and 24 mg per ml
Oral solution — 0.5 mg per 0.5 ml and 0.5 mg per 5 ml
Solution — 0.1%
Suspension — 0.1%

Dexamethasone

Tablets — 0.25 mg, 0.5 mg, 0.75 mg, 1 mg, 1.5 mg, 2 mg, 4 mg, 6 mg

▷ **Usual Adult Dosage Range:** Oral: 0.5 to 9 mg daily divided into 2 to 4 doses. Oral dose for children: 0.03 to 0.15 mg per kg per day divided into equal doses given every 6 to 12 hours. **Note: Actual dosage and administration schedule must be determined by the physician for each patient individually.**

Conditions Requiring Dosing Adjustments

Liver function: This drug is eliminated via the liver, however, no specific guidelines for dosing adjustments are available.

Kidney function: Used with caution as it can cause alkalosis (a change toward a more basic condition in the body's chemistry).

Obesity: Dosing on a mg per kg per day basis is recommended. Best to measure free urinary cortisol as well.

▷ **Dosing Instructions:** Tablet may be crushed and taken with or following food to prevent stomach irritation, preferably in the morning.

Usual Duration of Use: For acute disorders: 4 to 10 days. For chronic disorders: according to individual requirements. Length of therapy should not exceed the time needed to obtain adequate symptomatic relief in acute self-limiting conditions; or the time required to stabilize a chronic condition and permit gradual withdrawal. Because of its long duration of action, this drug is not appropriate for alternate day administration.

▷ **This Drug Should Not Be Taken If**
- you have had an allergic reaction to any dosage form of it previously.
- you have active peptic ulcer disease.
- you have an active herpes simplex infection of the eye.
- you have osteoporosis.
- you have a psychoneurosis or psychosis.
- you have active tuberculosis.

▷ **Inform Your Physician Before Taking This Drug If**
- you have had an unfavorable reaction to any cortisonelike drug.
- you have a history of peptic ulcer disease, thrombophlebitis or tuberculosis.
- you have: diabetes, glaucoma, high blood pressure, deficient thyroid function or myasthenia gravis.
- you plan to have surgery of any kind in the near future.

Possible Side-Effects (natural, expected and unavoidable drug actions)

Increased appetite, weight gain, retention of salt and water, excretion of potassium, increased susceptibility to infection.

▷ **Possible Adverse Effects** (unusual, unexpected and infrequent reactions)

If any of the following develop, consult your physician promptly for guidance.

Mild Adverse Effects
Allergic Reaction: Skin rash.
Headache, dizziness, insomnia.
Acid indigestion, abdominal distention.
Muscle cramping and weakness.
Acne, excessive growth of facial hair.

Serious Adverse Effects
Mental and emotional disturbances of serious magnitude.
Reactivation of latent tuberculosis.

Development of peptic ulcer.
Increased blood pressure.
Development of inflammation of the pancreas.
Thrombophlebitis (inflammation of a vein with the formation of blood clot)—pain or tenderness in thigh or leg, or swelling of the foot, ankle or leg.
Pulmonary embolism (movement of a blood clot to the lung)—sudden shortness of breath, pain in the chest, coughing, bloody sputum.
Low blood platelets.
Abnormal heart rhythm.
Cushing's syndrome.
Suppression of the adrenal gland.
High blood sugar.
Superinfections of the stomach.
Pancreatitis.
Increased pressure in the eye.
Cataracts.
Muscular weakness and myopathy.

▷ **Possible Effects on Sexual Function:** Altered timing and pattern of menstruation.

▷ **Adverse Effects That May Mimic Natural Diseases or Disorders**
Pattern of symptoms and signs resembling Cushing's syndrome.

Natural Diseases or Disorders That May Be Activated by This Drug
Latent diabetes, glaucoma, peptic ulcer disease, tuberculosis.

Possible Effects on Laboratory Tests
Blood amylase level: increased (possible pancreatitis).
Blood glucose level: increased.
Glucose tolerance test (GTT): decreased.
Blood potassium level: decreased.
Thyroid function tests: decreased.

CAUTION
1. Best to carry a card noting that you are taking this drug, if your course of treatment is to exceed 1 week.
2. Do not stop this drug abruptly if it is used for long-term treatment.
3. If vaccination against measles, rabies, smallpox or yellow fever is required, stop this drug 72 hours before vaccination and do not resume it for at least 14 days after vaccination.

Precautions for Use
By Infants and Children: Avoid prolonged use if possible. During long-term use, watch for suppression of normal growth and the possibility of increased intracranial pressure. Following long-term use, the child may be at risk for adrenal gland deficiency during stress for as long as 18 months after cessation.
By Those over 60 Years of Age: Avoid prolonged use of this drug. Continual use (even in small doses) can increase the severity of diabetes, enhance fluid retention, raise blood pressure, weaken resistance to infection, induce stomach ulcer and accelerate the development of cataract and osteoporosis.

Dexamethasone

▷ **Advisability of Use During Pregnancy**
Pregnancy Category: C. See Pregnancy Code at the back of this book.
Animal studies: Birth defects reported in mice, rats and rabbits.
Human studies: Adequate studies of pregnant women are not available.
Avoid completely during the first 3 months. Limit use during the last 6 months as much as possible. If used, examine infant for possible deficiency of adrenal gland function.

Advisability of Use if Breast-Feeding
Presence of this drug in breast milk: Yes.
Avoid drug or refrain from nursing.

Habit-Forming Potential: Use to suppress symptoms over an extended period of time may produce a state of functional dependence (see Glossary). In treating asthma and rheumatoid arthritis, it is best to keep the dose as small as possible and to attempt drug withdrawal after periods of reasonable improvement. Such procedures may reduce the degree of "steroid rebound"—the return of symptoms as the drug is withdrawn.

Effects of Overdosage: Fatigue, muscle weakness, stomach irritation, acid indigestion, excessive sweating, facial flushing, fluid retention, swelling of extremities, increased blood pressure.

Possible Effects of Long-Term Use: Increased blood sugar (possible diabetes), increased fat deposits on the trunk of the body ("buffalo hump"), rounding of the face ("moon face"), thinning and fragility of skin, loss of texture and strength of bones (osteoporosis, aseptic necrosis), cataracts, glaucoma, retarded growth and development in children.

Suggested Periodic Examinations While Taking This Drug (at physician's discretion)
Measurements of blood pressure, blood sugar and potassium levels.
Complete eye examinations at regular intervals.
Chest X-ray if history of tuberculosis.
Determination of the rate of development of the growing child to detect retardation of normal growth.

▷ **While Taking This Drug, Observe the Following**
Foods: No interactions expected. Ask physician about salt restriction or need for potassium-rich foods. During long-term use of this drug, it is advisable to eat a high-protein diet.
Nutritional Support: During long-term use, take a vitamin D supplement. During wound repair, take a zinc supplement.
Beverages: No restrictions. Drink all forms of milk liberally.
▷ *Alcohol:* No interactions expected. Caution if you are prone to peptic ulcer disease.
Tobacco Smoking: Nicotine increases the blood levels of naturally produced cortisone and related hormones. Heavy smoking may add to the expected actions of this drug and requires close observation for excessive effects.
Marijuana Smoking: May cause additional impairment of immunity.
▷ *Other Drugs*
Dexamethasone may *decrease* the effects of
- isoniazid (INH, Niconyl, etc.).
- salicylates (aspirin, sodium salicylate, etc.).

Dexamethasone *taken concurrently* with
- carbamazepine will reduce the effectiveness of dexamethasone.
- loop diuretics such as furosemide and bumetanide can result in additive potassium loss.
- oral anticoagulants may either increase or decrease their effectiveness; ask your doctor about prothrombin time testing and dosage adjustment.
- oral hypoglycemic agents (see Drug Classes) will decrease their effectiveness.

The following drugs may *decrease* the effects of dexamethasone
- antacids may reduce its absorption.
- barbiturates (Amytal, Butisol, phenobarbital, etc.).
- phenytoin (Dilantin, etc.).
- primidone.
- rifabutin.
- rifampin (Rifadin, Rimactane, etc.).

▷ *Driving, Hazardous Activities:* Usually no restrictions. Be alert to the rare occurrence of dizziness.

Aviation Note: The use of this drug *may be a disqualification* for piloting. Consult a designated Aviation Medical Examiner.

Exposure to Sun: No restrictions.

Occurrence of Unrelated Illness: This drug may decrease natural resistance to infection. Call your doctor if you develop an infection of any kind. It may also reduce your body's ability to respond to the stress of acute illness, injury or surgery. Keep your physician fully informed of any significant health changes.

Discontinuation: Do not stop this drug abruptly after chronic use. Ask your doctor for help regarding gradual withdrawal. For a period of 2 years after discontinuing this drug, it is essential in the event of illness, injury or surgery that you inform attending medical personnel that you have used this drug in the past.

DIAZEPAM (di AZ e pam)

Introduced: 1963 **Prescription:** USA: Yes; Canada: Yes **Available as Generic:** Yes **Class:** Mild tranquilizer, benzodiazepines **Controlled Drug:** USA: C-IV*; Canada: No

Brand Names: Diastat, ✦Apo-Diazepam, ✦Diazemuls, ✦Meval, ✦Novodipam, ✦Rival, Valium, Valrelease, Vazepam, ✦Vivol, Zetran

BENEFITS versus RISKS	
Possible Benefits	*Possible Risks*
RELIEF OF ANXIETY AND NERVOUS TENSION Wide margin of safety with therapeutic doses	Habit-forming potential with prolonged use Minor impairment of mental functions Very rare jaundice Very rare blood cell disorders

*See Schedules of Controlled Drugs at the back of this book.

Diazepam

▷ **Principal Uses**

As a Single Drug Product: Uses included in FDA approved labeling: (1) Provides short-term relief of mild to moderate anxiety; (2) relieves the symptoms of acute alcohol withdrawal: agitation, tremors, hallucinations, incipient delirium tremens; (3) eases skeletal muscle spasm; (4) provides short-term control of certain types of seizures (epilepsy and fever induced); (5) short-term relief of insomnia; (6) adjunctive use in endoscopic procedures; (7) decreases anxiety prior to electrical defibrillation of the heart (cardioversion).

Other (unlabeled) generally accepted uses: (1) Helps prevent LSD flashbacks; (2) short-term treatment of sleep walking; (3) treatment of persistent hiccups; (4) adjunctive treatment of catatonia.

How This Drug Works: By enhancing the nerve transmitter gamma-aminobutyric acid (GABA), this drug helps block higher brain centers and causes calming.

Available Dosage Forms and Strengths

Capsules, prolonged-action — 15 mg
Concentrate — 5 mg per ml
Injection — 5 mg per ml
Oral solution — 5 mg per ml, 5 mg per 5-ml teaspoonful
Tablets — 2 mg, 5 mg, 10 mg

▷ **Usual Adult Dosage Range:** 2 to 10 mg, 2 to 4 times daily. Dose may be increased cautiously as needed and tolerated. After 1 week of continual use, the total daily dose may be taken at bedtime. Total daily dose should not exceed 60 mg. **Note: Actual dosage and administration schedule must be determined by the physician for each patient individually.**

Conditions Requiring Dosing Adjustments

Liver function: The dose **must** be decreased by 50% in patients with liver compromise.

Kidney function: Caution—if 15 mg or more is given daily, diazepam metabolites may accumulate.

▷ **Dosing Instructions:** The tablet may be crushed and taken on empty stomach or with food or milk. The prolonged-action capsule should not be opened. Do not stop this drug abruptly if taken for more than 4 weeks.

Usual Duration of Use: Use on a regular schedule for 3 to 5 days is usually needed to see this drug's effectiveness in relieving moderate anxiety. Limit continual use to 1 to 3 weeks. Avoid uninterrupted and prolonged use.

▷ **This Drug Should Not Be Taken If**
- you have had an allergic reaction to any dosage form of it previously.
- you have acute narrow-angle glaucoma.
- it is prescribed for a child under 6 months of age.

▷ **Inform Your Physician Before Taking This Drug If**
- you are allergic to any benzodiazepine (see Drug Class Section).
- you have a history of alcoholism or drug abuse.
- you are pregnant or planning pregnancy.
- you have impaired liver or kidney function.
- you have a history of serious depression or mental disorder.
- you have: asthma, emphysema, epilepsy, or myasthenia gravis.

Diazepam

Possible Side-Effects (natural, expected and unavoidable drug actions)
Drowsiness (5%), lethargy, unsteadiness (0.2%), "hangover" effects on the day following bedtime use.

▷ **Possible Adverse Effects** (unusual, unexpected and infrequent reactions)
If any of the following develop, consult your physician promptly for guidance.

Mild Adverse Effects
Allergic Reactions: Rashes (0.4%), hives.
Dizziness, fainting, blurred or double vision, slurred speech, sweating, nausea.
Ringing in the ears.

Serious Adverse Effects
Allergic Reactions: Liver damage with jaundice (see Glossary), kidney damage, abnormally low blood platelet count, anaphylaxis.
Respiratory depression.
Bone marrow depression—low white blood cells, fever, sore throat.
Severe lowering of blood pressure, slow heart rate and cardiac arrest has been reported after rapid intravenous dosing.
Amnesia.
Obsessive-compulsive disorder following extended use and abrupt withdrawal.
Paradoxical responses of excitement, agitation, anger, rage.

▷ **Possible Effects on Sexual Function**
Altered timing and pattern of menstruation.
Small doses (2 to 5 mg/day) may help the anxiety seen in many cases of impotence in men and inhibited sexual responsiveness in women.
Larger doses (10 mg/day or more) can decrease libido, impair potency in men and inhibit orgasm in women.
Swelling and tenderness of male breast tissue (gynecomastia).

▷ **Adverse Effects That May Mimic Natural Diseases or Disorders**
Liver reaction with jaundice may suggest viral hepatitis.

Possible Effects on Laboratory Tests
White blood cell counts: decreased.
Blood thyroxine (T_4) level: decreased.
Liver function tests: increased liver enzymes (ALT/GPT, AST/GOT and alkaline phosphatase), increased bilirubin (all rare).
Urine sugar tests: no drug effect with TesTape; low test results with Clinistix and Diastix.
Urine screening tests for drug abuse: may be **positive**. (Test results depend upon amount of drug taken and testing method used.)

CAUTION
1. This drug should not be discontinued abruptly if it has been taken continually for more than 4 weeks.
2. Some over-the-counter drug products that contain antihistamines (allergy and cold preparations, sleep aids) can cause excessive sedation if combined with diazepam.

Precautions for Use
By Infants and Children: Safety and effectiveness for those under 6 months of age not established. This drug should not be used in hyperactive or psychotic children. Watch for excessive sedation and incoordination.
By Those over 60 Years of Age: Small doses are indicated. Observe for lethargy, indifference, fatigue, weakness, unsteadiness, disturbing dreams, nightmares and paradoxical reactions of excitement, agitation, anger, hostility and rage.

▷ **Advisability of Use During Pregnancy**
Pregnancy Category: D. See Pregnancy Code at the back of this book.
Animal studies: Cleft palate reported in mice; skeletal defects in rats.
Human studies: Available information is conflicting and inconclusive. Some findings of increased serious birth defects. Other studies have found no significant increase in birth defects.
Frequent use in late pregnancy can cause the "floppy infant" syndrome in the newborn: weakness, lethargy, unresponsiveness, depressed breathing, low body temperature.
Avoid use during entire pregnancy.

Advisability of Use if Breast-Feeding
Presence of this drug in breast milk: Yes.
Avoid drug or refrain from nursing.

Habit-Forming Potential: This drug can produce psychological and/or physical dependence (see Glossary) if used in large doses for an extended period of time.

Effects of Overdosage: Marked drowsiness, weakness, feeling of drunkenness, staggering gait, tremor, stupor progressing to deep sleep or coma.

Possible Effects of Long-Term Use: Psychological and/or physical dependence, rare blood cell disorders.

Suggested Periodic Examinations While Taking This Drug (at physician's discretion)
Complete blood cell counts during long-term use.

▷ **While Taking This Drug, Observe the Following**
Foods: No restrictions.
Beverages: Avoid excessive intake of caffeine-containing beverages: coffee, tea, cola. May be taken with milk.
▷ *Alcohol:* Avoid this combination. Alcohol increases the absorption of this drug and adds to its depressant effects on the brain. It is advisable to avoid alcohol completely—throughout the day and night—if it is necessary to drive or to engage in any hazardous activity.
Tobacco Smoking: Heavy smoking may reduce the calming action of this drug.
Marijuana Smoking: Increased sedation and impairment of intellectual and physical performance.
▷ *Other Drugs*
Diazepam may *increase* the effects of
- digoxin (Lanoxin), and cause digoxin toxicity.
- phenytoin (Dilantin), and cause phenytoin toxicity.

Diazepam may *decrease* the effects of
- levodopa (Sinemet, etc.), and reduce its effectiveness in treating Parkinson's disease.

Diazepam *taken concurrently* with
- narcotics or other centrally active medicines may cause additive respiratory depression or decreased levels of consciousness.

The following drugs may *increase* the effects of diazepam
- cimetidine (Tagamet).
- disulfiram (Antabuse).
- isoniazid (INH, Rifamate, etc.).
- oral contraceptives.
- sertraline (Zoloft).
- valproic acid (Depakene).

The following drugs may *decrease* the effects of diazepam
- ranitidine (Zantac).
- rifampin (Rimactane, etc.).
- rifabutin.
- theophylline (aminophylline, Theo-Dur, etc.).

▷ *Driving, Hazardous Activities:* This drug can impair mental alertness, judgment, physical coordination and reaction time. Avoid hazardous activities accordingly.

Aviation Note: The use of this drug *is a disqualification* for piloting. Consult a designated Aviation Medical Examiner.

Exposure to Sun: No restrictions.

Exposure to Heat: Because of reduced urine volume, this drug may accumulate in the body and produce effects of overdosage.

Discontinuation: Avoid sudden discontinuation if this drug has been taken for over 4 weeks without interruption. Dosage should be tapered gradually to prevent a withdrawal syndrome that could include depression, confusion, hallucinations, tremor, seizures, muscle cramping, sweating and vomiting.

DICLOFENAC (di KLOH fen ak)

Introduced: 1976 **Prescription:** USA: Yes; Canada: Yes **Available as Generic:** USA: No; Canada: No **Class:** Mild analgesic, anti-inflammatory **Controlled Drug:** USA: No; Canada: No
Brand Name: Apo-Diclo, Arthrotec, Cataflam, Novo-Difenac, Nu-Diclo, Voltaren, Voltaren Ophthalmic

Please see the acetic acid NSAIDs profile for further information.

DIDANOSINE (di DAN oh seen)

Other Names: Dideoxyinosine, DDI
Introduced: 1991 **Prescription:** USA: Yes; Canada: Yes **Available as Generic:** USA: No; Canada: No **Class:** Antiviral **Controlled Drug:** USA: No; Canada: No
Brand Name: Videx

BENEFITS versus RISKS	
Possible Benefits	**Possible Risks**
DELAYED PROGRESSION OF DISEASE IN HIV-INFECTED INDIVIDUALS WITH AIDS OR AIDS-RELATED COMPLEX	DRUG-INDUCED PANCREATITIS (10%) DRUG-INDUCED PERIPHERAL NEURITIS (34%) Drug-induced seizures (3%) Rare liver damage

▷ **Principal Uses**

As a Single Drug Product: Uses currently included in FDA approved labeling: (1) Treatment of human immunodeficiency virus (HIV) infections in adults and children (6 months of age or older) with advanced disease who cannot tolerate zidovudine or who have shown significant deterioration during zidovudine therapy. This drug is not a cure for AIDS, and it does not reduce the risk of transmission of HIV infection to others through sexual contact or contamination of blood.

Other (unlabeled) generally accepted uses: (1) Used in combination with hydroxyurea (Hydrea) to treat AIDS.

How This Drug Works: By interfering with essential HIV enzyme systems, this drug prevents growth and reproduction of HIV particles in infected cells, limiting the severity and extent of HIV infection.

Available Dosage Forms and Strengths

Pediatric oral solution — 10 mg/ml

Powder for oral solution — packets of 100 mg, 167 mg, 250 mg, 375 mg

Tablets, chewable/dispersible — 25 mg, 50 mg, 100 mg, 150 mg

Author's note: The company is actively investigating other formulations for this medicine.

▷ **Recommended Dosage Ranges** (Actual dosage and administration schedule must be determined by the physician for each patient individually.)

Infants and Children: For those 6 months of age or older, dosage is based on dosage form and body surface area:

Pediatric oral solution (reconstituted and admixed with buffers)—125 mg (12.5 ml)/12 hours for body surface area of 1.1–1.4 m^2, 94 mg (9.5 ml)/12 hours for body surface area of 0.8–1 m^2, 62 mg (6 ml)/12 hours for body surface area of 0.5–0.7 m^2, 31 mg (3 ml)/12 hours for body surface area of 0.4 m^2 or less.

Chewable/dispersible tablets—100 mg/12 hours for body surface area of 1.1–1.4 m^2, 75 mg/12 hours for body surface area of 0.8–1 m^2, 50 mg/12 hours for body surface area of 0.5–0.7 m^2, 25 mg/12 hours for body surface area of 0.4 m^2 or less. In children 1 year of age or older, each dose should consist of 2 tablets to ensure that adequate buffering is provided to prevent degradation of the drug in stomach acid secretions; in children younger than 1 year of age, 1 tablet will provide adequate buffering.

12 to 60 Years of Age: Dosing as follows:

Adult oral solution (buffered)—375 mg/12 hours for body weight of 75 kg or more, 250 mg/12 hours for body weight of 50–74 kg, 167 mg/12 hours for body weight of 35–49 kg.

Chewable/dispersible tablets—300 mg/12 hours for body weight of 75 kg or more, 200 mg/12 hours for body weight of 50–74 kg, 125 mg/12 hours for body weight of 35–49 kg. Each dose should consist of 2 tablets to ensure active drug is protected.

Over 60 Years of Age: Same as 12 to 60 group. Dose reduced in impaired liver or kidney function.

Conditions Requiring Dosing Adjustments

Liver function: Up to 60% of a given dose is changed by the liver to other compounds. There is an increased risk of liver toxicity if used in people with compromised livers. Dose must be decreased if used in liver failure.

Kidney function: Dose **must** be decreased in mild to moderate kidney failure. There is also an increased risk of magnesium toxicity and drug-induced pancreatitis in patients with kidney problems.

▷ **Dosing Instructions:** Best taken on an empty stomach, 2 hours before or 2 hours after eating.

The pediatric oral solution is first reconstituted with water and then combined with equal quantities of antacid (such as Mylanta or Maalox). This mixture must be shaken thoroughly before measuring each dose.

The adult oral solution is made by stirring 1 packet into 120 ml (4 ounces) of water until the powder is dissolved; this may take up to 3 minutes. The powder should not be mixed with fruit juice or other acidic liquid. The entire 4 ounce solution should be swallowed immediately.

The chewable/dispersible buffered tablets should be thoroughly chewed, crushed or dispersed in water before swallowing. To disperse the tablet(s), stir the prescribed number in at least 30 ml (1 ounce) of water until a uniform suspension is obtained. Swallow the entire preparation immediately.

Usual Duration of Use: Use on a regular schedule for several months is usually needed to see this drug's effectiveness in slowing AIDS progression. Long-term use (months to years) requires periodic physician evaluation.

Possible Advantages of This Drug

Does not cause serious bone marrow depression (production of blood cells).

Less frequent liver toxicity.

Less tendency for HIV to develop resistance to this drug.

▷ **This Drug Should Not Be Taken If**
- you have had an allergic reaction to it previously.
- you have active liver disease.
- you have had pancreatitis recently.

▷ **Inform Your Physician Before Taking This Drug If**
- you have had allergic reactions to any drugs in the past.
- you are taking any other drugs currently.
- you have a history of pancreatitis or peripheral neuritis.
- you have a history of gout or high blood uric acid level.
- you have a history of alcoholism.
- you have a history of diarrhea
- you have a history of phenylketonuria.
- you have a history of low blood platelets or blood disorder.
- you have a history of low blood potassium.

- you have a history of heart failure.
- you have a seizure disorder.
- you have impaired liver or kidney function.

Possible Side-Effects (natural, expected and unavoidable drug actions)
Mild decreases in red blood cell, white blood cell and platelet counts (1–5%).
Mild increases in blood uric acid levels (6%).

▷ **Possible Adverse Effects** (unusual, unexpected and infrequent reactions)
If any of the following develop, consult your physician promptly for guidance.

Mild Adverse Effects
Allergic Reactions: Skin rash and itching (25%).
Headache (36%), dizziness (8%), insomnia (25%), nervousness (3%), confusion (3%), rare visual disturbances.
Nausea, vomiting, stomach pain and diarrhea (34%), dry mouth and altered taste (16%), yeast infection of mouth (1%).
Asthma, cough.
Loss of hair (8%), muscle and joint pains (13%).

Serious Adverse Effects
Drug-induced pancreatitis (10%) usually seen in the first 6 months.
Drug-induced peripheral neuritis (see Glossary) (34%), usually occurring after 2 to 6 months of treatment.
Electrolyte imbalance (Low potassium, calcium or magnesium).
High blood sugar.
Serious skin rash (Stevens-Johnson syndrome).
Seizures (3%).
Optic neuritis and blindness (rare).
Rare liver damage.
Rare kidney damage.

▷ **Possible Effects On Sexual Function:** None reported.

▷ **Adverse Effects That May Mimic Natural Diseases or Disorders**
Drug-induced liver reaction may suggest viral hepatitis.

Possible Effects on Laboratory Tests
Complete blood cell counts: decreased red cells and white cells (3–5%); decreased platelets (1%).
Blood amylase level: increased (7–18%).
Blood uric acid level: increased (6%).
Blood Electrolytes: low calcium, potassium and magnesium.
Liver function tests: increased liver enzymes (ALT/GPT, AST/GOT and alkaline phosphatase), increased bilirubin (3–17%).

CAUTION
1. This drug does not cure HIV infection or reduce the risk of transmitting infection to others.
2. Report development of stomach pain with nausea and vomiting; this could indicate pancreatitis.
3. Report the development of pain, numbness, tingling or burning in the hands or feet; this could be peripheral neuritis. It may be necessary to stop this drug.

Precautions for Use
By Infants and Children: Safety and effectiveness for those under 6 months of age not established. Children are also at risk for developing pancreatitis and peripheral neuritis. It is recommended that detailed eye examinations be performed every 6 months and at any time that visual disturbance occurs.

By Those over 60 Years of Age: Reduced kidney function may require dosage reduction.

▷ Advisability of Use During Pregnancy
Pregnancy Category: B. See Pregnancy Code at the back of this book.
Animal studies: Rat and rabbit studies show no birth defects.
Human studies: Adequate studies of pregnant women not available.
Consult your physician for specific guidance.

Advisability of Use if Breast-Feeding
Presence of this drug in breast milk: Unknown.
Avoid drug or refrain from nursing.
Note: HIV has been found in human breast milk. Breast-feeding may result in transmission of HIV infection to the nursing infant.

Habit-Forming Potential: None.

Effects of Overdosage:
Nausea, vomiting, stomach pain, diarrhea, pain in hands and feet, irritability, confusion.

Possible Effects of Long-Term Use:
Peripheral neuritis (see Glossary).

Suggested Periodic Examinations While Taking This Drug (at physician's discretion)
Complete blood cell counts before starting treatment and weekly thereafter until tolerance is established.
Electrolytes.
Blood amylase levels, fractionated for salivary gland and pancreatic origin.
Liver and kidney function tests.

▷ While Taking This Drug, Observe the Following
Foods: High fat foods can decrease didanosine absorption and lower therapeutic benefit.
Beverages: No restrictions.
▷ *Alcohol:* No interactions expected.
Tobacco Smoking: No interactions expected.
▷ *Other Drugs*

Didanosine may *increase* the effects of
- zidovudine (Retrovir), and enhance its antiviral effect against HIV.

Didanosine may *decrease* the effects of
- dapsone, and render it ineffective; avoid concurrent use.
- ketoconazole, if taken at the same time; take ketoconazole at least 2 hours before taking didanosine.
- ciprofloxacin (Cipro), if taken at the same time; take ciprofloxacin at least 2 hours before taking didanosine.
- itraconazole. Separate dosing by at least two hours.
- tetracyclines (see Drug Class Section), if taken at the same time; take tetracyclines at least 2 hours before taking didanosine.

Didanosine *taken concurrently* with
- antacids will decrease didanosine absorption and lower its therapeutic benefit.
- histamine (H-2) blocking drugs (see Drug Class Section)—cimetidine, etc.,—may increase didanosine toxicity.
- pentamidine or sulfamethoxazole may increase the risk of drug-induced pancreatitis; watch for significant symptoms.
- triazolam (Halcion), may cause confusion.
- zalcitabine (Hivid), will cause increased neurotoxicity.

The following drug may *increase* the effects of didanosine
- ribavirin may enhance its antiviral effects.

▷ **Driving, Hazardous Activities:** This drug may cause dizziness and impaired vision. Restrict activities as necessary.

Aviation Note: The use of this drug *is a disqualification* for piloting. Consult a designated Aviation Medical Examiner.

Exposure to Sun: No restrictions.

Discontinuation: Do not stop this drug without your physician's knowledge and guidance.

DIFLUNISAL (di FLU ni sal)

Introduced: 1977 **Prescription:** USA: Yes; Canada: Yes **Available as Generic:** No **Class:** Mild analgesic, anti-inflammatory **Controlled Drug:** USA: No; Canada: No

Brand Name: Dolobid

Please see the new combined nonsteroidal (similar in composition to propionic acids) anti-inflammatory profile.

DIGITOXIN (di ji TOX in)

Introduced: 1942 **Prescription:** USA: Yes; Canada: Yes **Available as Generic:** Yes **Class:** Digitalis preparations **Controlled Drug:** USA: No; Canada: No

Brand Names: Crystodigin, ♦Digitaline

Please see the digoxin profile for further information.

DIGOXIN (di JOX in)

Introduced: 1934 **Prescription:** USA: Yes; Canada: No **Available as Generic:** Yes **Class:** Digitalis preparations **Controlled Drug:** USA: No; Canada: No

Brand Names: Lanoxicaps, Lanoxin, ♦Novodigoxin, Sk-Digoxin

Digoxin

BENEFITS versus RISKS	
Possible Benefits	**Possible Risks**
EFFECTIVE HEART STIMULANT IN CONGESTIVE HEART FAILURE	NARROW TREATMENT RANGE (treatment dose is 60% of toxic dose)
EFFECTIVE PREVENTION AND TREATMENT OF CERTAIN HEART RHYTHM DISORDERS	Frequent and sometimes serious disturbances of heart rhythm

▷ **Principal Uses**

As a Single Drug Product: Uses in current FDA approved labeling: (1) treatment of congestive heart failure; (2) restoration and maintenance of normal heart rate and rhythm in cases of atrial fibrillation, atrial flutter, PAT and atrial/supraventricular tachycardia.

Other (unlabeled) generally accepted uses: (1) post-operative arrhythmias; (2) helps to increase left ventricular function in patients with pacemakers; (3) may have a role in Wolff-Parkinson-White Syndrome.

How This Drug Works: Increases force of heart muscle contraction by increasing calcium. Slows the pacemaker and delays electrical transmission through the heart and helps restore normal rate and rhythm.

Available Dosage Forms and Strengths

Elixir, pediatric — 0.05 mg per ml
Capsules — 0.05 mg, 0.1 mg, 0.2 mg
Injection — 0.1 mg per ml and 0.25 mg per ml
Tablets — 0.125 mg, 0.25 mg, 0.5 mg

▷ **Usual Adult Dosage Range:** Rapid digitalization—1 to 1.5 mg divided into 2 or 3 doses given every 6 to 8 hours in 1 day. Slow digitalization—0.125 to 0.5 mg/day for 7 days. Maintenance—0.125 to 0.5 mg/day. Total daily dosage should not exceed 2 mg. **Note: Actual dosage and administration schedule must be determined by the physician for each patient individually.**

Conditions Requiring Dosing Adjustments

Liver function: Used with caution and blood levels should be obtained more frequently.

Kidney function: Dose **must** be adjusted in kidney compromise. Smaller doses and some cases of dosing every other day may be needed.

▷ **Dosing Instructions:** Tablet may be crushed, and best taken at the same time each day on an empty stomach. Can be taken with or following food if desired; milk and dairy products may delay absorption but do not reduce the amount of drug absorbed. The capsule should be swallowed whole.

Usual Duration of Use: Use on a regular schedule for 7 to 10 days is needed to see this drug's effectiveness in relieving heart failure or controlling heart rhythm disorders. Long-term use requires physician supervision and periodic assessment of continued need.

▷ **This Drug Should Not Be Taken If**
- you have had an allergic reaction to any dosage form of it previously.

▷ **Inform Your Physician Before Taking This Drug If**
- you have had an unfavorable reaction to a digitalis preparation.
- you have taken any digitalis preparation within the past 2 weeks.

- you now take (or have recently taken) any diuretic (urine-producing) drug.
- you have a history of severe lung disease.
- you have sustained damage to the heart muscle (myocardium).
- you have a history of low blood potassium or magnesium.
- you have impaired liver or kidney function.
- you have a history of thyroid function disorder.

Possible Side-Effects (natural, expected and unavoidable drug actions)
Slow heart rate, rare enlargement or sensitivity of the male breast.

▷ **Possible Adverse Effects** (unusual, unexpected and infrequent reactions)
If any of the following develop, consult your physician promptly for guidance.

Mild Adverse Effects
Allergic Reactions: Skin rash, hives.
Headache, drowsiness, lethargy, confusion, changes in vision: "halo" effect, blurring, spots, double vision, yellow-green vision.
Nightmares.
Loss of appetite, nausea, vomiting, diarrhea—early signs of adult toxicity.

Serious Adverse Effects
Idiosyncratic Reactions: Hallucinations, facial neuralgias, peripheral neuralgias, blindness (very rare).
Low blood platelets (rare).
Rare psychosis and hallucinations.
Serious skin rash (Stevens-Johnson syndrome).
Disorientation, most common in the elderly.
Heart rhythm disturbances.

▷ **Possible Effects on Sexual Function**
Decreased libido and impotence in 35% of male users.
Enlargement and tenderness of male breasts (gynecomastia).
Both effects are attributed to digoxin's estrogenlike action.

▷ **Adverse Effects That May Mimic Natural Diseases or Disorders**
Drug-induced mental changes may be mistaken for senile dementia or psychosis.

Possible Effects on Laboratory Tests
White blood cell counts: decreased.
Blood testosterone level: decreased 30% in men with long-term use.

CAUTION
1. Adhere strictly to prescribed dosage schedules. Do not raise or lower the dose without first consulting your doctor.
2. If you take calcium supplements, ask your physician for help. Avoid large doses.
3. Best to carry a card that says you are taking this drug.
4. Avoid taking over-the-counter antacids and cold, cough and allergy remedies without consulting your physician.

Precautions for Use
By Infants and Children: Observe carefully for indications of toxicity: slow heart rate (below 60 beats/minute), irregular heart rhythms.
By Those over 60 Years of Age: You may have reduced drug tolerance; smaller

Digoxin

doses are advisable. Watch for early toxicity: headache, dizziness, fatigue, weakness, lethargy, depression, confusion, nervousness, agitation, delusions, difficulty with reading. Promptly call your doctor if these happen.

▷ **Advisability of Use During Pregnancy**
Pregnancy Category: C. See Pregnancy Code at the back of this book.
Animal studies: No birth defects reported.
Human studies: Adequate studies of pregnant women not available. However, no birth defects from the therapeutic use of this drug have been reported.
Use this drug only if clearly needed. Overdosage can be harmful to the fetus.

Advisability of Use if Breast-Feeding
Presence of this drug in breast milk: Yes.
Monitor nursing infant closely and discontinue drug or nursing if adverse effects develop.

Habit-Forming Potential: None.

Effects of Overdosage: Loss of appetite, excessive saliva, nausea, vomiting, diarrhea, serious disturbances of heart rate and rhythm, intestinal bleeding, drowsiness, headache, confusion, delirium, hallucinations, convulsions.

Possible Effects of Long-Term Use: None reported.

Suggested Periodic Examinations While Taking This Drug (at physician's discretion)
Measurements of blood levels of digoxin, calcium, magnesium and potassium; electrocardiograms.
Time to sample blood for digoxin level: 6–8 hours after last dose, or just before next dose.
Recommended therapeutic range: 0.5–2.0 ng/ml.

▷ **While Taking This Drug, Observe the Following**
Foods: Consult physician regarding the advisability of eating high-potassium foods. The peak concentration and absorption rate will be decreased.
Beverages: Avoid excessive amounts of caffeine-containing beverages: coffee, tea, cola. May be taken with milk.
▷ *Alcohol:* No interactions expected.
Tobacco Smoking: Nicotine can cause heart muscle irritability and predispose to serious rhythm disturbances. Best to abstain from all forms of tobacco.
Marijuana Smoking: Possible accentuation of heart failure; reduced digoxin effect; possible changes in electrocardiogram, confusing interpretation.

▷ *Other Drugs*
Digoxin *taken concurrently* with
- diuretics (other than spironolactone and triamterene) can cause serious heart rhythm disturbances due to excessive loss of potassium.
- quinidine may result in decreased digoxin effectiveness and increased digoxin toxicity; careful dosage adjustments are necessary.
- propranolol or other beta blocking medicines (see Drug Class) may cause very slow heart rate.

The following drugs may *increase* the effects of digoxin
- amiodarone (Codarone).
- amphotericin B.

- benzodiazepines (Librium, Valium, etc.; see Drug Class Section).
- captopril (Capoten, Capazide).
- cyclosporine.
- diltiazem (Cardizem) and other calcium channel blockers (see Drug Class).
- disopyramide (Norpace).
- erythromycin (EES, Erythrocin, etc.), clarithromycin and azithromycin.
- ethacrynic acid.
- flecainide (Tambocor).
- hydroxychloroquine.
- ibuprofen (Advil, Medipren, Motrin, Nuprin, etc.).
- indomethacin (Indocin).
- itraconazole.
- methimazole (Tapazole).
- nifedipine (Adalat, Procardia).
- propylthiouracil (Propacil).
- quinine.
- tetracyclines (see Drug Class Section).
- tolbutamide (Orinase).
- verapamil (Isoptin).

The following drugs may *decrease* the effects of digoxin
- aluminum-containing antacids (Amphojel, Maalox, etc.).
- bleomycin (Blenoxane).
- carmustine (Bicnu).
- cholestyramine (Questran).
- colestipol (Colestid).
- cyclophosphamide (Cytoxan).
- cytarabine (Cytosar).
- doxorubicin (Adriamycin).
- methotrexate (Mexate).
- metoclopramide (Reglan).
- neomycin.
- penicillamine (Cuprimine, Depen).
- procarbazine (Matulane).
- rifampin or rifabutin.
- sulfa antibiotics or sulfasalazine.
- thyroid hormones.
- vincristine (Oncovin).

▷ *Driving, Hazardous Activities:* Usually no restrictions. However, this drug may cause drowsiness, vision changes and nausea. Restrict activities as necessary.

Aviation Note: Heart function disorders ***are a disqualification*** for piloting. Consult a designated Aviation Medical Examiner.

Exposure to Sun: No restrictions.

Occurrence of Unrelated Illness: Vomiting or diarrhea can seriously alter this drug's effectiveness. Notify your physician promptly.

Discontinuation: This drug may be continued indefinitely. Do not stop it without consulting your physician.

DILTIAZEM (dil TI a zem)

Introduced: 1977 **Prescription:** USA: Yes; Canada: Yes **Available as Generic:** No **Class:** Antianginal, antihypertensive, calcium channel blocker **Controlled Drug:** USA: No; Canada: No

Brand Names: ◆Apo-Diltiaz, Cardizem, Cardizem CD, Cardizem SR, Dilacor XR, Diltiazem, ◆Nu-Diltiaz, ◆Syn-Diltiazem

BENEFITS versus RISKS	
Possible Benefits	*Possible Risks*
EFFECTIVE PREVENTION OF BOTH MAJOR TYPES OF ANGINA	Depression, confusion
	Low blood pressure
	Heart rhythm disturbance (2%)
EFFECTIVE CONTROL OF MILD TO MODERATE HYPERTENSION	Fluid retention (2.4%)
	Liver damage (very rare)
	Rare muscle damage

▷ **Principal Uses**

As a Single Drug Product: Uses currently included in FDA approved labeling: treats (1) angina pectoris due to coronary artery spasm (Prinzmetal's variant angina) that occurs spontaneously or is associated with exertion; (2) classical angina-of-effort (due to atherosclerotic disease); (3) mild to moderate hypertension.

Other (unlabeled) generally accepted uses: (1) unstable angina; (2) congestive heart failure; (3) migraine prophylaxis; (4) prevention of abnormal protein excreation in the urine; (5) treatment of abnormal heart rhythms; (6) treatment of build up of abnormal plaques on the inside of blood vessels (atherosclerosis); (7) may help prevent abnormal growth of the left side of the heart (left ventricular hypertrophy) in patients who have suffered a heart attack; (8) can be of benefit in patients with esophageal disorders; (9) may have a role in helping ease the symptoms of an overactive thyroid gland (hyperthyroidism); (10) can ease symptoms of Raynaud's phenomena; (11) can have a role in preserving function in kidney and heart transplant patients.

How This Drug Works: By blocking normal calcium movement through certain cell walls (needed for nerve and muscle tissue), this drug slows electrical activity in the conduction system of the heart and inhibits the contraction of coronary arteries and peripheral arterioles. As a result of these combined effects, this drug

- prevents spontaneous coronary artery spasm (Prinzmetal's angina).
- reduces the rate and contraction force of the heart during exertion, lowers the oxygen needs of heart muscle; and reduces the occurrence of effort-induced angina (classical angina pectoris).
- reduces contraction of peripheral arterial walls, resulting in relaxation and consequent lowering of blood pressure. This further reduces heart work load during exertion and helps prevent angina.

Available Dosage Forms and Strengths

Tablets (immediate release) — 30 mg, 60 mg, 90 mg, 120 mg
Capsules (extended release) — 120 mg, 180 mg, 240 mg, 300 mg
Capsules (sustained release) — 60 mg, 90 mg, 120 mg

▷ **Usual Adult Dosage Range:** Initially 30 mg, 3 or 4 times daily. Dose may be increased gradually at 1 to 2 day intervals as needed and tolerated. Total daily dosage should not exceed 360 mg. **Note: Actual dosage and administration schedule must be determined by the physician for each patient individually.**

Conditions Requiring Dosing Adjustments

Liver function: Maximum daily dose in patients with liver compromise should be 90 mg. Rarely causes hepatoxicity, and a benefit to risk decision must be made.

Kidney function: May be one of the best to use in kidney compromise since it has such a large percentage of liver metabolism and fecal excretion. Caution must still be used however, as the drug can be a rare cause of kidney compromise.

▷ **Dosing Instructions:** Tablet may be crushed and is best taken before meals and at bedtime.

Usual Duration of Use: Use on a regular schedule for 2 to 4 weeks is required to see this drug's effectiveness in decreasing frequency and severity of angina and in lowering elevated blood pressure. The smallest effective dose should be used in long-term therapy (months to years).

Possible Advantages of This Drug

Often effective as single drug therapy.
Does not reduce blood supply to kidneys.
Does not raise blood cholesterol levels.
Does not induce asthma in susceptible individuals.

▷ **This Drug Should Not Be Taken If**
- you have had an allergic reaction to it previously.
- you have "sick sinus" syndrome (and do not have an artificial pacemaker).
- you have second-degree or third-degree heart block.
- you have low blood pressure—systolic pressure below 90.
- you have advanced stenosis of the aorta.

▷ **Inform Your Physician Before Taking This Drug If**
- you had an unfavorable response to any calcium blocker drug.
- you currently take any form of digitalis or a beta blocker (see Drug Class Section).
- you have a history of congestive heart failure.
- you have impaired liver or kidney function.
- you have a history of drug-induced liver damage.

Possible Side-Effects (natural, expected and unavoidable drug actions)
Fatigue (1.2%), light-headedness, heart rate and rhythm changes in some people (1.1%).

▷ **Possible Adverse Effects** (unusual, unexpected and infrequent reactions)
If any of the following develop, consult your physician promptly for guidance.

Mild Adverse Effects

Allergic Reactions: Skin rash (1.3%), hives, itching.
Headache (2.1%), drowsiness, dizziness (1.5%), nervousness, insomnia, depression, confusion, hallucinations.
Flushing, palpitations, fainting, slow heart rate, low blood pressure.
Nausea (1.9%), indigestion, heartburn, vomiting, diarrhea, constipation.

Serious Adverse Effects
   Serious disturbances of heart rate and/or rhythm, fluid retention (edema) (2.4%), congestive heart failure.
   Drug-induced myopathy or liver damage (very rare).

▷ **Possible Effects on Sexual Function:** Impotence is reported in less than 1% of users.

Possible Effects on Laboratory Tests
   Blood total cholesterol and triglyceride levels: no effects.
   Blood HDL cholesterol level: increased.
   Blood LDL and VLDL cholesterol levels: no effects.

CAUTION
1. Tell all physicians and dentists or other people who provide health care that you take this drug. Note the use of this drug on your card of personal identification.
2. You may use nitroglycerin and other nitrate drugs as needed to relieve acute angina pain. However, if your angina attacks become more frequent or intense, call your doctor promptly.

Precautions for Use
   By Infants and Children: Safety and effectiveness for those under 12 years of age not established.
   By Those over 60 Years of Age: May be more likely to have weakness, dizziness, fainting and falling. Take necessary precautions to prevent injury. Report promptly any changes in your pattern of thirst and urination.

▷ **Advisability of Use During Pregnancy**
   Pregnancy Category: C. See Pregnancy Code at the back of this book.
      Animal studies: Embryo and fetal deaths and skeletal birth defects reported in mice, rats and rabbits.
      Human studies: Adequate studies of pregnant women not available.
      Avoid this drug during the first 3 months.
      Use during the last 6 months only if clearly needed. Ask physician for help.

Advisability of Use if Breast-Feeding
   Presence of this drug in breast milk: Yes.
   Avoid drug or refrain from nursing.

Habit-Forming Potential: None.

Effects of Overdosage: Weakness, light-headedness, fainting, slow pulse, low blood pressure, shortness of breath, congestive heart failure.

Possible Effects of Long-Term Use: None reported.

Suggested Periodic Examinations While Taking This Drug (at physician's discretion)
   Evaluations of heart function, including electrocardiograms; liver and kidney function tests, with long-term use.

▷ **While Taking This Drug, Observe the Following**
   Foods: May increase absorption and cause a 30% increase in blood levels. Avoid excessive salt intake.
   Beverages: No restrictions. May be taken with milk.
▷ *Alcohol:* Use with caution. Alcohol may exaggerate the drop in blood pressure.
   Tobacco Smoking: Nicotine may reduce the effectiveness of this drug. Follow your physician's advice regarding smoking.

Marijuana Smoking: Possible reduced effectiveness of this drug; mild to moderate increase in angina; possible changes in electrocardiogram, confusing interpretation.

▷ *Other Drugs*
Diltiazem **taken concurrently** with
- aspirin can result in prolonged bleeding time or hemorrhage.
- beta blocker drugs or digitalis preparations (see Drug Classes Section) may affect heart rate and rhythm. Careful physician monitoring is necessary if these drugs are combined.
- carbamazepine (Tegretol) may result in toxicity and seizures.
- cyclosporine (Sandimmune) may result in cyclosporine toxicity and kidney failure.
- digoxin can result in digoxin toxicity.
- lithium can result in psychosis and neurotoxicity.
- phenytoin decreases phenytoin metabolism and causes phenytoin toxicity.
- rifampin may result in decreased diltiazem effectiveness.
- rifabutin may decrease diltiazem blood levels.

The following drugs may **increase** the effects of diltiazem
- cimetidine (Tagamet).
- ranitidine (Zantac).

▷ *Driving, Hazardous Activities:* Usually no restrictions. This drug may cause drowsiness or dizziness. Limit activities as necessary.

Aviation Note: Coronary artery disease **is a disqualification** for piloting. Consult a designated Aviation Medical Examiner.

Exposure to Sun: This drug may cause photosensitivity (see Glossary).

Exposure to Heat: Caution advised. Hot environments can exaggerate the blood-pressure-lowering effects of this drug. Observe for light-headedness or weakness.

Heavy Exercise or Exertion: This drug may improve ability to be more active without angina pain. Use caution and avoid excessive exercise that could impair heart function in the absence of warning pain.

Discontinuation: Do not stop this drug abruptly. Ask your doctor about gradual withdrawal.

DIPHENHYDRAMINE (di fen HI dra meen)

Introduced: 1946 **Prescription:** USA: Varies; Canada: No **Available as Generic:** Yes **Class:** Hypnotic, antihistamines **Controlled Drug:** USA: No*; Canada: No

Brand Names: Acetaminophen-PM, Allerdryl, Allergy capsules, Allergy formula, Allermax, ✦Ambenyl Expectorant [CD], Ambenyl Syrup [CD], Anacin P.M. Aspirin free, Banophen, Bayer Select, Beldin Syrup, Bena-D, Benahist, Benadryl, Benadryl 25, Benylin, ✦Benylin Decongestant [CD], ✦Benylin Pediatric Syrup, ✦Benylin Syrup w/Codeine [CD], ✦Caladryl [CD], Caldyphen lotion, Complete Allergy Medication, Compoz, Dermar-

---

*Ambenyl Syrup is C-V. See Schedules of Controlled Drugs at the back of this book.

Diphenhydramine

est, Di-Delamine, Dihydrex, Diphendryl, Diphenhist, Dormarex 2, ♦Ergodryl [CD], Excedrin P.M. [CD], Extra Strength Tylenol PM, Gecil, Genahist, Gen-D-Phen, Hydramine, ♦Insomnal, Kolex, ♦Mandrax [CD], Medi-Phedryl, Midol-PM, Nervine Nightime Sleep, Nidryl Elixir, Nighttime Cold Medicine [CD], Nite-Time, Noradryl [CD], Noradryl 25, Nytol, Pain Relief PM [CD], Pathadryl, ♦PMS-Diphenhydramine, Sinutab Maximum Strength, Sleep, Sleep-Eze 3, ♦Sleep-Eze D, Sominex, Sominex 2, Twilite, Unisom Sleepgels, Valdrene, Valu-dryl Allergy Medicine [CD], Wal-ben, Wal-dryl, Wehydryl

---

BENEFITS versus RISKS

Possible Benefits	*Possible Risks*
EFFECTIVE RELIEF OF ALLERGIC RHINITIS AND ALLERGIC SKIN DISORDERS	Marked sedation
	Atropinelike effects
EFFECTIVE, NONADDICTIVE SEDATIVE AND HYPNOTIC	Accentuation of prostatism (see Glossary)
Treatment of anaphylaxis	Rare blood cell disorders: abnormally low white blood cell and platelet counts
Prevention and relief of motion sickness	
Partial relief of symptoms of Parkinson's disease	

▷ **Principal Uses**

As a Single Drug Product: Uses currently included in FDA approved labeling: (1) Prevention or treatment of motion sickness (control of dizziness, nausea and vomiting); (2) the relief of symptoms associated with Parkinson's disease; (3) treatment of drug-induced parkinsonian reactions, especially in children or the elderly.

(4) treatment of conditions caused by histamine release (such as allergic drug reactions); (5) used as a short-term sleep aid.

Other (unlabeled) generally accepted uses: (1) cough supression; (2) eases the symptoms of the common cold; (3) can have a role in easing the discomfort of mucositis caused by radiation therapy.

As a Combination Drug Product [CD]: This drug may have a mild suppressant effect on coughing. It is combined with expectorants and codeine or dextromethorphan in some cough products.

How This Drug Works: This drug blocks the action of histamine after it has been released. Its natural side-effects are used to advantage: sedative action is used to induce drowsiness and sleep; its atropinelike action is used in motion sickness and Parkinson-related disorders.

Available Dosage Forms and Strengths

Capsules — 25 mg, 50 mg
Cream — 1%
Elixir — 12.5 mg per 5-ml teaspoonful (14% alcohol)
Spray — 1%
Syrup — 12.5 mg, 13.3 mg per 5-ml teaspoonful
Tablets — 25 mg, 50 mg

▷ **Usual Adult Dosage Range:** 25 to 50 mg/4 to 6 hours. Total daily dosage should not exceed 300 mg. **Note: Actual dosage and administration** schedule must be determined by the physician for each patient individually.

Conditions Requiring Dosing Adjustments
Liver function: Caution—single doses are not expected to be a problem, however, the use of multiple doses in patients with liver compromise has not been studied.
Kidney function: In severe kidney failure, the dose is given every 12–18 hours.

▷ **Dosing Instructions:** Tablet may be crushed and capsule may be opened, and best taken with or following food.

Usual Duration of Use: Use on a regular schedule for 2 to 3 days is needed to see effectiveness in relieving the symptoms of allergic rhinitis and dermatosis. If not effective after 5 days, this drug should stopped. As a bedtime sedative (hypnotic), use only as needed. Avoid long-term use without interruption.

▷ **This Drug Should Not Be Taken If**
- you have had an allergic reaction to any dosage form of it previously.
- you are taking, or have taken during the past 2 weeks, any monoamine oxidase (MAO) type A inhibitor drug (see Drug Class Section).
- you have chicken pox.

▷ **Inform Your Physician Before Taking This Drug If**
- you have had an unfavorable response to any antihistamine drug.
- you have narrow-angle glaucoma.
- you have peptic ulcer disease, with any degree of pyloric obstruction.
- you have prostatism (see Glossary).
- you are subject to bronchial asthma or seizures (epilepsy).
- you have dificulty urinating.
- you have G-6-PD deficiency.

Possible Side-Effects (natural, expected and unavoidable drug actions)
Drowsiness; weakness; dryness of nose, mouth and throat; constipation.

▷ **Possible Adverse Effects** (unusual, unexpected and infrequent reactions)
If any of the following develop, consult your physician promptly for guidance.
Mild Adverse Effects
Allergic Reactions: Skin rash, hives.
Headache, dizziness, inability to concentrate, nervousness, blurred or double vision, difficult urination.
Reduced tolerance for contact lenses.
Nausea, vomiting, diarrhea.
Serious Adverse Effects
Allergic Reaction: Anaphylactic reaction (see Glossary).
Idiosyncratic Reactions: Insomnia, excitement, confusion.
Hemolytic anemia (see Glossary).
Reduced white blood cell count—fever, sore throat, infections.
Blood platelet destruction (see Glossary)—abnormal bleeding or bruising.
Movement disorders (dyskinesias).
Porphyria.

Diphenhydramine

▷ **Possible Effects on Sexual Function:** Shortened menstrual cycle (early arrival of expected menstrual onset).

Natural Diseases or Disorders That May Be Activated by This Drug
Latent epilepsy, glaucoma, prostatism.

Possible Effects on Laboratory Tests
Red blood cell counts and hemoglobin: decreased.
Urine screening tests for drug abuse: *initial* test result may be falsely **positive**; *confirmatory* test result will be **negative**. (Test results depend upon amount of drug taken and testing method used.)

CAUTION
1. Stop this drug 5 days before diagnostic skin testing procedures in order to prevent false negative test results.
2. Do not use if you have active bronchial asthma, bronchitis or pneumonia.

Precautions for Use
By Infants and Children: This drug should not be used in premature or full-term newborn infants. Doses for children should be small, as the young child is especially sensitive to the effects of antihistamines on the brain and nervous system. Avoid the use of this drug in the child with chicken pox or a flulike infection—may adversely affect Reye syndrome if it develops.
By Those over 60 Years of Age: Increased risk of drowsiness, dizziness and unsteadiness, and impairment of thinking, judgment and memory. Can increase the degree of impaired urination associated with prostate enlargement (prostatism). Sedative effects may be misinterpreted as senility or emotional depression.

▷ **Advisability of Use During Pregnancy**
Pregnancy Category: B by the manufacturer and C by one researcher. See Pregnancy Code at the back of this book.
Animal studies: No birth defects reported in rats or rabbits.
Human studies: Information from studies of pregnant women indicates no significant increase in birth defects in 2948 exposures to this drug. A withdrawal syndrome of tremor and diarrhea has been reported in a 5-day-old infant whose mother used this drug (150 mg daily) during pregnancy.
Avoid drug during the last 3 months. Use sparingly during the first 6 months only if clearly needed.

Advisability of Use if Breast-Feeding
Presence of this drug in breast milk: Yes.
Avoid drug or refrain from nursing.

Habit-Forming Potential: None.

Effects of Overdosage: Marked drowsiness, confusion, incoordination, unsteadiness, muscle tremors, stupor, coma, seizures, fever, flushed face, dilated pupils, weak pulse, shallow breathing.

Possible Effects of Long-Term Use: The development of tolerance (see Glossary) and reduced effectiveness of drug.

Suggested Periodic Examinations While Taking This Drug (at physician's discretion)
Complete blood cell counts.

▷ **While Taking This Drug, Observe the Following**
Foods: No restrictions.
Beverages: No restrictions. May be taken with milk.

▷ *Alcohol:* Use extreme caution. The combination of alcohol and antihistamines can cause rapid and marked sedation.
Tobacco Smoking: No interactions expected.
Marijuana Smoking: Increased drowsiness and mouth dryness; accentuation of impaired thinking.

▷ Other Drugs
Diphenhydramine may *increase* the effects of
- amitriptyline and cause increased urinary retention.
- all drugs with a sedative effect such as benzodiazepines, tricyclic antidepressants, and narcotics (see Drug Classes), and cause oversedation.
- atropine and atropinelike drugs (see Drug Class Section).

The following drugs may *increase* the effects of diphenhydramine
- monoamine oxidase (MAO) type A inhibitor drugs (see Drug Class Section) delay elimination, exaggerating and prolonging its action.

Diphenhydramine *taken concurrently* with
- phenothiazines (see Drug Class) may result in increased difficulty urinating, intestinal obstruction or glaucoma, especially in those over 70 years old.
- temazepam in pregnancy results in increased death of the fetus.
- tricyclic antidepressants (see Drug Class) may cause increased risk of urinary retention.

▷ *Driving, Hazardous Activities:* This drug may impair mental alertness, judgment, physical coordination and reaction time. Restrict activities as necessary.
Aviation Note: The use of this drug *is a disqualification* for piloting. Consult a designated Aviation Medical Examiner.
Exposure to Sun: Caution—this drug may cause photosensitivity (see Glossary).
Exposure to Environmental Chemicals: The insecticides Aldrin, Dieldrin and Chlordane may decrease the effectiveness of this drug. Sevin may increase the sedative effects of this drug.

DIPYRIDAMOLE (di peer ID a mohl)

Introduced: 1959 **Prescription:** USA: Yes; Canada: No **Available as Generic:** USA: Yes; Canada: No **Class:** Platelet inhibitor **Controlled Drug:** USA: No; Canada: No

Brand Names: ✦Apo-Dipyridamole, ✦Asasantine [CD], ✦Novo-Diradol, Persantine, Pyridamole, SK-Dipyridamole

Dipyridamole

BENEFITS versus RISKS	
Possible Benefits	*Possible Risks*
EFFECTIVE PREVENTION OF THROMBOEMBOLISM (BLOOD CLOTS) FOLLOWING HEART VALVE SURGERY	Mild low blood pressure with dizziness and fainting (infrequent) Mild indigestion

▷ **Principal Uses**
   As a Single Drug Product: Uses currently included in FDA approved labeling: (1) Adjunctively with coumarin anticoagulants in the prevention of thromboembolism (blood clot formation and migration) following heart valve surgery; (2) intravenously as an alternative to exercise in heart imaging (thalium) and stress testing (thalium stress) in patients unable to tolerate exercise.
   Other (unlabeled) generally accepted uses: None at present.

How This Drug Works: By inhibiting the actions of certain enzymes, this drug prevents the aggregation of blood platelets (see Glossary) and thereby reduces the tendency to blood clot formation.

Available Dosage Forms and Strengths
   Tablets — 25 mg, 50 mg, 75 mg

▷ **Usual Adult Dosage Range:** 50 to 100 mg, 3 or 4 times daily. Total daily dosage should not exceed 400 mg. **Note: Actual dosage and administration schedule must be determined by the physician for each patient individually.**

Conditions Requiring Dosing Adjustments
   Liver function: Used with caution in patients with liver compromise, and in decreased dose.
   Kidney function: The kidneys are minimally involved in the elimination of this drug.

▷ **Dosing Instructions:** The tablet may be crushed and is best taken with a full glass of water on an empty stomach, 1 hour before or 2 hours after eating. However, it may be taken with or following food to reduce stomach irritation.

Usual Duration of Use: Reduction in platelet aggregation is thought to occur in 1 week. Long-term use (months to years) requires physician supervision.

▷ **This Drug Should Not Be Taken If**
   • you have had an allergic reaction to it previously.
   • you have just experienced an acute heart attack (myocardial infarction).
   • you have an allergy to tartrazine dye.
   • you have uncontrolled high blood pressure.

▷ **Inform Your Physician Before Taking This Drug If**
   • you have low blood pressure.
   • you have impaired liver function.
   • you have any type of bleeding disorder.
   • you are having angioplasty (percutaneous transluminal).

Possible Side-Effects (natural, expected and unavoidable drug actions)
   Flushing, light-headedness, weakness.

Dipyridamole

▷ **Possible Adverse Effects** (unusual, unexpected and infrequent reactions)
If any of the following develop, consult your physician promptly for guidance.
Mild Adverse Effects
Allergic Reaction: Skin rash.
Headache, dizziness, fainting.
Stomach irritation, nausea, taste disorders, diarrhea.
Serious Adverse Effects
Significant low blood pressure with large doses.
Paradoxical increase in angina on starting treatment (infrequent).
Aggravation of migraine headaches.
Bleeding from hemorrhoids.
Gallstones.
Spasm of the bronchi of the lung (bronchospsam).
Slow heart beats.
Lowered oxygen to the heart (myocardial ischemia).
May result in heart attack when used in patients with unstable angina who are given thallium stress tests.

▷ **Possible Effects on Sexual Function:** None reported.

Possible Effects on Laboratory Tests
Blood platelet counts: increased.

CAUTION
1. This drug may *increase* the frequency or severity of preexisting angina. If this response occurs, inform your physician promptly.
2. Anyone with low blood pressure should avoid large doses of this drug.

Precautions for Use
By Infants and Children: Observe closely for indications of excessively low blood pressure.
By Those over 60 Years of Age: Small starting doses (25 mg twice daily) are indicated. Avoid doses that cause excessively low blood pressure. Watch for tendency to develop hypothermia (see Glossary) in cold environments.

▷ **Advisability of Use During Pregnancy**
Pregnancy Category: B by the manufacturer, C by one researcher. See Pregnancy Code at the back of this book.
Animal studies: Mouse, rat and rabbit studies show no birth defects due to this drug.
Human studies: Few data are available, however, an early report of eight patients receiving dipyridamole plus aspirin experienced two abortions, 5 healthy babies and one child with a fifth finger on each hand that curved inward. Adequate studies of pregnant women are not available.
Use this drug only if clearly needed. If possible, avoid use during the last month of pregnancy and during labor and delivery because of possible prolongation of bleeding following delivery.

Advisability of Use if Breast-Feeding
Presence of this drug in breast milk: Yes, in small amounts.
Monitor nursing infant closely and discontinue drug or nursing if adverse effects develop.

Habit-Forming Potential: None.

Effects of Overdosage: Flushing, stomach irritation, nausea, vomiting, stomach cramps, diarrhea, rapid heart rate, low blood pressure, weakness, fainting, arrhythmia, myocardial ischemia.

Possible Effects of Long-Term Use: None reported.

Suggested Periodic Examinations While Taking This Drug (at physician's discretion)

Measurements of blood pressure in lying, sitting and standing positions.

▷ **While Taking This Drug, Observe the Following**

Foods: No restrictions.

Beverages: No restrictions. May be taken with milk.

▷ *Alcohol:* Use with caution. Alcohol may enhance the ability of this drug to lower blood pressure.

Tobacco Smoking: Nicotine can reduce the effectiveness of this drug. Follow physician's advice regarding smoking.

Marijuana Smoking: Possible reduced effectiveness of this drug; mild to moderate increase in angina; possible changes in electrocardiogram, confusing interpretation.

▷ *Other Drugs*

Dipyridamole may *increase* the effects of
- oral anticoagulants (warfarin, etc.), when doses of dipyridamole approach or exceed 400 mg/day; observe for abnormal bleeding or bruising.
- other drugs that inhibit platelet activity; observe for abnormal bleeding or bruising.

Dipyridamole *taken concurrently* with
- adenosine can result in adenosine toxicity because of reduced adenosine metabolism.
- aspirin makes it possible to reduce the dose of dipyridamole and thus lessen any side-effects that may occur.
- heparin can result in bleeding (hemorrhage).
- NSAIDs may result in water retention.
- theophylline may block dipyridamole opening of the coronary arteries and give a false negative result of thallium imaging of the heart.
- may help keep doxorubicin, etoposide and vinblastine inside cells.
- zidovudine may help zidovudine fight the HIV virus.

▷ *Driving, Hazardous Activities:* This drug may cause light-headedness or dizziness. Restrict activities as necessary.

Aviation Note: The use of this drug **may be a disqualification** for piloting. Consult a designated Aviation Medical Examiner.

Exposure to Sun: No restrictions.

Exposure to Heat: Use caution. Hot environments can cause significant drop in blood pressure.

Exposure to Cold: Use caution. This drug may increase the risk of hypothermia (see Glossary) in the elderly.

Discontinuation: Following long-term use, this drug should not be stopped abruptly. It should be withdrawn gradually over a period of 2 to 3 weeks. Ask your physician for guidance.

DISOPYRAMIDE (di so PEER a mide)

Introduced: 1969 **Prescription:** USA: Yes; Canada: Yes **Available as**
Generic: USA: Yes; Canada: No **Class:** Antiarrhythmic **Controlled**
Drug: USA: No; Canada: No
Brand Names: Napamide, Norpace, Norpace CR, Pisopyramide, ◆Rythmodan, ◆Rythmodan-LA

BENEFITS versus RISKS	
Possible Benefits	*Possible Risks*
EFFECTIVE TREATMENT OF SELECTED HEART RHYTHM DISORDERS	NARROW TREATMENT RANGE FREQUENT ADVERSE EFFECTS LOW BLOOD PRESSURE CONGESTIVE HEART FAILURE AGRANULOCYTOSIS Peripheral neuropathy Liver toxicity Heart conduction and rhythm abnormalities Frequent atropinelike side-effects

▷ **Principal Uses**
 As a Single Drug Product: Uses currently included in FDA approved labeling: (1) This drug is used to treat abnormal rhythms in the ventricles of the heart. It is classified as a Type 1 antiarrhythmic agent, similar to procainamide and quinidine in its actions.
 Other (unlabeled) generally accepted uses: (1) It is used to abolish and prevent the recurrence of premature beats arising in the atria (upper chambers) and the ventricles (lower chambers) of the heart; (2) also useful in the treatment and prevention of abnormally rapid heart rates (tachycardia) that originate in the atria or the ventricles; (3) eases arrhythmias and abnormal pressures in the heart arising from cardiomyopathy or subaortic stenosis.

How This Drug Works: By slowing the activity of the pacemaker and delaying the transmission of electrical impulses through the conduction system and muscle of the heart, this drug assists in restoring normal heart rate and rhythm.

Available Dosage Forms and Strengths
 Capsules — 100 mg, 150 mg
 Capsules, prolonged-action — 100 mg, 150 mg
  — 250 mg LA (in Canada)

▷ **Usual Adult Dosage Range:** 100 to 200 mg/6 hours. Dosage should not exceed 200 mg/6 hours or 800 mg/24 hours (1600 mg/24 hours have been used occasionally). **Note: Actual dosage and administration schedule must be determined by the physician for each patient individually.**

Conditions Requiring Dosing Adjustments
 Liver function: The dose should be decreased in patients with liver compromise by 25 to 50%.
 Kidney function: The dose **must** be adjusted in kidney compromise. In moder-

ate to severe kidney failure, the immediate release form usual dose is only given every 12–24 hours. This drug may cause urine retention and should be used with caution in patients with urinary outflow problems.

▷ **Dosing Instructions:** The regular capsules may be opened to take them, and are best taken on an empty stomach, 1 hour before or 2 hours after eating. However, it may be taken with or following food to reduce stomach irritation. The prolonged-action capsules should not be opened, chewed or crushed.

Usual Duration of Use: Use on a regular schedule for 2 to 4 days is needed to see this drug's effectiveness in correcting or preventing rhythm disorders. Long-term use requires physician supervision and periodic evaluation.

▷ **This Drug Should Not Be Taken If**
- you have had an allergic reaction to it previously.
- you have second-degree or third-degree heart block.
- you have sick sinus syndrome

▷ **Inform Your Physician Before Taking This Drug If**
- you have had unfavorable reactions to other antiarrhythmic drugs.
- you have heart disease of any kind, especially "heart block."
- you have a history of atrial fibrillation.
- you have a history of low blood potassium.
- you have a history of low blood pressure.
- you have a history of low white blood cells.
- you have impaired liver or kidney function.
- you have glaucoma, a family history of glaucoma or myasthenia gravis.
- you have an enlarged prostate gland.
- you take any form of digitalis or any diuretic drug that can cause loss of body potassium (ask your doctor).

Possible Side-Effects (natural, expected and unavoidable drug actions)
Drop in blood pressure in susceptible individuals.
Dry mouth (32%), constipation (11%), blurred vision (3–9%), impaired urination (14%).

▷ **Possible Adverse Effects** (unusual, unexpected and infrequent reactions)
If any of the following develop, consult your physician promptly for guidance.

Mild Adverse Effects
Allergic Reactions: Skin rash (1–3%), itching.
Headache, nervousness, fatigue, muscular weakness, mild aches.
Loss of appetite, indigestion, nausea, vomiting, diarrhea.
Lowered blood sugar level (hypoglycemia).

Serious Adverse Effects
Idiosyncratic Reaction: Acute psychotic behavior (rare).
Severe drop in blood pressure, fainting.
Blurred vision.
Progressive heart weakness, predisposing to congestive heart failure.
Inability to empty urinary bladder, prostatism (see Glossary).
Abnormal heart rhythms.
Peripheral neuropathy.
Low blood sugar (glucose).

Jaundice (see Glossary).
Abnormally low white blood cell count (rare).

▷ **Possible Effects on Sexual Function:** Rare impotence (300 mg/day); enlargement and tenderness of male breasts.

▷ **Adverse Effects That May Mimic Natural Diseases or Disorders**
Reversible jaundice may suggest viral hepatitis.

Natural Diseases or Disorders That May Be Activated by This Drug
Glaucoma, myasthenia gravis.

Possible Effects on Laboratory Tests
White blood cell counts: decreased.
Liver function tests: increased liver enzymes (ALT/GPT, AST/GOT and alkaline phosphatase), increased bilirubin.

CAUTION
1. Thorough heart exam (including electrocardiograms) is critical prior to using this drug.
2. Periodic heart exams are needed to follow drug responses. Some people may have heart rhythmn or function declines. Close monitoring of heart rate, rhythm and overall performance is essential.
3. Dosage must be individualized. Do not change your dosage without the knowledge and supervision of your physician.
4. Do not take any other antiarrhythmic drug while taking this drug unless directed to do so by your doctor.

Precautions for Use
By Infants and Children: Safety and effectiveness for those under 12 years of age not established. Initial use of this drug requires hospitalization and supervision by a qualified pediatrician.
By Those over 60 Years of Age: Reduced kidney function may require dose reductions. This drug can aggravate existing prostatism (see Glossary) and promote constipation. Observe carefully for light-headedness, dizziness, unsteadiness and tendency to fall.

▷ **Advisability of Use During Pregnancy**
Pregnancy Category: C. See Pregnancy Code at the back of this book.
Animal studies: No birth defects reported in rats and rabbits.
Human studies: Adequate studies of pregnant women are not available. It has been reported that this drug can cause contractions of the pregnant uterus.
Use this drug only if clearly needed. Ask your physician for guidance.

Advisability of Use if Breast-Feeding
Presence of this drug in breast milk: Yes.
Avoid drug or refrain from nursing.

Habit-Forming Potential: None.

Effects of Overdosage: Dryness of eyes, nose, mouth and throat; impaired urination; constipation; marked drop in blood pressure; abnormal heart rhythms; congestive heart failure.

Possible Effects of Long-Term Use: None reported.

Suggested Periodic Examinations While Taking This Drug (at physician's discretion)
Electrocardiograms, complete blood counts, potassium blood levels.

Disopyramide

▷ **While Taking This Drug, Observe the Following**

Foods: No restrictions. Ask physician regarding need for salt restriction and advisability of eating potassium-rich foods.

Beverages: No restrictions. May be taken with milk.

▷ *Alcohol:* Use caution. Alcohol can increase the blood-pressure-lowering effects and the blood-sugar-lowering effects of this drug.

Tobacco Smoking: Nicotine can cause irritability of the heart and reduce the effectiveness of this drug. Follow physician's advice regarding smoking.

▷ *Other Drugs*

Disopyramide may *increase* the effects of
- antihypertensive drugs, and cause excessive lowering of blood pressure.
- atropinelike drugs (see Drug Class Section).
- warfarin (Coumadin, etc.); check prothrombin times, adjust dosing.

Disopyramide may *decrease* the effects of
- ambenonium (Mytelase).
- neostigmine (Prostigmin).
- pyridostigmine (Mestinon).

Benefits of these three drugs in treating myasthenia gravis may be reduced.

Disopyramide *taken concurrently* with
- amiodarone may result in Torsades de Pointes.
- beta blockers (see Drug Class) may result in abnormally low heart rates.
- digoxin can cause digoxin toxicity.
- erythromycins (azithromycin, clarithromycin and EES) can cause increased disopyramide blood concentrations and abnormal heart effects.
- insulin or oral hypoglycemic (see Drug Class) agents may result in abnormally low blood sugars.
- phenobarbital may result in loss of disopyramide effectiveness.
- phenytoin can result in decreased disopyramide effectiveness and accumulation of a metabolite of phenytoin which causes a severe increase in anticholinergic (see Glossary) effects.
- potassium supplements may result in elevated potassium levels which can lead to disopyramide toxicity.
- quinidine can cause increases in disopyramide blood levels and decrease in quinidine levels.
- verapamil can precipitate or worsen congestive heart failure.
- warfarin may cause increased risk of bleeding. INR should be checked more frequently if these medicines are combined.

The following drugs may *decrease* the effects of disopyramide
- all diuretics that promote potassium loss.
- rifampin (Rimactane, Rifadin).
- rifabutin.

▷ *Driving, Hazardous Activities:* May cause dizziness or blurred vision. Limit activities as needed.

Aviation Note: The use of this drug *may be a disqualification* for piloting. Consult a designated Aviation Medical Examiner.

Exposure to Sun: Use caution. This drug causes photosensitization (see Glossary).

Exposure to Heat: Use caution. The use of this drug in hot environments may increase the risk of heat stroke.

Occurrence of Unrelated Illness: Vomiting, diarrhea or dehydration can affect this drug's action adversely. Report such developments promptly.

Discontinuation: This drug should not be stopped abruptly following long-term use. Ask your doctor for help regarding gradual dose reduction.

DISULFIRAM (di SULF i ram)

Introduced: 1948 **Prescription:** USA: Yes; Canada: Yes **Available as Generic:** USA: Yes; Canada: No **Class:** Antialcoholism **Controlled Drug:** USA: No; Canada: No

Brand Name: Antabuse

BENEFITS versus RISKS	
Possible Benefits	*Possible Risks*
EFFECTIVE ADJUNCT IN THE TREATMENT OF CHRONIC ALCOHOLISM	DANGEROUS REACTIONS WITH ALCOHOL INGESTION Acute psychotic reactions (uncommon) Drug-induced liver damage (rare) Drug-induced optic and/or peripheral neuritis (rare) Low blood platelets (rare)

▷ **Principal Uses**

As a Single Drug Product: Uses currently included in FDA approved labeling: (1) Deter abusive drinking of alcoholic beverages. It does not abolish the craving or impulse to drink.

Other (unlabeled) generally accepted uses: (1) limited use in helping skin problems (dermatitis) causes by nickel exposure; (2) some data increasing infection fighting cells in AIDS.

How This Drug Works: After alcohol is taken, this drug blocks normal liver enzyme activity after the conversion of alcohol to acetaldehyde. This causes excessive accumulation of acetaldehyde, and produces the disulfiram (Antabuse) reaction (see Glossary).

Available Dosage Forms and Strengths
Tablets — 250 mg, 500 mg

▷ **Usual Adult Dosage Range:** Once all signs of alcoholic intoxication are gone and no less than 12 hours after the last alcohol containing drink, treatment is started with 500 mg/day for 1 to 2 weeks. This is followed by a maintenance dose of 250 mg/day. The range of the maintenance dose is 125 mg to 500 mg/day and is individually determined. Total daily dosage should not exceed 1000 mg. **Note: Actual dosage and administration schedule must be determined by the physician for each patient individually.**

Conditions Requiring Dosing Adjustments

Liver function: This drug is a benefit to risk decision in mild liver compromise. Disulfiram is clearly contraindicated in portal hypertension and active hepatitis.

Kidney function: Dosing adjustments are not indicated.

Lung disease Accumulation of a metabolite may occur in severe lung problems. Drug levels or dose reduction will be needed.

▷ **Dosing Instructions:** The tablet may be crushed and taken with or following food to decrease stomach irritation.

Usual Duration of Use: Use on a regular schedule for several months is needed to see this drug's effectiveness in deterring alcohol use. If tolerated well, use should continue until permanent self-control and sobriety is seen.

▷ **This Drug Should Not Be Taken If**
- you have had a severe allergic reaction to disulfiram. (Note: The interaction of disulfiram and alcohol is ***not an allergic*** reaction.)
- you have taken any form of alcohol within the past 12 hours.
- you are pregnant.
- you have a history of psychosis.
- you have significant exposure to ethylene bromide where you live or work. Disulfiram inhibits the removal of this chemical and enhances the ability of ethylene bromide to cause cancer.
- you are taking (or have taken recently) metronidazole (Flagyl).
- you have coronary heart disease or a serious heart rhythm disorder.

▷ **Inform Your Physician Before Taking This Drug If**
- you have used disulfiram in the past.
- you do not intend to avoid alcohol completely while taking this drug.
- you do not understand what will happen if you drink alcohol while taking this drug.
- you are planning pregnancy in the near future.
- you have a history of diabetes, epilepsy, kidney or liver disease.
- you take oral anticoagulants, digitalis, isoniazid, paraldehyde or phenytoin (Dilantin).
- you have a history of low thyroid function (hypothyroidism).
- you have a history of lung disease.
- you plan to have surgery under general anesthesia while taking this drug.

Possible Side-Effects (natural, expected and unavoidable drug actions)
Drowsiness, lethargy during early use.
Offensive breath and body odor.

▷ **Possible Adverse Effects** (unusual, unexpected and infrequent reactions)
If any of the following develop, consult your physician promptly for guidance.
Mild Adverse Effects
Allergic Reactions: Skin rash, hives.
Headache, dizziness, restlessness, tremor.
Metallic or garliclike taste, indigestion (usually subsides in 2 weeks).
Serious Adverse Effects
Allergic Reactions: Severe skin rashes, drug-induced hepatitis (rare).
Idiosyncratic Reaction: Acute toxic effect on brain including abnormal movements and psychotic behavior.
Optic or peripheral neuritis (see Glossary).
Seizures.

Low thyroid function.
Low blood platelets (extremely rare).
Decreased or increased blood pressure.
Carpal tunnel syndrome.

▷ **Possible Effects on Sexual Function:** Decreased libido and/or impaired erection in 30% of users taking recommended doses of 125 to 500 mg/day.

▷ **Adverse Effects That May Mimic Natural Diseases or Disorders**
Liver reaction may suggest viral hepatitis.
Brain toxicity may suggest spontaneous psychosis.

Possible Effects on Laboratory Tests
Blood cholesterol level: increased.
Prothrombin time: increased (taken concurrently with warfarin).
Liver function tests: liver enzymes increased (ALT/GPT, AST/GOT and alkaline phosphatase), increased bilirubin.

CAUTION
1. Never taken by anyone who is in a state of alcoholic intoxication.
2. The patient must be fully informed about the purpose and actions of this drug *before* treatment is started.
3. Long-term use requires exam for reduced thyroid function.
4. Carry a personal identification card noting you are taking this drug.

Precautions for Use
By Infants and Children: Safety and effectiveness for those under 12 years of age not established.
By Those over 60 Years of Age: Watch for excessive sedation when the drug is started. *Do not* perform an "alcohol trial" to see the effects of this drug.

▷ **Advisability of Use During Pregnancy**
Pregnancy Category: C. See Pregnancy Code at the back of this book.
Animal studies: No defects reported in rats and hamsters.
Human studies: Two reports indicate that 4 of 8 fetuses exposed had serious birth defects. Adequate studies of pregnant women not available.
Avoid this drug completely if possible.

Advisability of Use if Breast-Feeding
Presence of this drug in breast milk: Unknown.
Avoid drug or refrain from nursing.

Habit-Forming Potential: None.

Effects of Overdosage: Marked lethargy, impaired memory, altered behavior, confusion, unsteadiness, weakness, stomach pain, nausea, vomiting, diarrhea.

Possible Effects of Long-Term Use: Decreased function of thyroid gland.

Suggested Periodic Examinations While Taking This Drug (at physician's discretion)
Visual acuity, liver function tests.

▷ **While Taking This Drug, Observe the Following**
Foods: Avoid all foods prepared with alcohol, including sauces, marinades, vinegars, desserts, etc. Ask when dining out about use of alcohol in cooking food.

Disulfiram

Beverages: Avoid all punches, fruit drinks, etc., that may contain alcohol. This drug may be taken with milk.

▷ *Alcohol:* ***Avoid completely in all forms*** while taking this drug and for 14 days following the last dose. Combination of disulfiram and alcohol—even in small amounts—produces the disulfiram (Antabuse) reaction. This starts in 5 to 10 minutes after ingesting alcohol and consists of: intense flushing, severe headache, shortness of breath, chest pains, nausea, repeated vomiting, sweating and weakness. If large amounts of alcohol are taken, the reaction may progress to blurred vision, vertigo, confusion, marked drop in blood pressure and loss of consciousness. Severe reactions may lead to convulsions and death. The reaction may last from 30 minutes to several hours, depending upon the amount of alcohol and disulfiram in the body.

Tobacco Smoking: No interactions expected.

Marijuana Smoking: Possible increase in drowsiness and lethargy.

▷ *Other Drugs*

Disulfiram may *increase* the effects of
- oral anticoagulants (warfarin, etc.), and increase the risk of bleeding; dosage adjustments may be necessary.
- barbiturates, and cause oversedation (see Drug Class Section).
- chlordiazepoxide (Librium) and diazepam (Valium), and cause oversedation.
- paraldehyde, and cause excessive depression of brain function.
- phenytoin (Dilantin), and cause toxicity; dosage must be decreased.

Disulfiram may *decrease* the effects of
- perphenazine (Tilafon, etc.).

Disulfiram *taken concurrently* with
- isoniazid (INH, etc.) may cause acute mental problems and incoordination.
- metronidazole (Flagyl) may cause acute mental and behavioral disturbances, making it necessary to stop treatment.
- OTC cough syrups, tonics, etc., containing alcohol may cause a disulfiram (Antabuse) reaction; avoid concurrent use. (See OTC Drugs in Glossary.)
- theophylline can lead to theophylline toxicity because the metabolism of theophylline is decreased.
- warfarin will result in an increased risk of bleeding.

The following drugs may *increase* the effects of disulfiram
- amitriptyline (Elavil) may enhance the disulfiram + alcohol interaction; avoid concurrent use of these drugs.

▷ *Driving, Hazardous Activities:* This drug may cause drowsiness or dizziness. Limit activities as necessary.

Aviation Note: Alcoholism ***is a disqualification*** for piloting. Consult a designated Aviation Medical Examiner.

Exposure to Sun: No restrictions.

Exposure to Environmental Chemicals: Thiram, a pesticide, and carbon disulfide, a pesticide and industrial solvent, can have additive toxic effects. Watch for toxic effects on the brain and nervous system.

Discontinuation: Drug treatment is only part of your total program. Do not stop it without the knowledge and guidance of your physician. If it must be stopped abruptly, there are no symptoms. However, no alcohol should be ingested for 14 days following discontinuation.

DORNASE ALPHA (DOOR nase AL fa)

Introduced: 1994 **Prescription:** USA: Yes; Canada: Yes **Available as Generic:** USA: No; Canada: No **Class:** Respiratory inhalant, Recombinant human deoxyribonuclease **Controlled Drug:** USA: No; Canada: No
Brand Names: Pulmozyme

BENEFITS versus RISKS	
Possible Benefits	*Possible Risks*
DECREASED MUCOUS VISCOCITY	Hoarseness
IMPROVED LUNG FUNCTION	Antibodies to DNA
DECREASED OCCURENCE OF RESPIRATORY INFECTIONS	Facial swelling (edema)
DECREASED HOSPITALIZATION	

▷ **Principal Uses**
As a Single Drug Product: Uses currently included in FDA approved labeling: (1) Management of cystic fibrosis in conjunction with standard therapies. Other (unlabeled) generally accepted uses: (1) may have a role in chronic bronchitis.

How This Drug Works: The sputum of people with cystic fibrosis contains large amounts of DNA and is much thicker than normal. Dornase breaks the DNA down, making the sputum easier to remove. Other undiscovered mechanisms may also account for its benefits.

Available Dosage Forms and Strengths
Solution — 2.5 ml ampules of 1.0 mg/ml dornase alpha (2.5 mg)

How To Store
This drug should be stored at 36–40 degrees and should be protected from light. Unused ampules should be stored in their protective pouch.

▷ **Recommended Dosage Ranges (Actual dosage and administration schedule must be determined by the physician for each patient individually.)**
Infants and Children:: Safety and efficacy for those under 5 not established.
5 to 60 Years of Age: One 2.5 mg dose administered by one of the tested nebulizers each day. Some selected patients may benefit from twice daily dosing (older patients).
Over 60 Years of Age: Same as 12 to 60 years of age.

Conditions Requiring Dosing Adjustments
Liver function: Not defined.
Kidney function: Not defined.

▷ **Dosing Instructions:** The solution must be kept in the refrigerator and protected from strong light. The drug should not be used if it is cloudy or discolored. Do **not** mix dornase with other medications. Clinical trials have only been conducted with the Hudson T Up-draft ll, Marquest Acorn ll and Pulmo-Aide compressor. The reusable PARI LC Jet nebulizer and PARI PRONEB compressor were also tested. Do **not** use with other equipment.

Usual Duration of Use: Use on a regular schedule for eight days usually determines effectiveness in cystic fibrosis. Long-term use (up to 12 months has

Dornase Alpha

been studied) requires periodic physician evaluation of response and dosage adjustment.

Possible Advantages of This Drug
Reduction in number of infections, use of antibiotics and hospitalizations with minimal side effects.

▷ **This Drug Should Not Be Taken If**
- you have had an allergic reaction to any dosage form of it previously.

▷ **Inform Your Physician Before Taking This Drug If**
- you had a rash after the last dose was taken.
- you are uncertain how to use the nebulizer or compressor.
- you are uncertain of how much dornase alpha to take or how often to take it.

Possible Side-Effects (natural, expected and unavoidable drug actions)
Hoarseness.

▷ **Possible Adverse Effects** (unusual, unexpected and infrequent reactions)
If any of the following develop, consult your physician promptly for guidance.
Mild Adverse Effects
Allergic Reactions: Rash (10–12%).
Pharyngitis (36–40%).
Laryngitis (3–4%).
Conjunctivitis (4–5%).
Facial swelling (rare).
Serious Adverse Effects
Allergic Reactions: None defined at present.
Chest pain (18–21%).
Antibodies to DNA (2–4%).

▷ **Possible Effects on Sexual Function:** None reported.

Possible Delayed Adverse Effects: None reported.

Possible Effects on Laboratory Tests
Antibodies to DNA.

CAUTION
1. This drug should only be used with one of the studied nebulizers and compressors.
2. Do not use the drug if it is cloudy or discolored.

Precautions for Use
By Infants and Children:
Safety and effectiveness for those under 5 years of age not established.
By Those over 60 Years of Age: No changes or precautions indicated.

▷ **Advisability of Use During Pregnancy**
Pregnancy Category: B. See Pregnancy Code at the back of this book.
Animal studies: Studies in rats and rabbits at up to 600 times the usual human dose have not revealed any harm to the fetus.
Human studies: Adequate studies of pregnant women are not available.
Ask your doctor for guidance.

Advisability of Use if Breast-Feeding
   Presence of this drug in breast milk: Unknown.
   Avoid drug or refrain from nursing.
Habit-Forming Potential: None.
Effects of Overdosage: Single doses of up to 180 times the usual human dose in rats and monkeys have been well tolerated.
Possible Effects of Long-Term Use: Unknown.
Suggested Periodic Examinations While Taking This Drug (at physician's discretion)
   Periodic pulmonary function tests.

▷ **While Taking This Drug, Observe the Following**
   Foods: No restrictions.
   Nutritional Support: Continued enzyme and nutritional support is still needed.
   Beverages: No specific restrictions.
▷ *Alcohol:* Follow your doctor's advice relative to alcohol use.
   Tobacco Smoking: Follow your doctor's advice regarding smoking.
▷ *Other Drugs*
   Clinical studies have revealed that dornase is compatible with medications typically used in management of cystic fibrosis. Specific adverse drug interactions are not documented at present.
▷ *Driving, Hazardous Activities:* Specific limitations because of drug effects are not defined at present.
   Aviation Note: The use of this drug **may be a disqualification** for piloting. Consult a designated Aviation Medical Examiner.
   Exposure to Sun: No restrictions.
   Discontinuation: This drug must be continued indefinitely to derive any benefit.
   Special Storage Instructions: This medicine should be stored in the refrigerator in its protective pouch.

DOXAZOSIN (dox AY zoh sin)

Introduced: 1986   **Prescription:** USA: Yes   **Available as Generic:** No   **Class:** Antihypertensive   **Controlled Drug:** USA: No
Brand Name: Cardura

BENEFITS versus RISKS	
Possible Benefits	*Possible Risks*
EFFECTIVE TREATMENT OF MILD TO MODERATE HYPERTENSION when used alone or in combination with other antihypertensive drugs	"First dose" drop in blood pressure, but without fainting (4%) Dizziness (19%) Fluid retention (4.0%) Rapid heart rate (0.3%)

▷ **Principal Uses**
   As a Single Drug Product: Uses currently included in FDA approved labeling:
      (1) A "step 1" antihypertensive drug to start treatment of mild to moderate hypertension.

Other (unlabeled) generally accepted uses: (1) used in conjunction with other drugs to treat congestive heart failure; (2) used to treat pheochromocytoma; (3) used in hypertension in diabetics; (4) useful in prostate problems (symptomatic benign prostatic hyperplasia).

How This Drug Works: By blocking certain actions of the sympathetic nervous system, this drug causes direct relaxation of blood vessel walls and lower blood pressure.

Decreases the peak pressure of the detrusor muscle, prevents alpha-1 receptor stimulation and, as such occurs, prevents smooth muscle contractions in the prostatic urethra and bladder neck and helps urine outflow.

Available Dosage Forms and Strengths
Tablets — 1 mg, 2 mg, 4 mg, 8 mg

▷ **Usual Adult Dosage Range:** Started with a "test dose" of 1 mg to check patient's response within the first 6 hours. If tolerated, dose is increased cautiously (as needed and tolerated) by doubling it every 2 weeks and taking as a single dose at bedtime. Doses in excess of 4 mg may increase the occurrence of light-headedness or dizziness, indicating low blood pressure. Total daily dosage should not exceed 16 mg. **Note: Actual dosage and administration schedule must be determined by the physician for each patient individually.**

Conditions Requiring Dosing Adjustments
Liver function: Extreme caution and lower doses **must** be used if the drug is used in patients with liver compromise.
Kidney function: Doses of 1–8 mg have been used. In one study of kidney compromise, one mg decreased the blood pressure for three days.

▷ **Dosing Instructions:** The tablet may be crushed and is best taken at bedtime to avoid orthostatic hypotension (see Glossary). May be taken without regard to food.

Usual Duration of Use: Use on a regular schedule for 6 to 8 weeks is needed to see this drug's benefit in controlling hypertension. Long-term use (months to years) requires physician supervision and evaluation.

Possible Advantages of This Drug
May be used to initiate treatment.
Effective with once-a-day dosage.
Causes depression or impotence infrequently.
Lowers blood cholesterol and sugar levels.
Does not lose effectiveness with long-term use.

▷ **This Drug Should Not Be Taken If**
- you have had an allergic reaction to this drug or to prazosin (Minipress) or terazosin (Hytrin).
- you are experiencing mental depression.
- you have active liver disease.
- you have angina (active coronary artery disease) and you are not taking a beta-blocking drug. (Consult your physician.)

▷ **Inform Your Physician Before Taking This Drug If**
- you have had orthostatic hypotension (see Glossary) when using other antihypertensive drugs.
- you have a history of mental depression.

- you have impaired circulation to the brain, or a history of stroke.
- you have coronary artery disease.
- you are taking other medicine to help lower your blood pressure.
- you have had a stroke and have high blood pressure.
- you have a history of low white blood cells.
- you have active liver disease or impaired liver function.
- you have impaired kidney function.
- you plan to have surgery under general anesthesia in the near future.

Possible Side-Effects (natural, expected and unavoidable drug actions)
Orthostatic hypotension (0.3%), drowsiness (5%), salt and water retention (4%), dry mouth (2%), nasal congestion (3%), constipation (1%).

▷ **Possible Adverse Effects** (unusual, unexpected and infrequent reactions)
If any of the following develop, consult your physician promptly for guidance.
Mild Adverse Effects
Allergic Reaction: Skin rash (1%), itching (1%)
Headache (14%), dizziness (19%), fatigue (12%), weakness (1%), nervousness (2%), numbness and tingling (1%), blurred vision (2%).
Palpitation (2%), rapid heart rate (0.3%), shortness of breath (1%).
Nausea (3%), diarrhea (2%), indigestion (1%).
Increased urination (2%).
Serious Adverse Effects
Mental depression (1%).
Low white blood cell counts.

▷ **Possible Effects on Sexual Function:** Impotence (2%).

Natural Diseases or Disorders That May Be Activated by This Drug
Latent coronary artery insufficiency.

Possible Effects on Laboratory Tests
White blood cell counts: rare occurrence of mild decrease while taking drug.
Blood lipid tests: decreased total cholesterol, LDL-cholesterol and cholesterol/HDL ratio; decreased triglycerides.
Blood sugar level: small decrease.

CAUTION
1. Watch for "first dose" response of precipitous drop in blood pressure, with or without fainting; this usually happens in the first 6 hours. Starting dose is 1 mg taken at bedtime for the first week; remain supine after taking these trial doses.
2. Impaired liver function will increase drug level and require smaller than usual doses.
3. Ask your doctor or pharmacist before you take over-the-counter remedies for allergic rhinitis or head colds; these preparations contain drugs that may interact with doxazosin.

Precautions for Use
By Infants and Children: Safety and effectiveness for those under 12 years of age not established.
By Those over 60 Years of Age: Therapy is started with no more than 1 mg/day for the first week. Subsequent increases in dose must be very gradual. Orthostatic hypotension can cause unexpected falls and injury; sit or lie

down promptly if you feel light-headed or dizzy. Report dizziness or chest pain promptly.

▷ **Advisability of Use During Pregnancy**
Pregnancy Category: B. See Pregnancy Code at the back of this book.
Animal studies: No birth defects found in rat or rabbit studies.
Human studies: Adequate studies of pregnant women not available.
Use this drug only if clearly needed. Ask your physician for guidance.

Advisability of Use if Breast-Feeding
Presence of this drug in breast milk: Unknown.
Watch nursing infant closely and discontinue drug or nursing if adverse effects develop.

Habit-Forming Potential: None.

Effects of Overdosage: Orthostatic hypotension, headache, generalized flushing, rapid heart rate, extreme weakness, irregular heart rhythm, circulatory collapse.

Possible Effects of Long-Term Use: None reported.

Suggested Periodic Examinations While Taking This Drug (at physician's discretion)
Measurements of blood pressure in lying, sitting and standing positions.
Measurements of body weight to detect fluid retention.

▷ **While Taking This Drug, Observe the Following**
Foods: No restrictions. Avoid excessive salt intake.
Beverages: No restrictions. May be taken with milk.
▷ *Alcohol:* Use with extreme caution. Alcohol can exaggerate the blood-pressure-lowering actions of this drug and cause excessive reduction.
Tobacco Smoking: Nicotine can contribute to this drug's ability to intensify coronary insufficiency. All forms of tobacco should be avoided.
▷ *Other Drugs*
The following drugs may *increase* the effects of doxazosin
• beta-adrenergic-blocking drugs (see Drug Class Section); severity and duration of the "first dose" response may be increased.
The following drugs may *decrease* the effects of doxazosin
• estrogens.
• indomethacin (Indocin) and other NSAIDs.
▷ *Driving, Hazardous Activities:* This drug may cause dizziness or drowsiness. Restrict activities as necessary.
Aviation Note: The use of this drug *is a disqualification* for piloting. Consult a designated Aviation Medical Examiner.
Exposure to Sun: No restrictions.
Exposure to Cold: Use caution. Cold environments may increase coronary insufficiency (angina) and hypothermia (see Glossary).
Heavy Exercise or Exertion: Excessive exertion can augment this drug's ability to induce angina.
Discontinuation: If you are taking this drug for congestive heart failure, do not stop it abruptly. Ask your physician for guidance.

DOXEPIN (DOX e pin)

Introduced: 1969 **Prescription:** USA: Yes; Canada: Yes **Available as Generic:** USA: Yes; Canada: No **Class:** Antidepressant **Controlled Drug:** USA: No; Canada: No

Brand Names: Adapin, Sinequan, ✦Triadapin, Zonalon

BENEFITS versus RISKS	
Possible Benefits	*Possible Risks*
EFFECTIVE RELIEF OF ENDOGENOUS DEPRESSION	ADVERSE BEHAVIORAL EFFECTS: Confusion, disorientation, hallucinations, delusions
EFFECTIVE RELIEF OF ANXIETY AND NERVOUS TENSION	CONVERSION OF DEPRESSION TO MANIA in manic-depressive disorder
Possibly beneficial in other depressive disorders	Aggravation of schizophrenia and paranoia
	Rare blood cell disorders
	Rare liver toxicity
	Low blood pressure on standing

▷ **Principal Uses**

As a Single Drug Product: Uses currently included in FDA aproved labeling: (1) To relieve the symptoms associated with spontaneous (endogenous) depression, refractory depression, neurotic depression, mixed depression anxiety and depression and anxiety in alcoholism; (2) helps treat sleep disturbances; (3) treats depression and anxiety associated with alcoholism.

Other (unlabeled) generally accepted uses: (1) Helps decrease the frequency of urination at night in cocaine addiction; (2) has a role in pain management in cancer patients; (3) can ease the extent of lowered blood glucose (postprandial hypoglycemia) which occurs after meals in some patients; (4) may help in the management of posttraumatic stress disorder; (5) helps people troubled by itching and swelling of unknown cause (idiopathic urticaria); (6) may help ease the craving which occurs when people try to stop smoking.

How This Drug Works: Relieves depression by slowly restoring to normal levels chemicals (norepinephrine and serotonin) that transmit nerve impulses.

Available Dosage Forms and Strengths
  Capsules — 10 mg, 25 mg, 50 mg, 75 mg, 100 mg, 150 mg
  Oral concentrate — 10 mg per ml
  Topical Cream — 50 mg per gram

▷ **Usual Adult Dosage Range:** Initially 25 mg 2 to 4 times daily. Dose may be increased cautiously as needed and tolerated by 10 to 25 mg daily at intervals of 1 week. Usual maintenance dose is 75 to 150 mg/24 hours. Total dose should not exceed 300 mg/24 hours. When the optimal requirement is determined, it may be taken at bedtime as one dose. **Note: Actual dosage and administration schedule must be determined by the physician for each patient individually.**

Doxepin

Conditions Requiring Dosing Adjustments
  Liver function: Doxepine has rarely caused hepatitis. This drug should be used with caution and in reduced dose in patients with liver compromise.
  Kidney function: Used with caution in patients with compromised kidneys and urine outflow problems.

▷ **Dosing Instructions:** May be taken without regard to meals. Capsule may be opened for administration.

Usual Duration of Use: Some benefit may be apparent within to 2 weeks, but adequate response may require continual use for 10 to 12 weeks or longer. Long-term use should not exceed 6 months without evaluation regarding the need for continuation of the drug. Consult your physician on a regular basis.

▷ **This Drug Should Not Be Taken If**
  • you have had an allergic reaction to it previously.
  • you are taking or have taken within the past 14 days any monoamine oxidase (MAO) type A inhibitor drug (see Drug Class Section).
  • you are recovering from a recent heart attack.
  • you have significant urine retention.
  • you have narrow-angle glaucoma.

▷ **Inform Your Physician Before Taking This Drug If**
  • you are allergic or sensitive to any other tricyclic antidepressant (see Drug Class Section).
  • you have a history of any of the following: Diabetes, epilepsy, glaucoma, heart disease, liver compromise, prostate gland enlargement or overactive thyroid function.
  • you are pregnant or are breast feeding.
  • you plan to have surgery under general anesthesia in the near future.

Possible Side-Effects (natural, expected and unavoidable drug actions)
  Drowsiness, blurred vision, dry mouth, constipation, impaired urination.

▷ **Possible Adverse Effects** (unusual, unexpected and infrequent reactions)
  If any of the following develop, consult your physician promptly for guidance.
  Mild Adverse Effects
    Allergic Reactions: Skin rash, hives, swelling of face or tongue, drug fever (see Glossary).
    Blurred vision.
    Stinging or burning of the skin with application of doxepin cream.
    Headache, dizziness, drowsiness, weakness, fainting, unsteady gait, tremors.
    Weight gain.
    Peculiar taste, irritation of tongue or mouth, nausea, indigestion.
    Fluctuation of blood sugar levels.
  Serious Adverse Effects
    Allergic Reactions: Hepatitis, with or without jaundice (see Glossary).
    Confusion, hallucinations, agitation, restlessness, delusions.
    Bone marrow depression (see Glossary)—fatigue, weakness, fever, sore throat, abnormal bleeding or bruising (reported for other drugs of this class).

Peripheral neuritis (see Glossary)—numbness, tingling, pain, loss of strength in arms and legs.
Ringing in the ears (rare).
Rare elevations in temperature.
Seizures (rare).
Rare kidney damage.
Low blood pressure on standing (3–4%).
Parkinson-like disorders (see Glossary)—usually mild and infrequent; more likely to occur in the elderly.
Abnormal heart rhythm or rate.

▷ **Possible Effects on Sexual Function:** Female breast enlargement with milk production; swelling of testicles.
Enlargement and tenderness of male breast tissue (gynecomastia).
Ejaculation disorder.
Painful and persistant erection (priapism).

▷ **Adverse Effects That May Mimic Natural Diseases or Disorders**
Liver toxicity may suggest viral hepatitis.

Natural Diseases or Disorders That May Be Activated by This Drug
Latent diabetes, epilepsy, glaucoma, impaired urination due to prostate gland enlargement (prostatism, see Glossary).

Possible Effects on Laboratory Tests
White blood cell and platelet counts: Decreased.

CAUTION
1. Dosage must be adjusted for each person individually. Report for follow-up evaluation and laboratory tests as directed by your physician.
2. It is advisable to withhold this drug if electroconvulsive therapy (ECT, "shock" treatment) is to be used to treat your depression.

Precautions for Use
By Infants and Children: Safety and effectiveness for those under 12 years of age not established.
By Those over 60 Years of Age: During the first 2 weeks of treatment, watch for development of confusion, agitation, forgetfulness, disorientation, delusions and hallucinations. Reduction of dosage or discontinuation may be necessary. Unsteadiness may predispose to falling and injury. This drug can increase the degree of impaired urination associated with prostate gland enlargement (prostatism).

▷ **Advisability of Use During Pregnancy**
Pregnancy Category: C. See Pregnancy Code at the back of this book.
Animal studies: No birth defects reported in rats, rabbits, dogs or monkeys.
Human studies: Adequate studies of pregnant women are not available.
Use this drug only if clearly needed. If possible, avoid use during the first 3 months and the last month. Ask physician for guidance.

Advisability of Use if Breast-Feeding
Presence of this drug in breast milk: Yes.
Monitor nursing infant very closely and discontinue drug or nursing if adverse effects develop.

Habit-Forming Potential: None.

Effects of Overdosage: Confusion, hallucinations, marked drowsiness, heart palpitations, dilated pupils, tremors, stupor, deep sleep, coma, convulsions.

Suggested Periodic Examinations While Taking This Drug (at physician's discretion)
Complete blood cell counts, liver function tests, serial blood pressure readings and electrocardiograms.

▷ **While Taking This Drug, Observe the Following**
Foods: No restrictions. This drug may increase the appetite and cause excessive weight gain.
Beverages: No restrictions. May be taken with milk.
▷ *Alcohol:* Avoid completely. This drug can markedly increase the intoxicating effects of alcohol and accentuate its depressant action on brain function.
Tobacco Smoking: May hasten the elimination of this drug. Higher doses may be necessary.
▷ *Other Drugs*
Doxepin may *increase* the effects of
- atropinelike drugs (see Drug Class Section).
- dicumarol, and increase the risk of bleeding; dosage adjustments may be necessary.
- phenytoin (Dilantin).
- thyroid hormones.

Doxepin may *decrease* the effects of
- clonidine (Catapres).
- guanethidine (Ismelin).

Doxepin *taken concurrently* with
- monoamine oxidase (MAO) type A inhibitor drugs may cause high fever, delirium and convulsions (see Drug Class Section).
- carbamazepine (Tegretol) may decrease the effectiveness of doxepin.
- cimetidine (Tagamet) may result in doxepin toxicity (urine retention, dry mouth).
- epinephrine will result in an exaggerated increase in blood pressure.
- fluoxetine (Prozac) can result in doxepin toxicity.
- methylphenidate (Ritalin) can result in doxepin toxicity.
- pseudoephedrine will result in abnormal increases in blood pressure and should not be combined in therapy.
- propoxyphene (Darvon) can result in doxepin toxicity.
- quinidine (Quinaglute) can result in doxepin toxicity.
- warfarin will result in prolonged action of the anticoagulant. More frequent INR testing is needed.

▷ *Driving, Hazardous Activities:* This drug may impair mental alertness, judgment, physical coordination and reaction time. Avoid hazardous activities.
Aviation Note: The use of this drug *is a disqualification* for piloting. Consult a designated Aviation Medical Examiner.
Exposure to Sun: Use caution until sensitivity to sun has been determined. This drug may cause photosensitivity (see Glossary).

Exposure to Heat: This drug can inhibit sweating and impair the body's adaptation to hot environments, increasing the risk of heat stroke. Avoid saunas.
Exposure to Cold: The elderly should use caution and avoid conditions conducive to hypothermia (see Glossary).
Discontinuation: It is advisable to discontinue this drug gradually. Abrupt withdrawal after long-term use can cause headache, malaise and nausea.

DOXYCYCLINE (dox ee SI kleen)

Introduced: 1967   **Prescription:** USA: Yes; Canada: Yes   **Available as Generic:** USA: Yes; Canada: No   **Class:** Antibiotic, tetracyclines   **Controlled Drug:** USA: No; Canada: No

Brand Names: Apo-Doxy, Apo-Doxy-Tabs, ✦Doryx, Doryx, Doxy 100, 200, Doxy Caps, Doxychel, ✦Doxycin, Doxy-Lemmon, Novopharm, Vibramycin, Vibra-Tabs, ✦Vibra-Tabs C-Pak

BENEFITS versus RISKS	
Possible Benefits	*Possible Risks*
EFFECTIVE TREATMENT OF INFECTIONS due to susceptible microorganisms	ALLERGIC REACTIONS, mild to severe
	Liver reaction with jaundice (rare)
	Kidney toxicity
	Fungal superinfections
	Drug-induced colitis
	Blood cell disorders

▷ **Principal Uses**
As a Single Drug Product: Uses currently included in FDA approved labeling: (1) Treats a broad range of infections caused by susceptible bacteria and protozoa; (2) treats and prevents "traveler's diarrhea"; (3) treat syphilis in people who are penicillin allergic; (4) helps prevent malaria in travelers. Other (unlabeled) generally accepted uses: (1) treatment of early Lyme disease; (2) treatment of sexual assault victims; (3) treatment of prostatitis.

How This Drug Works: Prevents growth and multiplication of susceptible bacteria by interfering with formation of essential proteins and causing leaky cell walls.

Available Dosage Forms and Strengths
Capsules — 50 mg, 100 mg
Capsules, coated pellets — 100 mg
Injection — 100 mg per vial and 200 mg per vial
Oral suspension — 25 mg per 5-ml teaspoonful
Syrup — 50 mg per 5-ml teaspoonful
Tablets — 50 mg, 100 mg

▷ **Usual Adult Dosage Range:** 100 mg/12 hours the first day; then 100 to 200 mg once daily or 50 to 100 mg/12 hours. Total daily dosage should not exceed 300 mg. **Note: Actual dosage and administration schedule must be determined by the physician for each patient individually.**

Doxycycline

Conditions Requiring Dosing Adjustments

Liver function: Patients with both liver and kidney compromise should have the dose decreased. This drug can cause liver problems, and a benefit to risk decision should be made in patients with liver compromise.

Kidney function: Patients with moderate to severe kidney failure should be given the usual dose, but only every 12–24 hours.

Malnutrition: Lower than expected levels may occur in patients with malnutrition. If clinical progress is not as expected, the dose may need to be increased.

▷ **Dosing Instructions:** The tablet may be crushed and the capsule opened, then best taken on an empty stomach, 1 hour before or 2 hours after eating. If stomach irritation occurs, it may be taken with food or milk. (Unlike other tetracyclines, the doxycycline absorption is not significantly changed by food or milk.) Take at same time each day, with a full glass of water or milk. Take the full course prescribed.

Usual Duration of Use: The time needed to control the infection and be free of fever and symptoms for 48 hours. This varies with the nature of the infection.

▷ **This Drug Should Not Be Taken If**
- you are allergic to any tetracycline drug (see Drug Class Section).
- you are pregnant or breast-feeding.
- you have severe liver disease.

▷ **Inform Your Physician Before Taking This Drug If**
- it is prescribed for a child under 8 years of age.
- you have a history of liver or kidney disease.
- you have systemic lupus erythematosus.
- you are taking any penicillin drug.
- you are taking any anticoagulant drug.
- you plan to have surgery under general anesthesia in the near future.

Possible Side-Effects (natural, expected and unavoidable drug actions)

Superinfections (see Glossary), often due to yeast organisms. These can occur in the mouth, intestinal tract, rectum and/or vagina, resulting in rectal and vaginal itching.

▷ **Possible Adverse Effects** (unusual, unexpected and infrequent reactions)

If any of the following develop, consult your physician promptly for guidance.

Mild Adverse Effects

Allergic Reactions: Skin rash, hives, itching of hands and feet, swelling of face or extremities.

Loss of appetite, nausea, vomiting, diarrhea.

Irritation of mouth or tongue, "black tongue," sore throat, abdominal cramping or pain.

Increased eosinophils.

Distortion of smell, perception of foul odors.

Serious Adverse Effects

Allergic Reactions: Anaphylactic reaction (see Glossary), asthma, fever, swollen joints, abnormal bleeding or bruising, jaundice (see Glossary).

Permanent discoloration and/or malformation of teeth when taken by children under 8 years of age, including unborn child and infant.

Ulceration of the esophagus.
Liver toxicity.
Kidney toxicity.
Skin reactions (erythema multiforme or Stevens-Johnson syndrome).

▷ **Possible Effects on Sexual Function:** None reported.

Natural Diseases or Disorders That May Be Activated by This Drug
Systemic lupus erythematosus.

Possible Effects on Laboratory Tests
Complete blood cell counts: decreased red cells, hemoglobin, white cells and platelets; increased eosinophils (allergic reaction).
Prothrombin time: increased.
Kidney function tests: increased blood creatinine and urea nitrogen (BUN) levels; increased urine protein (kidney damage).

CAUTION
1. Antacids and preparations containing aluminum, bismuth, iron, magnesium or zinc can prevent adequate drug absorption.
2. Troublesome and persistent diarrhea can occur. If diarrhea persists for more than 24 hours, stop this drug and call your doctor.

Precautions for Use
By Infants and Children: If possible, tetracyclines should not be given to those under 8 years old because of the risk of permanent tooth discoloration and deformity. Rarely, infants may develop increased intracranial pressure within the first 4 days of receiving this drug. Tetracyclines may inhibit normal bone growth and development.
By Those over 60 Years of Age: Natural skin changes may predispose to severe and prolonged itching reactions in the genital and anal regions.

▷ **Advisability of Use During Pregnancy**
Pregnancy Category: D. See Pregnancy Code at the back of this book.
Animal studies: Tetracycline causes limb defects in rats, rabbits and chickens.
Human studies: Information from studies of pregnant women indicates that drugs of this class can cause impaired development and discoloration of teeth and other developmental defects.
It is advisable to avoid this drug completely during entire pregnancy.

Advisability of Use if Breast-Feeding
Presence of this drug in breast milk: Yes.
Avoid drug or refrain from nursing.

Habit-Forming Potential: None.

Effects of Overdosage: Nausea, vomiting, diarrhea, acute liver damage (rare).

Possible Effects of Long-Term Use: Superinfections (see Glossary), prolongation of prothrombin time.

Suggested Periodic Examinations While Taking This Drug (at physician's discretion)
Complete blood cell counts, liver and kidney function tests.
During extended use, sputum and stool examinations may detect early superinfection due to yeast organisms.

330   Enalapril

▷ **While Taking This Drug, Observe the Following**
  Foods: Avoid meats and iron-fortified cereals and supplements for 2 hours before and after taking this drug. Avoid combination with dairy products.
  Beverages: No restrictions. May be taken with milk or carbonated beverages.
▷ *Alcohol:* Shortened half life and decreased antibiotic benefit. Best avoided if you have active liver disease.
  Tobacco Smoking: No interactions expected.
▷ *Other Drugs*
  Doxycycline may *increase* the effects of
  • oral anticoagulants such as warfarin, and make it necessary to reduce their dosage.
  • digoxin (Lanoxin), and cause digitalis toxicity.
  • lithium (Eskalith, Lithane, etc.), and increase the risk of lithium toxicity.
  Doxycycline may *decrease* the effects of
  • birth control pills (oral contraceptives), and impair their effectiveness.
  • penicillins, and impair their effectiveness in treating infections.
  The following drugs may *decrease* the effects of doxycycline
  • antacids (aluminum and magnesium preparations, sodium bicarbonate, etc.) may reduce drug absorption.
  • barbiturates (see Drug Class Section).
  • bismuth preparations (Pepto-Bismol, etc.).
  • carbamazepine (Tegretol).
  • cimetidine (Tagamet).
  • phenobarbital.
  • phenytoin (Dilantin).
  • iron and mineral preparations may reduce drug absorption.
▷ *Driving, Hazardous Activities:* Usually no restrictions. Watch for nausea or diarrhea.
  Aviation Note: The use of this drug **may be a disqualification** for piloting. Consult a designated Aviation Medical Examiner.
  Exposure to Sun: Use caution—tetracyclines can cause photosensitivity (see Glossary).

ENALAPRIL (e NAL a pril)

Introduced: 1981   **Prescription:** USA: Yes   **Available as Generic:** No   **Class:** Antihypertensive, ACE inhibitor   **Controlled Drug:** USA: No
Brand Names: ◆Vaseretic (also available in US) [CD], Vasotec

BENEFITS versus RISKS	
Possible Benefits	*Possible Risks*
EFFECTIVE CONTROL OF MILD TO SEVERE HIGH BLOOD PRESSURE	Headache (4.8%), dizziness (4.6%), fatigue (2.8%)
Possibly beneficial as adjunctive treatment in selected cases of congestive heart failure	Low blood pressure (2.3%)
	Bone marrow depression (rare)
	Allergic swelling of face, tongue or vocal cords (0.2%)
	Increased blood potassium (1%)

Enalapril

▷ **Principal Uses**
  As a Single Drug Product
    Uses currently included in FDA approved labeling: (1) treatment of all degrees of high blood pressure; (2) adjunctive treatment of symptomatic congestive heart failure.
    Other (unlabeled) generally accepted uses: (1) angina therapy; (2) captopril induced protein in the urine; (3) kidney failure in diabetics; (4) pheochromocytoma (a rare tumor which increases blood pressure).
  How This Drug Works: By blocking certain enzyme systems (angiotensin converting enzymes—ACE) that influence arterial function, this drug contributes to relaxation of arterial walls and lowers blood pressure. This reduces the workload of the heart and improves its performance.
  Available Dosage Forms and Strengths
    Tablets — 2.5 mg, 5 mg, 10 mg, 20 mg
▷ **Usual Adult Dosage Range:** For high blood pressure: Initially 5 mg once daily for weeks. Usual maintenance dose is 10 to 40 mg/day in a single dose or in 2 divided doses. Total daily dose should not exceed 40 mg if kidney function is impaired.
    For heart failure: 2.5 to 10 mg once or twice daily. Usually combined with other medications. Maximum is 40 mg daily. **Note: Actual dosage and administration schedule must be determined by the physician for each patient individually.**
  Conditions Requiring Dosing Adjustments
    Liver function: In patients with liver compromise, the dose may need to be **increased** because less of the drug is activated.
    Kidney function: Patients with mild to moderate kidney failure can be given 5 mg per day. In severe kidney failure, maximum dose is 2.5 mg per day.
    Diabetes: Patients with diabetes with decreased creatinine clearance and protein in the urine (proteinuria) should be given decreased doses.
▷ **Dosing Instructions:** Tablet may be crushed and taken on an empty stomach or with food, at same time each day.
  Usual Duration of Use: Use on a regular schedule for several weeks is needed to see this drug's effectiveness in controlling high blood pressure. Treatment of high blood pressure usually requires the long-term therapy.
▷ **This Drug Should Not Be Taken If**
  - you have had an allergic reaction to it previously.
  - you are pregnant (last 6 months).
  - you currently have a blood cell or bone marrow disorder.
  - you have active liver disease.
  - you have an abnormally high level of blood potassium.
▷ **Inform Your Physician Before Taking This Drug If**
  - you have had an allergic reaction (or other adverse effect) from any other ACE inhibitor (see Drug Class Section).
  - you are planning pregnancy.
  - you have severe liver disease.
  - you take immunosupressant medicines.
  - you have a history of kidney disease or impaired kidney function.

- you have scleroderma or systemic lupus erythematosus.
- you have any form of heart disease.
- you have renal artery stenosis.
- you have diabetes.
- you are taking other antihypertensives, diuretics, nitrates or potassium supplements.
- you have an autoimmune disease.
- you have swelling of the face or tongue. Call your doctor immediately if this occurs.
- you plan to have surgery under general anesthesia in the near future.

Possible Side-Effects (natural, expected and unavoidable drug actions)
Dizziness, light-headedness, fainting (excessive drop in blood pressure).

▷ **Possible Adverse Effects** (unusual, unexpected and infrequent reactions)
If any of the following develop, consult your physician promptly for guidance.
Mild Adverse Effects
Allergic Reactions: Skin rash, itching.
Headache, fatigue, drowsiness, nervousness, numbness and tingling, insomnia.
Rapid heart rate, palpitation.
Indigestion, taste disorders, stomach pain, nausea, vomiting, diarrhea.
Vulvovaginal itching.
Excessive sweating, muscle cramps.
Cough.
Ringing in the ears.
Baldness (rare).
Insomnia.

Serious Adverse Effects
Allergic Reactions: Swelling (angioedema) of face, tongue and/or vocal cords: Can be life threatening.
Bone marrow depression—fatigue, weakness, fever, sore throat, abnormal bleeding or bruising (very rare).
Problems with blood clotting.
Excessively low blood pressure.
Pancreatitis (rare).
Kidney toxicity.
Liver toxicity.
Laryngeal edema (rare).
Depression (rare).
Hallucinations (rare).
Elevated blood potassium.

▷ **Possible Effects on Sexual Function:** Rare report of impotence. Rare itching of the vulva and vagina.

Possible Effects on Laboratory Tests
Blood eosinophil counts: increased (allergic reaction).
Blood creatinine level: increased.
Blood potassium level: increased.
Blood uric acid level: decreased.

CAUTION
1. Consult your physician regarding the advisability of discontinuing other antihypertensive drugs (especially diuretics) for 1 week before starting this drug.
2. **Inform your physician immediately if you become pregnant.** This drug should not be taken beyond the first 3 months of pregnancy.
3. **Report promptly** any signs of infection (fever, sore throat), or water retention (weight gain, puffiness, swollen feet or ankles).
4. Do not use a salt substitute without your physician's knowledge and approval. (Many salt substitutes contain potassium.)
5. Blood counts and urine analyses are needed **before** starting this drug.

Precautions for Use
By Infants and Children: Safety and effectiveness for those in this age group not established.
By Those over 60 Years of Age: Small starting doses are advisable. Sudden or excessive lowering of blood pressure can predispose to stroke or heart attack.

▷ **Advisability of Use During Pregnancy**
Pregnancy Category: D during the last six months (second and third trimesters). See Pregnancy Code at the back of this book.
Animal studies: No birth defects found in rat or rabbit studies.
Human studies: Use of ACE inhibitor drugs during the last 6 months of pregnancy is known to possibly cause very serious injury and possible death to the fetus; skull and limb malformations, lung defects, and kidney failure have been reported in over 50 cases worldwide.
Avoid this drug completely during the last 6 months. During the first 3 months of pregnancy, ask your physician for help.

Advisability of Use if Breast-Feeding
Presence of this drug in breast milk: Yes.
Watch nursing infant closely and discontinue drug or nursing if adverse effects develop.

Habit-Forming Potential: None.

Effects of Overdosage: Excessive drop in blood pressure—light-headedness, dizziness, fainting.

Possible Effects of Long-Term Use: Gradual increase in blood potassium level.

Suggested Periodic Examinations While Taking This Drug (at physician's discretion)
Before starting drug: Complete blood cell counts; urine analysis with measurement of protein content; blood potassium level.
During use of drug: Blood cell counts; measurements of blood potassium.

▷ **While Taking This Drug, Observe the Following**
Foods: Consult physician regarding salt intake.
Nutritional Support: **Do not take** potassium supplements unless directed by your physician.
Beverages: No restrictions. May be taken with milk.
▷ *Alcohol:* Use caution until combined effect has been determined. Alcohol may enhance the blood-pressure-lowering effect of this drug.

Tobacco Smoking: No interactions expected.

▷ *Other Drugs*

Enalapril *taken concurrently* with
- allopurinol can result in serious skin reactions.
- aspirin or other NSAIDs (see Drug Class) can lessen therapeutic benefit of enalapril.
- azathioprine can cause severe impairment of blood formation (myelosuppression).
- cyclosporine can cause acute kidney failure.
- ethacrynic acid can cause excessive lowering of blood pressure.
- lithium can lead to lithium toxicity.
- loop diuretics (see Drug Class) and cause severe lowering of blood pressure upon standing up from a sitting position.
- phenothiazines (see Drug Class) can cause additive lowering of blood pressure.
- potassium preparations (K-Lyte, Slow-K, etc.) may cause increased blood levels of potassium with risk of serious heart rhythm disturbances.
- potassium-sparing diuretics: amiloride (Moduretic), spironolactone (Aldactazide), triamterene (Dyazide) may cause increased potassium with risk of serious heart rhythm disturbances.
- rifampin or rifabutin may cause decreased therapeutic benefit from enalapril.

▷ *Driving, Hazardous Activities:* Usually no restrictions. Be aware of possible drops in blood pressure with resultant dizziness or faintness.

Aviation Note: The use of this drug *may be a disqualification* for piloting. Consult a designated Aviation Medical Examiner.

Exposure to Sun: Caution advised. A similar drug of this class can cause photosensitivity.

Exposure to Heat: Caution advised. Avoid excessive perspiring with resultant loss of body water and drop in blood pressure.

Occurrence of Unrelated Illness: Promptly report any nausea, vomiting or diarrhea. Fluid and chemical imbalances must be corrected as soon as possible.

EPINEPHRINE (ep i NEF rin)

Other Name: Adrenaline

Introduced: 1900 **Prescription:** USA: Varies; Canada: No **Available as Generic:** USA: Yes; Canada: No **Class:** Antiasthmatic, antiglaucoma, decongestant **Controlled Drug:** USA: No; Canada: No

Brand Names: Adrenalin, Adrenomist, Ana-Kit, Asthmahaler, Asthmanephrine, Bronkaid Mist, ✦Bronkaid Mistometer, ✦Citanest Forte, Duranest [CD], ✦Dysne-Inhal, Epifrin, E-Pilo Preparations [CD], Epinal Ophthalmic, EpiPen, Epitrate, Glaucon, Marcaine, Medihaler-Epi Preparations, Micronephrine, Natulan, Norocaine, Octocaine, Primatene Mist, Propine Ophthalmic, Sensoricaine, Sus-Phrine, Thalfed [CD], Therex [CD], ✦Ultracaine, Vaponefrin, Xylocaine

Epinephrine

BENEFITS versus RISKS	
Possible Benefits	**Possible Risks**
EFFECTIVE RELIEF OF SEVERE ALLERGIC (ANAPHYLACTIC) REACTIONS	Significant increase in blood pressure (in sensitive individuals)
TEMPORARY RELIEF OF ACUTE BRONCHIAL ASTHMA	Idiosyncratic Reaction: pulmonary edema (fluid formation in lungs)
Reduction of internal eye pressure (treatment of glaucoma)	Heart rhythm disorders (in sensitive individuals)
Relief of allergic congestion of the nose and sinuses	

▷ **Principal Uses**

As a Single Drug Product: Uses currently included in FDA approved labeling: (1) inhalation to relieve acute attacks of bronchial asthma; (2) as a decongestant for symptomatic relief of allergic nasal congestion and as eye drops in the management of glaucoma; (3) used in treatment of anaphylactic shock; (4) used in emergency situations to treat abnormal heart rhythmns and in cardio-pulmonary resuscitation; (5) used as an aid to increase the beneficial effects of topical anesthetics.

Other (unlabeled) generally accepted uses: (1) septic shock; (2) wheezing in infants; (3) croup; (4) can have a role in easing painful erections (priapism).

How This Drug Works: By stimulating some nerve terminals (sympathetic), this drug acts to
- contract blood vessel walls and raise the blood pressure.
- inhibit release of histamine into skin and internal organs.
- dilate constricted bronchial tubes, increasing the size of the airways and improving the ability to breathe.
- decrease fluid formation in the eye, increase its outflow from the eye and reduce internal eye pressure.
- decrease the amount of blood in the nose, shrinking swelling (decongestion) and expanding the nasal airway.

Available Dosage Forms and Strengths

Aerosol — 0.2 mg, 0.27 mg, 0.3 mg per spray
Eye drops — 0.1%, 0.25%, 0.5%, 1% and 2%
Injection — 0.01 mg, 0.1 mg, 1 mg, 5 mg per ml
Nose drops — 0.1%
Solution for nebulizer — 1%, 1.25% and 2.25%

▷ **Usual Adult Dosage Range:** Aerosols: 1 inhalation, repeated in 1 to 2 minutes if needed; wait 4 hours before next inhalation. Eye drops: 1 drop/12 hours. Dosage may vary with product; follow printed instructions and label directions. **Note: Actual dosage and administration schedule must be determined by the physician for each patient individually.**

Conditions Requiring Dosing Adjustments

Liver function: Dosage reduction is not needed in liver compromise.
Kidney function: Dosage adjustment is not defined in kidney compromise.

▷ **Dosing Instructions:** Aerosols and inhalation solutions: After first inhalation, wait 1 to 2 minutes to determine if a second inhalation is necessary. If relief does not occur within 20 minutes of use, and difficult breathing persists, stop this drug and seek medical attention promptly. Avoid prolonged and excessive use. Eye drops: During instillation of drops and for 2 minutes following, press finger against the tear sac (inner corner of eye) to prevent rapid absorption of drug into body circulation.

Usual Duration of Use: According to individual needs. Long-term use requires physician supervision.

▷ **This Drug Should Not Be Taken If**
- you have had an allergic reaction to any dosage form of it previously.
- you have narrow-angle glaucoma.
- you are in shock.
- your heart is dilated and you have a coronary deficiency.
- you have experienced a recent stroke or heart attack.

▷ **Inform Your Physician Before Taking This Drug If**
- you have any degree of high blood pressure.
- you have any form of heart disease, especially coronary heart disease (with or without angina), or a heart rhythm disorder.
- you have diabetes or overactive thyroid function (hyperthyroidism).
- you have a history of stroke.
- you have a chronic lung disease
- you take: monoamine oxidase (MAO) type A inhibitors, phenothiazines (see Drug Classes Section), digitalis preparations or quinidine.

Possible Side-Effects (natural, expected and unavoidable drug actions)
In some people—restlessness, anxiety, headache, tremor, palpitation, cold hands and feet, dryness of mouth and throat (with use of aerosol).

▷ **Possible Adverse Effects** (unusual, unexpected and infrequent reactions)
If any of the following develop, consult your physician promptly for guidance.

Mild Adverse Effects
Allergic Reactions: Skin rash; eye drops may cause redness, swelling and itching of the eyelids.
Weakness, dizziness, pallor.

Serious Adverse Effects
Idiosyncratic Reaction: Sudden development of excessive fluid in the lungs (pulmonary edema).
In predisposed individuals—excessive rise in blood pressure with risk of stroke (cerebral hemorrhage).
Rapid heart rate and arrhythmias.
Seizures (rare).
Pulmonary edema.
Pigmentation of the eye.
Kidney toxicity (rare).
Porphyria (rare).

▷ **Possible Effects on Sexual Function:** May be of help in painful and abnormally prolonged erections (priapism).

Possible Effects on Laboratory Tests
Complete blood counts: red cells and white cells increased; eosinophils decreased.
Blood glucose level: increased.

Urine sugar tests: false low or negative results with Clinistix; true positive with Benedict's or Fehling's solution.

Acidosis.

CAUTION

1. Medication failure can result from frequent repeat use at short intervals. If this develops, avoid use for 12 hours, and a normal response should return.
2. Excessive use of aerosol preparations in asthmatics has been associated with sudden death.
3. This drug can cause significant irritability of the nerve pathways (conduction system) and muscles of the heart, predisposing to serious heart rhythm disorders. Consult your doctor if you have a heart disorder.
4. This drug can increase blood sugar level. If you have diabetes, test for sugar often to detect significant changes.
5. If you become unresponsive to this drug and you substitute isoproterenol (Isuprel), allow an interval of 4 hours between drugs.
6. Promptly discard this drug if a pink to red to brown or cloudiness (precipitation) occurs.

Precautions for Use

By Infants and Children: Use cautiously in small doses until tolerance is determined. Watch for any indications of weakness, light-headedness or inclination to faint.

By Those over 60 Years of Age: Small doses are indicated. Observe for: Nervousness, headache, tremor, rapid heart rate. If you have hardening of the arteries (arteriosclerosis), heart disease, high blood pressure, Parkinson's disease or prostatism (see Glossary), this drug may aggravate your disorder. Ask your doctor for help.

▷ **Advisability of Use During Pregnancy**

Pregnancy Category: C. See Pregnancy Code at the back of this book.

Animal studies: Birth defects reported in rats.

Human studies: Adequate studies of pregnant women are not available.

This drug can cause significant reduction of oxygen supply to the fetus. Use it only if clearly needed and in small, infrequent doses. Avoid during the first 3 months and during labor and delivery.

Advisability of Use if Breast-Feeding

Presence of this drug in breast milk: Yes.

Avoid drug or refrain from nursing.

Habit-Forming Potential: Tolerance to this drug can develop with frequent use (see Glossary), but dependence does not occur.

Effects of Overdosage: Nervousness, throbbing headache, dizziness, tremor, palpitation, disturbance of heart rhythm, difficult breathing, abdominal pain, vomiting of blood.

Possible Effects of Long-Term Use: "Epinephrine-fastness": loss of ability to respond to this drug's bronchodilator effect. With long-term treatment of glaucoma: Pigment deposits on eyeball and eyelids, possible damage to retina, impaired vision, blockage of tear ducts.

Suggested Periodic Examinations While Taking This Drug (at physician's discretion)

Blood pressure measurements; blood or urine sugar measurements in diabetics; vision testing and measurement of internal eye pressure in glaucoma.

▷ **While Taking This Drug, Observe the Following**
Foods: No restrictions, except those that cause you to have asthma.
Beverages: No restrictions.
▷ *Alcohol:* Alcoholic beverages can increase the urinary excretion of this drug.
Tobacco Smoking: No interactions expected. Follow physician's advice regarding smoking as it affects the condition under treatment.
▷ *Other Drugs*
Epinephrine *taken concurrently* with
- some beta blockers (carteolol, nadolol, propranolol) may cause increased blood pressure and decreased heart rate.
- chlorpromazine (Thorazine) or other phenothiazines (see Drug Class) may cause decreased blood pressure and increased heart rate.
- furazolidone (Furoxone) may cause increased blood pressure.
- guanethidine (Esimil, Ismelin) may cause increased blood pressure.
- halothane may cause abnormal heartbeats.
- pilocarpine (Ocusert) may cause increased myopia.
- tricyclic antidepressants (amitriptyline, etc.) may cause increased blood pressure and heart rhythm disturbances.
▷ *Driving, Hazardous Activities:* This drug may cause dizziness or nervousness. Limit activities as necessary.
Aviation Note: The use of this drug **may be a disqualification** for piloting. Consult a designated Aviation Medical Examiner.
Exposure to Sun: No restrictions.
Heavy Exercise or Exertion: No interactions expected. However, exercise can induce asthma in sensitive individuals.
Occurrence of Unrelated Illness: Use caution in presence of severe burns. This drug can increase drainage from burned tissue and cause significant loss of tissue fluids and blood proteins.
Discontinuation: If this drug fails to provide relief after an adequate trial, stop it and call your doctor. It is dangerous to increase the dosage or frequency.
Special Storage Instructions: Protect drug from exposure to air, light and heat. Keep in a cool place, preferably in the refrigerator.

ERGOTAMINE (er GOT a meen)

Introduced: 1926 **Prescription:** USA: Yes; Canada: Yes **Available as Generic:** No **Class:** Antimigraine, ergot preparations **Controlled Drug:** USA: No; Canada: No

Brand Names: ✦Bellergal [CD], Bellergal-S [CD], ✦Bellergal Spacetabs [CD], Cafergot [CD], Cafergot P-B [CD], Cafetrate [CD], Ercaf [CD], ✦Ergodryl [CD], Ergomar, Ergostat, Genergen, ✦Gravergol [CD], ✦Gynergen, Medihaler Ergotamine, ✦Megral [CD], Spastrin [CD], Wigraine [CD], Wigrettes

Ergotamine

BENEFITS versus RISKS	
Possible Benefits	*Possible Risks*
PREVENTION AND RELIEF OF VASCULAR HEADACHES: MIGRAINE, MIGRAINELIKE AND HISTAMINE HEADACHES	GANGRENE OF THE FINGERS, TOES OR INTESTINE AGGRAVATION OF CORONARY ARTERY DISEASE (ANGINA) ABORTION

▷ **Principal Uses**

As a Single Drug Product: Uses currently included in FDA approved labeling: (1) This drug is used primarily in the treatment of vascular headaches, especially migraine and "cluster" headaches. It is often effective in terminating the headache if taken within the first hour following the onset of pain. It may be used on a short-term basis in an attempt to prevent or abort "cluster" headaches during the period of their occurrence. The inhalation form provides rapid onset of action.

Other (unlabeled) generally accepted uses: (1) Helps to ease the symptoms of narcolepsy; (2) may have a role in patients who have a C5 quadriplegia in helping to treat excessive lowering of blood pressure which occurs on rising from a sitting position.

As a Combination Drug Product [CD]: This drug is combined with caffeine to take advantage of caffeine's ability to enhance its absorption. This makes a smaller dose of ergotamine effective, and reduces the risk of adverse effects with repeated use. This drug is also combined with belladonna (atropine) and one of the barbiturates to provide preparations that help premenstrual tension and the menopausal syndrome: nervousness, nausea, hot flushes and sweating.

How This Drug Works: By constricting the walls of blood vessels in the head, this drug prevents or relieves the excessive expansion (dilation) that causes the pain of migrainelike headaches.

Available Dosage Forms and Strengths
Aerosol — 9 mg per ml (0.36 mg/inhalation)
Suppositories — 2 mg (in combination with caffeine)
Tablets, sublingual — 2 mg

▷ **Usual Adult Dosage Range:** Inhalation: 1 spray (0.36 mg) at the onset of headache; repeat 1 spray every 5 to 10 minutes as needed for relief, up to a maximum of 6 sprays/24 hours. Do not exceed 15 sprays/week. Sublingual tablets: Dissolve 1 mg under tongue at the onset of headache; repeat 1 mg every 30 to 60 minutes as needed, up to a maximum of 5 mg/attack. Do not exceed 5 mg/24 hours or 10 mg/week. Try to determine the optimal dose required (up to 5 mg) that will abort the headache when taken as a single dose at the onset of pain. **Note: Actual dosage and administration schedule must be determined by the physician for each patient individually.**

Conditions Requiring Dosing Adjustments
Liver function: Should be used with caution in patients with liver compromise.
Kidney function: This drug is a rare cause of acute renal failure, and should be used with caution in patients with compromised kidneys.

Ergotamine

▷ **Dosing Instructions:** Follow written instructions and doses carefully. The regular tablets (combination drug) may be crushed for administration; the sustained-release tablets should be taken whole (not crushed). Sublingual tablets should be dissolved under the tongue, not swallowed.

Usual Duration of Use: Use on a regular schedule for several episodes of headache is often needed to see this drug's effectiveness in aborting or relieving the pain of vascular headache. Do not exceed recommended dosage schedules. If headaches are not controlled after several trials of maximal doses, ask your doctor about other treatments.

▷ **This Drug Should Not Be Taken If**
- you have had an allergic reaction to any dosage form.
- you are pregnant.
- you have a severe infection.
- you have any of the following conditions:
    angina pectoris (coronary artery disease)
    Buerger's disease
    hardening of the arteries (arteriosclerosis)
    high blood pressure (severe hypertension)
    thrombophelbitis
    ischemic heart disease
    peptic ulcer
    kidney disease or impaired kidney function
    liver disease or impaired liver function
    Raynaud's phenomenon
    thrombophlebitis
    severe itching

▷ **Inform Your Physician Before Taking This Drug If**
- you are allergic or overly sensitive to *any* ergot preparation.
- you are planning to have a face lift (rhytidectomy). This drug may cause serious skin flap plroblems.

Possible Side-Effects (natural, expected and unavoidable drug actions)
Usually infrequent and mild with recommended doses.
Some people may have cold hands and feet, with mild numbness and tingling.

▷ **Possible Adverse Effects** (unusual, unexpected and infrequent reactions)
If any of the following develop, consult your physician promptly for guidance.

Mild Adverse Effects
Allergic Reactions: Localized swellings (angioedema), itching.
Headache, drowsiness, dizziness, confusion.
Chest pain, numbness and tingling of fingers and toes, muscle pains in arms or legs.
Nausea, vomiting, diarrhea.

Serious Adverse Effects
Gangrene of the extremities—coldness; numbness; pain; dark discoloration; eventual loss of fingers, toes or feet.
Gangrene of the intestine—severe abdominal pain and swelling; emergency surgery required.
Retroperitoneal fibrosis.

Fibrous changes in the lung (pleuropulmonary fibrosis).
Pain syndromes (reflex sympathetic dystrophy).
Insufficient blood flow to the heart (myocardial ischemia).
Arrhythmias.
Fibrous changes in the heart (myocardial fibrosis).
Porphyria.
Lesions of the rectum or anus (anorectal lesions).
Kidney failure.

▷ **Possible Effects on Sexual Function:** None reported.

Natural Diseases or Disorders That May Be Activated by This Drug
Angina pectoris (coronary artery insufficiency), Buerger's disease, Raynaud's syndrome.

Possible Effects on Laboratory Tests
None reported.

CAUTION
1. Excessive use of this drug can provoke migraine headache and increase the frequency of its occurrence.
2. Do not exceed a total dose of 5 mg/24 hours or 10 mg/week.
3. Individual drug sensitivity varies greatly. Some may have early toxic effects while taking recommended doses. Promptly report: Numbness in fingers or toes, muscle cramping, chest pain.

Precautions for Use
By Infants and Children: Safety and effectiveness for those under 12 years of age not established.
By Those over 60 Years of Age: Natural circulation changes may make you more susceptible to adverse effects of this drug. See the preceding list of disorders that are contraindications for the use of this drug.

▷ **Advisability of Use During Pregnancy**
Pregnancy Category: X. See Pregnancy Code at the back of this book.
Animal studies: Fetal deaths reported due to this drug.
Human studies: Information from studies of pregnant women indicates that this drug can cause abortion.
This drug should be avoided during the entire pregnancy.

Advisability of Use if Breast-Feeding
Presence of this drug in breast milk: Yes.
Avoid drug or refrain from nursing.

Habit-Forming Potential: None.

Effects of Overdosage: Manifestations of "ergotism": coldness of skin, severe muscle pains, tingling and burning pain in hands and feet, loss of blood supply to extremities resulting in tissue death (gangrene) in fingers and toes. Acute ergot poisoning: nausea, vomiting, diarrhea, cold skin, numbness of extremities, confusion, seizures, coma.

Possible Effects of Long-Term Use: A form of functional dependence (see Glossary) may develop, resulting in withdrawal headaches when the drug is discontinued.

Suggested Periodic Examinations While Taking This Drug (at physician's discretion)
  Evaluation of circulation (blood flow) to the extremities.

▷ **While Taking This Drug, Observe the Following**
  Foods: No interactions expected. Avoid all foods to which you are allergic; some migraine headaches are due to food allergies.
  Beverages: No restrictions.
▷ *Alcohol:* Best avoided; alcohol can intensify vascular headache.
  Tobacco Smoking: Best avoided; nicotine can further reduce the restricted blood flow produced by this drug.
  Marijuana Smoking: Best avoided; additive effects can increase the coldness of hands and feet.
▷ *Other Drugs*
  Ergotamine may *decrease* the effects of
  • nitroglycerin, and reduce its effectiveness in preventing or relieving angina pain.
  The following drugs may *increase* the effects of ergotamine
  • beta blockers (see Drug Class).
  • erythromycins: Clarithromycin, azithromycin, E-Mycin, Eryc, etc.
  • sumatriptan (Imitrex) can also result in extended vasospastic reactions.
  • troleandomycin (TAO).
▷ *Driving, Hazardous Activities:* This drug may cause drowsiness or dizziness. Restrict activities as necessary.
  Aviation Note: Vascular headache *is a disqualification* for piloting. Consult a designated Aviation Medical Examiner.
  Exposure to Sun: No restrictions.
  Exposure to Cold: Avoid as much as possible. Cold further reduces restricted blood flow to the extremities.
  Discontinuation: Following long-term use, it may be necessary to withdraw this drug gradually to prevent withdrawal headache. Ask physician for guidance.

ERYTHROMYCIN (er ith roh MY sin)

Introduced: 1952   **Prescription:** USA: Yes; Canada: Yes   **Available as Generic:** Yes   **Class:** Antibiotic, erythromycins   **Controlled Drug:** USA: No; Canada: No

Brand Names: AK-Mycin Ophthalmic, Akne-Mycin, ✦Apo-Erythro Base, ✦Apo-Erythro E-C, ✦Apo-Erythro-ES, ✦Apo-Erythro-S, A/T/S, Benzamycin [CD], C-Solve 2, EES, Emgel, E-Mycin, E-Mycin E, E-Mycin 333, Eramycin, ✦Erybid, Eryc, Erycette, Eryderm, Erygel, Erymax, Erypar, EryPed, Ery-Tab, Erythrocin, ✦Erythromid, E-Solve 2, ETS-2%, Ilosone, Ilotycin, ✦Novorythro, PCE, Pediamycin, ✦Pediazole [CD], ✦PMS-Erythromycin, Robimycin, Sans-Acne, SK-Erythromycin, Staticin, ✦Stievamycin, T-Stat, Wyamycin E, Wyamycin S

Erythromycin

BENEFITS versus RISKS	
Possible Benefits	*Possible Risks*
EFFECTIVE TREATMENT OF INFECTIONS DUE TO SUSCEPTIBLE MICROORGANISMS	Allergic reactions, mild and infrequent Liver reaction (most common with erythromycin estolate) Drug-induced colitis (rare) Superinfections (rare)

▷ **Principal Uses**

As a Single Drug Product: Uses currently included in FDA approved labeling: Treatment of (1) skin and skin structure infections; (2) upper and lower respiratory tract infections, including "strep" throat, diphtheria and several types of pneumonia; (3) gonorrhea and syphilis; (4) amebic dysentery; (5) Legionnaire's disease and (5) long-term prevention of recurrences of rheumatic fever. Effective use requires the precise identification of the causative organism and determination of its sensitivity to erythromycin; (6) treatment of mycoplasma pneumonia; (7) listeriosis; (8) neonatal conjunctivitis; (9) pertussis; (10) urethritis.

Other (unlabeled) generally accepted uses: (1) Treatment of early Lyme disease; (2) treatment of Campylobacter jejuni infections; (3) used in chancroid; (4) helps sterilize the bowel before surgical procedures; (5) may help threatened preterm labor if the cause is ureaplasma organisms; (6) helps impetigo; (7) may have a role in Ogilvie's syndrome in restoring normal bowel function.

How This Drug Works: This drug prevents the growth and multiplication of susceptible organisms by interfering with their formation of essential proteins.

Available Dosage Forms and Strengths

Capsules — 125 mg, 250 mg
Capsules, enteric-coated — 125 mg, 250 mg
Drops — 100 mg per ml
Eye ointment — 5 mg per gram
Gel — 2%
Oral suspension — 125 mg, 250 mg per 5-ml teaspoonful
Skin ointment — 2%
Tablets — 250 mg, 500 mg
Tablets, chewable — 125 mg, 200 mg, 250 mg
Tablets, enteric-coated — 250 mg, 333 mg, 500 mg
Tablets, film-coated — 250 mg, 500 mg
Topical solution — 1.5% and 2%

▷ **Usual Adult Dosage Range:** 250 to 1000 mg/6 hours, according to nature and severity of infection. Total daily dosage should not exceed 8 grams. For endocarditis prophylaxis: 1 gram 2 hours before procedure and 500 mg 6 hours later.

Pediatrics: oral erythromycin is usually given at a dose of 30 to 50 mg per kilogram per day and is divided into three or four doses. **Note: Actual dosage and administration schedule must be determined by the physician for each patient individually.**

Erythromycin

Conditions Requiring Dosing Adjustments
Liver function: This drug is metabolized in the liver, and will accumulate in patients with liver compromise. Decreased doses may be needed. It should be used with caution in patients with biliary tract disease.

Kidney function: Patients with severe kidney failure can be given 50–75% of the usual dose at the usual time. It is a rare cause of interstitial nephritis (inflammation of a specific part of the kidney).

▷ **Dosing Instructions:** Nonenteric-coated preparations should be taken 1 hour before or 2 hours after eating. Enteric-coated preparations may be taken without regard to food. Regular uncoated capsules may be opened and tablets may be crushed for administration; coated and prolonged-action preparations should be swallowed whole. Ask pharmacist for guidance.

Usual Duration of Use: Use on a regular schedule for 3 to 5 days is necessary to determine this drug's effectiveness in controlling infections. For streptococcal infections: Not less than 10 consecutive days (without interruption) to reduce the possibility of developing rheumatic fever or glomerulonephritis. The duration of use should not exceed the time required to eliminate the infection.

▷ **This Drug Should Not Be Taken If**
- you have had an allergic reaction to any form of erythromycin previously.
- you have active liver disease.
- you are taking terfenadine or astemizole.

▷ **Inform Your Physician Before Taking This Drug If**
- you have a history of a previous "reaction" to erythromycin.
- you are allergic by nature: Hay fever, asthma, hives, eczema.
- you have a blood disorder.
- you have an abnormal heart rhythm.
- you have a history of porphyria.
- you have a history of kidney disorder.
- you have myasthenia gravis.
- you have a hearing disorder.
- you have taken the estolate form of erythromycin previously.

Possible Side-Effects (natural, expected and unavoidable drug actions)
Superinfections (see Glossary).

▷ **Possible Adverse Effects** (unusual, unexpected and infrequent reactions)
If any of the following develop, consult your physician promptly for guidance.

Mild Adverse Effects
Allergic Reactions: Skin rash, hives, itching.
Nausea, vomiting, diarrhea, abdominal cramping.

Serious Adverse Effects
Allergic Reaction: Rare anaphylactic reaction (see Glossary).
Idiosyncratic Reactions: Liver reaction—nausea, vomiting, fever, jaundice (usually but not exclusively associated with erythromycin estolate).
Decreased white blood cells (rare).
Abnormal heart rhythm (rare).
Worsening of myasthenia gravis.
Low body temperature (hypothermia)(rare).
Pseudomembranous colitis (rare).
Pancreatitis (rare).

Kidney problems (interstitial nephritis).
Hearing loss (ototoxicity).

▷ **Possible Effects on Sexual Function:** None reported.

▷ **Adverse Effects That May Mimic Natural Diseases or Disorders**
Liver toxicity may resemble acute gallbladder disease or viral hepatitis.

Possible Effects on Laboratory Tests
Complete blood cell counts: white cells may increase or decrease; eosinophils increased (allergic reaction); platelets decreased.
Prothrombin time: increased (drug taken concurrently with warfarin).
Liver function tests: liver enzymes increased (ALT/GPT, AST/GOT and alkaline phosphatase), increased bilirubin.

CAUTION
1. Take the full dosage prescribed to help prevent resistant bacteria.
2. If you have a history of liver disease or impaired liver function, avoid any form of erythromycin estolate.
3. If diarrhea develops and continues for more than 24 hours, consult your physician promptly.

Precautions for Use
By Infants and Children: Watch allergic children closely for indications of developing allergy to this drug. Observe also for evidence of gastrointestinal irritation.
By Those over 60 Years of Age: Watch for itching reactions in the genital and anal regions, often due to yeast superinfections. Observe also for evidence of hearing loss. Report such developments promptly.

▷ **Advisability of Use During Pregnancy**
Pregnancy Category: B. See Pregnancy Code at the back of this book.
Animal studies: Studies of rats are inconclusive.
Human studies: No increase in birth defects reported in 230 exposures. Information from adequate studies of pregnant women is not available.
Generally thought to be safe during entire pregnancy, *except for erythromycin estolate*; this form of erythromycin can cause toxic liver reactions during pregnancy and should be avoided.

Advisability of Use if Breast-Feeding
Presence of this drug in breast milk: Yes.
Watch nursing infant closely and discontinue drug or nursing if adverse effects develop.

Habit-Forming Potential: None.

Effects of Overdosage: Possible nausea, vomiting, diarrhea and abdominal discomfort.

Possible Effects of Long-Term Use: Superinfections (see Glossary).

Suggested Periodic Examinations While Taking This Drug (at physician's discretion)
Liver function tests if the estolate form is used.

▷ **While Taking This Drug, Observe the Following**
Foods: New formulation absorption is decreased by more than 70% (especially high fat meals) and effectiveness may be seriously compromised.
Beverages: Avoid fruit juices and carbonated beverages for 1 hour after taking any nonenteric-coated preparation. May be taken with milk.

▷ *Alcohol:* Avoid if you have impaired liver function or are taking the estolate form.
Tobacco Smoking: No interactions expected.
▷ *Other Drugs*
Erythromycin may *increase* the effects of
- carbamazepine (Tegretol), and cause toxicity.
- digoxin (Lanoxin), and cause toxicity.
- ergotamine (Cafergot, Ergostat, etc.), and cause impaired circulation to extremities.
- methylprednisolone (Medrol), and cause excess steroid effects.
- theophylline (aminophylline, Theo-Dur, etc.), and cause toxicity.
- warfarin (Coumadin), and increase the risk of bleeding.

Erythromycin may *decrease* the effects of
- clindamycin.
- lincomycin.
- penicillins.

Erythromycin *taken concurrently* with
- astemizole may cause serious arrhythmias.
- birth control pills (oral contraceptives) can cause loss of effectiveness and result in pregnancy.
- disopyramide may cause heart (cardiac) arrhythmias.
- lovastatin can cause rhabdomyolysis.
- midazolam may lead to excessive central nervous system depression.
- terfenadine can cause cardiac (heart) arrhythmias.
- triazolam may cause toxicity.
- trimexate decreases trimexate metabolism and leads to toxicity.
- valproic acid can lead to toxic blood levels.

▷ *Driving, Hazardous Activities:* This drug may cause nausea and/or diarrhea. Restrict activities as necessary.
Aviation Note: The use of this drug *may be a disqualification* for piloting. Consult a designated Aviation Medical Examiner.
Exposure to Sun: No restrictions.
Special Storage Instructions: Keep liquid forms refrigerated.
Observe the Following Expiration Times: Freshly mixed oral suspension—14 days. Premixed oral suspension—18 months. Ask pharmacist for help.

ESTROGENS (ES troh jenz)

Other Names: Chlorotrianisene, conjugated estrogens, esterified estrogens, estradiol, estriol, estrone, estropipate, quinestrol

Introduced: 1933 **Prescription:** USA: Yes; Canada: Yes **Available as Generic:** USA: Yes; Canada: No **Class:** Female sex hormones **Controlled Drug:** USA: No; Canada: No

Brand Names: ✦C.E.S., ✦Climestrone, ✦Congest, Delestrogen, DV, Estinyl, Estrace, Estraderm, Estraguard, Estratab, Estrovis, Feminone, ✦Femogen, ✦Femogex, Gynetone, Gynogen LA, Menest, Menrium [CD], Milprem [CD], ✦Minestrin, ✦Neo-Pause, ✦Oestrilin, Ogen, PMB [CD], PMS-Estradiol, Premarin, Progynon Pellet, TACE, Valergen-10, White Premarin

BENEFITS versus RISKS	
Possible Benefits	*Possible Risks*
EFFECTIVE RELIEF OF MENOPAUSAL HOT FLUSHES AND NIGHT SWEATS	INCREASED RISK OF CANCER OF THE UTERUS with 3syears of continual use
PREVENTION OR RELIEF OF ATROPHIC VAGINITIS, ATROPHY OF THE VULVA AND URETHRA	INCREASED RISK OF BREAST CANCER (EVEN IF COMBINED WITH A PROGESTERONE)
PREVENTION OF OSTEOPOROSIS	Increased frequency of gallstones
Prevention of thinning of the skin	Accelerated growth of preexisting fibroid tumors of the uterus
Mental tonic effect	Fluid retention
Prevention of postmenopausal cardiovascular disease	Postmenopausal bleeding
	Deep vein thrombophlebitis and thromboembolism (less likely with conjugated estrogens, more likely with synthetic unconjugated hormones)
	Increased blood pressure (rare)
	Decreased sugar tolerance (rare)

▷ **Principal Uses**

As a Single Drug Product: This widely used hormone is very effective when administered in proper dosage and carefully supervised. Its primary use is supplemental ("replacement" therapy) when used to treat the following conditions: (1) ovarian failure or removal in the young woman; (2) the menopausal syndrome; (3) postmenopausal atrophy of genital tissues; and (4) postmenopausal osteoporosis. It is also used in selected cases of breast cancer and prostate cancer.

As a Combination Drug Product [CD]: Estrogen is available in combination with chlordiazepoxide (Librium) and with meprobamate (Equanil, Miltown). These mild tranquilizers are added to provide a calming effect that makes the combination more effective in treating selected cases of the menopausal syndrome. See the Drug Profile of the Oral Contraceptives for a discussion of the combination of estrogens and progestins.

How This Drug Works: When used to correct hormonal deficiency states, estrogens restore normal cellular activity by increasing nuclear material and protein synthesis. The frequency and intensity of menopausal symptoms are reduced when normal tissue levels of estrogen are restored.

Available Dosage Forms and Strengths
   Capsules — 12 mg, 25 mg, 72 mg (TACE)
   Tablets — 0.02 mg, 0.05 mg, 0.1 mg, 0.3 mg, 0.5 mg, 0.625 mg, 0.9 mg, 1.25 mg, 2.5 mg, 5 mg
   Transdermal patch — 0.05 mg (4 mg) and 0.1 mg (8 mg)
      — 2 mg (only in Canada)
   Vaginal cream — 0.1 mg, 0.625 mg, 1.5 mg per gram

▷ **Usual Adult Dosage Range:** For conjugated and esterified estrogens: 0.3 to 1.25 mg daily for 21 days. Omit for 7 days. Repeat cyclically as needed. For other forms of estrogen: consult your physician. **Note: Actual dosage and** administration schedule must be determined by the physician for each patient individually.

Conditions Requiring Dosing Adjustments

Liver function: The dose should be decreased in mild liver disease. Estrogens should not be used in acute or severe liver compromise. This drug can be lithogenic (capable of causing stones) in the bile.

Kidney function: No expected dosing changes in kidney compromise.

▷ **Dosing Instructions:** The tablets may be crushed and may be taken without regard to food. The capsules should be taken whole.

Usual Duration of Use: Use on a regular schedule for 10 to 20 days is needed to see this drug's effectiveness in menopausal symptoms. Long-term use requires supervision and periodic evaluation by your physician every 6 months.

▷ **This Drug Should Not Be Taken If**
- you have had an allergic reaction to any form of it previously.
- you have a history of thrombophlebitis, embolism, heart attack or stroke.
- you have seriously impaired liver function.
- you have abnormal and unexplained vaginal bleeding.
- you have sickle cell disease.
- you have or are suspected to have breast cancer; (may be used to treat some kinds of breast cancer).
- you are pregnant.

▷ **Inform Your Physician Before Taking This Drug If**
- you have had an unfavorable reaction to estrogen therapy previously.
- you have a history of cancer of the breast or reproductive organs.
- you have: Fibrocystic breast changes, fibroid tumors of the uterus, endometriosis, migrainelike headaches, epilepsy, asthma, heart disease, high blood pressure, gallbladder disease, diabetes or porphyria.
- you smoke tobacco on a regular basis.
- you have a history of blood-clotting disorders.
- you plan to have surgery in the near future.

Possible Side-Effects (natural, expected and unavoidable drug actions)

Fluid retention, weight gain, "breakthrough" bleeding (spotting in middle of menstrual cycle), altered menstrual pattern, resumption of menstrual flow (bleeding from the uterus) after a period of natural cessation (postmenopausal bleeding), increased susceptibility to yeast infection of the genital tissues.

▷ **Possible Adverse Effects** (unusual, unexpected and infrequent reactions)

If any of the following develop, consult your physician promptly for guidance.

Mild Adverse Effects

Allergic Reactions: Skin rash, hives, itching.

Headache, nervous tension, irritability, accentuation of migraine headaches.

Nausea, vomiting, bloating, diarrhea.

Tannish pigmentation of the face.

Serious Adverse Effects

Idiosyncratic Reaction: Cutaneous porphyria—fragility and scarring of the skin.

Emotional depression, rise in blood pressure (in susceptible individuals).
Gallbladder disease, benign liver tumors, jaundice, rise in blood sugar.
Erosion of uterine cervix, enlargement of uterine fibroid tumors.
Thrombophlebitis (inflammation of a vein with formation of blood clot)—pain or tenderness in thigh or leg, with or without swelling of foot or leg.
Pulmonary embolism (movement of blood clot to lung)—sudden shortness of breath, pain in chest, coughing, bloody sputum.
Benign liver tumors.
Systemic lupus erythematosus (rare).
Stroke (blood clot in brain)—headaches, blackout, sudden weakness or paralysis of any part of the body, severe dizziness, altered vision, slurred speech, inability to speak.
Endometrial cancer.
Porphyria (rare).
Retinal thrombosis (blood clot in eye vessels)—sudden impairment or loss of vision.
Heart attack (blood clot in coronary artery)—sudden pain in chest, neck, jaw or arm; weakness; sweating; nausea.
Increased risk of breast cancer (even if combined with a progesterone).

▷ **Possible Effects on Sexual Function**
Swelling and tenderness of breasts, milk production.
Increased vaginal secretions.

Possible Delayed Adverse Effects: Estrogens taken during pregnancy can predispose the female child to the later development of cancer of the vagina or cervix following puberty.

▷ **Adverse Effects That May Mimic Natural Diseases or Disorders**
Liver reactions may suggest viral hepatitis.

Natural Diseases or Disorders That May Be Activated by This Drug
Latent hypertension, diabetes mellitus, acute intermittent porphyria.

Possible Effects on Laboratory Tests
Red blood cells, hemoglobin and platelets: decreased.
Blood calcium level: increased.
Blood total cholesterol level: decreased (treatment effect); increased in postmenopausal women.
Blood LDL cholesterol level: decreased in postmenopausal women.
Blood triglyceride level: no drug effect in postmenopausal women.
Blood glucose level: increased.
Glucose tolerance test (GTT): decreased.
Blood thyroid hormone (T_3 and T_4) levels: increased.
Blood uric acid level: decreased.
Liver function tests: increased liver enzymes (ALT/GPT, AST/GOT and alkaline phosphatase), increased bilirubin.

CAUTION
1. To avoid prolonged (uninterrupted) stimulation of breast and uterine tissues, estrogen should be taken in cycles of 3 weeks on and 1 week off of medication.
2. The estrogen in estrogen vaginal creams is absorbed systemically. It may also be absorbed through the penis during sexual intercourse and can cause enlargement and tenderness of male breast tissue.

Estrogens

Precautions for Use

By Those over 60 Years of Age: Very limited usefulness after 60. Restricted to women who are at increased risk for osteoporosis. In this age group, it is advisable to attempt relief of hot flushes with nonestrogenic medications. During use, report promptly any indications of impaired circulation: speech disturbances, altered vision, sudden hearing loss, vertigo, sudden weakness or paralysis, angina, leg pains.

▷ **Advisability of Use During Pregnancy**

Pregnancy Category: X. See Pregnancy Code at the back of this book.

Animal studies: Genital defects reported in mice and guinea pigs; cleft palate reported in rodents.

Human studies: Information from studies of pregnant women indicates that estrogens can masculinize the female fetus. In addition, limb defects and heart malformations have been reported.

It is now known that estrogens taken during pregnancy can predispose the female child to the development of cancer of the vagina or cervix following puberty. *Avoid estrogens completely during entire pregnancy.*

Advisability of Use if Breast-Feeding

Presence of this drug in breast milk: Yes, in minute amounts.

Estrogens in large doses can suppress milk formation.

Breast-feeding is considered to be safe during the use of estrogens.

Malnourished mothers may have unacceptable decreases in protein and nitrogen in their breast milk if this drug is used while breast-feeding.

Habit-Forming Potential: None.

Effects of Overdosage: Headache, drowsiness, nausea, vomiting, fluid retention, abnormal vaginal bleeding, breast enlargement and discomfort.

Possible Effects of Long-Term Use: High blood pressure, gallbladder disease with gallstone formation, increased growth of benign fibroid tumors of the uterus. Several reports suggest possible association between the long-term use (3+ years) of estrogens and the development of cancer of the lining of the uterus. Further studies are needed to establish a definite cause-and-effect relationship (see Glossary). Prudence dictates that women with uterus intact should use estrogens only when symptoms justify it and with proper supervision.

Suggested Periodic Examinations While Taking This Drug (at physician's discretion)

Regular (every 6 months) evaluation of the breasts and pelvic organs, including Pap smears. Liver function tests as indicated.

▷ **While Taking This Drug, Observe the Following**

Foods: Avoid excessive use of salt if fluid retention occurs.

Beverages: No restrictions. May be taken with milk.

▷ *Alcohol:* No interactions expected.

Tobacco Smoking: Recent studies indicate that heavy smoking (15 or more cigarettes daily) in association with the use of estrogen-containing oral contraceptives significantly increases the risk of heart attack (coronary thrombosis). Avoid heavy smoking during long-term estrogen therapy.

▷ *Other Drugs*

Estrogens *taken concurrently* with
- antidiabetic drugs may cause unpredictable fluctuations of blood sugar.

- oral hypoglycemic agents may cause loss of glucose control and high blood sugars.
- thyroid hormones may increase the bound (inactive) drug and require an increase in thyroid dose.
- tricyclic antidepressants (Elavil, Sinequan, etc.) may enhance their adverse effects and reduce their antidepressant effectiveness.
- warfarin (Coumadin) may cause unpredictable alterations of prothrombin activity.

The following drugs may *decrease* the effects of estrogens
- carbamazepine (Tegretol).
- phenobarbital.
- phenytoin (Dilantin).
- primidone (Mysoline).
- rifampin (Rifadin, Rimactane).

▷ *Driving, Hazardous Activities:* Usually no restrictions. Consult your physician for assessment of individual risk and for guidance regarding specific restrictions.

Aviation Note: Usually no restrictions. However, watch for the rare occurrence of disturbed vision and to restrict activities accordingly. Consult a designated Aviation Medical Examiner.

Exposure to Sun: Use caution—these drugs can cause photosensitivity (see Glossary).

Discontinuation: Best to stop estrogens periodically to see if they are still needed. The dose is reduced gradually to prevent acute withdrawal hot flushes. Avoid continual, uninterrupted use of large doses. Stop altogether when a definite need for replacement therapy has ended. Ask your doctor for help.

ETHAMBUTOL (eth AM byu tohl)

Introduced: 1971   **Prescription:** USA: Yes; Canada: Yes   **Available as Generic:** USA: No; Canada: No   **Class:** Anti-infective, antimycobacterial
Controlled Drug: USA: No; Canada: No
Brand Names: ◆Etibi, Myambutol

BENEFITS versus RISKS	
Possible Benefits	*Possible Risks*
EFFECTIVE ADJUNCTIVE TREATMENT OF PULMONARY TUBERCULOSIS	RARE OPTIC NEURITIS WITH IMPAIRMENT OR LOSS OF VISION
EFFECTIVE ADJUNCTIVE TREATMENT OF AIDS-RELATED M. AVIUM-INTRACELLULARE INFECTIONS	Rare peripheral neuritis (see Glossary)
	Activation of gout
Possibly effective treatment of tuberculous meningitis	

▷ **Principal Uses**

As a Single Drug Product: Uses currently included in FDA approved labeling: Treatment of pulmonary tuberculosis, in combination with other antitubercular drugs.

Ethambutol

Other (unlabeled) generally accepted uses: (1) Treatment of tuberculous meningitis; (2) Treatment of AIDS-related Mycobacterium avium-intracellulare (MAI) infections, in combination with other antimycobacterial drugs.

How This Drug Works: It enters mycobacterial cells that are actively dividing, and keeps them from reproducing by interfering with nuclear material (RNA).

Available Dosage Forms and Strengths
Tablets — 100 mg, 400 mg

▷ **Recommended Dosage Ranges** (Actual dosage and administration schedule must be determined by the physician for each patient individually.)

Infants and Children: Dosage not established. Some authorities recommend that children under 6 years of age not be given this drug.

13 to 60 Years of Age: For initial treatment of tuberculosis—15 mg/kg of body weight, once daily. The total daily dose should not exceed 500–1500 mg.

For retreatment of tuberculosis—25 mg/kg of body weight, once daily for 60 days; then 15 mg/kg of body weight. The total daily dose should not exceed 900–2500 mg.

For tuberculous meningitis or AIDS-related MAI infections—15 to 25 mg/kg of body weight, once daily.

Over 60 Years of Age: Same as 13 to 60 years of age.

Conditions Requiring Dosing Adjustments

Liver function: No dose decreases are anticipated in mild to moderate liver compromise.

Kidney function: For mild to moderate kidney failure, the usual dose can be given every 24–36 hours. Severe kidney failure only requires a dose every 48 hours.

▷ **Dosing Instructions:** The tablet may be crushed and taken with food to reduce stomach irritation. Take full course prescribed.

Usual Duration of Use: Use on a regular schedule for 4 to 6 weeks is needed necessary to determine this drug's effectiveness in controlling infections. Long-term use (6 months to 2 or more years) requires periodic physician evaluation.

▷ **This Drug Should Not Be Taken If**
- you have had an allergic reaction to it previously.
- you currently have optic neuritis or peripheral neuritis.
- you currently have active gout.

▷ **Inform Your Physician Before Taking This Drug If**
- you have a history of gout.
- you have a history of optic neuritis or peripheral neuritis.
- you have diabetes or a history of alcoholism; these conditions predispose to eye problems (optic neuritis).
- you have impaired kidney function.

Possible Side-Effects (natural, expected and unavoidable drug actions)
Increased blood level of uric acid (50–66% of users).

▷ **Possible Adverse Effects** (unusual, unexpected and infrequent reactions)
If any of the following develop, consult your physician promptly for guidance.

Mild Adverse Effects
  Allergic Reactions: Skin rash, itching, fever.
  Headache, confusion, disorientation.
  Loss of appetite, nausea, vomiting, stomach pain.
Serious Adverse Effects
  Allergic Reactions: Severe skin reactions, painful joints.
  Optic neuritis (one or both eyes): Eye pain, blurred vision, red-green color blindness.
  Peripheral neuritis (see Glossary): Numbness, tingling, burning, pain and/or weakness in hands or feet.
  Low blood platelets or white blood cells.
  Hallucinations.
  Porphyria (rare).
  Gouty arthritis.
▷ **Possible Effects on Sexual Function:** None reported.
Possible Delayed Adverse Effects: Optic neuritis may not happen until many months of therapy. Visual loss may continue for up to a year after stopping this drug, and may be permanent.
Natural Diseases or Disorders That May Be Activated by This Drug
  Latent gout.
Possible Effects on Laboratory Tests
  Complete blood cell counts: decreased white cells and platelets.
  Blood uric acid levels: increased.
  Liver function tests: increased liver enzymes (ALT/GPT, AST/GOT).
  Kidney function tests: increased blood urea nitrogen (BUN) and creatinine (rare kidney damage).
CAUTION
  1. Promptly report any vision changes; this could be the start of optic neuritis. Immediate evaluation is mandatory.
  2. Report promptly any unusual sensations in the hands or feet; these could indicate the onset of peripheral neuritis.
Precautions for Use
  By Infants and Children: Safety and effectiveness for those under 13 years of age not established.
  By Those over 60 Years of Age: Confusion or disorientation more likely. Age-related decrease in kidney function may require decreased doses.
▷ **Advisability of Use During Pregnancy**
  Pregnancy Category: B. See Pregnancy Code at the back of this book.
    Animal studies: Mouse and rabbit studies confirm multiple drug-induced birth defects.
    Human studies: Adequate studies of pregnant women are not available.
    Use this drug only if clearly needed. Ask your physician for guidance.
Advisability of Use if Breast-Feeding
  Presence of this drug in breast milk: Yes.
  Avoid drug or refrain from nursing.
Habit-Forming Potential: None.
Effects of Overdosage: Nausea, vomiting, stomach discomfort, confusion, possible blurred vision.

Possible Effects of Long-Term Use: Optic neuritis with significant visual impairment.

Suggested Periodic Examinations While Taking This Drug (at physician's discretion)
Complete eye examinations (including visual fields and color vision) should be performed before treatment is started and monthly during therapy.
Blood uric acid levels.
Liver and kidney function tests.

▷ **While Taking This Drug, Observe the Following**
Foods: Follow physician's advice regarding high-purine foods.
Beverages: Avoid excessive caffeinated coffee.
▷ *Alcohol:* No interactions expected.
Tobacco Smoking: No interactions expected.
▷ *Other Drugs*
The following drugs may *decrease* the effects of ethambutol
- antacids containing aluminum salts can slow and reduce absorption.

Ethambutol *taken concurrently* with
- BCG vaccine may blunt the immune response which could have been given by the vaccine.

▷ *Driving, Hazardous Activities:* This drug may cause confusion, disorientation and impaired vision. Restrict activities as necessary.
Aviation Note: The use of this drug *is a disqualification* for piloting. Consult a designated Aviation Medical Examiner.
Exposure to Sun: No restrictions.
Discontinuation: This drug is generally used for long-term treatment—months to years. Ask your doctor about the appropriate time to stop this medicine.

ETHANOL (ETH an all)

Other Names: Prescription: None
Non-prescription: Moonshine, alcohol, jack, white lightning, wine, beer, whiskey, vodka, others.

Introduced: 1980 (Prescription), 10 BC (Non-prescription) **Prescription:** USA: Yes (IV); Canada: Yes (IV)   **Available as Generic:** USA: Yes; Canada: Yes   **Class:** Central nervous system depressant, antianxiety agent (non-prescription form)   **Controlled Drug:** USA: No; Canada: No

Brand Names: Prescription: Tuss-Ornade (5%), Vicks Formula 44D, Temaril (5.7%), Nyquil Nightime Cold Medicine, Novahistine DMX Liquid, Eskaphen B, ✦Dilusol (38.7%), Non-prescription: Robert Alison Chardonnay (12% by volume), Bud Dry, Glenlivet, Smirnoff (40% by volume), others,

Warning: The clinical use of this medication is limited to intravenous treatment of methanol and antifreeze (ethylene glycol) poisoning, and as a preservative. Past use has included treatment of premature labor (tocolytic).
This drug, though widely used in its non-prescription form as an anti-anxiety agent is **not** an ideal anti-anxiety agent. Some people may not experience any mental or physical changes even though a breath or blood alcohol says they are "legally drunk."

Ethanol

BENEFITS versus RISKS	
Possible Benefits	*Possible Risks*
EFFECTIVE TREATMENT OF POISONING	WITHDRAWAL SYMPTOMS SEIZURES LIVER DAMAGE (with prolonged use) Pancreatitis Encephalopathy Low white blood cell counts and anemia Myopathy

▷ **Principal Uses**

As a Single Drug Product: Uses currently included in FDA approved labeling: (1) Supplementation of caloric intake intravenously in very specific cases.

Other (unlabeled) generally accepted uses: (1) Treatment of methanol or antifreeze (ethylene Glycol) poisoning; (2) adjunctive treatment of cancer pain; (3) intravenous treatment of DTs (delirium tremens); (4) used to sclerose esophageal varicies and stop bleeding; (5) treatment of hepatocellular cancer where severe liver problems preclude surgery; (6) used to sclerose thyroid cysts; (7) used to destroy nerve tissue (neurolytic block) in chronic pain therapy; (8) widely used in non-prescription form as an antianxiety agent, however, this is not recommended.

As a Combination Drug Product [CD]: Uses currently included in FDA approved labeling: (1) Widely present in elixirs and other liquid vehicles for drugs as a preservative, and partial drug action enhancer.

How This Drug Works: In overdose situations, this drug provides a less toxic alternative, and lets the body remove the antifreeze or methanol. When used in its non-prescription form, it depresses nerve function and leads to emotional changes and disturbances of perception, coordination and intoxication.

Available Dosage Forms and Strengths
 Intravenous — 5%, 10% and 95%
 Non-prescription — Each ounce of 100 proof whiskey has 15 ml of ethanol
  — 6 ounces (12%) wine has 22 ml of ethanol
  — 12 ounces of beer (4.9%) has 18 ml of ethanol

▷ **Recommended Dosage Ranges (Actual dosage and administration schedule must be determined by the physician for each patient individually.)**

Infants and Children: Methanol or ethylene glycol poisoning: 40 ml per kg per day.

18 to 60 Years of Age: Methanol or ethylene glycol poisoning: A loading dose of 0.6 mg per kg is given, and followed by 109 to 125 mg per kg per hour to maintain a blood level of 100 mg/dl.

Over 60 Years of Age: Same as 12 to 60 years of age for poisonings. The amount consumed versus the collective mental and physical effects may decrease in older people for the non-prescription products. It will generally take less of a dose to cause an equal or greater change in cordination or mental ability. There is also an increased risk of hypothermia.

356 Ethanol

Conditions Requiring Dosing Adjustments
Liver function: Ethanol is extensively metabolized in the liver to acetaldehyde and acetyl co-A. The drug is also a clear cause of liver toxicity. The dose must be decreased in liver compromise.
Kidney function: Minimal involvement of the kidney in the elimination of this drug.

▷ **Dosing Instructions:** If methanol or ethylene glycol poisoning is suspected: The nearest poison control center should be contacted, and oral dosing (use of a strong vodka mixed in orange juice) may be of benefit depending on your distance from a hospital or free-standing emergency center.

For non-prescription antianxiety use: The specific dose of this drug and the resulting blood level of alcohol depends on many factors, however, the more important ones are: The weight of the person, the metabolic activity of the liver, food content in the stomach, the strength of the alcohol in the consumed beverage, the number of "drinks" consumed over a given period of time, and how well hydrated (has there been extreme exercise and fluid loss) you are. Again, although a blood or breath alcohol may be a marker for mental or physical changes, some people may not have physical or mental changes and have a blood or breath alcohol which is in the state-defined range that constitutes being "legally drunk." Specific levels of blood or breath alcohol do not absolutely predict impairment.

Each 10 ml of ethanol increases the blood ethanol level of an average 150 lb (70 kg) man by 16.6 mg percent (3.6 mm/liter). The legal definition of intoxication is a blood alcohol level of 0.10 or 100 mg/dl. "Under the influence" in Maryland is .07 or 70 mg/dl. Driving impairment **may** occur at blood levels of 0.05% (50 mg/dl) or lower.

Usual Duration of Use: Use on a regular schedule for 48 hours determines effectiveness in methanol overdose. Long-term use as an antianxiety agent is **not** recommended.

▷ **This Drug Should Not Be Taken If**
- you have had an allergic reaction to any dosage form of it previously.
- you have epilepsy.
- you have a history of alcohol addiction.
- you are in diabetic coma.

▷ **Inform Your Physician Before Taking This Drug If**
- you have liver or kidney compromise.
- you have gout.
- you are a diabetic.
- you have congestive heart failure.

Possible Side-Effects (natural, expected and unavoidable drug actions)
Intoxication, perception, coordination and mood changes.

▷ **Possible Adverse Effects** (unusual, unexpected and infrequent reactions)
If any of the following develop, consult your physician promptly for guidance.
Mild Adverse Effects
Allergic Reactions: Itching, rash, hives and flushing.
Headache. "Hangover": Nausea, headache, malaise.

Sedation (dose dependent).
Disorientation.
Color blindness (with chronic use).
Neuropathy (tingling, burning or numbness).
Memory loss.
Vitamin deficiency.
Stomach irritation.
Myopathy (with chronic use).

Serious Adverse Effects
Allergic Reactions: Anaphylaxis: rash, swelling of tongue, breathing problems, flushing.
Bronchospasm (asthmatics at increased risk).
Respiratory depression.
Elevated or decreased white blood cell count.
Increased or decreased platelets.
Anemia (megaloblastic with chronic use).
Heart dysfunction (myopathy with chronic use).
High blood pressure.
Abnormal heart rhythms (atrial and ventricular).
Chest pain (angina).
Liver toxicity (cirrhosis with chronic use).
Osteoporosis (with chronic use).
Pancreatitis.
Encephalopathy (with chronic use).
Cerebrovascular bleeding (dose dependent).
Low blood sugar (especially if meals are missed).
Ketoacidosis (with chronic use).
Vitamin deficiency with chronic use (folic acid, vitamin B1 and B6).
Low magnesium (with chronic use).
Low potassium (especially with acute intoxication in children).
Gout (precipitated by alcohol use in those with gout).
Tolerance (with chronic use).
Withdrawal: Nausea, fever, rapid heart rate, halucinations.
May progress to DTs (5%): profound confusion, hallucinations, etc.

▷ **Possible Effects on Sexual Function:** Decreased libido, impotence (with excesive chronic use). Difficulty achieving an erection in males and decreased vaginal dilation in females. Chronic alcohol use may lead to tenderness and swelling of male and female breast tissue, testicular atrophy, low sperm counts, decreased menstrual blood flow and diminished capability for orgasm in females.

Possible Delayed Adverse Effects: Liver toxicity, anemia, low or high platelets, vitamin deficiency.

▷ **Adverse Effects That May Mimic Natural Diseases or Disorders**
Alcoholic cirrhosis may mimic hepatitis.

Natural Diseases or Disorders That May Be Activated by This Drug
Peptic ulcer disease.

Ethanol

Possible Effects on Laboratory Tests
    Liver function tests: elevated ALT.
    Complete blood count: decreased white blood cells, decreased hemoglobin, increased or decreased platelets.
    Amylase: elevated.
    Sperm count: decreased with chronic use.
    Magnesium: decreased with chronic use.

CAUTION

1. This drug in its non-prescription form may cause fatal increases in blood pressure if combined with cocaine.
2. With high doses (nearly pure "grain" alcohol) or many drinks (frequent dosing) over a short period of time, fatal blood alcohol levels may be reached with the non-prescription form.

Precautions for Use
  By Infants and Children:
    Safety and effectiveness for those under 12 years of age not established. Accidental and unsupervised drinking of the non-prescription form may result in severe consequences in children. Seriously low blood sugar may happen and be delayed up to 6 hours after drinking. Low potassium may also occur with high ethanol levels. Therapy is guided by blood sugar, potassium and blood alcohol (ethanol) levels. Fatality caused by low blood sugar was reported in a 4 year old child who drank 12 ounces of a mouthwash which contained 10% ethanol.
  By Those over 60 Years of Age: Poisoning with methanol or ethylene glycol is an emergency situation, and while there may be an increased sensitivity to effects, dosing is adjusted to blood levels. The non-prescription form dosing (number of drinks) tolerated would be expected to decrease with increasing age.

▷ **Advisability of Use During Pregnancy**
  Pregnancy Category: D, X if used for long periods. See Pregnancy Code at the back of this book.
  Human studies: Fetal alcohol syndrome, a collection of limb, neurological and behavioral defects occur with excessive alcohol use.
  Avoid use of this drug during your **entire** pregnancy.

Advisability of Use if Breast-Feeding
  Presence of this drug in breast milk: Yes.
  Avoid drug or refrain from nursing.

Habit-Forming Potential: Clearly defined alcoholism exists and occurs.

Effects of Overdosage: Toxic levels result in ataxia, loss of consciousness progressing to coma, anesthesia, respiratory failure and death. Levels of 150 to 300 mg/dl may result in exaggerated emotional states, confusion and incoordination. Fatalities most often result with blood concentrations greater than 400 mg/dl. Fatal blood levels vary greatly, however, and death has been reported following levels as low as 260 mg/dl. Once again, some people will not have any mental or physical changes with an alcohol level that is in the "legally drunk" range.

Possible Effects of Long-Term Use: Liver toxicity, anemia, esophageal varicies, low white blood cell counts, compromised heart function, high blood pressure, arrhythmias, depression, peripheral neuropathy, seizures, cerebrovascular accident (with acute high levels), water intoxication, vitamin deficiency, electrolyte disturbances, gastritis or ulcers, pancreatitis, muscle pain, osteoporosis, tolerance and withdrawal on discontinuation.

Suggested Periodic Examinations While Taking This Drug (at physician's discretion)

Blood alcohol levels and methanol or ethylene glycol levels guide therapy in poisonings.

Chronic alcohol abuse: Complete blood counts, liver function tests, amylase and lipase, electrocardiograms.

▷ **While Taking This Drug, Observe the Following**

Foods: No restrictions.

Nutritional Support: Vitamin support, particularly thiamine (B1), folic acid and B6 are needed with chronic use. Magnesium replacement is also needed.

Tobacco Smoking: No interactions expected.

Marijuana Smoking: Additive central nervous system depression.

▷ *Other Drugs*

Ethanol may *increase* the effects of
- Central nervous system depressants such as benzodiazepines, barbiturates, opioids and anesthetic agents.
- chlorpromazine (Thorazine) will result in increased sedation.
- cocaine and result in dangerous increases in blood pressure.
- diphenhydramine (Benadryl, others) will increase sedation.

Ethanol may *decrease* the effects of
- phenytoin (Dilantin) by reducing blood phenytoin levels.
- propranolol (Inderal) by increasing propranolol elimination.

Ethanol *taken concurrently* with
- acetaminophen (Tylenol) poses an increased risk of liver damage.
- oral hypoglycemic agents pose an increased risk of serious low glucose levels.
- aspirin may result in increased blood loss from the stomach.
- cefamandole (Mandol), cefotetan (Cefotan), metronidazole (Flagyl) and cefoperazone (Cefobid) may result in disulfiram-like reaction (see Glossary).
- disulfiram (Antabuse) will result in severe vomiting and intolerance.
- insulin may result in potential severe hypoglycemia.
- isoniazid may result in elevated isoniazid levels.
- lithium (Lithobid) may result in worsened impairment of coordination and intoxication.
- nitroglycerin (Nitrostat, others) may result in excessive decreases in blood pressure.
- tricyclic antidepressants may result in increased antidepressant levels and toxicity.

▷ *Driving, Hazardous Activities:* This drug may cause drowsiness, mental impairment and coordination problems.

Driving skill may be imparied at very low blood levels with the perception that capabilities are **not** reduced. Drinking and driving is **not** recommended. Restrict activities as necessary.

Aviation Note: The use of this drug *is a disqualification* for piloting. Consult a designated Aviation Medical Examiner.
Exposure to Sun: May result in additive dehydration.
Heavy Exercise or Exertion: May worsen the adverse effects of this drug.
Discontinuation: Abrupt discontinuation after chronic use may result in a serious withdrawal syndrome known as DTs or delirium tremens.

ETHOSUXIMIDE (eth oh SUX i mide)

Introduced: 1960 **Prescription:** USA: Yes; Canada: Yes **Available as Generic:** Yes **Class:** Anticonvulsant, succinimides **Controlled Drug:** USA: No; Canada: No

Brand Name: Zarontin

BENEFITS versus RISKS

Possible Benefits	*Possible Risks*
EFFECTIVE CONTROL OF ABSENCE SEIZURES (PETIT MAL EPILEPSY) in 70% of cases	RARE APLASTIC ANEMIA (See Aplastic Anemia and Bone Marrow Depression in Glossary)
EFFECTIVE CONTROL OF MYOCLONIC AND AKINETIC EPILEPSY in some individuals	Rare decrease in white blood cells and blood platelets

---

▷ **Principal Uses**

As a Single Drug Product: Uses currently included in FDA improved labeling:
(1) Used to treat petit mal epilepsy and is a drug of choice in absence seizures

Other (unlabeled) generally accepted uses: None at present.

How This Drug Works: By altering certain nerve impulses, this drug suppresses abnormal electrical activity that causes absence seizures of petit mal epilepsy.

Available Dosage Forms and Strengths
Capsules — 250 mg
Syrup — 250 mg per 5-ml teaspoonful

▷ **Usual Adult Dosage Range:** 20 to 40 mg per kilogram of body weight/24 hours. Initially 500 mg/24 hours.

Dosage may be increased cautiously by 250 mg every 4 to 7 days until satisfactory control is achieved. The total daily dosage should not exceed 1500 mg. **Note: Actual dosage and administration schedule must be determined by the physician for each patient individually.**

Conditions Requiring Dosing Adjustments
Liver function: Blood levels are recommended if this medication is used in liver compromise.
Kidney function: In severe kidney failure, 75% of the usual dose should be given at the usual interval.

▷ **Dosing Instructions:** Capsule may be opened and taken with food to reduce stomach irritation.

Ethosuximide 361

Usual Duration of Use: Use on a regular schedule for 1 to 2 weeks is usually needed to see this drug's effectiveness in reducing the frequency of absence seizures. Long-term use requires physician supervision.

▷ **This Drug Should Not Be Taken If**
- you are allergic to this or any succinimide (See Drug Class Section).
- you have active liver disease.
- you currently have a blood cell or bone marrow disorder.

▷ **Inform Your Physician Before Taking This Drug If**
- you have a history of liver or kidney disease.
- you have any type of blood disorder, especially one caused by drugs.
- you have a history of serious depression or other mental illness.

Possible Side-Effects (natural, expected and unavoidable drug actions)
Drowsiness, lethargy, fatigue.

▷ **Possible Adverse Effects** (unusual, unexpected and infrequent reactions)
If any of the following develop, consult your physician promptly for guidance.

Mild Adverse Effects
Allergic Reactions: Skin rash, hives.
Headache, dizziness, unsteadiness, euphoria, impaired vision, numbness and tingling in extremities.
Loss of appetite, nausea, vomiting, hiccups, stomach pain, diarrhea.
Excessive growth of hair.

Serious Adverse Effects
Allergic Reaction: Swelling of tongue.
Thickening and overgrowth of gums.
Nervousness, hyperactivity, disturbed sleep, night terrors.
Aggravation of emotional depression and paranoid mental disorders.
Severe bone marrow depression—fatigue, weakness, fever, sore throat, abnormal bleeding or bruising.
Porphyria (rare).
Myasthenia gravis (rare).
Systemic lupus erythematosus (rare).

▷ **Possible Effects on Sexual Function:** Increased libido (questionable); nonmenstrual vaginal bleeding.

Natural Diseases or Disorders That May Be Activated by This Drug
Latent psychosis, systemic lupus erythematosus.

Possible Effects on Laboratory Tests
Complete blood cell counts: decreased red cells, hemoglobin, white cells and platelets; increased eosinophils.
Blood aspartate aminotransferase (AST) level: increased in 33% of users.
Blood bilirubin level: increased (rare liver damage).
Blood lupus erythematosus (LE) cells: positive (rare).
Kidney function tests: increased blood urea nitrogen (BUN) level, increased urine protein content.

CAUTION
1. May increase the frequency of grand mal seizures in people with mixed seizure disorders.
2. Periodic blood counts and other tests are mandatory.

Ethosuximide

Precautions for Use
> *By Infants and Children:* If a single daily dose causes nausea or vomiting, give in 2 or 3 divided doses 8 to 12 hours apart. Large differences in response occur, and require blood levels. Watch for a lupuslike reaction: Fever, rash, arthritis.
>
> *By Those over 60 Years of Age:* Rarely used in this age group.

▷ **Advisability of Use During Pregnancy**
> *Pregnancy Category:* C. See Pregnancy Code at the back of this book.
> Animal studies: Bone defects reported in rodents.
> Human studies: Three instances of birth defects have been reported. Adequate studies of pregnant women are not available.
> Avoid during first 3 months. Use only if clearly needed during the last 6 months.

Advisability of Use if Breast-Feeding
> Presence of this drug in breast milk: Yes.
> Watch nursing infant closely and discontinue drug or nursing if adverse effects develop. If mother requires high doses, refrain from nursing. Ask doctor for help.

Habit-Forming Potential: None.

Effects of Overdosage: Increased drowsiness, lethargy, weakness, dizziness, unsteadiness, nausea, vomiting, stupor progressing to coma.

Possible Effects of Long-Term Use: Systemic lupus erythematosus.

Suggested Periodic Examinations While Taking This Drug (at physician's discretion)
> Complete blood counts every 2 weeks during the first months of use, then monthly thereafter; liver and kidney function tests.

▷ **While Taking This Drug, Observe the Following**
> *Foods:* No restrictions.
> *Beverages:* No restrictions. May be taken with milk.
▷ > *Alcohol:* Use caution—this drug may increase the sedative effects of alcohol. Excessive alcohol may precipitate seizures.
> *Tobacco Smoking:* No interactions expected.
▷ > *Other Drugs*
> Ethosuximide may *increase* the effects of
> - phenytoin (Dilantin), by slowing its elimination.
>
> Ethosuximide *taken concurrently* with
> - carbamazepine (Tegretol) may change ethosuximide blood levels.
> - valproic acid (Depakene) may unpredictably alter ethosuximide effects.
>
> The following drugs may *increase* the effects of ethosuximide
> - isoniazid (INH, Niconyl, etc.).
▷ > *Driving, Hazardous Activities:* This drug may cause drowsiness, dizziness, unsteadiness and impaired vision. Restrict activities as necessary.
> *Aviation Note:* Seizure disorders and the use of this drug *are disqualifications* for piloting. Consult a designated Aviation Medical Examiner.
> *Exposure to Sun:* No restrictions.
> *Discontinuation:* Do not stop taking this drug abruptly. Ask your physician for help with gradual dose reduction.

ETIDRONATE (e ti DROH nate)

Introduced: 1976 **Prescription:** USA: Yes; Canada: Yes **Available as Generic:** USA: No; Canada: No **Class:** Calcium regulator **Controlled Drug:** USA: No; Canada: No

Brand Name: Didronel

BENEFITS versus RISKS

Possible Benefits	*Possible Risks*
PARTIAL RELIEF OF SYMPTOMS OF PAGET'S DISEASE OF BONE	Increased bone pain
	Bone fractures
EFFECTIVE PREVENTION AND TREATMENT OF ABNORMAL CALCIFICATION	Kidney failure
	Focal Osteomalacia
Effective adjunctive treatment of abnormally high blood calcium levels (associated with malignant disease)	
Treatment of postmenopausal osteoporosis	

▷ **Principal Uses**

As a Single Drug Product: Uses currently included in FDA approved labeling: (1) treatment of symptomatic Paget's disease of bone (excessive bone growth of skull, spine and long bones); (2) prevention and treatment of abnormal bone formation (ossification) following total hip replacement or spinal cord injury; (3) adjunctive treatment of excessively high blood calcium levels due to malignant bone disease.

Other (unlabeled) generally accepted uses: (1) treatment of Paget's disease of bone that is not yet causing symptoms; (2) treatment of postmenopausal osteoporosis; (3) treatment of abnormal calcium levels which may result from prolonged immobilization; (4) helps hyperparathyroidism; (5) helps pulmonary alveolar microlithiasis (PAM).

How This Drug Works: This drug attaches to the surface of bone and slows the abnormally accelerated processes of "bone turnover" that occur in Paget's disease. In malignant bone disease, this drug slows bone destruction and reduces excessive transfer of calcium from bone to blood.

Available Dosage Forms and Strengths
Injection — 50 mg per ml
Tablets — 200 mg, 400 mg

▷ **Recommended Dosage Ranges** (Actual dosage and administration schedule must be determined by the physician for each patient individually.)

Infants and Children: Dosage not established.

12 to 60 Years of Age: For Paget's disease—Initially 5 mg/kg of body weight daily, as a single dose, for 6 months. Discontinue for a drug-free period of 6 months. As needed, repeat alternating 6 month courses of drug treatment and abstention.

For ossification associated with hip replacement—20 mg/kg of body weight daily for 1 month before and 3 months after surgery.

Etidronate

For ossification associated with spinal cord injury—Initially 20 mg/kg of body weight daily for 2 weeks after injury; then decrease dose to 10 mg/kg of body weight daily for an additional 10 weeks.

For high blood calcium associated with malignant bone disease—20 mg/kg of body weight daily for 30 days; if needed and tolerated, continue for a maximum of 90 days.

The total daily dose should not exceed 20 mg/kg of body weight.

Over 60 Years of Age: Same as 12 to 60 years of age.

Conditions Requiring Dosing Adjustments

Liver function: This drug is not known to be metabolized in the liver.

Kidney function: The drug should be used with caution if at all in patients with steady state creatinines (a measure of kidney function) greater than 2.5. Etidronate should never be used in patients with steady state creatinines greater than 5.0.

▷ **Dosing Instructions:** The tablet may be crushed and taken with water on an empty stomach, 2 hours before or after food; suggested times: On arising, midmorning, or at bedtime. Do not take with milk. If nausea or diarrhea occurs, the daily dose may be divided into 2 or 3 portions.

Usual Duration of Use: Use on a regular schedule for 1 to 3 months will determine this drug's effectiveness in relieving the symptoms of Paget's disease. If effective, the standard course of treatment is 6 months. Long-term use (months to years) requires periodic physician evaluation.

Possible Advantages of This Drug

Effective orally, with once-a-day dosage.

Less expensive than calcitonin.

Currently a "Drug of Choice"

for managing Paget's disease of bone.

▷ **This Drug Should Not Be Taken If**
- you have had an allergic reaction to it previously.
- you recently fractured a bone that has not healed completely.

▷ **Inform Your Physician Before Taking This Drug If**
- you have a history of heart disease, especially congestive heart failure.
- you have impaired kidney function.
- you are subject to enterocolitis, or recurrent diarrhea.

Possible Side-Effects (natural, expected and unavoidable drug actions)

Increased bone pain or tenderness (usually starts 4 to 6 weeks after begining treatment).

▷ **Possible Adverse Effects** (unusual, unexpected and infrequent reactions)

If any of the following develop, consult your physician promptly for guidance.

Mild Adverse Effects

Allergic Reactions: Skin rash, hives, itching.

Nausea, diarrhea.

Taste disorders.

Serious Adverse Effects

Allergic Reactions: Angioedema (swelling of face, lips, tongue, throat, and/or vocal cords); may be life-threatening.

Osteomalacia (thinning and weakening of bone) with fractures.
Pseudomembranous colitis.
Ulcers (rare).
Kidney failure.

▷ **Possible Effects on Sexual Function:** None reported.

Natural Diseases or Disorders That May Be Activated by This Drug
Senile osteomalacia.

Possible Effects on Laboratory Tests
Blood alkaline phosphatase levels: decreased.
Blood calcium levels: decreased.
Blood phosphate levels: increased.
Urine hydroxyproline values: decreased.

CAUTION
1. Maintain a well-balanced diet with adequate calcium and vitamin D.
2. Mineral supplements and drugs containing aluminum, calcium, iron, or magnesium can prevent etidronate absorption; separate doses by at least 2 hours.
3. Tell your doctor if nausea or diarrhea persists; dosage adjustment (multiple small doses) can help.
4. Call your physician if bone pain persists or increases.

Precautions for Use
By Infants and Children: Avoid large doses or prolonged use to reduce the risk of inducing rickets.
By Those over 60 Years of Age: Watch fluid balance carefully if this drug is given intravenously to lower blood calcium levels.

▷ **Advisability of Use During Pregnancy**
Pregnancy Category: C. See Pregnancy Code at the back of this book.
Animal studies: Rat and rabbit studies reveal no drug-induced birth defects.
Human studies: Adequate studies of pregnant women are not available.
Use this drug only if clearly needed. Ask your doctor for help.

Advisability of Use if Breast-Feeding
Presence of this drug in breast milk: Unknown.
Avoid drug or refrain from nursing.

Habit-Forming Potential: None.

Effects of Overdosage: Nausea, vomiting, diarrhea.

Possible Effects of Long-Term Use: Development of osteomalacia (softening and weakening of bone structure).

Suggested Periodic Examinations While Taking This Drug (at physician's discretion)
Measurements of blood calcium, phosphate, and alkaline phosphatase levels.
Measurement of urine hydroxyproline content.
Kidney function tests.

▷ **While Taking This Drug, Observe the Following**
Foods: Avoid all foods, especially dairy products, for 2 hours before and after taking this drug.

Nutritional Support: Ensure adequate intake of calcium and vitamin D.

Beverages: Take this drug with water. Avoid all forms of milk for 2 hours before and after taking this drug.

▷ *Alcohol:* No interactions expected.

Tobacco Smoking: No interactions expected.

▷ *Other Drugs*

The following drugs may *decrease* the effects of etidronate
- all antacids containing aluminum, calcium, or magnesium.
- all iron preparations.

Etidronate *taken concurrently* with
- foscarnet (Foscavir) may lead to additive decreases in calcium.
- plicamycin can lead to additive calcium decreases.

▷ *Driving, Hazardous Activities:* No restrictions.

Aviation Note: The use of this drug *may be a disqualification* for piloting. Consult a designated Aviation Medical Examiner.

Exposure to Sun: No restrictions.

Discontinuation: Take this medicine exactly as prescribed. Your doctor should decide when to stop this drug.

ETODOLAC (E TOE do lak)

Introduced: 1986 **Prescription:** USA: Yes **Available as Generic:** USA: No **Class:** NSAID, mild analgesic **Controlled Drug:** USA: No

Brand Names: Lodine

BENEFITS versus RISKS	
Possible Benefits	*Possible Risks*
EFFECTIVE TREATMENT OF MILD TO MODERATE INFLAMMATION AND PAIN	Gastrointestinal pain, ulceration or bleeding (rare)
DECREASED GASTROINTESTINAL BLEEDING RISK	Rare blood cell disorders: Low platelet counts, anemia
	Fluid retention
	Rare kidney damage
	Rare liver damage
	Hearing toxicity (ototoxicity) (2%)

Please see the acetic acid nonsteroidal anti-inflammatory drug profile for further information.

ETRETINATE (e TRET i nayt)

Introduced: 1976 **Prescription:** USA: Yes; Canada: Yes **Available as Generic:** USA: No; Canada: No **Class:** Antipsoriasis **Controlled Drug:** USA: No; Canada: No

Brand Name: Tegison

Etretinate

BENEFITS versus RISKS	
Possible Benefits	*Possible Risks*
EFFECTIVE TREATMENT FOR SEVERE, RESISTANT PSORIASIS	MAJOR DRUG-INDUCED BIRTH DEFECTS
	RARE DRUG-INDUCED HEPATITIS
	Adverse effects on eyes and vision
	Adverse effects on musculoskeletal structures
	Adverse effects on blood cholesterol and triglycerides
	Increased intracranial pressure (very rare)
	Extended PTT
	Increased triglycerides

▷ **Principal Uses**

As a Single Drug Product: Uses currently included in FDA approved labeling: (1) Treatment of severe, generalized forms of psoriasis (and related skin disorders) that have failed to respond to conventional, less hazardous treatments.

Other (unlabeled) generally accepted uses: (1) Treatment of acne; (2) local treatment of warts; (3) treatment of cutaneous neoplasia in kidney transplant patients; (4) eases symptoms of Darier's disease; (5) can help symptoms in a variety of abnormal keratin conditions; (6) eases cutaneous systemic lupus erythematosus; (7) helps Reiter's syndrome in AIDS patients.

How This Drug Works: Regulates cell differentiation in the skin; this results in a more normal pattern of cell growth, with reduction of inflammation and scale formation.

Available Dosage Forms and Strengths
Capsules — 10 mg, 25 mg

▷ **Usual Adult Dosage Range:** Initially 0.75 to 1 mg/kg/day, in divided doses, until satisfactory response is obtained (usually 8 to 16 weeks). Maintenance: 0.5 to 0.75 mg/kg/day, beginning after initial response. Total daily dosage should not exceed 75 mg. **Note: Actual dosage and administration schedule must be determined by the physician for each patient individually.**

Conditions Requiring Dosing Adjustments

Liver function: This drug is a rare cause of hepatitis. It should be used with caution in liver compromise, and the dose should be decreased.

Kidney function: The kidneys are not a significant factor in the elimination of this drug. Etretinate is a rare cause of kidney toxicity, and it should be used with caution in patients with compromised kidneys.

▷ **Dosing Instructions:** Take with or immediately following meals, preferably with whole milk. Do not suck or chew the capsule; swallow it whole.

Usual Duration of Use: Use on a regular schedule for 2 to 4 weeks is usually necessary to see this drug's benefit in reversing the skin changes of psoriasis. The full effect of treatment may not be apparent for 2 to 3 months of continual use. Long-term use (months to years) requires periodic physi-

Etretinate

cian evaluation. Due to the potential for accumulation and toxicity with long-term use, this drug should be temporarily discontinued after 18 months of treatment; it may be resumed as needed. Consult your physician on a regular basis.

Possible Advantages of This Drug: When used in conjunction with other antipsoriasis drugs and procedures, this drug can enhance the therapeutic response and reduce the total dosage and length of treatment required for satisfactory management.

▷ **This Drug Should Not Be Taken If**
- you have had an allergic reaction to any dosage form of it previously.
- you are pregnant or breast-feeding.
- you currently take vitamin A therapy.
- you plan to donate blood in the near future.

▷ **Inform Your Physician Before Taking This Drug If**
- you are allergic to vitamin A or other vitamin A derivatives: isotretinoin (Accutane), tretinoin (Retin-A).
- you are allergic to parabens (preservatives).
- you have cerebral or coronary artery disease.
- you have high blood cholesterol or triglyceride levels.
- you have diabetes.
- you have impaired liver or kidney function.
- you have alcoholism.
- you have a history of Crohn's disease or ulcerative colitis.

Possible Side-Effects (natural, expected and unavoidable drug actions)
Dry nose, nosebleed, dry lips, sore mouth and tongue, bleeding gums.
Loss of hair, skin peeling of hands and feet, dry skin, itching, bruising, nail deformities.
Thickening of bone (hyperostosis), calcification of tendons and ligaments, bone and joint pain.

▷ **Possible Adverse Effects** (unusual, unexpected and infrequent reactions)
If any of the following develop, consult your physician promptly for guidance.

Mild Adverse Effects
Allergic Reactions: Skin rash, hives, itching.
Headache, dizziness, fatigue, fever, emotional irritability.
Eye irritation, blurred or double vision, sensitivity to bright light, decreased tolerance for contact lenses, earache, impaired hearing.
Altered taste, loss of appetite, nausea, stomach pain, constipation, diarrhea.
Muscle cramps.
Painful urination.

Serious Adverse Effects
Increased intracranial pressure (less than 1%): Headache, nausea, vomiting, visual disturbances.
Hepatitis (1.5%); 4 reported deaths worldwide.
Kidney damage (nephrotoxicity) (very rare).
Eye reactions: corneal erosion, abrasion, staining; cataract; retinal hemorrhage; visual field defects; reduced night vision.
Inflammatory bowel disease (Crohn's disease), rare.
Altered blood fat levels: increased triglycerides (45%), increased total cho-

lesterol (16%), decreased HDL cholesterol (37%); any of these changes may increase the risk for the development of atherosclerotic heart disease.

Muscle damage (rare).

Abnormal bone changes (premature epiphyseal closure, periosteal thickening).

Ototoxicity.

Extended PTT.

Low blood platelets (rare).

▷ **Possible Effects on Sexual Function:** Altered timing and pattern of menstruation. Loss of libido. Erectile dysfunctions.

Possible Delayed Adverse Effects: This drug has been found in the blood 2.9 years following termination of its use and has the potential for inducing birth defects during this time. It has not been determined how long pregnancy should be avoided after therapy has been stopped.

▷ **Adverse Effects That May Mimic Natural Diseases or Disorders**

Increased intracranial pressure may suggest brain tumor.

Liver reactions may suggest viral hepatitis.

Joint pains due to calcification of ligaments and tendons may suggest the onset of arthritis.

Natural Diseases or Disorders That May Be Activated by This Drug

Angina may start in the people with coronary artery heart disease. Heart attack (myocardial infarction) has been associated with this drug.

Possible Effects on Laboratory Tests

Red blood cell counts: decreased.

Blood eosinophil counts: increased.

Blood total cholesterol, LDL cholesterol and triglyceride levels: increased.

Liver function tests: increased liver enzymes (ALT/GPT, AST/GOT and alkaline phosphatase.

PTT: increased.

CAUTION

1. *This drug should not be taken during pregnancy.* A pregnancy test should be performed within 2 weeks prior to taking this drug. In the absence of pregnancy, the drug should be started on the second or third day of the next normal menstrual period. An effective form of contraception should be used for 1 month before the drug is started, during the entire period of treatment, and for an indefinite period (minimum of 3 years) after the drug is discontinued. If pregnancy does occur, stop this drug immediately and consult your physician.

2. *Do not donate blood to a blood bank if you are taking this drug.* Blood containing this drug could pose a serious risk to the developing fetus of a pregnant patient who received it. Avoid blood donation for a minimum of 3 years if use of the blood is beyond your control.

3. *Comply fully with your physician's recommendations for periodic examinations before, during and following treatment with this drug.* These are mandatory for safe and effective use.

4. Avoid concurrent use of vitamin A supplements.

5. Call your doctor promptly if you have significant eye reactions or altered vision.

6. Your psoriasis may appear to worsen during the early period of treatment with this drug. Call your doctor if symptoms become severe or prolonged.
7. If dry mouth or sore and bleeding gums persist, consult your dentist.

Precautions for Use

By Infants and Children: This drug should be used only after all less-hazardous treatments have failed. Best to obtain pretreatment X-rays to determine bone age and to monitor bone growth and development by yearly X-ray studies. This drug can impair normal bone maturation.

By Those over 60 Years of Age: Watch for development of anemia, impaired kidney function and fluctuation of blood potassium levels.

▷ **Advisability of Use During Pregnancy**

Pregnancy Category: X. See Pregnancy Code at the back of this book.

Animal studies: No information available.

Human studies: Major birth defects occur in association with the use of this drug: Malformations of the skull, vertebrae, face, extremities, brain and spinal cord.

Avoid this drug completely during entire pregnancy. See *CAUTION*.

Advisability of Use if Breast-Feeding

Presence of this drug in breast milk: Unknown.

Avoid drug or refrain from nursing.

Habit-Forming Potential: None.

Effects of Overdosage: Severe headache, irritability, drowsiness, itching, nausea, vomiting.

Possible Effects of Long-Term Use: Hyperostosis (84%): abnormal thickening of bone (pelvis), calcification of ligaments and tendons (knees and ankles).

Suggested Periodic Examinations While Taking This Drug (at physician's discretion)

Complete blood counts; tests of blood sugar, potassium, sodium and chloride.

Blood cholesterol profiles, before and during treatment.

Liver and kidney function tests.

Complete eye examinations.

Bone X-rays, especially for children.

▷ **While Taking This Drug, Observe the Following**

Foods: No restrictions. High-fat foods increase absorption of this drug.

Beverages: No restrictions. Whole milk increases absorption of this drug.

▷ *Alcohol:* No interactions expected. Use moderately; excessive intake can increase blood triglyceride levels.

Tobacco Smoking: No interactions expected.

▷ *Other Drugs*

Etretinate may *increase* the effects of
- vitamin A and its derivatives (isotretinoin and tretinoin) and increase the risk of vitamin A toxicity.

Etretinate *taken concurrently* with
- carbamazepine (Tegretol) may result in decreased etretinate effectiveness.

- methotrexate may increase the risk of liver toxicity.
- tetracyclines may increase the risk of elevated intracranial pressure.
- warfarin (Coumadin) may cause a decreased effectiveness of warfarin.

▷ *Driving, Hazardous Activities:* This drug may cause dizziness and blurred vision. Limit activities as necessary.

Aviation Note: The use of this drug **may be a disqualification** for piloting. Consult a designated Aviation Medical Examiner.

Exposure to Sun: Use caution. This drug can cause photosensitivity (see Glossary).

Discontinuation: If this drug is not significantly beneficial after 4 months of continual use, it should be stopped. If response is adequate to justify its long-term use, it should be discontinued temporarily ("drug holiday") after 18 months of continual treatment. Once the skin has cleared satisfactorily, this drug should be stopped. Most people have some degree of recurrence by the end of 2 months. Subsequent treatment courses of 4 to 9 months can be started as required.

FAMCICLOVIR (Fam SEYE klo veer)

Introduced: June 1994 **Prescription:** USA: Yes **Available as Generic:** USA: No **Class:** Antiviral **Controlled Drug:** USA: No
Brand Names: Famvir

BENEFITS versus RISKS	
Possible Benefits	*Possible Risks*
EFFECTIVE TREATMENT OF HERPES ZOSTER (SHINGLES) TREATS AN INFECTION WHICH MAY BE LIFE THREATENING IN AIDS AND MARROW TRANSPLANT PATIENTS	Diarrhea Purpura Paresthesias

▷ **Principal Uses**

As a Single Drug Product: Uses currently included in FDA approved labeling: (1) Treatment of acute herpes zoster (shingles).

Other (unlabeled) generally accepted uses: May have a role in treating genital herpes.

How This Drug Works: This drug is changed in the body to the active penciclovir. Penciclovir inhibits the virus by blocking DNA synthesis and viral reproduction (replication).

Available Dosage Forms and Strengths
Tablets — 500 mg

▷ **Recommended Dosage Ranges (Actual dosage and administration schedule must be determined by the physician for each patient individually.)**

Infants and Children: Safety and efficacy for those under 18 not established.

18 to 60 Years of Age: 500 mg is given every 8 hours for seven days. It is important to start this medicine promptly after the diagnosis is made.

Over 60 Years of Age: Same as 12 to 60 years of age, except for those with compromised livers or kidneys.

Famciclovir

Conditions Requiring Dosing Adjustments
Liver function: No dose changes are needed in well-compensated liver impairment.
Kidney function: In people with mild kidney compromise (creatinine clearance greater than 60), 500 mg is given every 8 hours. People with mild to moderate compromise (creatinine clearance 40 to 59) receive 500 mg every 12 hours. Patients with moderate to severe kidney compromise (creatinine clearance 20 to 39) receive 500 mg every 24 hours.

Usual Duration of Use: Use on a regular schedule for two days usually determines effectiveness in treating Herpes zoster, and the medicine is typically continued for seven days. Physician evaluation is needed to determine when this medicine should be stopped.

▷ **This Drug Should Not Be Taken If**
- you have had an allergic reaction to any dosage form of it previously.

▷ **Inform Your Physician Before Taking This Drug If**
- you are uncertain how much famciclovir to take or how often to take it.
- you have a history of kidney or liver problems.
- your immune system is compromised.

▷ **Possible Adverse Effects** (unusual, unexpected and infrequent reactions)
If any of the following develop, consult your physician promptly for guidance.
Mild Adverse Effects
Allergic Reactions: Itching.
Diarrhea (7.7%).
Headache (22.7%).
Nausea (12.5).
Fatigue (4.4%).
Serious Adverse Effects
Allergic Reactions: Unknown.
Not defined at present
Purpura (2.8%).
Paresthesias (2.6%).
Rigors (1.5%).

▷ **Possible Effects on Sexual Function:** None reported.

Possible Delayed Adverse Effects: Unknown.

Possible Effects on Laboratory Tests
Unknown.

CAUTION
1. The best effect is achieved with this medicine if it is started very soon after the condition is diagnosed.

Precautions for Use
By Infants and Children:
Safety and effectiveness for those under 18 years of age not established.
By Those over 60 Years of Age: Specific adjustments or precautions are not defined except for those with compromised livers or kidneys.

▷ **Advisability of Use During Pregnancy**
Pregnancy Category: B. See Pregnancy Code at the back of this book.
Human studies: Adequate studies of pregnant women are not available.
Ask your doctor for guidance.

Advisability of Use if Breast-Feeding
Presence of this drug in breast milk: Unknown.
Stop nursing or discontinue the drug.

Effects of Overdosage: Unknown.

▷ **While Taking This Drug, Observe the Following**
Foods: No restrictions.
Tobacco Smoking: No interactions expected.
▷ *Driving, Hazardous Activities:* This drug may cause dizziness or fatigue. Restrict activities as necessary.
Aviation Note: The use of this drug **may be a disqualification** for piloting. Consult a designated Aviation Medical Examiner.
Exposure to Sun: No restrictions.

FAMOTIDINE (fa MOH te deen)

Introduced: 1986   **Prescription:** USA: Yes   **Available as Generic:** USA: No   **Class:** Antiulcer, H-2 receptor blocker   **Controlled Drug:** USA: No

Author's note: This drug was approved in 1995 as Pepcid AC. This is a nonprescription form of famotidine.

Brand Name: Pepcid, Pepcid AC (nonprescription)

BENEFITS versus RISKS	
Possible Benefits	*Possible Risks*
EFFECTIVE TREATMENT OF PEPTIC ULCER DISEASE: relief of symptoms, acceleration of healing, prevention of recurrence CONTROL OF HYPERSECRETORY STOMACH DISORDERS Beneficial in treatment of reflux esophagitis	Headache, dizziness

Please see the new histamine (H2) blocking drug profile for further information.

FELBAMATE (FELL ba mate)

Introduced: July 1993   **Prescription:** USA: Yes; Canada: approval is pending   **Available as Generic:** USA: No   **Class:** Anticonvulsant   **Controlled Drug:** USA: No

Brand Names: Felbatol

Warning: THIS DRUG HAS RECENTLY BEEN FOUND TO CAUSE APLASTIC ANEMIA, WHICH MAY BE FATAL. THIS DRUG MAY ALSO CAUSE ACUTE LIVER FAILURE, WHICH MAY ALSO BE FATAL. The drug presently remains on the market, reserved only for those people in whom the benefit outweighs the risk of felbamate. This drug should **not** be stopped abruptly because the risk of seizures will be increased—unless a suitable drug which prevents seizures has been started and appropriately covers

Felbamate

the specific seizure type which was being treated. If this drug is combined with phenytoin (Dilantin), serious increases in phenytoin levels may occur unless the phenytoin dose is adjusted.

BENEFITS versus RISKS	
Possible Benefits	*Possible Risks*
CONTROLS VARIOUS SEIZURE FORMS OF LENNOX-GASTAUT SYNDROME	FATAL APLASTIC ANEMIA
	LOW WHITE BLOOD CELL COUNTS AND PLATELETS (RARE)
CONTROLS SEIZURES REFRACTORY TO CARBAMAZEPINE OR PHENYTOIN	ACUTE LIVER FAILURE
	Stevens-Johnson syndrome (serious rash—rare)
	Agitation

▷ **Principal Uses**

As a Single Drug Product: Uses currently included in FDA approved labeling: (1) Used in combination therapy to help control seizures of Lennox-Gastaut syndrome; (2) effective in controlling refractory partial seizures; (3) used in combination treatment of partial seizures not controlled by appropriate levels of carbamazepine or phenytoin.

Other (unlabeled) generally accepted uses: May be used as a replacement for phenytoin in a variety of seizure disorders where phenytoin has not been tolerated. USE IS RESTRICTED TO THOSE PATIENTS IN WHOM THE BENEFIT OUTWEIGHS THE RISK OF FELBAMATE THERAPY.

How This Drug Works: This drug is chemically related to meprobamate (Equanil, Miltown). It is thought to decrease the spread of seizures and increase the stimulus required to produce a seizure (seizure threshold).

Available Dosage Forms and Strengths

Tablets — 400 mg, 600 mg

▷ **Recommended Dosage Ranges (Actual dosage and administration schedule must be determined by the physician for each patient individually.)**

Infants and Children: In children with Lennox-Gastaut syndrome, felbamate is started at 15 mg/kg/day taken in 3 or 4 divided doses. Concurrent anticonvulsants are decreased by 20%. Felbamate is subsequently increased as needed and tolerated by 15 mg/kg/day at weekly intervals to a maximum dose of 45 mg/kg/day. Other anticonvulsant drugs used concomitantly are adjusted based on drug levels or side effects. Safety and efficacy in infants or in children who do not have Lennox-Gastaut syndrome not established.

12 to 60 Years of Age: Dosing is started with 400 mg three times daily (1200 mg a day). Felbamate can be increased by 600 mg a day at two week intervals to a maximum dose of 3600 mg daily in people who have not previously been treated.

Monotherapy: Starting dose of 1200 mg daily and reduction of other anticonvulsant doses by one third. Felbamate is then increased weekly as needed and tolerated by 1200 mg per day to the 3600 mg per day maximum. Other anticonvulsants are decreased by one third with each increase in felbamate dose until they are stopped.

Adjunctive therapy: Felbamate is started at 400 mg three times a day (1200 mg a day) with a concomitant 20% reduction of other anticonvulsant drugs. Felbamate is subsequently increased as needed and tolerated to the maximum 3600 mg daily dose. Other anticonvulsant doses are adjusted according to drug levels or side effects.

Over 60 Years of Age: Use with caution, particularly in those with compromised livers or kidneys.

Conditions Requiring Dosing Adjustments

Liver function: Dosing of this drug should be adjusted based on blood levels in patients with compromised livers. THIS DRUG MAY CAUSE FATAL LIVER FAILURE.

Kidney function: Most of this drug is eliminated unchanged in the kidney, and dosing should be adjusted based on blood levels in people with kidney compromise.

▷ **Dosing Instructions:** Tablet may be crushed and taken with food to help prevent stomach upset. This medication should **not** be stopped abruptly.

Usual Duration of Use: Use on a regular schedule for two weeks usually determines effectiveness in controllng seizures. Long-term use (months to years) requires aggressive physician evaluation of response, potential adverse effects and dosage adjustment.

Possible Advantages of This Drug
Control of refractory seizures with fewer side effects than other available agents.

▷ **This Drug Should Not Be Taken If**
- you have had an allergic reaction to any dosage form of it previously.
- your seizures can be controlled by safer medicines.
- you have an active blood or bone marrow disorder.
- you have liver disease.

▷ **Inform Your Physician Before Taking This Drug If**
- you have a history of blood disorders.
- you take other anticonvulsants.
- you have impaired liver or kidney function.
- you have a history of alcoholism.
- you take other prescription or non-prescription medicines which were not discussed with your doctor when felbamate was prescribed.

▷ **Possible Adverse Effects** (unusual, unexpected and infrequent reactions)
If any of the following develop, consult your physician promptly for guidance.

Mild Adverse Effects
Allergic Reactions: Skin rash, itching.
Headache (6.9%) and somnolence (6.9%).
Insomnia (8.6%).
Anorexia (1.6%) and diarrhea (5.2%).
Constipation (6.9%).
Weight loss (1.1%).
Visual disturbances (diplopia).
Increased heart rate.

Serious Adverse Effects
Allergic Reactions: Anaphylactoid reaction.
Ataxia (3.5%).
Agitation or aggressive reaction (frequent).

Felbamate

Stevens-Johnson syndrome (rare).
Low phosphorous (3.4%).
Low sodium, magnesium and potassium (infrequent).
Low white blood cell count and platelets (infrequent).
FATAL APLASTIC ANEMIA (21 reported cases).
FATAL LIVER FAILURE.

▷ **Possible Effects on Sexual Function:** None reported.

Possible Effects on Laboratory Tests
Blood urea nitrogen (BUN): decreased levels.
Complete blood counts: decreased white blood cells and platelets.
Antinuclear antibody: positive test.
Electrolytes: decreased potassium, magnesium, sodium and phosphorous.

CAUTION
1. This drug should **not** be stopped abruptly as an increase in seizure activity may occur.
2. Promptly call your doctor if you develop abnormal bleeding or bruising or sore throat, fever and chills.

Precautions for Use
By Infants and Children:
Safety and effectiveness for those under 18 years of age (except children with Lennox-Gastaut syndrome have not been established.
By Those over 60 Years of Age: Starting doses should be conservative. Adjustment must be made in liver or kidney compromise.

▷ **Advisability of Use During Pregnancy**
Pregnancy Category: C. See Pregnancy Code at the back of this book.
Animal studies: No effects in rat pups at 6.9 times the human dose.
Human studies: Adequate studies of pregnant women are not available.
Ask your doctor for guidance.

Advisability of Use if Breast-Feeding
Presence of this drug in breast milk: Yes.
Avoid drug or refrain from nursing.

Habit-Forming Potential: Rats given 8.3 times the human dose have not demonstrated physical dependence or withdrawal.

Effects of Overdosage: Mild increases in heart rate and stomach upset.

Suggested Periodic Examinations While Taking This Drug (at physician's discretion)
Liver function tests.
Blood sodium, potassium and phosphorous.
Complete blood counts.
Felbamate levels.
Levels of other concomitantly used anticonvulsants.

▷ **While Taking This Drug, Observe the Following**
Foods: No restrictions.
Beverages: No specific restrictions defined at present.
▷ *Alcohol:* There are no documented drug interactions with felbamate and alcohol, however, alcohol can lower the amount of stimulus needed to cause a seizure (seizure threshold). Follow your doctor's advice regarding alcohol use.

Tobacco Smoking: No interactions expected.
Marijuana Smoking: May worsen fatigue.
▷ **Other Drugs**
Felbamate may *increase* the effects of
- valproic acid (Depakote).
- phenobarbital.
- phenytoin (Dilantin).

Felbamate may *decrease* the effects of
- carbamazepine (Tegretol).

Felbamate *taken concurrently* with
- other medications toxic to the liver may worsen this effect.
- other medications which cause aplastic anemia may worsen this effect.
- phenytoin (Dilantin) results in a large decrease in felbamate levels. Dosage adjustments must be made.
- carbamazepine (Tegretol) results in a large decrease in felbamate levels. Dosage adjustments will be needed.
- warfarin (Coumadin) may result in serious bleeding.

▷ *Driving, Hazardous Activities:* This drug may cause drowsiness. Restrict activities as necessary.

Aviation Note: The use of this drug *is a disqualification* for piloting. Consult a designated Aviation Medical Examiner.

Exposure to Sun: Use caution. This drug may cause photosensitivity.

Discontinuation: This drug should **not** be stopped abruptly. Ask your doctor for help regarding a gradual discontinuation schedule.

FELODIPINE (fe LOH di peen)

Introduced: 1986　**Prescription:** USA: Yes　**Available as Generic:** No　**Class:** Antihypertensive, calcium channel blocker　**Controlled Drug:** USA: No
Brand Name: Plendil

BENEFITS versus RISKS	
Possible Benefits	*Possible Risks*
EFFECTIVE TREATMENT OF MILD TO MODERATE HYPERTENSION	Peripheral edema (fluid retention in feet and ankles) 22%

▷ **Principal Uses**
As a Single Drug Product: Uses currently included in FDA approved labeling: Treatment of mild to moderate hypertension.

Other (unlabeled) generally accepted uses: (1) Treatment of angina; (2) treatment of arrhythmias; (3) adjunctive treatment of congestive heart failure; (4) useful in inhibiting the progression of atherosclerosis.

How This Drug Works: Controversial, however, by blocking the normal passage of calcium through certain cell walls (which is necessary for the function of nerve and muscle tissue), this drug slows the spread of electrical activity and reduces contraction of peripheral arterial walls, lowering the blood pressure.

Felodipine

Available Dosage Forms and Strengths
  Tablets (sustained release) — 5 mg, 10 mg

▷ **Recommended Dosage Ranges** (Actual dosage and administration schedule must be determined by the physician for each patient individually.)
  Infants and Children: Dosage not established.
  12 to 60 Years of Age: Initially 5 mg, once daily. Increase dose as needed and tolerated at intervals of 2 weeks. The usual dosage range is 5 to 10 mg, once daily. The total daily dose should not exceed 20 mg, once daily.
  Over 60 Years of Age: Same as 12 to 60 years of age. The total daily dose should not exceed 10 mg, once daily.

Conditions Requiring Dosing Adjustments
  Liver function: When felodipine is used in patients with liver compromise, the starting dose should be 5 mg per day with a maximum of 10 mg per day.
  Kidney function: The kidneys are not significantly involved in elimination of felodipine.

▷ **Dosing Instructions:** May be taken with or following food to reduce stomach irritation. The tablet should be swallowed whole; do not crush or chew.

Usual Duration of Use: Use on a regular schedule for 2 to 4 weeks is needed to determine this drug's effectiveness in controlling hypertension. The smallest effective dose should be used in long-term (months to years) therapy. Supervision and periodic physician visits are essential.

Possible Advantages of This Drug
  Gradual onset and prolonged duration of action, permitting effective once-a-day treatment.

▷ **This Drug Should Not Be Taken If**
  - you have had an allergic reaction to it previously.
  - you have active liver disease.
  - you have advanced aortic stenosis.
  - you have uncorrected congestive heart failure.

▷ **Inform Your Physician Before Taking This Drug If**
  - you have had an unfavorable response to any calcium blocker drug.
  - you currently take any form of digitalis or a beta blocker drug (see Drug Class Section).
  - you are taking any other drugs that lower blood pressure.
  - you have a history of congestive heart failure, heart attack or stroke.
  - you are subject to disturbances of heart rhythm.
  - you have circulatory impairment to the fingers.
  - you have muscular dystrophy.
  - you have myasthenia gravis.
  - you have a history of impaired liver or kidney function.

Possible Side-Effects (natural, expected and unavoidable drug actions)
  Swelling of feet and ankles (22%), flushing and sensation of warmth (6%).

▷ **Possible Adverse Effects** (unusual, unexpected and infrequent reactions)
  If any of the following develop, consult your physician promptly for guidance.

Mild Adverse Effects
    Allergic Reactions: Skin rash (1.5%).
    Headache (18%), dizziness (5%), fatigue (4%).
    Indigestion (2%), nausea (2%), stomach pain (2%), constipation or diarrhea (1%).
    Palpitations (up to 23%).
    Peripheral edema (22%).
    Sleep disorders.
    Pharyngitis (2%).
    Abnormal growth of the gums (gingival hyperplasia) (0.5%).
Serious Adverse Effects
    Allergic Reactions: None reported.
    Idiosyncratic Reactions: None reported.
    Tachycardia (up to 23%).
    Aggravation of angina.
    Decreased hemoglobin, hematocrit and red blood cell count.

▷ **Possible Effects on Sexual Function:** None reported.

▷ **Adverse Effects That May Mimic Natural Diseases or Disorders**
    An allergic rash and swelling of the legs may resemble erysipelas.

Possible Effects on Laboratory Tests
    None reported.

CAUTION
1. Tell all of your health care providers that you are taking this drug. Carry a note that says you take felodipine.
2. You may use nitroglycerin and other nitrate drugs as needed to relieve acute episodes of angina pain. However, if your angina attacks are becoming more frequent or intense, call your doctor promptly.

Precautions for Use
    By Infants and Children: Safety and effectiveness for those under 12 years of age not established.
    By Those over 60 Years of Age: You may be more susceptible to the development of weakness, dizziness, fainting and falling. Take necessary precautions to prevent injury.

▷ **Advisability of Use During Pregnancy**
    Pregnancy Category: C. See Pregnancy Code at the back of this book.
    Animal studies: No information available.
    Human studies: Adequate studies of pregnant women are not available.
    Avoid this drug during the first 3 months. Use during the last 6 months only if clearly needed. Ask physician for guidance.

Advisability of Use if Breast-Feeding
    Presence of this drug in breast milk: Unknown.
    Avoid drug or refrain from nursing.

Habit-Forming Potential: None.

Effects of Overdosage: Weakness, light-headedness, fainting, fast pulse, low blood pressure, shortness of breath, flushed and warm skin, tremors.

Possible Effects of Long-Term Use: None reported.

Suggested Periodic Examinations While Taking This Drug (at physician's discretion)
Evaluations of heart function, including electrocardiograms; measurements of blood pressure in supine, sitting and standing positions.

▷ **While Taking This Drug, Observe the Following**
Foods: No restrictions. Avoid excessive salt intake.
Beverages: Grapefruit juice can cause a serious increase in the absorption of this drug. Levels may be increased by over 400%. Do **not** take this drug with grapefruit juice. May be taken with milk.

▷ *Alcohol:* Use with caution—alcohol may exaggerate the drop in blood pressure experienced by some individuals.
Tobacco Smoking: Nicotine may reduce the effectiveness of this drug. Follow your physician's advice regarding smoking.

▷ *Other Drugs*
Felodipine *taken concurrently* with
- beta blocker drugs or digitalis preparations (see Drug Classes) may affect heart rate and rhythm adversely. Careful monitoring by your physician is necessary if these drugs are taken concurrently.
- digoxin may increase digoxin levels and result in toxicity.
- magnesium (particularly in high doses) can cause low blood pressure.
- phenobarbital can cause decreased felodipine benefits.
- phenytoin may cause decreased phenytoin levels.

The following drug may *increase* the effects of felodipine
- cimetidine (Tagamet).

▷ *Driving, Hazardous Activities:* Usually no restrictions. This drug may cause dizziness. Restrict activities as necessary.
Aviation Note: Hypertension *is a disqualification* for piloting. Consult a designated Aviation Medical Examiner.
Exposure to Sun: No restrictions.
Exposure to Heat: Caution advised. Hot environments can exaggerate the blood-pressure-lowering effects of this drug. Observe for light-headedness or weakness.
Discontinuation: Do not stop this drug abruptly. Ask your physician about gradual withdrawal. Watch for development of rebound hypertension.

FENAMATES
(Nonsteroidal Antiinflammatory Drugs)

Meclofenamate (MEK low fen a mate) **Mefenamic acid** (MEF en amik a sid)

Introduced: 1977, 1966 **Prescription:** USA: Yes; Canada: Yes **Available as Generic:** Yes **Class:** NSAID, mild analgesic **Controlled Drug:** USA: No; Canada: No

Brand Names: Meclodium, Meclomen, Meclodium, Ponstel, ✦Ponstan

BENEFITS versus RISKS	
Possible Benefits	*Possible Risks*
EFFECTIVE RELIEF OF MILD TO MODERATE PAIN AND INFLAMMATION	Gastrointestinal pain, ulceration, bleeding (rare) Rare kidney damage Rare fluid retention Rare bone marrow depression Rare hemolytic anemia (mefenamic acid) Rare systemic lupus erythematosus (mefenamic acid) Rare pancreatitis (mefenamic acid)

▷ **Principal Uses**
  As a Single Drug Product: Uses currently included in FDA approved labeling: (1) Meclofenamate is used to relieve pain of osteoarthritis and rheumatoid arthritis; (2) Mefenamic acid is used to relieve chronic pain; painful menstruation (dysmenorrhea) and postoperative pain.
  Other (unlabeled) generally accepted uses: (1) Meclofenamate is used to treat temperal arteritis and the nephrotic syndrome; (2) Mefenamic acid is used to treat PMS, osteoarthritis (maximum one week) and temperal arteritis.

How These Drugs Work: These drugs reduce tissue levels of prostaglandins (and related substances), chemicals involved in the production of inflammation and pain.

Available Dosage Forms and Strengths
  Meclofenamate (Meclomen):
  Capsules — 50 mg, 100 mg
  Mefenamic acid (Ponstel)
  Capsule — 250 mg

▷ **Usual Adult Dosage Range:** Meclofenamate:
  200 to 400 mg daily, in 3 or 4 divided doses. Total daily dosage should not exceed 400 mg.
  Mefenamic acid:
  500 mg initially, then 250 mg every 6 hours taken with food.
  Note: Actual dosage and administration schedule must be determined by the physician for each patient individually.

Conditions Requiring Dosing Adjustments
  Liver function: Changes in dosing are not presently recommended in liver compromise.
  Kidney function: Meclofenamate is kidney eliminated, however specific dosing guidelines have not been elaborated. Mefenamic acid should **not** be used in patients with compromised kidneys.

▷ **Dosing Instructions:** Take with food or milk to prevent stomach irritation. Take with a full glass of water and remain upright (do not lie down) for 30 minutes. The capsule may be opened for administration.

Usual Duration of Use: Meclofenamate: Use on a regular schedule for 2 to 3 weeks usually determines effectiveness in arthritis therapy. Long-term use (months to years) requires physician supervision and periodic evaluation.
Mefenamic acid: Peak levels occur in up to 4 hours. Use beyond seven days is not recommended.

▷ **These Drugs Should Not Be Taken If**
- you have had an allergic reaction to them previously.
- you are subject to asthma or nasal polyps caused by aspirin.
- you have active peptic ulcer disease, regional enteritis, ulcerative colitis or any form of gastrointestinal bleeding.
- you have a bleeding disorder or a blood cell disorder.
- you have severe impairment of kidney function.
- you have systemic lupus erythematosus (mefenamic acid)
- you have recently had pancreatitis (mefenamic acid).

▷ **Inform Your Physician Before Taking These Drugs If**
- you are allergic to aspirin or to other aspirin substitutes.
- you have a history of peptic ulcer disease, regional enteritis or ulcerative colitis.
- you have a history of any type of bleeding disorder.
- you have impaired liver or kidney function.
- you have high blood pressure or a history of heart failure.
- you take: acetaminophen, aspirin or other aspirin substitutes, anticoagulants, oral antidiabetic drugs or cortisonelike drugs.

Possible Side-Effects (natural, expected and unavoidable drug actions)
Ringing in ears, fluid retention.

▷ **Possible Adverse Effects** (unusual, unexpected and infrequent reactions)
If any of the following develop, consult your physician promptly for guidance.

Mild Adverse Effects
Allergic Reactions: Skin rash, hives, itching.
Headache, dizziness, altered or blurred vision, depression.
Mouth sores, indigestion, nausea, vomiting (11%), diarrhea (10% to 33%, sometimes severe).

Serious Adverse Effects
Allergic Reactions: Severe skin reactions, drug fever (see Glossary).
Active peptic ulcer, with or without bleeding.
Kidney damage with painful urination, bloody urine, reduced urine formation.
Rare bone marrow depression (see Glossary)—fatigue, weakness, fever, sore throat, abnormal bleeding or bruising.
Mefenamic acid: Also causes rare hemolytic anemia, seizures, porphyria, liver damage, pancreatitis and systemic lupus erythematosus.

▷ **Possible Effects on Sexual Function**
None reported.

Possible Delayed Adverse Effects: Mild anemia due to "silent" blood loss from the stomach (less than that caused by aspirin).

Natural Diseases or Disorders That May Be Activated by These Drugs
Peptic ulcer disease, ulcerative colitis.

Possible Effects on Laboratory Tests
Complete blood cell counts: decreased red cells, hemoglobin, white cells and platelets (all rare). For mefenamic acid also add SLE test.

CAUTION
1. Dosage should always be limited to the smallest amount that produces reasonable improvement.
2. This drug may mask early indications of infection. Inform your physician if you think you are developing an infection of any kind.
3. Mefenamic acid should be used for a maximum of seven days.

Precautions for Use
By Infants and Children: Safety and effectiveness for those under 14 years of age have not been established for meclofenamate and 18 years of age for mefenamic acid.

By Those over 60 Years of Age: Small doses are advisable until tolerance is determined. Observe for any indications of liver or kidney toxicity, fluid retention, dizziness, confusion, impaired memory, stomach bleeding or diarrhea.

▷ **Advisability of Use During Pregnancy**
Pregnancy Category: Meclofenamate: B, normally and D in the last three months of pregnancy. Mefenamic acid: C. See Pregnancy Code at the back of this book.

Animal studies: Some minor birth defects reported in rodents for meclofenamate. Increased fetal resorption in rabbits with 2.5 times the human mefanamic acid dose.

Human studies: Adequate studies of pregnant women are not available.

Avoid meclofenamate during the first and last 3 months. Ask physician for guidance regarding use during the second 3 months.

The manufacturer does not recommend the use of meclofenamate during pregnancy.

Use of mefenamic acid is late pregnancy should be avoided. Ask your doctor for help regarding mefenamic acid use in pregnancy.

Advisability of Use if Breast-Feeding
Presence of these drugs in breast milk: Yes.
Avoid drug or refrain from nursing.

Habit-Forming Potential: None.

Effects of Overdosage: Drowsiness, nausea, vomiting, diarrhea, marked agitation, irrational behavior, metabolic acidosis and seizures.

Possible Effects of Long-Term Use: None identified.

Suggested Periodic Examinations While Taking These Drugs (at physician's discretion)
Complete blood cell counts, kidney function tests, complete eye examinations if vision is altered in any way.

▷ **While Taking These Drugs, Observe the Following**
Foods: No restrictions.
Beverages: No restrictions. May be taken with milk.
▷ *Alcohol:* Use with caution. The irritant action of alcohol on the stomach lining, added to the irritant action of this drug in sensitive individuals, can increase the risk of stomach ulceration and/or bleeding.

Tobacco Smoking: No interactions expected.
▷ *Other Drugs*
Meclofenamate may *increase* the effects of
- acetaminophen (Tylenol, etc.), and increase the risk of kidney damage; avoid prolonged use of this combination.
- anticoagulants (Coumadin, etc.), and increase the risk of bleeding; monitor prothrombin time, adjust dose accordingly.

Meclofenamate *taken concurrently* with the following drugs may increase the risk of bleeding; avoid these combinations:
- aspirin.
- dipyridamole (Persantine).
- sulfinpyrazone (Anturane).
- valproic acid (Depakene).

Mefenamic acid *taken concurrently with*
- magnesium containing antacids may result in rapid mefenamic acid toxicity.
- anticoagulants (Coumadin, etc.) will displace the drugs from binding sites and increase bleeding risk.
- aspirin, dipyridamole or sulfinpyrazone may result in increased bleeding risk.

Meclofenamate or mefenamic acid *taken concurrently with*
- diuretics (see Drug Class) may result in decreased effectiveness of the diuretic in controlling blood pressure.
- lithium will increase blood lithium levels over time and may result in toxicity.
- methotrexate will result in serious methotrexate toxicity.

▷ *Driving, Hazardous Activities:* This drug may cause dizziness or altered vision. Restrict activities as necessary.

Aviation Note: The use of these drugs *may be a disqualification* for piloting. Consult a designated Aviation Medical Examiner.

Exposure to Sun: No restrictions.

FENOPROFEN (fen oh PROH fen)

Introduced: 1976 **Prescription:** USA: Yes; Canada: Yes **Available as Generic:** Yes **Class:** Mild analgesic, anti-inflammatory **Controlled Drug:** USA: No; Canada: No
Brand Name: Nalfon

BENEFITS versus RISKS	
Possible Benefits	*Possible Risks*
EFFECTIVE RELIEF OF MILD TO MODERATE PAIN AND INFLAMMATION	Gastrointestinal pain, ulceration, bleeding (rare) Rare liver or kidney damage Rare fluid retention Rare bone marrow depression

Please see the propionic-acid, nonsteroidal anti-inflammatory drug profile for further information.

FENTANYL TRANSDERMAL (FEN ta nil Tranz dur mull)

Introduced: 1991 **Prescription:** USA: Yes; Canada: Yes **Available as Generic:** USA: No; Canada: No **Class:** Narcotic analgesic **Controlled Drug:** USA:C-ll*
Brand Names: Duragesic

BENEFITS versus RISKS	
Possible Benefits	*Possible Risks*
EFFECTIVE PAIN RELIEF WITH A PATCH APPLIED TO THE SKIN	Habit-forming potential with prolonged use
PATCH APPLICATION NEEDED ONLY ONCE EVERY THREE DAYS	Impaiment of mental function
	Methemoglobinemia (rare)
	Respiratory depression

▷ **Principal Uses**
    As a Single Drug Product: Uses currently included in FDA approved labeling:
        (1) Treatment of chronic pain.
    Other (unlabeled) generally accepted uses: None.
How This Drug Works: This drug acts at specific pain receptors (Mu agonist) to block pain.
Available Dosage Forms and Strengths
    Transdermal patch — 2.5 mg, 5 mg, 7.5 mg, 10 mg
▷ **Recommended Dosage Ranges (Actual dosage and administration schedule must be determined by the physician for each patient individually.)**
    Infants and Children: Safety and efficacy for those under 12 years of age not established.
    18 to 60 Years of Age: Not indicated for patients 18 years old who weigh less than 50 kg (110 lbs).
    In patients who have not been using opiods such as morphine, the 25 mcg/hr (2.5 mg) patch should be used.
    In people who have been given opiods previously, the amount needed to control pain on a 24 hour basis is calculated, converted to an equal amount of morphine (morphine equianalgesic dose), and then converted to fentanyl.
    Over 60 Years of Age: These people should receive the 25 mcg/hr (2.5 mg) patch, unless they were already receiving the equivalent of 135 mg of oral morphine daily. Intravenous fentanyl has been cleared more slowly in this population than in younger patients, and careful observation for overdose should be made.
Conditions Requiring Dosing Adjustments
    Liver function: The dose must be decreased in liver compromise.
    Kidney function: In moderate to severe kidney failure, 75% of the usual dose should be given.
    In severe kidney failure, the dose should be reduced by 50%.
▷ **Dosing Instructions:** The patch should be removed from its protective pouch, and the stiff protective liner removed from the sticky side of the patch. Do

*See schedules of Controlled Drugs at the back of this book.

not cut or damage the system. The sticky side of the patch should be applied to a non-hairy, dry area such as the back, chest, flank or upper arm. Avoid any skin which is burned, irritated or excessively oily. Wash your hands once you have successfully applied the patch. Once the patch has been worn for three days, a new patch should be applied to a different area. The exhausted patch should be folded onto itself and flushed down the toilet. Avoid exposing the patch to external heat sources such as electric blankets or heating pads.

Usual Duration of Use: Use on a regular schedule for one to three days usually determines effectiveness in controlling pain. An immediate release form of morphine or similar opioid should be available for pain control while this drug reaches its peak effect. Long-term use (months) requires periodic physician evaluation of response and dosage adjustment of both the patch and an immediate release form of morphine or similar drug.

Possible Advantages of This Drug

Effective pain relief with patch placement once every three days and no injections.

▷ **This Drug Should Not Be Taken If**
- you have had an allergic reaction to any dosage form of it previously.
- you have mild or intermittent pain.
- you have acute or postoperative pain without opportunity for proper dose adjustment.

▷ **Inform Your Physician Before Taking This Drug If**
- you have liver or kidney compromise.
- you have chronic lung disease.
- you have an abnormally slow heart beat or other heart disease.
- you develop a high fever.
- you take a MAO inhibitor (see Drug Classes).
- you have a brain tumor.
- you are anemic.
- you have a history of alcoholism or drug abuse.
- you take other prescription or non-prescription medicines which were not discussed with your doctor when transdermal fentanyl was prescribed.

Possible Side-Effects (natural, expected and unavoidable drug actions)

Constipation, dry mouth and sleepiness (10% or greater).

▷ **Possible Adverse Effects** (unusual, unexpected and infrequent reactions)

If any of the following develop, consult your physician promptly for guidance.

Mild Adverse Effects

Allergic Reactions: Skin rash and itching.
Nausea and vomiting (10%).
Sleepiness and confusion (10% or greater).
Sweatiness and constipation (10% or greater).
Blurred vision.
Tremor.
Amblyopia ($<1\%$).

Serious Adverse Effects

Allergic Reactions: Exfoliative dermatitis and/or anaphylactoid reactions.
Arrhythmias (rare).
Paranoid reaction (rare).

Depersonalization and stupor (dose related or rare).
Seizures (rare).
Hallucinations (3–10%).
Methemoglobinemia.
Parasthesias (1%).
Urinary retention (3–10%).
Porphyrias (rare).
Respiratory depression (3–10%).

▷ **Possible Effects on Sexual Function:** Impotence and blunted orgasm sensation in men. Irregular menstrual periods and blunted orgasm sensation in women.

Possible Delayed Adverse Effects: Dependence and tolerance.

Possible Effects on Laboratory Tests
Methemoglobinemia.

CAUTION
1. Extreme caution should be used if this drug is combined with other opioids, narcotic drugs, benzodiazepines or alcohol.
2. May cause serious constipation in older patients.
3. Do not expose the patch site to external sources of heat such as heating pads or electric blankets as an increased rate of drug release may occur.

Precautions for Use
By Infants and Children:
Safety and effectiveness for those under 12 years of age not established.
By Those over 60 Years of Age: The 25 mcg patch should be used as a starting dose unless you are already taking more than 135 mg of morphine daily. Those with cardiac, respiratory kidney or liver compromise should be given low doses and be carefully monitored.

▷ **Advisability of Use During Pregnancy**
Pregnancy Category: C, D if used in high doses when the baby is born or for prolonged periods. See Pregnancy Code at the back of this book.
Animal studies: Some fetal death data with intravenous use in rats.
Human studies: Adequate studies of pregnant women are not available.
Ask your doctor for guidance.

Advisability of Use if Breast-Feeding
Presence of this drug in breast milk: Yes.
Avoid drug or refrain from nursing.

Habit-Forming Potential: Fentanyl is a schedule two narcotic and can cause dependence resembling morphine dependence. Physical and psychological dependence and tolerance can occur with repeated use.

Effects of Overdosage: Dizziness, amnesia and stupor. Respiratory depression and apnea may occur.

Possible Effects of Long-Term Use: Tolerance and physical or psychological dependence.

Suggested Periodic Examinations While Taking This Drug (at physician's discretion)
Liver function tests.

▷ **While Taking This Drug, Observe the Following**
Foods: No restrictions.
Beverages: No restrictions.

▷ *Alcohol:* Avoid the combination. Additive results in loss of mental status, respiratory depression and confusion.
Tobacco Smoking: No interactions expected.
Marijuana Smoking: Additive adverse effects; however, marijuana may block the vomiting effect of fentanyl.

▷ *Other Drugs*
Fentanyl may *increase* the effects of
- benzodiazepines such as diazepam (Valium) and alprazolam (Xanax).
- central nervous system depressants such as opiates, barbiturates, tranquilizers, and tricyclic antidepressants.

Fentanyl *taken concurrently* with
- amiodarone (Codarone) may result in heart (cardiac) toxicity.
- MAO inhibitors (see Drug Class) may worsen the lowering of blood pressure and depression of breathing seen with fentanyl.

▷ *Driving, Hazardous Activities:* This drug may cause drowsiness, sedation and respiratory depression. Restrict activities as necessary.
Aviation Note: The use of this drug *is a disqualification* for piloting. Consult a designated Aviation Medical Examiner.
Exposure to Sun: No restrictions.
Discontinuation: The patch may be removed if the drug is not tolerated or is to be stopped. Once the patch is removed, fentanyl will still continue to be released from the patch site for 17 hours or more. Ideally, if pain medicine is still needed, the chosen alternative should be substituted, and fentanyl transdermal slowly tapered.

FILGRASTIM (Phil GRA stem)

Other Names: Recombinant G-CSF

Introduced: 1991 **Prescription:** USA: Yes; Canada: Yes **Available as Generic:** USA: No; Canada: No **Class:** Hematopoietic agent **Controlled Drug:** USA: No; Canada: No

Brand Names: Neupogen

BENEFITS versus RISKS	
Possible Benefits	*Possible Risks*
PREVENTION OF INFECTIONS DUE TO LOWERED WHITE BLOOD CELL COUNTS: FOLLOWING CHEMOTHERAPY FOLLOWING BONE MARROW TRANSPLANT IN PATIENTS WITH CHRONIC OR CYCLIC NEUTROPENIA INCREASED WHITE BLOOD CELLS IN AIDS PATIENTS CORRECTION OF DRUG-INDUCED LOWERING OF WHITE BLOOD CELLS	Bone pain Changes in heart waves (rare)

Filgrastim

▷ **Principal Uses**

As a Single Drug Product: Uses currently included in FDA approved labeling: (1) Used to help white blood cell counts recover after chemotherapy and bone marrow transplants; (2) used subcutaneously or intravenously to reduce or prevent low white blood cell counts which occur after cancer chemotherapy; (3) treats patients who have an absence of white blood cells at birth; (4) used to help patients with Kostman's syndrome have improved white blood cell counts; (5) used to help patients who have low white blood cell counts (neutropenia) of unknown cause (idiopathic).

Other (unlabeled) generally accepted uses: (1) Helps patients recover from a particular kind of lack of white blood cells (agranulocytosis) which has been caused by medications (drug-induced); (2) used in AIDS patients to help restore white blood cell counts; (3) used to treat patients with severe long-term (chronic) low white blood cell counts; (4) used to treat patients with abnormally low white blood cell and neutrophil counts (myelodysplastic syndrome).

How This Drug Works: This drug is made by recombinant technology and is one of the many acknowledged hematopoietic growth factors. Filgrastin regulates the proliferation and release of early (progenitor) forms of white blood cells. This medicine also can tell the bone marrow to increase the rate at which it makes white blood cells. Filgrastim may also work with other factors to increase the production of blood platelets.

Available Dosage Forms and Strengths

Solution for injection — 300 mcg per ml (supplied as a 300 or 480 mcg vial)

How To Store

The prepared solution should be stored at 36 to 46 degrees Fahrenheit (2 to 8 degrees Centigrade). This medicine **should not** be frozen. Some centers draw up a seven-day supply of syringes which are then stored in a refirgerator.

▷ **Recommended Dosage Ranges (Actual dosage and administration schedule must be determined by the physician for each patient individually.)**

Infants and Children: The medicine has been studied in this population and doses of 0.6 to 120 mcgs per kilogram per day for up to three years have been well tolerated. These doses have been used in children 3 months to 18 years of age. In chronic low white blood cell counts (chronic neutropenia), doses of 5 to 10 mcg per kilogram per day have been used.

18 to 60 Years of Age: Patients receiving therapy which destroys the bone marrow (myeloablative treatment) and then are given a bone marrow transplant should wait 24 hours after the chemotherapy was given and 24 hours after bone marrow transplant, then receive 10 mcg per kg per day as a starting dose. This dose is adjusted depending on the degree of increase of white blood cells (absolute neutrophil count).

Patients receiving medicine which suppresses the bone marrow: Should wait until 24 hours after or 24 hours before the chemotherapy is given. In this population, filgrastim therapy is started with 5 mcg per kilogram per day. Doses may be increased by 5 mcg per kg per day for each cycle of chemotherapy based on the severity of the lowering of white blood cell count (nadir) and how long the lowered white cell (absolute neutrophil) count lasts. This drug can be given daily for up to 14 days.

Over 60 Years of Age: Same as 12 to 60 years of age.

Conditions Requiring Dosing Adjustments
Liver function: Not significantly involved in the elimination of this drug.
Kidney function: Roughly 90% of a given filgrastim dose is eliminated by the kidneys. Changes in dosing are not defined.

▷ **Dosing Instructions:** The solution in the reconstituted vial should be colorless and clear. Once your doctor or nurse has taught you how to inject the medicine:
1. Make certain the solution has not expired (check the expiration date).
2. Make certain you have the correct kind of syringe (insulin syringes are commonly used).
3. Follow the provided patient instructions carefully.
4. If your are using a syringe, make certain you inject the medicine under the skin, not into a vein.
5. This medicine can also be given intravenously over a period of 15 to 30 minutes.

Usual Duration of Use: Continual use on a regular schedule for up to two weeks (10 to 14 days) may be needed to determine this drug's effectiveness in correcting low white blood (absolute neutrophil) count after chemotherapy. Bone marrow transplant patients may take still longer to respond. Long-term problems with white blood cells (such as chronic neutropenia) may require years of therapy. Long-term use requires periodic evaluation of response and dosage adjustment. Consult your physician on a regular basis.

Possible Advantages of This Drug
Effective recombinant product with few side effects.

▷ **This Drug Should Not Be Taken If**
- you have had an allergic reaction to any dosage form of it previously.
- known allergy to E. coli (a bacteria) derived products.

▷ **Inform Your Physician Before Taking This Drug If**
- you have a history of gout.
- you have a history of psoriasis.
- you have received chemotherapy within the last 24 hours.
- you have a history of heart problems.
- you have a history of leukemia (myeloid type). This safety and efficacy of this medicine is not established in that condition.
- you have a history of cancer (with myeloid characteristics). There is a possibility that this drug may act as a growth factor for these tumors. Use, however, in a small number of leukemia patients has not resulted in worsening of their leukemia.
- you are uncertain of how much filgrastim to take or how often to take it.

Possible Side-Effects (natural, expected and unavoidable drug actions)
Pain on injection.
Bone pain (up to 22% in Phase Three studies).

▷ **Possible Adverse Effects** (unusual, unexpected and infrequent reactions)
If any of the following develop, consult your physician promptly for guidance.
Mild Adverse Effects
Allergic Reactions: Skin rash or itching.
Mild decreases in blood pressure.

Mild increases in uric acid.
Nausea and anorexias (rare).
Bone pain (mild to moderate) (up to 22%).
Enlargement of the spleen (reported in patients with chronic lowering of the white blood cells (chronic neutropenia).
Serious Adverse Effects
Allergic Reactions: Anaphylaxis (rare).
Depression of part of the heart action (ST depression) (rare).
Sweet syndrome (acute neutrophilic dermatosis).
Worsening of psoriasis.
Potential (though not yet reported) for this medicine to act as a growth factor for certain cancers (malignancies of the myeloid type).

▷ **Possible Effects on Sexual Function:** None reported.

Possible Delayed Adverse Effects: Increased uric acid.

▷ **Adverse Effects That May Mimic Natural Diseases or Disorders**
None reported.

Natural Diseases or Disorders That May Be Activated by This Drug
Gout.

Possible Effects on Laboratory Tests
Absolute neutrophil count: increased.
Alkaline phosphatase: increased.
Uric acid: increased mildly.
Lactate dehydrogenase (LDH): increased.

CAUTION
1. Bone pain may be prevented by taking acetaminophen (Tylenol, others) before this medicine is injected.
2. Call your doctor if you have chills, fever or any other sign of infection.
3. Be certain to follow up with your laboratory testing as scheduled.
4. The solution in the vial should be clear. Do **not** inject any discolored or cloudy solution.
5. Make sure you have the correct kind of syringe before you inject this medicine.
6. This medicine can be given intravenously when it is appropriately prepared. If your doctor has instructed you on how to give yourself an injection using a syringe, the medicine should be given under the skin. Be certain you understand the technique.
7. Always change the site in which you inject this medicine as your doctor instructed.

Precautions for Use
By Infants and Children:
This medicine has been used in children with long-term lowering of white blood cell counts (chronic neutropenia) in doses of 5 to 10 mcg per kg per day.
By Those over 60 Years of Age: No specific precautions.

▷ **Advisability of Use During Pregnancy**
Pregnancy Category: C. See Pregnancy Code at the back of this book.
Animal studies: In rabbits given 80 mcg per kg per day (very high doses), increased abortion and death of embryos were observed.

Human studies: Information from adequate studies of pregnant women is not available. Ask your doctor for help with this benefit to risk decision.

Advisability of Use if Breast-Feeding
Presence of this drug in breast milk: Unknown.
Ask your doctor for guidance.

Habit-Forming Potential: None.

Effects of Overdosage: No maximum tolerated dose has been identified.

Possible Effects of Long-Term Use: Enlarged spleens may occur in up to 25% of patients (splenomegaly) with severe chronic neutropenia. Skin rashes may occur in up to 6% of patients.

Suggested Periodic Examinations While Taking This Drug (at physician's discretion)
Complete blood cell counts and platelet counts should be obtained prior to chemotherapy and twice weekly during filgrastim therapy.

▷ **While Taking This Drug, Observe the Following**
Foods: No restrictions.
Beverages: No restrictions.
▷ *Alcohol:* No restrictions.
Tobacco Smoking: No interactions expected.
▷ *Other Drugs*
Filgrastim *taken concurrently* with
- lithium (Lithobid, others) may (in theory) result in additive release of white blood cells.

▷ *Driving, Hazardous Activities:* No restrictions presently attributed to this medicine.
Aviation Note: The use of this drug *is probably not a disqualification* for piloting. Consult a designated Aviation Medical Examiner.
Exposure to Sun: No restrictions.
Occurrence of Unrelated Illness: Report development of chills, fever or other signs or symptoms of infection immediately to your doctor.
Discontinuation: In patients receiving medicine which suppresses the bone marrow: the drug is usually stopped if a white count (absolute neutrophil count) reaches 10,000 per cubic millimeter after the expected lowest white blood cell count is reached specific to the chemotherapy which was given.
In people receiving medicine which destroys the bone marrow and subsequently have a bone marrow transplant: The drug is started as described earlier. If the white blood cell count reaches 1,000 per cubic millimeter, the dose is decreased to 5 mcg per kilogram per day. Once the white blood cell count reaches 1,000 per cubic millimeter for six consecutive days, filgrastim can be stopped.
Special Storage Instructions: This drug should be stored at 36 to 46 degrees Fahrenheit once it has been reconstituted. Care should be taken *not to shake* the prepared drug as it may lose activity. Care should also be taken *not to freeze* the prepared medicine as it will clump and lose therapeutic activity.
Observe the Following Expiration Times: Once the medicine is prepared, it is stable for one day (24 hours) if it is refrigerated. If the drug is stored at room temperature, it is stable for 24 hours. Medicine left at room temperature for more than 24 hours should be returned.

FINASTERIDE (Fin ES tur ide)

Introduced: 1992 **Prescription:** USA: Yes; Canada: Yes **Available as Generic:** USA: No; Canada: No **Class:** 5-alpha reductase inhibitor
Controlled Drug: USA: No; Canada: No
Brand Name: Proscar

BENEFITS versus RISKS	
Possible Benefits	*Possible Risks*
NONSURGICAL TREATMENT OF SYMPTOMATIC BENIGN PROSTATIC HYPERPLASIA, shrinkage of prostatic tissue, and increase in urine flow.	IMPOTENCE (3.7%) Decreased libido (3.3%)

▷ **Principal Uses**
As a Single Drug Product: Uses currently included in FDA approved labeling: Treatment of symptomatic benign prostatic hyperplasia (BPH). Maximum shrinkage of the prostate has occurred after six months of therapy. Other (unlabeled) generally accepted uses: A study of 200 men showed 58% had clinically significant hair growth after one year of use.

How This Drug Works: Finasteride blocks an enzyme (chemical responsable for helping a chemical reaction take place) called 5-alpha reductase. This effect blocks the conversion of testosterone to dihydrotestosterone in the liver and tissues; when the dihydrotestosterone hormone is not available, the prostate shrinks. When the prostate shrinks, symptoms such as urgency and difficulty in urination improve.

Available Dosage Forms and Strengths
Finasteride (Proscar) tablets — 5 mg

How To Store
Keep at room temperature. Avoid exposure to extreme humidity.

▷ **Recommended Dosage Ranges (Actual dosage and administration schedule must be determined by the physician for each patient individually.)**
Infants and Children: Not indicated.
12 to 60 Years of Age: Symptomatic benign prostatic hyperplasia often does not occur in the younger end of this adult dosing range; however, the dose for this age range is—
5 (five) mg each day taken by mouth.
Over 60 Years of Age: Same as 12 to 60 years of age, unless liver function has decreased.

Conditions Requiring Dosing Adjustments
Liver function: Extensive metabolism occurs in the liver, however, specific guidelines for decreases in doses are not available. People with abnormal liver function tests should be followed more closely by their physicians.
Kidney function:
No dose decreases needed for mild to moderate kidney failure.

▷ **Dosing Instructions:** This medicine is best taken on an empty stomach. Food changes the peak blood concentration that is reached, and may decrease the total amount absorbed.

Usual Duration of Use: Use on a regular schedule for at least 6 (six) months is needed to see this drug's effectiveness in shrinking the prostate and decreasing symptoms.

Possible Advantages of This Drug
May give you symptomatic relief of benign prostatic hyperplasia (BPH) without surgery.

Currently a "Drug of Choice"
for people who have symptomatic BPH and are not candidates for surgery.

▷ **This Drug Should Not Be Taken If**
- you have had an allergic reaction to any dosage form of it previously.

▷ **Inform Your Physician Before Taking This Drug If**
- have a history of impaired liver function or liver disease.
- you have kidney problems of any nature.
- your sexual partner is pregnant.

Possible Side-Effects (natural, expected and unavoidable drug actions)
Usually increases testosterone levels; however, the significance of this effect is not known.

▷ **Possible Adverse Effects** (unusual, unexpected and infrequent reactions)
If any of the following develop, consult your physician promptly for guidance.
Mild Adverse Effects
Allergic Reactions: Rare skin rash, hives.
Increased plasma testosterone.
Serious Adverse Effects
Allergic Reactions: Rare hypersensitivity reactions.

▷ **Possible Effects on Sexual Function:** Impotence (3.7%).
Decreased libido (3.3%).
Decreased volume of ejaculate (2.8%).
Adverse sexual effects may resolve in more than 60% of patients who continue this medication.

Possible Delayed Adverse Effects: Not defined at present.

Possible Effects on Laboratory Tests
Decreased PSA (prostate specific antigen).

CAUTION
1. You should have a digital rectal examination and other examinations for prostate cancer before this medicine is started.
2. If you have a change in liver function, inform your doctor.
3. If your sexual partner is pregnant, avoid exposing your partner to your semen. Exposure to finasteride containing semen may cause genital abnormalities in male offspring.

Precautions for Use
By Infants and Children:
Safety and effectiveness for infants and children not established.
By Those over 60 Years of Age: No specific precautions other than changes related to decreased liver function.

▷ **Advisability of Use During Pregnancy**
Pregnancy Category: X. See Pregnancy Code at the back of this book.
Animal studies: When administered to pregnant rats, the male offspring developed hypospadias. The offspring experienced decreased prostatic and seminal vesicular weight, slow preputial separation and transient nipple problems.
Human studies: Contraindicated in women who are pregnant or who plan to become pregnant. Women who are pregnant must avoid exposure to crushed tablets, and exposure to semen of a sexual partner who is on finasteride.
Ask your physician for guidance.

Advisability of Use if Breast-Feeding
Refrain from nursing if you have been exposed to finasteride or finasteride containing semen.

Habit-Forming Potential: None.

Effects of Overdosage: Multiple doses of up to 80 mg per day have been taken without adverse effect.

Possible Effects of Long-Term Use: Adverse effects of long term use are similar to short-term use effects.

Suggested Periodic Examinations While Taking This Drug (at physician's discretion)
Patients should be monitored for signs and symptoms of hypersensitivity.
Patients should be monitored for improvement in symptoms of BPH.

▷ **While Taking This Drug, Observe the Following**
Foods: This medicine is best taken on an empty stomach.
Beverages: No restrictions.
▷ *Alcohol:* No restrictions.
Tobacco Smoking: No interactions expected.
Marijuana Smoking: No interactions expected.
▷ *Other Drugs*
Finasteride may *decrease* the effects of
• theophylline.
Driving, Hazardous Activities: No restrictions.
Aviation Note: No restrictions.
Exposure to Sun: No restrictions.

FLUCONAZOLE (flu KOHN a zohl)

Introduced: 1985 **Prescription:** USA: Yes; Canada: Yes **Available as Generic:** USA: No; Canada: No **Class:** Antifungal **Controlled Drug:** USA: No; Canada: No

Brand Name: Diflucan

Fluconazole

BENEFITS versus RISKS	
Possible Benefits	**Possible Risks**
EFFECTIVE TREATMENT AND SUPPRESSION OF CRYPTOCOCCAL MENINGITIS	Severe skin reactions (rare)
EFFECTIVE TREATMENT OF CANDIDA INFECTIONS OF THE MOUTH, THROAT AND ESOPHAGUS	Possible liver damage (rare)
EFFECTIVE TREATMENT OF SYSTEMIC CANDIDA INFECTIONS	
Effective one-dose treatment of vaginal yeast infections	

▷ **Principal Uses**

As a Single Drug Product: Uses currently included in FDA approved labeling: (1) Treatment of Candida (yeast) infections of the mouth, throat and esophagus (may be AIDS-related); (2) therapy of systemic Candida infections—pneumonia, peritonitis, urinary tract infections (may be AIDS-related).

Other (unlabeled) generally accepted uses: (1) Prevention of yeast infections in patients with low white blood cell counts, cancer or those taking steroids; (2) treatment and suppression of Cryptococcal meningitis; (3) treatment of some fungal eye infections (endopthalmitis); (4) one dose treatment of vaginal yeast infections; (5) treatment of Aspergillus pneumonia; (6) treatment of candidal urinary tract infections; (7) used to treat some fungal infections which may occur in people who have received transplanted organs.

How This Drug Works: By damaging cell walls and blocking essential cell enzymes, this drug inhibits cell growth and reproduction (with low drug concentrations) and destroys fungal cells (with high drug concentrations).

Available Dosage Forms and Strengths

    Injection — 200 mg in 100 ml and 400 mg in 200 ml
    Tablets — 50 mg, 100 mg, 150 mg, 200 mg
Oral suspension — 50 mg per 5 ml
    — 200 mg per 5 ml

▷ **Recommended Dosage Ranges** (Actual dosage and administration schedule must be determined by the physician for each patient individually.)

Infants and Children: From 3 to 13 years of age—3–6 mg/kg of body weight daily.

13 to 60 Years of Age: For treatment of Cryptococcal meningitis—400 mg once daily until significant improvement occurs; then 200 to 400 mg once daily for 10 to 12 weeks after the cerebrospinal fluid (CSF) culture becomes negative.

For suppression of Cryptococcal meningitis—200 mg once daily.

For treatment of Candida infections of mouth and throat—200 mg on the first day; then 100 mg once daily for 2 weeks.

For treatment of Candida infection of the esophagus—200 mg on the first day; then 100 mg once daily for at least 3 weeks; continue treatment for 2 weeks after all signs of infection are gone. If needed, doses up to 400 mg once daily may be used.

For treatment of systemic Candida infections—400 mg on the first day; then 200 mg once daily for at least 4 weeks; continue treatment for 2 weeks after clearance of all symptoms of infection.

Over 60 Years of Age: Same as 13 to 60 years of age. Dose must be adjusted for impaired kidneys.

Conditions Requiring Dosing Adjustments

Liver function: This drug is a rare cause of hepatitis and should be used with caution in patients with liver compromise.

Kidney function: In mild to moderate kidney failure, 50% of the usual dose should be given every 48 hours. In severe kidney failure, 25% of the usual dose should be given every 48 hours.

▷ **Dosing Instructions:** The tablet may be crushed, and is best taken on an empty stomach; may be taken with or after food to reduce stomach upset.

Usual Duration of Use: Use on a regular schedule for 2 to 4 weeks is usually needed to see this drug's benefit in controlling Candidal or Cryptococcal infections. Actual cures or long-term suppression often require continual treatment for many months. May be continuous therapy in AIDS.

Currently a "Drug of Choice"
for maintenance therapy to prevent relapse following control of AIDS-related Candidal esophagitis.

▷ **This Drug Should Not Be Taken If**
- you have had an allergic reaction to it previously.
- you have active liver disease.

▷ **Inform Your Physician Before Taking This Drug If**
- you are allergic to: clotrimazole, itraconazole, ketoconazole or miconazole.
- you have impaired liver or kidney function.
- you are taking any other drugs currently.
- you tend to have low blood potassium.

▷ **Possible Adverse Effects** (unusual, unexpected and infrequent reactions)
If any of the following develop, consult your physician promptly for guidance.

Mild Adverse Effects
Allergic Reactions: Skin rash (1.8%).
Headache (1.9%).
Nausea (3.7%), vomiting (1.7%), stomach pain (1.7%), diarrhea (1.5%).

Serious Adverse Effects
Allergic Reactions: Severe dermatitis (Stevens Johnson Syndrome) (very rare). Anaphylactoid reactions.
Liver toxicity (rare).
Abnormally low blood platelet counts: Abnormal bruising or bleeding.
Low white blood cell counts.
Seizures (rare).
Adrenal suppression (rare).
Low blood potassium.

▷ **Possible Effects on Sexual Function:** Amenorrhea.

Possible Delayed Adverse Effects: None reported.

▷ **Adverse Effects That May Mimic Natural Diseases or Disorders**
Possible liver reaction may suggest viral hepatitis.

Possible Effects on Laboratory Tests
Blood platelet counts: decreased.
Liver function tests: increased liver enzymes (ALT/GPT, AST/GOT and alkaline phosphatase), increased bilirubin.

Precautions for Use
By Infants and Children: Safety and effectiveness for those under 13 years of age not established.
By Those over 60 Years of Age: Age-related decrease in kidney function may require adjustment of dosage.

▷ **Advisability of Use During Pregnancy**
Pregnancy Category: C. See Pregnancy Code at the back of this book.
Animal studies: Rat studies revealed significant abnormalities in bone growth and development.
Human studies: Adequate studies of pregnant women not available.
Use this drug only if clearly needed. Ask your doctor for help.

Advisability of Use if Breast-Feeding
Presence of this drug in breast milk: Unknown.
Avoid drug or refrain from nursing.

Habit-Forming Potential: None.

Effects of Overdosage: Possible nausea, vomiting, diarrhea.

Possible Effects of Long-Term Use: None reported.

Suggested Periodic Examinations While Taking This Drug (at physician's discretion)
Liver and kidney function tests.

▷ **While Taking This Drug, Observe the Following**
Foods: No restrictions.
Beverages: No restrictions. May be taken with milk.
▷ *Alcohol:* No interactions expected.
Tobacco Smoking: No interactions expected.

▷ *Other Drugs*
Fluconazole may *increase* the effects of
- oral antidiabetic drugs (chlorpropamide, glipizide, glyburide, tolbutamide), and cause hypoglycemia; check glucose levels carefully.
- cyclosporine (Sandimmune).
- phenytoin (Dilantin, etc.), and cause phenytoin toxicity; monitor phenytoin blood levels.
- warfarin (Coumadin), and cause unwanted bleeding; monitor prothrombin times as necessary.

The following drug may *decrease* the effects of fluconazole
- rifampin (Rifadin, Rimactane, etc.).

Fluconazole ***taken concurrently*** with
- astemizole (Hismanal) may result in fatal toxicity to the heart.
- loratidine (Claritin) may result in toxicity to the heart.
- terfenadine (Seldane) may result in toxicity to the heart.
- trimexate may increase trimexate toxicity.

▷ *Driving, Hazardous Activities:* No restrictions.
Aviation Note: The use of this drug is probably not a disqualification for piloting. Consult a designated Aviation Medical Examiner.
Exposure to Sun: No restrictions.
Discontinuation: Take the full course prescribed. Continual treatment for several months may be necessary. Consult your physician regarding the appropriate time to consider discontinuation.

FLUCYTOSINE (flu SI toh seen)

Other Names: 5-fluorocytosine, 5-FC
Introduced: 1977 **Prescription:** USA: Yes; Canada: Yes **Available as Generic:** USA: No; Canada: No **Class:** Antifungal **Controlled Drug:** USA: No; Canada: No
Brand Names: Ancobon, ✦Ancotil

BENEFITS versus RISKS	
Possible Benefits	*Possible Risks*
EFFECTIVE ADJUNCTIVE TREATMENT OF CERTAIN INFECTIONS CAUSED BY CANDIDA, CRYPTOCOCCUS FUNGI and Aspergillus	BONE MARROW DEPRESSION (8 to 13%)
	DRUG-INDUCED LIVER DAMAGE (10 to 25%)
	Peripheral neuritis
Effective adjunctive treatment of chromomycosis infection.	Ulcerative colitis (rare)

▷ **Principal Uses**
As a Single Drug Product: Uses currently included in FDA approved labeling: (1) Treatment of endocarditis, osteomyelitis, arthritis, meningitis, pneumonia, septicemia and urinary tract infections caused by Candida; (2) treatment of meningitis, pneumonia, septicemia, endocarditis and urinary tract infections caused by Cryptococcus. These infections are often AIDS-related.
Other (unlabeled) generally accepted uses: (1) Treatment of disseminated Candidiasis, Chromomycosis and Cryptococcosis. These infections may be AIDS-related; (2) treatment of general fungal infections.
Note: Flucytosine is usually used together with amphotericin B to treat disseminated fungal infections.
How This Drug Works: This drug goes into fungal cells and blocks production of RNA and DNA, thus inhibiting fungal development and reproduction.
Available Dosage Forms and Strengths
Capsules — 250 mg, 500 mg
▷ **Recommended Dosage Ranges** (Actual dosage and administration schedule must be determined by the physician for each patient individually.)
Infants and Children: 12.5 to 37.5 mg/kg of body weight, every 6 hours; or 375 to 562.5 mg/M^2 of body surface, every 6 hours.
12 to 60 Years of Age: 12.5 to 37.5 mg/kg of body weight, every 6 hours.
Over 60 Years of Age: Same as 12 to 60 years of age. If kidney function is impaired, dosage reduction is mandatory.

Conditions Requiring Dosing Adjustments

Liver function: In mild to moderate hepatic compromise, changes in dosage do not presently appear to be needed. Flucytosine has been associated with liver toxicity (especially with blood levels greater than 100 mcg/ml), and should be used with caution in patients with liver compromise.

Kidney function: In mild to moderate kidney failure, the usual dose can be given every 12–24 hours. In severe kidney failure, the usual dose can be given every 24–48 hours.

▷ **Dosing Instructions:** If a single dose requires more than one capsule, space administration over a period of 15 minutes to reduce stomach irritation and nausea. The capsule may be opened and taken with or after food.

Usual Duration of Use: Use on a regular schedule for 4 to 6 weeks is needed to see effectiveness in controlling candida or cryptococcal infection. Long-term use (months to years) requires periodic physician evaluation.

Currently a "Drug of Choice"
for treatment of Cryptococcal meningitis, taken together with amphotericin B.

▷ **This Drug Should Not Be Taken If**
- you have had an allergic reaction to it previously.
- you have an active blood cell or bone marrow disorder.
- you have active liver disease.

▷ **Inform Your Physician Before Taking This Drug If**
- you have a history of drug-induced bone marrow depression.
- you have a history of peripheral neuritis.
- you have impaired liver or kidney function.

Possible Side-Effects (natural, expected and unavoidable drug actions)
None.

▷ **Possible Adverse Effects** (unusual, unexpected and infrequent reactions)
If any of the following develop, consult your physician promptly for guidance.

Mild Adverse Effects
Allergic Reactions: Skin rash, itching.
Headache, dizziness, drowsiness, confusion, hallucinations.
Loss of appetite, nausea, vomiting, stomach pain, diarrhea.

Serious Adverse Effects
Allergic Reactions: Anaphylactoid reactions.
Bone marrow depression (see Glossary): fatigue, weakness, fever, sore throat, abnormal bleeding or bruising.
Liver damage, with or without jaundice (see Glossary).
Peripheral neuritis (see Glossary).
Bowel perforation (rare).
Kidney damage (rare).

▷ **Possible Effects on Sexual Function:** None reported.

▷ **Adverse Effects That May Mimic Natural Diseases or Disorders**
Drug-induced hepatitis may suggest viral hepatitis.

Natural Diseases or Disorders That May Be Activated by This Drug
Crohn's disease, ulcerative colitis.

Possible Effects on Laboratory Tests
Complete blood counts: decreased red cells, hemoglobin, white cells and platelets.
Liver function tests: increased liver enzymes (ALT/GPT, AST/GOT and alkaline phosphatase), increased bilirubin.
Kidney function tests: increased blood urea nitrogen (BUN) and creatinine.

CAUTION
1. When this drug is used alone, resistance can occur rapidly; it is usually used concurrently with amphotericin B (given intravenously).

Precautions for Use
By Infants and Children: No information available.
By Those over 60 Years of Age: If necessary, adjust dosage for age-related decrease in kidney function.

▷ **Advisability of Use During Pregnancy**
Pregnancy Category: C. See Pregnancy Code at the back of this book.
Animal studies: Rat studies reveal drug-induced birth defects.
Human studies: Adequate studies of pregnant women not available.
Use this drug only if clearly needed. Ask your physician for guidance.

Advisability of Use if Breast-Feeding
Presence of this drug in breast milk: Yes.
Avoid drug or refrain from nursing.

Habit-Forming Potential: None.

Effects of Overdosage: Nausea, vomiting, stomach pain, diarrhea, confusion.

Possible Effects of Long-Term Use: Bone marrow depression, liver or kidney damage.

Suggested Periodic Examinations While Taking This Drug (at physician's discretion)
Measurement of blood levels of flucytosine.
Complete blood cell counts.
Liver and kidney function tests.

▷ **While Taking This Drug, Observe the Following**
Foods: No restrictions.
Beverages: No restrictions. May be taken with milk.
▷ *Alcohol:* No interactions expected.
Tobacco Smoking: No interactions expected.
▷ *Other Drugs*
The following drug may *decrease* the effects of flucytosine
- cytarabine (Cytosar).
- antacids.

Flucytosine *taken concurrently* with
- amphotericin B may result in increased risk of kidney toxicity.

▷ *Driving, Hazardous Activities:* This drug may cause dizziness, drowsiness or confusion. Limit activities as necessary.
Aviation Note: The use of this drug *may be a disqualification* for piloting. Consult a designated Aviation Medical Examiner.
Exposure to Sun: Use caution—this drug may cause photosensitivity (see Glossary).
Discontinuation: This drug may be needed for an extended period of time. Your physician should determine the appropriate time to stop it.

FLUNISOLIDE (flu NIS oh lide)

Introduced: 1980 **Prescription:** USA: Yes; Canada: Yes **Available as Generic:** No **Class:** Antiasthmatic, cortisonelike drugs **Controlled Drug:** USA: No; Canada: No

Brand Names: Aerobid, Aerobid-M, ✦Bronalide, Nasalide, ✦Rhinalar

---

BENEFITS versus RISKS

Possible Benefits	Possible Risks
EFFECTIVE CONTROL OF SEVERE, CHRONIC BRONCHIAL ASTHMA	Yeast infections of mouth and throat Increased susceptibility to respiratory tract infections Localized areas of "allergic" pneumonia

---

▷ **Principal Uses**
 As a Single Drug Product: Uses currently included in FDA approved labeling: (1) Treats chronic bronchial asthma in people who require cortisonelike drugs for asthma control. This inhalation dosage form is better than cortisone taken by mouth (swallowed) or by injection in that it works locally on the respiratory tract. (2) treatment of various kinds of allergic rhinitis. Other (unlabeled) generally accepted uses: (1) Treatment of nasal polyps; (2) treatment of bronchopulmonary dysplasia.

How This Drug Works: By increasing cyclic AMP, this drug may increase epinephrine, which is an effective bronchodilator and antiasthmatic. An additional benefit is reduction of local allergic reaction and inflammation.

Available Dosage Forms and Strengths
 Inhalation aerosol — 0.25 mg (250 mcg) per metered spray
 Nasal solution — 25 mcg per actuation

▷ **Recommended Dosage Ranges** (Actual dosage and administration schedule must be determined by the physician for each patient individually.)
 Infants and Children: Up to 4 years of age—Dosage not established.
  4 years of age and older—0.5 mg (2 metered sprays) 2 times a day, morning and evening. Limit total daily dosage to 1 mg.
 15 to 60 Years of Age: Oral inhalation: 0.5 to 1 mg (2 to 4 metered sprays) 2 times a day, morning and evening. Limit total daily dose to 2 mg.
 Nasal inhalation: 2 sprays per nostril twice daily.
 Over 60 Years of Age: Same as 15 to 60 years of age.

Conditions Requiring Dosing Adjustments
 Liver function: Specific guidelines not available for dosage adjustment in liver compromise.
 Kidney function: No specific changes are recommended in patients with compromised kidneys.

▷ **Dosing Instructions:** May be used as needed without regard to eating. Shake the container well before using. Carefully follow the printed patient instructions provided with the unit. Rinse the mouth and throat (gargle) with water thoroughly after each inhalation.

Usual Duration of Use: Use on a regular schedule for 1 to 4 weeks is necessary to see effectiveness in controlling severe, chronic asthma. Long-term use requires physician supervision and guidance.

▷ **This Drug Should Not Be Taken If**
- you have had an allergic reaction to it previously.
- you are experiencing severe acute asthma or status asthmaticus that requires more intense treatment for prompt relief.
- you have a form of nonallergic bronchitis with asthmatic features.

▷ **Inform Your Physician Before Taking This Drug If**
- you are now taking or have recently taken any cortisone-related drug (including ACTH by injection) for any reason (see Drug Class Section).
- you have a history of tuberculosis.
- you have Herpes simplex infection of the eye.
- you have chicken pox.
- you have chronic bronchitis or bronchiectasis.
- you think you may have an active infection of any kind, especially a respiratory infection.

Possible Side-Effects (natural, expected and unavoidable drug actions)
Yeast infections (thrush) of the mouth and throat.
Unpleasant taste.

▷ **Possible Adverse Effects** (unusual, unexpected and infrequent reactions)
If any of the following develop, consult your physician promptly for guidance.

Mild Adverse Effects
Allergic Reactions: Skin rash, hives, itching.
Headache, dizziness, nervousness, loss of smell or taste.
Upper respiratory infections, cough.
Heart palpitation, increased blood pressure, swelling of feet and ankles.
Loss of appetite, indigestion, nausea, vomiting, stomach pain, diarrhea.
Sore throat (20%).
Nasal irritation.
Insomnia.

Serious Adverse Effects
Allergic Reaction: Localized areas of "allergic" pneumonitis (lung inflammation).
Bronchospasm, asthmatic wheezing (rare).
Tachycardia (1–3%).
Hypertension (1–3%).

▷ **Possible Effects on Sexual Function:** None reported.

Natural Diseases or Disorders That May Be Activated by This Drug
Cortisone-related drugs (used by inhalation) that produce systemic effects can impair immunity and lead to reactivation of "healed" or quiescent tuberculosis. People with a history of tuberculosis should be watched closely during use of cortisonelike drugs by inhalation.

Possible Effects on Laboratory Tests
None reported.

CAUTION
1. This drug does not act primarily as a brochodilator and should not be used for immediate relief of acute asthma.
2. If you were using any cortisone-related drugs for treatment of your asthma *before* changing to this inhaler drug, you may need to resume the cortisone-related drug if you are injured, have an infection or if you

require surgery. Be sure to tell your doctor physician about prior use of cortisone-related drugs taken either by mouth or by injection.
3. If severe asthma returns while using this drug, call your physician immediately so that supportive treatment can be provided as needed.
4. If you have used cortisone-related drugs in the past year, carry a card that says this has happened. During periods of stress it may be necessary to resume cortisone treatment in adequate dosage.
5. Five to 10 minutes should separate the inhalation of bronchodilators such as albuterol, epinephrine, pirbuterol, etc., (which should be used first) and the inhalation of this drug. This lets more flunisolide reach the bronchial tubes, and reduces risk of adverse effects from the propellants used in the two inhalers.

Precautions for Use
By Infants and Children: Safety and effectiveness for those under 4 years of age not established. To obtain maximal benefit, the use of a spacer device is recommended for inhalation therapy in children.
By Those over 60 Years of Age: People with chronic bronchitis or bronchiectasis should be watched closely for the development of lung infections.

▷ **Advisability of Use During Pregnancy**
Pregnancy Category: C. See Pregnancy Code at the back of this book.
Animal studies: Rat and rabbit studies reveal significant birth defects due to this drug.
Human studies: Adequate studies of pregnant women not available.
Avoid drug during the first 3 months. Use infrequently and only as clearly needed during the last 6 months.

Advisability of Use if Breast-Feeding
Presence of this drug in breast milk: Unknown.
Avoid drug or refrain from nursing.

Habit-Forming Potential: With recommended dosage, a state of functional dependence (see Glossary) is not likely to develop.

Effects of Overdosage: Indications of cortisone excess (due to systemic absorption)—fluid retention, flushing of the face, stomach irritation, nervousness.

Possible Effects of Long-Term Use: Development of acne, cataracts, altered menstrual pattern.

Suggested Periodic Examinations While Taking This Drug (at physician's discretion)
Inspection of mouth and throat for evidence of yeast infection.
Check of adrenal function in people who have used cortisone-related drugs for an extended period of time before using this drug.
X-ray of the lungs of people with a prior history of tuberculosis.

▷ **While Taking This Drug, Observe the Following**
Foods: No specific restrictions beyond those advised by your physician.
Beverages: No specific restrictions.
▷ *Alcohol:* No interactions expected.
Tobacco Smoking: No interactions expected. However, smoking can worsen asthma and reduce the effectiveness of this drug. Follow your physician's advice.

▷ *Other Drugs*
  The following drugs may *increase* the effects of flunisolide
  - inhalant bronchodilators—albuterol, bitolterol, epinephrine, etc.
  - oral bronchodilators—aminophylline, ephedrine, terbutaline, theophylline, etc.

  Flunisolide *taken concurrently* with
  - Stanazolol may result in increased risk of acne or edema.

▷ *Driving, Hazardous Activities:* No restrictions.
  Aviation Note: The use of this drug and the disorder for which this drug is prescribed *may be disqualifications* for piloting. Consult a designated Aviation Medical Examiner.
  Exposure to Sun: No restrictions.
  Occurrence of Unrelated Illness: Acute infections, serious injuries or surgical procedures can create an urgent need for cortisone-related drugs given by mouth and/or injection. Call your doctor immediately in the event of new illness or injury.
  Discontinuation: If this drug has made it possible to reduce or discontinue cortisonelike drugs by mouth, *do not* stop this drug abruptly. If you must stop this drug, consult your physician promptly. Cortisone preparations and other measures may be necessary.
  Special Storage Instructions: Store at room temperature. Avoid exposure to temperatures above 120 degrees F (49 degrees C). Do not store or use this inhaler near heat or open flame.

FLUOXETINE (flu OX e teen)

Introduced: 1978 **Prescription:** USA: Yes **Available as Generic:** USA: No **Class:** Antidepressant **Controlled Drug:** USA: No
Brand Name: Prozac

BENEFITS versus RISKS	
Possible Benefits	*Possible Risks*
EFFECTIVE TREATMENT OF MAJOR DEPRESSIVE DISORDERS in 60% to 75% of cases	Serious allergic reactions (4%) Conversion of depression to mania in manic-depressive disorders (1%)
Possibly effective in relieving the symptoms of obsessive-compulsive disorder	

▷ **Principal Uses**
  As a Single Drug Product: Uses currently included in FDA approved labeling: (1) Treatment of major forms of depression that have not responded well to other therapies. This drug should not be used to treat the symptoms of mild and transient (reactive) depression; (2) obsessive-compulsive disorder.
  Author's note: The FDA granted approvable status for use of fluoxetine in the treatment of bulimia. Final approval is still pending.
  Other (unlabeled) generally accepted uses: (1) refractory bulimia; (2) refractory diabetic neuropathy; (3) may help control kleptomania; (4) can be of

help in treating obesity, especially when obesity is accompanied by depression; (5) eases symptoms of panic attacks, (6) may be given only during the premenstrual period (based on a Canadian study) to treat premenstrual syndrome (PMS).

How This Drug Works: It slowly restores normal levels of a nerve transmitter (serotonin).

Available Dosage Forms and Strengths
Capsules — 20 mg
Syrup — 20 mg per ml

▷ **Usual Adult Dosage Range:** Started at 20 mg every 1 to 3 days as a single morning dose; if no improvement after 4 weeks of treatment, the dose may be increased by 20 mg/day as needed and tolerated. Doses over 20 mg/day should be taken in 2 divided doses, early morning and noon. Maximum daily dosage is 80 mg. **Note: Actual dosage and administration schedule must be determined by the physician for each patient individually.**

Conditions Requiring Dosing Adjustments
Liver function: The dose should be decreased or the dosing interval lengthened in patients with liver compromise. It is also a rare cause of hepatoxicity, and should be used with caution in this patient population.
Kidney function: The dose should be decreased in severe renal compromise.

▷ **Dosing Instructions:** The capsule may be opened and the contents mixed with any convenient food. To make smaller doses, the contents may be mixed with orange juice or apple juice and refrigerated; doses of 5 mg to 10 mg may prove effective and better tolerated.

Usual Duration of Use: Use on a regular schedule for as little as 1 to 2 weeks may reveal the begining of improvement in depression. Up to 4 to 8 weeks may be needed to determine (1) this drug's effectiveness in relieving depression; (2) the pattern of both favorable and unfavorable effects. Long-term use (months to years) requires periodic physician evaluation.

Possible Advantages of This Drug
Does not cause weight gain, a common side-effect of tricyclic antidepressants. May actually cause weight loss.
Less likely to cause dry mouth, constipation, urinary retention, orthostatic hypotension (see Glossary) and heart rhythm disturbances than tricyclic antidepressants.
Does not cause Parkinson-like reactions.

▷ **This Drug Should Not Be Taken If**
- you have had an allergic reaction to any dosage form of it previously.
- you currently take or have taken within the past 14 days any monoamine oxidase (MAO) type A inhibitor (see Drug Class Section).

▷ **Inform Your Physician Before Taking This Drug If**
- you have had any adverse effects from antidepressant drugs.
- you have impaired liver or kidney function.
- you have Parkinson's disease.
- you have a seizure disorder.
- you have a history of psychosis.
- you have a history of SIADH.
- you are pregnant or plan pregnancy while taking this drug.

Possible Side-Effects (natural, expected and unavoidable drug actions)
   Decreased appetite (8.7%), weight loss (13%).
▷ **Possible Adverse Effects** (unusual, unexpected and infrequent reactions)
   If any of the following develop, consult your physician promptly for guidance.
   Mild Adverse Effects
   Allergic Reactions: Skin rash (2.7%), hives (2%), itching (2.4%).
   Headache (20%), nervousness (14%), insomnia (13%), drowsiness (11%), tremor (7%), dizziness (5%), fatigue (4%), impaired concentration (1.5%).
   Altered taste (1.8%), nausea (21%), vomiting (2.4%), diarrhea (12%).
   Hair loss (rare).
   Blurred vision.
   Excessive sweating (30%).
   Serious Adverse Effects
   Allergic Reactions: Serum sickness-like syndrome (2% to 3%): fever, weakness, joint pain and swelling, swollen lymph glands, fluid retention, skin rash and/or hives.
   Drug-induced seizures (0.2%).
   Worsening of Parkinson's disease.
   Intense suicidal preoccupation in severe depression that does not respond to this drug. (See Current Controversies at the end of this Profile.)
   Low blood pressure on standing (orthostatic hypotension).
   Mania or hypomania (1%).
   Psychosis.
   Abnormal and excessive urination (SIADH).
   Liver toxicity (rare).
▷ **Possible Effects on Sexual Function:** Impaired erection (1.9%), inhibition of ejaculation, and inhibited orgasm in men and women.

Natural Diseases or Disorders That May Be Activated by This Drug
   Latent epilepsy.

Possible Effects on Laboratory Tests
   Blood glucose level: decreased.
   Blood sodium level: decreased.

CAUTION
   1. If any skin reaction develops (rash, hives, etc.), stop this drug and inform your physician promptly.
   2. If dry mouth develops and persists for more than 2 weeks, consult your dentist for help.
   3. Ask your doctor or pharmacist before taking any other prescription or over-the-counter drug while taking fluoxetine.
   4. If you must start any monoamine oxidase (MAO) type A inhibitor (see Drug Class Section), allow an interval of 5 weeks after stopping this drug before starting the MAO inhibitor.
   5. This drug should be withheld if electroconvulsive therapy (ECT, "shock" treatment) is to be used.

Precautions for Use
   By Infants and Children: Safety and effectiveness for those under 12 years of age are not established.
   By Those over 60 Years of Age: Total daily dosage should not exceed 60 mg.

Fluoxetine

▷ **Advisability of Use During Pregnancy**
Pregnancy Category: B. See Pregnancy Code at the back of this book.
Animal studies: No birth defects due to this drug found in rat or rabbit studies.
Human studies: Adequate studies of pregnant women are not available.
Use this drug only if clearly needed.

Advisability of Use if Breast-Feeding
Presence of this drug in breast milk: Yes.
Avoid drug or refrain from nursing.

Habit-Forming Potential: Reports have surfaced of patients using excess doses of fluoxetine or combining the drug with alcohol have surfaced. It appears possible that a euphoric effect and abuse potential exists.

Effects of Overdosage: Agitation, restlessness, excitement, nausea, vomiting, seizures.

Possible Effects of Long-Term Use: None reported.

Suggested Periodic Examinations While Taking This Drug (at physician's discretion)
None.

▷ **While Taking This Drug, Observe the Following**
Foods: No restrictions.
Beverages: No restrictions. May be taken with milk.
▷ *Alcohol:* Avoid completely.
Tobacco Smoking: No interactions expected.
▷ *Other Drugs*
Fluoxetine may *increase* the effects of
- diazepam (Valium).
- digitalis preparations (digitoxin, digoxin).
- warfarin (Coumadin) and related oral anticoagulants.
- phenytoin (Dilantin) by increasing the drug level.

Fluoxetine *taken concurrently* with
- antidiabetic drugs (insulin, oral hypoglycemics) may increase the risk of hypoglycemic reactions; monitor blood sugar levels carefully.
- monoamine oxidase (MAO) type A inhibitor drugs may cause confusion, agitation, high fever, seizures and dangerous elevations of blood pressure. Avoid combining these drugs.
- carbamazepine (Tegretol) will increase the carbamazepine level. Drug levels are critical if the drugs are combined.
- lithium (Lithobid, etc.) will result in increased lithium levels and increased risk of neurotoxicity. Avoid the combination.
- tryptophan will result in central nervous system toxicity. Avoid the combination.
- any tricyclic antidepressant (amitriptyline, nortriptyline, etc.) will result in increased antidepressant drug levels that will persist for weeks. Avoid the combination.
- haloperidol (Haldol) will increase haloperidol levels. Dosage decrease and blood levels are needed.
- buspirone (Buspar) may increase underlying anxiety. Avoid the combination.

- astemizole (Hismanal), loratidine (Claritin) or terfenadine (Seldane), or similar drugs may result in increased terfenadine levels and risk of heart arrhythmias. Avoid combining.
- selegiline (Eldepryl) can result in serotonin toxicity syndrome. Avoid this combination.

▷ *Driving, Hazardous Activities:* This drug may cause drowsiness, dizziness, impaired judgment and delayed reaction time. Restrict activities as necessary.

Aviation Note: The use of this drug *is a disqualification* for piloting. Consult a designated Aviation Medical Examiner.

Exposure to Sun: No restrictions.

Discontinuation: Slow drug elimination makes withdrawal effects unlikely. However, call your doctor if you plan to stop this drug for any reason.

Current Controversies in Drug Management

In 1990 it was reported that six patients being treated with fluoxetine experienced the onset of intense and violent suicidal preoccupation. All six had severe depression that had not responded to the use of fluoxetine for 2 to 7 weeks. For most of them, suicidal mentality persisted for 2 to 3 months after discontinuation of the drug.

The resultant adverse publicity suggested that this experience may be somewhat characteristic of fluoxetine in contrast to other antidepressant drugs. A review of relevant literature on this subject reveals that the development or intensification of suicidal thoughts during treatment (regardless of the severity of depression) has been documented repeatedly for many antidepressant drugs in wide use. Suicidal thinking may emerge during treatment with any antidepressant. Recent reports establish that some patients who become suicidal while taking one antidepressant can be switched to fluoxetine and experience cessation of suicidal thinking and satisfactory relief of depression.

This is another example of the marked variability of individual response to drug therapy. The choice of a drug to treat many serious disorders remains an experiment of trial and error. Successful management requires clinical judgment (based on experience), close monitoring and appropriate doses.

FLUPHENAZINE (flu FEN a zeen)

Introduced: 1959   **Prescription:** USA: Yes; Canada: Yes   **Available as Generic:** USA: No; Canada: Yes   **Class:** Strong tranquilizer, phenothiazines
Controlled Drug: USA: No; Canada: No

Brand Names: ✤Apo-Fluphenazine, ✤Modecate, ✤Moditen, Permitil, PMS-Fluphenazine, Prolixin

Fluphenazine

BENEFITS versus RISKS	
Possible Benefits	*Possible Risks*
EFFECTIVE CONTROL OF ACUTE MENTAL DISORDERS	SERIOUS TOXIC EFFECTS ON BRAIN with long-term use
Beneficial effects on thinking, mood and behavior	Liver damage with jaundice (less than 0.5%)
	Rare blood cell disorders: abnormally low white blood cell counts

▷ **Principal Uses**

As a Single Drug Product: Uses currently included in FDA approved labeling: (1) treatment of schizophrenia.

Other (unlabeled) currently accepted uses: (1) combination treatment of refractory neuropathy; (2) an alternative neuroleptic drug in treating Tourette's syndrome in combination with clonidine; (3) therapy of Alzheimer's disease.

How This Drug Works: By inhibiting the action of dopamine, this drug acts to correct an imbalance of nerve impulse transmissions.

Available Dosage Forms and Strengths
 Concentrate — 5 mg per ml (1% alcohol)
   Elixir — 2.5 mg per 5-ml teaspoonful (14% alcohol)
   Injection — 2.5 mg per ml
   Tablets — 1 mg, 2.5 mg, 5 mg 10 mg

▷ **Usual Adult Dosage Range:** 0.5 to 2.5 mg 1 to 4 times/day; adjust dosage as needed and tolerated. Total daily dosage should not exceed 20 mg. **Note: Actual dosage and administration schedule must be determined by the physician for each patient individually.**

Conditions Requiring Dosing Adjustments

Liver function: Used with caution in patients with both liver and kidney compromise.

Kidney function: Used with caution in patients with compromised kidneys and livers.

▷ **Dosing Instructions:** Regular tablets can be crushed and taken with or following meals to reduce stomach irritation. Prolonged-action tablets should be swallowed whole (not crushed). The concentrate must be diluted in 4 to 6 ounces of water, milk, fruit juice or carbonated beverage.

Usual Duration of Use: Use on a regular schedule for several weeks is needed to determine effectiveness in controlling psychotic disorders. If not of benefit in 6 weeks, it should be stopped. Long-term use (months to years) requires periodic physician evaluation.

▷ **This Drug Should Not Be Taken If**
- you are allergic to any of the drugs bearing the brand names listed.
- you have a history of brain damage.
- you have active liver disease.
- you have cancer of the breast.
- you have an active blood dyscrasia.
- you have a current blood cell or bone marrow disorder.

▷ **Inform Your Physician Before Taking This Drug If**
- you are allergic or sensitive to any phenothiazine (see Drug Class Section).
- you have impaired liver or kidney function.
- you have any type of seizure disorder.
- you have diabetes, glaucoma, heart disease or chronic lung disease.
- you have a history of lupus erythematosus.
- you have a history of depressed white blood cell counts of the granulocytic series (agranulocytosis).
- you have a history of neuroleptic malignant syndrome.
- you are taking large doses of other medicines which can depress the central nervous system.
- you are taking any drug with sedative effects.
- you will have surgery under general or spinal anesthesia soon.

Possible Side-Effects (natural, expected and unavoidable drug actions)
Drowsiness (usually during the first 2 weeks), orthostatic hypotension (see Glossary), blurred vision, dry mouth, nasal congestion, constipation, impaired urination (all mild).

▷ **Possible Adverse Effects** (unusual, unexpected and infrequent reactions)
If any of the following develop, consult your physician promptly for guidance.

Mild Adverse Effects
Allergic Reactions: Skin rash, hives, itching.
Lowering of body temperature, especially in the elderly.
Headache, dizziness, weakness, excitement, restlessness, unusual dreaming.
Increased appetite and weight gain.

Serious Adverse Effects
Allergic Reactions: Hepatitis with jaundice (see Glossary), usually between second and fourth week; anaphylactic reaction (see Glossary).
Idiosyncratic Reaction: Neuroleptic malignant syndrome (see Glossary).
Impaired production of white blood cells—fever, sore throat, infections.
Parkinson-like disorders (see Glossary); muscle spasms of face, jaw, neck, back, extremities.
Liver toxicity.
Porphyria.
Abnormal heart beats (rare).
Seizures (rare).
Prolonged drop in blood pressure with weakness, perspiration and fainting.

▷ **Possible Effects on Sexual Function**
Decreased male libido; increased female libido.
Impaired erection (38% to 42%); complete impotence.
Inhibited male orgasm (58%); inhibited female orgasm (22% to 33%).
Inhibited ejaculation (46%).
Altered timing and pattern of menstruation (91%).
Female breast enlargement and milk production.
Prolonged and painful erection.
Male breast enlargement and tenderness.
May help treat sexual hyperactivity.

▷ **Adverse Effects That May Mimic Natural Diseases or Disorders**
Nervous system reactions may suggest Parkinson's disease.
Liver reactions may suggest viral hepatitis.
Reactions resembling systemic lupus erythematosus may occur.

Natural Diseases or Disorders That May Be Activated by This Drug
Latent epilepsy, glaucoma, prostatism (see Glossary).

Possible Effects on Laboratory Tests
Complete blood counts: decreased red cells, hemoglobin, white cells and platelets; increased eosinophils (allergic reaction).
Liver function tests: increased liver enzymes (ALT/GPT, AST/GOT and alkaline phosphatase), increased bilirubin.
Urine pregnancy tests: false positive results.
Urine screening test for drug abuse: initial test may be falsely **positive** for barbiturates; the confirmatory test will be **negative**.

CAUTION
1. Many over-the-counter medications (see OTC Drugs in Glossary) for allergies, colds and coughs can interact unfavorably with this drug. Ask your physician or pharmacist help before using any such medications.
2. Antacids containing aluminum and/or magnesium can prevent absorption.
3. Obtain prompt evaluation of any change or disturbance of vision.

Precautions for Use
By Infants and Children: Do not use this drug in infants under 6 months of age, or in children of any age with symptoms suggestive of Reye syndrome (see Glossary). Monitor carefully for blood cell changes.
By Those over 60 Years of Age: Small starting doses are advisable. Increased risk of drowsiness, lethargy, constipation, lowering of body temperature (hypothermia) and orthostatic hypotension (see Glossary). This drug can enhance existing prostatism (see Glossary). You may also be more susceptible to the development of Parkinson-like reactions and/or tardive dyskinesia (see discussion of these terms in Glossary).

▷ **Advisability of Use During Pregnancy**
Pregnancy Category: C. See Pregnancy Code at the back of this book.
Animal studies: Significant birth defects reported in mice.
Human studies: Adequate studies of pregnant women are not available.
Avoid drug during the first 3 months and during the last month because of possible effects on the newborn infant.

Advisability of Use if Breast-Feeding
Presence of this drug in breast milk: Unknown.
Avoid drug or refrain from nursing.

Habit-Forming Potential: None.

Effects of Overdosage: Marked drowsiness, weakness, tremor, agitation, unsteadiness, deep sleep, coma, convulsions.

Possible Effects of Long-Term Use: Tardive dyskinesia (see Glossary); eye changes—cataracts and pigmentation of retina; gray to violet pigmentation of skin in exposed areas, more common in women.

Suggested Periodic Examinations While Taking This Drug (at physician's discretion)
   Complete blood counts, especially between 4 to 10 of therapy.
   Liver function tests, electrocardiograms.
   Complete eye examinations—eye structures and vision.
   Careful tongue exam for evidence of fine, involuntary, wavelike movements that could be the beginning of tardive dyskinesia.

▷ **While Taking This Drug, Observe the Following**
   Foods: No restrictions.
   Beverages: No restrictions. May be taken with milk.
▷ *Alcohol:* Avoid completely. Alcohol can increase phenothiazine sedation and accentuate depressant effects on brain function and blood pressure. Phenothiazines can increase the intoxicating effects of alcohol.
   Tobacco Smoking: Possible reduction of drowsiness from drug.
   Marijuana Smoking: Moderate increase in drowsiness; accentuation of orthostatic hypotension; increased risk of precipitating latent psychoses, confusing the interpretation of mental status and drug responses.
▷ *Other Drugs*
   Fluphenazine may *increase* the effects of
   • all sedative drugs, and cause excessive sedation.
   • all atropinelike drugs, and cause nervous system toxicity.
   Fluphenazine may *decrease* the effects of
   • guanethidine (Ismelin, Esimil), and reduce its effectiveness in lowering blood pressure.
   Fluphenazine *taken concurrently* with
   • beta blocker drugs (see Drug Class Section) may cause increased effects of both drugs; watch drug effects—may need smaller doses.
   • lithium can cause increase toxicity to the nerves.
   • MAO inhibitors (see Drug Class) can cause very low blood pressure and worsening of the central nervous system and respiratory depression effects.
   The following drugs may *decrease* the effects of fluphenazine
   • antacids containing aluminum and/or magnesium.
   • benztropine (Cogentin).
   • trihexyphenidyl (Artane).
▷ *Driving, Hazardous Activities:* This drug can impair mental alertness, judgment and physical coordination. Avoid hazardous activities.
   Aviation Note: The use of this drug *is a disqualification* for piloting. Consult a designated Aviation Medical Examiner.
   Exposure to Sun: Use caution—some phenothiazines can cause photosensitivity (see Glossary).
   Exposure to Heat: Use caution and avoid excessive heat. This drug may impair the regulation of body temperature and increase heat stroke risk.
   Exposure to Cold: Use caution and dress warmly. Increased risk of hypothermia in the elderly.
   Discontinuation: After long-term use, do not stop this drug suddenly. Gradual withdrawal over 2 to 3 weeks under physician supervision is needed. Do not stop this drug without your doctor's knowledge and approval. The relapse rate of schizophrenia after discontinuation is 50–60%.

FLURAZEPAM (floor AZ e pam)

Introduced: 1970 **Prescription:** USA: Yes; Canada: Yes **Available as Generic:** USA: Yes; Canada: Yes **Class:** Hypnotic, benzodiazepines
Controlled Drug: USA: C-IV*; Canada: No
Brand Names: ♦Apo-Flurazepam, Dalmane, Durapam, ♦Novoflupam, ♦Somnol, ♦Som-Pam

---

BENEFITS versus RISKS

Possible Benefits	*Possible Risks*
EFFECTIVE HYPNOTIC after 4 weeks of continual use	Habit-forming potential with long-term use
NO SUPPRESSION OF REM (RAPID EYE MOVEMENT) SLEEP	Minor impairment of mental functions ("hangover" effect)
NO REM SLEEP REBOUND after discontinuation	Very rare jaundice
	Very rare blood cell disorder
Wide margin of safety with therapeutic doses	Suppression of stage-4 sleep with reduced "quality" of sleep

---

▷ **Principal Uses**

As a Single Drug Product: Uses currently included in FDA approved labeling: Short-term treatment of insomnia consisting of difficulty in falling asleep, frequent nighttime awakenings, and/or early morning awakenings.

Other (unlabeled) generally accepted uses: May be of benefit in patients who have undergone herniorrhaphy in helping them sleep.

How This Drug Works: By enhancing the action of the nerve transmitter gamma-aminobutyric acid (GABA), arousal of higher brain centers is blocked and helps sleep occur.

Available Dosage Forms and Strengths
Capsules — 15 mg, 30 mg (U.S., Canada)
Tablets — 15 mg, 30 mg (Canada)

▷ **Recommended Dosage Ranges** (Actual dosage and administration schedule must be determined by the physician for each patient individually.)

Infants and Children: Up to 15 years of age—use not recommended.
15 to 60 Years of Age: Initially 15 mg at bedtime; increase to 30 mg only if needed and tolerated.
Over 60 Years of Age: Same as 15 to 60 years of age. Usually 15 mg is adequate; use higher doses with caution.

Conditions Requiring Dosing Adjustments
Liver function: The dose **must** be decreased in patients with liver compromise. Flurazepam is also a rare cause of hepatocellular and cholestatic jaundice, and must be used as a benefit to risk decision in patients with compromised livers.
Kidney function: Changes in dosage are not usually needed.

▷ **Dosing Instructions:** The capsule may be opened and taken on an empty stomach or with food or milk. Do not stop this drug abruptly if taken for more than 4 weeks.

*See Schedules of Controlled Drugs at the back of this book.

Usual Duration of Use: Use for 3 nights is usually needed to see this drug's benefit in relieving insomnia. If possible, this drug should be used for periods of 3 to 5 nights intermittently, repeated as needed with appropriate dosage adjustment. Avoid uninterrupted and prolonged use. Duration of use should not exceed 2 weeks without reappraisal of continued need.

▷ **This Drug Should Not Be Taken If**
- you have had an allergic reaction to it previously.
- you are pregnant.
- you have sleep apnea.
- you have acute narrow-angle glaucoma.

▷ **Inform Your Physician Before Taking This Drug If**
- you are allergic to any benzodiazepine (see Drug Class Section).
- you have a history of alcoholism or drug abuse.
- you are planning pregnancy.
- you have impaired liver or kidney function.
- you are an alcoholic.
- you have a history of serious depression or mental disorder.
- you are taking other drugs with sedative effects.
- you have: asthma, emphysema, epilepsy, or myasthenia gravis.

Possible Side-Effects (natural, expected and unavoidable drug actions)
"Hangover" effects on arising: drowsiness, lethargy and unsteadiness.

▷ **Possible Adverse Effects** (unusual, unexpected and infrequent reactions)
If any of the following develop, consult your physician promptly for guidance.

Mild Adverse Effects
Allergic Reactions: Skin rash, hives, burning eyes, swelling of tongue.
Dizziness, fainting, blurred vision, double vision, slurred speech, nausea, indigestion.
Taste disorders.

Serious Adverse Effects
Allergic Reactions: Rare liver damage with jaundice (see Glossary).
Idiosyncratic Reactions: Nervousness, talkativeness, irritability, apprehension, euphoria, excitement, hallucinations.
Rare bone marrow depression—impaired production of white blood cells, fever, sore throat.
Liver toxicity (rare).
Intraocular pressure increase.
Sleep apnea.
Increased risk of hip fracture (from falls) if used in those over 60.

▷ **Possible Effects on Sexual Function:** None reported.

▷ **Adverse Effects That May Mimic Natural Diseases or Disorders**
Liver reaction with jaundice may suggest viral hepatitis.

Possible Effects on Laboratory Tests
Liver function tests: increased liver enzymes (ALT/GPT, AST/GOT and alkaline phosphatase, increased bilirubin.
Urine sugar tests: no drug effect with TesTape; false low results with Clinistix and Diastix; false positive result with Benedict's solution.

Flurazepam

Urine screening tests for drug abuse: may be **positive**. (Test results depend upon amount of drug taken and testing method used.)

CAUTION
1. This drug should not be stopped abruptly if it has been taken continually for more than 4 weeks.
2. Some over-the-counter drug products that contain antihistamines (allergy and cold preparations, sleep aids) can cause excessive sedation.
3. Regular nightly use of any hypnotic drug should be avoided.
4. This drug is transformed by the liver into long-acting forms that can persist in the body for 24 hours or more. With continual use of this drug daily, these active drug forms accumulate and produce increasing sedation. If you experience a "hangover" effect, avoid hazardous activities (driving, etc.) and the use of alcohol.

Precautions for Use
By Infants and Children: Safety and effectiveness for those under 15 years of age not established.

By Those over 60 Years of Age: Starting doses are reduced and given less often. Watch for lethargy, indifference, fatigue, weakness, unsteadiness, disturbing dreams, nightmares and paradoxical reactions (excitement, agitation, anger and rage.)

Because this is a long-acting benzodiazepine, it may cause residual sluggishness and unsteadiness with increased risk of falls. This drug may also increase the number of periods of sleep apnea in this age group.

▷ **Advisability of Use During Pregnancy**
Pregnancy Category: X. See Pregnancy Code at the back of this book.
Animal studies: No birth defects reported in rat and rabbit studies.
Human studies: Adequate studies of pregnant women are not available.
Several studies indicate an increased risk of birth defects if drugs of this class (benzodiazepines) are used during the first 3 months.
Frequent use in late pregnancy can cause the "floppy infant" syndrome in the newborn: weakness, lethargy, unresponsiveness, depressed breathing, low body temperature.
Avoid use during entire pregnancy.

Advisability of Use if Breast-Feeding
Presence of this drug in breast milk: Probably yes.
Avoid drug or refrain from nursing.

Habit-Forming Potential: This drug can produce psychological and/or physical dependence (see Glossary) if used in large doses for an extended period of time. Avoid continual use.

Effects of Overdosage: Marked drowsiness, weakness, feeling of drunkenness, staggering gait, tremor, stupor progressing to deep sleep or coma.

Possible Effects of Long-Term Use: Psychological and/or physical dependence, impaired liver function.

Suggested Periodic Examinations While Taking This Drug (at physician's discretion)
Complete blood cell counts and liver function tests during long-term use.

▷ **While Taking This Drug, Observe the Following**
  Foods: No restrictions.
  Beverages: Avoid excessive intake of caffeine-containing beverages (coffee, tea, cola) within 4 hours of taking this drug. May be taken with milk.
▷ *Alcohol:* Use with extreme caution—alcohol may increase the absorption of this drug and add to its depressant effects on the brain. It is advisable to avoid alcohol completely—throughout the day and night—if it is necessary to drive or to engage in any hazardous activity.
  Tobacco Smoking: Heavy smoking may reduce the hypnotic action of this drug.
  Marijuana Smoking: Increased sedation and significant impairment of intellectual and physical performance.
▷ *Other Drugs*
  Flurazepam may *increase* the effects of
  • digoxin (Lanoxin), and cause digoxin toxicity.
  • lithium and cause additive drowsiness.
  • phenytoin (Dilantin), and cause phenytoin toxicity.
  Flurazepam may *decrease* the effects of
  • levodopa (Sinemet, etc.), and reduce its effectiveness in treating Parkinson's disease.
  The following drugs may *increase* the effects of flurazepam
  • cimetidine (Tagamet).
  • disulfiram (Antabuse).
  • isoniazid (INH, Rifamate, etc.).
  • oral contraceptives.
  • valproic acid (Depakene).
  The following drugs may *decrease* the effects of flurazepam
  • rifampin (Rimactane, etc.).
  • theophylline (aminophylline, Theo-Dur, etc.).
▷ *Driving, Hazardous Activities:* This drug can impair mental alertness, judgment, physical coordination and reaction time. Avoid hazardous activities accordingly.
  Aviation Note: The use of this drug *is a disqualification* for piloting. Consult a designated Aviation Medical Examiner.
  Exposure to Sun: No restrictions.
  Exposure to Heat: Use caution until the effect of excessive perspiration is determined. Because of reduced urine volume, this drug may accumulate in the body and produce effects of overdosage.
  Discontinuation: Avoid sudden discontinuation if this drug has been taken for over 4 weeks without interruption. Dosage should be tapered gradually to prevent a withdrawal syndrome that could include depression, confusion, hallucinations, tremor, seizures, muscle cramping, sweating and vomiting.

FLURBIPROFEN (flur BI pro fen)

Introduced: 1977 **Prescription:** USA: Yes; Canada: Yes **Available as Generic:** USA: No; Canada: No **Class:** Mild analgesic, anti-inflammatory **Controlled Drug:** USA: No; Canada: No
Brand Names: Ansaid, ✦Froben, ✦Froben-SR, Ocufen

BENEFITS versus RISKS	
Possible Benefits	*Possible Risks*
EFFECTIVE RELIEF OF SYMPTOMS ASSOCIATED WITH MAJOR TYPES OF ARTHRITIS	PEPTIC ULCER DISEASE (1% to 4%) with associated bleeding and perforation
Effective relief of symptoms associated with bursitis, tendinitis and related conditions	Liver toxicity with jaundice (less than 1%)
Effective relief of menstrual cramps	Water retention
	Rare kidney toxicity
	Rare aplastic anemia (see Glossary)

Please see the propionic acid nonsteroidal anti-inflammatory drug profile for further information.

FLUTAMIDE FLU ta mide

Introduced: 1983 **Prescription:** USA: Yes; Canada: Yes **Available as Generic:** USA: No; Canada: No **Class:** Antiandrogen, antineoplastic
Controlled Drug: USA: No; Canada: No
Brand Names: ◆Euflex, Eulexin

BENEFITS versus RISKS	
Possible Benefits	*Possible Risks*
EFFECTIVE ADJUNCTIVE TREATMENT OF PROSTATE CANCER	Rare drug-induced hepatitis (less than 1%)
	Breast enlargement and tenderness
	Hot flashes

▷ **Principal Uses**
  As a Single Drug Product: Uses currently included in FDA approved labeling: Treatment of metastatic prostate cancer, used concurrently with leuprolide (given by injection).
  Other (unlabeled) generally accepted uses: None.

How This Drug Works: Flutamide is an antiandrogenic drug; it suppresses the biological effects of the male sex hormone (testosterone, an androgen) by blocking its uptake and binding in target tissues (such as the prostate gland). It is used in conjunction with leuprolide, a hormonelike drug that suppresses the production of testosterone by the testicles (by damping the pituitary gland's stimulation of the testicles). The combination of these two drug actions—chemical castration by leuprolide and testosterone blockage by flutamide—significantly reduces hormonal stimulation of cancerous prostate tissue.

Available Dosage Forms and Strengths
  Capsules — 125 mg (U.S.)
  Tablets — 250 mg (Canada)

▷ **Recommended Dosage Ranges** (Actual dosage and administration schedule must be determined by the physician for each patient individually.)
  Infants and Children: Not used in this age group.

12 to 60 Years of Age: 250 mg every 8 hours. Flutamide is to be taken concurrently with leuprolide; the usual dose of leuprolide is 7.5 mg given by injection once a month.
Over 60 Years of Age: Same as 12 to 60 years of age.

Conditions Requiring Dosing Adjustments
Liver function: It should be used with caution in patients with liver compromise. It is also a rare cause of cholestatic jaundice.
Kidney function: Used with caution in kidney compromise.

▷ **Dosing Instructions:** May be taken without regard to food. The capsule may be opened and the tablet may be crushed for administration.

Usual Duration of Use: Use on a regular schedule for 2 to 3 months is usually needed to see this drug's effectiveness in controlling prostate cancer. Long-term use (months to years) requires periodic physician evaluation.

Possible Advantages of This Drug
Ease of use.
Significantly less toxicity than chemotherapeutic drugs.

Currently a "Drug of Choice"
for the management of prostate cancer (in combination with leuprolide).

▷ **This Drug Should Not Be Taken If**
- you have had an allergic reaction to it previously.

▷ **Inform Your Physician Before Taking This Drug If**
- you have a history of liver disease or impaired liver function.
- you have hypertension.
- you have a history of anemia, low white blood cells or low blood platelets.
- you have a history of lupus erythematosus.

Possible Side-Effects (natural, expected and unavoidable drug actions)
Hot flashes (61%), loss of libido (36%), impotence (33%), breast enlargement and tenderness (9%).

▷ **Possible Adverse Effects** (unusual, unexpected and infrequent reactions)
If any of the following develop, consult your physician promptly for guidance.
Mild Adverse Effects
Allergic Reactions: Skin rash (3%).
Drowsiness, nervousness (1%).
Indigestion (6%), nausea/vomiting (11%), diarrhea (12%).
Fluid retention (edema) of legs (4%).
Serious Adverse Effects
Drug-induced hepatitis with jaundice (see Glossary) (less than 1%).
Low blood platelets (1%).
Low white blood cells (3%).
Anemia (6%).
Rare heart attack.

▷ **Possible Effects on Sexual Function**
See Possible Side-Effects above.

▷ **Adverse Effects That May Mimic Natural Diseases or Disorders**
Drug-induced hepatitis may suggest viral hepatitis.

Flutamide

Possible Effects on Laboratory Tests
  Complete blood counts: decreased red and white cells, hemoglobin and platelets.
  Liver function tests: increased liver enzymes (ALT/GPT, AST/GOT and alkaline phosphatase), increased bilirubin.
  Sperm counts: decreased.
  Testosterone levels: decreased.

CAUTION
  1. For best results, flutamide and leuprolide should be started together and continued for the duration of therapy.
  2. During combination therapy with flutamide and leuprolide, symptoms of prostate cancer (difficult urination, bone pain, etc.) may worsen temporarily; these are transient and not significant.

Precautions for Use
  By Those over 60 Years of Age: This drug is more slowly excreted. If digestive symptoms or edema are troublesome, ask your doctor about adjusting your dose.

▷ **Advisability of Use During Pregnancy**
  Pregnancy Category: D. See Pregnancy Code at the back of this book.
  Animal studies: Rat studies reveal malformation of bone structures and feminization of male fetuses.
  Human studies: Adequate studies of pregnant women are not available.

Habit-Forming Potential: None.

Effects of Overdosage: Possible drowsiness, unsteadiness, nausea, vomiting.

Possible Effects of Long-Term Use: None reported.

Suggested Periodic Examinations While Taking This Drug (at physician's discretion)
  Prostatic specific antigen (PSA) assays.
  Complete blood cell counts.
  Liver function tests.

▷ **While Taking This Drug, Observe the Following**
  Foods: No restrictions.
  Beverages: No restrictions. May be taken with milk.
▷ *Alcohol:* No interactions expected.
  Tobacco Smoking: No interactions expected.
▷ *Other Drugs:* Flutamide **taken concurrently** with
   • influenza, pneumococcal or yellow fever vaccine may result in blunting of immune response to the vaccine.
▷ *Driving, Hazardous Activities:* This drug may cause drowsiness. Restrict activities as necessary.
  Aviation Note: The use of this drug **may be a disqualification** for piloting. Consult a designated Aviation Medical Examiner.
  Exposure to Sun: This drug may cause photosensitivity (see Glossary).
  Discontinuation: To be determined by your physician.

FLUTICASONE (flew tick a zone)

Introduced: 1994 **Prescription:** USA: Yes; Canada: Yes **Available as Generic:** USA: No; Canada: No **Class:** corticosteroid **Controlled Drug:** USA: No; Canada: No

Brand Names: Flonase, Cutivate

> Author's note: This profile will focus on the aqueous nasal form of this medicine.

Warning: Even though this medicine is a nasal spray, there is still a remote risk of suppression of the hypothalamic pituitary adrenal (HPA) axis.

BENEFITS versus RISKS	
Possible Benefits	*Possible Risks*
EFFECTIVE, ONCE A DAY RELIEF OF SEASONAL ALLERGIC RHINITIS	Reversible adrenal gland suppression Irritation of the nose

▷ **Principal Uses**

As a Single Drug Product: Uses currently included in FDA approved labeling: (1) Management of perennial and seasonal allergic or nonallergic rhinitis in adults or children who are 12 years of age or older.

Other (unlabeled) generally accepted uses: None.

How This Drug Works: This medicine belongs to a new class of corticosteroids. The exact mechanism of action of this medicine is not known, however, halomethyl carbothionates have very potent anti-inflammatory and blood vessel contracting (vasoconstrictive) activity.

Available Dosage Forms and Strengths

Amber Glass Bottle — 16 gram (120 actuations) and 9 gram (60 actuations)

▷ **Recommended Dosage Ranges (Actual dosage and administration schedule must be determined by the physician for each patient individually.)**

Infants and Children: Safety and efficacy for those less than 12 years of age have not yet been defined.

12 to 60 Years of Age: Dosing is started with two sprays (50 mcg in each spray) in each nostril once daily. The same dose can also be given as 100 mcg twice daily (8 AM and 8 PM). After a few days, the dose can often be decreased to 100 mcg (one spray in each nostril) daily.

Over 60 Years of Age: Same as 12 to 60 years of age.

Conditions Requiring Dosing Adjustments

Liver function: This drug is extensively changed in the liver, however, no specific dosing changes are defined in patients with comrpomised livers.

Kidney function: No changes in dosing needed.

▷ **Dosing Instructions:** A patient instruction sheet will always accompany this medicine. The instructions should be followed closely. Your doctor should be called if the condition worsens or does not improve.

Usual Duration of Use: Continual use on a regular schedule for several days is usually necessary to determine this drug's effectiveness in treating seasonal and perennial allergic rhinitis. Long-term use (months to years) requires periodic evaluation of response and dosage adjustment. Consult your physician on a regular basis.

Fluticasone

Possible Advantages of This Drug
Once a day dosing.

▷ **This Drug Should Not Be Taken If**
- you have had an allergic reaction to any dosage form of it previously.

▷ **Inform Your Physician Before Taking This Drug If**
- you are already taking systemic prednisone.
- you are exposed to measles or chicken pox.
- you are uncertain of how much fluticasone to take or how often to take it.
- you take other prescription or non-prescription medicines which were not discussed with your doctor when fluticasone was prescribed.
- you have signs or symptoms of an infection in your nose.
- your allergic rhinitis does not improve or worsens.

Possible Side-Effects (natural, expected and unavoidable drug actions)
Irritation of the nose (1–3%). Systemic steroid effects (possible).

▷ **Possible Adverse Effects** (unusual, unexpected and infrequent reactions)
If any of the following develop, consult your physician promptly for guidance.
Mild Adverse Effects
Allergic Reactions: Contact dermatitis.
Nosebleeds.
Nasal burning (3–6%).
Dizziness.
Unpleasant taste, nausea or vomiting (less than 1%).
Serious Adverse Effects
Allergic Reactions: Anaphylaxis.
Suppression of the HPA axis (rare).
Increased risk from viral infections.
Yeast infections of the nose (rare).
Cushing's syndrome (with excessive doses or very sensitive patients).

▷ **Possible Effects on Sexual Function:** None defined.

Possible Delayed Adverse Effects: Yeast infections of the nose (rare).

▷ **Adverse Effects That May Mimic Natural Diseases or Disorders**
None defined.

Natural Diseases or Disorders That May Be Activated by This Drug
If systemic effects occur, the patient may be more susceptible to infections, or dormant infections may become active.

Possible Effects on Laboratory Tests
Cortisol levels: decreased.

CAUTION
1. Call your doctor if you are exposed to measles or chicken pox.
2. Long-term use requires periodic evaluation for yeast infection of the nose.
3. Call your doctor if your condition does not improve or worsens.

Precautions for Use
By Infants and Children:
Safety and effectiveness for use by those under 12 years of age have not been established.
By Those over 60 Years of Age: No specific precautions.

▷ **Advisability of Use During Pregnancy**
Pregnancy Category: C. See Pregnancy Code at the back of this book.
Animal studies: High dose studies in rats revealed fetal toxicity consistant with changes caused by other steroids.
Human studies: Information from adequate studies of pregnant women is not available. Ask your doctor for guidance.

Advisability of Use if Breast-Feeding
Presence of this drug in breast milk: Unknown.
Monitor nursing infant closely and discontinue drug or nursing if adverse effects develop.

Habit-Forming Potential: Not defined.

Effects of Overdosage: Not defined.

Possible Effects of Long-Term Use: Rare nasal yeast infections.

Suggested Periodic Examinations While Taking This Drug (at physician's discretion)
Nasal exams.

▷ **While Taking This Drug, Observe the Following**
Foods: No restrictions.
Beverages: No restrictions.
▷ *Alcohol:* No interactions expected.
Tobacco Smoking: No interactions expected.
▷ *Other Drugs*
Fluticasone *taken concurrently* with
- Systemic steroids (such as prednisone) may increase the likelihood of suppression of the HPA axis.

▷ *Driving, Hazardous Activities:* This drug may cause dizziness. Restrict activities as necessary.
Aviation Note: The use of this drug **may be a disqualification** for piloting. Consult a designated Aviation Medical Examiner.
Exposure to Sun: No restrictions.
Discontinuation: This medicine should not be stopped abruptly. Talk with your doctor before stopping this drug.

FLUVOXAMINE (FLEW vox a mean)

Introduced: 1995   **Prescription:** USA: Yes; Canada: Yes   **Available as Generic:** USA: No; Canada: No   **Class:** Antidepressant, selective serotonin reuptake inhibitor   **Controlled Drug:** USA: No; Canada: No

Brand Names: Luvox

Warning: Do **not** combine this medicine with a MAO (see Drug Classes) inhibitor.

BENEFITS versus RISKS	
Possible Benefits	*Possible Risks*
TREATMENT OF OBSESSIVE-COMPULSIVE DISORDER	Nausea and vomiting (resolves with time)

Fluvoxamine

▷ **Principal Uses**
As a Single Drug Product: Uses currently included in FDA approved labeling: (1) Treatment of obsessive compulsive disorder.
Other (unlabeled) generally accepted uses: (1) May have a role in helping alcohol induced organic brain syndrome; (2) can have a role in treating depression; (3) may be useful in eating problems where binging is a key difficulty; (4) can help panic attacks; (5) could have a role in weight reduction.

How This Drug Works: This medicine inhibits the reuptake of a certain neurotransmitter (5-HT). This effect then has its beneficial change in the treated behaviors or conditions.

Available Dosage Forms and Strengths
Tablets — 50 mg 100 mg

▷ **Recommended Dosage Ranges (Actual dosage and administration schedule must be determined by the physician for each patient individually.)**
Infants and Children: Safety and efficacy have not been established in those under 18 years old.
18 to 60 Years of Age: Therapy is started with 50 mg which is given at bedtime. The dose may then be increased as needed and tolerated by 50 mg intervals every 7 days. The maximum dose is 300 mg daily. The prescriber should remember that the drug may take from 4 to 14 days to begin to work. If a patient does need a daily dose greater than 100 mg, the dose should be divided into two equal amounts which are then given twice daily.
Over 60 Years of Age: This medicine is removed 50% more slowly than in younger patients. Plasma concentrations are also roughly 40% higher than in younger patients. Slower time frames for any increases beyond the starting dose and lower maintenance doses are indicated.

Conditions Requiring Dosing Adjustments
Liver function: This drug is extensively changed by the liver. If it is used in patients with liver disease, lower starting doses, slow dose increases and careful patient monitoring is indicated.
Kidney function: A low starting dose and careful patient monitoring is needed.

▷ **Dosing Instructions:** Take this medicine exactly as prescribed and at the same time. This medicine may be taken with or without food. Call your doctor if vomiting (a possible side effect) continues for more than two days after you start treatment.

Usual Duration of Use: Continual use on a regular schedule for 4 to 14 days is usually necessary to determine this drug's effectiveness in heping obsessive-compulsive disorder. Long-term use (months to years) requires periodic evaluation of response and dosage adjustment. Consult your physician on a regular basis.

Possible Advantages of This Drug
Requires one daily dosing and has a good side effect profile.

▷ **This Drug Should Not Be Taken If**
- you have had an allergic reaction to any dosage form of it previously.
- you have taken a MAO inhibitor (see Drug Classes) within the last 14 days.
- you have taken terfenadine or astemizole.

Fluvoxamine

▷ **Inform Your Physician Before Taking This Drug If**
- you have continued to have a problem with vomiting two days after starting this medicine.
- you feel light headed when you get up from a sitting position.
- you are uncertain of how much fluvoxamine to take or how often to take it.
- you have a history of heart problems.
- you take other prescription or non-prescription medicines which were not discussed with your doctor when fluvoxamine was prescribed.

Possible Side-Effects (natural, expected and unavoidable drug actions)
Nausea and vomiting (usually stops after a few days of treatment).

▷ **Possible Adverse Effects** (unusual, unexpected and infrequent reactions)
If any of the following develop, consult your physician promptly for guidance.

Mild Adverse Effects
Allergic Reactions: Skin rash.
Somnolence and dry mouth (26%).
Headache or agitation (22% and 16%).
Sleep disorders.
Constipation (18%).
Anorexia (15%).

Serious Adverse Effects
Allergic Reactions: Anaphylactoid reaction.
Liver toxicity (rare).
Seizures (rare).
Mania.
Excessive urination (SIADH) (rare).
Serious skin rash (Toxic epidermal necrolysis) (rare).

▷ **Possible Effects on Sexual Function:** Delayed or absent orgasm.

Possible Delayed Adverse Effects: Not reported.

▷ **Adverse Effects That May Mimic Natural Diseases or Disorders**
Not reported.

Natural Diseases or Disorders That May Be Activated by This Drug
None defined.

Possible Effects on Laboratory Tests
Liver function tests: increased.
Melatonin level: increased.

CAUTION
1. This medicine has several drug-drug interactions. Be certain to tell any health care professionals who provide care for you that you take this medicine.
2. If nausea and vomiting continue for more than two days after you start this medicine, call your doctor.

Precautions for Use
By Infants and Children:
Safety and effectiveness for use by those under 18 years of age have not been established.

By Those over 60 Years of Age: Lowering starting and maintenance doses are indicated.

Fluvoxamine

▷ **Advisability of Use During Pregnancy**
Pregnancy Category: C. See Pregnancy Code at the back of this book.
   Animal studies: Consistent with category C.
   Human studies: Information from adequate studies of pregnant women is not available. Ask your doctor for help.

Advisability of Use if Breast-Feeding
   Presence of this drug in breast milk: Yes, in small amounts.
   Monitor nursing infant closely and discontinue drug or nursing if adverse effects develop.

Habit-Forming Potential: None, but a withdrawal syndrome has been reported if the medicine is stopped abruptly.

Effects of Overdosage: Nausea, vomiting, seizures.

Possible Effects of Long-Term Use: Not defined.

Suggested Periodic Examinations While Taking This Drug (at physician's discretion)
   Liver function tests.

▷ **While Taking This Drug, Observe the Following**
   Foods: No restrictions.
   Beverages: No restrictions.
▷ *Alcohol:* No significant interaction. Ask your doctor for guidance.
   Tobacco Smoking: No interactions expected.
   Marijuana Smoking: Additive somnolence.
▷ *Other Drugs*
   Fluvoxamine *taken concurrently* with
   - amitriptyline can result in amitriptyline toxicity.
   - astemizole (Hismanal) may cause serious heart arrhythmias. Do not combine.
   - benzodiazepines (see Drug Classes) may result in benzodiazepine toxicity.
   - beta blockers (see Drug Classes) may result in decreased drug clearance and toxicity.
   - carbamazepine (Tegretol) may cause toxicity.
   - clomipramine may cause toxicity.
   - clozapine can result in higher clozapine levels and toxicity.
   - imipramine may result in imipramine toxicity.
   - lithium can cause serotonin syndrome.
   - MAO inhibitors (see Drug Classes) can cause toxicity. Do **not** combine.
   - maprotiline can cause maprotiline toxicity.
   - methadone may result in increased opioid effects.
   - terfenadine (Seldane) may cause serious heart arrhythmias. Do not combine.
   - theophylline may result in theophylline toxicity.
   - warfarin (Coumadin) can result in bleeding.
▷ *Driving, Hazardous Activities:* This drug may cause drowsiness. Restrict activities as necessary.
   Aviation Note: The use of this drug **is probably a disqualification** for piloting. Consult a designated Aviation Medical Examiner.

Exposure to Sun: No restrictions.
Discontinuation: A withdrawal syndrome has been reported if this medicine is abruptly stopped. The doses should be slowly tapered.

FOSCARNET (Fos KAR net)

Introduced: 1992 **Prescription:** USA: Yes **Available as Generic:** USA: No **Class:** Antiviral **Controlled Drug:** USA: No
Brand Name: Foscavir

BENEFITS versus RISKS	
Possible Benefits	*Possible Risks*
TREATMENT OF CYTOMEGALOVIRUS (CMV) RETINITIS IN PATIENTS WITH ACQUIRED IMMUNODEFICIENCY SYNDROME (AIDS), AND SIGNIFICANT DELAY IN PROGRESSION OF OCCULAR DISEASE	SEIZURES (10%) FEVER (65%) ENCEPHALOPATHY (RARE) DEPRESSION (5% OR GREATER) CARDIAC ARREST (RARE) SIGNIFICANT RENAL (KIDNEY) IMPARIMENT (up to 33%) ELECTROLYTE ABNORMALITIES INCLUDING: HYPOKALEMIA (low blood potassium) (16%), HYPOCALCEMIA (low blood calcium) (16%), HYPOMAGNESEMIA (low blood magnesium) (15%), HYPOPHOSPHATEMIA (low blood phosphorous) (8%), and HYPERPHOSPHATEMIA (high blood phosphorous) (6%), ACIDOSIS (1–5%), THROMBOCYTOPENIA (1–5%) BRONCHOSPASM (1–5%) Anemia

▷ **Principal Uses**

As a Single Drug Product: Uses currently included in FDA approved labeling: (1) Single drug treatment of CMV retinitis in patients with AIDS; (2) combination therapy with ganciclovir of resistant CMV retinitis in AIDS patients; (3) treatment of acyclovir resistant Herpes simplex virus infections in patients with compromised immune systems (such as AIDS).

Other (unlabeled) generally accepted uses: (1) Therapy of acyclovir resistant Herpes simplex infections in AIDS patients; (2) therapy of CMV pneumonia or pneumonitis in AIDS patients; (3) helps Varicella-zoster (shingles) resistant to acyclovir.

How This Drug Works: This drug blocks the ability of viruses to reproduce. Foscarnet accomplishes this effect by blocking genetic material (DNA) polymerases. This specific mechanism may allow foscarnet to be effective against strains of CMV that are resistant to ganciclovir or other agents.

Foscarnet

Available Dosage Forms and Strengths

Foscarnet (Foscavir) for intravenous infusion:
  250 ml bottles in cases of 12—NDC # 0186190501
  500 ml bottles in cases of 12—NDC # 0186190601

The final solution should be colorless and free of particulates or precipitation. Never use an IV solution which is not colorless or has visible elements in it. The standard 24 mg/ml solution can be used without dilution if it is infused into a central line (central venous catheter). If a peripheral vein (for example a vein in the arm) is used, the standard solution must be diluted to 12 mg/ml. The IV bag should say 0.9% NaCl (normal saline) or D5W (5% dextrose in water) as these are compatible solutions.

How To Store

Store at room temperature (59–86 degrees) and protect from heat or freezing. Once the bottle is opened, prepared solutions should be used within 24 hours.

▷ **Recommended Dosage Ranges (Actual dosage and administration schedule must be determined by the physician for each patient individually.)**

Infants and Children: Safety and effectiveness in this population have **not** been established.

18 to 60 Years of Age: For induction:

In adults with normal renal function, the initial dose is 60 mg/kg. This dose must be given intravenously, and is to be infused at a constant rate (controlled by an infusion pump) over a minimum of 1 hour and repeated every 8 hours. This dose and schedule is to be repeated for 2 to 3 weeks depending on clinical response or occurrence of side effects. It is recommended by the manufacturer that adequate hydration be used (if there are no clinical contraindications) to establish a diuresis (outflow of urine) both prior to and during treatment. This is important because it can help decrease renal (kidney) toxicity.

For maintenance treatment:

Once the induction period is successfully completed, the recommended maintenance dose is 90–120 mg/kg/day for people with normal renal function. If renal function is compromised, the dose **must** be adjusted. Each dose must be given over a 2 hour period. Because of potential toxicity, the 90 mg/kg/day dose is recommended as the starting maintenance dose. If the retinitis progresses, dosing can increase to the 120 mg/kg/day level. If patients tolerate foscarnet well, they may benefit from an escalation to the 120 mg/kg/day dose earlier than usual. Once again, (unless clinically contraindicated) hydration sufficient to cause a diuresis both prior to and during treatment is suggested to help limit toxicity. It is critical that an infusion pump be used to infuse all doses. If your retinitis progresses while you are being treated with foscavir, you can be retreated with the induction and maintenance dosing schedules.

Over 65 Years of Age: Studies have not been conducted in this age group. Logically, since people over 65 tend to have age related decreases in renal (kidney) function, particular attention should be paid to adjusting the initial dose to the degree of renal compromise. Assessment of renal function during therapy should occur more frequently in this age group, if the drug is used at all.

Conditions Requiring Dosing Adjustments
Liver function: Abnormal liver function has been associated with foscarnet administration, however, compromised liver function is typically not a criteria for initial dosing adjustments.

Kidney function: Both the induction dose and maintenance dose of foscarnet must be individualized according to the status of kidney function. Once therapy is started, creatinine clearance (a measure of kidney function) should either be estimated from the Cockcroft and Gault equation (a specific calculation using a single blood creatinine) or measured 2 to 3 times a week during the induction phase.

Creatinine clearance should be determined at least every 1 to 2 weeks during maintenance therapy. Doses during the induction or maintenance phase **must** be adjusted to changes in kidney function, and take body weight in kg into account. A complete chart is provided by the manufacturer which outlines appropriate steps to take.

▷ **Dosing Instructions:** In order to minimize renal toxicity, it is important to have enough IV fluid given to you to make you urinate both before and during the foscarnet infusion. It is very probable that you may have two IVs infusing (running) at the same time—one containing the foscarnet and one for fluids.

Usual Duration of Use: Use on a regular schedule for the 2 to 3 week induction phase and initiation of the maintenance phase is usually needed to see this drug's effectiveness in helping the retinitis. During this time, regular ophthalmologic exams will be needed. Long-term use requires physician evaluation of response and dosage adjustment. Periodic interruptions of therapy because of side effects are not unusual.

Possible Advantages of This Drug
Has a higher effectiveness in CMV retinitis and a better averse effect profile than other medicines currently available to treat this disease.

Currently a "Drug of Choice"
for initial treatment and maintenance treatment of cytomegalovirus retinitis in patients with AIDS.

▷ **This Drug Should Not Be Taken If**
- you have had an allergic reaction to any dosage form of it previously.
- your renal (kidney) function is compromised to the extent that your creatinine clearance is less than 50 ml/min or your creatinine is greater than 2.8 mg/dl.

▷ **Inform Your Physician Before Taking This Drug If**
- you are pregnant or plan to become pregnant.
- you are taking other prescription or non-prescription drugs which were not discussed when foscarnet was prescribed.
- you do not understand when and how often the medicine is to be given.
- you have a neurologic (especially a seizure disorder) or cardiac disorder that he or she is not aware of.
- you tend to have low serum electrolytes.
- you have kidney disease or an anemia that he or she is not aware of.
- you have previously been treated for depression.
- you have abnormal heartbeats and are being treated by a cardiologist.
- you have high blood pressure.
- you have a liver disease that he or she is not aware of.

Foscarnet

Possible Side-Effects (natural, expected and unavoidable drug actions)
Antidiuretic hormone disorders (a hormone that effects the kidney which leads to increased urine output if it is decreased, decreased urine output if it is increased), decreased gonadotropins (substances which stimulate the ovaries or testicles), swelling of male breast tissue.

▷ **Possible Adverse Effects** (unusual, unexpected and infrequent reactions)
If any of the following develop, consult your physician promptly for guidance.
Mild Adverse Effects
Allergic Reactions: Rash (less than 5%). Maculopapular rash, itching (1-5%).
Nausea (47%), vomiting and headache (26%), myalgias and conjunctivitis (1-5%) and aggravated psoriasis (less than 1%).
Serious Adverse Effects
Allergic Reactions: Bronchospasm (1-5%), pneumonitis and lung effusions (less than 1%).
Fever (65%), seizure (10%), perioral (around the mouth) numbness (occurs as a symptom with electrolyte depletion), aggressive reaction (1-5%), meningitis (1-5%), aphasia (1-5%).
Encephalopathy and coma (less than 1%).
Malignant hyperpyrexia, cerebral edema, and psychosis (rare).
ECG abnormalities and hypertension (1-5%).
Anemia (33%), declines in renal function including ARF, and decreased creatinine clearance (27%), acute renal failure (1-5%), glomerulonephritis (less than 1%).
Thrombosis (1-5%), thrombocytopenia (1-5%), pneumothorax (1-5%), pulmonary embolism (less than 1%), pancytopenia (less than 1%), acidosis, hypercalcemia.
Abnormal liver function (1-5%), hepatitis (less than 1%), jaundice (less than 1%), hepatosplenomegaly (less than 1%).
Colitis, duodenal ulcer, enterocolitis, abnormal glucose tolerance, vocal cord paralysis (less than 1%), respiratory depression, deafness, blindness, antidiuretic hormone disorders, and paralysis, (less than 1%).
Rare deaths have been reported.

▷ **Possible Effects on Sexual Function:** Swelling of the breast in men, decreased gonadotropins (substances which stimulate the ovary or testicle), penile inflammation, perineal pain in women.

Possible Delayed Adverse Effects: None defined to date.

▷ **Adverse Effects That May Mimic Natural Diseases or Disorders**
The drug induced fever associated with foscarnet may mimic a variety of infectious processes. Acute renal failure due to foscarnet mimics ARF due to other causes. Seizures seen secondary to foscarnet mimic those with organic (natural) causes. Hepatitis caused by foscavir mimics infectious viral hepatitis. Hypertension from foscarnet mimics labile hypertension due to other causes. Depression is similar to depression due to natural causes.

Natural Diseases or Disorders That May Be Activated by This Drug
Chronic renal failure, seizure disorders, labile or stabile hypertension, cardiac conduction problems, anemias.

Possible Effects on Laboratory Tests

Complete blood counts: Increased white blood cells, decreased hemoglobin and hematocrit, decreased white blood cells, decreased platelets, decreased granulocytes (a specific kind of white blood cell).

Decreased coagulation (blood clotting) factors

Increased serum creatinine and BUN, and decreased creatinine clearance.

Increased phosphorous.

Decreased potassium, chloride, calcium, magnesium and phosphorous.

Increased liver enzymes (SGPT, LDH and SGOT).

CAUTION

1. Do not administer this drug by rapid IV (bolus or all at once) injection.
2. Do not exceed the recommended frequency, dosage or infusion rate.
3. Do not administer without an infusion pump.
4. Do not use any IV solution which has visible particles or precipitates or is colored.
5. Check the outdate on the IV bag. Do not use outdated solutions.
6. Tell your doctor at once if mouth tingling or numbness begins.

Precautions for Use

By Infants and Children: Safety and effectiveness for infants and children not established.

By Those over 65 Years of Age: Studies have not been conducted in this age group. Because of age-related declines in kidney function, increased testing is needed.

▷ **Advisability of Use During Pregnancy**

Pregnancy Category: C. See Pregnancy Code at the back of this book.

Animal studies: When daily subcutaneous doses of up to 75 mg/kg of foscarnet were given to female rats prior to and during mating as well as during pregnancy and 21 days after birth, a slight increase in the number of skeletal defects was observed. Rabbit doses of 75 mg/kg and rat doses of 150 mg/kg during pregnancy caused an increase in skeletal defects. These doses are not sufficient to determine the effects of foscarnet at typical human therapeutic doses.

Human studies: Adequate studies of pregnant women are not available. Ask your physician for guidance.

Advisability of Use if Breast-Feeding

Presence of this drug in breast milk: No information is available regarding presence of foscarnet in human breast milk. Animal data (rats) where 75 mg/kg was given resulted in foscarnet maternal milk levels that were 3 times higher than those in the maternal circulation. Avoid drug or refrain from nursing.

Habit-Forming Potential: None.

Effects of Overdosage: Overdosage was reported in 10 patients in controlled clinical trials. One patient died after receiving a total daily dose of 12.5 grams for 3 days (instead of the 10.9 grams which was ordered). The patient experienced a grand mal seizure and died 3 days later. Nine other patients were given 1.14–8.0 times their ordered doses. Three patients had renal function impairment, 3 had seizures, 4 had perioral or limb paresthesias, and 5 patients had disturbances in electrolytes which primarily involved phosphate and calcium.

Possible Effects of Long-Term Use: Declines in renal function, electrolyte imbalances and hematological disturbances.

Suggested Periodic Examinations While Taking This Drug (at physician's discretion)

Baseline (before foscarnet therapy is started) measured or estimated creatinine clearance should be determined, followed by testing 2 to 3 times weekly during induction, and determinations once every 1 to 2 weeks thereafter. Some patients (especially those with preexisting renal compromise may need more frequent testing. Baseline and periodic creatinine clearances are needed. Foscarnet therapy should be stopped if the creatinine clearance falls below 0.4 ml/min/kg.

The same schedule for creatinine clearance should be used for tests of serum calcium, magnesium, phosphorous and potassium. Patients with preexisting heart or nerve disease may need more frequent testing. Patients who receive medications which deplete or increase any of the previously mentioned electrolytes should also be watched more closely. Patients with seizures or perioral (around the mouth) numbness should have immediate electrolyte testing.

▷ **While Taking This Drug, Observe the Following**

Foods: No restrictions.

Beverages: No restrictions.

▷ *Alcohol:* May increase the potential for liver damage. Avoid alcohol.

Tobacco Smoking: No interactions expected.

Marijuana Smoking: May cause additive respiratory problems, additive difficulty in concentration and additive tachycardia may also occur. Potentiation of seizures is possible. Swelling of the breast in males may increase in incidence. Increased risk for decreases in gonadotropins.

▷ *Other Drugs*

Foscavir *taken concurrently* with
- aminoglycosides such as: gentamicin, tobramicin and amikacin, may increase the risk of renal (kidney) toxicity.
- amphotericin B can cause increased risk of kidney toxicity.
- ciprofloxacin can cause increased risk of seizures.
- edetate disodium, pamidronate, plicamycin and etidronate may cause an increase in the drop of ionized calcium.
- kidney toxic drugs such as amphotericin B should be avoided if possible due to additive toxicity.
- pentamidine may cause additive hypocalcemia (low calcium).
- zidovudine may cause increased risk of anemia.

▷ *Driving, Hazardous Activities:* This drug may cause confusion, and is only administered intravenously. Restrict activities as necessary.

Aviation Note: The use of this drug *may be a disqualification* for piloting. Consult a designated Aviation Medical Examiner.

Exposure to Sun: No restrictions.

Discontinuation: Dosing of foscarnet **must** be interrupted if the creatinine clearance falls below 0.4 ml/min/kg.

Observe the Following Expiration Times: Discard any prepared solutions (those removed from the sealed bottle) 24 hours after the bottle was opened. Never use any solution which has visible particles or precipitates or is colored.

FOSINOPRIL (FOH sin oh pril)

Introduced: 1986 **Prescription:** USA: Yes **Available as Generic:** No **Class:** Antihypertensive, ACE inhibitor **Controlled Drug:** USA: No
Brand Name: Monopril

BENEFITS versus RISKS	
Possible Benefits	*Possible Risks*
EFFECTIVE CONTROL OF MILD TO MODERATE HIGH BLOOD PRESSURE	Headache (3.2%), dizziness (1.6%), fatigue (1.5%) Low blood pressure (less than 1%) Allergic swelling of face, tongue, throat, vocal cords (less than 1%)

▷ **Principal Uses**
As a Single Drug Product: Uses currently included in FDA approved labeling: Treatment of mild to moderate high blood pressure, alone or concurrently with a thiazide diuretic.
Other (unlabeled) generally accepted uses: (1) Combination with other drugs (digoxin and diuretics) to treat congestive heart failure; (2) may help decrease enlargement of the left side of the heart; (3) can have a role in stopping the progression of atherosclerosis; (4) reduces abnormal elimination of protein by the kidneys.

How This Drug Works: By blocking an enzyme system (angiotensin-converting enzyme, ACE), this drug relaxes arterial walls and lowers blood pressure. This, in turn, reduces the workload of the heart and improves its performance.

Available Dosage Forms and Strengths
Tablets — 10 mg, 20 mg

▷ **Recommended Dosage Ranges** (Actual dosage and administration schedule must be determined by the physician for each patient individually.)
Infants and Children: Dosage not established.
18 to 60 Years of Age: Initially 10 mg once daily for those not taking a diuretic; 5 mg once daily for those taking a diuretic. Usual maintenance dose is 20 to 40 mg/day taken in a single dose. Total daily dosage should not exceed 80 mg.
Over 60 Years of Age: Same as 18 to 60 years of age.

Conditions Requiring Dosing Adjustments
Liver function: Fosinopril is a prodrug, and is changed into fosinoprilat (the active form) by the liver. It should be used with caution and in lower doses in patients with liver compromise. Fosinopril can also be a rare cause of hepatitis.
Kidney function: This drug undergoes dual hepatobiliary (liver and bile) and renal (via the kidneys) elimination. Patients with renal compromise (especially those with renal artery stenosis) should be started on a decreased dose, and the dose should be increased slowly and only if needed.

▷ **Dosing Instructions:** The tablet may be crushed, and taken on an empty stomach or with food, at the same time each day.

Usual Duration of Use: Use on a regular schedule for 2 to 3 weeks determines effectiveness in controlling high blood pressure. Long-term use of effective medicines and periodic physician evaluation is needed in high blood pressure.

Possible Advantages of This Drug
Usually controls blood pressure effectively with one daily dose.
Relatively low incidence of adverse effects.
No adverse influence on asthma, cholesterol blood levels or diabetes.
Sudden withdrawal does not result in a rapid increase in blood pressure.

▷ **This Drug Should Not Be Taken If**
- you have had an allergic reaction to it previously.
- you are pregnant (last 6 months).
- you currently have a blood cell or bone marrow disorder.
- you have an abnormally high level of blood potassium.

▷ **Inform Your Physician Before Taking This Drug If**
- you have had an allergic reaction (or other adverse effect) to any ACE inhibitor (see Drug Class Section).
- you are planning pregnancy.
- you have a history of kidney disease or impaired kidney function.
- you have scleroderma or systemic lupus erythematosus.
- you have cerebral artery disease.
- you have any form of heart disease.
- you are taking: Other antihypertensives, diuretics, nitrates or potassium supplements.
- you plan to have surgery under general anesthesia in the near future.

Possible Side-Effects (natural, expected and unavoidable drug actions)
Dizziness (1.6%), orthostatic hypotension (1.4%) (see Glossary), increased blood potassium level (2.6%).

▷ **Possible Adverse Effects** (unusual, unexpected and infrequent reactions)
If any of the following develop, consult your physician promptly for guidance.
Mild Adverse Effects
Allergic Reactions: Skin rash, hives, itching (less than 1.0%).
Headache (3.2%), fatigue (1.5%), drowsiness, numbness and tingling, weakness (less than 1%).
Chest pain, palpitation (less than 1.0%), cough (2.2%).
Indigestion, nausea and vomiting (1.2%), diarrhea (1.5%).
Serious Adverse Effects
Allergic Reactions: Swelling (angioedema) of face, tongue and/or vocal cords (less than 0.1%); can be life-threatening.
Impairment of kidney function (less than 1.0%).
Decreased white blood cells have been reported with similar medicines.
Symptomatic hypotension.
Compromise of kidney function, especially in those with severe congestive heart failure.

▷ **Possible Effects on Sexual Function:** Decreased libido (less than 1%).

Possible Effects on Laboratory Tests
   Blood potassium level: increased.
   Liver function tests: increased liver enzymes (ALT/GPT, AST/GOT and alkaline phosphatase), increased bilirubin.
   Kidney function tests: increased blood urea nitrogen (BUN) and creatinine.
   May give a falsely low test for digoxin levels.

CAUTION
   1. Ask your doctor if you should stop other antihypertensive drugs (especially diuretics) for 1 week before starting this drug.
   2. **Inform your physician immediately if you become pregnant.** This drug should not be taken beyond the first 3 months of pregnancy.
   3. **Report promptly** any indications of infection (fever, sore throat), or water retention (weight gain, puffiness, swollen feet or ankles).
   4. Do not use a salt substitute without your physician's knowledge and approval. (Many salt substitutes contain potassium.)
   5. It is advisable to obtain blood cell counts and urine analyses **before** starting this drug.

Precautions for Use
   By Infants and Children: Safety and effectiveness for those under 18 years of age not established.
   By Those over 60 Years of Age: Small starting doses are advisable. Sudden and excessive lowering of blood pressure can predispose to stroke or heart attack in impaired brain circulation or coronary artery heart disease.

▷ **Advisability of Use During Pregnancy**
   Pregnancy Category: D. See Pregnancy Code at the back of this book.
   Animal studies: Significant birth defects associated with this drug.
   Human studies: The use of ACE inhibitor drugs during the last 6 months of pregnancy is known to possibly cause very serious injury and possible death to the fetus; skull and limb malformations, lung defects, and kidney failure have been reported in over 50 cases worldwide.
   Avoid this drug completely during the last 6 months. During the first 3 months of pregnancy, use this drug only if clearly needed. Ask your physician for guidance.

Advisability of Use if Breast-Feeding
   Presence of this drug in breast milk: Yes.
   Avoid drug or refrain from nursing.

Habit-Forming Potential: None.

Effects of Overdosage: Excessive drop in blood pressure, light-headedness, dizziness, fainting.

Possible Effects of Long-Term Use: Gradual increase in blood potassium level.

Suggested Periodic Examinations While Taking This Drug (at physician's discretion)
   Before starting drug: Complete blood counts; urine analysis with measurement of protein content; blood potassium level.
   During use of drug: Blood cell counts; measurements of blood potassium.

▷ **While Taking This Drug, Observe the Following**
Foods: Consult physician regarding salt intake.
Nutritional Support: **Do not take** potassium supplements unless directed by your physician.
Beverages: No restrictions. May be taken with milk.
▷ *Alcohol:* Use caution—alcohol may enhance the blood-pressure-lowering effect.
Tobacco Smoking: No interactions expected.
▷ *Other Drugs*
Fosinopril *taken concurrently* with
- cyclosporine (Sandimmune) may cause acute kidney failure.
- lithium causes increased lithium blood levels and toxicity; blood levels and dosage decreases are critical.
- potassium preparations (K-Lyte, Slow-K, etc.) may cause increased blood levels of potassium with risk of serious heart rhythm disturbances.
- potassium-sparing diuretics: amiloride (Moduretic), spironolactone (Aldactazide), triamterene (Dyazide) may cause increased blood levels of potassium with risk of serious heart rhythm disturbances.
- chlorpromazine (thorazine) can cause large and undesirable decreases in blood pressure. Avoid this combination.
- cyclosporine (Sandimmune) can cause a large decrease in kidney function.
- loop diuretics—furosemide or bumetanide (Lasix, Bumex) can cause marked lowering of blood pressure on standing (postural hypotension).
▷ *Driving, Hazardous Activities:* Usually no restrictions. Be aware of possible drops in blood pressure with resultant dizziness or faintness.
Aviation Note: The use of this drug *may be a disqualification* for piloting. Consult a designated Aviation Medical Examiner.
Exposure to Sun: Caution advised. A similar drug of this class can cause photosensitivity.
Exposure to Heat: Caution advised. Avoid excessive perspiring with resultant loss of body water and drop in blood pressure.
Occurrence of Unrelated Illness: Promptly report any nausea, vomiting or diarrhea. Fluid and chemical imbalances must be corrected as soon as possible.
Discontinuation: This drug may be stopped abruptly without causing a sudden increase in blood pressure. However, you should ask your physician before stopping this drug for any reason.

FUROSEMIDE (fur OH se mide)

Introduced: 1964 **Prescription:** USA: Yes; Canada: Yes **Available as Generic:** USA: Yes; Canada: Yes **Class:** Antihypertensive, diuretic
Controlled Drug: USA: No; Canada: No

Brand Names: ✦Albert Furosemide, ✦Apo-Furosemide, Fumide MD, Furocot, ✦Furoside, Lasaject, Lasimide, Lasix, ✦Lasix special, Lo-Aqua, Luramide, Myrosemide, Ro-Semide, SK-Furosemide, ✦Uritol

BENEFITS versus RISKS	
Possible Benefits	*Possible Risks*
PROMPT, EFFECTIVE, RELIABLE DIURETIC	WATER AND ELECTROLYTE DEPLETION with excessive use
MODEST ANTIHYPERTENSIVE IN MILD TO MODERATE HYPERTENSION	Excessive potassium loss Increased blood sugar level Increased blood uric acid level
ENHANCES EFFECTIVENESS OF OTHER ANTIHYPERTENSIVES	Decreased blood calcium level Rare liver damage Rare blood cell disorder

▷ **Principal Uses**

As a Single Drug Product: Uses currently included in FDA approved labeling: (1) Used to increase urine and remove excessive water (edema) that is seen in: (a) congestive heart failure (b) some forms of liver, lung and kidney disease; (2) it is used in the treatment of high blood pressure, but usually is combined with other drugs.

Other (unlabeled) generally accepted uses: (1) Inhaled furosemide may help protect the lungs in people with asthma; (2) can have a role in helping infants with chronic bronchopulmonary dysplasia.

How This Drug Works: By increasing the elimination of salt and water through increased urine production, this drug reduces fluid in the blood and body tissues. These changes also contribute to lowering blood pressure.

Available Dosage Forms and Strengths
Injection — 10 mg per ml
Solution — 10 mg per ml and 40 mg per 5-ml teaspoonful
Tablets — 20 mg, 40 mg, 80 mg

▷ **Usual Adult Dosage Range:** As antihypertensive: 40 mg/12 hours initially; increase dose as needed and tolerated. As diuretic: 20 to 80 mg in a single dose initially; if necessary, increase the dose by 20 to 40 mg/6 to 8 hours. The smallest effective dose should be used, and total daily dose should not exceed 600 mg. **Note: Actual dosage and administration schedule must be determined by the physician for each patient individually.**

Conditions Requiring Dosing Adjustments

Liver function: Larger doses may be needed in patients with liver compromise, and extreme care must be used to maintain critical electrolytes.

Kidney function: Larger initial doses may be needed before any benefit is seen. Furosemide is also capable of causing kidney stones and protein in urine.

Cystic fibrosis: Patients with this disease may be more sensitive to the drug, and smaller starting doses are indicated.

▷ **Dosing Instructions:** The tablet may be crushed and taken with or following meals to reduce stomach irritation. Best taken in the morning to avoid nighttime urination.

Usual Duration of Use: Use on a regular schedule for 2 to 3 weeks is best to see effectiveness in lowering high blood pressure. Long-term use (months to years) requires periodic physician evaluation of response.

▷ **This Drug Should Not Be Taken If**
- you have had an allergic reaction to any dosage form of it previously.
- your kidneys are not making urine.

▷ **Inform Your Physician Before Taking This Drug If**
- you are allergic to any form of "sulfa" drug.
- you are pregnant or planning pregnancy.
- you have a history of kidney or liver disease.
- you have diabetes, gout or lupus erythematosus.
- you have impaired hearing.
- you have low blood potassium.
- you take any form of cortisone, digitalis, oral antidiabetic drug or insulin.
- you plan to have surgery under general anesthesia in the near future.

Possible Side-Effects (natural, expected and unavoidable drug actions)
Light-headedness on arising from sitting or lying position (see Orthostatic Hypotension in Glossary).
Increase in blood sugar level, affecting control of diabetes.
Increase in blood uric acid level, affecting control of gout.
Decrease in blood potassium level, causing muscle weakness and cramping.

▷ **Possible Adverse Effects** (unusual, unexpected and infrequent reactions)
If any of the following develop, consult your physician promptly for guidance.

Mild Adverse Effects
Allergic Reactions: Skin rashes, hives, drug fever.
Headache, dizziness, blurred or yellow vision, ringing in ears, numbness and tingling.
Reduced appetite, indigestion, nausea, vomiting, diarrhea.
Metabolic alkalosis.

Serious Adverse Effects
Allergic Reactions: Hepatitis with jaundice (see Glossary), anaphylactic reaction (see Glossary), severe skin reactions.
Idiosyncratic Reaction: Fluid accumulation in lungs.
Temporary hearing loss.
Inflammation of the pancreas—severe abdominal pain.
Bone marrow depression (see Glossary)—fatigue, weakness, fever, sore throat, abnormal bleeding or bruising.
Low blood pressure on standing.
Abnormal heart beats (arrhythmias).
Excessive activity of the parathyroid gland (hyperparathyroidism).
Low blood potassium or magnesium.
Vitamin deficiency (thiamine).
Pancreatitis (rare).
Kidney stones (calcium containing) (rare).
Liver toxicity (cholestatic jaundice).
Skin lesions (Erythema multiforme).
Skin syndromes (Stevens-Johnson syndrome).
Hip fractures (may increase risk).

▷ **Possible Effects on Sexual Function:** Impotence (5%) using recommended dosage of 20 to 80 mg/day.

▷ **Adverse Effects That May Mimic Natural Diseases or Disorders**
Liver reaction may suggest viral hepatitis.

Natural Diseases or Disorders That May Be Activated by This Drug
Diabetes, gout, systemic lupus erythematosus.

Possible Effects on Laboratory Tests
Complete blood counts: reduced red cells, hemoglobin, white cells and platelets.
Blood amylase and lipase levels: increased (possible pancreatitis).
Blood sodium and chloride levels: decreased.
Blood levels of total cholesterol, LDL and VLDL cholesterol, and triglycerides: increased.
Blood glucose level: increased.
Glucose tolerance test (GTT): decreased.
Blood potassium level: decreased.
Blood thyroid hormone (T_3 and T_4) levels: decreased.
Blood uric acid level: increased.
Blood urea nitrogen (BUN): increased.
Urine sugar tests: no drug effect with TesTape; false low results with Clinistix and Diastix.

CAUTION
1. Take exactly the dose which was prescribed. Increased doses can cause serious loss of sodium and potassium, with resultant loss of appetite, nausea, fatigue, weakness, confusion and tingling in the extremities.
2. If you take a digitalis preparation (digitoxin, digoxin), ensure an adequate intake of high-potassium foods to prevent potassium deficiency. (See Table of High Potassium Foods)

Precautions for Use
By Infants and Children: Avoid overdosage that could cause serious dehydration. Significant potassium loss can occur within the first 2 weeks of drug use.
By Those over 60 Years of Age: Small starting doses are critical. Increased risk of impaired thinking, orthostatic hypotension, potassium loss and blood sugar increase. Overdosage and extended use of this drug can cause excessive loss of body water, thickening (increased viscosity) of the blood and an increased tendency for the blood to clot—predisposing to stroke, heart attack or thrombophlebitis (vein inflammation with blood clot).

▷ **Advisability of Use During Pregnancy**
Pregnancy Category: C. See Pregnancy Code at the back of this book.
Animal studies: Significant birth defects have been reported.
Human studies: Adequate studies of pregnant women are not available.
It should not be used during pregnancy unless a very serious complication occurs for which this drug is significantly beneficial. Avoid completely during the first 3 months. Ask physician for guidance.

Advisability of Use if Breast-Feeding
Presence of this drug in breast milk: Yes.
Avoid drug or refrain from nursing.

Habit-Forming Potential: None.

440   Furosemide

Effects of Overdosage: Dry mouth, thirst, lethargy, weakness, muscle cramping, nausea, vomiting, drowsiness progressing to stupor or coma.

Possible Effects of Long-Term Use: Impaired water, salt and potassium balance; dehydration and increased blood coagulability, with risk of blood clots. Development of diabetes in predisposed individuals.

Suggested Periodic Examinations While Taking This Drug (at physician's discretion)
Complete blood counts, measurements of blood levels of sodium, potassium, chloride, sugar and uric acid.
Kidney and liver function tests.

▷ **While Taking This Drug, Observe the Following**
Foods: Ask your doctor about eating foods rich in potassium. If so advised, see the Table of High Potassium Foods. Follow physician's advice regarding the use of salt. Food decreases absorption of furosemide by up to 30%. Take this medicine 1 hour before or 2 hours after a meal.
Beverages: No restrictions. This drug may be taken with milk.
▷ *Alcohol:* Use with caution—alcohol may exaggerate the blood-pressure-lowering effects of this drug and cause orthostatic hypotension.
Tobacco Smoking: No interactions expected. Follow physician's advice.
▷ *Other Drugs*
Furosemide may *increase* the effects of
• other antihypertensive drugs; dosage adjustments may be necessary to prevent excessive lowering of blood pressure.
• digoxin and result in digoxin toxicity.
• lithium, and cause lithium toxicity.
Furosemide may *decrease* the effects of
• oral antidiabetic drugs (sulfonylureas); dosage adjustments may be necessary for proper control of blood sugar.
Furosemide *taken concurrently* with
• amikacin, gentamicin, tobramycin or other aminoglycosides may cause hearing toxicity (ototoxicity).
• cholestyramine may cause loss of furosemide effectiveness.
• colestipol may cause loss of furosemide effectiveness.
• corticosteroids (see Drug Class) may cause additive loss of potassium.
• cyclosporine may cause elevated uric acid levels (hyperuricemia) and gout.
• digitalis preparations (digitoxin, digoxin) require blood tests or dose changes to maintain potassium levels and avoid heart rhythm problems.
• NSAIDs (see Drug Class) may cause loss of diuretic effectiveness.
The following drug may *decrease* the effects of furosemide
• indomethacin (Indocin).
▷ *Driving, Hazardous Activities:* Use caution until the possible occurrence of orthostatic hypotension, dizziness or impaired vision has been determined.
Aviation Note: The use of this drug **may be a disqualification** for piloting. Consult a designated Aviation Medical Examiner.
Exposure to Sun: Use caution—this drug may cause photosensitivity (see Glossary).

Exposure to Heat: Avoid excessive perspiring, which could cause additional loss of salt and water from the body.

Heavy Exercise or Exertion: Avoid exertion that produces light-headedness, excessive fatigue or muscle cramping. Isometric exercises—the "overload" technique for strengthening individual muscles—can raise blood pressure significantly. Ask physician for guidance regarding participation in this form of exercise.

Occurrence of Unrelated Illness: Vomiting or diarrhea can produce a serious imbalance of important body chemistry. Ask your doctor for guidance.

Discontinuation: It may be advisable to discontinue this drug 5 to 7 days before major surgery. Ask your physician, surgeon and/or anesthesiologist for guidance regarding dosage adjustment or drug withdrawal.

GANCICLOVIR (Ganz EYE klo veer)

Introduced: 1995 (tablet)   **Prescription:** USA: Yes; Canada: Yes   **Available as Generic:** USA: No; Canada: No   **Class:** Antiviral   **Controlled Drug:** USA: No; Canada: No

Brand Names: Cytovene

Warning: The oral form of this medicine should only be used in patients who are not candidates for intravenous administration and in whom the risk of more rapid disease progression is outweighed by the benefit of avoiding the intravenous route.

BENEFITS versus RISKS	
Possible Benefits	*Possible Risks*
Oral or IV treatment of CMV retinitis	More rapid progression of CMV disease
Decreased side effects with the oral form	Bone marrow suppression
Transition to an oral form following intravenous induction	

▷ **Principal Uses**

As a Single Drug Product: Uses currently included in FDA approved labeling: (1) Treatment of Cytomegalolvirus retinitis; (2) prevention of CMV retinitis in a variety of patients such as: Liver, kidney, lung, bone marrow and heart transplant patients.

Other (unlabeled) generally accepted uses: (1) Treatment of pediatric CMV; (2) may have a role in treating Epstein Barr virus infection; (3) can have a role in leukoplakia.

How This Drug Works: This medicine is changed into an active triphosphate form by cells infected with cytomegalovirus. This active form interferes with synthesis of DNA and the ability of the virus to survive.

Available Dosage Forms and Strengths
Capsules — 250 mg
Intravenous — 500 mg per 10 ml

How To Store

The intravenous solution should be stored at 4 degrees centigrade and used within 12 hours after it has been reconstituted.

Ganciclovir

▷ **Recommended Dosage Ranges (Actual dosage and administration schedule must be determined by the physician for each patient individually.)**

Infants and Children: **Author's note—this drug has potential for reproductive toxicity and the risk of causing cancer. It is used in children only after careful evaluation and with extreme caution.**

Induction: 2.5 mg per kg given intravenously three times daily.

Maintenance: 6.5 mg per kg given intravenously once daily 5 to 7 times a week.

12 to 60 Years of Age: Induction: 5 mg per kg intravenously (infused over 1 hour) every 12 hours for 14 to 21 days.

Maintenance dose: 5 mg per kg infused into a vein over 1 hour each day. Some centers have used 6 mg per kg given once daily 5 days weekly. If retinitis progresses, the patient can be restarted on the twice daily dosing approach.

Oral: Once the intravenous induction dosing has been accomplished, oral ganciclovir is given 1000 mg 3 times daily. Some centers have opted for 500 mg 6 times per day, given every 3 hours while the patient is awake. If retinitis progresses, intravenous induction therapy should be given.

Intravitreous: An experimental slow release device was used in a small number of patients with good results. This used a 6 mg pellet which lasted 4 months.

Over 60 Years of Age: Kidney function must be assessed and the dose appropriately adjusted.

Conditions Requiring Dosing Adjustments

Liver function: The liver is only minimally involved in the elimination of this drug, and dosing changes in liver compromise are not needed.

Kidney function: The dose **must** be decreased in kidney compromise. This adjustment is accomplished based on creatinine clearance (see Glossary):

Induction—

70 or higher: 5 mg per kg every 12 hours; 50–69: 2.5 mg per kg every 12 hours; 25–49: 2.5 mg per kg every 24 hours; 10–24: 1.25 mg per kg every 24 hours; less than 10: 1.25 mg per kg 3 times weekly.

Maintenance—

70 or higher: 5 mg per kg every 24 hours; 50–69: 2.5 mg per kg every 24 hours; 25–49: 1.25 mg per kg every 24 hours; 10–24: 0.625 mg per kg every 24 hours; less than 10: 0.625 mg per kg 3 times weekly.

▷ **Dosing Instructions:** This medicine should be taken with food if taken by mouth (orally). It is best to take the medicine at the same time each day. If you are taking the capsule form and your vision declines, call your doctor immediately.

Usual Duration of Use: Continual use on a regular schedule for up to 16 days is usually necessary to determine this drug's effectiveness in treating retinitis. Because of a very high frequency of relapse, most centers recommend ongoing maintenance therapy. Long-term use (months to years) requires periodic evaluation of response and dosage adjustment. Consult your physician on a regular basis.

Possible Advantages of This Drug

Transition from the intravenous form to the oral form (if successful in treatment) offers a clear quality of life advantage.

Currently a "Drug of Choice"
for patients with kidney failure.

▷ **This Drug Should Not Be Taken If**
- you have had an allergic reaction to any dosage form of it previously.
- your absolute neutrophil count (a specific kind of white blood cell) is less than 500 per cubic millimeter.
- your platelet count is less than 25,000 per cubic millimeter.

▷ **Inform Your Physician Before Taking This Drug If**
- you think you are dehydrated (this drug is primarily removed by the kidneys).
- you have a sore throat or fever.
- you have a history of blood cell disorders.
- you are planning pregnancy.
- you are male and are planning pregnancy (attempted conception should be avoided for at least 3 months after ganciclovir therapy.
- you are uncertain of how much ganciclovir to take or how often to take it.
- you take other prescription or non-prescription medicines which were not discussed with your doctor when ganciclovir was prescribed. This includes natural extracts or herbal remedies and underground therapies for AIDS.

Possible Side-Effects (natural, expected and unavoidable drug actions)
Pain at the injection site with the IV form.

▷ **Possible Adverse Effects** (unusual, unexpected and infrequent reactions)
If any of the following develop, consult your physician promptly for guidance.

Mild Adverse Effects
Allergic Reactions: Skin rash and itching.
Confusion, headache and nervousness (3–4%).
Tremor, somnolence, abnormal dreams and ataxia (5%).
Rapid heart rate (tachycardia) (rare).
Pins and needles sensations of the hands (paresthesias).
Fever (2%).
Decreased blood glucose (1%).
Nausea, vomiting or diarrhea (up to 5%).
Phlebitis.

Serious Adverse Effects
Allergic Reactions: Anaphylactoid reaction.
Bone marrow suppression (25%).
Arrhythmias (rare).
Coma or psychosis (5%).
Phlebitis.
Seizures (rare).
Liver toxicity (2%).
Retinal detachment (1%).
This drug is a potential cancer causing (carcinogenic) agent (no percentage defined).

▷ **Possible Effects on Sexual Function:** Reversible infertility in men.

Ganciclovir

Possible Delayed Adverse Effects: Not defined.

▷ **Adverse Effects That May Mimic Natural Diseases or Disorders**
Increased liver enzymes may mimic hepatitis.

Natural Diseases or Disorders That May Be Activated by This Drug
None defined.

Possible Effects on Laboratory Tests
Liver enzymes: increased.
Serum bilirubin: increased.
Serum creatinine: increased.
Blood glucose: decreased.

CAUTION
1. The oral form may be less effective than the intravenous form. Call your doctor immediately if your vision declines.
2. This drug can cause bone marrow suppression. Call your doctor if you develop a sore throat, start to bruise easily or develop a fever.

Precautions for Use
By Infants and Children:
Safety and effectiveness for use by those under 18 years of age have not been established. The drug has been used selectively in patients as young as 36 weeks.
By Those over 60 Years of Age: Because of the age-related decline in kidney function, a creatinine clearance should be obtained and dosing adjusted appropriately.

▷ **Advisability of Use During Pregnancy**
Pregnancy Category: C. See Pregnancy Code at the back of this book.
Animal studies: Rabbits have developed cleft palate, exhibited poorly developed organs and have experienced fetal death.
Human studies: Information from adequate studies of pregnant women is not available. Use of this drug during pregnancy is not recommended.

Advisability of Use if Breast-Feeding
Presence of this drug in breast milk: Unknown.
Avoid drug or refrain from nursing.

Habit-Forming Potential: None.

Effects of Overdosage: Nausea and vomiting, excessive salivation, increased liver function tests, bone marrow suppression and kidney failure.

Possible Effects of Long-Term Use: Not defined.

Suggested Periodic Examinations While Taking This Drug (at physician's discretion)
Platelet counts and complete blood counts: every 2 days during induction and weekly thereafter.
Liver function tests: monthly.
Kidney function tests: every 2 weeks.
Eye (ophthalmologic) exams: weekly during induction and every two weeks thereafter. These exams may be needed more frequently if the optic nerve or macula of the eye is involved.

▷ **While Taking This Drug, Observe the Following**
Foods: No restrictions—the oral form should be taken with food.
Beverages: No restrictions.

▷ *Alcohol:* No restrictions, however, alcohol may blunt the immune system.
Tobacco Smoking: No interactions expected.
Marijuana Smoking: May increase somnolence.
▷ *Other Drugs*
Ganciclovir **taken concurrently** with
- amphotericin B may result in increased bone marrow suppression.
- cancer chemotherapy may result in additive bone marrow suppression.
- cotrimoxazole may result in added bone marrow suppression problems.
- cyclosporine (Sandimune) can result in increased kidney toxicity.
- dapsone is a benefit to risk decision as additive bone marrow suppression may occur.
- flucytosine can cause additive bone marrow toxicity.
- imipenem/cilastatin (Primaxin) can cause seizures.
- pentamidine may result in additive bone marrow suppression.
- zidovudine will cause a serious increase in bone marrow suppression.

The following drugs may **increase** the effects of ganciclovir
- probenecid, by interfering with elimination by the kidney.

▷ *Driving, Hazardous Activities:* This drug may cause somnolence. Restrict activities as necessary.
Aviation Note: The use of this drug **may be a disqualification** for piloting. Consult a designated Aviation Medical Examiner.
Exposure to Sun: No restrictions.
Discontinuation: Talk with your doctor before stopping this medicine.
Special Storage Instructions: The intravenous form should be stored at 4 degrees centigrade.
Observe the Following Expiration Times: The intravenous form will be stamped or labeled with a specific expiration time if this has been provided by a home infusion company.

GEMFIBROZIL (jem FI broh zil)

Introduced: 1976   **Prescription:** USA: Yes; Canada: Yes   **Available as Generic:** USA: Yes; Canada: No   **Class:** Anticholesterol   **Controlled Drug:** USA: No; Canada: No
Brand Name: Lopid

BENEFITS versus RISKS	
Possible Benefits	*Possible Risks*
EFFECTIVE REDUCTION OF TRIGLYCERIDE BLOOD LEVELS AND ELEVATION OF HIGH DENSITY (HDL) CHOLESTEROL BLOOD LEVELS (40% to 50% reduction of triglycerides; 25% to 30% elevation of HDL cholesterol)	May elevate total cholesterol levels in one third of users Gallstone formation with long-term use Increased susceptibility to viral and bacterial infections

▷ **Principal Uses**
As a Single Drug Product: Uses currently included in FDA approved labeling: (1) reduces abnormally high blood levels of triglycerides in Types II and

Gemfibrozil

IV blood lipid (fat) disorders; (2) decreases risk for developing coronary artery heart disease.

Other (unlabeled) generally accepted uses: (1) used in diabetics as combination therapy with oral hypoglycemic agents to further increase desirable HDLs.

How This Drug Works: Reduces blood levels of triglycerides by inhibiting their production in the liver. Decreases VLDL and LDL. Causes a larger increase in desirable HDL than clofibrate.

Available Dosage Forms and Strengths
Capsules — 300 mg
Tablets — 600 mg

▷ **Usual Adult Dosage Range:** 1200 to 1600 daily in 2 divided doses. The average dose is 1200 mg/24 hours. Dose increases should be made gradually over a period of 2 to 3 months. **Note: Actual dosage and administration schedule must be determined by the physician for each patient individually.**

Conditions Requiring Dosing Adjustments

Liver function: This drug is contraindicated in primary billiary cirrhosis and severe liver failure.

Kidney function: In patients with moderate kidney failure, 50% of the usual dose should be given at the usual interval. Patients with severe kidney failure should be given 25% of the usual dose at the usual dosing interval.

▷ **Dosing Instructions:** The capsule may be opened and taken 30 minutes before the morning and evening meals.

Usual Duration of Use: Use on a regular schedule for 4 to 8 weeks determines effectiveness in reducing blood levels of triglycerides. Long-term use (months to years) requires periodic physician evaluation.

Currently a "Drug of Choice"
for initiating treatment of elevated LDL cholesterol and VLDL triglycerides.

▷ **This Drug Should Not Be Taken If**
- you have had an allergic reaction to it previously.
- you have biliary cirrhosis of the liver.
- you have severe kidney compromise.

▷ **Inform Your Physician Before Taking This Drug If**
- you have impaired liver or kidney function.
- you have gallbladder disease or gallstones.
- you are a diabetic.
- you have an underactive thyroid (hypothyroidism).

Possible Side-Effects (natural, expected and unavoidable drug actions)
Moderate increase in blood sugar levels.

▷ **Possible Adverse Effects** (unusual, unexpected and infrequent reactions)
If any of the following develop, consult your physician promptly for guidance.

Mild Adverse Effects
Allergic Reactions: Skin rash, hives, itching.
Headache, dizziness, blurred vision, fatigue, muscle aches and cramps.
Indigestion, excessive gas, stomach discomfort (6%), nausea (4%), vomiting (1.6%), diarrhea (5%).
Paresthesias (very rare).

Serious Adverse Effects
> Abnormally low white blood cell count: Fever, chills, sore throat.
> Formation of gallstones with long-term use.
> Raynaud's phenomenon (rare).
> Low blood potassium.
> Liver toxicity.
> Myopathy (muscle weakness and tenderness).
> Rhabdomyolosis (inability to walk, muscle weakness).

▷ **Possible Effects on Sexual Function:** Decreased libido. Impotence.

Natural Diseases or Disorders That May Be Activated by This Drug
Latent diabetes, latent urinary tract infections.

Possible Effects on Laboratory Tests
Complete blood counts: decreased red cells, hemoglobin, white cells and platelets.
Blood HDL cholesterol levels: increased.
Blood triglyceride levels: decreased.
Liver function tests: increased liver enzymes (ALT/GPT, AST/GOT and alkaline phosphatase, increased bilirubin.

CAUTION
1. Gemfibrozil is used only after diet has been ineffective in lowering triglyceride levels.
2. If you used the drug clofibrate (Atromid-S) in the past, inform your physician fully regarding your experience.
3. Periodic triglyceride and cholesterol levels are critical.

Precautions for Use
By Infants and Children: Safety and effectiveness for those under 12 years of age not established.
By Those over 60 Years of Age: Watch for increased tendency to infection; treat all infections promptly.

▷ **Advisability of Use During Pregnancy**
Pregnancy Category: C. See Pregnancy Code at the back of this book.
Animal studies: Produces adverse effects in rabbits and rats.
Human studies: Adequate studies of pregnant women are not available.
Ask your physician for guidance.

Advisability of Use if Breast-Feeding
Presence of this drug in breast milk: Unknown.
Avoid drug or refrain from nursing.

Habit-Forming Potential: None.

Effects of Overdosage: Abdominal pain, nausea, vomiting, diarrhea.

Possible Effects of Long-Term Use: Formation of gallstones.

Suggested Periodic Examinations While Taking This Drug (at physician's discretion)
Complete blood cell counts.
Measurements of blood levels of total cholesterol, HDL and LDL cholesterol fractions, triglycerides and sugar.
Liver function tests.

448 Glipizide

▷ **While Taking This Drug, Observe the Following**
 Foods: Follow the diet prescribed by your physician.
 Beverages: No restrictions. May be taken with milk.
▷ *Alcohol:* No interactions expected.
 Tobacco Smoking: No interactions expected.
▷ *Other Drugs*
 Gemfibrozil may *increase* the effects of
 • glyburide and other oral hypoglycemic agents (see Drug Classes).
 • lovastatin if taken at the same time and results in myopathy.
 • warfarin (Coumadin), and increase the risk of bleeding; prothrombin time measurements and dose changes are critical.
 Gemfibrozil may *decrease* the effects of
 • chenodiol (Chenix), reducing its benefit in gallstone therapy.
▷ *Driving, Hazardous Activities:* This drug may cause dizziness and blurred vision. Restrict activities as necessary.
 Aviation Note: The use of this drug **is usually not a disqualification** for piloting. Consult a designated Aviation Medical Examiner.
 Exposure to Sun: No restrictions.
 Discontinuation: If triglyceride lowering does not occur after 3 months, this drug should be stopped.

GLIPIZIDE (GLIP i zide)

Introduced: 1972   **Prescription:** USA: Yes   **Available as Generic:** No   **Class:** Antidiabetic, sulfonylureas   **Controlled Drug:** USA: No
Brand Name: Glucotrol

BENEFITS versus RISKS	
Possible Benefits	*Possible Risks*
Help in regulating blood sugar in noninsulin-dependent diabetes (adjunctive to appropriate diet and weight control)	HYPOGLYCEMIA, severe and prolonged INCREASED CARDIOVASCULAR MORTALITY Allergic skin reactions (some severe) Rare blood cell and bone marrow disorders

▷ **Principal Uses**
 As a Single Drug Product: Uses currently included in FDA approved labeling: (1) Better control of mild to moderate type II diabetes mellitus (adult, maturity-onset) that does not require insulin, but is not adequately controlled by diet alone.
 Other (unlabeled) generally accepted uses: (1) delay of abnormal metabolism and blood vessel disease if given early in diabetes.
How This Drug Works: This drug (1) stimulates the secretion of insulin; and (2) enhances the utilization of insulin by appropriate tissues.
Available Dosage Forms and Strengths
 Tablets — 5 mg, 10 mg
▷ **Usual Adult Dosage Range:** Initially 5 mg daily with breakfast. At 7-day intervals the dose may be increased by increments of 2.5 to 5 mg daily as

needed and tolerated. Total daily dosage should not exceed 40 mg. A "loading" or priming dose is not necessary and should not be given. **Note: Actual dosage and administration schedule must be determined by the physician for each patient individually.**

Conditions Requiring Dosing Adjustments
Liver function: Patients with liver failure should be given a starting dose of 2.5 mg, and closely monitored.

Kidney function: Glipizide is contraindicated in severe renal compromise. Patients should be monitored closely if the drug is used in mild to moderate renal (kidney) compromise. It is a rare cause of kidney stones.

▷ **Dosing Instructions:** If the daily maintenance dose is found to be 15 mg or more, the total dose should be divided into 2 equal doses—the first taken with the morning meal, the second with the evening meal. The tablet may be crushed for administration.

Usual Duration of Use: Use on a regular schedule for 1 to 2 weeks determines effectiveness in controlling diabetes. Failure to respond to maximal doses within 1 month constitutes a primary failure. Up to 10% of those who respond initially may develop secondary failure. Blood sugars must be measured, and your doctor will decide if the drug should be continued.

Possible Advantages of This Drug
Effective with once-daily dosing.
Onset of action within 30 minutes.
Near-normal insulin response to eating.
Well tolerated by the elderly diabetic.

Currently a "Drug of Choice"
for starting therapy in noninsulin-dependent diabetes when diet and weight control fail.

▷ **This Drug Should Not Be Taken If**
- you have had an allergic reaction to it previously.
- you have severe impairment of liver or kidney function.
- you have diabetic ketoacidosis.
- you are pregnant.

▷ **Inform Your Physician Before Taking This Drug If**
- you are allergic to other sulfonylurea drugs or to "sulfa" drugs.
- your diabetes has been unstable or "brittle" in the past.
- you do not know how to recognize or treat hypoglycemia (see Glossary).
- you are pregnant.
- you have a history of congestive heart failure, peptic ulcer disease, cirrhosis of the liver, bone marrow depression, hypothyroidism or porphyria.

Possible Side-Effects (natural, expected and unavoidable drug actions)
If drug dosage is excessive or if meals are missed or inadequate, abnormally low blood sugar (hypoglycemia) will occur as a drug effect.

▷ **Possible Adverse Effects** (unusual, unexpected and infrequent reactions)
If any of the following develop, consult your physician promptly for guidance.

Glipizide

Mild Adverse Effects
  Allergic Reactions: Skin rash, hives, itching.
  Headache (1.25%), drowsiness (1.75%), dizziness (2.25%), fatigue (2.13%), sweating (1.25%).
  Indigestion, nausea (1.38%), vomiting, diarrhea (1.25%).

Serious Adverse Effects
  Allergic Reactions: Hepatitis with jaundice (see Glossary), severe skin reactions.
  Idiosyncratic Reaction: Hemolytic anemia (see Glossary).
  Disulfiramlike reaction with concurrent use of alcohol (see Glossary), infrequent with this drug.
  Low blood sodium.
  Drug-induced urinary stones.
  Bone marrow depression (see Glossary)—fatigue, weakness, fever, sore throat, abnormal bleeding or bruising.
  Increased risk of cardiovascular mortality (based on University Group Diabetes Program UGDP).

▷ **Possible Effects on Sexual Function:** None reported.

▷ **Adverse Effects That May Mimic Natural Diseases or Disorders**
  Liver reactions may suggest viral hepatitis.

Possible Effects on Laboratory Tests
  Complete blood counts: decreased red cells, hemoglobin, white cells and platelets.
  Blood glucose levels: decreased.
  Liver function tests: increased liver enzymes (ALT/GPT, AST/GOT and alkaline phosphatase), increased bilirubin.

CAUTION
  1. This drug is only one part of a total diabetes program. It is not a substitute for a proper diet and regular exercise.
  2. Over time (usually several months), this drug may not work. Periodic follow-up examinations are necessary.

Precautions for Use
  By Infants and Children: This drug does not work in type (juvenile, growth-onset) insulin-dependent diabetes.
  By Those over 60 Years of Age: Used with caution, and started with 2.5 mg/day. Dose is increased slowly and glucose checked often. Repeated hypoglycemia in the elderly can cause brain damage.

▷ **Advisability of Use During Pregnancy**
  Pregnancy Category: C. See Pregnancy Code at the back of this book.
  Animal studies: No birth defects reported in rats and rabbits.
  Human studies: Adequate studies of pregnant women are not available.
  Because uncontrolled blood sugar levels during pregnancy are associated with a higher incidence of birth defects, many experts recommend that insulin (instead of an oral agent) be used as necessary to control diabetes during the entire pregnancy.

Advisability of Use if Breast-Feeding
  Presence of this drug in breast milk: Unknown.
  Avoid drug or refrain from nursing.

Habit-Forming Potential: None.

Effects of Overdosage: Symptoms of mild to severe hypoglycemia: Headache, light-headedness, faintness, nervousness, confusion, tremor, sweating, heart palpitation, weakness, hunger, nausea, vomiting, stupor progressing to coma.

Possible Effects of Long-Term Use: Reduced thyroid function (hypothyroidism). Increased frequency and severity of heart and blood vessel diseases with long-term use of this class of drugs are highly controversial and inconclusive. A direct cause-and-effect relationship (see Glossary) is tenuous. Ask your physician for help.

Suggested Periodic Examinations While Taking This Drug (at physician's discretion)
Complete blood cell counts, liver function tests, thyroid function tests, periodic evaluation of heart and circulatory system.

▷ **While Taking This Drug, Observe the Following**
Foods: Follow the diabetic diet prescribed by your physician.
Beverages: As directed in the diabetic diet. May be taken with milk.

▷ *Alcohol:* Use with extreme caution—alcohol can prolong this drug's hypoglycemic effect. This drug can also cause a disulfiramlike reaction (see Glossary): Facial flushing, sweating, palpitation.

Tobacco Smoking: No interactions expected.

▷ *Other Drugs*
The following drugs may *increase* the effects of glipizide
- aspirin, and other salicylates.
- cimetidine (Tagamet).
- clofibrate (Atromid S).
- fenfluramine (Pondimin).
- monoamine oxidase (MAO) type A inhibitors (see Drug Class Section).
- NSAIDs (see Drug Class).
- ranitidine (Zantac).
- sulfa drugs such as Septra.

The following drugs may *decrease* the effects of glipizide
- beta blocker drugs (see Drug Class Section).
- bumetanide (Bumex).
- diazoxide (Proglycem).
- ethacrynic acid (Edecrin).
- furosemide (Lasix).
- phenytoin (Dilantin).
- rifampin.
- thiazide diuretics (see Drug Class Section).

Glipizide *taken concurrently* with
- cyclosporine (Sandimmune) may result in cyclosporine toxicity.
- warfarin (Coumadin) can cause an increased hypoglycemic effect.

▷ *Driving, Hazardous Activities:* Dosing schedule, eating schedule and physical activities must be coordinated to prevent hypoglycemia. Know the early symptoms of hypoglycemia so you can avoid hazardous activities and take corrective measures.

Aviation Note: Diabetes *is a disqualification* for piloting. Consult a designated Aviation Medical Examiner.

Exposure to Sun: Some drugs of this class can cause photosensitivity (see Glossary).

Occurrence of Unrelated Illness: Acute infections, vomiting or diarrhea, serious injuries and surgical procedures can worsen diabetic control and may require insulin. If any of these conditions occur, call your doctor.

Discontinuation: Because of secondary failures, the continued benefit of this drug should be evaluated every 6 months.

GLYBURIDE (GLI byoor ide)

Other Name: Glibenclamide

Introduced: 1970   **Prescription:** USA: Yes; Canada: Yes   **Available as Generic:** Yes   **Class:** Antidiabetic, sulfonylureas   **Controlled Drug:** USA: No; Canada: No

Brand Names: ✦Albert-Glyburide, ✦Apo-Glyburide, DiaBeta, ✦Euglucon, ✦Gen-Glybe, Glubate, Glynase Prestab, Micronase, ✦Novo-Glyburide

BENEFITS versus RISKS	
Possible Benefits	*Possible Risks*
Help in regulating blood sugar in noninsulin-dependent diabetes (adjunctive to appropriate diet and weight control)	HYPOGLYCEMIA, severe and prolonged INCREASED RISK OF CARDIOVASCULAR MORTALITY Allergic skin reactions (some severe) Rare liver damage Rare blood cell and bone marrow disorders

▷ **Principal Uses**

As a Single Drug Product: Uses currently included in FDA approved labeling: (1) helps control mild to moderate type II diabetes mellitus (adult, maturity-onset) that does not require insulin, but can't be adequately controlled by diet alone.

Other (unlabeled) generally accepted uses: None.

How This Drug Works: This drug (1) stimulates the secretion of insulin, (2) decreases glucose production in the liver, and (3) enhances insulin use.

Available Dosage Forms and Strengths
Tablets — 1.25 mg, 2.5 mg, 5 mg

▷ **Usual Adult Dosage Range:** Initially 2.5 to 5 mg daily with breakfast. At 7-day intervals the dose may be increased by increments of 2.5 mg daily as needed and tolerated. Total daily dosage should not exceed 20 mg. A "loading" or priming dose is not necessary and should not be given. **Note: Actual dosage and administration schedule must be determined by the physician for each patient individually.**

Conditions Requiring Dosing Adjustments

Liver function: Glyburide may cause catastrophic hypoglycemia (low blood sugar) if it is used in patients with liver disease. Should **not** be used in these patients. It is also a rare cause of hepatitis and cholestatic jaundice.

Glyburide

Kidney function: Glyburide should be used with caution in mild renal compromise, with low initial doses and careful patient monitoring. The drug is relatively contraindicated in severe kidney failure.

▷ **Dosing Instructions:** If the daily maintenance dose is found to be 10 mg or more, the total dose should be divided into 2 equal doses: the first taken with the morning meal, the second with the evening meal. The tablet may be crushed for administration.

Usual Duration of Use: Use on a regular schedule for 1 to 2 weeks determines effectiveness in controlling diabetes. No response to peak doses in 1 month constitutes a primary failure. Up to 10% of those who respond initially may develop secondary failure. The duration of effective use can only be determined by periodic measurement of the blood sugar.

▷ **This Drug Should Not Be Taken If**
- you have had an allergic reaction to it previously.
- you have severe impairment of liver and kidney function.
- you have diabetic ketoacidosis.
- you are pregnant.

▷ **Inform Your Physician Before Taking This Drug If**
- you are allergic to other sulfonylurea drugs or to "sulfa" drugs.
- your diabetes has been unstable or "brittle" in the past.
- you do not know how to recognize or treat hypoglycemia (see Glossary).
- you have a history of problems with blood clotting.
- you have G6PD deficiency.
- you have a history of congestive heart failure, peptic ulcer disease, cirrhosis of the liver, hypothyroidism or porphyria.

Possible Side-Effects (natural, expected and unavoidable drug actions)

If drug dosage is excessive or food intake is delayed or inadequate, abnormally low blood sugar (hypoglycemia) will occur as a predictable drug effect.

▷ **Possible Adverse Effects** (unusual, unexpected and infrequent reactions)

If any of the following develop, consult your physician promptly for guidance.

Mild Adverse Effects

Allergic Reactions: Skin rash, hives, itching.
Headache, drowsiness, dizziness, fatigue.
Indigestion, heartburn, nausea.
Bed wetting at night (nocturnal enuresis) (especially in young adults).
Abnormally frequent urination.

Serious Adverse Effects

Allergic Reactions: Hepatitis with jaundice (see Glossary), severe skin reactions (exfoliative dermatitis).
Idiosyncratic Reaction: Hemolytic anemia (see Glossary).
Disulfiramlike reaction with concurrent use of alcohol (see Glossary), infrequent with this drug.
Bone marrow depression (see Glossary)—fatigue, weakness, fever, sore throat, abnormal bleeding or bruising.
Liver toxicity (cholestatic jaundice).
Blood clotting defects (coagulation).

Glyburide

Cardiovascular mortality (increased) (based on the University Group Diabetes Program (UGDP).
Drug-induced urinary tract stones.

▷ **Possible Effects on Sexual Function:** None reported.

▷ **Adverse Effects That May Mimic Natural Diseases or Disorders**
Liver reactions may suggest viral hepatitis.

Possible Effects on Laboratory Tests
Blood platelet counts: decreased.
Blood cholesterol and triglyceride levels: decreased.
Blood glucose levels: decreased.
Liver function tests: increased liver enzymes (ALT/GPT, AST/GOT and alkaline phosphatase), rare and transient.

CAUTION
1. This drug is only part of the program for management of your diabetes. It is not a substitute for a proper diet and regular exercise.
2. Over time (usually several months), this drug may not work. Periodic follow-up examinations are necessary.

Precautions for Use
By Infants and Children: This drug does not work in type (juvenile, growth-onset) insulin-dependent diabetes.
By Those over 60 Years of Age: Used with caution and started with 1.25 mg/day. Dose is slowly increased and glucose closely followed. Repeated hypoglycemia in the elderly can cause brain damage.

▷ **Advisability of Use During Pregnancy**
Pregnancy Category: B. See Pregnancy Code at the back of this book.
Animal studies: No birth defects reported in rats and rabbits.
Human studies: Adequate studies of pregnant women are not available.
Uncontrolled blood sugar levels during pregnancy are associated with a higher incidence of birth defects, so many experts recommend insulin (instead of an oral agent) to control diabetes during the entire pregnancy.

Advisability of Use if Breast-Feeding
Presence of this drug in breast milk: Unknown.
Avoid drug or refrain from nursing.

Habit-Forming Potential: None.

Effects of Overdosage: Symptoms of mild to severe hypoglycemia: headache, light-headedness, faintness, nervousness, confusion, tremor, sweating, heart palpitation, weakness, hunger, nausea, vomiting, stupor progressing to coma.

Possible Effects of Long-Term Use: Reduced thyroid gland function (hypothyroidism). Reports of increased frequency and severity of heart and blood vessel diseases associated with long-term use of this class of drugs are highly controversial and inconclusive. A direct cause-and-effect relationship (see Glossary) is tenuous. Ask your physician for guidance.

Suggested Periodic Examinations While Taking This Drug (at physician's discretion)
Complete blood cell counts, liver function tests, thyroid function tests, periodic evaluation of heart and circulatory system.

▷ **While Taking This Drug, Observe the Following**
  Foods: Follow the diabetic diet prescribed by your physician.
  Beverages: As directed in the diabetic diet. May be taken with milk.
▷ *Alcohol:* Use with extreme caution—alcohol can exaggerate this drug's hypoglycemic effect. This drug can cause a disulfiramlike reaction (see Glossary): facial flushing, sweating, palpitation.
  Tobacco Smoking: No interactions expected.
▷ *Other Drugs*
  The following drugs may *increase* the effects of glyburide
  • aspirin, and other salicylates.
  • cimetidine (Tagamet).
  • clofibrate (Atromid S).
  • fenfluramine (Pondimin).
  • monoamine oxidase (MAO) type A inhibitors (see Drug Classes).
  • phenylbutazone (Butazolidin).
  • ranitidine (Zantac).
  The following drugs may *decrease* the effects of glyburide
  • beta blocker drugs (see Drug Class Section).
  • bumetanide (Bumex).
  • diazoxide (Proglycem).
  • ethacrynic acid (Edecrin).
  • furosemide (Lasix).
  • phenytoin (Dilantin).
  • rifampin.
  • thiazide diuretics (see Drug Class Section).
  Glyburide *taken concurrently* with
  • Warfarin (Coumadin) may result in bleeding.
▷ *Driving, Hazardous Activities:* Regulate dosing, eating and physical activities carefully to prevent hypoglycemia. Know the early symptoms of hypoglycemia so you can avoid hazardous activities and take corrective measures.
  Aviation Note: Diabetes **is a disqualification** for piloting. Consult a designated Aviation Medical Examiner.
  Exposure to Sun: Use caution until sensitivity has been determined. Some drugs of this class can cause photosensitivity (see Glossary).
  Occurrence of Unrelated Illness: Acute infections, vomiting or diarrhea, serious injuries and surgical procedures can worsen diabetic control and may require insulin. If any of these conditions occur, consult your physician promptly.
  Discontinuation: Because of the possibility of secondary failure, it is advisable to evaluate the continued benefit of this drug every 6 months.

GRISEOFULVIN (gri see oh FUL vin)

Introduced: 1959 **Prescription:** USA: Yes; Canada: Yes **Available as Generic:** USA: No; Canada: No **Class:** Antifungal **Controlled Drug:** USA: No; Canada: No

Brand Names: Fulvicin P/G, Fulvicin U/F, Grifulvin V, Grisactin, Grisactin Ultra, ✦Grisovin-FP, Gris-PEG, Nasatab-LA, Ultramiclosize Griseofulvin

Griseofulvin

BENEFITS versus RISKS	
Possible Benefits	**Possible Risks**
EFFECTIVE TREATMENT OF ALL TYPES OF TINEA INFECTION	Rare drug-induced hepatitis Rare peripheral neuritis Decreased white blood cell counts Disulfiram-like reactions

▷ **Principal Uses**

As a Single Drug Product: Uses currently included in FDA approved labeling: Treatment of tinea (ringworm) infections of the beard (tinea barbae), scalp (tinea capitis), body (tinea corporis), groin (tinea cruris, jock itch), feet (tinea pedis, athlete's foot), fingernails and toenails (tinea unguium).

Other (unlabeled) generally accepted uses: (1) Eases symptoms of lichen planus; (2) may help retard the progression of systemic sclerosis; (3) pain relief in Herpes Zoster (shingles).

Note: This drug works against species of fungus that are sensitive to it. It is not effective against yeasts, bacteria or viruses. It should not be used for minor fungus infections.

How This Drug Works: By disrupting fungal reproduction, this drug prevents the growth and multiplication of susceptible fungi. This drug is deposited primarily in the skin, hair and nails—the sites of tinea infection.

Available Dosage Forms and Strengths
Microsize formulations
    Capsules — 125 mg, 250 mg
    Oral suspension — 125 mg per 5-ml teaspoonful
    Tablets — 250 mg, 500 mg
Ultramicrosize formulations
    Tablets — 125 mg, 165 mg, 250 mg, 330 mg

▷ **Recommended Dosage Ranges** (Actual dosage and administration schedule must be determined by the physician for each patient individually.)

Infants and Children: 14 to 23 kg—62.5 to 125 mg every 12 hours; or 125 to 250 mg once daily.

23 kg and over—125 to 250 mg every 12 hours; or 250 to 500 mg once daily.

For microsize formulations—10 to 11 mg/kg of body weight daily, in single or divided doses.

For ultramicrosize formulations—(over 2 years of age) 7.3 mg/kg of body weight daily, in single or divided doses.

12 to 60 Years of Age: For tinea pedis and nail infections—500 mg every 12 hours.

For tinea barbae, capitis, corporis and cruris—250 mg every 12 hours, or 500 mg once daily.

For microsize formulations—500 to 1000 mg daily, in single or divided doses.

For ultramicrosize formulations—330 to 375 mg daily, in single or divided doses.

Over 60 Years of Age: Same as 12 to 60 years of age.

Conditions Requiring Dosing Adjustments

Liver function: Contraindicated in hepatocellular (loss of functional cells) liver failure.

Griseofulvin

Kidney function: The kidney is not involved in the elimination of this drug.

▷ **Dosing Instructions:** The tablet can be crushed and the capsule opened and taken with or following meals to reduce stomach upset; fatty foods increase absorption of this drug. Shake the oral suspension well before measuring the dose.

Usual Duration of Use: Use on a regular schedule is critical until the infecting fungus is totally eliminated from infected tissues. Usual treatment periods are as follows: for tinea capitis—10 to 12 weeks; for tinea barbae—4 to 6 weeks; for tinea corporis and cruris—4 to 6 weeks; for tinea pedis—6 to 8 weeks; for tinea unguium—6 to 8 months for fingernails and 8 to 12 months for toenails.

Currently a "Drug of Choice"
for tinea capitis (fungus infection of scalp and hair), tinea barbae (fungus infection of the beard), and tinea unguium (fungus infection of fingernails and toenails).

▷ **This Drug Should Not Be Taken If**
- you have had an allergic reaction to it previously.
- you have active liver disease.
- you have porphyria.
- you have a mild fungus infection that will respond to local therapy.
- you are pregnant.

▷ **Inform Your Physician Before Taking This Drug If**
- you are allergic to any form of penicillin.
- you have impaired liver function.
- you have a history of porphyria.
- you have lupus erythematosus.
- you are planning pregnancy.
- you are taking oral birth control pills that contain estrogen.
- you are currently taking an anticoagulant drug.

Possible Side-Effects (natural, expected and unavoidable drug actions)
Mild lowering of blood pressure.
Superinfections (see Glossary): thrush (yeast) infection of the mouth, tongue or gums.

▷ **Possible Adverse Effects** (unusual, unexpected and infrequent reactions)
If any of the following develop, consult your physician promptly for guidance.
Mild Adverse Effects
Allergic Reactions: Skin rash, hives, itching.
Headache, dizziness, lethargy, blurred vision, insomnia, confusion.
Nausea, vomiting, stomach pain, diarrhea.
Taste disorders.
Serious Adverse Effects
Allergic Reactions: Anaphylactic reaction (see Glossary). Severe skin reactions (Stevens-Johnson syndrome, erythema multiforme or Toxic epidermal necrolysis).
Idiosyncratic Reactions: Lupus-like syndrome—fever; painful, swollen joints; aching muscles; enlarged lymph glands.

Rare drug-induced hepatitis: yellow skin and eyes, light-colored stools, dark urine.
Peripheral neuritis (see Glossary): Numbness and tingling, burning pain in hands and feet.
Hallucinations.
Deficiency of white blood cells.

▷ **Possible Effects on Sexual Function:** Rare enlargement of male breast tissue.

▷ **Adverse Effects That May Mimic Natural Diseases or Disorders**
Drug-induced hepatitis may suggest viral hepatitis.

Natural Diseases or Disorders That May Be Activated by This Drug
Systemic lupus erythematosus, porphyria.

Possible Effects on Laboratory Tests
Complete blood cell counts: decreased white cells (neutrophils).
Lupus erythematosus (LE) cells: positive.
Prothrombin time: decreased.
Blood uric acid level: decreased.
Liver function tests: increased liver enzymes (ALT/GPT, AST/GOT and alkaline phosphatase), increased bilirubin.
Kidney function tests: increased blood urea nitrogen (BUN) and creatinine.

CAUTION
1. Not used for minor infections that will respond to local therapy.
2. This drug is not recommended for use during pregnancy. If you are using an oral contraceptive that contains estrogen, you should also use an additional method of contraception while taking this drug and for 1 month after discontinuing it.
3. Persistent diarrhea can develop in some people. If diarrhea persists more than 24 hours, call your doctor promptly.

Precautions for Use
By Infants and Children: Safety and effectiveness for those under 2 years of age not established.
By Those over 60 Years of Age: No information available.

▷ **Advisability of Use During Pregnancy**
Pregnancy Category: C. See Pregnancy Code at the back of this book.
Animal studies: Rat and dog studies reveal significant birth defects associated with use of this drug.
Human studies: Adequate studies of pregnant women are not available.
It is recommended that this drug not be used during any period of pregnancy.

Advisability of Use if Breast-Feeding
Presence of this drug in breast milk: Unknown, but expected.
Avoid drug or refrain from nursing.

Habit-Forming Potential: None.

Effects of Overdosage: Possible nausea, vomiting, diarrhea, fainting.

Possible Effects of Long-Term Use: Superinfections, especially due to yeast organisms.
Decreased white blood cells.
Liver damage.
Peripheral neuritis (see Glossary).

Suggested Periodic Examinations While Taking This Drug (at physician's discretion)
  Complete blood cell counts.
  Liver and kidney function tests (during extended use).
▷ **While Taking This Drug, Observe the Following**
  Foods: No restrictions. High-fat foods enhance absorption of this drug.
  Beverages: No restrictions. Preferably taken with milk.
▷ *Alcohol:* Use with caution—this drug can increase the intoxicating effects of alcohol and a disulfiramlike reaction (see Glossary) can occur.
  Tobacco Smoking: No interactions expected.
▷ *Other Drugs*
  Griseofulvin may *decrease* the effects of
   • birth control pills (oral contraceptives), resulting in breakthrough bleeding and unwanted pregnancy.
   • warfarin (Coumadin); monitor prothrombin times and adjust dosing.
  The following drugs may *decrease* the effects of griseofulvin
   • barbiturates.
   • primidone (Mysoline).
▷ *Driving, Hazardous Activities:* This drug may cause dizziness, confusion or impaired vision. Restrict activities as necessary.
  Aviation Note: The use of this drug *may be a disqualification* for piloting. Consult a designated Aviation Medical Examiner.
  Exposure to Sun: Use caution until sensitivity is determined. This drug may cause photosensitivity (see Glossary).
  Discontinuation: Some fungal infections require long-term treatment. Your doctor should decide when it is appropriate to stop this drug.

GUANFACINE (GWAHN fa seen)

Introduced: 1980 **Prescription:** USA: Yes **Available as Generic:** USA: No **Class:** Antihypertensive **Controlled Drug:** USA: No
Brand Name: Tenex

BENEFITS versus RISKS	
Possible Benefits	*Possible Risks*
EFFECTIVE ANTIHYPERTENSIVE in mild to moderate high blood pressure	Amnesia, confusion, mental depression (3% or less)

▷ **Principal Uses**
  As a Single Drug Product: Uses currently included in FDA approved labeling: (1) Used in the treatment of mild to moderate high blood pressure. Generally added when a "step 1" drug proves to be inadequate. It may also be used as a "step 3" or "step 4" drug in place of drugs that cause orthostatic hypotension (see Glossary).
  Other (unlabeled) generally acceptd uses: (1) heroin withdrawal; (2) may be useful in problem pregnancies.
How This Drug Works: By reducing sympathetic nervous system output (by affecting brain alpha two receptors), this drug causes relaxation of blood vessel walls and lowering of blood pressure.

Guanfacine

Available Dosage Forms and Strengths
Tablets — 1 mg
— 2 mg

▷ **Usual Adult Dosage Range:** Initially 1 mg once daily taken at bedtime. The dose may be increased after 3 to 4 weeks to 2 mg daily, as needed and tolerated. If needed, the dose may be increased again after 3 to 4 weeks to 3 mg daily. The total daily requirement may be taken in 2 divided doses if necessary for stable blood pressure control. **Note: Actual dosage and administration schedule must be determined by the physician for each patient individually.**

Conditions Requiring Dosing Adjustments
Liver function: It should be used with caution in patients with liver compromise.
Kidney function: Used with caution, but can be removed by non-kidney mechanisms.

▷ **Dosing Instructions:** Tablets may be crushed and taken without regard to eating. It is recommended that the daily dose be taken at bedtime to reduce the side-effect of daytime drowsiness.

Usual Duration of Use: Continual use on a regular schedule for 4 to 6 weeks is usually necessary to determine this drug's effectiveness in controlling high blood pressure. Long-term use (months to years) requires supervision and guidance by the physician. Consult your physician on a regular basis.

▷ **This Drug Should Not Be Taken If**
- you have had an allergic reaction to it previously.

▷ **Inform Your Physician Before Taking This Drug If**
- you have a circulatory disorder of the brain.
- you have angina or coronary artery disease.
- you have or have had serious emotional depression.
- you have impaired liver or kidney function.
- you are a diabetic.
- you have a history of orthostatic hypotension.
- you are taking any sedative or hypnotic drugs or an antidepressant.
- you plan to have surgery under general anesthesia in the near future.

Possible Side-Effects (natural, expected and unavoidable drug actions)
Drowsiness (21%), dry nose and mouth (30%), constipation (10%), decreased heart rate, mild orthostatic hypotension (see Glossary).

▷ **Possible Adverse Effects** (unusual, unexpected and infrequent reactions)
If any of the following develop, consult your physician promptly for guidance.
Mild Adverse Effects
Allergic Reactions: Skin rash, itching.
Headache (4%), dizziness (11%), fatigue (9%), insomnia (4%).
Sedation (5–30%).
Indigestion, nausea, diarrhea.
Leg cramps
Serious Adverse Effects
Abnormally low blood pressure on standing (orthostatic hypotension).
Slow heartbeat (bradycardia).

Liver toxicity (rare).
Rebound hypertension (if abruptly stopped).

▷ **Possible Effects on Sexual Function:** Decreased libido, impotence.

Possible Effects on Laboratory Tests
Blood cholesterol and triglyceride levels: decreased.

CAUTION
1. ***Do not discontinue this drug suddenly.*** Sudden withdrawal can produce anxiety, nervousness, tremors, fast or irregular heart action, nausea, stomach cramps, vomiting and rebound hypertension.
2. Hot weather and fever can reduce blood pressure significantly. Dosage adjustments may be necessary.
3. Report the development of any tendency to emotional depression.

Precautions for Use
By Infants and Children: Safety and effectiveness for use by those under 12 years of age have not been established.
By Those over 60 Years of Age: **Proceed cautiously**. Pressure should be reduced without creating the risks associated with excessively low blood pressure. Watch for light-headedness, dizziness, unsteadiness, fainting and falling. Sedation and dry mouth occur commonly in elderly users. Report promptly any changes in mood or behavior: depression, delusions, hallucinations.

▷ **Advisability of Use During Pregnancy**
Pregnancy Category: B. See Pregnancy Code at the back of this book.
Animal studies: No birth defects due to this drug reported in rat and rabbit studies.
Human studies: Adequate studies of pregnant women are not available.
Use this drug only if clearly needed. Ask your physician for guidance.

Advisability of Use if Breast-Feeding
Presence of this drug in breast milk: Probably yes.
Avoid drug or refrain from nursing.

Habit-Forming Potential: None.

Effects of Overdosage: Marked drowsiness, weakness, dry mouth, slow pulse, low blood pressure, vomiting, stupor progressing to coma.

Possible Effects of Long-Term Use: Development of tolerance (see Glossary) with loss of drug effectiveness.

Suggested Periodic Examinations While Taking This Drug (at physician's discretion)
Blood pressure measurements.

▷ **While Taking This Drug, Observe the Following**
Foods: Avoid excessive salt, and ask your doctor about degree of salt restriction.
Beverages: No restrictions. May be taken with milk.
▷ *Alcohol:* Use with extreme caution—combined effects can cause marked drowsiness and exaggerated reduction of blood pressure.
Tobacco Smoking: No interactions expected. Follow your physician's advice about tobacco.

▷ *Other Drugs:* Guanfacine *taken concurrently* with
  • amitriptyline can cause decreased effectiveness as an antihypertensive.
  • desipramine and other tricyclic antidepressants can cause loss of therapeutic benefits of guanfacine.
  • phenobarbital can lead to loss of therapeutic effect of guanfacine.

▷ *Driving, Hazardous Activities:* Use caution. This drug can cause drowsiness and can impair mental alertness, judgment and coordination.

Aviation Note: Hypertension (high blood pressure) *is a disqualification* for piloting. Consult a designated Aviation Medical Examiner.

Exposure to Sun: No restrictions.

Exposure to Heat: Use caution. Hot environments may reduce the blood pressure significantly; be alert to the possibility of orthostatic hypotension (see Glossary).

Heavy Exercise or Exertion: Use caution. Isometric exercises can raise blood pressure significantly. This drug may intensify the hypertensive response to isometric exercise. Ask physician for guidance.

Occurrence of Unrelated Illness: Fever may lower blood pressure significantly. Vomiting may prevent regular use of this drug and result in acute withdrawal reactions. Call your doctor.

Discontinuation: **Do not stop this drug suddenly.** Withdrawal reactions occur within 2 to 7 days after the last dose. Best to reduce dose gradually (over 3 to 4 days), with periodic monitoring of the blood pressure.

HALOPERIDOL (hal oh PER i dohl)

Introduced: 1958 **Prescription:** USA: Yes; Canada: Yes **Available as Generic:** USA: Yes; Canada: Yes **Class:** Strong tranquilizer, butyrophenones **Controlled Drug:** USA: No; Canada: No

Brand Names: ✦Apo-Haloperidol, Haldol, ✦Haldol LA, Halperon, ✦Novo-Peridol, ✦Peridol

BENEFITS versus RISKS	
Possible Benefits	*Possible Risks*
EFFECTIVE CONTROL OF ACUTE FREQUENT PSYCHOSES: beneficial effects on thinking, mood and behavior	FREQUENT PARKINSON-LIKE SIDE-EFFECTS
	SERIOUS TOXIC EFFECTS ON BRAIN with long-term use
EFFECTIVE CONTROL OF SOME CASES OF TOURETTE'S DISORDER	Rare blood cell disorders
	Abnormally low white blood cell count
Beneficial in management of some hyperactive children	

▷ **Principal Uses**

As a Single Drug Product: Uses currently included in FDA improved labeling: (1) Helps control psychotic thinking and abnormal behavior associated with acute psychosis of unknown nature, acute schizophrenia, paranoid states and the manic phase of manic-depressive disorders; (2) helps control outbursts of aggression and agitation; (3) used to treat Gilles de la Tourette's syndrome.

Other (unlabeled) generally accepted uses: (1) Helps control refractory hiccups; (2) used to lessen delirium in LSD flashbacks and phencyclidine intoxication; (3) used as combination (adjuvant) therapy in chronic pain syndromes; (4) may be helpful in autistic patients; (5) may have a role in refractory vomiting caused by cancer chemotherapy; (6) can ease symptoms in refractory sneezing; (5) may be helpful as adjunctive therapy in stuttering.

How This Drug Works: By interfering with a nerve impulse transmitter (dopamine) in the brain, this drug reduces anxiety and agitation, improves coherence and organization of thinking and abolishes delusions and hallucinations.

Available Dosage Forms and Strengths
  Concentrate — 2 mg per ml
    Injection — 5 mg per ml and 50 mg per ml
    Tablets — 0.5 mg, 1 mg, 2 mg, 5 mg, 10 mg, 20 mg

▷ **Usual Adult Dosage Range:** Initially 0.5 to 2 mg 2 or 3 times daily. Dose may be increased by 0.5 mg/day at 3- to 4-day intervals as needed and tolerated. The usual dosage range is 0.5 to 30 mg/24 hours. The total daily dosage should not exceed 100 mg. **Note: Actual dosage and administration schedule must be determined by the physician for each patient individually.**

Conditions Requiring Dosing Adjustments
  Liver function: The dose, dosing interval and titration interval (time taken to adjust the medication to the desired effect) should be adjusted with liver compromise.
  Kidney function: High doses of haloperidol should be used with caution in kidney compromise.

▷ **Dosing Instructions:** The tablet may be crushed and taken with or following food to reduce stomach irritation. The concentrate may be diluted in 2 ounces of water or fruit juice; do not add it to coffee or tea.

Usual Duration of Use: Use on a regular schedule for several weeks determines this drug's effectiveness in controlling psychotic behavior. If it doesn't provide significant benefit in 6 weeks, it should be stopped. Long-term use requires supervision and periodic physician evaluation.

▷ **This Drug Should Not Be Taken If**
  - you have had an allergic reaction to any dosage form of it previously.
  - you are experiencing severe mental depression.
  - you have any form of Parkinson's disease.
  - you have cancer of the breast.
  - you have severe active liver disease.
  - you currently have a bone marrow or blood cell disorder.

▷ **Inform Your Physician Before Taking This Drug If**
  - you are allergic or abnormally sensitive to phenothiazine drugs.
  - you have a history of mental depression.
  - you have any type of heart disease.
  - you have impaired liver or kidney function.
  - you have thyroid disease.
  - you are allergic to the dye tartrazine.
  - you are pregnant or are planning pregnancy.

Haloperidol

- you have a history of neuroleptic malignant syndrome.
- you have low blood pressure, epilepsy or glaucoma.
- you are taking any drugs with a sedative effect.
- you plan to have surgery and general or spinal anesthesia soon.

Possible Side-Effects (natural, expected and unavoidable drug actions)
Mild drowsiness, low blood pressure, blurred vision, dry mouth, constipation, marked and frequent Parkinson-like reactions (see Glossary).

▷ **Possible Adverse Effects** (unusual, unexpected and infrequent reactions)
If any of the following develop, consult your physician promptly for guidance.
Mild Adverse Effects
Allergic Reactions: Skin rash, hives.
Dizziness, weakness, agitation, insomnia.
Loss of appetite, indigestion, nausea, vomiting, diarrhea.
Urinary retention.
Serious Adverse Effects
Allergic Reactions: Rare liver reaction with jaundice, asthma, spasm of vocal cords.
Idiosyncratic Reactions: Neuroleptic malignant syndrome (see Glossary).
Depression, disorientation, eye damage (deposits in cornea, lens and retina).
Blood cell disorders: anemia, fluctuation in number of white blood cells.
Nervous system reactions: rigidity of extremities, tremors, restlessness, constant movement, facial grimacing, eye-rolling, spasm of neck muscles, tardive dyskinesia (see Glossary).
Abnormal heart beats (premature ventricular contractions).
Seizures.
Worsening of psychosis.
Low blood sugar.
Abnormal and frequent urination (SIADH).
Liver toxicity.
Abnormal eye orientations (oculogyric crisis).
Bronchospasm (rare).
Myasthenia gravis (rare).

▷ **Possible Effects on Sexual Function**
Decreased libido; impotence (10–20%); painful ejaculation; priapism (see Glossary).
Tender and enlarged breast tissue in men; breast enlargement with milk production in women.
Altered timing and pattern of menstruation.

▷ **Adverse Effects That May Mimic Natural Diseases or Disorders**
Liver reaction may suggest viral hepatitis.
Nervous system reactions may suggest Parkinson's disease or Reye syndrome.

Natural Diseases or Disorders That May Be Activated by This Drug
Latent epilepsy, glaucoma, diabetes.

Possible Effects on Laboratory Tests
Complete blood counts: decreased red cells, hemoglobin and white cells; increased eosinophils.

Prothrombin time: decreased.
Blood cholesterol level: decreased.
Blood glucose level: increased.
Liver function tests: increased liver enzymes (ALT/GPT, AST/GOT and alkaline phosphatase), increased bilirubin.

CAUTION
1. The smallest effective dose should be used for long-term therapy.
2. Used with extreme caution in epilepsy; can alter seizure patterns.
3. People with lupus erythematosus and those taking prednisone are more susceptible to nervous system reactions.
4. Levodopa should **not** be used to treat Parkinson-like reactions; it can cause agitation and worsening of the psychotic disorder.
5. Obtain prompt evaluation of any change or disturbance in vision.

Precautions for Use
By Infants and Children: This drug should not be used in children under 3 years of age or 15 kg in weight. Avoid this drug in the presence of symptoms suggestive of Reye syndrome. Children are quite susceptible to nervous system reactions induced by this drug.

By Those over 60 Years of Age: Small doses are indicated when therapy is started. This drug can cause significant changes in mood and behavior; watch for confusion, disorientation, agitation, restlessness, aggression and paranoia. You may be more susceptible to the development of drowsiness, lethargy, orthostatic hypotension (see Glossary), hypothermia (see Glossary), Parkinson-like reactions and prostatism (see Glossary).

▷ **Advisability of Use During Pregnancy**
Pregnancy Category: C. See Pregnancy Code at the back of this book.
Animal studies: Cleft palate reported in mouse studies.
Human studies: No increase in birth defects reported in 100 exposures. Adequate studies of pregnant women are not available.
Avoid during the first trimester. Use only if clearly needed. Ask physician for guidance.

Advisability of Use if Breast-Feeding
Presence of this drug in breast milk: Yes.
Monitor nursing infant closely and discontinue drug or nursing if adverse effects develop.

Habit-Forming Potential: Reports of recreational use have been filed. If the drug is stopped suddenly, patient may experience a withdrawal syndrome.

Effects of Overdosage: Marked drowsiness, weakness, tremor, unsteadiness, agitation, stupor, coma, convulsions.

Possible Effects of Long-Term Use: Eye damage—deposits in cornea, lens or retina; tardive dyskinesia (see Glossary).

Suggested Periodic Examinations While Taking This Drug (at physician's discretion)
Complete blood counts, liver function tests, eye examinations, electrocardiograms.
The tongue should be watched for fine, involuntary, wavelike movements that could be the beginning of tardive dyskinesia.

Haloperidol

▷ **While Taking This Drug, Observe the Following**
Foods: No restrictions.
Beverages: No restrictions. May be taken with milk.
▷ *Alcohol:* Avoid completely. Alcohol can increase the sedative action of haloperidol and accentuate its depressant effects on brain function. Haloperidol can increase the intoxicating effects of alcohol.
Tobacco Smoking: No interactions expected.
Marijuana Smoking: Moderate increase in drowsiness; accentuation of orthostatic hypotension; increased risk of precipitating latent psychosis, confusing interpretation of mental status and of drug response.
▷ *Other Drugs*
Haloperidol may *increase* the effects of
- all drugs with sedative actions, and cause excessive sedation.
- some antihypertensive drugs and cause excessive lowering of blood pressure; monitor the combined effects carefully.

Haloperidol may *decrease* the effects of
- guanethidine (Esimil, Ismelin), and reduce its antihypertensive effect.

Haloperidol *taken concurrently* with
- anticholinergic drugs (see Drug Classes) can cause additive anticholinergic effects (dry mouth, constipation or sedation.)
- beta blocker drugs may cause excessive lowering of blood pressure.
- fluoxetine (Prozac) can result in an increased risk of haloperidol toxicity.
- lithium may cause toxic effects on the brain and nervous system.
- methyldopa (Aldomet) may cause serious dementia.

The following drugs may *decrease* the effects of haloperidol
- antacids containing aluminum and/or magnesium may reduce its absorption.
- barbiturates.
- benztropine (Cogentin).
- carbamazepine (Tegretol).
- phenytoin (Dilantin).
- rifampin (Rifater, others).
- trihexyphenidyl (Artane).

▷ *Driving, Hazardous Activities:* This drug may impair mental alertness, judgment and physical coordination. Restrict activities as necessary.
Aviation Note: The use of this drug *is a disqualification* for piloting. Consult a designated Aviation Medical Examiner.
Exposure to Sun: Use caution—this drug can cause photosensitivity.
Exposure to Heat: Use caution in hot environments. This drug may impair the regulation of body temperature and increase the risk of heat stroke.
Exposure to Cold: This drug can increase the risk of hypothermia (see Glossary) in the elderly.
Discontinuation: This drug should not be stopped abruptly following long-term use. Gradual withdrawal over a period of 2 to 3 weeks is advised. Ask doctor for help.

HISTAMINE (H-2) BLOCKING DRUGS

Cimetidine (si MET i deen)   **Ranitidine** (ra NI te deen)   **Famotidine** (fa MOH te deen)   **Nizatidine** (ni ZA te deen)
Introduced: 1977, 1983, 1986, 1988   **Prescription:** USA: Yes; Canada: Yes
Available as Generic: USA: No; Canada: Yes   **Class:** Histamine (H-2) Blocking Drugs   **Controlled Drug:** USA: No; Canada: No
Brand Names: ✦Apo-Cimetidine, ✦Enlon, ✦Novo-Cimetine, ✦Nu-Cimet ✦Peptol, Tagamet, Tagamet HB (nonprescription form is now available), Zantac, ✦Zantac-C, ✦Apo-Ranitidine, Novo-Ranidine, Nu-Ranit, Pepcid, Pepcid AC (nonprescription form is FDA approved), Axid

Warning: The brand names Zantac and Xanax are similar and can be mistaken. These are very different drugs, and can lead to serious problems. Check the color chart and verify that you are taking the correct drug.

BENEFITS versus RISKS	
Possible Benefits	*Possible Risks*
EFFECTIVE TREATMENT OF PEPTIC ULCER DISEASE: relief of symptoms, acceleration of healing, prevention of recurrence	Drug-induced hepatitis (rare)
	Bone marrow depression (rare)
	Confusion (particularly in compromised elderly)
CONTROL OF HYPERSECRETORY STOMACH DISORDERS	Low blood platelet counts (rare)
TREATMENT OF REFLUX ESOPHAGITIS	

▷ **Principal Uses**

As a Single Drug Product: Uses currently included in FDA approved labeling: (1) Treatment and prevention of recurrence of peptic ulcer. (2) Cimetidine, ranitidine and famotidine are used for both duodenal and gastric ulcers as well as conditions where extreme production (Zollinger-Ellison syndrome) of stomach acid occurs. (3) All four medications are used to control excess acid moving from the stomach into the lower throat (gastroesophageal reflux disease—GERD). (4) Cimetidine is approved for use in preventing upper stomach/intestinal bleeding. (5) Cimetidine, ranitidine, famotidine and nizatidine have been used as combination treatment with antibiotics and bismuth compounds (Pepto Bismol and others) in refractory ulcers where the organism Helicobacter pylori has been found.

Other (unlabeled) generally accepted uses: (1) Ranitidine, famotidine and nizatidine have been used in the prevention of upper stomach/intestinal bleeding. (2) Cimetidine has been used prior to surgery to prevent aspiration pneumonitis caused by anesthesia, and ranitidine has shown some benefit here as well. (3) Cimetidine, ranitidine and famotidine have been used to help prevent ulcers which may occur in acutely and seriously ill patients.

How These Drugs Work: These drugs block the action of histamine, and by doing this, inhibit the ability of the stomach to make acid. Once the acid production is decreased, the body is able to heal itself. Ulcers which are resistant to healing have now been shown to have an infectious compo-

Histamine (H-2) Blocking Drugs

nent, and antibiotics combined with a histamine (H-2) blocking drug can work.

Available Dosage Forms and Strengths
Cimetidine (Tagamet):
- Injection — 300 mg per 2 ml
  - 300 mg per 50 ml (single dose in 0.9% sodium chloride)
- Liquid — 300 mg per 5 ml (2.8% alcohol)
- Tablets — 200 mg, 300 mg, 400 mg, 800 mg (see color chart)

Ranitidine (Zantac):
- Injection — 0.5 mg per ml (single dose in 100 ml)
  - 25 mg per ml (in 2, 10 and 40 ml vials and 2 ml syringes)
- Syrup — 15 mg per ml (7.5 % alcohol)
- Tablets — 150 mg, 300 mg (see color chart)
- GELdose Capsules — 150 mg, 300 mg.

Famotidine (Pepcid):
- Injection — 10 mg per ml (in 2 ml and 4 ml vials)
- Oral Suspension — 40 mg per 5 ml
- Tablets — 20 mg, 40 mg (see color chart)

Nizatidine (Axid):
- Pulvules (capsules) — 150 and 300 mg (see color chart)

▷ **Recommended Dosage Ranges (Actual dosage and administration schedule must be determined by the physician for each patient individually.)**

Infants and Children: Safety and effectiveness for those under 16 years of age not established.

16 to 60 Years of Age: Peptic ulcer and hypersecretory states:
- cimetidine: 300 mg by mouth four times daily—taken with meals and at bedtime
- ranitidine: 150 mg by mouth twice daily. Up to 6 grams in hypersecretory states.
- famotidine: 40 mg by mouth at bedtime. Up to 640 mg daily for hypersecretory states.
- nizatidine: 300 mg by mouth at bedtime. Not used for hypersecretory states.

Over 60 Years of Age: Cimetidine: Half the usual adult dose to start. Ranitidine, famotidine and nizatidine: Same dose as 16 to 60 years of age. All pose a risk for formation of masses (phytobezoars) of undigested vegetable fibers. Watch for nervousness, confusion, loss of appetite, stomach fullness, nausea and vomiting.

Conditions Requiring Dosing Adjustments:

Liver function: Cimetidine and famotidine are most dependent on the liver for elimination. Dose must be decreased in liver failure.

Kidney function: All histamine blockers are primarily eliminated by the kidneys. Doses **must** be decreased in moderate kidney failure.

▷ **Dosing Instructions:** Cimetidine and ranitidine should be taken immediately after meals to obtain the longest decrease in stomach acid when treating peptic ulcers. Cimetidine, ranitidine and famotidine should be taken after meals when used in hypersecretory states.

Histamine (H-2) Blocking Drugs

Usual Duration of Use: Use on a regular schedule for 4 to 6 weeks usually determines effectiveness in healing active peptic ulcer disease. Long-term use (months to years) for prevention requires periodic individualized consideration by your physician. Continual use for 6 to 12 weeks is needed to heal the esophagus when cimetidine, ranitidine famotidine or nizatidine is used in GERD.

Possible Advantages of These Drugs
Famotidine and nizatidine offer effective treatment of peptic ulcer disease with once a day dosing.

▷ **These Drugs Should Not Be Taken If**
- you have had an allergic reaction to any dosage form of it previously.

▷ **Inform Your Physician Before Taking This Drug If**
- you have impaired liver or kidney function.
- you have a low sperm count (cimetidine).
- you are taking any anticoagulant drug.
- you have had low white blood cell counts.
- you are taking propranolol or quinidine (cimetidine).

Possible Side-Effects (natural, expected and unavoidable drug actions)
None reported.

▷ **Possible Adverse Effects** (unusual, unexpected and infrequent reactions)
If any of the following develop, consult your physician promptly for guidance.

Mild Adverse Effects
Allergic Reactions: Skin rash and hives.
Headache: ranitidine and famotidine rare, cimetidine 1%, and famotidine 4.7%.
Diarrhea: ranitidine and nizatidine rare, cimetidine 1%, and famotidine 1.7%.
Arthralgia: cimetidine, ranitidine and famotidine are rare causes.

Serious Adverse Effects
Allergic Reactions: Cimetidine and ranitidine can be rare causes of pancreatitis and anemia. Cimetidine and nizatidine can cause exfoliative dermatitis.
Idiosyncratic Reactions: Nervousness, confusion, hallucinations.
Liver damage: cimetidine, ranitidine and nizatidine (rare).
Abnormal heart rhythmn/arrest: cimetidine, ranitidine and nizatidine (rare).
Bone marrow depression: cimetidine and ranitidine are rare causes.
Decreased platelets: cimetidine, ranitidine, famotidine and nizatidine (rare).
Bronchspasm: cimetidine and famotidine are rare causes.

▷ **Possible Effects on Sexual Function:** Impotence: ranitidine, famotidine and nizatidine (rare), cimetidine (1%).
Libido loss: ranitidine, famotidine and nizatidine (rare).
Male breast enlargement: ranitidine and nizatidine (rare), cimetidine (3–4%).

Histamine (H-2) Blocking Drugs

Possible Delayed Adverse Effects: Male breast enlargement (ranitidine, nizatidine and cimetidine as above).
Famotidine may impair vitamin B-12 absorption and lead to deficiency.

▷ **Adverse Effects That May Mimic Natural Diseases or Disorders**
Liver changes may mimic viral hepatitis.

Possible Effects on Laboratory Tests
Blood Platelet counts: may be decreased by all histamine (H-2) blockers.
Complete blood counts: rare white blood cell (granulocytes) decrease by cimetidine and ranitidine.
Urine protein tests (Multistix): False-positive with ranitidine use.
Urine urobilinogen: False-positive with nizatidine.
Thyroid hormones: T4 and free T4 are decreased with ranitidine use.
Liver enzymes (SGPT,OT etc.): Can be increased with liver damage.
Sperm count: Decreased with cimetidine.

CAUTION
1. Ulcer rebound/perforation can occur if you stop these drugs abruptly.
2. Once medicine is stopped, call your doctor promptly if symptoms recur.
3. Some of cimetidine is removed by hemodialysis. Redose is needed.

Precautions for Use
By Infants and Children:
Safety and effectiveness by those under 16 not established.
By Those over 60 Years of Age: Increased risk of masses of partially digested vegetable fibers (phytobezoars), especially in people who can't chew well. Watch closely for decreased appetite, stomach fullness, nausea and vomiting.

▷ **Advisability of Use During Pregnancy**
Pregnancy Category: B for cimetidine, ranitidine and famotidine. C for nizatidine. See Pregnancy Code at the back of this book.
Animal studies: No birth defects for cimetidine, ranitidine and famotidine. Rabbit studies of nizatidine showed heart, brain/spinal cord defects.
Human studies: Adequate studies of pregnant women are not available.
Use cimetidine, ranitidine or famotidine only if clearly needed. Ask your doctor for advice.
Nizatidine must be avoided during the first 3 months of pregnancy. Ask your doctor for guidance.

Advisability of Use if Breast-Feeding
Presence of this drug in breast milk: Yes.
Avoid drugs or refrain from nursing.

Habit-Forming Potential:
None.

Effects of Overdosage: Confusion, mild slowing of the heart (bradycardia), sweating, drowsiness, muscle twitching, seizures, cardiac arrest, coma.

Possible Effects of Long-Term Use: Rare liver damage with cimetidine, ranitidine and nizatidine. Swelling and tenderness of breast tissue with cimetidine, ranitidine and nizatidine.

Suggested Periodic Examinations While Taking This Drug (at physician's discretion)
Complete blood counts, liver and kidney function tests, more frequent tests

Histamine (H-2) Blocking Drugs 471

of prothrombin times if an anticoagulant is also taken, and sperm counts (cimetidine).

▷ **While Taking This Drug, Observe the Following**
Foods: Protein-rich foods increase stomach acid secretion. Ask doctor for advice.
Nutritional Support: Cimetidine may decrease vitamin B-12 over time and require supplements.
Beverages: No restrictions. May take these medicines with milk.
▷ *Alcohol:* No interactions; however, stomach acidity is increased by alcohol—avoid use.
Tobacco Smoking: Smoking is a clear risk factor for peptic ulcer disease. Stop if possible.
Marijuana Smoking: Possible additive reduction in sperm counts with cimetidine use.

▷ *Other Drugs*
Cimetidine may *increase* the effects of
- oral anticoagulants—with increased risk of bleeding.
- benzodiazepines (Librium, etc.)—see Drug Class Section.
- carbamazepine (Tegretol) with increased toxicity.
- meperidine (Demerol, others) and result in toxicity with potential respiratory depression and low blood pressure.
- metoprolol (Lopressor, others) and result in very slow heartbeat and excessively low blood pressure.
- morphine (MS Contin, MSIR others) and result in central nervous system depression and respiratory depression.
- phenytoin (Dilantin).
- procainamide (Procan, Pronestyl).
- propranolol (Inderal).
- quinidine (Quiniglute).
- theophylline (Theo-Dur, etc.).
- warfarin (Coumadin).

Ranitidine may *increase* the effects of
- diazepam (Valium).
- procainamide (Procan, Pronestyl).
- glipizide (Glucotrol).
- theophylline (Theo-Dur, etc.).
- warfarin (Coumadin).

Nizatidine may *increase* the effects of
- high dose aspirin (increased level and toxicity risk).

Cimetidine ***taken concurrently*** with
- carmustine (BCNU) may cause severe bone marrow depression.
- chloroquine will result in toxicity and may cause cardiac arrest.
- cisapride (Propulcid) will result in increased cisapride levels and a potential serious increase in heart rate.
- oral hypoglycemic agents such as glipizide (Glucotrol), glyburide (DiaBeta, Micronase), and tolbutamide (Tolinase, others) and may result in severe low blood sugars and seizures.

Cimetidine, ranitidine famotidine and nizatidine ***taken concurrently*** with
- antacids will result in a decreased histamine blocker level.

Cimetidine *may decrease the effects of*
- iron salts, by decreasing absorption.
- indomethacin, by decreasing absorption.
- ketoconazole, itraconazole and fluconazole.
- tetracyclines, by decreasing absorption.

▷ *Driving, Hazardous Activities:* Use caution until the degree of confusion, dizziness or other effect is seen.

Aviation Note: The use of these drugs **may be a disqualification** for piloting. Consult a designated Aviation Medical Examiner.

Exposure to Sun: No restrictions.

Occurrence of Unrelated Illness: Idiopathic thrombocytopenic purpura (ITP), a rare lowering of blood platelets is a contraindication for use of any of these medications. Aplastic anemia, whatever the cause may be worsened by cimetidine.

Discontinuation: **Do not** stop these medicines suddenly if they are being taken for peptic ulcer disease. Ask your doctor for withdrawal instructions. Be alert to the recurrence of ulcers any time after these drugs are stopped. Recurrent or refractory ulcers may also represent an infectious disease caused by Helicobacter pylori. If this is the case, combination therapy with an antibiotic may be indicated.

HYDRALAZINE (hi DRAL a zeen)

Introduced: 1950 **Prescription:** USA: Yes; Canada: Yes **Available as Generic:** USA: Yes; Canada: No **Class:** Antihypertensive **Controlled Drug:** USA: No; Canada: No

Brand Names: Alazine, Apo-Hydralazine, Apresazide [CD], Apresoline, Apresoline-Esidrix [CD], Dralzine, H-H-R, H.H.R., Hydroserpine [CD], Novo-Hylazin, Nu-Hydral, Ser-Ap-Es [CD], Serpasil-Apresoline [CD], Unipres [CD]

BENEFITS versus RISKS	
Possible Benefits	*Possible Risks*
EFFECTIVE STEP 2 OR 3 ANTIHYPERTENSIVE FOR MODERATE TO SEVERE HYPERTENSION when used adjunctively with other antihypertensive drugs Possibly beneficial in the management of severe congestive heart failure	DRUG-INDUCED LUPUS ERYTHEMATOSUSLIKE SYNDROME (up to 13%) Intensification of angina pectoris Rare blood cell disorders Rare liver damage

▷ **Principal Uses**

As a Single Drug Product: Uses currently included in FDA approved labeling: (1) as a step 2 or antihypertensive drug in combination with other drugs for treatment of moderate to severe high blood pressure or hypertensive crisis; (2) therapy of hypertension caused by abnormal changes in kidney blood vessels.

Other (unlabeled) generally accepted uses: (1) Therapy for aortic or mitral heart valve insufficiency—providing support until surgery can be performed; (2) treatment of acute congestive heart failure in combination with dobutamine; (3) help in anorexia or cachexia; (4) therapy of high blood pressure in pregnancy; (5) sickle cell priapism.

As a Combination Drug Product [CD]: Available combined with hydrochlorothiazide (a diuretic) and with reserpine (another type of antihypertensive). When used in combination, several different types of drug action occur at the same time and result in a more beneficial decrease in blood pressure.

How This Drug Works: By causing direct relaxation of arterial walls (mechanism unknown), this drug lowers blood pressure. The dilation of blood vessels can also help in some cases of heart failure by reducing the workload and increasing the output of the heart. Combination therapy with a diuretic reduces the amount of sodium and water in the body, and combination with reserpine reduces the rate and force of contraction of the heart and increases blood vessel expansion.

Available Dosage Forms and Strengths
Tablets — 10 mg, 25 mg, 50 mg, 100 mg

▷ **Usual Adult Dosage Range:** Initially 10 mg 4 times daily for 2 to 4 days; then increase to 25 mg 4 times daily for the balance of the first week. During the second week the dose may be increased to 50 mg 4 times daily if needed and tolerated. The total daily dosage should not exceed 300 mg for fast acetylators or 200 mg for slow acetylators. Ask your physician for guidance. **Note: Actual dosage and administration schedule must be determined by the physician for each patient individually.**

Conditions Requiring Dosing Adjustments
Liver function: Hydralazine can cause hepatitis, hepatic necrosis and noncancerous growths. It should be used with caution in patients with liver compromise.
Kidney function: In mild to moderate kidney failure the usual dose can be given every eight hours. In severe kidney failure and people with slow hydralazine metabolism the usual dose is given every 12 to 24 hours and 200 mg per day is a maximum. This medication should be used with caution.

▷ **Dosing Instructions:** The tablet may be crushed and the capsule [CD] may be opened and best taken with or following meals to help absorption and reduce stomach upset.

Usual Duration of Use: Use on a regular schedule for several weeks determines effectiveness in lowering blood pressure. Long-term use requires physician supervision.

▷ **This Drug Should Not Be Taken If**
- you have had an allergic reaction to it previously.
- you have rheumatic heart disease.
- you have coronary artery disease.
- you have mitral valvular heart disease.

▷ **Inform Your Physician Before Taking This Drug If**
- you have a history of any type of heart disease.
- you have lupus erythematosus.

Hydralazine

- you have active angina pectoris.
- you have impaired brain circulation.
- you are subject to migraine headaches.
- you have impaired kidney function.
- you have systemic lupus erythematosus.
- you have a history of liver sensitivity to other drugs.
- you plan to have surgery under general anesthesia in the near future.

Possible Side-Effects (natural, expected and unavoidable drug actions)
Orthostatic hypotension (see Glossary), nasal congestion, constipation, delayed or impaired urination, increased heart rate of 10 to 25 beats/minute.

▷ **Possible Adverse Effects** (unusual, unexpected and infrequent reactions)
If any of the following develop, consult your physician promptly for guidance.

Mild Adverse Effects
Allergic Reactions: Skin rash, hives, itching, drug fever.
Headache, dizziness, flushing of face, palpitation.
Loss of appetite, nausea, vomiting, diarrhea.
Taste or smell disorders.
Tremors, muscle cramps.
Reflex tachycarida.

Serious Adverse Effects
Allergic Reactions: Liver reaction, with or without jaundice.
Idiosyncratic Reactions: Behavioral changes: nervousness, confusion, emotional depression. Bleeding into lung tissue: densities found on X-ray. A syndrome resembling rheumatoid arthritis or lupus erythematosus (see Glossary).
Intensification of coronary artery disease.
Peripheral neuropathy (see Glossary): weakness, numbness and/or pain in extremities.
Serious skin rashes (Stevens-Johnson syndrome).
Drug-induced periarteritis nodosa.
Drug-induced porphyria.
Drug-induced gastrointestinal bleeding.
Glomerulonephritis.
Drug-induced gallstones.
Congestive heart failure (rare).
ST segment depression on ECG.
Excessive lowering of the blood pressure.
Rare bone marrow depression (see Glossary): fatigue, weakness, fever, sore throat, abnormal bleeding or bruising.

▷ **Possible Effects on Sexual Function:** Rare reports of impotence and priapism (see Glossary).

▷ **Adverse Effects That May Mimic Natural Diseases or Disorders**
Drug fever may suggest systemic infection. Liver reaction may suggest viral hepatitis. Skin and joint symptoms may suggest lupus erythematosus.

Natural Diseases or Disorders That May Be Activated by This Drug
Latent coronary artery disease.

Possible Effects on Laboratory Tests
Complete blood cell counts: decreased red cells, hemoglobin, white cells and platelets.
Blood antinuclear antibodies (ANA): positive.
Blood cholesterol level: decreased.
Blood lupus erythematosus (LE) cells: positive.
Blood urea nitrogen (BUN) level: increased (kidney damage).
Liver function tests: increased liver enzymes (ALT/GPT, AST/GOT and alkaline phosphatase), increased bilirubin.

CAUTION
1. Increased risk of toxicity with large doses. Follow prescribed doses exactly and keep appointments for follow-up examinations.
2. Report the development of any tendency to emotional depression.
3. May cause salt and water retention if not taken with a diuretic.
4. This drug can provoke migraine headache.

Precautions for Use
By Infants and Children: Dosage is based upon age, weight and kidney function status. Watch for development of a lupus erythematosuslike reaction.

By Those over 60 Years of Age: Low doses are indicated. Unacceptably high blood pressure should be slowly reduced, avoiding the risks associated with excessively low blood pressure. Sudden, rapid and excessive reduction of blood pressure can predispose to stroke or heart attack. Watch for dizziness, unsteadiness, fainting or falling. Headache, palpitation and rapid heart rates are more common in the elderly and can mimic acute anxiety states.

▷ **Advisability of Use During Pregnancy**
Pregnancy Category: C. See Pregnancy Code at the back of this book.
Animal studies: Birth defects of head and facial bones reported in mice.
Human studies: Adequate studies of pregnant women are not available.
Avoid use during the first and last 3 months; if taken late in pregnancy, this drug can cause low blood platelets (see Glossary) in the newborn.

Advisability of Use if Breast-Feeding
Presence of this drug in breast milk: Yes.
Avoid drug or refrain from nursing.

Habit-Forming Potential: None, but sudden stopping of this medicine may result in congestive heart failure.

Effects of Overdosage: Marked light-headedness, dizziness, headache, flushing of skin, nausea, vomiting, collapse of circulation; loss of consciousness, cold and sweaty skin, weak and rapid pulse, irregular heart rhythm.

Possible Effects of Long-Term Use: An acute or subacute syndrome resembling rheumatoid arthritis or lupus erythematosus, usually seen in slow acetylators taking daily doses of over 200 mg.

Suggested Periodic Examinations While Taking This Drug (at physician's discretion)
Complete blood counts, liver function tests, blood tests for evidence of lupus erythematosus.

While Taking This Drug, Observe the Following

Foods: May decrease hydralazine absorption and lessen its therapeutic effect.

Nutritional Support: Watch for peripheral neuropathy and take pyridoxine (vitamin B-6) as needed. Ask physician for guidance.

Beverages: No restrictions. May be taken with milk.

▷ *Alcohol:* Use with extreme caution—alcohol can exaggerate the blood-pressure-lowering effect of this drug and cause excessive reduction.

Tobacco Smoking: Avoid completely. Nicotine can contribute significantly to this drug's ability to intensify angina in susceptible individuals.

▷ *Other Drugs*

Hydralazine may *increase* the effects of
- metoprolol (Lopressor) and other beta blocking medicines.
- oxprenolol (Trasicor).
- propranolol (Inderal).

Hydralazine *taken concurrently* with
- NSAIDs may blunt hydralazine's benefit in lowering blood pressure.

▷ *Driving, Hazardous Activities:* May cause light-headedness or dizziness. Limit activities as necessary.

Aviation Note: Hypertension and the use of this drug *are disqualifications* for piloting. Consult a designated Aviation Medical Examiner.

Exposure to Sun: No restrictions.

Exposure to Heat: Caution advised. Hot environments may reduce blood pressure significantly.

Exposure to Cold: Caution advised. Cold environments may increase this drug's ability to cause angina in susceptible individuals.

Heavy Exercise or Exertion: Caution advised. Exertion can increase this drug's ability to cause angina. Also, isometric exercises can raise blood pressure significantly.

HYDROCHLOROTHIAZIDE (hi droh klor oh THI a zide)

Introduced: 1959 **Prescription:** USA: Yes; Canada: Yes **Available as Generic:** USA: Yes; Canada: Yes **Class:** Antihypertensive, diuretic, thiazides **Controlled Drug:** USA: No; Canada: No

Brand Names: Aldactazide [CD], Aldoril-15/25 [CD], Aldoril D30/D50 [CD], ◆Apo-Hydro, ◆Apo-Methazide [CD], ◆Apo-Triazide [CD], Apresazide [CD], Apresoline-Esidrix [CD], Capozide [CD], ◆Co-Betaloc [CD], Diaqua, Dyazide [CD], Esidrix, H-H-R, H.H.R., HydroDIURIL, Hydro-Chlor, Hydromal, Hydropres [CD], Hydro-T, Hydro-Z-50, Inderide [CD], Inderide LA [CD], ◆Ismelin-Esidrix [CD], Lopressor HCT [CD], Maxzide [CD], Maxzide-25 [CD], M Dopazide, Mictrin, ◆Moduret [CD], Moduretic [CD], ◆Natrimax, ◆Neo-Codema, Normozide [CD], ◆Novo-Noparil [CD], ◆Novohydrazide, ◆Novospirozine [CD], ◆Novotriamzide [CD], ◆Nu-Amilzide, ◆Nu-Triazide, Oretic, Oreticyl [CD], ◆PMS Dopazide [CD], Prinzide [CD], Ser-Ap-Es [CD], Serpasil-Esidrix [CD], SK-Hydrochlorothiazide, Thiuretic, Timolide [CD], Trandate HCT [CD], Unipres [CD], ◆Urozide, Vaseretic [CD], ◆Viskazide [CD], Zestoretic [CD], Zide, Ziac

Warning: Recent studies have shown that doses of 50 mg may increase risk of sudden heart (cardiac) death by 70%. Doses greater than 100 mg may increase risk of sudden cardiac death by 400%. This effect is thought to be due to loss of magnesium and potassium from the body. Ask your doctor for guidance.

BENEFITS versus RISKS	
Possible Benefits	*Possible Risks*
EFFECTIVE, WELL-TOLERATED DIURETIC	LOSS OF BODY POTASSIUM AND MAGNESIUM ESPECIALLY WITH DOSES OVER 25 MG
POSSIBLY EFFECTIVE IN MILD HYPERTENSION	SUDDEN CARDIAC DEATH SECONDARY TO ELECTROLYTE LOSS
ENHANCES EFFECTIVENESS OF OTHER ANTIHYPERTENSIVES	
Beneficial in treatment of diabetes insipidus	Increased blood sugar
	Increased blood uric acid
	Increased blood calcium
	Rare blood cell disorders

Please see the thiazide diuretic profile for further information.

HYDROCODONE (hi droh KOH dohn)

Other Name: Dihydrocodeinone
Introduced: 1951 **Prescription:** USA: Yes; Canada: Yes **Available as Generic:** USA: Yes; Canada: No **Class:** Analgesic, narcotic; cough suppressant **Controlled Drug:** USA: C-III*; Canada: Yes

Brand Names: Allay [CD], Anaplex, Anexsia [CD], Anexsia 7.5 [CD], Azdone [CD], Ban-Tuss-HC [CD], ✦Biohisdex DHC [CD], ✦Biohisdine DHC [CD], Chemdal-HD [CD], Detussin [CD], DHC Plus, Dimetane Expectorant-DC [CD], Duocet [CD], Duratuss HD [CD], Endagen HD [CD], Endal-HD, Histussin HC [CD], ✦Hycodan, Hycodan [CD], ✦Hycomine [CD], Hycomine Compound [CD], Hycomine Pediatric Syrup [CD], ✦Hycomine-S [CD], Hycomine Syrup [CD], Hycotuss Expectorant [CD], Lorcet-HD [CD], Lorcet Plus [CD], Lortab [CD], Lortab ASA [CD], Medipain 5, Norcet 7 [CD], ✦Novahistex DH [CD], ✦Novahistine DH [CD], ✦Robidone, T-Gesic [CD], Triaminic Expectorant DH [CD], ✦Tussaminic Expectorant DH [CD], Tussend [CD], Tussend Expectorant [CD], Tussionex [CD], Tycolet [CD], Vanex [CD], Vicodin [CD], Vicodin ES [CD], Zydone [CD]

BENEFITS versus RISKS	
Possible Benefits	*Possible Risks*
EFFECTIVE RELIEF OF MILD TO MODERATE PAIN	Mild allergic reactions (infrequent)
	Nausea, constipation
EFFECTIVE CONTROL OF COUGH	Potential for addiction

▷ **Principal Uses**
As a Single Drug Product: Uses currently included in FDA approved labeling: (1) controls cough; (2) relieves mild to moderate pain.

*See Schedules of Controlled Drugs at the back of this book.

Hydrocodone

Other (unlabeled) generally accepted uses: May be a benefit in some patients with chronic obstructive lung disease.

As a Combination Drug Product [CD]: Hydrocodone is often added to cough mixtures containing antihistamines, decongestants and expectorants to make these "shotgun" preparations more effective in reducing cough. It is also combined with milder analgesics, such as acetaminophen and aspirin, to enhance pain relief.

How This Drug Works: Depresses some brain functions, decreasing pain perception, calming emotional responses to pain and reducing cough reflex sensitivity.

Available Dosage Forms and Strengths
Syrup — 5 mg per 5-ml teaspoonful
Tablets — 5 mg

▷ **Usual Adult Dosage Range:** As analgesic—5 to 10 mg/4 to hours as needed. For cough—5 mg/4 to 6 hours as needed. Total daily dosage should not exceed 60 mg. **Note: Actual dosage and administration schedule must be determined by the physician for each patient individually.**

Conditions Requiring Dosing Adjustments

Liver function: Used with caution in patients with severe liver compromise with decreases in dose or longer dosing intervals.

Kidney function: This drug may cause urinary retention, and a benefit to risk decision should be made in patients with renal (kidney) outflow problems. Up to 20% of this drug is eliminated by the kidneys. Consideration for reduced doses should be given, especially for longer term therapy.

▷ **Dosing Instructions:** Tablet may be crushed and taken with or following food to reduce stomach irritation or nausea.

Usual Duration of Use: As required, to control pain or cough. Continual use should not exceed 5 to 7 days without interruption and reassessment of need.

▷ **This Drug Should Not Be Taken If**
- you have had an allergic reaction to any dosage form of it previously.
- you have a lesion in your head (intracranial) which causes increased pressure.
- you are having an acute attack of asthma.

▷ **Inform Your Physician Before Taking This Drug If**
- you have had an unfavorable reaction to any narcotic drug in the past.
- you have a history of drug abuse or alcoholism.
- you have chronic lung disease with impaired breathing.
- you have impaired liver or kidney function.
- you have gallbladder disease, a seizure disorder or an underactive thyroid gland.
- you have difficulty emptying the urinary bladder.
- you are taking any other drugs that have a sedative effect.
- you plan to have surgery under general anesthesia in the near future.

Possible Side-Effects (natural, expected and unavoidable drug actions)
Drowsiness, light-headedness, dry mouth, urinary retention, constipation.

▷ **Possible Adverse Effects** (unusual, unexpected and infrequent reactions)
   If any of the following develop, consult your physician promptly for guidance.
   Mild Adverse Effects
   Allergic Reactions: Skin rash, hives, itching.
   Dizziness, impaired concentration, sensation of drunkenness, confusion, depression, blurred or double vision, facial flushing, sweating.
   Nausea, vomiting.
   Abnormal constriction of the pupils of the eye (miosis).
   Serious Adverse Effects
   Allergic Reactions: Anaphylaxis (rare), severe skin reactions.
   Idiosyncratic Reactions: Delirium, hallucinations, excitement, increased sensitivity to pain after the analgesic effect has worn off.
   Seizures (rare).
   Impaired breathing.
   Refractory constipation.
   Liver toxicity.
   Kidney toxicity.
   Psychological and physical dependence.

▷ **Possible Effects on Sexual Function:** Blunting of sexual response or drive.

▷ **Adverse Effects That May Mimic Natural Diseases or Disorders**
   Paradoxical behavioral disturbances may suggest psychotic disorder.

Possible Effects on Laboratory Tests
   Blood amylase and lipase levels: increased (natural side-effect).
   Urine screening tests for drug abuse: *initial* test result may be falsely **positive**; *confirmatory* test result will be **negative**. (Test results depend upon amount of drug taken and testing method used.)

CAUTION
   1. Patients with asthma, chronic bronchitis or emphysema may have significant respiratory problems with excessive use of this drug because of thickening of bronchial secretions and suppression of coughing.
   2. Combination of this drug with atropinelike drugs can increase the risk of urinary retention and reduced intestinal function.
   3. Do not take this drug following acute head injury.

Precautions for Use
   By Infants and Children: Do not use this drug in children under 2 years of age because of their vulnerability to life-threatening respiratory depression.
   By Those over 60 Years of Age: Small doses and short-term treatment are indicated. May be increased susceptibility to drowsiness, dizziness, unsteadiness, falling, urinary retention and constipation (often leading to fecal impaction).

▷ **Advisability of Use During Pregnancy**
   Pregnancy Category: C. See Pregnancy Code at the back of this book.
   Animal studies: Birth defects reported in hamster studies.
   Human studies: Adequate studies of pregnant women are not available.

Hydrocodone taken repeatedly during the last few weeks before delivery may cause withdrawal symptoms in the newborn infant.
Use this drug only if clearly needed and in small, infrequent doses.

Advisability of Use if Breast-Feeding
Presence of this drug in breast milk: Unknown.
Monitor nursing infant closely and discontinue drug or nursing if adverse effects develop. Ask physician for guidance.

Habit-Forming Potential: Psychological and/or physical dependence can develop with use of large doses for an extended period of time. True dependence is infrequent and unlikely with prudent use.

Effects of Overdosage: Drowsiness, restlessness, agitation, nausea, vomiting, dry mouth, vertigo, weakness, lethargy, stupor, coma, seizures.

Possible Effects of Long-Term Use: Psychological and physical dependence, chronic constipation.

Suggested Periodic Examinations While Taking This Drug (at physician's discretion)
Liver function tests.

▷ **While Taking This Drug, Observe the Following**
Foods: No restrictions.
Beverages: No restrictions. May be taken with milk.
▷ *Alcohol:* Use extreme caution. Hydrocodone can intensify the intoxicating effects of alcohol, and alcohol can intensify the depressant effects of hydrocodone on brain function, breathing and circulation.
Tobacco Smoking: No interactions expected.
Marijuana Smoking: Increased drowsiness and pain relief; impaired mental and physical status.
▷ *Other Drugs*
Hydrocodone may *increase* the effects of
- other drugs with sedative effects.
- atropinelike drugs, and increase the risk of constipation and urinary retention.

▷ *Driving, Hazardous Activities:* This drug can impair mental alertness, judgment, reaction time and physical coordination. Avoid hazardous activities accordingly.
Aviation Note: The use of this drug ***is a disqualification*** for piloting. Consult a designated Aviation Medical Examiner.
Exposure to Sun: No restrictions.
Discontinuation: Best limited to short-term use. If used for extended periods, discontinuation should be gradual to minimize withdrawal (usually mild with this drug).

HYDROXYCHLOROQUINE (hi drox ee KLOR oh kwin)

Introduced: 1967 **Prescription:** USA: Yes; Canada: Yes **Available as Generic:** USA: No; Canada: No **Class:** Antimalarial, lupus suppressant, rheumatoid arthritis suppressant **Controlled Drug:** USA: No; Canada: No
Brand Name: ◆Dermoplast, Plaquenil

Hydroxychloroquine

BENEFITS versus RISKS	
Possible Benefits	*Possible Risks*
EFFECTIVE PREVENTION AND TREATMENT OF CERTAIN FORMS OF MALARIA	INFREQUENT BUT SERIOUS DAMAGE OF CORNEAL AND RETINAL EYE TISSUES
Possibly effective in the management of acute and chronic rheumatoid arthritis and juvenile arthritis	RARE BUT SERIOUS BONE MARROW DEPRESSION: aplastic anemia, deficient white blood cells and platelets
Possibly effective in the management of chronic discoid and systemic lupus erythematosus	Rare heart muscle damage
	Rare ear damage: hearing loss, ringing in ears

▷ **Principal Uses**

As a Single Drug Product: Uses currently included in FDA approved labeling: (1) Prevention and therapy of acute attacks of certain types of malaria; (2) reduces disease activity in rheumatoid arthritis; (3) suppresses disease activity in chronic discoid and systemic lupus erythematosus.

Other (unlabeled) generally accepted uses: (1) Treatment of Sjogren's syndrome which is characterized by marked immune problems; (2) treatment of refractory Lyme arthritis; (3) therapy of sarcoidosis, polymorphous light eruption, porphyria, solar urticaria and chronic vasculitis; (4) may have a role in helping decrease steroid requirements in patients with asthma; (5) can help decrease insulin needs in patients who take an oral hypoglycemic agent with insulin; (6) part of a combination regimen in treating Weber-Christian Syndrome.

How This Drug Works: As an anti-infective in treating malaria, it is thought that this drug binds to and impairs the function of DNA in the organisms.

As an antiarthritic and antilupus drug, it is thought to act as a mild immunosuppressant. It accumulates in white blood cells and inhibits many enzymes involved in tissue destruction.

Available Dosage Forms and Strengths
Tablets — 200 mg

▷ **Usual Adult Dosage Range:** For malaria suppression: 400 mg once every 7 days.

For malaria treatment: (1) 800 mg as a single dose; or (2) initially 800 mg, followed by 400 mg in 6 to 8 hours; then 400 mg once a day on the second and third days.

For pediatric malaria treatment: 10 mg per kg followed in 6 hours by 5 mg per kg with 5 mg per kg given 18 hours after the second dose and finally 5 mg per kg taken 24 hours after the first dose was given.

For rheumatoid arthritis: Up to 6.5 mg per kilogram of lean body weight daily.

For lupus erythematosus: Up to 6.5 mg per kilogram of lean body weight daily.

Note: Actual dosage and administration schedule must be determined by the physician for each patient individually.

Conditions Requiring Dosing Adjustments

Liver function: It should be used with caution and as a benefit to risk decision in patients with liver compromise or who are already taking liver toxic drugs.

Kidney function: Used with caution in kidney compromise.

▷ **Dosing Instructions:** Take with food or milk to reduce stomach irritation. The tablet may be crushed and mixed with jam, jelly or jello for administration. Take full course of treatment as prescribed.

Note: For malaria prevention, begin medication 2 weeks before entering malarious area; continue medication while in the area and for 4 weeks after leaving the area.

For treating arthritis and lupus, take medication on a regular schedule daily; continual use for 6 months may be necessary to determine maximal benefit.

Usual Duration of Use: Use on a regular schedule for 2 weeks before exposure, during period of exposure, and 4 weeks after exposure determines this drug's effectiveness in preventing attacks of malaria. Use on a regular schedule for up to 6 months may be required to evaluate benefits in reducing rheumatoid arthritis and lupus erythematosus. If significant improvement is not achieved, this drug should be stopped. Long-term use (months to years) requires periodic physician evaluation of response and dosage adjustment.

Possible Advantages of This Drug
Considered to have less potential for retinal toxicity than chloroquine.

Currently a "Drug of Choice"
for the treatment of chronic discoid and systemic lupus erythematosus.

▷ **This Drug Should Not Be Taken If**
- you have had an allergic reaction to chloroquine or hydroxychloroquine.
- you have an active bone marrow or blood cell disorder.
- should not be used for long-term treatment in children.

▷ **Inform Your Physician Before Taking This Drug If**
- you are pregnant or planning pregnancy.
- you have had bone marrow depression or a blood cell disorder.
- you have a deficiency of glucose-6-phosphate dehydrogenase.
- you have any disorder of the eyes, especially disease of the cornea or retina, or visual field changes.
- you have impaired hearing or ringing in the ears.
- you have a seizure disorder of any kind.
- you have a history of peripheral neuritis.
- you have low blood pressure or a heart rhythm disorder.
- you have peptic ulcer disease, Crohn's disease or ulcerative colitis.
- you have impaired liver or kidney function.
- you have a history of porphyria.
- you have any form of psoriasis.
- you are taking antacids, cimetidine, digoxin or penicillamine.

Possible Side-Effects (natural, expected and unavoidable drug actions)
Light-headedness (low blood pressure); blue-black discoloration of skin, fingernails, or mouth lining with long-term use.

▷ **Possible Adverse Effects** (unusual, unexpected and infrequent reactions)
If any of the following develop, consult your physician promptly for guidance.
Mild Adverse Effects
Allergic Reactions: Skin rash, itching (more common in African-Americans).
Loss of hair color, loss of hair.
Headache, blurring of near vision (reading), ringing in ears.
Loss of appetite, nausea, vomiting, stomach cramps, diarrhea.
Dizziness.
Serious Adverse Effects
Allergic Reactions: Severe skin rash, exfoliative dermatitis.
Idiosyncratic Reactions: Hemolytic anemia in those with glucose-6-phosphate dehydrogenase deficiency in red blood cells.
Emotional or psychotic mental changes; seizures.
Loss of hearing.
Porphyria.
Excessive muscle weakness.
Eye tissue damage, specifically cornea and retina, with significant impairment of vision.
Heart rhythm abnormalities.
Aplastic anemia (see Glossary): Abnormally low red blood cell counts (fatigue and weakness), abnormally low white blood cell counts (fever, sore throat, infections), abnormally low platelet counts (abnormal bruising or bleeding).

▷ **Possible Effects on Sexual Function:** None reported.

Possible Delayed Adverse Effects: Irreversible retinal damage has developed 7 years after discontinuation of chloroquine, a closely related drug. Retinal damage is more likely to occur following high-dose and/or long-term use.

▷ **Adverse Effects That May Mimic Natural Diseases or Disorders**
Central nervous system toxicity may suggest unrelated neuropsychiatric disorder. Seizures may suggest the onset of epilepsy.

Natural Diseases or Disorders That May Be Activated by This Drug
Porphyria, psoriasis.

Possible Effects on Laboratory Tests
Complete blood cell counts: decreased red cells, hemoglobin, white cells and platelets.
Liver function tests: increased liver enzymes (ALT/GPT, AST/GOT and alkaline phosphatase), increased bilirubin.
Electrocardiogram: conduction abnormalities, prolonged QRS interval, T-wave changes, heart block have all been reported for chloroquine, a closely related drug.

CAUTION
1. This drug does not prevent relapses in certain types of malaria.
2. High-dose and/or long-term use of this drug may cause irreversible retinal damage, significant visual impairment or hearing loss due to nerve damage. Report promptly any changes in vision or hearing so appropriate evaluation can be made.

Hydroxychloroquine

Precautions for Use

By Infants and Children: This age group is very sensitive to the effects of this drug. Dosages should be determined and therapy should be monitored by a qualified pediatrician.

By Those over 60 Years of Age: Tolerance for this drug may be reduced. Watch for behavioral changes, low blood pressure, heart rhythm disturbances, muscle weakness and changes in vision or hearing.

▷ **Advisability of Use During Pregnancy**

Pregnancy Category: D. See Pregnancy Code at the back of this book.
Animal studies: No information available.
Human studies: Adequate studies of pregnant women are not available. However, closely related drugs of this class are known to cause abnormal retinal pigmentation and hemorrhage and congenital deafness in the fetus.
Avoid use during pregnancy except for the suppression or treatment of malaria.

Advisability of Use if Breast-Feeding

Presence of this drug in breast milk: Yes.
Avoid drug or refrain from nursing.

Habit-Forming Potential: None.

Effects of Overdosage: Drowsiness, headache, blurred vision, excitability, low blood pressure, seizures, coma.

Possible Effects of Long-Term Use: Irreversible eye damage (cornea and retina), hearing loss, muscle weakness, aplastic anemia.

Suggested Periodic Examinations While Taking This Drug (at physician's discretion)

Complete blood cell counts; liver and kidney function tests.
Serial blood pressure readings and electrocardiograms.
Neurological examinations for significant muscle weakness.
Complete eye examinations before starting high-dose and/or long-term treatment and every 3 to 6 months during drug use.
Hearing tests as indicated.

▷ **While Taking This Drug, Observe the Following**

Foods: No restrictions.
Beverages: No restrictions. May be taken with milk.
▷ *Alcohol:* Use sparingly to minimize stomach irritation.
Tobacco Smoking: No interactions expected.
▷ *Other Drugs*

Hydroxychloroquine may *increase* the effects of
- digoxin (Lanoxin), and increase its toxic potential.
- penicillamine (Cuprimine, Depen), and increase its toxic potential.

The following drug may *increase* the effects of hydroxychloroquine
- cimetidine (Tagamet).

The following drugs may *decrease* the effects of hydroxychloroquine
- magnesium salts and antacids.

▷ *Driving, Hazardous Activities:* This drug may cause light-headedness, blurred vision or impaired hearing. Restrict activities as necessary.

Aviation Note: The use of this drug **may be a disqualification** for piloting. Consult a designated Aviation Medical Examiner.

Exposure to Sun: Use caution until sensitivity has been determined. Closely related drugs of this class may cause photosensitivity (see Glossary).

Discontinuation: This drug should be stopped and prompt evaluation should be made if any of the following develop—any changes in vision or hearing, seizures, unusual muscle weakness, indications of infection (fever, sore throat, etc.), abnormal bruising or bleeding.

HYDROXYUREA (Hi DROXEE yur ia)

Introduced: 1995 (AIDS or Sickle Cell) **Prescription:** USA: Yes; Canada: Yes **Available as Generic:** USA: No; Canada: No **Class:** Anti-AIDS, anticancer, antisickle-cell **Controlled Drug:** USA: No; Canada: No
Brand Names: Hydrea
Warning: This drug is a cytoxic agent. Appropriate precautions must be taken.

BENEFITS versus RISKS	
Possible Benefits	*Possible Risks*
COMBINATION TREATMENT OF AIDS	BONE MARROW SUPPRESSION
DECREASED SEVERITY AND FREQUENCY OF SICKLE CELL CRISES	Hepatitis
Treatment of chronic myelocytic leukemia	
Treatment of melanoma	
Treatment of other cancers	

▷ **Principal Uses**

As a Single Drug Product: Uses currently included in FDA approved labeling: (1) Blast crisis; (2) chronic myelogenous leukemia; (3) head and neck cancers; (4) chronic leukemias; (5) cancers of certain cell types (squamous cell).

Other (unlabeled) generally accepted uses: (1) Used to decrease the frequency and severity of sickle cell crises; (2) used to treat certain diseases of the red blood cells (Polycythemia vera); (3) used in combination with didanosine to treat AIDS patients.

How This Drug Works: When used in cancer, this medicine is a cell cycle specific drug. It works in the S phase of mitosis.

When used in AIDS patients, the exact mechanism of action is not fully understood.

When used in sickle cell patients, the specific mechanism has not been identified.

Available Dosage Forms and Strengths

Capsule — 500 mg

▷ **Recommended Dosage Ranges (Actual dosage and administration schedule must be determined by the physician for each patient individually.)**

Infants and Children: Safety and effectiveness have not been defined in this age group.

18 to 60 Years of Age: All doses are decided based on ideal or actual weight, whichever is less.
  Oral dosing: Usual oral doses range from 20 to 30 mg per kilogram per day which is given as a single daily dose. Some centers give 80 mg per kg every third day. If a patient is in blast crisis, up to 12 grams per day has been given to rapidly decrease white blood cell counts.
  In the sickle cell studies: Patients were started on 15 mg per kg and had their dose increased by 5 mg per kg every 12 weeks unless toxicity occurred or the maximum dose of 35 mg per kg per day was reached.
Over 60 Years of Age: Same as 18 to 60 years of age.

Conditions Requiring Dosing Adjustments
Liver function: No changes in dosing are anticipated.
Kidney function: The dose must be decreased in patients with kideny compromise. Decreases of up to 50% are needed in severe compromise.

▷ **Dosing Instructions:** This medicine is best taken on an empty stomach. Call your doctor if you vomit after taking this medicine.

Usual Duration of Use: Continual use on a regular schedule for up to 16 weeks may be needed to treat cancers of the head and neck. Treatment in sickle cell disease is ongoing, using the lowest effective dose. Treatment in AIDS is yet to be defined.
  Long-term use (months to years) requires periodic evaluation of response and dosage adjustment. Consult your physician on a regular basis.

Currently a "Drug of Choice"
  for reducing the frequency and severity of sickle cell crises in patients with sickle cell disease.

▷ **This Drug Should Not Be Taken If**
  - you have had an allergic reaction to any dosage form of it previously.
  - you have severly depressed bone marrow. This is seen in very low white blood cell, platelet or hemoglobins.

▷ **Inform Your Physician Before Taking This Drug If**
  - you have signs or symptoms of cancer.
  - you are considering pregnancy (males or females).
  - you have had chemotherapy or radiation therapy previously.
  - you have compromised kidneys.
  - you have Herpes zoster (shingles).
  - you have recently been exposed to chicken pox.
  - you are having unusual brusing or bleeding.
  - you are unsure of how to appropriately dispose of urine or vomit.
  - you are uncertain of how much hydroxyurea to take or how often to take it.
  - you take other prescription or non-prescription medicines which were not discussed with your doctor when hydroxyurea was prescribed.

Possible Side-Effects (natural, expected and unavoidable drug actions)
  Hair loss, painful mouth sores, sensitivity to the sun.

▷ **Possible Adverse Effects** (unusual, unexpected and infrequent reactions)
  If any of the following develop, consult your physician promptly for guidance.

Mild Adverse Effects
  Allergic Reactions: Skin rash and itching.
  Headaches (rare).
  Nausea, vomiting or diarhea (up to 25%).
  Dizziness or disorientation (rare).
  Loss of appetite.
  Difficulty urinating (rare).
  Ulceration of the skin (rare).
Serious Adverse Effects
  Allergic Reactions:
  Idiosyncratic Reactions:
  Bone marrow suppression.
  Convulsions (rare).
  Hepatitis (rare).
  Drug-induced lupus erythematosus (rare).
  Lung problems (acute interstitial lung disease) (rare).
  Hallucinations (rare).

▷ **Possible Effects on Sexual Function:**   None reported.

Possible Delayed Adverse Effects: Bone marrow suppression.

▷ **Adverse Effects That May Mimic Natural Diseases or Disorders**
  Liver toxicity may be similar to acute hepatitis.

Natural Diseases or Disorders That May Be Activated by This Drug
  Not defined.

Possible Effects on Laboratory Tests
  Liver function tests: increased.
  Complete blood counts: decreases in several components.

CAUTION
  1. This medicine is toxic to cells. Be certain your doctor has carefully explained how to dispose of urine or vomit.
  2. Call your doctor at once if you have a seizure.
  3. Both women and men should avoid conception for several months after taking this medicine.
  4. Wash your hands after taking this medicine **before** you touch your eyes or your nose.

Precautions for Use
  By Infants and Children:
    Safety and effectiveness for use by those under 18 years of age have not been established.
  By Those over 60 Years of Age: Natural declines in kidney function may require decreases in doses.

▷ **Advisability of Use During Pregnancy**
  Pregnancy Category: D. See Pregnancy Code at the back of this book.
  Animal studies: This drug is known to cause birth defects in animals.
  Human studies: Information from adequate studies of pregnant women is not available. Ask your doctor for help in making this benefit to risk decision.

Advisability of Use if Breast-Feeding
    Presence of this drug in breast milk: Yes.
    Avoid drug or refrain from nursing.

Habit-Forming Potential: None.

Effects of Overdosage: Bone marrow depression, increased heart rate, liver cell damage, testicular damage.

Possible Effects of Long-Term Use: Bone marrow depression.

Suggested Periodic Examinations While Taking This Drug (at physician's discretion)
    Dental exams, complete blood counts.

▷ **While Taking This Drug, Observe the Following**
    Foods: No restrictions.
    Beverages: No restrictions.
▷   *Alcohol:* Do not drink alcohol.
    Tobacco Smoking: No interactions expected.
▷   *Other Drugs*
      Hydroxyurea *taken concurrently* with
      • fluorouracil may increase toxicity to nerves.
      • other medicines which cause bone marrow suppression (see Drug Tables) may result in additive bone marrow suppression.
▷   *Driving, Hazardous Activities:* This drug may cause dizziness or hallucinations. Restrict activities as necessary.
    Aviation Note: The use of this drug **is probably a disqualification** for piloting. Consult a designated Aviation Medical Examiner.
    Exposure to Sun: Use extreme caution. Extreme reactions to the sun have been reported.
    Occurrence of Unrelated Illness: Call your doctor at once if you develop fever or chills.
    Discontinuation: Do not stop this medicine without first discussing this with your doctor.

IBUPROFEN (i BYU proh fen)

Introduced: 1969   **Prescription:** USA: Varies; Canada: Yes   **Available as Generic:** Yes   **Class:** Mild analgesic, anti-inflammatory   **Controlled Drug:** USA: No; Canada: No

Brand Names: Aches-N-Pain, ✦Actiprofen, Advil, ✦Amersol, ✦Apo-Ibuprofen, Bayer Select, Children's Advil, Children's Motrin, Children's Motrin (nonprescription strength), CoAdvil [CD], Dimetapp Sinus [CD], Dologesic, Dristan Sinus, Genpril, Guildprofen, Haltran, Ibuprin, Ibuprohm, Ibu-Tab, Medipren, Medi-Profen, Midol-IB, Motrin, Motrin IB, ✦Novoprofen, Nuprin, PediaProfen, Rufen, Superior Pain Medicine, Supreme Pain Medicine

BENEFITS versus RISKS	
Possible Benefits	*Possible Risks*
EFFECTIVE RELIEF OF MILD TO MODERATE PAIN AND INFLAMMATION	Gastrointestinal pain, ulceration, bleeding (rare) Rare kidney damage Rare fluid retention Rare bone marrow depression (less than 1%)

Please see the propionic acid nonsteroidal anti-inflammatory drug profile for further information.

IMIPRAMINE (im IP ra meen)

Introduced: 1955 **Prescription:** USA: Yes; Canada: Yes **Available as Generic:** USA: Yes; Canada: Yes **Class:** Antidepressant **Controlled Drug:** USA: No; Canada: No

Brand Names: ◆Apo-Imipramine, ◆Impril, Janimine, ◆Novopramine, ◆PMS Imipramine, Sk-pramine, Tipramine, Tofranil, Tofranil-PM

BENEFITS versus RISKS	
Possible Benefits	*Possible Risks*
EFFECTIVE RELIEF OF NEUROTIC AND PSYCHOTIC DEPRESSIVE STATES of various causes and degree EFFECTIVE TREATMENT FOR CHILDHOOD BEDWETTING (enuresis) Possibly effective in the management of chronic, severe pain; in aiding cocaine withdrawal; in relieving symptoms of attention deficit disorder; in preventing panic attacks; in controlling binge eating and purging in bulimia	ADVERSE BEHAVIORAL EFFECTS: confusion, delirium, disorientation, hallucinations, delusions CONVERSION OF DEPRESSION TO MANIA in manic-depressive disorders Aggravation of schizophrenia and paranoia Induction of serious heart rhythm abnormalities Abnormally low white blood cell and platelet counts (rare)

▷ **Principal Uses**

   As a Single Drug Product: Uses currently included in FDA approved labeling: (1) Relieves severe emotional depression and to initiate gradual restoration of normal mood; (2) aid in the prevention of childhood bedwetting in children over 6 years of age; (3) used to treat delusions.
   Other (unlabeled) generally accepted uses: (1) Helps treat agoraphobia; (2) some case evidence of help in treating aspermia; (3) can be of help in chronic pain syndromes; (4) eases diabetic neuropathy; (5) Inappropriate emotionalism (such as pathological crying) can be controlled by this drug; (6) of use in globus hystericus syndrome; (7) may have a role in treating panic disorder; (8) can help post traumatic stress disorder; (9) may help

control retrograde ejaculation; (10) can be of adjunctive benefit in helping control schizophrenia; (11) shows some benefit in patients who fail ENT surgery or weight reduction as treatment of sleep apnea.

How This Drug Works: Not completely established. It is thought that by increasing brain tissue concentrations of certain nerve impulse transmitters (norepinephrine and seratonin), this drug relieves the symptoms associated with depression. Beneficial effects in treating bedwetting are thought to be due partially to this drug's atropinelike action.

Available Dosage Forms and Strengths
 Capsules — 75 mg, 100 mg, 125 mg, 150 mg
 Injection — 25 mg per 2 ml
 Tablets — 10 mg, 25 mg, 50 mg, 75 mg

▷ **Usual Adult Dosage Range:** Initially 75 mg daily, divided into 3 doses. Dose may be increased cautiously as needed and tolerated by 10 mg to 25 mg daily at intervals of 1 week. The usual maintenance dose is 50 mg to 150 mg/24 hours. The total daily dosage should not exceed 200 mg for outpatient therapy. (When determined, the optimal daily requirement may be given at bedtime as a single dose.) **Note: Actual dosage and administration schedule must be determined by the physician for each patient individually.**

Conditions Requiring Dosing Adjustments
 Liver function: This drug is significantly metabolized in the liver to active and inactive metabolites. It should be used with caution and in decreased dose in patients with liver compromise. It is also a rare cause of hepatic necrosis.
 Kidney function: The kidneys are not appreciably involved in the elimination of imipramine. No changes in dosage are presently anticipated in renal compromise.

▷ **Dosing Instructions:** May be taken without regard to meals. If necessary, may be taken with food to reduce stomach irritation. The capsule may be opened and the tablet may be crushed for administration. Note: Tofranil-PM capsules should not be used to treat childhood bedwetting.

Usual Duration of Use: Continual use on a regular schedule for 3 to 4 weeks is usually necessary to determine this drug's effectiveness in relieving depression; optimal response may require 3 or more months of use. Long-term use (months to years) requires periodic evaluation of response and dosage adjustment. Consult your physician on a regular basis.

Possible Advantages of This Drug
 Less likely to increase the heart rate than other tricyclic antidepressants.
 Less hazardous and more easily managed than monoamine oxidase (MAO) inhibitor antidepressants.

Currently a "Drug of Choice"
 for adjunctive use in treating childhood bedwetting when organic causes for this disorder have been eliminated.

▷ **This Drug Should Not Be Taken If**
 • you have had an allergic reaction to it previously.
 • you are taking, or have taken within the past 14 days, any monoamine oxidase (MAO) type A inhibitor drug (see Drug Class Section).
 • you have had a recent heart attack (myocardial infarction).

- you have angina, abnormal heart beats or congestive heart failure.
- you are pregnant.
- you have narrow-angle glaucoma.

▷ **Inform Your Physician Before Taking This Drug If**
- you have had an adverse reaction to any other antidepressant drug.
- you have any type of seizure disorder.
- you have increased internal eye pressure.
- you have any type of heart disease, especially coronary artery disease or a heart rhythm disorder.
- you are subject to bronchial asthma.
- you have impaired liver or kidney function.
- you have any type of thyroid disorder or are taking thyroid medication.
- you have diabetes or sugar intolerance.
- you have prostatism (see Glossary).
- you have a history of alcoholism.
- you plan to have surgery under general anesthesia in the near future.

Possible Side-Effects (natural, expected and unavoidable drug actions)
Moderate drowsiness, light-headedness (low blood pressure), blurred vision, dry mouth, constipation, impaired urination.

▷ **Possible Adverse Effects** (unusual, unexpected and infrequent reactions)
If any of the following develop, consult your physician promptly for guidance.

Mild Adverse Effects

Allergic Reactions: Skin rash, hives, swelling of face or tongue, drug fever (see Glossary).

Headache, dizziness, nervousness, weakness, unsteadiness, tremors, fainting.

Increased appetite, weight gain.

Sleep disturbances.

Irritation of tongue or mouth, dry mouth (xerostomia), dental cavities, altered taste, indigestion, nausea.

Fluctuations of blood sugar.

Serious Adverse Effects

Allergic Reactions: Drug-induced hepatitis, with or without jaundice; anaphylactoid reaction (see terms in Glossary).

Idiosyncratic Reactions: Neuroleptic malignant syndrome (see Glossary).

Adverse behavioral effects: confusion, delirium, disorientation, delusions, hallucinations.

Abnormally low blood pressure on standing (orthostatic hypotension).

Tourette's syndrome (rare).

Porphyria (rare).

Liver or kidney toxicity (rare).

Drug-induced Myasthenia Gravis (rare).

Abnormal urine excretion (SIADH).

Spasm of blood vessels.

Seizures; reduced control of epilepsy.

Eye changes (glaucoma, ophthalmoplegia).

Aggravation of paranoid psychoses and schizophrenia.

Heart rhythm disturbances.

Abnormally low white blood cell and platelet counts: Fever, sore throat, infections, abnormal bleeding or bruising.

▷ **Possible Effects on Sexual Function**

Decreased libido, increased libido (antidepressant effect), impaired erection (43%), impaired ejaculation (28%), impotence, inhibited male orgasm (20%), inhibited female orgasm (27%), male breast enlargement and tenderness, female breast enlargement with milk production, swelling of testicles.

▷ **Adverse Effects That May Mimic Natural Diseases or Disorders**

Liver toxicity may suggest viral hepatitis.

Natural Diseases or Disorders That May Be Activated by This Drug

Latent diabetes, epilepsy, glaucoma, prostatism.

Possible Effects on Laboratory Tests

Complete blood cell counts: decreased white cells and platelets; increased eosinophils (allergic reaction).

Blood glucose levels: increased and decreased (fluctuations).

Liver function tests: increased liver enzymes (ALT/GPT, AST/GOT and alkaline phosphatase), increased bilirubin.

CAUTION

1. Observe for early indications of toxicity or overdosage: confusion, agitation, rapid heart rate, heart irregularity. Measurement of the blood level of the drug will clarify the situation.
2. Use with caution in treating depression associated with schizophrenia. Observe closely for any deterioration of thinking or behavior.
3. It is advisable to withhold this drug if electroconvulsive therapy is to be used to treat the depression in the near future.

Precautions for Use

By Infants and Children: Safety and effectiveness for use by those under 6 years of age have not been established. Recent experience indicates that children (6 to 12 years of age) may be more susceptible than adults to heart toxicity from this and related drugs. Dosage and management should be supervised by a properly trained pediatrician.

By Those over 60 Years of Age: Initiate treatment with 25 mg at bedtime. Dosage may be increased gradually as needed and tolerated to 100 mg daily in divided doses. During the first 2 weeks of treatment, observe for behavioral reactions: Restlessness, agitation, forgetfulness, disorientation, delusions or hallucinations. Also observe for unsteadiness and instability that may predispose to falling. This drug may aggravate prostatism.

▷ **Advisability of Use During Pregnancy**

Pregnancy Category: D. See Pregnancy Code at the back of this book.

Animal studies: Skeletal defects reported in rabbit studies. No defects reported in mouse, rat and monkey studies.

Human studies: Information from adequate studies of pregnant women is not available. Case reports of fetal respiraratory distress, convulsions.

Ask your doctor for guidance.

Advisability of Use if Breast-Feeding
Presence of this drug in breast milk: Yes, in small amounts.
Monitor nursing infant closely and discontinue drug or nursing if adverse effects develop.

Habit-Forming Potential: Psychological or physical dependence is possible. A withdrawal syndrome has been described.

Effects of Overdosage: Confusion, hallucinations, drowsiness, tremors, heart irregularity, seizures, stupor, hypothermia (see Glossary) early, fever later.

Possible Effects of Long-Term Use: Neuroleptic malignant syndrome (see Glossary): Fever, fast or irregular heartbeat, fast breathing, sweating, weakness, muscle stiffness, seizures, loss of bladder control.

Suggested Periodic Examinations While Taking This Drug (at physician's discretion)
Monitoring of blood drug levels as appropriate.
Complete blood cell counts; liver and kidney function tests.
Serial blood pressure readings and electrocardiograms.
Measurement of internal eye pressure.

▷ **While Taking This Drug, Observe the Following**
Foods: No specific restrictions. May need to limit food intake to avoid excessive weight gain.
Beverages: No restrictions. May be taken with milk.
▷ *Alcohol:* Avoid completely. This drug can markedly increase the intoxicating effects of alcohol; the combination can depress brain function significantly.
Tobacco Smoking: May accelerate the elimination of this drug and require increased dosage.
Marijuana Smoking: Increased drowsiness and mouth dryness; possible reduced effectiveness of this drug. Excessive increases in heart rate.

▷ *Other Drugs*
Imipramine may *increase* the effects of
- all drugs with sedative effects; observe for excessive sedation.
- all drugs with atropinelike effects (see Drug Class Section).
- norepinephrine.
- phenytoin (Dilantin).
- warfarin (Coumadin) and require more frequent INR testing.

Imipramine may *decrease* the effects of
- clonidine (Catapres).
- guanadrel (Hylorel).
- guanethidine (Ismelin, Esimil).
- guanfacine (Tenex).

Imipramine *taken concurrently* with
- anticonvulsants requires careful monitoring for changes in seizure patterns and need to adjust anticonvulsant dosage.
- ethchlorvynol (Placidyl) may cause delirium; avoid concurrent use.
- monoamine oxidase (MAO) type A inhibitor drugs (see Drug Class Section) may cause high fever, seizures and excessive rise in blood pressure; avoid concurrent use of these drugs and provide periods of 14 days between administration of either.

- stimulant drugs (amphetamine, cocaine, epinephrine, phenylpropanolamine, etc.) may cause severe high blood pressure and/or high fever.
- thyroid preparations may increase the risk of heart rhythm disorders.

The following drugs may *increase* the effects of imipramine
- cimetidine (Tagamet).
- estrogens.
- fluoxetine (Prozac)
- labetalol.
- methylphenidate (Ritalin).
- oral contraceptives.
- phenothiazines (see Drug Class Section).
- quinidine.
- ranitidine (Zantac).

The following drugs may *decrease* the effects of imipramine
- barbiturates (see Drug Class, Section Four).
- carbamazepine (Tegretol).
- chloral hydrate (Noctec, Somnos, etc.).
- lithium (Lithobid, Lithotab, etc.).
- reserpine (Serpasil, Ser-Ap-Es, etc.).

▷ *Driving, Hazardous Activities:*
This drug may impair mental alertness, judgment, physical coordination and reaction time. Restrict activities as necessary.

Aviation Note:
The use of this drug **is a disqualification** for piloting. Consult a designated Aviation Medical Examiner.

Exposure to Sun: Use caution until sensitivity has been determined. This drug may cause photosensitivity (see Glossary).

Exposure to Heat: Use caution. This drug can inhibit sweating and impair the body's adaptation to hot environments, increasing the risk of heat stroke. Avoid saunas.

Exposure to Cold: The elderly should use caution and avoid conditions conducive to hypothermia (see Glossary).

Exposure to Environmental Chemicals: This drug may mask the symptoms of poisoning due to handling certain insecticides (organophosphorus types). Read their labels carefully.

Discontinuation: It is advisable to discontinue this drug gradually over a period of 3 to 4 weeks. Abrupt withdrawal after prolonged use may cause nausea, vomiting, diarrhea, headache, malaise, disturbed sleep and vivid dreaming. When this drug is stopped, it may be necessary to adjust the dosages of other drugs taken concurrently.

INDAPAMIDE (in DAP a mide)

Introduced: 1974 **Prescription:** USA: Yes; Canada: Yes **Available as Generic:** No **Class:** Antihypertensive, diuretic **Controlled Drug:** USA: No; Canada: No

Brand Names: ◆Lozide, Lozol

Indapamide

BENEFITS versus RISKS	
Possible Benefits	*Possible Risks*
EFFECTIVE ONCE-A-DAY TREATMENT OF MILD TO MODERATE HYPERTENSION	Excessive loss of blood potassium (14%)
EFFECTIVE, MILD DIURETIC	Increased blood sugar level
	Increased blood uric acid level

▷ **Principal Uses**

As a Single Drug Product: Uses currently included in FDA approved labeling: (1) Increases urine output (diuresis) to correct fluid retention seen in congestive heart failure (edema); (2) used as starting therapy in high blood pressure (hypertension).

Other (unlabeled) generally accepted uses: (1) Helps ease the excessive elimination of calcium in the urine (hypercalciuria); (2) May help protect the heart after blood-flow problems (preserves ischemic heart from reperfusion injury).

How This Drug Works: Increases elimination of salt and water (through increased urine production). Relaxes the walls of smaller arteries and decreases pressure reactions (angiotensin two). The combined effects lower blood pressure.

Available Dosage Forms and Strengths

Tablets — 2.5 mg

▷ **Usual Adult Dosage Range:** Started with 2.5 mg/day, as a single dose in the morning. If needed, the dose may be increased to 5 mg/day after 1 week (for diuresis) or after 4 weeks (for hypertension). Maximum total daily dose is 5 mg. (In Canada, the total daily dosage limit is given as 2.5 mg.) **Note: Actual dose and dosing schedule must be individually determined by your doctor.**

Conditions Requiring Dosing Adjustments

Liver function: Used with caution and in decrease dose in patients with liver problems. Blood chemistry (electrolytes) should be closely followed.

Kidney function: Must be stopped if kidney failure progresses after indapamide is started.

▷ **Dosing Instructions:** The tablet may be crushed and taken with or following food to reduce stomach upset. Take in the morning to avoid nighttime urination.

Usual Duration of Use: Use on a regular schedule for 2 to 4 weeks determines peak effect in lowering blood pressure. Long-term use (months to years) requires periodic physician evaluation.

Possible Advantages of This Drug

Causes no significant increase in blood cholesterol levels.
Less likely to cause significant loss of potassium.

▷ **This Drug Should Not Be Taken If**
- you have had an allergic reaction to it previously.
- your kidneys are not making any urine.

▷ **Inform Your Physician Before Taking This Drug If**
- you are allergic to any form of "sulfa" drug.
- you are pregnant or planning pregnancy.

- you have a history of kidney or liver disease.
- you have diabetes, gout or lupus erythematosus.
- you take any form of cortisone, digoxin, oral antidiabetic drug or insulin.
- you have had a sympathectomy.
- you plan to have surgery under general anesthesia in the near future.

Possible Side-Effects (natural, expected and unavoidable drug actions)
Light-headedness on arising from sitting or lying position (see Orthostatic Hypotension in Glossary).
Increase in blood sugar level, affecting control of diabetes.
Increase in blood uric acid level, affecting control of gout.
Decrease in blood potassium level, causing muscle weakness and cramping.
Low blood sodium and magnesium.

▷ **Possible Adverse Effects** (unusual, unexpected and infrequent reactions)
If any of the following develop, consult your physician promptly for guidance.

Mild Adverse Effects
Allergic Reactions: Skin rashes, hives, itching.
Headache, dizziness, drowsiness, weakness, lethargy, visual disturbance.
Reduced appetite, indigestion, nausea, vomiting, diarrhea.
Paresthesias.
Increased uric acid may blunt gout control.
Urination at night.

Serious Adverse Effects
Abnormally low blood pressure on standing (orthostatic hypotension).
Abnormal heart beats (premature ventricular contractions) (rare).
Worsening of glucose intolerance.
Low blood potassium.
Low blood sodium.
Liver toxicity (rare).
Serious skin rashes (Stevens-Johnson syndrome, Toxic epidermal necrolysis).

▷ **Possible Effects on Sexual Function:** Decreased libido (4%); impotence (less than 1%).

Natural Diseases or Disorders That May Be Activated by This Drug
Diabetes, gout, systemic lupus erythematosus.

Possible Effects on Laboratory Tests
Total cholesterol and LDL cholesterol levels: no effect or slightly increased.
Blood HDL cholesterol level: no effect or slightly decreased.
Blood potassium level: slightly decreased.
Blood uric acid level: increased.

CAUTION
1. Take exactly as prescribed—excessive doses can cause excessive sodium and potassium loss, with decrease in appetite, nausea, fatigue, weakness, confusion and tingling in the extremities.
2. If you take a digitalis preparation (digitoxin, digoxin), ensure intake of high-potassium foods to help avoid digitalis toxicity. (See Table of High Potassium Foods.)

Precautions for Use
By Infants and Children: Safety and effectiveness for those under 12 years of age not established.
By Those over 60 Years of Age: Best to start with small doses. You may be more susceptible to impaired thinking, orthostatic hypotension, potassium loss and blood sugar increase. Overdosage or extended use causes excessive loss of body water, thickening (increased viscosity) of blood and an increased tendency for the blood to clot—predisposing to stroke, heart attack or thrombophlebitis (vein inflammation with blood clot).

▷ **Advisability of Use During Pregnancy**
Pregnancy Category: B. See Pregnancy Code at the back of this book.
Animal studies: No birth defects reported.
Human studies: Data from studies of pregnant women is not available.
This drug should not be used during pregnancy unless a very serious complication occurs for which this drug is significantly beneficial. Ask physician for guidance.

Advisability of Use if Breast-Feeding
Presence of this drug in breast milk: Unknown.
Avoid drug or refrain from nursing.

Habit-Forming Potential: None.

Effects of Overdosage: Dry mouth, thirst, lethargy, weakness, muscle cramping, nausea, vomiting, drowsiness progressing to stupor or coma.

Possible Effects of Long-Term Use: Impaired balance of water, salt and potassium in blood and body tissues. Development of diabetes in predisposed individuals.

Suggested Periodic Examinations While Taking This Drug (at physician's discretion)
Measurements of blood levels of sodium, potassium, chloride, sugar and uric acid.

▷ **While Taking This Drug, Observe the Following**
Foods: Ask about a high potassium diet. If so advised, see the Table of High Potassium Foods in Section Six. Follow doctor's advice about salt use.
Beverages: No restrictions. This drug may be taken with milk.
▷ *Alcohol:* Alcohol may exaggerate the blood-pressure-lowering effects of this drug and cause orthostatic hypotension.
Tobacco Smoking: No interactions expected. Follow physician's advice.
▷ *Other Drugs*
Indapamide may *increase* the effects of
- other antihypertensive drugs; dosage adjustments may be necessary to prevent excessive lowering of blood pressure.
- lithium, and cause lithium toxicity.

Indapamide may *decrease* the effects of
- oral antidiabetic drugs (sulfonylureas); dose adjustments may be needed for proper control of blood sugar.

Indapamide *taken concurrently* with
- digitalis preparations (digitoxin, digoxin) must be followed closely and adjustments made to prevent fluctuations of blood potassium levels and serious disturbances of heart rhythm.

- NSAIDs (see Drug Classes) may blunt the therapeutic benefit of indapamide.

The following drugs may *decrease* the effects of indapamide
- cholestyramine (Cuemid, Questran) may interfere with its absorption.
- colestipol (Colestid) may interfere with its absorption.

Take cholestyramine and colestipol 1 hour before any oral diuretic.

▷ *Driving, Hazardous Activities:* Use caution until the possible occurrence of orthostatic hypotension, drowsiness, dizziness or impaired vision has been determined.

Aviation Note: The use of this drug *may be a disqualification* for piloting. Consult a designated Aviation Medical Examiner.

Exposure to Sun: No restrictions.

Exposure to Heat: Excessive perspiring could cause additional loss of salt and water.

Heavy Exercise or Exertion: Isometric exercises can raise blood pressure significantly. Ask physician for help.

Occurrence of Unrelated Illness: Vomiting or diarrhea can produce a serious imbalance of important body chemistry. Consult your physician for guidance.

Discontinuation: It may be advisable to discontinue this drug 5 to 7 days before major surgery. Ask your physician, surgeon and/or anesthesiologist for guidance.

INDOMETHACIN (in doh METH a sin)

Introduced: 1963 **Prescription:** USA: Yes; Canada: Yes **Available as Generic:** USA: Yes; Canada: No **Class:** Mild analgesic, anti-inflammatory
Controlled Drug: USA: No; Canada: No
Brand Names: ✦Apo-Indomethacin, Indameth, ✦Indocid, ✦Indocid PDA, Indocin, Indocin-SR, Indo-Lemmon, ✦Novomethacin, ✦Nu-Indo, Zendole

BENEFITS versus RISKS	
Possible Benefits	*Possible Risks*
EFFECTIVE RELIEF OF MILD TO MODERATE PAIN AND INFLAMMATION	Gastrointestinal pain, ulceration, bleeding (rare)
	Rare liver or kidney damage
	Rare fluid retention
	Rare bone marrow depression
	Mental depression, confusion

Please see acetic acid nonsteroidal anti-inflammatory drug profile for further information.

INFLUENZA VACCINE (IN flew en za)

Other Names: Flu vaccine

Introduced: Specific formulation for each year **Prescription:** USA: Yes; Canada: Yes **Available as Generic:** USA: No; Canada: No **Class:** Antiviral **Controlled Drug:** USA: No; Canada: No

Brand Names: Fluogen, Flu-Shield, Fluzone

Author's note: The three virus strains for the 1995 flu vaccines are: A/Texas, A/Johannesburg, and B/Harbin (Beijing-like).

Warning: Since the vaccine is formulated to contain the viral strains expected to cause the most serious problems in a given year, the side effects or adverse effects may differ annually.

BENEFITS versus RISKS

Possible Benefits	*Possible Risks*
PREVENTION OF INFLUENZA CAUSED BY THE MOST SERIOUS OR PREVALENT VIRAL STRAINS IDENTIFIED FOR A GIVEN YEAR	GUILLAIN-BARRE SYNDROME (questionable causation) Fever, aches and malaise Hypersensitivity (rare)

▷ **Principal Uses**

As a Single Drug Product: Uses currently included in FDA approved labeling: (1) Prevention of influenza.

Other (unlabeled) generally accepted uses: (1) Used in patients with compromised immune systems (such as HIV positive, cancer patients and bone marrow transplant patients); (2) can be of use in isolated outbreaks such as in nursing homes or military camps; (3) may decrease the number of middle ear infections in children who attend day-care centers.

How This Drug Works: This vaccine is made of purified parts of the surface of the virus, split virus or whole virus which has been inactivated. When it is injected, it stimulates the immune system to make antibodies. These antibodies (which are created and the production knowledge stored in immune cells roughly two weeks after vaccination) act to reduce disease severity or decrease the probability of infection by the expected flu viruses.

Available Dosage Forms and Strengths

Typical split virus: 15 mcg per 0.5 ml of each of the three selected strains

How To Store

This vaccine is ideally stored in the refrigerator. If this is how storage is accomplished, the outdate specified by the manufacturer is valid. If the vaccine is stored at room temperature, it is stable for up to seven days.

▷ **Recommended Dosage Ranges (Actual dosage and administration schedule must be determined by the physician for each patient and each flu season individually.)**

Infants and Children: 6 to 35 months old should be given 0.25 ml of a split dose vaccine. If this is the first vaccination, two doses should be given one month apart. Split dose is suggested for children because it tends to cause fewer undesirable effects.

Influenza Vaccine

Children 3 to 8 years old should be given 0.5 ml of the selected split virus vaccine. Children in this age range who have not been previously vaccinated should be given two vaccinations, one month apart.

Children 9 years old or older should be given a single vaccination of 0.5 ml of split virus vaccine in the deltoid muscle.

13 to 60 Years of Age: Should be given 0.5 ml of whole or split virus vaccine in the deltoid muscle.

Over 60 Years of Age: Same as 13 to 60 years of age.

Conditions Requiring Dosing Adjustments
Liver function: Not involved.
Kidney function: Not involved.

▷ **Dosing Instructions:** Prior vaccination does **not** mean you are immune to the current year virus strains. Some tenderness at the injection site is possible. Fever and muscular aches or pains are also possible and may be treated with acetaminophen (Tylenol, others).

Usual Duration of Use: Single vaccination confers relative immunity to the expected viral strains in two weeks. This does **not** confer immunity to all strains of virus capable of causing an influenza-like (flu-like) syndrome. Annual vaccination is strongly suggested.

Possible Advantages of This Drug
Allows the prevention of a viral syndrome which can cause loss of several weeks of work in younger otherwise healthy patients or serious illness in older or compromised patients.

Currently a "Drug of Choice"
for prevention of type A influenza due to the viral strains which are of the greatest concern in the current flu season.

▷ **This Drug Should Not Be Taken If**
- you have had an allergic reaction to any dosage form of it previously.
- you are allergic to eggs (the virus is grown on eggs).
- you have an acute illness and a fever.

▷ **Inform Your Physician Before Taking This Drug If**
- you are HIV positive.
- you have a history of blood disorders.
- you have had Guillain-Barre syndrome.
- you have a history of seizures.
- you have been receiving cancer therapy (chemotherapy).

Possible Side-Effects (natural, expected and unavoidable drug actions)
Pain at the vaccination site. Muscle aches, fever or bothersome tiredness (malaise). This is **not** the flu. The vaccine contains viral fragments or noninfectious virus. These symptoms are a reaction to the components of the vaccine.

▷ **Possible Adverse Effects** (unusual, unexpected and infrequent reactions)
If any of the following develop, consult your physician promptly for guidance.
Mild Adverse Effects
Allergic Reactions: Swelling and redness.
Muscle aches or fever.

Fatigue, nausea and headache.
Vasculitis (joint pain, weakness, fever and rash) (rare).
Serious Adverse Effects
Allergic Reactions: Anaphylactoid reactions.
Low blood platelets (extremely rare).
Pericarditis (very rare).
Guillain-Barre syndrome (rare and of questionable causation).
Kidney toxicity (very rare).
Vision changes (very rare).

▷ **Possible Effects on Sexual Function:**   None reported.

Possible Delayed Adverse Effects: None reported.

▷ **Adverse Effects That May Mimic Natural Diseases or Disorders**
Reaction to vaccine contents may mimic the flu.

Natural Diseases or Disorders That May Be Activated by This Drug
None reported.

Possible Effects on Laboratory Tests
Hepatitis B test: false positive.
Hepatitis C test: false positive.
HTLV-1 test: false positive.

CAUTION
1. The fact that a patient has had the vaccine in the previous year does **not** confer immunity to the flu in following years.
2. The flu vaccine typically confers immunity to the virus types that are predicted to cause the most problems in a particular flu season. The vaccine does not confer immunity to all strains of virus which are capable of causing a flu-like syndrome.
3. If muscle aches or fever occur after vaccination, acetaminophen (Tylenol, others) is recomended. Do **not** take aspirin to address these symptoms if they occur after vaccination.
4. Call your doctor immediately if you develop hives, facial swelling or difficulty breathing after the vaccination.

Precautions for Use
By Infants and Children:
Safety and effectiveness for use by those under 6 months of age have not been established.
By Those over 60 Years of Age: The vaccine may be especially valuable in this age group as the effects of the flu may be very challenging.

▷ **Advisability of Use During Pregnancy**
Pregnancy Category: C. See Pregnancy Code at the back of this book.
Animal studies: Animal studies have not been conducted.
Human studies: Information from adequate studies of pregnant women is not available. Ask your doctor for guidance.

Advisability of Use if Breast-Feeding
Presence of this drug in breast milk: Not defined.
Monitor nursing infant closely and contact your doctor if adverse effects develop. The CDC has not listed breast-feeding as a precaution against receiving this vaccine.

Habit-Forming Potential: None.

Effects of Overdosage: No specific cases reported. Treatment would be consistent with any symptoms the patient presents.

Possible Effects of Long-Term Use: Not indicated for long-term use.

Suggested Periodic Examinations While Taking This Drug (at physician's discretion)
None indicated.

▷ **While Taking This Drug, Observe the Following**
  Foods: No restrictions.
  Beverages: No restrictions.
▷ *Alcohol:* No restrictions.
  Tobacco Smoking: No interactions expected.
▷ *Other Drugs*
  Influenza vaccine may *increase* the effects of
  • carbamazepine (Tegretol) by decreasing the elimination of the drug.
  • phenobarbital by increasing the half life of the drug.
  • theophylline (Theo-Dur, others) by increasing the blood level of the drug.
  • warfarin (Coumadin) and pose an increased risk of bleeding.
  Influenza vaccine *taken concurrently* with
  • cyclosporine (sandimmune) can cause blunting of the immune response to the vaccine.
  • immunosuppressive agents (chemotherapy, corticosteroids) may be associated with an impaired or blunted immune response to the vaccine.
  • methotrexate can result in blunting of the immune response to this vaccine
  • phenytoin (Dilantin) has had variable effects on the blood levels of this drug.
▷ *Driving, Hazardous Activities:* This drug may cause excessive tiredness and muscle aches. Restrict activities as necessary.
  Aviation Note: The use of this drug **may be a short-term disqualification** for piloting. Consult a designated Aviation Medical Examiner.
  Exposure to Sun: No restrictions.
  Exposure to Heat: Since this vaccine may cause short duration fevers, it is wise to avoid hot environments for a day after vaccination.
  Heavy Exercise or Exertion: A fever may result from this vaccination and it is wise to avoid strenuous exercise for a day after vaccination.
  Author's note: There is now a Vaccine Adverse Event Reporting System (VAERS). The toll free number is 1–800-822–7967.

INSULIN (IN suh lin)

Introduced: 1922 **Prescription:** USA: No; Canada: No **Available as Generic:** Yes **Class:** Antidiabetic **Controlled Drug:** USA: No; Canada: No

Brand Names: Humulin BR, Humulin L, Humulin N, Humulin R, Humulin U, Humulin U Ultralente, Humulin 70/30, Iletin I NPH, Iletin II Pork, ✦Initard, Insulatard NPH, ✦Insulin-Toronto, Lente Iletin I, Lente Iletin II Beef, Lente Iletin II Pork, Lente Insulin, Lente Purified Pork, Mixtard, Mixtard Human 70/30, Novolin L, Novolin N, NovolinPen, Novolin R,

◆Novolin-Lente, ◆Novolin-NPH, Novolin-70/30, ◆Novolin-Toronto, ◆Novolin-Ultralente, ◆Novolinset, NPH Iletin I, NPH Iletin II Beef, NPH Iletin II Pork, NPH Insulin, NPH Purified Pork, Protamine, Zinc & Iletin I, Protamine, Zinc & Iletin II Beef, Protamine, Zinc & Iletin II Pork, Regular Concentrated Iletin II, Regular Iletin I, Regular Iletin II Beef, Regular Iletin II Pork, Regular Iletin II U-500, Regular Insulin, Regular Purified Pork Insulin, Semilente Iletin I, Semilente Insulin, Semilente Purified Pork, Ultralente Iletin I, Ultralente Insulin, Ultralente Purified Beef, Velosulin, ◆Velosulin Cartridge, Velosulin Human

---

BENEFITS versus RISKS

Possible Benefits	*Possible Risks*
EFFECTIVE CONTROL OF TYPE I (INSULIN-DEPENDENT) DIABETES MELLITUS	HYPOGLYCEMIA WITH EXCESSIVE DOSAGE Infrequent allergic reactions

---

▷ **Principal Uses**

As a Single Drug Product: Uses currently included in FDA approved labelling: (1) Used in diabetes mellitus which is insulin-dependent, and in people who have noninsulin-dependent diabetes who are experiencing stress such as illness; (2) used to control blood sugar in critically ill patients who are being fed by intravenous nutrient mixtures.

Other (unlabeled) generally accepted uses: (1) Controls blood sugar in pregnancy (gestational diabetes); (2) insulin in combination with glucagon has been used in alcoholic hepatitis; (3) may have a role in combination therapy with an oral hypoglycemic agent in some diabetics; (4) helps diabetic ketoacidosis; (5) can help diabetic neuropathy and retinopathy; (6) can be of help in critically ill patients with maple syrup urine disease.

How This Drug Works: Insulin helps sugar through the cell wall to the inside of the cell (by direct action on cell membranes) where it is used for energy.

Available Dosage Forms and Strengths
  Injections — 40 units, 100 units and 500 units per ml
  PenFil cartridges — 150 units

▷ **Usual Adult Dosage Range:** According to individual requirements for the optimal regulation of blood sugar on a 24-hour basis. **Note: Actual dosage and administration schedule must be determined by the physician for each patient individually.**

Conditions Requiring Dosing Adjustments

Liver function: Specific adjustment guidelines are not available.

Kidney function: Caution should be used in patients with compromised kidneys.

Thyrotoxicosis: Glucose utilization is typically increased and insulin requirements may actually decrease.

▷ **Dosing Instructions:** Inject insulin subcutaneously according to the schedule prescribed by your physician. The timing and frequency of injections will vary with the type of insulin precribed. The following table of insulin actions (according to type) will help you understand the treatment schedule prescribed for you.

Insulin

Insulin Type	Action Onset	Peak	Duration
Regular	0.5–1 hr	2–4 hrs	5–7 hrs
Isophane (NPH)	3–4 hrs	6–12 hrs	18–28 hrs
Regular 30%/NPH 70%	0.5 hr	4–8 hrs	24 hrs
Semilente	1–3 hrs	2–8 hrs	12–16 hrs
Lente	1–3 hrs	8–12 hrs	18–28 hrs
Ultralente	4–6 hrs	18–24 hrs	36 hrs
Protamine Zinc	4–6 hrs	14–24 hrs	36 hrs

Usual Duration of Use: In Type I insulin-dependent (juvenile-onset) diabetes mellitus, insulin therapy is usually required for life. Type II noninsulin-dependent (maturity-onset) diabetes may be controlled by oral antidiabetic drugs and/or diet but can require insulin for adequate control. Such occasions include serious infections, injuries, burns, surgical procedures and other physical stress. Insulin is used as needed on a temporary basis to regulate the body's use of sugar until recovery is complete. Consult your physician on a regular basis.

▷ **This Drug Should Not Be Taken If**
- the need for insulin and its correct dosage schedule has not been established by a properly qualified physician.

▷ **Inform Your Physician Before Taking This Drug If**
- you have an insulin allergy.
- you do not know how to recognize and treat abnormally low blood sugar (see Hypoglycemia in Glossary).
- you are pregnant.
- you take: aspirin, beta blockers, fenfluramine (Pondimin), monoamine oxidase (MAO) type A inhibitors (see Drug Classes Section).

Possible Side-Effects (natural, expected and unavoidable drug actions)
In stable diabetes, no side-effects occur when insulin dose, diet and physical activity are correctly balanced and maintained.
In unstable ("brittle") diabetes, unexpected drops in blood sugar levels can occur, resulting in hypoglycemia (see Glossary).

▷ **Possible Adverse Effects** (unusual, unexpected and infrequent reactions)
If any of the following develop, consult your physician promptly for guidance.
Mild Adverse Effects
Allergic Reactions: Local redness, swelling and itching at site of injection. Occasional hives.
Taste disorders.
Thinning of subcutaneous tissue at sites of injection.
Serious Adverse Effects
Allergic Reaction: Anaphylactic reactions (see Glossary).
Severe, prolonged hypoglycemia.
Inflammation of the parotid (parotitis).
Hemolytic anemia (rare).
Arrhythmias (associated with hypoglycemia).
Very fast heart rate (with intravenous use).
Porphyria (rare).

▷ **Possible Effects on Sexual Function:** May resolve sexual dysfunction in patients who have this prior to starting insulin therapy. May also cause decrease in libido and erective dysfunction.

▷ **Adverse Effects That May Mimic Natural Diseases or Disorders**
The early signs of hypoglycemia may be mistaken for alcoholic intoxication.

Possible Effects on Laboratory Tests
Blood cholesterol level: decreased.
Blood glucose level: decreased.
Blood potassium level: decreased.

CAUTION
1. Carry with you a card of personal identification with a notation that you have diabetes and are taking insulin.
2. Know how to recognize hypoglycemia and how to treat it. Always carry a readily available form of sugar, such as hard candy or sugar cubes. Report all episodes of hypoglycemia to your doctor.
3. Your vision may improve during the first few weeks of insulin therapy. Postpone eye exams for glasses for 6 weeks after starting insulin.
4. Insulin is absorbed more quickly or slowly depending on where it is injected. Absorption is 80% greater from the abdominal wall than from the leg, and 30% greater than from the arm. It is advisable to rotate the injection site within the same body region than from one site to another.

Precautions for Use
By Infants and Children: Insulin dosages and schedules are modified according to patient size. Adhere strictly to the physician's prescribed routine.
By Those over 60 Years of Age: Insulin needs may change with age. Periodic individual evaluation is needed to identify the best dose and schedule. The aging brain adapts well to higher blood sugar levels. Rigid attempts at "tight" sugar control may result in hypoglycemia that shows as confusion and abnormal behavior. Repeated hypoglycemia (especially if severe) may cause brain damage.

▷ **Advisability of Use During Pregnancy**
Pregnancy Category: B. See Pregnancy Code at the back of this book.
Animal studies: Inconclusive.
Human studies: Adequate studies of pregnant women are not available. Birth defects occur 2 to 4 times more frequently in infants of diabetic mothers than in infants of mothers who do not have diabetes. The exact causes of this are not known.
Insulin is the drug of choice for managing diabetes during pregnancy. To preserve the health of the mother and fetus, every effort must be made to establish the best dose of insulin necessary for "good control" and to prevent episodes of hypoglycemia.

Advisability of Use if Breast-Feeding
Presence of this drug in breast milk: No.
Insulin treatment of the mother has no adverse effect on the nursing infant.
Breast-feeding may decrease insulin requirements; dosage adjustment may be necessary.

Habit-Forming Potential: None; however cases of surreptitious insulin injection have been reported.

Effects of Overdosage: Hypoglycemia: fatigue, weakness, headache, nervousness, irritability, sweating, tremors, hunger, confusion, delirium, abnormal behavior (resembling alcoholic intoxication), loss of consciousness, seizures.

Possible Effects of Long-Term Use: Thinning of subcutaneous fat tissue at sites of insulin injection.

Suggested Periodic Examinations While Taking This Drug (at physician's discretion)
Checking of urine sugar content when you are ill. Measurement of blood sugar levels at intervals recommended by physician.

▷ **While Taking This Drug, Observe the Following**
Foods: Follow your diabetic diet conscientiously. Do not omit snack foods in midafternoon or at bedtime if they help prevent hypoglycemia.
Beverages: According to prescribed diabetic diet.
▷ *Alcohol:* Used excessively, alcohol can cause severe hypoglycemia, resulting in brain damage.
Tobacco Smoking: Regular smoking can decrease insulin absorption and increase insulin requirements by 30%. It is advisable to stop smoking altogether.
Marijuana Smoking: Possible increase in blood sugar levels.
▷ *Other Drugs*
The following drugs may *increase* the effects of insulin
- aspirin, and other salicylates.
- some beta blocker drugs (especially the nonselective ones) may prolong insulin-induced hypoglycemia. (See Drug Class Section).
- clofibrate.
- fenfluramine (Pondimin).
- monoamine oxidase (MAO) type A inhibitors (see Drug Class Section).

The following drugs may *decrease* the effects of insulin (by raising blood sugar levels)
- chlorthalidone (Hygroton).
- cortisonelike drugs (see Drug Classes).
- furosemide (Lasix).
- oral contraceptives.
- phenytoin (Dilantin, etc.).
- thiazide diuretics (see Drug Classes).
- thyroid preparations.

▷ *Driving, Hazardous Activities:* Be prepared to stop and take corrective action if hypoglycemia develops.
Aviation Note: Diabetes and the use of this drug **are disqualifications** for piloting. Consult a designated Aviation Medical Examiner.
Exposure to Sun: No restrictions.
Exposure to Heat: Use caution. Sauna baths can signficantly increase the rate of insulin absorption and cause hypoglycemia.
Heavy Exercise or Exertion: Use caution. Periods of unusual or unplanned heavy physical activity will use up sugar more quickly and predispose to hypoglycemia.
Occurrence of Unrelated Illness: Omission of meals as a result of nausea, vomiting or injury may lead to hypoglycemia. Infections can increase insulin needs. Ask doctor for help.

Discontinuation: Do not stop this drug without asking your doctor. Omission of insulin may result in life-threatening coma.

Special Storage Instructions: Keep in a cool place, preferably in the refrigerator. Protect from freezing. Protect from strong light and high temperatures when not refrigerated.

Observe the Following Expiration Times: Do not use this drug if it is older than the expiration date on the vial. Always use fresh, "within date" insulin.

IODOQUINOL (i oh doh KWIN ohl)

Other Name: di-iodohydroxyquin

Introduced: No data **Prescription:** USA: Yes; Canada: Yes **Available as Generic:** USA: Yes; Canada: No **Class:** Anti-infective, antiprotozoal

Controlled Drug: USA: No; Canada: No

Brand Names: ◆Diodoquin, Diquinol, Vytone, Yodoxin

BENEFITS versus RISKS	
Possible Benefits	*Possible Risks*
EFFECTIVE TREATMENT OF CARRIERS OF INTESTINAL AMEBA (cyst passers) Effective adjunctive treatment of invasive amebic infections	OPTIC NERVE DAMAGE Peripheral neuritis Drug-induced goiter

▷ **Principal Uses**

As a Single Drug Product: Uses currently included in FDA approved labeling: (1) Treatment of carriers of amebic cysts in the intestinal tract who have no symptoms of infection; (2) treatment of resistant skin conditions such as seborrhea.

Other (unlabeled) generally accepted uses: (1) Combination therapy of active, invasive amebic infection concurrently with metronidazole; (2) treatment of intestinal infection caused by Balantidium coli; (3) may have a role in helping to treat Aspergillosis infections in the lungs.

How This Drug Works: This drug kills ameba by interfering with essential enzyme systems. Since the drug is poorly absorbed, it reaches high concentrations at the sites of intestinal infection.

Available Dosage Forms and Strengths
Tablets — 210 mg, 650 mg

▷ **Recommended Dosage Ranges** (Actual dosage and administration schedule must be determined by the physician for each patient individually.)

Infants and Children: 10 to 13.3 mg/kg of body weight, 3 times a day for 20 days. The total daily dose should not exceed 1.95 grams.

12 to 60 Years of Age: Tablet: 630 or 650 mg, 3 times a day for 20 days. Maximum daily dose is 2 grams.

Iodoquinol-hydrocortisone cream: Applied to the affected area four times a day.

Over 60 Years of Age: Same as 12 to 60 years of age.

Note: If needed, the course of therapy may be repeated after a drug-free interval of 2 to 3 weeks.

Iodoquinol

Conditions Requiring Dosing Adjustments
Liver function: This drug is contraindicated in liver compromise.
Kidney function: Iodoquinol is contraindicated in kidney compromise.

▷ **Dosing Instructions:** The tablet may be crushed and is best taken after meals to reduce stomach upset.

Usual Duration of Use: Use on a regular schedule for 3 weeks determines this drug's effectiveness in controlling or eliminating amebic infections. Long-term use requires periodic physician evaluation.

▷ **This Drug Should Not Be Taken If**
- you have had an allergic reaction to it previously.
- you have active optic neuritis or peripheral neuritis.
- you are a child with chronic diarrhea (increased risk of optic atrophy and vision loss).
- you have active liver disease.

▷ **Inform Your Physician Before Taking This Drug If**
- you are allergic to chloroxine, iodine, pamaquine, pentaquine, primaquine or related drugs.
- you have a history of optic neuritis or peripheral neuritis.
- you have a history of thyroid disease or dysfunction.
- you have impaired liver or kidney function.

Possible Side-Effects (natural, expected and unavoidable drug actions)
Thyroid gland enlargement (goiter).

▷ **Possible Adverse Effects** (unusual, unexpected and infrequent reactions)
If any of the following develop, consult your physician promptly for guidance.
Mild Adverse Effects
Allergic Reactions: Skin rash, hives, itching.
Headache, fever, chills.
Nausea, vomiting, stomach pain, diarrhea, rectal itching.
Serious Adverse Effects
Optic neuritis: blurred vision, eye pain.
Peripheral neuritis (see Glossary).
Seizures (rare).
Thyroid gland enlargement.

▷ **Possible Effects on Sexual Function:** None reported.

▷ **Adverse Effects That May Mimic Natural Diseases or Disorders**
Thyroid gland enlargement may suggest a natural, spontaneous goiter.

Possible Effects on Laboratory Tests
Thyroid function tests: decreased I-131 uptake. This may persist for up to 6 months after discontinuation of this drug.

CAUTION
1. Not to be used to treat chronic, nonspecific diarrheas of unknown cause. Positive identification of Entameba histolytica in patient stools is mandatory for use of this drug.
2. Avoid long-term use if possible, especially in children. Although this drug is poorly absorbed (approximately 8%), long-term use can cause serious adverse effects.

3. Promptly report any visual changes while taking this drug, and arrange for thorough eye examinations as soon as possible.

Precautions for Use
By Infants and Children: Avoid prolonged use and high doses; children are more susceptible to optic neuritis and peripheral neuritis.
By Those over 60 Years of Age: No information available.

▷ **Advisability of Use During Pregnancy**
Pregnancy Category: C. See Pregnancy Code at the back of this book.
Animal studies: No information available.
Human studies: Adequate studies of pregnant women are not available.
Use this drug only if clearly needed. Ask your physician for guidance.

Advisability of Use if Breast-Feeding
Presence of this drug in breast milk: Unknown.
Avoid drug or refrain from nursing.

Habit-Forming Potential: None.

Effects of Overdosage: Nausea, vomiting, stomach pain, diarrhea.

Possible Effects of Long-Term Use: Optic neuritis, peripheral neuritis.

Suggested Periodic Examinations While Taking This Drug (at physician's discretion)
Thyroid function status.

▷ **While Taking This Drug, Observe the Following**
Foods: No restrictions.
Beverages: No restrictions. May be taken with milk.
▷ *Alcohol:* Use sparingly.
Tobacco Smoking: No interactions expected.
▷ *Other Drugs*
Iodoquinol *taken concurrently* with
• lithium may increase the possibility of drug-induced hypothyroidism.
▷ *Driving, Hazardous Activities:* No restrictions.
Aviation Note: The use of this drug *may be a disqualification* for piloting. Consult a designated Aviation Medical Examiner.
Exposure to Sun: No restrictions.
Discontinuation: To be determined by your physician. Do not use this drug for nonspecific diarrhea. Do not use this drug for extended periods of time.

IPRATROPIUM (i pra TROH pee um)

Introduced: 1975   **Prescription:** USA: Yes; Canada: Yes   **Available as Generic:** USA: No; Canada: No   **Class:** Bronchodilator   **Controlled Drug:** USA: No; Canada: No

Brand Name: Atrovent

Ipratropium

BENEFITS versus RISKS	
Possible Benefits	**Possible Risks**
EFFECTIVE BRONCHODILATOR FOR TREATMENT OF CHRONIC BRONCHITIS AND EMPHYSEMA	Mild and infrequent adverse effects (see below)
Possibly effective as adjunctive treatment in some cases of bronchial asthma	

▷ **Principal Uses**

As a Single Drug Product: Helps prevent or relieve episodes of difficult breathing in chronic bronchitis and emphysema. Should not be used to treat acute attacks of asthma because it takes a while to work.

How This Drug Works: This drug is a derivative of atropine. Through its atropinelike (anticholinergic) action, it blocks bronchial constriction and opens them up.

Available Dosage Forms and Strengths
Inhalation aerosol — 14 gram metered dose inhaler; 18 mcg per inhalation
Nebulizer — 250 mcg/ml solution
Nasal inhaler — 20 mcg per actuation

▷ **Usual Adult Dosage Range:** Initially 2 inhalations (36 mcg) 4 times a day, 4 hours apart. If needed, the dose may be increased to 4 inhalations (80 mcg) at one time to get optimal relief. Maintain 4 hour intervals between doses. Maximum daily dose is 12 inhalations (216 mcg). **Note: Actual dose and dosing schedule must be determined by the physician for each patient individually.**

Conditions Requiring Dosing Adjustments
Liver function: Specific guidelines for doasge decreases have not been elaborated.
Kidney function: Used with caution in patients with bladder neck obstructions.

▷ **Dosing Instructions:** Carefully follow the patient instructions provided with the inhaler. Shake well before using.

Usual Duration of Use: Continual use on a regular schedule for 48 to 72 hours is usually necessary to determine this drug's effectiveness. Long-term use (months to years) requires check of response and dosage adjustment. See your doctor.

Possible Advantages of This Drug
Produces a greater degree of bronchodilation than theophylline in patients with chronic bronchitis and emphysema.
Causes minimal adverse effects.
Repeated use does not lead to tolerance and loss of effectiveness.
Suitable for long-term maintenance therapy.

Currently a "Drug of Choice"
for difficult breathing associated with chronic bronchitis and emphysema.

Ipratropium

▷ **This Drug Should Not Be Taken If**
- you have had an allergic reaction to it previously.
- you are allergic to atropine or to aerosol propellants (fluorocarbons).

▷ **Inform Your Physician Before Taking This Drug If**
- you have had an adverse effect from any belladonna derivative previously.
- you have a history of glaucoma.
- you have any form of urinary retention or prostatism (see Glossary).

Possible Side-Effects (natural, expected and unavoidable drug actions)
Throat dryness (5%), cough (3%), irritation from aerosol (1.6%), blurred vision (1.2%), dry mouth (2.4%), impaired urination (1%).

▷ **Possible Adverse Effects** (unusual, unexpected and infrequent reactions)
If any of the following develop, consult your physician promptly for guidance.

Mild Adverse Effects
Allergic Reactions: Skin rash (1.2%), hives (rare).
Headache (2%), dizziness (1%), nervousness (3%).
Lip and mouth ulcers, unpleasant taste, indigestion (2.4%), nausea (2.8%).
Palpitations (rare).

Serious Adverse Effects
Abnormal heartbeats (supraventricular tachycardia) (rare).
Intraocular pressure changes (rare).

▷ **Possible Effects on Sexual Function**
None reported.

Natural Diseases or Disorders That May Be Activated by This Drug
Angle-closure glaucoma, prostatism (see Glossary).

Possible Effects on Laboratory Tests
None reported.

CAUTION
1. Won't start to work for 5 to 15 minutes. It should **not** be used alone to treat acute attacks of asthma needing a fast result.
2. When used as combination therapy with beta-adrenergic antiasthmatic drugs (albuterol, terbutaline, metaproterenol, etc.), the beta-adrenergic aerosol should be used about 5 minutes before using ipratropium to prevent fluorocarbon toxicity.
3. When used as an adjunct to steroid or cromolyn aerosols (beclomethasone, Intal), ipratropium should be used about 5 minutes before using the steroid or cromolyn aerosol to prevent fluorocarbon toxicity.
4. Contact with the eyes can cause temporary blurring of vision.

Precautions for Use
By Infants and Children: Safety and effectiveness for those under 12 years of age not established.
By Those over 60 Years of Age: Watch for possible development of prostatism and adjust dosage as necessary.

▷ **Advisability of Use During Pregnancy**
Pregnancy Category: B. See Pregnancy Code at the back of this book.
Animal studies: No drug-induced birth defects in mice, rat or rabbit studies.

Human studies: Adequate studies of pregnant women are not available. Use this drug only if clearly needed.

Advisability of Use if Breast-Feeding
Presence of this drug in breast milk: Possibly yes, but in very small amounts. Watch nursing infant closely and stop drug or nursing if adverse effects start.

Habit-Forming Potential: None.

Effects of Overdosage: This drug is not well absorbed into the circulation when it is taken by aerosol inhalation. No systemic effects of overdose are expected.

Possible Effects of Long-Term Use: No adverse effects reported.

Suggested Periodic Examinations While Taking This Drug (at physician's discretion)
Internal eye pressure measurements if appropriate.

▷ **While Taking This Drug, Observe the Following**
Foods: No restrictions.
Beverages: No restrictions.
▷ *Alcohol:* No interactions expected.
Tobacco Smoking: No interactions expected. However, smoking should be avoided completely if you have chronic bronchitis or emphysema.
▷ *Other Drugs*
Ipratropium may *increase* the effects of
• other atropinelike drugs (see Drug Class Section).
▷ *Driving, Hazardous Activities:*
May may cause dizziness or blurred vision. Restrict activities as necessary.
Aviation Note: The use of this drug **may be a disqualification** for piloting. Consult a designated Aviation Medical Examiner.
Exposure to Sun: No restrictions.
Exposure to Cold: Inhaling cold air may cause bronchospasm and induce asthmatic breathing and cough; dosage adjustment of this drug may be necessary.
Heavy Exercise or Exertion: This drug is not considered to be consistently effective in preventing or treating exercise-induced asthma.
Discontinuation: Ask your doctor for help. Substitute medication may be advisable.

ISONIAZID (i soh NI a zid)

Other Names: Isonicotinic acid hydrazide, INH

Introduced: 1956   **Prescription:** USA: Yes; Canada: Yes   **Available as Generic:** USA: Yes; Canada: Yes   **Class:** Antitubercular   **Controlled Drug:** USA: No; Canada: No

Brand Names: INH, ♦Isotamine, Laniazid, Nydrazid, P-I-N Forte [CD], ♦PMS Isoniazid, Rifamate [CD], Rifater [CD], Rimactane/INH Dual Pack [CD], Teebaconin, Teebaconin and Vitamin B-6 [CD]

Isoniazid

BENEFITS versus RISKS	
Possible Benefits	*Possible Risks*
EFFECTIVE PREVENTION AND TREATMENT OF ACTIVE TUBERCULOSIS	ALLERGIC LIVER REACTION (1% to 2%) Peripheral neuropathy (see Glossary) Bone marrow depression (see Glossary) Mental and behavioral disturbances

▷ **Principal Uses**

As a Single Drug Product: Uses currently included in FDA approved labeling: (1) Used alone to prevent the development of tuberculous infection in people who are at high risk because of exposure to infection or recent conversion of a negative tuberculin skin test to positive; (2) used in combination with other drugs to treat tuberculosis in a variety of body sites.

Other (unlabeled) generally accepted uses: (1) May have a role in treating atypical mycobacteria which can be associated with Crohn's disease; (2) can have a role in combination treatment of cutaneous Leishmaniasis.

As a Combination Drug Product [CD]: Available in combination with rifampin, another antitubercular drug that works in a different way. This combination is more effective than either drug used alone. Isoniazid can cause low pyridoxine (vitamin B-6); for this reason, a combination of the two drugs is available in tablet form.

How This Drug Works: By interfering with metabolism or cell walls, this drug kills (bactericidal) or inhibits (bacteristatic) susceptible tuberculosis organisms.

Available Dosage Forms and Strengths
  Injection — 100 mg per ml
   Syrup — 50 mg per 5-ml teaspoonful
   Tablets — 50 mg, 100 mg, 300 mg

▷ **Usual Adult Dosage Range:** For prevention: 300 mg once daily. For treatment: 5 mg per kilogram of body weight daily. The total daily dosage should not exceed 600 mg. **Note: Actual dose and dosing schedule must be determined on an individual basis by the physician.**

Conditions Requiring Dosing Adjustments

Liver function: Should **not** be used in acute liver disease. It should be discontinued if the liver function tests become increased to three times the normal value.

Kidney function: Should be used with caution in kidney compromise—a rare cause of nephrosis.

▷ **Dosing Instructions:** The tablet may be crushed and taken with food to prevent stomach irritation.

Usual Duration of Use: Use on a regular schedule for 1 or more years is often necessary, depending upon the nature of the infection. Shorter courses of intermittent high doses may work. See your doctor on a regular basis.

▷ **This Drug Should Not Be Taken If**
  • you have had an allergic reaction (especially a liver reaction) to any dosage form of it previously.
  • you have active liver disease.

▷ **Inform Your Physician Before Taking This Drug If**
- you have serious impairment of liver or kidney function.
- you drink an alcoholic beverage daily.
- you are an alcoholic.
- you have a seizure disorder.
- you take other drugs on a long-term basis, especially phenytoin (Dilantin).
- you plan to have surgery under general anesthesia in the near future.

Possible Side-Effects (natural, expected and unavoidable drug actions)
None.

▷ **Possible Adverse Effects** (unusual, unexpected and infrequent reactions)
If any of the following develop, consult your physician promptly for guidance.

Mild Adverse Effects

Allergic Reactions: Skin rash, fever, swollen glands, painful muscles and joints.

Dizziness, indigestion, nausea, vomiting.

Serious Adverse Effects

Allergic Reactions: Drug-induced hepatitis (see Glossary): Loss of appetite, nausea, fatigue, fever, itching, dark-colored urine, yellow discoloration of eyes and skin, hypersensitvity meningitis.

Severe skin reactions (Stevens-Johnson syndrome, Pellegra).

Peripheral neuritis (see Glossary): numbness, tingling, pain, weakness in hands and/or feet.

Acute mental and behavioral disturbances, psychosis, impaired vision, increase in epileptic seizures.

High or low blood sugars (hyperglycemia or hypoglycemia).

Porphyria.

Kidney toxicity (nephrotoxicity) (very, very rare).

Bone marrow depression (see Glossary): fatigue, weakness, fever, sore throat, abnormal bleeding or bruising.

Abnormal muscle changes (rhabdomyolysis) (very, very rare).

▷ **Possible Effects on Sexual Function:** Male breast enlargement and tenderness.

Possible Delayed Adverse Effects: An increase in the frequency of cirrhosis of the liver has been reported.

▷ **Adverse Effects That May Mimic Natural Diseases or Disorders**

Drug-induced hepatitis may suggest viral hepatitis. Collagen vascular changes may mimic rheumatoid arthritis or systemic lupus erythematosus. Pseudolymphoma may occur.

Natural Diseases or Disorders That May Be Activated by This Drug

Latent epilepsy, systemic lupus erythematosus (questionable).

Possible Effects on Laboratory Tests

Complete blood cell counts: decreased red cells, hemoglobin, white cells and platelets; increased eosinophils (allergic reaction).

Blood amylase level: increased (possible pancreatitis).

Blood antinuclear antibodies (ANA): positive.

Blood lupus erythematosus (LE) cells: positive.

Blood glucose level: increased (with large doses).

Liver function tests: increased liver enzymes (ALT/GPT, AST/GOT and alkaline phosphatase), increased bilirubin.

Urine sugar tests: increased; false positive results with Benedict's solution and Clinitest.

CAUTION
1. Ask your doctor about determining if you are a "slow" or "rapid" inactivator (acetylator) of isoniazid. This has a bearing on your predisposition to developing adverse effects.
2. Copper sulfate tests for urine sugar may give a false positive test result. (Diabetics please note.)

Precautions for Use

By Infants and Children: Use with caution in children with seizure disorders. "Slow acetylators" are more prone to adverse drug effects. It is advisable to give supplemental pyridoxine (vitamin B-6).

By Those over 60 Years of Age: There is a greater incidence of liver damage in this age group; and liver status should be closely watched. Observe for any indications of an "acute brain syndrome" consisting of confusion, delirium and seizures.

▷ **Advisability of Use During Pregnancy**

Pregnancy Category: C. See Pregnancy Code at the back of this book.

Animal studies: No birth defects reported in mice, rats or rabbits.

Human studies: Data from adequate studies of pregnant women is not available.

If clearly needed, this drug is now used at any time during pregnancy. Ask your physician for guidance.

Advisability of Use if Breast-Feeding

Presence of this drug in breast milk: Yes.

Avoid drug or refrain from nursing.

Habit-Forming Potential: None.

Effects of Overdosage: Nausea, vomiting, dizziness, blurred vision, hallucinations, slurred speech, stupor, coma, seizures.

Possible Effects of Long-Term Use: Peripheral neuritis due to a deficiency of pyridoxine (vitamin B-6).

Suggested Periodic Examinations While Taking This Drug (at physician's discretion)

Complete blood cell counts, liver function tests, complete eye examinations.

▷ **While Taking This Drug, Observe the Following**

Foods: Eat the following foods cautiously until your tolerance is determined: Swiss and Cheshire cheeses, tuna fish, skipjack fish and Sardinella species. These may interact with the drug to produce skin rash, itching, sweating, chills, headache, light-headedness or rapid heart rate. Taking this drug with food also acts to decrease absorption and lessen therapeutic benefits.

Nutritional Support: It is advisable to take a supplement of pyridoxine (vitamin B-6) to prevent peripheral neuritis. Ask your physician for dosage.

Beverages: No restrictions. May be taken with milk.

▷ *Alcohol:* Alcohol may reduce the effectiveness of this drug and increase the risk of liver toxicity.

Tobacco Smoking: No interactions expected.

▷ *Other Drugs*
   Isoniazid may *increase* the effects of
   • carbamazepine (Tegretol), and cause toxicity.
   • phenytoin (Dilantin), and cause toxicity.
   The following drugs may *decrease* the effects of isoniazid
   • cortisonelike drugs (see Drug Classes).
   Isoniazid *taken concurrently* with
   • acetaminophen (Tylenol) may increase the risk of hepatotoxicity.
   • BCG vaccine will result in decreased vaccine effectiveness.
   • ketoconazole, itraconazole or related compounds may result in decreased therapeutic benefit of the antifungal.
   • rifampin can result in a serious increased risk of liver toxicity.
   • theophylline may result in theophylline toxicity.
   • valproic acid (Depakene) can result in isoniazid or valproic acid toxicity.
   • warfarin (Coumadin) may result in increased bleeding risk.
▷ *Driving, Hazardous Activities:* This drug may cause dizziness. Restrict activities as necessary.
   Aviation Note: The use of this drug *may be a disqualification* for piloting. Consult a designated Aviation Medical Examiner.
   Exposure to Sun: No restrictions.
   Discontinuation: Long-term treatment is required. Do not stop this drug without asking your physician.

ISOSORBIDE DINITRATE (i soh SOHR bide di NI trayt)

Other Name: Sorbide nitrate
Introduced: 1959   **Prescription:** USA: Yes; Canada: No   **Available as Generic:** USA: Yes; Canada: No   **Class:** Antianginal, nitrates   **Controlled Drug:** USA: No; Canada: No
Brand Names: ✦Apo-ISDN, ✦Cedocard-SR, ✦Coradur, ✦Coronex, Dilatrate-SR, Iso-BID, Isonate, Isordil, Isordil Tembids, Isordil Titradose, Isotrate Timecells, ✦Novosorbide, Sorbitrate-SA, Sorbitrate
Warning: The brand names Isordil and Isuprel are similar and can be mistaken for each other; this can lead to serious medication errors. These names represent very different drugs. Isordil is the generic drug isosorbide dinitrate; used to treat angina. Isuprel is the generic drug isoproterenol; used for asthma. Verify that you are taking the correct drug.

BENEFITS versus RISKS	
Possible Benefits	*Possible Risks*
EFFECTIVE RELIEF AND PREVENTION OF ANGINA	Orthostatic hypotension (see Glossary)
EFFECTIVE ADJUNCTIVE TREATMENT IN SELECTED CASES OF CONGESTIVE HEART FAILURE	Rare skin reactions (severe peeling)

▷ **Principal Uses**
   As a Single Drug Product: Uses currently included in FDA approved labeling: (1) The sublingual (under-the-tongue) tablets and the chewable tablets are

Isosorbide Dinitrate

used to prevent and to relieve acute attacks of anginal pain; (2) the longer-acting tablets and capsules are used to prevent the development of angina, but are not effective in relieving acute episodes of anginal pain.

Other (unlabeled) generally accepted uses: (1) This drug is also used to improve heart function in selected cases of congestive heart failure; (2) can help ease the pressure in esophageal varices in alcoholics; (3) can help painful leg cramping (intermittent claudication); used after a heart attack intravenously to help address congestive heart failure.

How This Drug Works: By direct action on the muscle in blood vessel walls, this drug relaxes and dilates both arteries and veins. Its beneficial effects in treating angina and heart failure are due to (1) dilation of coronary arteries, and (2) dilation of systemic veins. The net effects are improved blood flow to the heart muscle and reduced work load of the heart.

Available Dosage Forms and Strengths
- Capsules — 40 mg
- Capsules, prolonged-action — 40 mg
- Tablets — 5 mg, 10 mg, 20 mg, 30 mg, 40 mg
- Tablets, chewable — 5 mg, 10 mg
- Tablets, prolonged-action — 40 mg
- Tablets, sublingual — 2.5 mg, 5 mg, 10 mg

▷ **Recommended Dosage Ranges** (Actual dosage and administration schedule must be determined by the physician for each patient individually.)

Infants and Children: Dosage not established.

12 to 60 Years of Age: Sublingual tablets: 5 to 10 mg dissolved under tongue every 2 to 3 hours; use for relief of acute attack and for prevention of anticipated attack.

Chewable tablets: Initially, 5 mg chewed to evaluate tolerance; increase dose to 5 or 10 mg every 2 to 3 hours as needed and tolerated; use for relief of acute attack and for prevention of anticipated attack.

Tablets: 5 to 30 mg 4 times daily to prevent acute attack; usual dose is 10 to 20 mg 4 times/day.

Prolonged-action capsules and tablets: 40 mg/6 to 12 hours as needed to prevent acute attacks.

The total daily dosage should not exceed 120 mg.

Over 60 Years of Age: Same as 12 to 60 years of age.

Conditions Requiring Dosing Adjustments

Liver function: It should be used with caution and in decreased dose in patients with liver compromise, as increased blood levels will occur.

Kidney function: No specific dosing changes are needed in compromised kidneys. This drug can discolor (brown to black) urine.

▷ **Dosing Instructions:** Capsules and tablets to be swallowed are best taken on an empty stomach to achieve maximal blood levels. Regular tablets may be crushed for administration; prolonged-action capsules and tablets should be taken whole.

Usual Duration of Use: Use on a regular schedule for 3 to 7 days is needed to (1) identify this drug's peak effect in preventing or relieving acute anginal pain, and (2) to find the optimal dosage shedule. Long-term use (months to years) requires physician supervision.

Isosorbide Dinitrate

▷ **This Drug Should Not Be Taken If**
- you have had an allergic reaction to any dosage form of it previously.
- you have severe anemia.
- you have increased intraocular pressure.
- you have an overactive thyroid gland.
- you have abnormal growth of the heart muscle (hypertrophic cardiomyopathy).
- you have had a very recent heart attack (myocardial infarction).

▷ **Inform Your Physician Before Taking This Drug If**
- you have had an unfavorable response to other nitrate drugs or vasodilators in the past.
- you have a history of low blood pressure.
- you have any form of glaucoma.
- you have had a cerebral hemorrhage recently.
- you are pregnant or are planning pregnancy.
- you are allergic to the dye tartrazine.
- you have a G6PD deficiency.

Possible Side-Effects (natural, expected and unavoidable drug actions)
Flushing of face, throbbing in head, palpitation, rapid heart rate, orthostatic hypotension (see Glossary).

▷ **Possible Adverse Effects** (unusual, unexpected and infrequent reactions)
If any of the following develop, consult your physician promptly for guidance.

Mild Adverse Effects
Allergic Reaction: Skin rash.
Headache (may be severe and persistent), dizziness, fainting.
Nausea, vomiting.
Urine discoloration.

Serious Adverse Effects
Allergic Reaction: Severe dermatitis with peeling of skin.
Transient ischemic attacks (TIAs) in presence of impaired circulation within the brain: dizziness, fainting, impaired vision or speech, localized numbness or weakness.
Anemia (in those with G6PD deficiency).
Abnormal heart rates or conduction.
Abnormally low blood pressure on standing (postural hypotension).

▷ **Possible Effects on Sexual Function:** None reported.

▷ **Adverse Effects That May Mimic Natural Diseases or Disorders**
Spells of low blood pressure (due to this drug) may mimic late-onset epilepsy.

Possible Effects on Laboratory Tests
None reported.

CAUTION
1. Tolerance (see Glossary) to long-acting forms of nitrates may cause sublingual tablets of nitroglycerin to be less effective in relieving acute anginal attacks. Antianginal effectiveness is restored after 1 week of abstinence from long-acting nitrates.
2. Many over-the-counter (OTC) medications for allergies, colds and

coughs contain drugs that may counteract the desired drug effects. Ask your physician or pharmacist for help before using such medications.

Precautions for Use

By Those over 60 Years of Age: Small starting doses are advisable. You may be more susceptible to the development of low blood pressure and associated "blackout" spells, fainting and falling. Throbbing headaches and flushing may be more apparent.

▷ **Advisability of Use During Pregnancy**

Pregnancy Category: C. See Pregnancy Code at the back of this book.
Animal studies: No information available.
Human studies: Adequate studies of pregnant women are not available.
Use this drug only if clearly needed.

Advisability of Use if Breast-Feeding

Presence of this drug in breast milk: Unknown.
If drug is thought to be necessary, monitor the nursing infant for low blood pressure and poor feeding.

Habit-Forming Potential: None.

Effects of Overdosage: Headache, dizziness, marked flushing of face and skin, vomiting, weakness, fainting, difficult breathing, coma.

Possible Effects of Long-Term Use: Development of tolerance with temporary loss of effectiveness at recommended doses. Development of abnormal hemoglobin (red blood cell pigment).

Suggested Periodic Examinations While Taking This Drug (at physician's discretion)

Measurement of internal eye pressure. Red cell counts and hemoglobin tests.

▷ **While Taking This Drug, Observe the Following**

Foods: No restrictions.

Beverages: No restrictions. May be taken with milk.

▷ *Alcohol:* Use extreme caution and avoid alcohol completely in the presence of any side-effects or adverse effects of this drug. Alcohol may exaggerate the blood-pressure-lowering effect of this drug.

Tobacco Smoking: Nicotine can reduce the benefits of this drug. Avoid all forms of tobacco.

Marijuana Smoking: Possible reduced effectiveness of this drug; mild to moderate increase in angina; possible changes in electrocardiogram, confusing interpretation.

▷ *Other Drugs*

Isosorbide dinitrate *taken concurrently* with
- antihypertensive drugs may cause excessive lowering of blood pressure; dosage adjustments may be necessary.

▷ *Driving, Hazardous Activities:* Usually no restrictions. This drug may cause dizziness or spells of low blood pressure. Restrict activities as necessary.

Aviation Note: Coronary artery disease *is a disqualification* for piloting. Consult a designated Aviation Medical Examiner.

Exposure to Sun: No restrictions.

Exposure to Heat: Use caution. Hot environments can cause significant drop in blood pressure.

Exposure to Cold: Cold environments can increase the need for this drug and limit its benefits.

Heavy Exercise or Exertion: This drug may improve your ability to be more active without anginal pain. Use caution and avoid excessive exertion.

Discontinuation: It is advisable to gradually withdraw this drug after long-term use. Dose and frequency of prolonged-action dosage forms should be reduced gradually over a period of 4 to 6 weeks.

ISOSORBIDE MONONITRATE (i soh SOHR bide mon oh NI trayt)

Introduced: 1983 **Prescription:** USA: Yes **Available as Generic:** USA: No **Class:** Antianginal, nitrates **Controlled Drug:** USA: No
Brand Name: Elan (Italy), Imdur, Ismo, Monoket

BENEFITS versus RISKS	
Possible Benefits	*Possible Risks*
EFFECTIVE PREVENTION OF ANGINA	Orthostatic hypotension (see Glossary) Headache (9%)

▷ **Principal Uses**

As a Single Drug Product: Uses currently included in FDA approved labeling: To reduce the frequency and severity of recurrent angina; not effective in acute anginal pain.

Other (unlabeled) generally accepted uses: (1) May have a role in treating congestive heart failure.

How This Drug Works: By direct action on the muscle in blood vessel walls, this drug relaxes and dilates both arteries and veins. Beneficial effects in treating angina are due to (1) dilation of coronary arteries, and (2) dilation of systemic veins. The net effects are improved blood flow to the heart muscle and reduced workload of the heart.

Available Dosage Forms and Strengths
Tablets — 20 mg Ismo
— 60 mg Imdur

▷ **Recommended Dosage Ranges** (Actual dosage and administration schedule must be determined by the physician for each patient individually.)

Infants and Children: Dosage not established.

12 to 60 Years of Age: Ismo: 20 mg (1 tablet), taken twice daily: take the first tablet on arising; take the second tablet 7 hours later. Do not take additional doses during the balance of the day.

The total daily dosage should not exceed 40 mg.

Imdur: 30 mg (one half tablet) or 60 mg (a whole tablet) once daily, taken in the morning when you get up.

The total daily dose should not exceed 250 mg.

Over 60 Years of Age: Same as 12 to 60 years of age.

Isosorbide Mononitrate

Conditions Requiring Dosing Adjustments
Liver function: This drug should be used with caution in patients with liver compromise, however, no specific guidelines for dosage reduction are available.
Kidney function: No dosing changes are recommended in renal compromise. Isosorbide monontrate may turn the urine brown to black in color.

▷ **Dosing Instructions:** The tablet may be crushed and is preferably taken on an empty stomach to achieve maximal blood levels.

Usual Duration of Use: Use on a regular schedule for 3 to 7 days determines this drug's effectiveness in preventing episodes of acute anginal pain. Long-term use (months to years) requires physician supervision.

Possible Advantages of This Drug
Designed to provide the best possible prevention of acute angina with minimal development of tolerance (loss of effectiveness). See the term *tolerance* in the Glossary. The nitrate-free interval during the evening and night prevents the development of tolerance.

▷ **This Drug Should Not Be Taken If**
- you have had an allergic reaction to it previously.
- you have had a very recent heart attack (myocardial infarction).
- you currently have congestive heart failure.
- you have a severe anemia.
- your thyroid is overactive.
- you have a hypertrophic cardiomyopathy.

▷ **Inform Your Physician Before Taking This Drug If**
- you have had an unfavorable response to other nitrate drugs or vasodilators in the past.
- you have a history of low blood pressure.
- you have had a cerebral hemorrhage recently.
- you are pregnant or are planning pregnancy.
- you have any form of glaucoma.

Possible Side-Effects (natural, expected and unavoidable drug actions)
Flushing of face, throbbing in head, palpitation, rapid heart rate, orthostatic hypotension (see Glossary).

▷ **Possible Adverse Effects** (unusual, unexpected and infrequent reactions)
If any of the following develop, consult your physician promptly for guidance.

Mild Adverse Effects
Allergic Reactions: Skin rash, itching (less than 1%).
Headache (9%), dizziness (1%), fainting (less than 1%).
Blurred vision.
Nausea, vomiting (3%).
Bad breath (Halitosis).

Serious Adverse Effects
Transient ischemic attacks (TIAs) in presence of impaired circulation within the brain: Dizziness, fainting, impaired vision or speech, localized numbness or weakness.
Bone marrow depression (less than 5%).
Anemia (in patients with G6PD deficiency).

Abnormally low blood pressure.
Abnormal heart beats (less than 1%).

▷ **Possible Effects on Sexual Function:** Decreased libido and impotence (less than 5%).

▷ **Adverse Effects That May Mimic Natural Diseases or Disorders**
Spells of low blood pressure with fainting (due to this drug) may be mistaken for late-onset epilepsy.

Possible Effects on Laboratory Tests
None reported.

CAUTION
1. Take this drug exactly as prescribed. If headaches are frequent or troublesome, call your doctor. Aspirin or acetaminophen may be taken to relieve headaches.
2. Many over-the-counter (OTC) medications for allergies, colds and coughs contain drugs that may counteract the desired effects of this drug. Ask your doctor or pharmacist for help before using such medications.

Precautions for Use
By Those over 60 Years of Age: Small starting doses are advisable. Increased risk of low blood pressure and associated "blackout" spells, fainting and falling. Throbbing headaches and flushing may be more apparent.

▷ **Advisability of Use During Pregnancy**
Pregnancy Category: C—Ismo. See Pregnancy Code at the back of this book. B—Imdur.
Animal Studies: Rat and rabbit studies reveal embryo deaths due to large doses of Ismo. Rat and rabbit studies did not reveal embryo deaths from Imdur.
Human studies: Adequate studies of pregnant women are not available.
Use this drug only if clearly needed. Ask your physician for guidance.

Advisability of Use if Breast-Feeding
Presence of this drug in breast milk: Unknown.
If drug is thought to be necessary, watch the nursing infant for low blood pressure and poor feeding.

Habit-Forming Potential: None.

Effects of Overdosage: Headache, dizziness, marked flushing of face and skin, vomiting, weakness, fainting, difficult breathing, coma.

Possible Effects of Long-Term Use: Development of abnormal hemoglobin (red blood cell pigment).

Suggested Periodic Examinations While Taking This Drug (at physician's discretion)
Measurement of internal eye pressure.

▷ **While Taking This Drug, Observe the Following**
Foods: No restrictions.
Beverages: No restrictions. May be taken with milk.
▷ *Alcohol:* Use extreme caution. Avoid alcohol completely in the presence of any side-effects or adverse effects of this drug. Alcohol may exaggerate the blood-pressure-lowering effect of this drug.

Tobacco Smoking: Nicotine can reduce the effectiveness of this drug. Avoid all forms of tobacco.

Marijuana Smoking: Possible reduced effectiveness of this drug; mild to moderate increase in angina; possible changes in electrocardiogram, confusing interpretation.

▷ **Other Drugs**

Isosorbide mononitrate *taken concurrently* with
- antihypertensive drugs may cause excessive lowering of blood pressure; dosage adjustments may be necessary.
- calcium channel-blocking drugs (see Drug Classes) may cause marked orthostatic hypotension (see Glossary).

▷ *Driving, Hazardous Activities:* Usually no restrictions. This drug may cause dizziness or spells of low blood pressure. Restrict activities as necessary.

Aviation Note: Coronary artery disease *is a disqualification* for piloting. Consult a designated Aviation Medical Examiner.

Exposure to Sun: No restrictions.

Exposure to Heat: Use caution. Hot environments can cause significant drop in blood pressure.

Exposure to Cold: Cold environments can increase the need for this drug and limit effectiveness.

Heavy Exercise or Exertion: This drug may improve your ability to be more active without anginal pain. Use caution and avoid excessive exertion.

Discontinuation: It is advisable to withdraw this drug gradually (over a period of 2 to 4 weeks) after long-term use.

ISOTRETINOIN (i soh TRET i noin)

Introduced: 1979 **Prescription:** USA: Yes; Canada: Yes **Available as Generic:** No **Class:** Antiacne **Controlled Drug:** USA: No; Canada: No
Brand Name: Accutane

BENEFITS versus RISKS	
Possible Benefits	*Possible Risks*
EFFECTIVE TREATMENT OF SEVERE CYSTIC ACNE	MAJOR BIRTH DEFECTS
	Initial worsening of acne (transient)
	Inflammation of lips (90%)
	Dry skin, nose and mouth
	Musculoskeletal discomfort
	Corneal opacities (rare)

▷ **Principal Uses**

As a Single Drug Product: Uses currently included in FDA approved labeling: (1) reserved to treat severe, disfiguring nodular and cystic acne that has failed to respond to all other forms of standard therapy. *It should not be used to treat mild forms of acne.* It is also used to treat some less common conditions of the skin that are due to disorders of keratin production.

Other (unlabeled) generally accepted uses: (1) May be helpful in refractory hypertrophic lupus erythematosus; (2) can help control resistant oral leukoplakia; (3) Apert syndrome facial treatment; (4) used adjunctively to surgery in some cervical cancers; (5) treats mycosis fungoides; (6) eases symptoms in Darier's disease; (7) may have a role in treating dysplastic nevi; (8) eases symptoms of Grover's disease; (9) can help treat the abnormal gum growth (gingival hyperplasia) which can occur with Phenytoin therapy; (10) treats severe and refractory rosacea; (11) has been combined with interferon alpha treatment in squamous cell skin cancer.

How This Drug Works: By an unknown action, this drug reduces the size of sebaceous glands and inhibits sebum (skin oil) production. This helps to correct the major feature of acne and its complications.

Available Dosage Forms and Strengths
Capsules — 10 mg, 20 mg, 40 mg

▷ **Usual Adult Dosage Range:** Starting dose is based on the patient's weight and severity of acne; the usual dose is 0.5 to 2 mg per kilogram of body weight daily, taken in 2 divided doses for 15 to 20 weeks. After weeks of treatment, the dose should be adjusted according to response of the acne and the development of adverse effects. **Note: Actual dosage and administration schedule must be determined by the physician for each patient individually.**

Conditions Requiring Dosing Adjustments
Liver function: The dose should be decreased when isotretinoin is used in patients with compromised livers.
Kidney function: Isotretinoin is used with caution in kidney compromise.

▷ **Dosing Instructions:** Begin treatment only on the second or third day of your next normal menstrual period. Take with meals (morning and evening) to achieve optimal blood levels. The capsule should not be opened for administration.

Usual Duration of Use: Use on a regular schedule for 15 to 20 weeks best determines effectiveness in clearing or improving severe cystic acne. The drug may be stopped earlier if the total cyst count is reduced by more than 70%. If a repeat course of treatment is necessary, it should not be started for 2 months. Long-term use (months to years) requires physician supervision.

▷ **This Drug Should Not Be Taken If**
- you have had an allergic reaction to it previously
- you are allergic to parabens, preservatives used in this drug product.
- you are pregnant, or planning pregnancy.

▷ **Inform Your Physician Before Taking This Drug If**
- you have had an allergic reaction to any form of vitamin A in the past.
- you have diabetes mellitus.
- you have a cholesterol or triglyceride disorder.
- you have a history of liver or kidney disease.

Possible Side-Effects (natural, expected and unavoidable drug actions)
Dryness of the nose and mouth (80%), inflammation of the lips (90%), dryness of the skin with itching (80%), peeling of the palms and soles (5%).

▷ **Possible Adverse Effects** (unusual, unexpected and infrequent reactions)
  If any of the following develop, consult your physician promptly for guidance.
  Mild Adverse Effects
    Allergic Reaction: Skin rash—may resemble pityriasis rosea (less than 10%).
    Thinning of hair, conjunctivitis, intolerance of contact lenses, decreased night vision, muscular and joint aches, headache, fatigue, indigestion.
  Serious Adverse Effects
    Skin infections, worsening of arthritis, inflammatory bowel disorders.
    Abnormal acceleration of bone development in children.
    Development of opacities in the cornea of the eye.
    Reduced red blood cell and white blood cell counts; increased blood platelet count.
    Seizures.
    Kidney toxicity (rare).
    Pancreatitis (rare).
    Abnormal blood glucose control.
    Increased pressure within the head, with associated headache, visual disturbances, nausea and vomiting.
    Drug-induced hepatitis.

▷ **Possible Effects on Sexual Function**
  Decreased male libido (7%), decreased female libido (13%) beginning after 1 month of drug use.
  Impotence (3%) beginning after 3 months of drug use.
  Decreased vaginal secretions (43%).
  Altered timing and pattern of menstruation (22%).
  Female breast discharge (rare).

Possible Effects on Laboratory Tests
  Complete blood cell counts: infrequently decreased red cells and white cells.
  Blood total cholesterol, LDL cholesterol, VLDL cholesterol and triglyceride levels: increased.
  Blood HDL cholesterol levels: decreased.
  Blood thyroid hormones (T_3, T_4 and free T_4 index): decreased.
  Liver function tests: infrequently increased liver enzymes (ALT/GPT, AST/GOT and alkaline phosphatase), increased bilirubin.

CAUTION
  1. This drug should not be used to treat mild forms of acne.
  2. Worsening of your acne may occur during the first few weeks of treatment; this will subside with continued use of the drug.
  3. Do not take any other form of vitamin A while taking this drug. (Observe contents of multiple vitamin preparations.)
  4. Women with potential for pregnancy should have a ***blood*** pregnancy test within 2 weeks before taking this drug and should use 2 effective forms of contraception simultaneously during its use. Contraception should be continued until normal menstruation resumes after discontinuing this drug.
  5. This drug may cause increased blood levels of cholesterol and triglycerides.

6. If repeated courses of this drug are prescribed, wait a minimum of 2 months between courses before resuming medication.

Precautions for Use
By Infants and Children: Long-term use (6 to 12 months) may cause abnormal acceleration of bone growth and development. Your physician can monitor this possibility by periodic X-ray examination of long bones.

▷ **Advisability of Use During Pregnancy**
Pregnancy Category: X. See Pregnancy Code at the back of this book.
Animal studies: Birth defects of skull, brain and vertebral column found in rats; skeletal birth defects found in rabbits.
Human studies: Adequate studies of pregnant women are not available. However, many serious birth defects (thought to be due to this drug) have been reported. These include major abnormalities of the head, brain, heart, blood vessels and hormone-producing glands.
Avoid this drug completely during entire pregnancy.

Advisability of Use if Breast-Feeding
Presence of this drug in breast milk: Unknown.
Avoid drug or refrain from nursing.

Habit-Forming Potential: None.

Effects of Overdosage: Increased blood pressure, lethargy, nausea, vomiting, mild gastrointestinal bleeding, elevated blood calcium, hallucinations and psychosis.

Suggested Periodic Examinations While Taking This Drug (at physician's discretion)
Complete blood cell counts, including platelet counts.
Measurements of blood cholesterol and triglyceride levels.
Complete eye examinations.
Liver and kidney function tests.

▷ **While Taking This Drug, Observe the Following**
Foods: Increases absorption and may be a good mechanism to maintain blood levels.
Beverages: No restrictions.
▷ *Alcohol:* No interactions expected.
Tobacco Smoking: No interactions expected.
▷ *Other Drugs:* Isotretinoin ***taken concurrently*** with
  • carbamazepine (Tegretol) may cause subtherapeutic carbamazepine levels.
  • tetracyclines may cause increased risk of pseudotumor cerebri.
▷ *Driving, Hazardous Activities:* No restrictions.
Exposure to Sun: Caution, this drug can cause photosensitivity (see Glossary).

ISRADIPINE (is RA di peen)

Introduced: 1984 **Prescription:** USA: Yes **Available as Generic:** USA: No **Class:** Antihypertensive, calcium channel blocker **Controlled Drug:** USA: No
Brand Name: DynaCirc

Isradipine 527

BENEFITS versus RISKS	
Possible Benefits	*Possible Risks*
EFFECTIVE TREATMENT OF MILD TO MODERATE HYPERTENSION	Headache (13.7%) Dizziness (7.3%) Fluid retention (7.2%) Palpitations (4.0%)

▷ **Principal Uses**
   As a Single Drug Product: Uses currently included in FDA approved labeling: (1) treats mild to moderate hypertension, alone or concurrently with thiazide-type diuretics.
   Other (unlabeled) generally accepted uses: (1) treatment of chronic, stable angina; (2) combination therapy of congestive heart failure; (3) may help resolve atherosclerosis; (4) could have a role in premature labor.

How This Drug Works: By blocking passage of calcium through cell walls (which is necessary for the function of nerve and muscle tissue), this drug inhibits the contraction of coronary arteries and peripheral arterioles. As a result of these effects, this drug
   • promotes dilation of the coronary arteries (antianginal effect).
   • reduces the degree of contraction of peripheral arterial walls, resulting in relaxation and consequent lowering of blood pressure. This further reduces the work load of the heart and helps prevent angina.

Available Dosage Forms and Strengths
   Capsules — 2.5 mg, 5 mg

▷ **Usual Adult Dosage Range:** Initially 2.5 mg 2 times daily, 12 hours apart, for a trial period of 2 to 4 weeks. If needed, the dose may be increased by 5 mg per day at intervals of 2 to 4 weeks. The usual maintenance dose is 5 to 10 mg daily. The total daily dosage should not exceed 20 mg. **Note: Actual dose and dosing schedule must be determined by the physician for each patient individually.**

Conditions Requiring Dosing Adjustments
   Liver function: Specific guidelines for dosage reduction are not available, yet empiric decreases in dosing are prudent in patients with compromised livers.
   Kidney function: Used with caution in kidney compromise.

▷ **Dosing Instructions:** May be taken with or following food to reduce stomach irritation. The capsule may be opened; mixed with food and swallowed promptly.

Usual Duration of Use: Use on a regular schedule for 2 to 4 weeks determines this drug's effectiveness in controlling hypertension or in reducing the frequency and severity of angina. The smallest effective dose should be used for long-term (months to years) therapy. Periodic physician evaluation is essential.

Possible Advantages of This Drug
   Does not cause orthostatic hypotension (see Glossary).
   No adverse effects on heart or kidney function.
   No adverse effects on blood cholesterol levels.

Isradipine

▷ **This Drug Should Not Be Taken If**
- you have had an allergic reaction to it previously.
- you have symptomatic low blood pressure (hypotension).
- you have advanced narrowing of the aorta.

▷ **Inform Your Physician Before Taking This Drug If**
- you have had an unfavorable response to any calcium blocker drug in the past (see Drug Classes).
- you are currently taking any beta blocker drug (see Drug Class Section).
- you are taking any drugs that lower blood pressure.
- you have a history of congestive heart failure, heart attack or stroke.
- you are subject to disturbances of heart rhythm.
- you have muscular dystrophy.
- you have myasthenia gravis.
- you have impaired liver or kidney function.
- you plan to have surgery under general anesthesia in the near future.

Possible Side-Effects (natural, expected and unavoidable drug actions)
Rapid heart rate (1.5%), swelling of the feet and ankles (7.2%), flushing and sensation of warmth (2.6%).

▷ **Possible Adverse Effects** (unusual, unexpected and infrequent reactions)
If any of the following develop, consult your physician promptly for guidance.

Mild Adverse Effects
Allergic Reactions: Skin rash (1.5%), hives, itching.
Headache (13.7%), dizziness (7.3%), weakness (1.2%), nervousness (1%), blurred vision (1%).
Decreased skin sensation (1.5%).
Palpitation (4%), shortness of breath (1.8%).
Indigestion (1.7%), nausea (1.8%), vomiting (1.1%), constipation (1%).
Cramps in legs and feet.
Weight loss.
Abnormal growth of the gums (gingival hyperplasia).

Serious Adverse Effects
Allergic Reactions: None reported.
Rare heart rhythm disturbances.
Increased frequency or severity of angina when therapy is started or following an increase in dose (2.4%).
Marked drop in blood pressure with fainting (1%).
Low white blood cell counts.

▷ **Possible Effects on Sexual Function:** Decreased libido, impotence (less than 1%).

▷ **Adverse Effects That May Mimic Natural Diseases or Disorders**
Flushing and warmth may resemble menopausal "hot flushes."

Possible Effects on Laboratory Tests
White blood cell counts: decreased (less than 1% of users).
Liver function tests: increased enzyme levels (infrequent).
Electrocardiogram: slight increase in QT interval

Isradipine

CAUTION
1. If you are monitoring your own blood pressure, check it just before each dose and 2 to 3 hours after each dose. This will detect excessive fluctuations between high and low readings.
2. Tell all physicians and dentists who care for you that you take this drug. Note the use of this drug on your personal identification card.
3. Nitroglycerin and other nitrate drugs may be used as needed to relieve acute episodes of angina pain. However, if your angina attacks are becoming more frequent or intense, notify your physician promptly.

Precautions for Use
By Infants and Children: Safety and effectiveness for those under 18 years of age not established.
By Those over 60 Years of Age: Usually well tolerated by this age group. However, watch for weakness, dizziness, fainting and falling. Take necessary precautions to prevent injury.

▷ **Advisability of Use During Pregnancy**
Pregnancy Category: C. See Pregnancy Code at the back of this book.
Animal studies: Embryo and fetal toxicity reported in small animals, but no birth defects due to this drug.
Human studies: Adequate studies of pregnant women are not available.
Avoid this drug during the first 3 months. Use during the last 6 months only if clearly needed. Ask physician for guidance.

Advisability of Use if Breast-Feeding
Presence of this drug in breast milk: Unknown.
Avoid drug or refrain from nursing.

Habit-Forming Potential: None.

Effects of Overdosage: Weakness, light-headedness, fainting, fast pulse, low blood pressure, shortness of breath, flushed and warm skin, tremors and abnormal heart beats.

Possible Effects of Long-Term Use: None reported.

Suggested Periodic Examinations While Taking This Drug (at physician's discretion)
Evaluations of heart function, including electrocardiograms; measurements of blood pressure in supine, sitting and standing positions.

▷ **While Taking This Drug, Observe the Following**
Foods: No restrictions. Avoid excessive salt intake.
Beverages: No restrictions. May be taken with milk.
▷ *Alcohol:* Use caution. Alcohol may exaggerate the drop in blood pressure in some people.
Tobacco Smoking: Nicotine may reduce the effectiveness of this drug. Follow your physician's advice regarding smoking.
Marijuana Smoking: Possible reduced effectiveness; mild to moderate increase in angina; possible changes in electrocardiogram, confusing interpretation.
▷ *Other Drugs*
Isradipine **taken concurrently** with
- beta blocker drugs or digitalis preparations (see Drug Classes) may affect

heart rate and rhythm adversely. Careful monitoring by your physician is needed if these drugs are taken concurrently.
- digloxin may cause an increased blood level. Laboratory testing of blood levels should be performed more often if these drugs are combined.
- magnesium, especially in doses used in premature labor can cause very low and abnormal blood pressure.

▷ *Driving, Hazardous Activities:* Usually no restrictions. This drug may cause drowsiness or dizziness. Restrict activities as necessary.

Aviation Note: Coronary artery disease and hypertension **are disqualifications** for piloting. Consult a designated Aviation Medical Examiner.

Exposure to Sun: No restrictions.

Exposure to Heat: Caution advised. Hot environments can exaggerate the blood-pressure-lowering effects of this drug. Observe for light-headedness or weakness.

Heavy Exercise or Exertion: This drug may improve your ability to be more active without resulting angina pain. Use caution and avoid excessive exercise that could impair heart function in the absence of warning pain.

Discontinuation: Do not stop this drug abruptly. Ask your doctor about gradual withdrawal. Watch for the development of rebound angina.

KETOCONAZOLE (kee toh KOHN a zohl)

Introduced: 1981 **Prescription:** USA: Yes; Canada: Yes **Available as Generic:** USA: No; Canada: No **Class:** Antifungal **Controlled Drug:** USA: No; Canada: No

Brand Name: Nizoral

BENEFITS versus RISKS	
Possible Benefits	*Possible Risks*
EFFECTIVE TREATMENT OF THE FOLLOWING FUNGUS INFECTIONS: Blastomycosis, Candidiasis, Chromomycosis, Coccidioidomycosis, Histoplasmosis, Paracoccidioidomycosis, Tinea (Ringworm)	SERIOUS DRUG-INDUCED LIVER DAMAGE (1 in 10,000) Rare but serious allergic reactions Low blood platelets and anemia (rare)
Beneficial short-term treatment of advanced prostate cancer	
Beneficial auxiliary treatment of Cushing's syndrome	

▷ **Principal Uses**

As a Single Drug Product: Uses currently included in FDA approved labeling: (1) Treatment of lung and systemic blastomycosis; (2) Treatment of Candida (yeast) infections of the skin, mouth, throat and esophagus (may be AIDS-related); (3) Treatment of systemic Candida infections—pneumonia, peritonitis, urinary tract infections (may be AIDS-related); (4) Auxiliary treatment of chromomycosis; (5) Treatment of lung and systemic coccidioidomycosis; (6) Treatment of lung and systemic histoplasmosis;

(7) Treatment of paracoccidioidomycosis; (8) Treatment of Tinea infections of the body, groin (jock itch), and feet (athlete's foot).

Other (unlabeled) generally accepted uses: (1) Treatment of Candida infections of the vulva and vagina; (2) short-term treatment of prostate cancer; (3) treatment of Cushing's syndrome (excessive adrenal hormones); (4) treatment of systemic sporotrichosis; (5) topical treatment of fungal dandruff; (6) therapy of fungal infections of the toe nails; (7) designated as an orphan drug in therapy kidney toxicity caused by cyclosporine; (8) treats visceral leishmaniasis.

How This Drug Works: As an antifungal: By damaging cell walls and impairing critical cell enzymes, this drug inhibits cell growth and reproduction (with low drug levels) and destroys fungal cells (with high drug concentrations).

In treating prostate cancer: This drug decreases testosterone (male hormone) levels; and prostate cancer cells need testosterone to grow.

In treating Cushing's syndrome: This drug suppresses the excessive production of adrenal corticosteroid hormones.

Available Dosage Forms and Strengths
>   Cream — 2% (For local application to Candida or Tinea skin infections)
>   Shampoo — 2% (For topical therapy of fungal dandruff)
> Oral suspension — 100 mg per 5-ml teaspoonful (Canada)
>   Tablets — 200 mg (U.S. and Canada)

▷ **Recommended Dosage Ranges** (Actual dosage and administration schedule must be determined by the physician for each patient individually.)

Infants and Children: Up to 2 years of age: Dosage not established.

Over 2 years of age: 3.3 to 10 mg/kg of body weight, once daily; the dosage depends upon the nature of the infection.

12 to 60 Years of Age: For fungus infections—200 to 400 mg once daily; 800 mg maximum daily dose.

For prostate cancer—400 mg 3 times a day; 1,200 mg maximum daily dose.

For Cushing's syndrome—600 to 1200 mg once daily; total daily dosage should not exceed 1200 mg.

Over 60 Years of Age: Same as 12 to 60 years of age.

Conditions Requiring Dosing Adjustments

Liver function: The dose should be empirically decreased in patients with liver compromise.

Kidney function: Decreased doses are not needed in kidney compromise.

▷ **Dosing Instructions:** The tablet may be crushed and is best taken with or after food to enhance absorption and reduce stomach irritation. Do not take with antacids. Take the full course prescribed.

Usual Duration of Use: Use on a regular schedule for 2 to 4 weeks determines effectiveness in controlling fungal infections. Actual cures or long-term suppression often require continual treatment for many months. Periodic physician evaluation of response and dosage adjustment are essential.

▷ **This Drug Should Not Be Taken If**
- you have had an allergic reaction to it previously.
- you have active liver disease.
- you take astemizole or tefenadine.

▷ **Inform Your Physician Before Taking This Drug If**
- you are allergic to related antifungal drugs: clotrimazole, fluconazole, itraconazole or miconazole.
- you have a history of liver disease or impaired liver function.
- you take loratadine.
- you have a history of adrenal insufficiency.
- you have a history of low blood platelets or anemia.
- you have a history of alcoholism.
- you have a deficiency of stomach hydrochloric acid.
- you are taking any other drugs currently.

Possible Side-Effects (natural, expected and unavoidable drug actions)
Suppression of testosterone and adrenal corticosteroid hormone production (more pronounced with high drug doses).

▷ **Possible Adverse Effects** (unusual, unexpected and infrequent reactions)
If any of the following develop, consult your physician promptly for guidance.

Mild Adverse Effects
Allergic Reactions: Skin rash, hives, itching (1.5%).
Headache, dizziness, drowsiness, photophobia (all less than 1%).
Nausea and vomiting (3-10%), stomach pain (1.2%), diarrhea (1%).
Increased blood pressure.
Hair loss.
Tinitis.
Muscle and joint aches.

Serious Adverse Effects
Allergic Reactions: Anaphylactic reaction (see Glossary).
Severe liver toxicity (very rare): Loss of appetite, nausea, fatigue, yellow skin and eyes, dark urine, light-colored stools. (See jaundice in Glossary.)
Suppression of the adrenal gland.
Low thyroid activity.
Rare mental depression.
Hemolytic anemia (rare).
Abnormally low blood platelet counts: Abnormal bruising or bleeding.

▷ **Possible Effects on Sexual Function:** Decreased testosterone blood levels: Reduced sperm counts, decreased libido, impotence, male breast enlargement and tenderness.
Altered menstrual patterns.

Possible Delayed Adverse Effects: Deficiency of adrenal corticosteroid hormones (cortisone-related); this could be serious during stress resulting from illness or injury.

▷ **Adverse Effects That May Mimic Natural Diseases or Disorders**
Drug-induced liver reaction may suggest viral hepatitis.

Possible Effects on Laboratory Tests
Complete blood cell counts: decreased red cells, white cells and platelets.
Liver function tests: increased liver enzymes (ALT/GPT, AST/GOT and alkaline phosphatase), increased bilirubin.
Adrenal corticosteroid blood levels: decreased.
Testosterone blood levels: decreased.

Precautions for Use
By Infants and Children: Safety and effectiveness for those under 2 years of age not established.
By Those over 60 Years of Age: No information available. It is advisable to avoid high doses.

▷ **Advisability of Use During Pregnancy**
Pregnancy Category: C. See Pregnancy Code at the back of this book.
Animal studies: Rat studies revealed significant embryo toxicity and birth defects due to this drug.
Human studies: Adequate studies of pregnant women are not available.
Use this drug only if clearly needed. Ask your physician for guidance.

Advisability of Use if Breast-Feeding
Presence of this drug in breast milk: Yes.
Avoid drug or refrain from nursing.

Habit-Forming Potential: None.

Effects of Overdosage: Possible nausea, vomiting, diarrhea.

Possible Effects of Long-Term Use: Suppression of adrenal corticosteroid hormone production, requiring replacement therapy during periods of stress.

Suggested Periodic Examinations While Taking This Drug (at physician's discretion)
Liver function tests should be obtained BEFORE long-term therapy is started and checked monthly during treatment.
Sperm counts.

▷ **While Taking This Drug, Observe the Following**
Foods: No restrictions.
Beverages: No restrictions. May be taken with milk.
▷ *Alcohol:* Avoid completely. Alcohol can cause a disulfiram-like reaction (see Glossary). In addition, alcohol may cause liver toxicity.
Tobacco Smoking: No interactions expected.
▷ *Other Drugs*
Ketoconazole may *increase* the effects of
- oral hypoglycemic agents (see Drug Class) and result in very low blood sugars.
- nonsedating antihistamines such as astemizole (Hismanal), terfenadine (Seldane) and loratadine (Claritin) and cause serious heart rhythm problems. Do not combine.
- cortisonelike drugs (prednisone, etc.).
- cyclosporine (Sandimmune).
- quinidine (Quinaglute) and cause toxicity. Blood levels are needed.
- warfarin (Coumadin), and cause bleeding; prothrombin times are needed.

Ketoconazole may *decrease* the effects of
- theophyllines (Aminophyllin, Theo-Dur, etc.).
- didanosine (Videx).

The following drugs may *decrease* the effects of ketoconazole
- antacids; if needed, take antacids 2 hours after ketoconazole.
- histamine H-2 blocking drugs: cimetidine, famotidine, nizatidine, ranitidine; if needed, take 2 hours after ketoconazole.
- isoniazid (Laniazid, Nydrazid, etc.).
- rifampin (Rifadin, Rifater, Rimactane, etc.).

Ketoconazole *taken concurrently* with
- phenytoin (Dilantin) may change the levels of both drugs.

▷ *Driving, Hazardous Activities:* This drug may cause dizziness or drowsiness. Restrict activities as necessary.

Aviation Note: The use of this drug *may be a disqualification* for piloting. Consult a designated Aviation Medical Examiner.

Exposure to Sun: This drug may cause photophobia; wear sun glasses if appropriate.

Discontinuation: Take the full course prescribed. Continual treatment for several months may be needed. Ask your doctor when the drug should be stopped.

KETOPROFEN (kee toh PROH fen)

Introduced: 1973　**Prescription:** USA: Yes; Canada: Yes　**Available as Generic:** Yes　**Class:** Mild analgesic, anti-inflammatory　**Controlled Drug:** USA: No; Canada: No

Brand Names: ✦Apo-Keto, ✦Apo-keto-E, Orudis, Orudis SR, ✦Orudis E-50, ✦Orudis E-100, Oruvail ER, ✦Oruvail SR, ✦Rhodis, ✦Rhodis EC

BENEFITS versus RISKS	
Possible Benefits	*Possible Risks*
EFFECTIVE RELIEF OF MILD TO MODERATE PAIN AND INFLAMMATION	Gastrointestinal pain, ulceration, bleeding (rare) Rare congestive heart failure Rare liver or kidney damage Rare fluid retention Rare bone marrow depression

Please see the propionic acid nonsteroidal anti-inflammatory drug profile for further information.

KETOROLAC (KEY tor o lak)

Introduced: 1991　**Prescription:** USA: Yes; Canada: Yes　**Available as Generic:** USA: No; Canada: No　**Class:** Nonsteroidal anti-inflammatory drug, analgesic　**Controlled Drug:** USA: No; Canada: No

Brand Name: Toradol, Acular

BENEFITS versus RISKS	
Possible Benefits	*Possible Risks*
EFFECTIVE LIMITED DURATION TREATMENT OF PAIN HABIT FORMING POTENTIAL AVOIDED RESPIRATORY DEPRESSION OF NARCOTICS AVOIDED Easy change from intramuscular (IM) to oral form	Mental depression (rare) Gastrointestinal ulceration and bleeding (rare) Rare kidney or liver damage Rare serious skin damage Rare edema and low blood pressure

▷ **Principal Uses**
As a Single Drug Product: Uses currently included in FDA approved labeling: (1) Short-term (5 days at most, regardless of route) use in pain management; (2) itchy eyes caused by seasonal allergies.

Other (unlabeled) generally accepted uses: (1) 0.5% solution used to manage postoperative inflammation after cataract surgery. The same solution has been used to reduce disruption of the blood-aqueous humor barrier, and for the treatment of chronic aphakic or pseudophakic macular edema; (2) used to decrease the total dose of narcotics needed when used in combination therapy of chronic pain; (3) eases the pain of pericarditis and reflex sympathetic dystrophy.

How This Drug Works: The pain relieving and anti-inflammatory effect comes from inhibition of prostaglandins and other chemicals that cause pain and inflammation.

Available Dosage Forms and Strengths
Ketorolac (Toradol) tablets — 10 mg
Ketorolac ophthalmic solution — 0.5% solution
Ketorolac (Toradol) injection — 15 mg: 15 mg/ml in a 1 ml syringe NDC # 0033-2443-40
— 30 mg: 30 mg/ml in a 1 ml syringe NDC # 0033-2434-40
— 60 mg: 30 mg/ml in a 2 ml syringe NDC # 0033-2444-40

How To Store
Store at room temperature and avoid exposure to intense light or humidity.

▷ **Recommended Dosage Ranges (Actual dosage and administration schedule must be determined by the physician for each patient individually.)**
Infants and Children: Not indicated for use.
12 to 60 Years of Age: 10 mg orally as needed for pain relief every 4 to 6 hours. Doses of 10 mg QID (four times daily) are not recommended long-term. When used for pain, it is best taken every 4 to 6 hours instead of taking it only when the pain returns. Maximum total daily IM or IV dose is 120 mg. Maximum total daily oral dose is 40 mg.
Over 65 Years of Age: Use of 5 to 10 mg every 6 hours—that is, the lowest effective dose given at the longest effective dosing interval is recommended. For patients who are over 65 and who weigh less than 110 pounds (50 kg) or have compromised kidneys, the maximum daily dose (IV or IM) is 60 mg.

Conditions Requiring Dosing Adjustments
Liver function: Should be used with caution in patients with liver impairment.
Kidney function: Ketorolac and similar drugs may further damage impaired kidneys, and must be used as a benefit to risk decision.

▷ **Dosing Instructions:** This drug can be taken with food or milk to help decrease stomach upset. This may, however, delay the peak pain relieving effect.

Usual Duration of Use: Ketorolac can only be used for five days when it is used intramuscularly. Oral ketorolac is indicated for limited duration (5 days) treatment of pain. Prolonged therapy, especially with the intramuscular injection can increase the frequency of side effects by 10–50%. Current labeling says that a total of 5 days is the maximum duration of therapy.

For example, if a patient receives one day of intravenous ketorolac, he or she can then only receive 4 days of oral therapy.

Possible Advantages of This Drug
Effective oral treatment of pain while avoiding the abuse or dependence potential and respiratory depression which can be seen with narcotic use.

Currently a "Drug of Choice"
for treatment of mild to moderate pain in people (with normal renal function) prone to the abuse potential of narcotics or who have lung disease, which would increase risk of narcotics respiratory depression.

▷ **This Drug Should Not Be Taken If**
- you have had an allergic reaction to any form of it previously.
- you have had an allergic reaction to any of the components of a ketorolac tablet.
- you have had an allergic reaction to aspirin or other NSAIDs.
- you have the partial or complete syndrome of angioedema, nasal polyps, bronchospastic activity (asthma) or other allergic reactions to NSAIDS.
- you have a history of or have active ulcer disease or gastrointestinal bleeding.
- you have a bleeding disorder or a blood cell disorder.
- your kidneys are seriously compromised.
- there is a suspicion of cerebrovascular bleeding.
- you are dehydrated (volume depleted).
- you are breast-feeding your infant.
- you are in labor or are delivering your baby.
- you are scheduled for major surgery.
- you take NSAIDs (see Drug Classes). Ask your doctor or pharmacist.

▷ **Inform Your Physician Before Taking This Drug If**
- you are pregnant or plan to become pregnant.
- you are allergic to aspirin or other NSAIDs.
- you have a history of ulcer disease or any type of bleeding problem.
- you have impaired kidney or liver function.
- you have high blood pressure or heart failure.
- you take: Valproic acid, methotrexate, probenecid, oral hypoglycemic agents, furosemide, anticoagulants or lithium.
- you are an alcoholic.
- you have systemic lupus erythematosus (SLE).
- you are uncertain of how much to take or when to take this medicine.

Possible Side-Effects (natural, expected and unavoidable drug actions)
Edema (fluid retention) and weight gain, dry mouth, headache, light headedness (low blood pressure).

▷ **Possible Adverse Effects** (unusual, unexpected and infrequent reactions)
If any of the following develop, consult your physician promptly for guidance.
Mild Adverse Effects
Allergic Reactions: Skin rash, itching, and swelling of the face or extremities.

Headache (17%), drowsiness or somnolence (3–14%), nervousness and abnormal dreams (1–4%), mouth sores (3–9%), nausea (12), diarrhea (3–9%), and increased sweating (3–9%).

Paresthesias (2%).

Ringing in the ears (tinitis).

Serious Adverse Effects

Allergic Reactions: Asthma, difficulty breathing, Stevens Johnson syndrome (a potentially fatal fulminant rash with high fever and Lyell syndrome.)

Tachycardia (fast heartbeat) and hypertension (rare).

Tachypnia (rapid breathing) and prostration.

Mental depression (rare).

Gastrointestinal ulceration and bleeding (1% or less).

Kidney damage with bloody urine, decreased urine formation and painful urination (1% or less).

Liver damage (rare).

▷ **Possible Effects on Sexual Function:** None reported.

Possible Delayed Adverse Effects: Mild anemia due to "silent" blood loss from the stomach. Peptic or duodenal ulceration. Positive stool occult blood. Kidney toxicity.

▷ **Adverse Effects That May Mimic Natural Diseases or Disorders**

Flank pain caused by drug induced acute renal failure may mimic urinary tract infection symptoms. Liver reaction may suggest viral hepatitis. Positive stool occult blood may mimic a variety of gastrointestinal disorders.

Natural Diseases or Disorders That May Be Activated by This Drug

Ulcerative colitis, peptic ulcer disease, asthma, clotting disorders.

Possible Effects on Laboratory Tests

Complete blood counts: decreased red cells, hemoglobin and hematocrit, white blood cell count and platelets.

Prothrobin time: may be increased if ketorolac is used with coumadin.

Bleeding time: can be prolonged for 24 to 48 hours after ketorolac is stopped.

Urinalysis: hematuria (blood in urine) and proteinuria (protein in urine).

Liver function tests: increased SGPT, and SGOT. Increased bilirubin may occur with progression of or more involved liver damage.

Kidney function tests: increased BUN (blood urea nitrogen) and creatinine.

Lithium levels: We recommend increased checks of lithium levels as other drugs of the same class have caused increased lithium levels.

Stool occult blood: This test may become positive.

CAUTION

1. This drug may hide early signs of infection. Inform your physician if you think you are developing an infection of any kind.
2. Long term use of oral ketorolac is associated with adverse gastrointestinal effects and is not recommended.
3. The probability of serious adverse effects increases with doses greater than 40 mg PO (by mouth) daily.
4. The bleeding time can be increased for 24 to 48 hours after ketorolac has been stopped.
5. Ketorolac should not be used before surgery since platelet (a blood component important to clotting) function is inhibited and sedation and anxiety may be increased.

6. Ketorolac should not be used in obstetrics because prostaglandin inhibition may affect fetal circulation and uterine contraction.
7. Do not take this medicine with other NSAIDs. Additive adverse effects can occur.
8. If you take lithium and ketorolac at the same time, lithium levels should be checked more frequently.

Precautions for Use
By Infants and Children:
Safety and effectiveness for those under 12 years of age are not established.
By Those over 65 Years of Age: An increased risk of gastrointestinal toxicity has not been clearly established, however, older patients are more likely to experience serious consequences from NSAID-induced (nonsteroidal anti-inflammatory drug—such as ketorolac) intestinal ulceration or bleeding. For these reasons, we recommend that ketorolac be used with caution and in the lower end of the defined dosing ranges.

▷ **Advisability of Use During Pregnancy**
Pregnancy Category: C. See Pregnancy Code at the back of this book.
Animal studies: Studies conducted in rabbits and rats did not reveal teratogenicity to the fetus. Oral doses administered after the seventeenth gestational day in rats caused dystocia and higher pup mortality.
Human studies: Adequate studies of pregnant women are not available. Ask your physician for guidance.

Advisability of Use if Breast-Feeding
Presence of this drug in breast milk: Yes.
Watch infant closely and discontinue drug or nursing if adverse effects develop.

Habit-Forming Potential: Although ketorolac is an analgesic (pain relieving medicine), it is not a narcotic and has not shown tolerance, physical dependence or any withdrawal upon abrupt discontinuation.

Effects of Overdosage: Single oral doses greater than 100mg/kg in mice, rats and monkeys has caused: Decreased activity, pallor, diarrhea, vomiting and labored breathing.

Possible Effects of Long-Term Use: Not indicated for long term use as the adverse effects may increase in incidence and severity.

Suggested Periodic Examinations While Taking This Drug (at physician's discretion)
Liver and kidney function tests. Complete blood counts.

▷ **While Taking This Drug, Observe the Following**
Foods: No restrictions, however the time it takes for ketorolac to reach its peak effect may be delayed if you take it with food.
Beverages: No restrictions, may be taken with milk.
▷ *Alcohol:* Additive sedation may occur. Additive irritation of the lining of the stomach or intestine can occur. Use of this drug with alcohol is not recommended.
Tobacco Smoking: No interactions expected, however smoking may make you more susceptible to the stomach and intestine irritating effect of ketorolac.
Marijuana Smoking: May cause additive drowsiness.

▷ *Other Drugs*
Ketorolac may *increase* the effects of
- anticoagulants such as coumadin or heparin.
- insulin and oral hypoglycemic agents.
- lithium and cause lithium toxicity.
- muscle relaxants such as pancuronium.
- nifedipine or verapamil.
- thrombolytic agents such as streptokinase or TPA.

Ketorolac may *decrease* the effects of
- antihypertensive (high blood pressure medication) such as beta blockers and captopril.
- diuretics such as hydrochlorothiazide.

Ketorolac *taken concurrently* with
- acetaminophen (Tylenol) can increase the risk of adverse kidney effects.
- alcohol, aspirin, methotrexate, steroids or potassium supplements may increase the risk of gastrointestinal side effects including ulceration and hemorrhage.
- gold compounds may increase renal (kidney) toxicity.
- other NSAIDS such as indomethacin can increase the risk of toxicity.
- probenecid may result in ketorolac toxicity.
- the following medications may increase the risk of bleeding: Aspirin, diflunisal, dipyridamole, sulfinpyrazone and valproic acid.

▷ *Driving, Hazardous Activities:* This drug may cause drowsiness and dizziness. Restrict activities as necessary.

Aviation Note: The use of this drug *may be a disqualification* for piloting. Consult a designated Aviation Medical Examiner.

Exposure to Sun: Use caution, and minimize exposure time if you appear to be more sensitive than usual. Report any change in tolerance of sun exposure to your doctor, and he or she will report this to the FDA.

Occurrence of Unrelated Illness: Sudden worsening of asthma or acute swelling of the ankles should be reported to your doctor promptly.

Discontinuation: This drug should only be used short-term. This drug should be stopped, and prompt medical evaluation made if there is: Sudden occurrence of bleeding from the nose or gums, flank pain and decreased urination, black or tarry stools, difficulty breathing, and skin rash with or without sloughing of the skin.

This medication is also discussed in the acetic acid nonsteroidal anti-inflammatory drug profile.

LABETALOL (la BET a lohl)

Introduced: 1978 **Prescription:** USA: Yes; Canada: Yes **Available as Generic:** No **Class:** Antihypertensive, alpha- and beta-adrenergic blocker **Controlled Drug:** USA: No; Canada: No

Brand Names: Normodyne, Normozide [CD], Trandate, Trandate HCT [CD]

Labetalol

BENEFITS versus RISKS	
Possible Benefits	*Possible Risks*
EFFECTIVE, WELL-TOLERATED ANTIHYPERTENSIVE in mild to moderate high blood pressure	CONGESTIVE HEART FAILURE in advanced heart disease
	Worsening of angina in coronary heart disease (if drug is abruptly withdrawn)
	Masking of low blood sugar (hypoglycemia) in drug-treated diabetes
	Liver toxicity

▷ **Principal Uses**

As a Single Drug Product: Uses currently included in FDA approved labeling: (1) Therapy of mild to moderate high blood pressure. May be used alone in combination.

Other (unlabeled) generally acepted uses: (1) Combination therapy of hypertension in heart attacks (acute MI); (2) treatment of cocaine overdose; (3) therapy of phobic anxiety reactions; (4) treatment of angina; (5) therapy of pheochromocytoma, a tumor that releases compounds which increase blood pressure.

How This Drug Works: By blocking part of the sympathetic nervous system, this drug
- reduces the rate and contraction force of the heart, thus lowering the ejection pressure of blood leaving the heart.
- reduces the degree of contraction of blood vessel walls, resulting in their expansion and lowering of blood pressure.

Available Dosage Forms and Strengths
Injection — 5 mg per ml
Tablets — 100 mg, 200 mg, 300 mg

▷ **Usual Adult Dosage Range:** Initially, 100 mg twice daily, 12 hours apart; the dose may be increased by 100 mg twice daily every 2 to 3 days as needed to reduce blood pressure. The usual maintenance dose is 200 to 400 mg twice daily. Maximum daily dose is 2400 mg/24 hours, given as 800 mg 3 times daily. **Note: Actual dose and dosing schedule must be determined individually by your doctor.**

Conditions Requiring Dosing Adjustments
Liver function: The dose **must** be decreased in patients with compromised livers. It is also a rare cause of severe liver (hepatocellular) injury.
Kidney function: Decreased doses are not thought to be needed in kidney compromise.

▷ **Dosing Instructions:** The tablet may be crushed and is best taken at the same times daily, ideally following morning and evening meals. Do not abruptly stop this drug.

Usual Duration of Use: Use on a regular schedule for 10 to 14 days determines effectiveness in lowering blood pressure. Long-term use (months to years) of this drug will be determined by your individual response to an overall treatment program (weight reduction, salt restriction, smoking cessation, etc.).

Possible Advantages of This Drug
Decreases blood pressure more promptly than other beta blocker drugs. Can be used to treat hypertensive emergencies.

▷ **This Drug Should Not Be Taken If**
- you have had an allergic reaction to it previously.
- you have active bronchial asthma.
- you have congestive heart failure.
- you are in cardiogenic shock.
- you have an abnormally slow heart rate or a serious form of heart block.

▷ **Inform Your Physician Before Taking This Drug If**
- you have had an adverse reaction to any beta blocker drug (see Drug Class Section).
- you have a history of serious heart disease.
- you have a history of hay fever (allergic rhinitis), asthma, chronic bronchitis or emphysema.
- you have a history of overactive thyroid function (hyperthyroidism).
- you have a history of low blood sugar (hypoglycemia).
- you are a diabetic.
- you have a history of spasms of the bronchi of the lungs.
- you have impaired liver or kidney function.
- you have intermittent claudication.
- you have diabetes or myasthenia gravis.
- you take any form of digitalis, quinidine or reserpine, or any calcium blocker drug (see Drug Classes).
- you plan to have surgery under general anesthesia in the near future.

Possible Side-Effects (natural, expected and unavoidable drug actions)
Lethargy and fatigability (11%), light-headedness in upright position (see Orthostatic Hypotension in Glossary).

▷ **Possible Adverse Effects** (unusual, unexpected and infrequent reactions)
If any of the following develop, consult your physician promptly for guidance.

Mild Adverse Effects
Allergic Reactions: Skin rash, itching.
Headache, drowsiness, dizziness (20%), scalp tingling (during early treatment).
Urine retention, difficulty urinating.
Vivid dreams, nightmares, depression.
Indigestion, nausea, diarrhea.
Joint and muscle discomfort, fluid retention (edema).

Serious Adverse Effects
Chest pain, shortness of breath, precipitation of congestive heart failure.
Induction of bronchial asthma (in asthmatic individuals).
Elevated blood glucose.
Lichen planus.
Abnormally low blood pressure on standing (postural hypotension).
Muscle toxicity (toxic myopathy).

542   Labetalol

Drug-induced systemic lupus erythematosus.
Aggravation of myasthenia gravis.
Liver damage with jaundice (rare).
Difficult urination (urinary bladder retention).

▷ **Possible Effects on Sexual Function**

Impotence (10%), inhibited ejaculation (10%), prolonged erection following orgasm (related to higher doses), Peyronie's disease (see Glossary).

Decreased vaginal secretions (with low doses), inhibited female orgasm (related to higher doses).

Possible Effects on Laboratory Tests

None reported.

CAUTION

1. ***Do not stop this drug suddenly*** without the knowledge and help of your doctor. Carry a note or wear a labetalol drug identification bracelet.
2. Ask your physician or pharmacist before using nasal decongestants usually present in over-the-counter cold preparations and nose drops. These can cause sudden increases in blood pressure if combined with labetalol.
3. Report the development of any tendency to emotional depression.

Precautions for Use

By Infants and Children: Safety and effectiveness for those under 12 years of age not established. However, if this drug is used, watch for low blood sugar (hypoglycemia) during periods of reduced food intake.

By Those over 60 Years of Age: Proceed *cautiously* with all antihypertensive drugs. Therapy should be started with small doses, with frequent checks of blood pressure. Sudden, rapid or excessive lowering of blood pressure can increase stroke or heart attack risk. Watch for dizziness, unsteadiness, tendency to fall, confusion, hallucinations, depression or urinary frequency.

▷ **Advisability of Use During Pregnancy**

Pregnancy Category: C. See Pregnancy Code at the back of this book.
Animal studies: No significant increase in birth defects found in rats or rabbits; some increase in fetal deaths reported.
Human studies: Adequate studies of pregnant women are not available.
Use this drug only if clearly needed. Ask physician for guidance.

Advisability of Use if Breast-Feeding

Presence of this drug in breast milk: Yes, in very small amounts.
Avoid drug or refrain from nursing.

Habit-Forming Potential: None.

Effects of Overdosage: Weakness, slow pulse, low blood pressure, fainting, cold and sweaty skin, congestive heart failure, possible coma and convulsions.

Possible Effects of Long-Term Use: Reduced heart reserve and eventual heart failure in susceptible individuals with advanced heart disease.

Suggested Periodic Examinations While Taking This Drug (at physician's discretion)

Measurements of blood pressure, evaluation of heart function.

▷ **While Taking This Drug, Observe the Following**
  Foods: May increase the absorption of labetalol and result in a larger than expected blood level. Patients taking this medicine should also avoid excessive salt intake.
  Beverages: No restrictions. May be taken with milk.
▷ *Alcohol:* Use with caution. Alcohol may exaggerate this drug's ability to lower blood pressure and may increase its mild sedative effect.
  Tobacco Smoking: Nicotine may reduce this drug's effectiveness in treating high blood pressure, and increase brochial constriction seen in regular smokers.
▷ *Other Drugs*
  Labetalol may *increase* the effects of
  - oral hypoglycemic agents (see Drug Class) and prolong recovery from any hypoglycemia (low blood sugar) which may occur.
  - other antihypertensive drugs and cause excessive lowering of blood pressure. Dosage adjustments may be necessary.

  Labetalol *taken concurrently* with
  - amiodarone may result in extremely slow heart rates and cardiac arrest.
  - cimetidine (Tagamet) and cause elevated labetalol levels and low blood pressure or heart rate.
  - clonidine (Catapres) must be closely watched for rebound high blood pressure if clonidine is withdrawn while labetalol is still being taken.
  - epinephrine may result in severe increases in blood pressure.
  - imipramine and other tricyclic antidepressants (TCAs) may result in increases in antidepressant blood levels and toxicity.
  - insulin must be watched for development of hypoglycemia (see Glossary).
  - NSAIDs may result in blunting of the therapeutic effect of labetalol.
▷ *Driving, Hazardous Activities:* Use caution until the full extent of fatigue, dizziness and blood pressure change has been determined.
  Aviation Note: The use of this drug *is a disqualification* for piloting. Consult a designated Aviation Medical Examiner.
  Exposure to Sun: No restrictions.
  Exposure to Heat: Caution advised. Hot environments can lower the blood pressure and exaggerate the effects of this drug.
  Exposure to Cold: Caution advised. Cold environments can increase blood flow problems in the extremities that may occur with beta blocker drugs. The elderly should take precautions to prevent hypothermia (see Glossary).
  Heavy Exercise or Exertion: It is advisable to avoid exertion that produces light-headedness, excessive fatigue or muscle cramping. The use of this drug may intensify the hypertensive response to isometric exercise.
  Occurrence of Unrelated Illness: Fever can lower the blood pressure and require decreased doses. Nausea or vomiting may interrupt scheduled doses. Ask your doctor for help.
  Discontinuation: If possible, gradual reduction of dose over a period of 2 to 3 weeks is recommended. Ask your physician for specific guidance.

LAMOTRIGINE (Lamb OH tri jean)

Introduced: 1995 **Prescription:** USA: Yes; Canada: Yes **Available as**
Generic: USA: No **Class:** Anticonvulsant, phenyltriazine **Controlled**
Drug: USA: No; Canada: No
Brand Names: Lamictal

Available Dosage Forms and Strengths
Tablets — 25 mg, 100 mg, 150 mg, 200 mg
Author's note: This profile will be further developed in subsequent editions of this book as more data become available.

LANSOPRAZOLE (Lan SO pra soul)

Introduced: 1995 **Prescription:** USA: Yes; Canada: Yes **Available as**
Generic: USA: No; Canada: No **Class:** Antiulcer, proton pump inhibitor
Controlled Drug: USA: No; Canada: No
Brand Names: Prevacid

BENEFITS versus RISKS	
Possible Benefits	*Possible Risks*
VERY EFFECTIVE TREATMENT OF CONDITIONS ASSOCIATED WITH EXCESSIVE PRODUCTION OF STOMACH (GASTRIC) ACID: ZOLLINGER-ELLISON SYNDROME, MASTOCYTOSIS ENDOCRINE ADENOMA VERY EFFECTIVE TREATMENT OF REFLUX ESOPHAGITIS VERY EFFECTIVE TREATMENT OF DUODENAL ULCER	Rare liver enzyme increases Rare protein in the urine

▷ **Principal Uses**
As a Single Drug Product: Uses currently included in FDA approved labeling: (1) Used to treat duodenal ulcers; (2) treats erosive esophagitis; (3) used in syndromes (such as Zollinger-Ellison) where excessive amounts of stomach acid are produced.
Other (unlabeled) generally accepted uses: (1) Treatment of gastric ulcers.

How This Drug Works: This drug inhibits a specific enzyme system (the H/K adenosine triphosphate) in the stomach (parietal cells) lining and stops the production of stomach acid. It thereby:
(1) eliminates the principal cause of the condition under treatment.
(2) creates an environment conducive to healing.

Available Dosage Forms and Strengths
Capsules — 15 mg 30 mg

▷ **Recommended Dosage Ranges (Actual dosage and administration schedule must be determined by the physician for each patient individually.)**
Infants and Children: Not studied in this age group.

18 to 60 Years of Age: For duodenal ulcer:
15 mg daily, taken before a meal. Four weeks of therapy are indicated.
For erosive esophagitis:
30 mg daily, taken before a meal. Up to eight weeks of treatment can be given. If healing does not occur, an additional 8 weeks may be considered.
For excessive acid production syndromes:
Dosing is started at 60 mg daily. The dose is increased as needed and tolerated. Doses up to 90 mg twice daily have been used.
Over 60 Years of Age: Same as 18 to 60 years of age.

Conditions Requiring Dosing Adjustments
Liver function: Decreases in doses should be considered.
Kidney function: No dosing changes needed.
Author's note: Since this medication has only been recently approved, further information will be provided in subsequent editions of this book.

LEVODOPA (lee voh DOH pa)

Introduced: 1967 **Prescription:** USA: Yes; Canada: Yes **Available as Generic:** USA: Yes; Canada: No **Class:** Antiparkinsonism **Controlled Drug:** USA: No; Canada: No

Brand Names: Bendopa, Dopar, Larodopa, ◆Prolopa [CD], Sinemet [CD], Sinemet CR [CD]

BENEFITS versus RISKS	
Possible Benefits	*Possible Risks*
EFFECTIVE RELIEF OF SYMPTOMS IN 80% OF CASES OF IDIOPATHIC PARKINSON'S DISEASE	Emotional depression, confusion, abnormal thinking and behavior Abnormal involuntary movements Heart rhythm disturbance Urinary bladder retention Induction of peptic ulcer (rare) Blood abnormalities: hemolytic anemia, reduced white blood cell count (both rare)

▷ **Principal Uses**
As a Single Drug Product: Uses currently included in FDA approved labeling: (1) Treats the major types of Parkinson's disease: paralysis agitans ("shaking palsy" of unknown cause), the type that follows encephalitis, the parkinsonism that develops with aging (associated with hardening of the brain arteries), and the forms of parkinsonism that follow poisoning by carbon monoxide or manganese.
Other (unlabeled) generally accepted uses: (1) May have a limited role in treating catatonic stupor; (2) can improve conscious level in coma caused by liver failure.
As a Combination Drug Product [CD]: This drug is available in combination with carbidopa, a chemical that prevents the breakdown of levodopa before it reaches its site of action. The addition of carbidopa reduces

Levodopa

levodopa requirements by 75%, and also decreases the frequency and severity of adverse effects.

How This Drug Works: Levodopa enters the brain tissue and is converted to dopamine. After sufficient dosage, this corrects the dopamine deficiency (thought to be the cause of parkinsonism) and restores a more normal brain chemistry.

Carbidopa blocks an enzyme (decarboxylase) that degrades levodopa before it reaches the brain. This allows a lower dose to have a greater benefit. Products containing carbidopa also have fewer adverse effects.

Available Dosage Forms and Strengths

Capsules — 100 mg, 250 mg, 500 mg
Tablets — 100 mg, 250 mg, 500 mg
Tablets, Sinemet — 10-100 mg, 25-100 mg, 25-250 mg
Tablets, Sinemet CR, sustained-release — 50-200 mg

▷ **Usual Adult Dosage Range:** Initially, 250 mg 2 to 4 times/day. The dose may be increased cautiously by increments of 100 to 750 mg at 3- to 7-day intervals as needed and tolerated. The total dosage should not exceed 8000 mg/24 hours. If the combination drug Sinemet is used, the total levodopa requirement will be considerably less. **Note: Actual dosage and administration schedule must be determined by the physician for each patient individually.**

Conditions Requiring Dosing Adjustments

Liver function: Dosing changes are not indicated in liver compromise.

Kidney function: Possible urine retention requires that patients with urine outflow problems should be closely watched. No dose decreases needed in kidney failure.

▷ **Dosing Instructions:** The tablet may be crushed and is best taken with or following carbohydrate foods to reduce stomach upset; when possible, do not take this drug with high-protein foods. Sustained-release tablet (Sinemet CR) may be cut in half, but it should not be crushed or chewed.

Usual Duration of Use: Use on a regular schedule for 3 to 6 weeks determines effectiveness in relieving the major symptoms of parkinsonism. Maximal effectiveness may require continual use for 6 months. Long-term use (months to years) requires physician supervision and periodic evaluation.

Possible Advantages of This Drug

The slow-release formulation of Sinemet CR allows a 25% to 50% reduction in dosing frequency. The wearing-off phenomenon and end-of-dose failure seen with standard Sinemet may be reduced or eliminated.

▷ **This Drug Should Not Be Taken If**
- you are allergic to any of the drugs bearing the brand names listed.
- you have narrow-angle glaucoma (inadequately controlled).
- you have a history of melanoma.
- you are taking, or have taken within the past 14 days, any monoamine oxidase (MAO) type A inhibitor drug (see Drug Class Section).

▷ **Inform Your Physician Before Taking This Drug If**
- you have diabetes, epilepsy, heart disease, high blood pressure or chronic lung disease.

- you have impaired liver or kidney function.
- you have problems making blood (hematopoiesis).
- you are taking medicines for blood pressure.
- you have had a heart attack and have some abnormal heart rhythms.
- you have a history of depression or other mental illness.
- you have a history of peptic ulcer disease or malignant melanoma.
- you plan to have surgery under general anesthesia in the near future.

Possible Side-Effects (natural, expected and unavoidable drug actions)
Fatigue, lethargy, altered taste, offensive body odor, orthostatic hypotension (see Glossary).
Pink to red colored urine, which turns black on exposure to air (of no significance).

▷ **Possible Adverse Effects** (unusual, unexpected and infrequent reactions)
If any of the following develop, consult your physician promptly for guidance.

Mild Adverse Effects
Allergic Reactions: Skin rash, itching.
Headache, dizziness, numbness, unsteadiness, insomnia, nightmares, blurred vision, double vision.
Loss of appetite, nausea, vomiting, dry mouth, difficult swallowing, excessive gas, diarrhea, constipation.
Loss of hair (rare).

Serious Adverse Effects
Idiosyncratic Reactions: Hemolytic anemia (see Glossary). Neuroleptic malignant syndrome (see Glossary).
Confusion, delusions, hallucinations, agitation, paranoia, depression, psychotic episodes, seizures.
Low blood pressure on standing (orthostatic hypotension).
Increased blood pressure.
Congestive heart failure (rare).
Mania (rare).
Abnormal involuntary movements of the head, face and extremities.
Disturbances of heart rhythm, high blood pressure (rare).
Development of peptic ulcer, gastrointestinal bleeding.
Urinary bladder retention.
Low blood platelets (rare).
Low white blood cell count—increased infection risk, fever, sore throat.

▷ **Possible Effects on Sexual Function:** Increased libido reported by both males and females (24% to 36%); inhibited ejaculation (rare); priapism (see Glossary).

▷ **Adverse Effects That May Mimic Natural Diseases or Disorders**
Mental reactions may resemble idiopathic psychosis.

Natural Diseases or Disorders That May Be Activated by This Drug
Latent peptic ulcer.

Possible Effects on Laboratory Tests
Complete blood cell counts: occasionally decreased white cells; occasionally increased eosinophils (without symptoms).
Blood thyroxine (T_4) level: increased.

Urine sugar tests: no effect with TesTape; false negative with Clinistix; false positive with Clinitest.

Urine ketone tests: false positive with Ketostix and Phenistix.

CAUTION
1. Advisable to begin treatment with small doses, and to increase dosage gradually until the desired response is achieved.
2. As improvement occurs, avoid excessive and hurried activity (which often causes falls and injury).

Precautions for Use

By Infants and Children: This drug can cause precocious puberty when taken by the prepubertal boy. Watch for hypersexual behavior and for premature growth of genital organs.

By Those over 60 Years of Age: Therapy should start with half the usual adult dose; and dose increases should be made in small increments as needed and tolerated. Watch for significant behavioral changes: Depression or inappropriate elation, acute confusion, agitation, paranoia, dementia, nightmares and hallucinations. Abnormal involuntary movements may also occur.

▷ **Advisability of Use During Pregnancy**

Pregnancy Category: C. See Pregnancy Code at the back of this book.

Animal studies: Significant birth defects reported in rodent studies.

Human studies: Adequate studies of pregnant women are not available.

Avoid use of drug during the first 3 months. Use only if clearly needed during the last 6 months.

Advisability of Use if Breast-Feeding

Presence of this drug in breast milk: Yes.

Avoid drug or refrain from nursing.

Habit-Forming Potential: None.

Effects of Overdosage: Muscle twitching, spastic closure of eyelids, nausea, vomiting, diarrhea, weakness, fainting, confusion, agitation, hallucinations.

Possible Effects of Long-Term Use: Development of abnormal involuntary movements involving the head, face, mouth and extremities. May be reversible and gradually subside as the drug is withdrawn.

Suggested Periodic Examinations While Taking This Drug (at physician's discretion)

Complete blood cell counts; measurements of internal eye pressure; blood pressure measurements in lying, sitting and standing positions.

▷ **While Taking This Drug, Observe the Following**

Foods: Insofar as possible, do not take concurrently with protein foods; proteins compete for absorption.

Nutritional Support: If taken alone (without carbidopa), watch for tingling of the extremities (peripheral neuritis). Small (10 mg or less) doses of pyridoxine (vitamin B-6) may help. Larger doses can decrease the effectiveness of levodopa. If taking Sinemet, supplemental pyridoxine is not required.

Beverages: No restrictions. May be taken with milk.

▷ *Alcohol:* No interactions expected.

Tobacco Smoking: No interactions expected.

Marijuana Smoking: Increased fatigue and lethargy; possible accentuation of orthostatic hypotension (see Glossary).
▷ *Other Drugs*
Levodopa **taken concurrently** with
- monoamine oxidase (MAO) type A inhibitor drugs (see Drug Class Section) can cause a dangerous rise in blood pressure and body temperature. Do not combine these drugs.

The following drugs may **decrease** the effects of levodopa
- chlordiazepoxide (Librium) or other benzodiazepines (see Drug Classes).
- iron salts.
- papaverine (Cerespan, Pavabid, Vasospan, etc.).
- phenytoin (Dilantin, etc.).
- pyridoxine (vitamin B-6).
- tricyclic antidepressants (see Drug Classes).

▷ *Driving, Hazardous Activities:* This drug may cause dizziness, impaired vision and orthostatic hypotension. Restrict activities as necessary.

Aviation Note: Parkinson's disease **is a disqualification** for piloting. Consult a designated Aviation Medical Examiner.

Exposure to Sun: No restrictions.

Exposure to Heat: Use caution. This drug can cause flushing and excessive sweating and predispose to heat exhaustion.

Occurrence of Unrelated Illness: Dark-colored skin lesions should be evaluated carefully by your doctor as they may be malignant melanoma. White blood cell counts should be closely followed if you develop an infection.

LEVOTHYROXINE (lee voh thi ROX een)

Other Names: L-thyroxine, thyroxine, T-4

Introduced: 1953 **Prescription:** USA: Yes; Canada: Yes **Available as Generic:** USA: Yes; Canada: No **Class:** Thyroid hormones **Controlled Drug:** USA: No; Canada: No

Brand Names: ✦Eltroxin, Euthroid [CD], L-Thyroxine, Levothroid, Levoxine, Syroxine, Synthroid, Thyrolar [CD], Thyroid USP

BENEFITS versus RISKS	
Possible Benefits	*Possible Risks*
EFFECTIVE REPLACEMENT THERAPY IN STATES OF THYROID HORMONE DEFICIENCY (HYPOTHYROIDISM)	Intensification of angina in presence of coronary artery disease
	Drug-induced hyperthyroidism (with excessive dosage)
EFFECTIVE TREATMENT OF SIMPLE GOITER AND CHRONIC THYROIDITIS	Spasm of the coronary vessels (rare)
EFFECTIVE TREATMENT OF THYROID GLAND CANCER	

▷ **Principal Uses**
As a Single Drug Product: Uses currently included in FDA approved labeling:
(1) Replacement therapy to correct thyroid deficiency (hypothyroidism);

Levothyroxine

(2) Treatment of simple (nonendemic) goiter and benign thyroid nodules; (3) Treatment of Hashimoto's thyroiditis; (4) Adjunctive prevention and treatment of thyroid cancer.

Other (unlabeled) generally accepted uses: (1) Helps amenorrhea caused (secondary to) low thyroid function; (2) may be helpful in helping fetal lung tissue mature in babies expected to be premature; (3) treatment of Grave's disease.

As a Combination Drug Product [CD]: This thyroid hormone is available in combination with the other principal thyroid hormone, liothyronine, in a preparation (generic name: liotrix) that resembles the natural hormone material produced by the thyroid gland.

How This Drug Works: By altering cellular chemistry that stores energy in an inactive (reserve) form, this drug makes more energy available and increases the rate of cellular metabolism of all tissues throughout the body. Thyroid hormones are essential to normal growth and development, especially the development of the infant's brain and nervous system.

Available Dosage Forms and Strengths
Injections — 100 mcg per ml and 500 mcg per ml
Tablets — 0.0125 mg, 0.025 mg, 0.05 mg, 0.075 mg, 0.1 mg, 0.112 mg, 0.125 mg, 0.15 mg, 0.175 mg, 0.2 mg, 0.3 mg

▷ **Recommended Dosage Ranges** (Actual dosage and administration schedule must be determined by the physician for each patient individually.)

Infants and Children: Up to 6 months of age—5 to 6 mcg/kg of body weight, in a single daily dose.
6 to 12 months of age—5 to 6 mcg/kg of body weight, in a single daily dose.
1 to 5 years of age—3 to 5 mcg/kg of body weight, in a single daily dose.
6 to 10 years of age—4 to 5 mcg/kg of body weight, in a single daily dose.
Over 10 years of age—2 to 3 mcg/kg of body weight, in a single daily dose, until the usual adult daily dose is reached: 150 to 200 mcg.

12 to 60 Years of Age: Starts at 0.05 mg as a single daily dose; increased by 0.025 to 0.05 mg at intervals of 2 to 3 weeks as needed and tolerated. Usual maintenance dose is 0.075 to 0.125 mg/day. Total daily dosage should not exceed 0.3 mg.

Over 60 Years of Age: Initially 0.0125 to 0.025 mg as a single daily dose; increase gradually at intervals of 3 to 4 weeks, as needed and tolerated. The usual maintenance dose is approximately 0.075 mg daily.

Conditions Requiring Dosing Adjustments
Liver function: Dosing changes are not indicated in patients with liver compromise.
Kidney function: Dosing changes are not indicated in kidney compromise.

▷ **Dosing Instructions:** The tablets may be crushed and are best taken in the morning on an empty stomach to ensure maximal absorption and uniform results.

Usual Duration of Use: Use on a regular schedule for 4 to 6 weeks determines effectiveness in correcting the symptoms of thyroid deficiency. Long-term use (months to years, possibly for life) requires physician supervision.

Currently a "Drug of Choice"
for the treatment of hypothyroidism.

Levothyroxine

▷ **This Drug Should Not Be Taken If**
- you have had an allergic reaction to it previously.
- you are recovering from a heart attack; ask your doctor for help.
- you have an adrenal insufficiency which has not been corrected.
- you are using it to lose weight and your thyroid function is normal (no deficiency).

▷ **Inform Your Physician Before Taking This Drug If**
- you have high blood pressure, any form of heart disease or diabetes.
- you have a history of Addison's disease or adrenal gland deficiency.
- you are taking any antiasthmatic medications.
- you are taking an anticoagulant.

Possible Side-Effects (natural, expected and unavoidable drug actions)
None if dosage is adjusted correctly.

▷ **Possible Adverse Effects** (unusual, unexpected and infrequent reactions)
If any of the following develop, consult your physician promptly for guidance.

Mild Adverse Effects
Allergic Reactions: Skin rash, hives.
Headache in sensitive individuals, even with proper dosage adjustment.

Serious Adverse Effects
Increased frequency or intensity of angina in people with coronary artery disease.
Spasm of the arteries which supply blood to the heart (rare).
Seizures.
Pseudotumor cerebri (rare).
Drug-induced porphyria (rare.
Decrease in IgA immune concentration.
May be a part of the development of osteoporosis.
Drug-induced Myasthenia Gravis (rare).
Note: Other adverse effects are manifestations of excessive dosage. See Effects of Overdosage category.

▷ **Possible Effects on Sexual Function**
Altered menstrual pattern during dosage adjustments.
Possibly beneficial in treating impaired sexual function that is associated with true hypothyroidism.

Natural Diseases or Disorders That May Be Activated by This Drug
Latent coronary artery insufficiency (angina), diabetes.

Possible Effects on Laboratory Tests
Prothrombin time: increased (when taken concurrently with warfarin).
Blood total cholesterol, HDL and LDL cholesterol levels: decreased.
Blood triglyceride levels: no effect.
Blood glucose level: increased.
Blood thyroid hormone levels: increased T_3, T_4 and free T_4.
Blood thyroid stimulating hormone (TSH) level: decreased.

CAUTION
1. Careful supervision of individual response is needed to identify correct dosage. Do not change dosing without asking your physician.
2. This drug should not be used to treat nonspecific fatigue, obesity, infer-

tility or slow growth. Such use is inappropriate and could be harmful.

Precautions for Use

By Infants and Children: Thyroid-deficient children often require higher doses than adults. Transient hair loss may occur during the early months of treatment. Follow the child's response to thyroid therapy by periodic measurements of bone age, growth, mental and physical development.

By Those over 60 Years of Age: Usually, requirements for thyroid hormone replacement are about 25% lower than in younger adults. Watch closely for any indications of toxicity.

▷ **Advisability of Use During Pregnancy**

Pregnancy Category: A. See Pregnancy Code at the back of this book.

Animal studies: Cataract formation reported in rat studies. Other defects reported in rabbit and guinea pig studies.

Human studies: Thyroid hormones do not reach the fetus (cross the placenta) in significant amounts. Clinical experience has shown that appropriate use of thyroid hormones causes no adverse effects on the fetus.

Use this drug only if clearly needed and with carefully adjusted dosage.

Advisability of Use if Breast-Feeding

Presence of this drug in breast milk: Yes, in minimal amounts.

Breast-feeding is considered safe with correctly adjusted dosage.

Habit-Forming Potential: None.

Effects of Overdosage: Headache, sense of increased body heat, nervousness, increased sweating, hand tremors, insomnia, rapid and irregular heart action, diarrhea, muscle cramping, weight loss, heart attack.

Possible Effects of Long-Term Use: Bone loss (osteoporosis) in the lumbar vertebrae (spine).

Suggested Periodic Examinations While Taking This Drug (at physician's discretion)

Measurement of thyroid hormone levels in blood.

▷ **While Taking This Drug, Observe the Following**

Foods: Enteral formulas for nutrition support which contain soybeans may increase the fecal elimination of thyroxine.

Beverages: No restrictions.

▷ *Alcohol:* No interactions expected.

Tobacco Smoking: No interactions expected.

▷ *Other Drugs*

Levothyroxine may *increase* the effects of
- warfarin (Coumadin), and increase the risk of bleeding; decreased anticoagulant dosage is usually needed. Prothrombin times are necessary.

Levothyroxine may *decrease* the effects of
- digoxin (Lanoxin), when correcting hypothyroidism; a larger dose of digoxin may be needed.

Levothyroxine *taken concurrently* with
- antacids may cause decreased levothyroxine absorption and a decreased therapeutic efect.
- all antidiabetic drugs (insulin and sulfonylureas) may require an in-

creased dose to obtain proper control of blood sugar levels. Once correct doses of both drugs have been identified, a reduction in the dose of thyroid may require a simultaneous reduction in the antidiabetic drug.
- benzodiazepines (Librium and others) can enhance the toxic or therapeutic effects of both drugs.
- tricyclic antidepressants (see Drug Class Section) may cause an increase in the activity of both drugs; watch for signs of overdosage.

The following drug may *decrease* the effects of levothyroxine
- cholestyramine (Cuemid, Questran) may reduce its absorption; intake of the two drugs should be separated by 5 hours.
- iron salts by decreasing absorption.
- lovastatin.
- phenytoin (Dilantin) can increase levothyroxine clearance.
- sodium polystyrene sulfonate.

▷ *Driving, Hazardous Activities:* No restrictions.

Aviation Note: The use of this drug is probably not a disqualification for piloting. Consult a designated Aviation Medical Examiner.

Exposure to Sun: No restrictions.

Exposure to Heat: This drug may decrease individual tolerance to warm environments, increasing discomfort due to heat. Consult your physician if you develop symptoms of overdosage during the warm months of the year.

Heavy Exercise or Exertion: Use caution if you have angina (coronary artery disease). This drug may increase the frequency or severity of angina during physical activity.

Discontinuation: This drug must be taken continually on a regular schedule to correct thyroid deficiency. Do not stop it without consulting your physician.

LIDOCAINE AND PRILOCAINE CREAM (Lie DO kane)
(PRY low kane)

Introduced: December 1992   **Prescription:** USA: Yes; Canada: Yes
Available as Generic: USA: No; Canada: No   **Class:** local anesthetic
Controlled Drug: USA: No; Canada: No

Brand Names: Emla cream

Warning: This cream should **not** be used in patients with congenital methemoglobinemia.
The maximum application area should **not** be exceeded. Do not put more on than a 3.9 inch by 3.9 inch (10 cm by 10 cm) area for those 10 kg or less.

BENEFITS versus RISKS	
Possible Benefits	*Possible Risks*
EFFECTIVE PAIN CONTROL	Systemic absorption and possible adverse effects
	Methemoglobinemia

Lidocaine and Prilocaine Cream

▷ **Principal Uses**
  As a Combination Drug Product [CD]: Uses currently included in FDA approved labeling: (1) Used on normal skin as a topical anesthetic for local pain relief.
  Other (unlabeled) generally accepted uses: None.
How This Drug Works: This combination cream releases lidocaine and prilocaine into the outermost layers of skin. These amide-type anesthetics inhibit normal nerve chemistry (ion fluxes) and prevent transfer of nerve information (pain).
Available Dosage Forms and Strengths
  Cream — 2.5% lidocaine and 2.5% prilocaine in 5 gram and 30 gram tubes.
▷ **Recommended Dosage Ranges (Actual dosage and administration schedule must be determined by the physician for each patient individually.)**
  Infants and Children: For body weight up to 10 kg: maximum application area in square centimeters is 100. For body weight of 10 to 20 kg: maximum application area in square centimeters is 600. For body weight above 20 kg: maximum application area in square centimeters is 2000.
  12 to 60 Years of Age: Estimated mean lidocaine absorption is 0.045 mg/cm squared/hour.
  Estimated mean absorption of prilocaine is 0.077 mg/cm squared/hour.
  Over 60 Years of Age: Same as 12 to 60 years of age except in those with liver or kidney compromise.
Conditions Requiring Dosing Adjustments
  Liver function: Prilocaine and lidocaine are metabolized in the liver, and consideration must be given to reduced application area in liver compromise.
  Kidney function: Dosing changes are not anticipated in kidney compromise.
▷ **Dosing Instructions:** Peak effect is reached in two to three hours.
Usual Duration of Use: Use for at least one hour is usually necessary to determine this drug's effectiveness in providing pain prevention. Peak effect is reached in two to three hours.
Possible Advantages of This Drug
  Simple application and lack of adverse effects
▷ **This Drug Should Not Be Taken If**
  - you have had an allergic reaction to any dosage form of it previously.
  - the skin the drug is to be applied on is open or abraded.
▷ **Inform Your Physician Before Taking This Drug If**
  - you have a history of glucose-6-phosphate deficiency (ask your doctor).
  - you have liver or kidney disease.
  - you have a history of methemoglobinemia.
  - you are pregnant.
Possible Side-Effects (natural, expected and unavoidable drug actions)
  Blanching (37%) or redness (30%) of the skin where the cream is applied.
▷ **Possible Adverse Effects** (unusual, unexpected and infrequent reactions)
  If any of the following develop, consult your physician promptly for guidance.
  Mild Adverse Effects
  Allergic Reactions: itching and edema.

Blanching (37%) and redness (30%) of the skin.
Altered temperature sensation (7%).
Serious Adverse Effects
Allergic Reactions: Anaphylactoid reaction.
Bronchospasm (rare).
Shock (rare).
Dose related bradycardia, hypotension and heart arrest (rare).

▷ **Possible Effects on Sexual Function:** None reported.

Possible Effects on Laboratory Tests
Methemoglobinemia.

CAUTION
1. Systemic absorption may occur with prolonged use or use on abraded skin.
2. May cause ear damage (ototoxicity) if applied to the middle ear.
3. Should **not** be applied to mucous membranes.

Precautions for Use
By Infants and Children:
Children under seven years of age may have less benefit from this drug than older children.
By Those over 60 Years of Age: Short-term and limited area use is indicated, especially in those with liver compromise or in people taking class one antiarrhythmic drugs such as tocainide or mexilitine.

▷ **Advisability of Use During Pregnancy**
Pregnancy Category: B. See Pregnancy Code at the back of this book.
Animal studies: Prilocaine and lidocaine studies on rats have revealed no harm to the fetus.
Human studies: Adequate studies of pregnant women are not available.

Advisability of Use if Breast-Feeding
Presence of this drug in breast milk: Yes.
Monitor nursing infant closely and discontinue drug or nursing if adverse effects develop.

Habit-Forming Potential: None.

Effects of Overdosage: Toxic levels of prilocaine (less than 6 ug/ml) and/or lidocaine (less than 5 ug/ml) cause decreases in mean arterial pressure, cardiac output and total peripheral resistance. Cardiovascular changes may lead to arrest. Typical levels achieved with topical application are far below toxic amounts.

Suggested Periodic Examinations While Taking This Drug (at physician's discretion)
Methemoglobin in those with a history of methemoglobinemia.
Glucose-6-phosphate dehydrogenase in those with family history.

▷ **While Taking This Drug, Observe the Following**
Foods: No restrictions.
Beverages: No restrictions.
▷ *Alcohol:* Because of low systemic levels achieved, significant interaction is not expected.
Tobacco Smoking: No interactions expected.

556 **Liothyronine**

▷ *Other Drugs*
   Lidocaine prilocaine cream may *increase* the effects of
   - class one antiarrhythmic drugs such as tocainide (Tonocard) and mexiletine (Mexitil).
▷ *Driving, Hazardous Activities:* Systemic effects are not expected from this drug.
   Aviation Note: The use of this drug **may be a disqualification** for piloting. Consult a designated Aviation Medical Examiner.
   Exposure to Sun: Temperature sensation may be blunted. Use caution.
   Exposure to Heat: Temperature sensation may be blunted. Use caution.
   Exposure to Cold: Temperature sensation may be blunted. Use caution.

LIOTHYRONINE (li oh THI roh neen)

Other Names: triiodothyronine, T-3
Introduced: 1956   **Prescription:** USA: Yes; Canada: Yes   **Available as Generic:** USA: Yes; Canada: No   **Class:** Thyroid hormones   **Controlled Drug:** USA: No; Canada: No
Brand Names: Cyronine, Cytomel, Euthroid [CD], Tyroid USP, Thyrolar [CD], Triostat

BENEFITS versus RISKS	
Possible Benefits	*Possible Risks*
EFFECTIVE REPLACEMENT THERAPY IN STATES OF THYROID HORMONE DEFICIENCY (HYPOTHYROIDISM)	Intensification of angina in presence of coronary artery disease
EFFECTIVE TREATMENT OF SIMPLE GOITER AND CHRONIC THYROIDITIS	Drug-induced hyperthyroidism (with excessive dosing)
EFFECTIVE TREATMENT OF THYROID GLAND CANCER	Rapid heart beat
	Heart attack (2%)

▷ **Principal Uses**
   As a Single Drug Product: Uses currently included in FDA approved labeling: (1) Replacement therapy to correct thyroid deficiency (hypothyroidism); (2) treatment of simple (nonendemic) goiter and benign thyroid nodules; (3) treatment of Hashimoto's thyroiditis; (4) adjunctive prevention and treatment of thyroid cancer; (5) therapy of cretinism; (6) used to help diagnose different kinds of thyroid problems.
   Other (unlabeled) generally accepted uses: (1) Can help infertility caused by low thyroid function; (2) thyroid replacement of choice in thyroid cancer.
   As a Combination Drug Product [CD]: This thyroid hormone is available in combination with the other principal thyroid hormone, levothyroxine, in a preparation (generic name: liotrix) that resembles the natural hormone material produced by the thyroid gland.
How This Drug Works: By altering cellular chemistry that stores energy reserves, this drug makes more energy available and increases cellular metabolism in all tissues of the body. Thyroid hormones are essential to

normal growth and development, especially the development of the infant's brain and nervous system.

Available Dosage Forms and Strengths
Injection — 10 mcg per ml
Tablets — 5 mcg, 25 mcg and 50 mcg

▷ **Recommended Dosage Ranges** (Actual dosage and administration schedule must be determined by the physician for each patient individually.)
Infants and Children: Use not recommended.
12 to 60 Years of Age: For mild hypothyroidism—Initially 25 mcg daily; increased by 12.5 to 25 mcg every 1 to 2 weeks as needed and tolerated. The usual maintenance dose is 20 to 50 mcg daily.
For severe hypothyroidism—Initially 2.5 to 5 mcg daily; increased by 5 to 10 mcg at intervals of 1 to 2 weeks. When a dose of 25 mcg is reached, increase by 12.5 to 25 mcg at intervals of 1 to 2 weeks, as needed and tolerated. The usual maintenance dose is 25 to 50 mcg daily.
For simple goiter—Initially 5 mcg daily; increase by 5 to 10 mcg at intervals of 1 to 2 weeks. When a dose of 25 mcg is reached, increase by 12.5 to 25 mcg at intervals of 1 week, as needed and tolerated. The usual maintenance dose is 50 to 100 mcg daily.
Over 60 Years of Age: Initially 5 mcg as a single daily dose; increase by 5 mcg at intervals of 2 weeks, as needed and tolerated. The usual maintenance dose is 12.5 to 37.5 mcg daily.

Conditions Requiring Dosing Adjustments
Liver function: Dosing changes are not indicated in patients with liver compromise.
Kidney function: Dosing changes are not indicated in renal compromise.

▷ **Dosing Instructions:** The tablets may be crushed and are preferably taken in the morning on an empty stomach to ensure maximal absorption and uniform results.

Usual Duration of Use: Use on a regular schedule for 2 to 4 days determines effectiveness in correcting the symptoms of thyroid deficiency. Long-term use (months to years, possibly for life) requires physician supervision.

▷ **This Drug Should Not Be Taken If**
- you have had an allergic reaction to it previously.
- you are recovering from a heart attack; ask your doctor for guidance.
- you have an uncorrected adrenal cortical deficiency.
- you are using it to lose weight and your thyroid function is normal (no deficiency).

▷ **Inform Your Physician Before Taking This Drug If**
- you have high blood pressure, any form of heart disease or diabetes.
- you have a history of Addison's disease or adrenal gland deficiency.
- you are taking any antiasthmatic medications.
- you take digoxin.
- you are taking an anticoagulant.

Possible Side-Effects (natural, expected and unavoidable drug actions)
None if dosage is adjusted correctly.

▷ **Possible Adverse Effects** (unusual, unexpected and infrequent reactions)
If any of the following develop, consult your physician promptly for guidance.

558   Liothyronine

Mild Adverse Effects
   Allergic Reactions: Skin rash, hives.
   Headache in sensitive individuals, even with proper dosage adjustment.
   Rapid heart rate (tachycardia).
Serious Adverse Effects
   Increased frequency or intensity of angina in the presence of coronary artery disease.
   Abnormal heart beats (6%).
   Lowering of blood pressure (2%).
   Heart attack (2%).
   Hyperthyroidism.
   Drug-induced Myasthenia Gravis (rare).
   Note: Other adverse effects are manifestations of excessive dosage. See Effects of Overdosage category.

▷ **Possible Effects on Sexual Function**
   Altered menstrual pattern during dosage adjustments.
   Possibly beneficial in treating impaired sexual function that is associated with true hypothyroidism.

Natural Diseases or Disorders That May Be Activated by This Drug
   Latent coronary artery insufficiency (angina), diabetes.

Possible Effects on Laboratory Tests
   Prothrombin time: increased (when taken concurrently with warfarin).
   Blood total cholesterol, HDL and LDL cholesterol levels: decreased.
   Blood triglyceride levels: no effect.
   Blood glucose level: increased.
   Blood thyroid hormone levels: increased T_3.
   Blood thyroid stimulating hormone (TSH) level: decreased.

CAUTION
1. Careful supervision of individual response is needed to identify correct dose. Do not change dosing schedule without asking your doctor.
2. This drug should not be used to treat nonspecific fatigue, obesity, infertility or slow growth. Such use is inappropriate and could be harmful.

Precautions for Use
   By Infants and Children: **Not** recommended for treatment of this age group. It must reach the brain and nervous system, and this drug may not do that. Levothyroxine is the drug of choice to treat thyroid deficiency in infants and children.
   By Those over 60 Years of Age: Requirements for thyroid hormone replacement are usually about 25% lower than in younger adults. Watch closely for any toxicity.

▷ **Advisability of Use During Pregnancy**
   Pregnancy Category: A. See Pregnancy Code at the back of this book.
   Animal studies: No information available.
   Human studies: Thyroid hormones do not reach the fetus (cross the placenta) in significant amounts. Clinical experience has shown that appropriate use of thyroid hormones causes no adverse effects on the fetus.
   Use this drug only if clearly needed and with carefully adjusted dosage.

Advisability of Use if Breast-Feeding
  Presence of this drug in breast milk: Yes, in minimal amounts.
  Breast-feeding is considered safe with correctly adjusted dosage.
Habit-Forming Potential: None.
Effects of Overdosage: Headache, sense of increased body heat, nervousness, increased sweating, hand tremors, insomnia, rapid and irregular heart action, diarrhea, muscle cramping, weight loss, heart attack.
Possible Effects of Long-Term Use: Bone loss (osteoporosis) in the lumbar vertebrae (spine).
Suggested Periodic Examinations While Taking This Drug (at physician's discretion)
  Measurement of thyroid hormone levels in blood.
▷ **While Taking This Drug, Observe the Following**
  Foods: No restrictions.
  Beverages: No restrictions.
▷ *Alcohol:* No interactions expected.
  Tobacco Smoking: No interactions expected.
▷ *Other Drugs*
  Liothyronine may *increase* the effects of
  • warfarin (Coumadin), and increase the risk of bleeding; decreased anticoagulant doses and more frequent prothrombin times are needed.
  Liothyronine may *decrease* the effects of
  • digoxin (Lanoxin), when correcting hypothyroidism; a larger dose of digoxin may be needed.
  Liothyronine *taken concurrently* with
  • all antidiabetic drugs (insulin and sulfonylureas) may require an increased dose to obtain proper control of blood sugar. Once correct doses of both drugs have been determined, if thyroid dose is decreased, a simultaneous reduction in the antidiabetic drug may be needed.
  • tricyclic antidepressants (see Drug Class Section) may cause an increase in the activity of both drugs; watch for signs of toxicity.
  The following drug may *decrease* the effects of liothyronine
  • cholestyramine (Cuemid, Questran) and perhaps other cholesterol lowering resins may reduce its absorption; intake of the two drugs should be separated by 5 hours.
▷ *Driving, Hazardous Activities:* No restrictions.
  Aviation Note: The use of this drug is probably not a disqualification for piloting. Consult a designated Aviation Medical Examiner.
  Exposure to Sun: No restrictions.
  Exposure to Heat: This drug may decrease individual tolerance to warm environments, increasing discomfort due to heat. Consult your physician if you develop symptoms of overdosage during the warm months of the year.
  Heavy Exercise or Exertion: Use caution if you have angina (coronary artery disease). This drug may increase the frequency or severity of angina during physical activity.
  Discontinuation: This drug must be taken continually on a regular schedule to correct thyroid deficiency. Do not stop it without consulting your physician.

LISINOPRIL (li SIN oh pril)

Introduced: 1988 **Prescription:** USA: Yes **Available as Generic:** No **Class:** Antihypertensive, ACE inhibitor **Controlled Drug:** USA: No
Brand Names: Prinivil, Prinzide [CD], Zestoretic [CD], Zestril

BENEFITS versus RISKS	
Possible Benefits	*Possible Risks*
EFFECTIVE CONTROL OF MILD TO SEVERE HIGH BLOOD PRESSURE	Headache (5.3%), dizziness (6.3%), fatigue (3.3%)
	Low blood pressure (1.8%)
	Allergic swelling of face, tongue, throat, vocal cords (0.1%)
	Kidney compromise
	Possible lowering of white blood cell counts

▷ **Principal Uses**

As a Single Drug Product: Uses currently included in FDA approved labeling: (1) Treats all degrees of high blood pressure. Mild to moderate high blood pressure usually responds to low doses; severe high blood pressure may require higher doses and the concurrent use of a thiazide or other class of antihypertensive drug; (2) helps improve survival in congestive heart failure.

Other (unlabeled) generally accepted uses: (1) Used after heart attacks to help reduce adverse effects; (2) helps patients with some kidney problems (nephrotic syndrome).

As a Combination Drug Product [CD]: Combined with the diuretic hydrochlorothiazide to enhance antihypertensive action.

How This Drug Works: By blocking certain enzyme systems, this drug helps relax arterial walls throughout the body and lowers the resistance to blood flow that causes high blood pressure. This, in turn, reduces the workload of the heart and improves its performance.

Available Dosage Forms and Strengths

Tablets — 5 mg, 10 mg, 20 mg, 40 mg
Prinzide Zestoretic — 20 mg lisinopril with 12.5 or 25 mg of hydrochlorothiazide

▷ **Recommended Dosage Ranges** (Actual dosage and administration schedule must be determined by the physician for each patient individually.)

Infants and Children: Dosage not established.

12 to 60 Years of Age: Initially 10 mg once daily for those not taking a diuretic; 5 mg once daily for those taking a diuretic. Usual maintenance dose is 20 to 40 mg/day taken in a single dose. Maximum total daily dosage is 80 mg.

Over 60 Years of Age: Same as 12 to 60 years of age.

Conditions Requiring Dosing Adjustments

Liver function: The liver is minimally involved in the elimination of this drug.

Kidney function: Patients with moderate kidney failure should be started on 5 mg daily. In severe kidney failure, the patient can be given 2.5 mg of lisinopril daily. Contraindicated in kidney blood flow problems (renal artery stenosis).

▷ **Dosing Instructions:** The tablet may be crushed and taken on an empty stomach or with food, at same time each day.

Usual Duration of Use: Use on a regular schedule for several weeks determines effectiveness in controlling high blood pressure. The proper treatment of high blood pressure usually requires the long-term use of effective medications.

Possible Advantages of This Drug
Controls blood pressure effectively with one daily dose.
Relatively low incidence of adverse effects.
No adverse influence on asthma, cholesterol blood levels or diabetes.
Sudden withdrawal does not result in a rapid increase in blood pressure.

▷ **This Drug Should Not Be Taken If**
- you have had an allergic reaction to it previously.
- you currently have a blood cell or bone marrow disorder.
- you are pregnant.
- you have an abnormally high level of blood potassium.

▷ **Inform Your Physician Before Taking This Drug If**
- you have a history of kidney disease or impaired kidney function.
- you have Myasthenia Gravis or a specific autoimmune disease.
- you have scleroderma or systemic lupus erythematosus.
- you have cerebral artery disease.
- you are taking another drug which can suppress the immune system.
- you have any form of heart disease.
- you are breast-feeding.
- you have swelling of the face, glottis or tongue. Call your doctor if this occurs after starting this medicine.
- you have a history of elevated potassium.
- you are taking any of the following drugs: other antihypertensives, diuretics, nitrates or potassium supplements.
- you plan to have surgery under general anesthesia in the near future.

Possible Side-Effects (natural, expected and unavoidable drug actions)
Dizziness (6.3%), orthostatic hypotension (1.4%) (see Glossary), increased blood potassium level (2.2%).

▷ **Possible Adverse Effects** (unusual, unexpected and infrequent reactions)
If any of the following develop, consult your physician promptly for guidance.
Mild Adverse Effects
Allergic Reactions: Skin rash (1.5%), itching (0.3% to 1.0%).
Headache (5.3%), fatigue (3.3%), numbness and tingling (0.8%), weakness (1.3%), insomnia.
Blurred vision (rare).
Sensation of mouth scalding.
Psoriasis (rare).
Chest pain (1.3%), palpitation (0.3% to 1.0%), cough (2.9%).
Indigestion (1.0%), nausea (2.3%), vomiting (1.3%), diarrhea (3.2%).

Lisinopril

Serious Adverse Effects
- Allergic Reactions: Swelling (angioedema) of face, tongue and/or vocal cords (less than 0.1%); can be life-threatening.
- Heart attack (myocardial infarction) (1.3%).
- Impairment of kidney function (0.3% to 1.0%).
- Orthostatic hypotension (1.4 %).
- Hepatitis (rare).
- Abnormal heart beats (rare).
- Hyperkalemia (4.8 %).
- Hyperuricemia and gout (rare).
- Hyperthermia, arthralgia and positive ANA titer (rare).
- Pancreatitis (rare).

▷ **Possible Effects on Sexual Function:** Decreased libido (0.2%), impotence (0.7%).

Possible Effects on Laboratory Tests
None reported.

CAUTION
1. Ask your doctor about the advisability of stopping other antihypertensive drugs (especially diuretics) for 1 week before starting this drug.
2. **Report promptly** any signs of infection (fever, sore throat), or water retention (weight gain, puffiness, swollen feet or ankles).
3. Do not use a salt substitute without your physician's knowledge and approval. (Many salt substitutes contain potassium.)
4. It is advisable to obtain blood cell counts and urine analyses **before** starting this drug.

Precautions for Use
By Infants and Children: Safety and effectiveness for use by those in this age group have not been established.
By Those over 60 Years of Age: Small starting doses indicated. Sudden and excessive lowering of blood pressure can predispose to stroke or heart attack in those with impaired brain circulation or coronary artery heart disease.

▷ **Advisability of Use During Pregnancy**
Pregnancy Category: D. See Pregnancy Code at the back of this book.
Animal studies: No birth defects found in mouse or rat studies. Impaired bone formation found in rabbit studies.
Human studies: May cause fetal or neonatal injury or death. May cause fetal death or injury if used during the last six months of pregnancy.

Advisability of Use if Breast-Feeding
Presence of this drug in breast milk: Unknown.
Avoid drug or refrain from nursing.

Habit-Forming Potential: None.

Effects of Overdosage: Excessive drop in blood pressure, light-headedness, dizziness, fainting.

Possible Effects of Long-Term Use: Gradual increase in blood potassium level.

Suggested Periodic Examinations While Taking This Drug (at physician's discretion)

Before starting drug: Complete blood cell counts; urine analysis with measurement of protein content; blood potassium level.
During use of drug: Blood cell counts; measurements of blood potassium.

▷ **While Taking This Drug, Observe the Following**
Foods: Consult physician regarding salt intake.
Nutritional Support: ***Do not take*** potassium supplements unless directed by your physician.
Beverages: No restrictions. May be taken with milk.

▷ *Alcohol:* Use caution until combined effect has been determined. Alcohol may enhance the blood-pressure-lowering effect of this drug.
Tobacco Smoking: No interactions expected.

▷ *Other Drugs*
Lisinopril ***taken concurrently*** with
- acetaminophen may cause increased blood pressure.
- allopurinol can result increased risk of hypersensitivity reactions.
- chlorpromazine (Thorazine) may cause low blood pressure.
- cyclosporine can cause acute kidney (renal) failure.
- lithium may cause lithium toxicity.
- loop diuretics (bumetanide and furosemide).
- NSAIDs can cause blunting of the therapeutic effect of lisinopril.
- potassium preparations (K-Lyte, Slow-K, etc.) may cause increased blood levels of potassium with risk of serious heart rhythm disturbances.
- potassium-sparing diuretics: amiloride (Moduretic), spironolactone (Aldactazide), triamterene (Dyazide) may cause increased blood levels of potassium with risk of serious heart rhythm disturbances.

▷ *Driving, Hazardous Activities:* Usually no restrictions. Be aware of possible drops in blood pressure with resultant dizziness or faintness.
Aviation Note: The use of this drug ***may be a disqualification*** for piloting. Consult a designated Aviation Medical Examiner.
Exposure to Sun: Caution advised. A similar drug of this class can cause photosensitivity.
Exposure to Heat: Caution advised. Avoid excessive perspiring with resultant loss of body water and drop in blood pressure.
Occurrence of Unrelated Illness: Report promptly any disorder that causes nausea, vomiting or diarrhea. Fluid and chemical imbalances must be corrected as soon as possible.
Discontinuation: This drug may be stopped abruptly without causing a sudden increase in blood pressure. However, ask your doctor before stopping this drug for any reason.

LITHIUM (LITH i um)

Introduced: 1949   **Prescription:** USA: Yes; Canada: Yes   **Available as Generic:** USA: Yes; Canada: No   **Class:** Antidepressant, antimanic
Controlled Drug: USA: No; Canada: No

Brand Names: ✦Carbolith, Cibalith-S, ✦Duralith, Eskalith, Eskalith CR, Lithane, ✦Lithizine, Lithobid, Lithonate, Lithotabs

Lithium

BENEFITS versus RISKS	
Possible Benefits	*Possible Risks*
RAPID REVERSAL OF ACUTE MANIA	VERY NARROW MARGIN BETWEEN TREATMENT AND TOXIC BLOOD LEVELS
STABILIZATION OF MOOD	
Prevention of recurrent depression in "responders"	POTENTIALLY FATAL TOXICITY with inadequate monitoring
	Infrequent induction of diabetes mellitus, hypothyroidism
	Diabetes insipiduslike syndrome (excessive dilute urine without sugar)

▷ **Principal Uses**

As a Single Drug Product: Uses currently included in FDA approved labeling: (1) Management of bipolar disorder. Promptly corrects acute mania, and also stabilizes these disorders by reducing the frequency and severity of recurrent manic-depressive mood swings; (2) used to treat mania; (3) helps control mania.

Other (unlabeled) generally accepted uses: (1) May be helpful in chronic hair pulling (trichotillomania); (2) can help prevent cluster headaches; (3) may help control aggressive behavior; (4) can have a role in Fanconi aplastic anemia; (5) could have an adjunctive role in AIDS patients who have low platelet and white blood cells; (6) may help patients who have mood problems which also effects their sex drive.

How This Drug Works: It is thought that lithium changes the way nerve signals are transmitted and interpreted, influencing emotional status and behavior.

Available Dosage Forms and Strengths

        Capsules — 150 mg, 300 mg, 600 mg
        Syrup — 8 mEq per 5-ml teaspoonful
        Tablets — 300 mg
        Tablets, prolonged-action — 300 mg, 450 mg

▷ **Usual Adult Dosage Range:** First day: 300 mg taken 3 times, 6 hours apart; second day and thereafter: Increase dose to 1200 mg/24 hours and later to 1800 mg/24 hours if needed and tolerated. The usual maintenance dose is 600 to 1200 mg/24 hours taken in 3 divided doses. The total daily dosage should not exceed 3600 mg. **Note: Actual dose and dosing schedule must be determined by the physician for each patient individually.**

Conditions Requiring Dosing Adjustments

Liver function: The liver is minimally involved in the elimination of lithium.
Kidney function: If the decision is made to use lithium in this patient population, frequent and careful monitoring and decreased dosing must be provided.

▷ **Dosing Instructions:** The capsules may be opened and the regular tablets crushed and taken with or after meals to reduce stomach upset. The prolonged-action tablets should be swallowed whole and not altered.

Usual Duration of Use: Use on a regular schedule for 1 to 3 weeks determines effectiveness in correcting acute mania; several months of continual treatment may be required to correct depression. Long-term use (months to years) requires physician supervision and periodic evaluation.

Currently a "Drug of Choice"
for the treatment of acute mania in bipolar manic-depressive disorders.

▷ **This Drug Should Not Be Taken If**
- you have had an allergic reaction to any dosage form of it previously.
- you have uncontrolled diabetes or uncorrected hypothyroidism.
- you are breast-feeding.
- you will be unable to comply with the need for regular monitoring of lithium blood levels.
- you have severe kidney failure.

▷ **Inform Your Physician Before Taking This Drug If**
- you have a history of a schizophreniclike thought disorder.
- you have any type of organic brain disease, or a history of grand mal epilepsy.
- you have diabetes, heart disease, hypothyroidism or impaired kidney function.
- you are on a salt-restricted diet.
- you are pregnant or planning pregnancy.
- you are taking any diuretic drug or a cortisonelike steroid preparation.
- you plan to have surgery under general anesthesia in the near future.

Possible Side-Effects (natural, expected and unavoidable drug actions)
Increased thirst and urine volume may occur in 60% of initial users and in 20% of long-term maintenance users. Weight gain may occur in first few months of use. Drowsiness and lethargy may occur in sensitive individuals.

▷ **Possible Adverse Effects** (unusual, unexpected and infrequent reactions)
If any of the following develop, consult your physician promptly for guidance.

Mild Adverse Effects
Allergic Reactions: Skin rashes, generalized itching.
Skin dryness, loss of hair.
Headache, dullness, joint pain, dizziness, weakness, blurred vision, ringing in ears, fine hand tremor, unsteadiness.
Metallic taste, loss of appetite, stomach irritation, nausea, vomiting, diarrhea.
Edema.
Incontinence.
Increased white blood cells—**not** a sign of infection, but an effect of lithium.

Serious Adverse Effects
"Blackout" spells, confusion, stupor, slurred speech, spasmodic movements of extremities, epilepticlike seizures.
Abnormal fixed eye position (oculogyric crisis).
Abnormal changes in heart rate, rhythm and wave forms.
Loss of bladder or rectal control.
Diabetes insipiduslike syndrome: Loss of kidney concentrating power, excessive dilute urine.
Abnormal movements (may be a sign of toxicity).

Cerebellar atrophy (rare).
Increased blood platelets.
Inflammation of the heart muscle (myocarditis) (rare).
Pseudotumor cerebri.
Drug-induced Myasthenia Gravis or Systemic Lupus Erythematosus.
Low thyroid function.
Abnormally high thyroid function.
Elevated blood calcium (rare).
Elevated blood sugar.
Hyperparathyroidism.
Poyrphyria.
Inflammation of the parotid gland.
Drug-induced low potassium.
Neuroleptic malignant syndrome (rare).

▷ **Possible Effects on Sexual Function:** Decreased libido (blood level of 0.7 to 0.9 meq/L); inhibited erection: 30% of users (0.6 to 0.8 meq/L); male infertility; female breast swelling with milk production.

▷ **Adverse Effects That May Mimic Natural Diseases or Disorders**
Painful discoloration and coldness of the hands and feet may resemble Raynaud's syndrome.

Natural Diseases or Disorders That May Be Activated by This Drug
Diabetes mellitus may be worsened. Psoriasis may be intensified. Myasthenia gravis may be induced (1 case).

Possible Effects on Laboratory Tests
White blood cell and platelet counts: increased.
Blood alkaline phosphatase (bone isoenzyme): markedly increased in 66% of users.
Blood cholesterol level: increased.
Blood parathyroid hormone level: increased.
Blood thyroid stimulating hormone (TSH) level: increased.
Blood thyroid hormone (T_3 and T_4) levels: decreased.
Blood uric acid level: decreased.
Blood bromide levels: increased.

CAUTION

1. The blood level of drug required to be effective is quite close to the level that can cause toxic effects. Periodic measurements of blood lithium levels are mandatory for appropriate adjustments of dosage. Follow instructions exactly regarding drug dosage and periodic blood tests.
2. Lithium should be stopped at the first signs of toxicity: drowsiness, sluggishness, unsteadiness, tremor, muscle twitching, vomiting or diarrhea.
3. The major causes of lithium toxicity are
   - accidental overdose (may be due to inadequate blood level checks).
   - impaired kidney function.
   - salt restriction.
   - inadequate fluid intake, dehydration.
   - concurrent use of diuretics.
   - intercurrent illness.

- childbirth (rapid decrease in kidney clearance of lithium).
- initiation of treatment with a new drug.
4. Over-the-counter preparations that contain iodides (some cough products and vitamin-mineral supplements) should be avoided because of the added antithyroid effect when taken with lithium.

Precautions for Use

By Infants and Children: Safety and effectiveness for those under 12 years of age not established. Follow physician's instructions exactly.

By Those over 60 Years of Age: Treatment should start with a "test" dose of 75 to 150 mg daily. Observe closely for early indications of toxic effects, especially if on a low-salt diet and using diuretics. Increased risk of Parkinsonian reactions (abnormal gait and movements); coma can develop without warning symptoms.

▷ **Advisability of Use During Pregnancy**

Pregnancy Category: D. See Pregnancy Code at the back of this book.

Animal studies: Cleft palate reported in mice; eye, ear and palate defects reported in rats.

Human studies: Adequate studies of pregnant women are not available. However, cardiovascular defects and goiter in newborn infants (of mothers using lithium) have been reported. If the infant's blood level of lithium approaches the toxic range before delivery, the newborn may suffer the "floppy infant" syndrome: weakness, lethargy, unresponsiveness, low body temperature, weak cry and poor feeding ability.

Avoid use of drug during the first 3 months. Use only if clearly necessary during the last 6 months. Monitor mother's blood lithium levels carefully to avoid possible toxicity.

Advisability of Use if Breast-Feeding

Presence of this drug in breast milk: Yes, in significant amounts.

Avoid drug or refrain from nursing.

Habit-Forming Potential: None.

Effects of Overdosage: Drowsiness, weakness, lack of coordination, nausea, vomiting, diarrhea, muscle spasms, blurred vision, dizziness, staggering gait, slurred speech, confusion, stupor, coma, seizures.

Possible Effects of Long-Term Use: Hypothyroidism (5%), goiter, reduced sugar tolerance, diabetes insipiduslike syndrome, serious kidney damage.

Suggested Periodic Examinations While Taking This Drug (at physician's discretion)

Regular determinations of blood lithium levels are absolutely essential.

Time to sample blood for lithium level: 12 hours after evening dose, or in the morning, just before next dose.

Recommended therapeutic range: 0.8 to 1.5 mEq/L acute and 0.6 to 1.2 maintenance.

Periodic evaluation of thyroid gland size and function.

Complete blood cell counts; kidney function tests.

▷ **While Taking This Drug, Observe the Following**

Foods: Maintain a normal diet; **do not** restrict your use of salt.

Beverages: No restrictions. Drink at least 8 to 12 glasses of liquids/24 hours. This drug may be taken with milk.

▷ *Alcohol:* Used with caution. May have an increased intoxicating effect. Avoid alcohol completely if any symptoms of lithium toxicity develop.
Tobacco Smoking: No interactions expected.
Marijuana Smoking: Possible increase in apathy, lethargy, drowsiness or sluggishness; accentuation of lithium-induced tremor; possible increased risk of precipitating psychotic behavior.

▷ *Other Drugs*
Lithium may *increase* the effects of
- tricyclic antidepressants (see Drug Classes).

Lithium *taken concurrently* with
- ACE inhibitors such as captopril (Capoten) may increase lithium levels by as much as three times the level prior to combination therapy.
- calcium channel blockers such as Diltiazem (see Drug Classes) may cause neurotoxicity or psychosis.
- carbamazepine (Tegretol) or with
- chlorpromazine (Thorazine, etc.), and other phenothiazines or with
- fluoxetine (Prozac) or with
- haloperidol (Haldol) or with
- methyldopa (Aldomet, etc.) is usually well tolerated; however, it may cause a severe neurotoxic reaction in susceptible individuals. These combinations should be used very cautiously.
- diazepam (Valium) may cause hypothermia.
- verapamil (Calan, Isoptin) may cause unpredictable effects; both lithium toxicity and decreased lithium blood levels have been reported.

The following drugs may *increase* the effects of lithium
- bumetanide (Bumex).
- ethacrynic acid (Edecrin).
- fluoxetine (Prozac).
- furosemide (Lasix, etc.).
- indomethacin (Indocin).
- piroxicam (Feldene) or any nonsteroidal anti-inflammatory drug (NSAID).
- thiazide diuretics (see Drug Class Section).

The following drugs may *decrease* the effects of lithium
- acetazolamide (Diamox, etc.).
- sodium bicarbonate.
- theophylline (Theo-Dur, etc.) and related drugs.

▷ *Driving, Hazardous Activities:* This drug may impair mental alertness, judgment, physical coordination and reaction time. Restrict activities as necessary.
Aviation Note: The use of this drug *is a disqualification* for piloting. Consult a designated Aviation Medical Examiner.
Exposure to Sun: No restrictions.
Exposure to Heat: Excessive sweating can cause significant depletion of salt and water and resultant lithium toxicity. Avoid sauna baths.
Occurrence of Unrelated Illness: Fever, sweating, vomiting or diarrhea can result in significant alterations of blood and tissue lithium concentrations. Close monitoring of your physical condition and blood lithium levels is needed to prevent serious toxicity.
Discontinuation: Sudden discontinuation does not cause withdrawal symp-

toms. Avoid premature discontinuation; some individuals may require continual treatment for up to a year to achieve maximal response. Discontinuation by "responders" may result in recurrence of either mania or depression. Lithium should be discontinued if symptoms of brain toxicity appear or if an uncorrectable diabetes insipiduslike syndrome develops.

LOMEFLOXACIN (loh me FLOX a sin)

Introduced: 1992 **Prescription:** USA: Yes **Available as Generic:** USA: No **Class:** Anti-infective **Controlled Drug:** USA: No
Brand Name: Maxaquin

Warning: Reports are being made for some drugs in this class which find tendon rupture as a rare adverse effect. Ask your doctor about limits on strenuous exercise while you are taking this medicine. A rare idiosyncratic reaction has also been reported which presents as mental confusion and disorientation. Use of this medicine after head trauma may be a risk factor. If you have suffered a fall, ask your doctor if a medicine in a different antibiotic class should be substituted. If you are taking this drug and notice a change in your thinking, call your doctor.

BENEFITS versus RISKS

Possible Benefits	Possible Risks
HIGHLY EFFECTIVE TREATMENT FOR SOME INFECTIONS OF THE LOWER RESPIRATORY TRACT and URINARY TRACT	Rare but serious allergic reactions
Rare seizures
Neurologic reactions (rare)
Tendon rupture (rare)
Effective prevention of postoperative infection of the lower urinary tract	Headache (3.2%), dizziness (2.3%)
Nausea (3.7%), diarrhea (1.4%)

▷ **Principal Uses**

As a Single Drug Product: Uses currently included in FDA approved labeling: Used primarily to treat responsive infections (in adults) of: (1) the lower respiratory tract (lungs and bronchial tubes); (2) the urinary tract (kidneys, bladder, urethra). Also used to prevent postoperative infection following transurethral surgical procedures.

Other (unlabeled) generally accepted uses: (1) Limited use in dermatologic infections.

How This Drug Works: By blocking the bacterial enzyme DNA gyrase (which is required for DNA synthesis and cell reproduction), this drug arrests bacterial growth (in low concentrations) and destroys bacteria (in high concentrations).

Available Dosage Forms and Strengths
 Tablets — 400 mg

▷ **Recommended Dosage Ranges** (Actual dosage and administration schedule must be determined by the physician for each patient individually.)
Infants and Children: Use not recommended.
18 to 60 Years of Age: For bronchitis—400 mg daily for 10 days.
For cystitis—400 mg daily for 10 days.

For complicated urinary tract infections—400 mg daily for 14 days.

For preoperative prevention of urinary tract infection—400 mg (single dose) taken 2 to 6 hours before surgery.

Over 60 Years of Age: Same as 18 to 60 years of age.

Conditions Requiring Dosing Adjustments

Liver function: No changes in dosing are indicated in patients with compromised livers.

Kidney function: Patients with mild to moderate kidney failure can be given a 400 mg loading dose to be followed by 200 mg daily. The same doses and less frequent dosing should be used in severe kidney failure.

▷ **Dosing Instructions:** The tablet may be crushed and taken without regard to food. Drink fluids liberally during the entire course of treatment. Avoid antacids containing aluminum or magnesium and supplements containing iron or zinc for 2 hours before and after dosing.

Usual Duration of Use: Use on a regular schedule for up to 10 days determines effectiveness in eradicating infection. The drug should be continued for at least 2 days after all indications of infection have disappeared.

Possible Advantages of This Drug

Very broad spectrum of antibacterial activity.

No significant effect on kidney function.

▷ **This Drug Should Not Be Taken If**
- you have had an allergic reaction to it previously.
- you are pregnant or breast-feeding.
- you have a seizure disorder that is not adequately controlled.
- it is prescribed for a person under 18 years of age.

▷ **Inform Your Physician Before Taking This Drug If**
- you are allergic to cinoxacin (Cinobac), nalidixic acid (NegGram), ciprofloxacin (Cipro), norfloxacin (Noroxin), ofloxacin (Floxin), or other related quinolone drugs.
- you have a seizure disorder or a circulatory disorder of the brain.
- you have a history of psychosis.
- you have a history of tendon disease.
- you have impaired kidney function.
- you are taking any form of probenecid, sucralfate, antacids or warfarin.

Possible Side-Effects (natural, expected and unavoidable drug actions)

Superinfections: yeast vaginitis (less than 1%). (See Superinfection in the Glossary.)

▷ **Possible Adverse Effects** (unusual, unexpected and infrequent reactions)

If any of the following develop, consult your physician promptly for guidance.

Mild Adverse Effects

Allergic Reactions: Rash, hives, itching (less than 1%).

Headache (3.2%), dizziness (2.3%), weakness, drowsiness, nervousness, insomnia, visual disturbances (less than 1%).

Nausea (3.7%), vomiting, indigestion, diarrhea (1.4%).

Serious Adverse Effects

Allergic Reactions: Anaphylactoid reactions (see Glossary).

Idiosyncratic Reactions: Rare and unpredictable central nervous system problems ranging from sleep disorders to extreme confusion to seizures have been reported.

Central nervous system stimulation: restlessness, tremor, hallucinations, aphasia and seizures (all very rare).

Tendon rupture (rare).

▷ **Possible Effects on Sexual Function:** Intermenstrual bleeding.

▷ **Natural Diseases or Disorders That May Be Activated by This Drug**
Latent epilepsy.

Possible Effects on Laboratory Tests
Liver function tests: rarely increased liver enzymes (ALT/GPT, AST/GOT).
Blood urea nitrogen (BUN): rarely increased.

CAUTION
1. With high doses or prolonged use of other drugs of this class, crystal formation in the kidney may occur. This can be prevented by drinking large amounts of water, up to 2 quarts/24 hours.
2. May decrease the formation of saliva and predispose to dental cavities or gum disease. Consult your dentist if dry mouth persists.
3. If a skin rash, hives or other indications of allergy develop, stop this drug and inform your physician promptly.
4. Avoid the use of iron and mineral supplements while taking this drug.
5. Experience with a drug in the same class says that it should be stopped immediately at the first sign of lightheadedness, restlessness or confusion. Call your doctor immediately if these problems develop.

Precautions for Use
By Infants and Children: Avoid the use of this drug completely. It can impair normal bone growth and development in immature animals.
By Those over 60 Years of Age: Impaired kidney function may require dosage reduction.

▷ **Advisability of Use During Pregnancy**
Pregnancy Category: C. See Pregnancy Code at the back of this book.
Animal studies: Mild skeletal defects due to this drug were found in rabbit studies; toxic effects on the fetus were shown in monkey studies. This drug can impair normal bone development in immature dogs.
Human studies: adequate studies of pregnant women are not available. However, the potential for adverse effects on fetal bone development contraindicates the use of this drug during entire pregnancy.

Advisability of Use if Breast-Feeding
Presence of this drug in breast milk: Unknown.
Avoid drug or refrain from nursing.

Habit-Forming Potential: None.

Effects of Overdosage: Hallucinations, nausea, vomiting, interstitial nephritis, seizures, precipitation of drug crystals in the kidney, joint and tendon toxicity, celebellar dysfunction.

Possible Effects of Long-Term Use: Superinfections (see Glossary).

Suggested Periodic Examinations While Taking This Drug (at physician's discretion)
None.

572   Loperamide

▷ **While Taking This Drug, Observe the Following**
  Foods: No restrictions.
  Beverages: No restrictions. May be taken with milk.
▷ *Alcohol:* No interactions expected.
  Tobacco Smoking: No interactions expected.
▷ *Other Drugs*
    Lomefloxacin may *increase* the effects of
    • warfarin (Coumadin), and increase the risk of bleeding; prothrombin times should be carefully followed.
    The following drug may *increase* the effects of lomefloxacin
    • probenecid (Benemid).
    The following drugs may *decrease* the effects of lomefloxacin
    • antacids containing aluminum or magnesium can reduce the absorption of lomefloxacin and lessen its effectiveness.
    • iron salts.
    • sucralfate (Carafate) can impair absorption of lomefloxacin. Take antacids and sucralfate 4 hours before or 2 hours after taking lomefloxacin.
▷ *Driving, Hazardous Activities:* This drug may cause drowsiness, dizziness and impaired vision. Restrict activities as necessary.
  Aviation Note: The use of this drug *may be a disqualification* for piloting. Consult a designated Aviation Medical Examiner.
  Exposure to Sun: This drug may rarely cause photosensitivity (see Glossary). Sunglasses are advised if eyes are overly sensitive to bright light.
  Discontinuation: If you experience no adverse effects from this drug, take the full course prescribed for best results. Ask your doctor when to stop the drug.

LOPERAMIDE (loh PER a mide)

Introduced: 1977   **Prescription:** USA: Yes; Canada: No   **Available as Generic:** No   **Class:** Antidiarrheal   **Controlled Drug:** USA: No; Canada: No
Brand Names: Anti-Diarrheal, Imodium, Imodium AD, Pepto Diarrhea Control

BENEFITS versus RISKS	
Possible Benefits	*Possible Risks*
EFFECTIVE RELIEF OF INTESTINAL CRAMPING AND DIARRHEA	Drowsiness Constipation Induction of toxic megacolon

▷ **Principal Uses**
  As a Single Drug Product: Uses currently included in FDA approved labeling: (1) Control of cramping and diarrhea associated with acute gastroenteritis and chronic enteritis and colitis; (2) Used to reduce the volume of discharge from ileostomies.
    Other (unlabeled) generally accepted uses: (1) Used in irritable bowel syndrome which has failed to respond to dietary supplements; (2) combination therapy of travelers diarrhea; (3) decreases unformed stools in Shigella diarrhea.

Loperamide

How This Drug Works: This drug acts directly on the nerve supply of the gastrointestinal tract, decreases secretions and helps relieve cramping and diarrhea.

Available Dosage Forms and Strengths
  Capsules — 2 mg
  Liquid — 1 mg per 5-ml teaspoonful (alcohol 5.25%)
  Tablets — 2 mg

▷ **Usual Adult Dosage Range:** For acute diarrhea: 4 mg initially, then 2 mg after each unformed stool until diarrhea is controlled. For chronic diarrhea: 4 to 8 mg/day in divided doses, taken 8 to 12 hours apart. Maximum daily dosage is 16 mg. **Note: Actual dosage and administration schedule must be determined by the physician for each patient individually.**

Conditions Requiring Dosing Adjustments
  Liver function: Dosing adjustments in patients with liver compromise are not needed.
  Kidney function: Changes in dosing are not indicated in kidney compromise.

▷ **Dosing Instructions:** The capsule may be opened and taken on an empty stomach or with food if stomach upset occurs.

Usual Duration of Use: Use on a regular schedule for 48 hours determines effectiveness in controlling acute diarrhea; continual use for 10 days may be needed to evaluate its effectiveness in controlling chronic diarrhea. If diarrhea persists, consult your physician.

▷ **This Drug Should Not Be Taken If**
  - you have had an allergic reaction to it previously.
  - it is prescribed for a child under 2 years of age.

▷ **Inform Your Physician Before Taking This Drug If**
  - you have a history of liver disease or impaired liver function.
  - you have regional enteritis or ulcerative colitis.
  - you have acute dysentery.

Possible Side-Effects (natural, expected and unavoidable drug actions)
  Drowsiness, constipation.

▷ **Possible Adverse Effects** (unusual, unexpected and infrequent reactions)
  If any of the following develop, consult your physician promptly for guidance.
  Mild Adverse Effects
  Allergic Reaction: Skin rash.
  Fatigue, dizziness.
  Reduced appetite, cramps, dry mouth, nausea, vomiting, stomach pain, bloating.
  Serious Adverse Effects
  "Toxic megacolon" (distended, immobile colon with fluid retention) may develop while treating acute ulcerative colitis.
  Parylitic ileus.

▷ **Possible Effects on Sexual Function:** None reported.

Possible Effects on Laboratory Tests
  None reported.

CAUTION
1. Do not exceed recommended doses.
2. If treating chronic diarrhea, promptly report development of bloating, abdominal distension, nausea, vomiting, constipation or abdominal pain.

Precautions for Use
By Infants and Children: Do not use in those under 2 years of age. Follow physician's instructions exactly regarding dosage. Watch for drowsiness, irritability, personality changes and altered behavior.
By Those over 60 Years of Age: Small starting doses are needed as you may be more sensitive to the sedative and constipating effects of this drug.

▷ **Advisability of Use During Pregnancy**
Pregnancy Category: B. See Pregnancy Code at the back of this book.
Animal studies: No birth defects found in rat and rabbit studies.
Human studies: Adequate studies of pregnant women are not available.
Use sparingly and only if clearly needed. Ask physician for guidance.

Advisability of Use if Breast-Feeding
Presence of this drug in breast milk: Unknown.
Avoid drug or refrain from nursing.

Habit-Forming Potential: None.

Effects of Overdosage: Drowsiness, lethargy, depression, dry mouth.

Possible Effects of Long-Term Use: None identified.

Suggested Periodic Examinations While Taking This Drug (at physician's discretion)
None required.

▷ **While Taking This Drug, Observe the Following**
Foods: No restrictions. Follow prescribed diet.
Beverages: No restrictions. May be taken with milk.
▷ *Alcohol:* Use with caution. This drug may increase the depressant action of alcohol on the brain.
Tobacco Smoking: No interactions expected.
▷ *Other Drugs:* No significant drug interactions reported.
▷ *Driving, Hazardous Activities:* This drug may cause drowsiness or dizziness. Restrict activities as necessary.
Aviation Note: The use of this drug *is a disqualification* for piloting. Consult a designated Aviation Medical Examiner.
Exposure to Sun: No restrictions.

LORATADINE (Lor AT a deen)

Introduced: 1992   **Prescription:** USA: Yes; Canada: Yes   **Available as**
Generic: USA: No; Canada: No   **Class:** nonsedating antihistamines
Controlled Drug: USA: No; Canada: No
Brand Names: Claritin, ✦Claritin Extra
Warning: This drug has some life-threatening drug—drug interactions with some antifungal drugs. Read the section in this profile on other drugs very carefully.

BENEFITS versus RISKS	
Possible Benefits	*Possible Risks*
Effective and long lasting relief of allergic rhinitis or allergic skin disorders	Rare heart rhythm disturbances

▷ **Principal Uses**
   As a Single Drug Product: Uses currently included in FDA approved labeling: (1) Used to treat allergic disorders such as seasonal rhinitis (hay fever) and rhinitis.
   Other (unlabeled) generally accepted uses: (1) Has a role in treating allergic swellings of unknown cause.

How This Drug Works: Medications in this class block the action of histamine, thereby stoping the development of symptoms (which are caused by histamine) such as swelling and itching of the eyes.

Available Dosage Forms and Strengths
   Tablet — 10 mg

▷ **Recommended Dosage Ranges (Actual dosage and administration schedule must be determined by the physician for each patient individually.)**
   Infants and Children: Not indicated.
   12 to 60 Years of Age: Dosing is started at 10 mg daily. The dose may subsequently be increased as needed or tolerated to a maximum of 40 mg daily.
   Over 60 Years of Age: This medicine may be more slowly removed by patients in this age range. Consideration must be given to less frequent dosing if symptoms of accumulation of this drug occur.

Conditions Requiring Dosing Adjustments
   Liver function: Patients with liver compromise may be given 10 mg every other day.
   Kidney function: Decreased doses or dosing intervals are indicated.

▷ **Dosing Instructions:** This medicine is best taken on an empty stomach.

Usual Duration of Use: Continual use on a regular schedule for 3 to 5 days is usually necessary to determine this drug's effectiveness in treating hay fever. Long-term use (months to years) requires periodic evaluation of response and dosage adjustment. See your doctor on a regular basis.

Possible Advantages of This Drug
   Less sedating than previously available antihistamines.
   Once a day dosing.

▷ **This Drug Should Not Be Taken If**
   - you have had an allergic reaction to any dosage form of it previously.
   - you are taking ketoconazole, itraconazole, fluconazole or macrolide (see Drug Classes) antibiotics.
   - you are presently being tested (using skin tests) for allergies.

▷ **Inform Your Physician Before Taking This Drug If**
   - you have asthma.
   - you are at risk for drowsiness or fainting.
   - you have a history of a heart rhythm disorder.
   - you have a history of liver or kidney compromise.
   - you are uncertain of how much loratadine to take or how often to take it.

Loratadine

- you take other prescription or non-prescription medicines which were not discussed with your doctor when loratadine was prescribed.

Possible Side-Effects (natural, expected and unavoidable drug actions)
Dry nose, mouth or throat.

▷ **Possible Adverse Effects** (unusual, unexpected and infrequent reactions)
If any of the following develop, consult your physician promptly for guidance.
Mild Adverse Effects
Allergic Reactions: Skin rash.
Headache, drowsiness or dizziness.
Serious Adverse Effects
Allergic Reactions: Not defined.
Idiosyncratic Reactions: Not reported.
Potential for heart rhythm disturbances.

▷ **Possible Effects on Sexual Function:** None reported.

Possible Delayed Adverse Effects: None reported.

▷ **Adverse Effects That May Mimic Natural Diseases or Disorders**
None reported.

Natural Diseases or Disorders That May Be Activated by This Drug
None reported.

Possible Effects on Laboratory Tests
Skin tests for allergies will be blunted and less diagnostic.

CAUTION
1. This medicine has some serious drug—drug interactions. Talk to your doctor or pharmacist before taking any medicines which were not discussed when loratadine was prescribed.
2. Report dizziness, heart palpitation or chest pain promptly.

Precautions for Use
By Infants and Children:
Safety and effectiveness for use by those under 12 years of age have not been established.
By Those over 60 Years of Age: Smaller starting and maintenance doses are needed. Longer dosing intervals may be needed as well.

▷ **Advisability of Use During Pregnancy**
Pregnancy Category: B. See Pregnancy Code at the back of this book.
Animal studies: No birth defects reported.
Human studies: Information from adequate studies of pregnant women is not available.

Advisability of Use if Breast-Feeding
Presence of this drug in breast milk: Yes.
Ask your doctor for guidance.

Habit-Forming Potential: None.

Effects of Overdosage: Dry mouth, serious heart rhythm disturbances.

Possible Effects of Long-Term Use: None defined.

Suggested Periodic Examinations While Taking This Drug (at physician's discretion)
Electrocardiogram (ECG), especially for those with heart conditions.

▷ **While Taking This Drug, Observe the Following**
   Foods: No restrictions.
   Beverages: No restrictions.
▷ *Alcohol:* May cause excessive drowsiness.
   Tobacco Smoking: No interactions expected.
   Marijuana Smoking: Additive drowsiness or lethargy.
▷ *Other Drugs*
   Loratadine **taken concurrently** with
   • ketoconazole, itraconazole or fluconazole may cause serious heart rhythm toxicity.
   • other nonsedating antihistamines have been reported to have toxic interactions with macrolide antibiotics such as azithromycin, clarithromycin or erythromycin.
▷ *Driving, Hazardous Activities:* This drug may cause drowsiness. Restrict activities as necessary.
   Aviation Note: The use of this drug **may be a disqualification** for piloting. Consult a designated Aviation Medical Examiner.
   Exposure to Sun: Rare cases of photosensitivity have been reported with other medicines in this class. Use Caution.

LORAZEPAM (Lor A za pam)

Introduced: 1977 **Prescription:** USA: Yes; Canada: Yes **Available as Generic:** USA: Yes; Canada: Yes **Class:** Mild tranquilizer, benzodiazepines
Controlled Drug: USA: C-IV*; Canada: No
Brand Names: Ativan, ✦Apo-Lorazepam, ✦Novo-Lorazepam, ✦Nu-Loraz, Lorazepam Intensol

BENEFITS versus RISKS	
Possible Benefits	*Possible Risks*
RELIEF OF ANXIETY AND NERVOUS TENSION	Habit-forming potential with prolonged use
NOT CHANGED SIGNIFICANTLY INTO ACTIVE DRUG FORMS IN THE LIVER	Minor impairment of mental functions
	Very rare blood cell disorders
Wide margin of safety with therapeutic doses	Very rare movement disorders
	Very rare liver disorders
	Dose related respiratory depression
	Withdrawal symptoms if abruptly stopped

▷ **Principal Uses**
   As a Single Drug Product: Uses currently included in FDA approved labeling: (1) Helps treat anxiety; (2) used to relieve insomnia; (3) used in surgical cases to help in delivering effective anesthesia; (4) used intravenously as a sedative.

*See schedules of Controlled Drugs at the back of this book.

Other (unlabeled) generally accepted uses: (1) Used to help prevent the severe symptoms of alcohol detoxification (Delirium tremens or DTs); (2) used under the tongue to treat serial seizures in children; (3) can be used to promote amnesia in patients who must take chemotherapy and have suffered vomiting.

How This Drug Works: This drug attaches to a specific site (GABA-A receptor) in the brain and enables gamma-aminobutyric acid to inhibit activity of nervous tissue. Drugs in this class also reduce the time it takes to fall asleep and the number of times people awaken during the night.

Available Dosage Forms and Strengths
>Tablet — 0.5 mg, 1 mg, 2 mg
Oral Solution — 2 mg per ml
Injection — 2 mg, 4 mg per ml

▷ **Recommended Dosage Ranges (Actual dose and dosing schedule must be determined by the physician for each patient individually.)**

Infants and Children: Safety and effectiveness in those under 18 years of age not established. Has been used in 1 to 4 mg doses under the tongue for treatment of serial seizures in children.

18 to 60 Years of Age: Sedation and anxiety: Therapy is started with 1 mg per day in 2 to 3 divided doses. Doses may be increased as needed and tolerated to the usual maintenance dose of 2 to 6 mg daily in divided doses. The maximum dose is 10 mg daily.

Insomnia: 2 to 4 mg at bedtime.

Over 60 Years of Age: Sedation and anxiety: therapy is started with 0.5 to 1 mg in divided doses. The initial dose should not exceed two mg daily.

Insomnia: 0.5 to 1 mg at bedtime.

Conditions Requiring Dosing Adjustments

Liver function: The dose **must** be decreased in liver compromise, and the drug should **not** be used in liver failure.

Kidney function: The drug should **not** be used in kidney failure. In mild to moderate kidney compromise, the dose **must** be decreased.

▷ **Dosing Instructions:** The tablet may be crushed and taken on an empty stomach or with milk or food. Do **not** stop this drug abruptly if it has been taken for more than 4 weeks.

Usual Duration of Use: Use on a regular schedule for 3 to 5 days usually determines effectiveness in relieving moderate anxiety or insomnia. Continual use should be limited to 1 to 3 weeks. Consult your physician on a regular basis.

Possible Advantages of This Drug
More direct elimination and lack of active forms may be of benefit in the elderly. Increased lipid solubility is of benefit when the drug is used to treat acute alcohol withdrawal.

▷ **This Drug Should Not Be Taken If**
- you have had an allergic reaction to any dosage form of it previously.
- you have a primary depression or psychosis.
- you have excessively low blood pressure.
- you have narrow-angle glaucoma.

▷ **Inform Your Physician Before Taking This Drug If**
- you are allergic to any benzodiazepine (see Drug Classes).
- you have a history of alcoholism or drug abuse.
- you are pregnant or planning pregnancy.
- you have impaired liver or kidney function.
- you have a history of low white blood cell counts.
- you have: asthma, emphysema, epilepsy or myasthenia gravis.
- you take other prescription or non-prescription medicines which were not discussed with your doctor when lorazepam was prescribed.

Possible Side-Effects (natural, expected and unavoidable drug actions)
Sedation (15%), dizziness (6.9%), unsteadiness (3.4%), "hangover" effects on the day following bedtime use.

▷ **Possible Adverse Effects** (unusual, unexpected and infrequent reactions)
If any of the following develop, consult your physician promptly for guidance.
Mild Adverse Effects
Allergic Reactions: Rashes (rare), hives.
Dizziness, insomnia, fainting, confusion, blurred vision, slurred speach, constipation and sweating.
Amnesia.
Ringing in the ears.
Serious Adverse Effects
Allergic Reactions: Liver damage with jaundice (see Glossary) (rare).
Low white blood cell counts (leukopenia—rare).
Paradoxical exictement and rage (rare).
Low blood pressure (rare).
Hallucinations.
Porphyria (rare).
Respiratory depression.
Respiratory depression (dose related).
Abnormal body movements (rare).
Seizures (rare).

▷ **Possible Effects on Sexual Function:** Extremely rare decreased male libido or impotence.

Possible Effects on Laboratory Tests
White blood cell counts: decreased.
Liver function tests: increased SGPT, SGOT and LDH.

CAUTION
1. This drug should **not** be stopped abruptly if it has been taken continually for more than 4 weeks.
2. Some over-the-counter medications containing antihistamines can cause excessive sedation if taken with lorazepam.
3. Lorazepam should **not** be combined with alcohol. Combination will worsen adverse mental and coordination decreases, and increase lorazepam levels.

Precautions for Use
By Infants and Children:
Safety and effectiveness for those under 18 years of age not established.

Lorazepam has been used under the tongue in children with serial seizures.

By Those over 60 Years of Age: Small doses are indicated. Watch for lethargy, fatigue, weakness and paradoxical agitation, anger, hostility and rage.

▷ **Advisability of Use During Pregnancy**
Pregnancy Category: D. See Pregnancy Code at the back of this book.
Animal studies: Cleft palate has been reported in mice; skeletal defects in rats with similar drugs in this class.
Human studies: Adequate studies of pregnant women are not available.
Frequent use in late pregnancy can result in "floppy infant" syndrome in the newborn: Weakness, lethargy, depressed breathing and low body temperature.
Avoid use during the entire pregnancy

Advisability of Use if Breast-Feeding
Presence of this drug in breast milk: Yes.
Avoid drug or refrain from nursing.

Habit-Forming Potential: This drug can cause psychological and/or physical dependence (see Glossary) if used in large doses for an extended period of time.

Effects of Overdosage: Marked drowsiness, weakness, feeling of drunkenness, staggering gait, depression of breathing, stupor progressing to coma.

Possible Effects of Long-Term Use: Psychological or physical dependence, rare liver toxicity.

Suggested Periodic Examinations While Taking This Drug (at physician's discretion)
Liver function tests and complete blood cell counts.

▷ **While Taking This Drug, Observe the Following**
Foods: No restrictions.
Beverages: Avoid exessive caffeine-containing beverages: coffee, tea and cola.
▷ *Alcohol:* Avoid this combination. Alcohol increases depression of mental function, further worsens coordination and causes increased lorazepam levels.
Tobacco Smoking: Heavy smoking may reduce the calming action of this drug.
Marijuana Smoking: Additive drowsiness, and impaired physical performance.
▷ *Other Drugs*
Lorazepam *taken concurrently* with
- lithium (Lithobid, others) may result in a lowering of body temperature (hypothermic reaction).
- oxycodone (Percocet, others) and other central nervous system depressants may result in additive CNS or respiratory depression.
- phenytoin may result in altered phenytoin or lorazepam levels.

The following drugs may *increase* the effects of lorazepam
- probenecid—and result in a 50% increased lorazepam level.

The following drugs may *decrease* the effects of lorazepam
- caffeine, amphetamines or other stimulants.
▷ *Driving, Hazardous Activities:* This drug can impair alertness and coordination. Restrict activities as necessary.

Aviation Note: The use of this drug *is a disqualification* for piloting. Consult a designated Aviation Medical Examiner.
Exposure to Sun: No restrictions.
Discontinuation: Do **not** stop this drug suddenly if it has been taken for over 4 weeks. Consult your doctor about a gradual tapering of dosage.

LOSARTAN (Low SAR tan)

Other Names: None.
Introduced: 1995 **Prescription:** USA: Yes; Canada: Yes **Available as Generic:** USA: No; Canada: No **Class:** Angiotensin II antagonist **Controlled Drug:** USA: No; Canada: No
Brand Names: Cozaar

BENEFITS versus RISKS	
Possible Benefits	*Possible Risks*
EFFECTIVE CONTROL OF HIGH BLOOD PRESSURE BY A NOVEL MECHANISM	Not clearly defined
Decreased cough versus ACE inhibitors	

▷ **Principal Uses**

As a Single Drug Product: Uses currently included in FDA approved labeling: (1) treatment of high blood pressure.
Other (unlabeled) generally accepted uses: None.
As a Combination Drug Product [CD]: This drug has been combined with hydrochlorothiazide in a new fixed dosage form. The drug is called Hyzaar, and it contains 12.5 mg of hydrochlorothiazide and 50 mg of losartan. The different ways in which these drugs work complement each other, making the combination a more effective hypertensive.
How This Drug Works: This drug and its active metabolite block the effects of angiotensin II by binding to a specific site (the AT1) receptor. This helps the blood vessels stay more open and thereby controls blood pressure. This drug and its metabolite also block the secretion of aldosterone.

Available Dosage Forms and Strengths
Tablet — 25 mg, 50 mg

▷ **Recommended Dosage Ranges (Actual dosage and administration schedule must be determined by the physician for each patient individually.)**
Infants and Children: Not recommended for use in this age group.
18 to 60 Years of Age: A starting dose of 50 mg daily is used. If the blood pressure response is not sufficient, the same dose may be divided into two equal doses and given twice daily. The dose may also be increased as needed and tolerated and is then given in two divided doses daily.
Over 60 Years of Age: Patients who are dehydrated or who have a decreased intravascular volume should be given 25 mg once daily as a starting dose.

Conditions Requiring Dosing Adjustments
Liver function: This drug is extensively changed (metabolized) in the liver to an active metabolite. The drug has not been studied in patients with liver

compromise, and liver compromise is considered a relative contraindication for this medicine.

Kidney function: This medicine has not been studied in patients with compromised kidneys. Kidney compromise is a relative contraindication for losartan.

▷ **Dosing Instructions:** Food slows the absorption of losartan, but does not decrease the total absorption of this medicine.

Usual Duration of Use: Continual use on a regular schedule for several weeks is usually necessary to determine this drug's effectiveness in controlling high blood pressure.

Long-term use (months to years) requires periodic evaluation of response and dosage adjustment. Consult your physician on a regular basis.

Possible Advantages of This Drug
A completely new mechanism of action.
Appears to avoid the cough effect typical of ACE inhibitors.

▷ **This Drug Should Not Be Taken If**
- you have had an allergic reaction to any dosage form of it previously.
- you are pregnant.

▷ **Inform Your Physician Before Taking This Drug If**
- you have a history of liver or kidney disease.
- you have a history of circulation problems in the brain.
- you have a history of disease in the blood vessels which supply the heart (coronary artery disease).
- you are uncertain of how much losartan to take or how often to take it.

Possible Side-Effects (natural, expected and unavoidable drug actions)
None.

▷ **Possible Adverse Effects** (unusual, unexpected and infrequent reactions)
If any of the following develop, consult your physician promptly for guidance.

Mild Adverse Effects
Allergic Reactions: Skin rash.
Dizziness or confusion.
Fatigue or muscle cramps.
Sleep disturbances.
Nausea and headache.

Serious Adverse Effects
Allergic Reactions: Not defined.
Swelling of the face and lips (angioedema) (rare).

▷ **Possible Effects on Sexual Function:** Decreased libido, impotence (both rare).

Possible Delayed Adverse Effects: None reported.

▷ **Adverse Effects That May Mimic Natural Diseases or Disorders**
None reported.

Natural Diseases or Disorders That May Be Activated by This Drug
None reported.

Possible Effects on Laboratory Tests
Liver function tests: increased.

CAUTION
1. This drug should **not** be taken in pregnancy.

Precautions for Use
By Infants and Children:
Safety and effectiveness for use by those under 18 years of age have not been established.
By Those over 60 Years of Age: People in this age group may be more sensitive to the effects of medicines which lower blood pressure. Lower starting doses are indicated in patients who are dehydrated.

▷ **Advisability of Use During Pregnancy**
Pregnancy Category: C in the first three months, D in the fourth month through birth. See Pregnancy Code at the back of this book.
Animal studies: Rat studies have produced kidney toxicity and death in fetuses.
Human studies: Information from adequate studies of pregnant women is not available. If pregnancy is detected, this medicine should be stopped as soon as possible.

Advisability of Use if Breast-Feeding
Presence of this drug in breast milk: Unknown, but expected.
Avoid drug or refrain from nursing.

Habit-Forming Potential: None.

Effects of Overdosage: Severe decreases in blood pressure. Increased heart rate.

Possible Effects of Long-Term Use: Not defined.

Suggested Periodic Examinations While Taking This Drug (at physician's discretion)
Periodic checks of blood pressure and liver function tests.

▷ **While Taking This Drug, Observe the Following**
Foods: Follow the diet that your doctor has prescribed.
Nutritional Support: Not indicated.
Beverages: Avoid excessive caffeine intake.
▷ *Alcohol:* Alcohol may intensify the blood pressure lowering effects of this medicine. Ask your doctor for guidance.
Tobacco Smoking: No interactions expected, however, tobacco smoke lessens the oxygen available to your body.
Marijuana Smoking: May increase the blood pressure lowering effects of this drug.
▷ *Other Drugs*
No specific drug–drug interactions have been identified with this medicine as yet.
▷ *Driving, Hazardous Activities:* This drug may cause confusion. Restrict activities as necessary.
Aviation Note: The use of this drug **may be a disqualification** for piloting. Consult a designated Aviation Medical Examiner.
Exposure to Sun: No restrictions.
Exposure to Heat: Caution. Excessive sweating (perspiration) may lead to

dehydration and to an excessive blood pressure lowering effect of this drug.
Discontinuation: Talk with your doctor before stopping this medicine for any reason.

LOVASTATIN (loh vah STA tin)

Introduced: 1987 **Prescription:** USA: Yes **Available as Generic:** USA: No **Class:** Anticholesterol **Controlled Drug:** USA: No
Brand Name: Mevacor

BENEFITS versus RISKS	
Possible Benefits	*Possible Risks*
EFFECTIVE REDUCTION OF TOTAL BLOOD CHOLESTEROL in selected individuals	Drug-induced hepatitis (without jaundice) 1.9%
SLOWS PROGRESSION OF CORONARY ATHEROSCLEROSIS	Drug-induced myositis (muscle inflammation) 0.5%
	Drug-induced stomach ulceration (rare)

▷ **Principal Uses**

As a Single Drug Product: Uses currently included in FDA approved labeling: (1) Reduces abnormally high total blood cholesterol levels in people with Type II hypercholesterolemia. It should not be used until a trial of non-drug methods for lowering cholesterol has proved to be inadequate; (2) Recently approved for use in slowing the progression of coronary (heart) atherosclerosis in patients with coronary heart disease.

Other (unlabeled) generally accepted uses: (1) May help decrease hypercholesterolemia in cholesterol ester storage disease prior to liver transplant.

How This Drug Works: This drug is converted in the body to mevolinic acid, which inhibits the liver enzyme that starts to make cholesterol. It decreases low-density lipoproteins (LDL), the fraction of total blood cholesterol that increases the risk of coronary heart disease. This drug also increases high-density lipoproteins (HDL), the cholesterol fraction that is thought to reduce the risk of heart disease.

Available Dosage Forms and Strengths
Tablets — 10 mg, 20 mg, 40 mg

▷ **Usual Adult Dosage Range:** Initially 20 mg once a day; dose may be increased up to 40 mg twice a day as needed and tolerated. Dosage adjustments should be made at 4-week intervals.

Limited data supports low dose therapy where some patients responded to 20 mg as a single evening dose. Maximum daily dosage should not exceed 80 mg. **Note: Actual dose and dosing schedule must be determined by the physician for each patient individually.**

Conditions Requiring Dosing Adjustments

Liver function: It should be used with caution in patients with liver compromise.

Kidney function: The kidney is not significantly involved in the elimination of lovastatin.

▷ **Dosing Instructions:** Take with food, preferably with the evening meal for maximal effectiveness. (The highest rates of cholesterol production occur between midnight and 5 A.M.). The tablet may be crushed for administration.

Usual Duration of Use: Use on a regular schedule for 4 to 6 weeks determines effectiveness in reducing blood levels of total and LDL cholesterol. Long-term use (months to years) requires periodic physician evaluation of response.

Possible Advantages of This Drug: Recent studies indicate that this drug is more effective and better tolerated than other drugs currently available for reducing total and LDL cholesterol. Its long-term effects are yet to be determined. See Cholesterol Disorders in Section Two.

▷ **This Drug Should Not Be Taken If**
- you have had an allergic reaction to it previously.
- you have active liver disease.
- you have active peptic ulcer disease.
- you are pregnant or breast-feeding.

▷ **Inform Your Physician Before Taking This Drug If**
- you have a history of liver disease or impaired liver function.
- you have had peptic ulcer disease or upper gastrointestinal bleeding.
- you are not using any method of birth control, or you are planning pregnancy.
- you have a history of kidney compromise.
- you regularly consume substantial amounts of alcohol.
- you have cataracts or impaired vision.
- you have any type of chronic muscular disorder.

Possible Side-Effects (natural, expected and unavoidable drug actions)
Development of abnormal liver function tests without associated symptoms.

▷ **Possible Adverse Effects** (unusual, unexpected and infrequent reactions)
If any of the following develop, consult your physician promptly for guidance.
Mild Adverse Effects
Allergic Reactions: Skin rash, itching (5.2%).
Headache (9.3%), dizziness (2.0%), blurred vision (1.5%), altered taste (0.8%).
Indigestion (3.9%), stomach pain (5.7%), nausea (4.7%), excessive gas (6.4%), constipation (4.9%), diarrhea (5.5%).
Insomnia.
Muscle cramps and/or pain (2.4%).
Serious Adverse Effects
Marked and persistent abnormal liver function tests with focal hepatitis (without jaundice) occurred in 1.9% after 1 year of use.
Acute myositis (muscle pain and tenderness) occurred in 0.5% during long-term use.
Cataracts were a concern based on some early data, however, long-term information fails to demonstrate any adverse effect on the lens of the eye.

Lovastatin

Stomach and duodenal ulceration with bleeding have been reported in a few cases.

Systemic lupus erythematosus-like syndrome (rare).

▷ **Possible Effects on Sexual Function:** None reported.

Possible Delayed Adverse Effects: None reported to date.

Natural Diseases or Disorders That May Be Activated by This Drug
Latent liver disease and peptic ulcer disease.

Possible Effects on Laboratory Tests
Blood alanine aminotransferase (ALT) enzyme level: increased (with higher doses of drug).
Blood total cholesterol, LDL cholesterol and triglyceride levels: decreased.
Blood HDL cholesterol level: increased.

CAUTION
1. Stop the drug immediately and call your doctor if you become pregnant.
2. Promptly report development of muscle pain or tenderness, especially if accompanied by fever or malaise.
3. Report promptly the development of altered or impaired vision so that appropriate evaluation can be made.

Precautions for Use
By Infants and Children: Safety and effectiveness for those under 20 years of age not established.
By Those over 60 Years of Age: Tell your doctor about any personal or family history of cataracts. Comply with periodic eye examinations. Promptly report any alterations in vision.

▷ **Advisability of Use During Pregnancy**
Pregnancy Category: X. See Pregnancy Code at the back of this book.
Animal studies: Mouse and rat studies reveal skeletal birth defects due to this drug.
Human studies: Adequate studies of pregnant women are not available.
This drug should be avoided during entire pregnancy.

Advisability of Use if Breast-Feeding
Presence of this drug in breast milk: Probably yes.
Avoid drug or refrain from nursing.

Habit-Forming Potential: None.

Effects of Overdosage: Increased indigestion, stomach distress, nausea, diarrhea.

Possible Effects of Long-Term Use: Abnormal liver function with focal hepatitis.

Suggested Periodic Examinations While Taking This Drug (at physician's discretion)
Blood cholesterol studies: total cholesterol, HDL and LDL fractions.
Liver function tests every 4 to 6 weeks during the first 15 months of use and periodically thereafter.
Complete eye examination at beginning of treatment and periodically thereafter. Ask your physician for guidance.

▷ **While Taking This Drug, Observe the Following**
Foods: Follow a standard low-cholesterol diet.
Beverages: No restrictions. May be taken with milk.

▷ *Alcohol:* No interactions expected. Use sparingly.
Tobacco Smoking: No interactions expected.
Other Drugs
Lovastin **taken concurrently** with
- clofibrate may result in a severe rhabdomyolosis.
- cyclosporine (Sandimmune) can cause a severe myopathy.
- erythromycin (EES) and perhaps other macrolide antibiotics (asithromycin and clarithromycin) may result in severe rhabdomyolysis.
- gemfibrozil may cause myopathy.
- niacin can cause myopathy.
- warfarin may result in bleeding.

▷ *Driving, Hazardous Activities:* This drug may cause dizziness or impaired vision. Restrict activities as necessary.
Aviation Note: The use of this drug **may be a disqualification** for piloting. Consult a designated Aviation Medical Examiner.
Exposure to Sun: No restrictions.
Discontinuation: Do not stop this drug without your physician's knowledge and guidance.

MAPROTILINE (ma PROH ti leen)

Introduced: 1974 **Prescription:** USA: Yes; Canada: Yes **Available as Generic:** No **Class:** Antidepressant **Controlled Drug:** USA: No; Canada: No
Brand Name: Ludiomil

BENEFITS versus RISKS	
Possible Benefits	*Possible Risks*
EFFECTIVE RELIEF OF ALL TYPES OF DEPRESSION	ADVERSE BEHAVIORAL EFFECTS: confusion, disorientation, hallucinations
	CONVERSION OF DEPRESSION TO MANIA in manic-depressive disorders
	Irregular heart rhythms
	Rare liver toxicity with jaundice
	Rare seizures with therapeutic doses
	Low white blood cells (rare)

▷ **Principal Uses**
As a Single Drug Product: Uses currently included in FDA approved labeling: (1) Relieves spontaneous (endogenous) depression and reactive depressions, and helps restore normal mood. This drug should be used only when a diagnosis of true depression of significant degree has been established. It should not be used to treat mild and transient despondency.
Other (unlabeled) generally accepted uses: (1) Adjunctive use in chronic pain; (2) helps decrease and control bed wetting; (3) may have a role in the combination therapy of bulimia and other eating disorders; (4) can help cocaine craving.

Maprotiline

How This Drug Works: It is thought that this drug relieves depression by slowly restoring the nerve impulse transmitter norepinephrine to normal levels within brain tissue.

Available Dosage Forms and Strengths
Tablets — 10 mg (in Canada), 25 mg, 50 mg, 75 mg

▷ **Usual Adult Dosage Range:** Initially 25 mg 3 times daily. Dose may be increased cautiously as needed and tolerated by 10 to 25 mg daily at intervals of 1 week. Usual maintenance dose is 50 to 100 mg/24 hours. The total daily dose should not exceed 150 mg. When the optimal requirement is determined, it may be taken at bedtime as one dose. **Note: Actual dosage and administration schedule must be determined by the physician for each patient individually.**

Conditions Requiring Dosing Adjustments
Liver function: It should be used with caution, and the dose empirically decreased in patients with liver compromise.
Kidney function: Dosage adjustments not indicated in kidney failure. The drug should be used with caution in patients with urine outflow problems as maprotaline may worsen the problem.

▷ **Dosing Instructions:** The tablet may be crushed and taken without regard to meals.

Usual Duration of Use: Some benefit may be apparent within to 2 weeks, but adequate response may require continual use for 4 to 6 weeks or longer. Long-term use should not exceed 6 months without reevaluation for continued use.

▷ **This Drug Should Not Be Taken If**
- you have had an allergic reaction to it previously.
- you are taking or have taken within the past 14 days any monoamine oxidase (MAO) type A inhibitor drug (see Drug Classes).
- you are recovering from a recent heart attack.

▷ **Inform Your Physician Before Taking This Drug If**
- you are allergic or overly sensitive to any tricyclic antidepressant (see Drug Class Section).
- you have a history of any of the following: Alcoholism, asthma, epilepsy, glaucoma, heart disease, paranoia, prostate gland enlargement, schizophrenia or overactive thyroid function.
- you have impaired liver or kidney function.
- you plan to have surgery under general anesthesia in the near future.
- you have an overactive thyroid gland.

Possible Side-Effects (natural, expected and unavoidable drug actions)
Drowsiness, blurred vision, dry mouth, constipation, impaired urination.

▷ **Possible Adverse Effects** (unusual, unexpected and infrequent reactions)
If any of the following develop, consult your physician promptly for guidance.
Mild Adverse Effects
Allergic Reactions: Skin rash, itching.
Insomnia, nervousness, palpitations, dizziness, unsteadiness, tremors, fainting, weakness.
Blurred vision.

Cavities.
Delayed urination.
Nausea, vomiting, acid indigestion, diarrhea.
Increased sweating.
Serious Adverse Effects
Behavioral effects: Anxiety, confusion, hallucinations.
Aggravation of paranoid psychosis and schizophrenia.
Aggravation of seizure disorders (epilepsy).
Abnormally low blood pressure.
Vasculitis.
Myoclonus (rare).
Liver toxicity with jaundice (see Glossary).
Decreased white blood cells (rare)

▷ **Possible Effects on Sexual Function:** Decreased libido, increased libido (antidepressant effect), impotence, male breast enlargement and tenderness, female breast enlargement with milk production, swelling of testicles.

▷ **Adverse Effects That May Mimic Natural Diseases or Disorders**
The development of jaundice may suggest viral hepatitis.

Natural Diseases or Disorders That May Be Activated by This Drug
Latent epilepsy, glaucoma, prostatism (see Glossary).

Possible Effects on Laboratory Tests
Liver function tests: Rarely increased liver enzymes (ALT/GPT and AST/GOT).

CAUTION
1. Dose must be individualized. Report for follow-up evaluation and laboratory tests as directed by your physician.
2. Observe for early indications of toxicity: confusion, agitation, rapid heartbeat.
3. It is advisable to withhold this drug if electroconvulsive therapy (ECT, "shock" treatment) is to be used to treat your depression.

Precautions for Use
By Infants and Children: Safety and effectiveness for use as an antidepressant by those under 18 years of age have not been established.
By Those over 60 Years of Age: During the first 2 weeks of treatment, watch for confusion, agitation, forgetfulness, disorientation, delusions and hallucinations. Reduction of dosage or discontinuation may be necessary. Unsteadiness may predispose to falling and injury. This drug can increase the degree of impaired urination associated with prostate gland enlargement (prostatism).

▷ **Advisability of Use During Pregnancy**
Pregnancy Category: B. See Pregnancy Code at the back of this book.
Animal studies: No birth defects found in mouse, rat or rabbit studies.
Human studies: Adequate studies of pregnant women are not available.
Avoid use of drug during first 3 months. Use during the last 6 months only if clearly needed.

Advisability of Use if Breast-Feeding
Presence of this drug in breast milk: Yes.

Watch nursing infant closely for drowsiness or failure to feed properly; discontinue drug or nursing if adverse effects develop.

Habit-Forming Potential: None.

Effects of Overdosage: Confusion, hallucinations, marked drowsiness, heart palpitations, dilated pupils, tremors, stupor, respiratory depression, deep sleep, coma, convulsions.

Suggested Periodic Examinations While Taking This Drug (at physician's discretion)
Complete blood cell counts, liver function tests, serial blood pressure readings and electrocardiograms.

▷ **While Taking This Drug, Observe the Following**
Foods: No restrictions.
Beverages: No restrictions. May be taken with milk.
▷ *Alcohol:* Avoid completely. This drug can markedly increase the intoxicating effects of alcohol and accentuate its depressant action on brain function.
Tobacco Smoking: No interactions expected.
Marijuana Smoking: Increased drowsiness and dryness of mouth; possible reduced effectiveness.

▷ *Other Drugs*
Maprotiline may *increase* the effects of
- atropinelike drugs (see Drug Class Section).
- all drugs with sedative effects, and cause excessive sedation.

Maprotiline may *decrease* the effects of
- clonidine (Catapres).
- guanethidine (Ismelin).
- methyldopa (Aldomet).
- reserpine (Serpasil, Ser-Ap-Es, etc.).

Maprotiline *taken concurrently* with
- amphetaminelike drugs may cause severe high blood pressure and/or high fever (see Drug Classes).
- antiseizure drugs requires careful monitoring for change in seizure patterns; dosage adjustments may be necessary.
- ethchlorvynol (Placidyl) may cause delirium; avoid concurrent use.
- monoamine oxidase (MAO) type A inhibitor drugs may cause high fever, delirium and convulsions (see Drug Class Section).
- thyroid preparations may impair heart rhythm and function.

Ask physician for guidance regarding adjustment of thyroid dose.
The following drugs may *decrease* the effects of maprotiline
- estrogens.
- oral contraceptives.

▷ *Driving, Hazardous Activities:* This drug may impair mental alertness, judgment, physical coordination and reaction time. Avoid hazardous activities.
Aviation Note: The use of this drug *is a disqualification* for piloting. Consult a designated Aviation Medical Examiner.
Exposure to Sun: Use caution. This drug may cause photosensitivity (see Glossary).
Exposure to Heat: This drug can inhibit sweating and impair the body's adaptation to hot environments, increasing the risk of heat stroke. Avoid saunas.

Exposure to Cold: The elderly should use caution and avoid conditions conducive to hypothermia (see Glossary).

Discontinuation: It is advisable to discontinue this drug gradually. Abrupt withdrawal after long-term use may cause headache, malaise and nausea.

MECLOFENAMATE (me kloh fen AM ayt)

Introduced: 1977 **Prescription:** USA: Yes **Available as Generic:** Yes **Class:** Mild analgesic, anti-inflammatory **Controlled Drug:** USA: No

Brand Names: Meclodium, Meclomen

BENEFITS versus RISKS	
Possible Benefits	*Possible Risks*
EFFECTIVE RELIEF OF MILD TO MODERATE PAIN AND INFLAMMATION	Gastrointestinal pain, ulceration, bleeding (rare) Rare kidney damage Rare fluid retention Rare bone marrow depression

Please see the fenamate nonsteroidal anti-inflammatory drug profile for further information.

MEDROXYPROGESTERONE (me DROX ee proh JESS te rohn)

Introduced: 1959 **Prescription:** USA: Yes; Canada: Yes **Available as Generic:** Yes **Class:** Female sex hormones, progestins **Controlled Drug:** USA: No; Canada: No

Brand Names: Amen, Cycrin, Curretab, Depo-Provera, Provera

BENEFITS versus RISKS	
Possible Benefits	*Possible Risks*
EFFECTIVE TREATMENT OF ABSENT OR ABNORMAL MENSTRUATION due to hormone imbalance EFFECTIVE CONTRACEPTION when given by injection Useful adjunctive therapy in selected cases of uterine and kidney cancer	Thrombophlebitis (rare) Pulmonary embolism (rare) Liver reaction with jaundice (rare) Drug-induced birth defects

▷ **Principal Uses**

As a Single Drug Product: Uses currently included in FDA approved labeling: (1) Used to initiate and regulate menstruation and to correct abnormal patterns of menstrual bleeding caused by hormonal imbalance (and not by organic disease); (2) used in combination to treat metastatic, inoperable or recurrent endometrial carcinoma; (3) treatment of renal cell carcinoma; (4) used as a contraceptive injected into the muscle once every three months; (5) helps dysfunctional uterine bleeding.

Medroxyprogesterone

Other (unlabelled) generally accepted uses: (1) Used as a part of combination therapy in breast, refractory prostate, lung and ovarian cancer; (2) Therapy of endometriosis; (3) undefined use in osteoporosis; (4) helps abnormal hair growth in women (hirsutism); (5) can help breast pain (mastalgia); (6) used in combination with estrogen to help symptoms of menopause; (7) can be of use in pelvic congestion and Pickwickian syndrome; (8) may help severe PMS; (9) can be of use in male hypersexuality.

How This Drug Works: By inducing and maintaining a lining in the uterus that resembles pregnancy, this drug can prevent uterine bleeding until it is withdrawn. By suppressing the release of the pituitary gland hormone that induces ovulation, and by stimulating the secretion of mucus by the uterine cervix (to resist the passage of sperm), this drug can prevent pregnancy.

Available Dosage Forms and Strengths
   Injection — 150 mg (single dose vials)
   Tablets — 2.5 mg, 5 mg, 10 mg

▷ **Usual Adult Dosage Range:** To initiate menstruation: 5 to 10 mg/day for 5 to 10 days, started at any time; to correct abnormal bleeding: 5 to 10 mg/day for 5 to 10 days, started on the sixteenth or twenty-first day of the menstrual cycle. Withdrawal bleeding usually begins within 3 to 7 days after stopping the drug.

As a contraceptive: Intramuscular injections of 150 mg every 3 months are needed. **Note: Actual dosage and administration schedule must be determined by the physician for each patient individually.**

Conditions Requiring Dosing Adjustments
   Liver function: It should be used with caution, and the dose empirically decreased in patients with liver compromise.
   Kidney function: The kidneys are not involved in the elimination of this medication.

▷ **Dosing Instructions:** The tablet may be crushed and taken on an empty stomach or with food to prevent nausea.

Usual Duration of Use: Use on a regular schedule for 2 or 3 menstrual cycles determines effectiveness in correcting abnormal patterns of menstrual bleeding. Consult your physician on a regular basis.

▷ **This Drug Should Not Be Taken If**
   - you have had an allergic reaction to it previously.
   - you are pregnant.
   - you have seriously impaired liver function.
   - you have a history of cancer of the breast or reproductive organs.
   - you have a history of thrombophlebitis, embolism or stroke.
   - you have abnormal and unexplained vaginal bleeding.

▷ **Inform Your Physician Before Taking This Drug If**
   - you have impaired kidney function.
   - you have any of the following disorders: asthma, diabetes, emotional depression, epilepsy, heart disease, migraine headaches.

Possible Side-Effects (natural, expected and unavoidable drug actions)
   Fluid retention, weight gain, changes in menstrual timing and flow, spotting between periods.

▷ **Possible Adverse Effects** (unusual, unexpected and infrequent reactions)
If any of the following develop, consult your physician promptly for guidance.
Mild Adverse Effects
Allergic Reactions: Skin rash, hives, itching.
Fatigue, weakness, nausea.
Acne, excessive hair growth.
Serious Adverse Effects
Liver toxicity with jaundice (see Glossary): yellow eyes and skin, dark-colored urine, light-colored stools.
Thrombophlebitis (inflammation of a vein with blood clot formation): pain or tenderness in thigh or leg, with or without swelling of the foot, ankle or leg.
Pulmonary embolism (movement of blood clot to lung): sudden shortness of breath, chest pain, cough, bloody sputum.
Stroke (blood clot in the brain): sudden headache, blackouts, sudden weakness or paralysis of any part of the body, severe dizziness, double vision, slurred speech, inability to speak.
Retinal thrombosis (blood clot in principal blood vessel to the eye): sudden impairment or loss of vision.
Drug-induced pseudotumor cerebri.
Pneumonitis, especially in patients who have received radiation therapy.

▷ **Possible Effects on Sexual Function**
Altered timing and pattern of menstruation.
Female breast tenderness and secretion.
Decreased vaginal secretions.

▷ **Adverse Effects That May Mimic Natural Diseases or Disorders**
Liver toxicity may suggest viral hepatitis.

Possible Effects on Laboratory Tests
Blood total cholesterol, HDL cholesterol, LDL cholesterol and triglyceride levels: decreased.
Glucose tolerance test (GTT): decreased.

CAUTION
1. There is an increased risk of birth defects in children whose mothers take this drug during the first 4 months of pregnancy.
2. Inform your physician promptly if you think you may be pregnant.
3. This drug should not be used as a test for pregnancy.

Precautions for Use
By Infants and Children: Not used in this age group.
By Those over 60 Years of Age: Used selectively as adjunctive therapy in treating cancer of the breast, uterus, prostate and kidney. Observe for excessive fluid retention.

▷ **Advisability of Use During Pregnancy**
Pregnancy Category: D. See Pregnancy Code at the back of this book.
Animal studies: Genital defects reported in rat and rabbit studies; masculinization of the female rodent fetus; various defects in chick embryo and rabbit.
Human studies: In a study of 1016 pregnancies, oral doses of 80–120 mg

daily used from the 5th to 7th week of pregnancy to the 18th week was not associated with teratogenic effects. Other data show masculinization of the female genitals: enlargement of the clitoris, fusion of the labia. Increased risk of heart, nervous system and limb defects when used in the second and third trimesters of pregnancy.

The drug is used as a benefit to risk decision in the first three months of pregnancy. Avoid this drug completely during the last six months of pregnancy.

Advisability of Use if Breast-Feeding
Presence of this drug in breast milk: Yes.
Avoid drug or refrain from nursing.

Habit-Forming Potential: None.

Effects of Overdosage: Nausea, vomiting, fluid retention, breast enlargement and discomfort, abnormal vaginal bleeding.

Possible Effects of Long-Term Use: May contribute to the development of osteoporosis.

Suggested Periodic Examinations While Taking This Drug (at physician's discretion)
Regular examinations (every 6 to 12 months) of the breasts and reproductive organs (pelvic examination of the uterus and ovaries, including Pap smear).

▷ **While Taking This Drug, Observe the Following**
Foods: No restrictions.
Beverages: No restrictions.
▷ *Alcohol:* No interactions expected.
Tobacco Smoking: It is advisable to smoke lightly or not at all.
▷ *Other Drugs*
The following drugs may *decrease* the effects of medroxyprogesterone
• rifampin (Rifadin, Rimactane, etc.) may hasten its elimination.
Medroxyprogesterone *taken concurrently* with
• warfarin (Coumadin) may increase the length of time needed to remove the warfarin by up to 71%. Increased lab INR testing is needed.
▷ *Driving, Hazardous Activities:* Usually no restrictions. Ask your doctor about your individual risk and for guidance regarding specific restrictions.
Aviation Note: The use of this drug *may be a disqualification* for piloting. Consult a designated Aviation Medical Examiner.
Exposure to Sun: No restrictions.

MEFENAMIC ACID (Me FEN am ik a sid)

Introduced: 1966 **Prescription:** USA: Yes; Canada: Yes **Available as Generic:** USA: Yes; Canada: Yes **Class:** NSAID, mild analgesic **Controlled Drug:** USA: No; Canada: No

Brand Names: ✦Ponstan, Ponstel

Warning: The use of mefenamic acid beyond one week is **not** recommended.

BENEFITS versus RISKS	
Possible Benefits	*Possible Risks*
Effective relief of mild to moderate pain and inflammation	Hemolytic anemia Low white blood cell counts (rare) Gastrointestinal pain, ulceration and bleeding (rare) Rare kidney damage Rare systemic lupus erythematosus Rare pancreatitis

Please see the fenamate nonsteroidal anti-inflammatory drug profile for further information.

MEPERIDENE (me PER i deen)

Other Name: Pethidine
Introduced: 1939   **Prescription:** USA: Yes; Canada: Yes   **Available as Generic:** Yes   **Class:** Strong analgesic, opioids   **Controlled Drug:** USA: C-II*; Canada: No
Brand Names: Demerol, Demerol APAP [CD], Pethadol

BENEFITS versus RISKS	
Possible Benefits	*Possible Risks*
EFFECTIVE RELIEF OF MODERATE TO SEVERE PAIN	POTENTIAL FOR HABIT FORMATION (DEPENDENCE) Weakness, fainting Disorientation, hallucinations Interference with urination

▷ **Principal Uses**
  As a Single Drug Product: Uses currently included in FDA approved labeling: (1) This potent analgesic is used by mouth or injection to relieve moderate to severe pain of any cause.
  Other (unlabeled) generally accepted uses: (1) Used to treat fevers caused by amphotericin-B; (2) can help porphyrias; (3) eases postanesthesia chills; (4) used in sickle cell disease pain.
  As a Combination Drug Product [CD]: This drug is available in combination with acetaminophen (APAP) to create a dosage form that utilizes two pain relievers, and also reduces fever.
How This Drug Works: Acting primarily as a depressant of certain brain functions, this drug suppresses the perception of pain and calms the emotional response to pain.
Available Dosage Forms and Strengths
  Injection — 10 mg per ml, 25 mg per ml, 50 mg per ml, 75 mg per ml and 100 mg per ml
  Syrup — 50 mg per 5-ml teaspoonful
  Tablets — 50 mg, 100 mg

*See Schedules of Controlled Drugs at the back of this book.

Meperidene

▷ **Usual Adult Dosage Range:** Taken by mouth: 50 to 150 mg/3 to 4 hours as needed to relieve pain; the usual dose is 100 mg. The total daily dosage should not exceed 900 mg. **Note: Actual dosage and dosing schedule must be determined by the physician for each patient individually.**

Conditions Requiring Dosing Adjustments

Liver function: The initial dose should be the same in liver compromise, however, subsequent doses should be decreased by 50% or the dosing interval doubled.

Kidney function: Patients with mild to moderate kidney failure should be given 75% of the usual dose at the usual interval. Patients with severe kidney failure should be given 50% of the usual dose at the usual time. **Multiple doses should be avoided** as a toxic (normeperidine) metabolite may accumulate and can cause severe central nervous system reactions.

▷ **Dosing Instructions:** The tablet may be crushed and taken with or following food to reduce stomach irritation or nausea. The syrup may be diluted in 4 ounces of water to reduce the numbing effect on the tongue and mouth tissues.

Usual Duration of Use: As required to control pain. Continual use should not exceed 5 to 7 days without interruption and reassessment of need.

▷ **This Drug Should Not Be Taken If**
- you have had an allergic reaction to any dosage form of it previously.
- you are having an acute attack of asthma.
- you have significant respiratory depression.
- you are taking, or have taken within the past 14 days, any monoamine oxidase (MAO) type A inhibitor drug (see Drug Classes).

▷ **Inform Your Physician Before Taking This Drug If**
- you have a history of drug abuse or alcoholism.
- you have impaired liver or kidney function.
- you have a history of asthma, epilepsy or glaucoma.
- you are taking any other drugs that have a sedative effect.
- you plan to have surgery under general anesthesia in the near future.

Possible Side-Effects (natural, expected and unavoidable drug actions)
Drowsiness, light-headedness, weakness, euphoria, dry mouth, urinary retention, constipation.

▷ **Possible Adverse Effects** (unusual, unexpected and infrequent reactions)
If any of the following develop, consult your physician promptly for guidance.

Mild Adverse Effects
Allergic Reactions: Skin rash, hives, itching.
Headache, dizziness, impaired concentration, sensation of drunkenness, confusion, depression, blurred or double vision.
Facial flushing, sweating, heart palpitation.
Nausea, vomiting, taste disorders.
Constipation.

Serious Adverse Effects
Allergic Reactions: Anaphylactic reactions.
Drop in blood pressure, causing severe weakness and fainting.
Disorientation, hallucinations, unstable gait, tremor, muscle twitching.

Slow heart beat.
Drug-induced myasthenia gravis.
Respiratory depression.
Urinary retention.
Kidney failure (rare).
Seizures, especially in patients with kidney failure who are given multiple doses.

▷ **Possible Effects on Sexual Function:** Blunting of sexual response. Retrograde ejaculation.

▷ **Adverse Effects That May Mimic Natural Diseases or Disorders**
Paradoxical behavioral disturbances may suggest psychotic disorder.

Possible Effects on Laboratory Tests
Blood alanine aminotransferase (ALT) and aspartate aminotransferase (AST) levels: increased (natural side-effects).
Blood amylase and lipase levels: increased (natural side-effects).

CAUTION
1. If you have asthma, chronic bronchitis or emphysema, excessive use of this drug may cause significant respiratory difficulty, thickening of bronchial secretions and suppression of coughing.
2. The concurrent use of this drug with atropinelike drugs can increase the risk of urinary retention and reduced intestinal function.
3. Do not take this drug following acute head injury.

Precautions for Use
By Infants and Children: Do not use this drug in infants under 1 year of age because of their vulnerability to life-threatening respiratory depression.
By Those over 60 Years of Age: Small doses initially and slow increases as needed and tolerated. Limit use to short-term treatment only if possible. There may be increased risk of drowsiness, dizziness, unsteadiness, falling, urinary retention and constipation (often leading to fecal impaction).

▷ **Advisability of Use During Pregnancy**
Pregnancy Category: B, D if used in higher doses or for a longer period of time, especially when the baby is due to be born. See Pregnancy Code at the back of this book.
Animal studies: Significant birth defects reported in hamster studies.
Human studies: Adequate studies of pregnant women are not available. However, no significant increase in birth defects was found in 1100 drug exposures.
Avoid during the first 3 months. Used sparingly and in small doses during the last 6 months only if clearly needed as it has clear effects on the breathing capabilities of the infant.

Advisability of Use if Breast-Feeding
Presence of this drug in breast milk: Yes.
Avoid drug or refrain from nursing.

Habit-Forming Potential: This drug can cause psychological and physical dependence (see Glossary).

Effects of Overdosage: Marked drowsiness, confusion, tremors, convulsions, stupor leading to coma.

Possible Effects of Long-Term Use: Psychological and physical dependence, chronic constipation.

Suggested Periodic Examinations While Taking This Drug (at physician's discretion)

Should assess bowel status if prone to constipation.

▷ **While Taking This Drug, Observe the Following**

Foods: No restrictions.

Beverages: No restrictions. May be taken with milk.

▷ *Alcohol:* Opioid analgesics can intensify the intoxicating effects of alcohol, and alcohol can intensify the depressant effects of opioids on brain function, breathing and circulation. Alcohol is best avoided.

Tobacco Smoking: No interactions expected.

Marijuana Smoking: Increase in drowsiness and pain relief; impairment of mental and physical performance.

▷ *Other Drugs*

Meperidine may *increase* the effects of
- other drugs with sedative effects.
- atropinelike drugs, and increase the risk of constipation and urinary retention.

Meperidine *taken concurrently* with
- cimetidine (Tagamet), famotidine, nizatidine, ranitidine and omeprazole act to increase alkalinity of the stomach and may result in increased meperidine levels and toxicity.
- intravenous acyclovir (Zovirax) can result in kidney and nerve problems.
- monoamine oxidase (MAO) type A inhibitor drugs (see Drug Classes) can cause the equivalent of an acute narcotic overdose: unconsciousness; severe breathing depression, slowed heart action and circulation. Can also cause excitability, convulsions, high fever and rapid heart action.
- phenothiazines (see Drug Class Section) can cause excessive and prolonged depression of brain functions, breathing and circulation.
- phenytoin (Dilantin) can result in decreased therapeutic effect of meperidine.

▷ *Driving, Hazardous Activities:* This drug can impair mental alertness, judgment, reaction time and physical coordination. Avoid hazardous activities.

Aviation Note: The use of this drug *is a disqualification* for piloting. Consult a designated Aviation Medical Examiner.

Exposure to Sun: No restrictions.

Discontinuation: Best limited to short-term use. If used for extended periods of time, discontinuation should be gradual to minimize withdrawal effects.

MERCAPTOPURINE (mer kap toh PYUR een)

Other Names: 6-mercaptopurine, 6-MP

Introduced: 1960   **Prescription:** USA: Yes; Canada: Yes   **Available as Generic:** USA: No; Canada: No   **Class:** Antineoplastic, immunosuppressant

Controlled Drug: USA: No; Canada: No

Brand Name: Purinethol

Mercaptopurine

BENEFITS versus RISKS	
Possible Benefits	*Possible Risks*
EFFECTIVE TREATMENT OF CERTAIN ACUTE AND CHRONIC LEUKEMIAS AND LYMPHOMAS	BONE MARROW DEPRESSION (see Glossary)
Effective treatment of polycythemia vera	DRUG-INDUCED LIVER DAMAGE
	Rare gastrointestinal ulceration
Possibly effective treatment of Crohn's disease and ulcerative colitis	
Possibly effective treatment of severe psoriatic arthritis	

▷ **Principal Uses**
   As a Single Drug Product: Uses currently included in FDA approved labeling: Combination treatment of (1) acute lymphocytic leukemia; (2) acute non-lymphocytic leukemia.
   Other (unlabeled) generally accepted uses: Treatment of (1) inflammatory bowel diseases (Crohn's disease and ulcerative colitis); (2) certain cases of severe psoriatic arthritis.

How This Drug Works: This drug interferes with specific stages of cell reproduction (tissue growth) by inhibiting the formation of DNA and RNA.

Available Dosage Forms and Strengths
   Tablets — 50 mg

▷ **Recommended Dosage Ranges** (Actual dosage and administration schedule must be determined by the physician for each patient individually.)
   Infants and Children: For leukemia—2.5 mg/kg of body weight (to the nearest 25 mg) daily, in single or divided doses.
   12 to 60 Years of Age: For leukemia—initially 2.5 mg/kg of body weight (to the nearest 25 mg) daily, in single or divided doses, for 4 weeks. If needed and tolerated, the dose may be increased to 5 mg/kg of body weight daily. For maintenance, 1.5 to 2.5 mg/kg of body weight daily.
   For inflammatory bowel disease—1.5 mg/kg of body weight daily. The dose is subsequently adjusted to keep the platelet count above 100,000 and the white blood cell count above 4500.
   Over 60 Years of Age: Same as 12 to 60 years of age.

Conditions Requiring Dosing Adjustments
   Liver function: Used with caution and in decreased doses in patients with liver compromise. It is also a rare cause of liver hepatoxicity.
   Kidney function: The dose should be decreased in patients with renal (kidney) compromise to avoid accumulation of drug. It is a rare cause of drug crystals in urine.

▷ **Dosing Instructions:** The tablet may be crushed and taken with or following food to reduce stomach upset.

Usual Duration of Use: Use on a regular schedule for 4 to 6 weeks determines effectiveness in inducing remission in leukemia; continual use for 2 to 3 months to determine benefit in treating inflammatory bowel disease. Long-term use (months to years) requires periodic physician evaluation.

Mercaptopurine

▷ **This Drug Should Not Be Taken If**
- you have had an allergic reaction to it previously.
- you have a solid tumor or lymphoma (this drug is **not** indicated).
- you are pregnant. (Ask your physician for guidance.)

▷ **Inform Your Physician Before Taking This Drug If**
- you have a history of drug-induced bone marrow depression.
- you have impaired liver or kidney function.
- you are not using any contraception.
- you have gout.
- you have inflammatory bowel disease.
- you have been exposed recently to chicken pox or herpes zoster (shingles).
- you are taking any of the following drugs: allopurinol, probenecid, sulfinpyrazone, anticoagulants, immunosuppressants.

Possible Side-Effects (natural, expected and unavoidable drug actions)
Bone marrow depression (see Glossary).
Abnormally increased blood uric acid levels; possible urate kidney stones.

▷ **Possible Adverse Effects** (unusual, unexpected and infrequent reactions)
If any of the following develop, consult your physician promptly for guidance.
Mild Adverse Effects
Allergic Reactions: Skin rash, itching.
Headache, weakness.
Loss of appetite, mouth and lip sores, nausea, vomiting, diarrhea.
Serious Adverse Effects
Liver damage with jaundice (see Glossary).
Kidney damage: fever, cloudy or bloody urine.
Gastrointestinal ulceration: stomach pain, bloody or black stools.

▷ **Possible Effects on Sexual Function:** Suppression of sperm production; cessation of menstruation.

Possible Delayed Adverse Effects: Bone marrow depression may not be apparent during early treatment.

▷ **Adverse Effects That May Mimic Natural Diseases or Disorders**
Drug-induced liver damage may suggest viral hepatitis.

Natural Diseases or Disorders That May Be Activated by This Drug
Latent gout, peptic ulcer disease, inflammatory bowel disease.

Possible Effects on Laboratory Tests
Complete blood cell counts: decreased red cells, hemoglobin, white cells and platelets.
Blood glucose levels: falsely increased with SMA testing.
Blood uric acid levels: increased.
Liver function tests: increased liver enzymes (ALT/GPT, AST/GOT and alkaline phosphatase), increased bilirubin.
Kidney function tests: increased blood urea nitrogen (BUN) and creatinine.
Sperm counts: decreased.

Mercaptopurine

CAUTION
1. Comply fully with all requests for periodic laboratory tests.
2. Call your doctor at the first sign of infection or abnormal bleeding or bruising.
3. Inform your physician promptly if you become pregnant.
4. It is best to avoid immunizations while taking this drug, and to avoid contact with people who have recently taken oral poliovirus vaccine.

Precautions for Use
By Infants and Children: No specific problems anticipated.
By Those over 60 Years of Age: Increased risk of bone marrow depression. Periodic blood counts are mandatory.

▷ **Advisability of Use During Pregnancy**
Pregnancy Category: D. See Pregnancy Code at the back of this book.
Animal studies: Rat studies reveal toxic effects on the embryo.
Human studies: Adequate studies of pregnant women are not available. This drug is known to cause abortions and premature births.
Avoid drug during entire pregnancy if possible. Use a nonhormonal method of contraception.

Advisability of Use if Breast-Feeding
Presence of this drug in breast milk: Unknown.
Avoid drug or refrain from nursing.

Habit-Forming Potential: None.

Effects of Overdosage: Headache, dizziness, abdominal pain, nausea.

Possible Effects of Long-Term Use: Development of new malignant diseases.

Suggested Periodic Examinations While Taking This Drug (at physician's discretion)
Complete blood cell counts.
Blood uric acid levels.
Liver and kidney function tests.

▷ **While Taking This Drug, Observe the Following**
Foods: No restrictions.
Beverages: No restrictions. Drink liquids liberally, up to 2 quarts daily.
▷ *Alcohol:* Avoid completely.
Tobacco Smoking: No interactions expected.
▷ *Other Drugs*
Mercaptopurine may *decrease* the effects of
- warfarin (Coumadin); the INR should be checked more frequently.

The following drug may *increase* the effects of mercaptopurine
- allopurinol (Zyloprim).

Mercaptopurine *taken concurrently* with
- methotrexate (Mexate) can result in mercaptopurine toxicity.

▷ *Driving, Hazardous Activities:* No restrictions.
Aviation Note: The use of this drug *may be a disqualification* for piloting. Consult a designated Aviation Medical Examiner.
Exposure to Sun: No restrictions.
Discontinuation: To be determined by your physician.

MESALAMINE (me SAL a meen)

Other Names:
Mesalazine
5-aminosalicylic acid
5-ASA

Introduced: 1982   **Prescription:** USA: Yes; Canada: Yes   **Available as Generic:** USA: No; Canada: No   **Class:** Bowel anti-inflammatory   **Controlled Drug:** USA: No; Canada: No

Brand Names: Asacol, Pentasa, Rowasa, ◆Salofalk

BENEFITS versus RISKS	
Possible Benefits	*Possible Risks*
EFFECTIVE SUPPRESSION OF INFLAMMATORY BOWEL DISEASE	Allergic reactions: acute intolerance syndrome Drug-induced kidney damage (very rare)

▷ **Principal Uses**

As a Single Drug Product: Uses currently included in FDA approved labeling: (1) Treatment of active mild to moderate ulcerative colitis, proctosigmoiditis, and proctitis.

Other (unlabeled) generally accepted uses: (1) May help improve semen quality which had been damaged by prior sulfasalazine treatment; (2) can ease canker sores (aphthous ulcers); (3) has a steroid sparing effect in Chron's disease; (4) used to maintain remission in ulcerative colitis.

How This Drug Works: This drug suppresses the formation of prostaglandins (and related compounds), tissue substances that induce inflammation, tissue destruction and diarrhea—the main problems in ulcerative colitis and proctitis.

Available Dosage Forms and Strengths
Rectal suspension — 4 grams per 60-ml unit
Suppositories — 250 mg (Canada) and 500 mg (U.S. and Canada)
Tablets, sustained-release — 400 mg

▷ **Recommended Dosage Ranges** (Actual dosage and administration schedule must be determined by the physician for each patient individually.)

Infants and Children: Dosage not established.

12 to 60 Years of Age: Rectal suspension—4 grams (as a retention enema) every night for 3 to 6 weeks.

Suppositories—500 mg (inserted into rectum) 2 or 3 times daily.

Tablets—400 to 800 mg (1 or 2 tablets by mouth) 3 times daily for 6 weeks. The total daily dose should not exceed 2400 mg.

Over 60 Years of Age: Same as 12 to 60 years of age.

Conditions Requiring Dosing Adjustments

Liver function: Specific guidelines for dosage adjustment in liver compromise not available.

Kidney function: This drug should be used with caution in kidney compromise.

Mesalamine 603

▷ **Dosing Instructions:** Rectal suspension—Use as a retention enema at bedtime; if possible, empty the rectum before inserting suspension; try to retain the suspension all night.

Tablets—Best taken with 8 ounces of water on an empty stomach, 1 hour before or 2 hours after eating. However, it may be taken with or following food to reduce stomach upset. The sustained-release tablet should be swallowed whole without alteration.

Usual Duration of Use: Use on a regular schedule for 1 to 3 weeks determines effectiveness in controlling ulcerative colitis. Long-term use (months to years) requires supervision and periodic physician evaluation.

Possible Advantages of This Drug
Does not cause bone marrow or blood cell disorders.
Does not inhibit sperm production or function.

▷ **This Drug Should Not Be Taken If**
- you have had an allergic reaction to it previously.
- you have severely impaired kidney function.
- you have active ulcer disease.

▷ **Inform Your Physician Before Taking This Drug If**
- you are allergic to aspirin (or other salicylates), olsalazine or sulfasalazine.
- you are allergic by nature: History of hay fever, asthma, hives, eczema.
- you have impaired liver or kidney function.
- you have a history of a blood clotting disorder.
- you have a history of low white blood cell counts.
- you are currently taking sulfasalazine (Azulfidine).

Possible Side-Effects (natural, expected and unavoidable drug actions)
Anal irritation (with use of rectal suspension or suppositories).

▷ **Possible Adverse Effects** (unusual, unexpected and infrequent reactions)
If any of the following develop, consult your physician promptly for guidance.

Mild Adverse Effects
Allergic Reactions: Skin rash.
Headache, hair loss (rare).
Blurred vision, ringing in the ears.
Paresthesias, neck and joint pain, dizziness, cough.
Nausea, stomach pain, excessive gas.

Serious Adverse Effects
Allergic Reactions: Acute intolerance syndrome: fever, skin rash, severe headache, severe stomach pain, bloody diarrhea.
Kidney damage (nephrosis, interstitial nephritis) (rare).
Peripheral neuropathy (rare).
Pancreatitis (rare).
Peptic ulcers (rare).
Low white blood cell, anemia and platelet counts (rare).
Myocarditis, pericarditis or pericardial effusions (rare).
Hepatitis (rare).

▷ **Possible Effects on Sexual Function:** None reported.

Metaproterenol

Possible Effects on Laboratory Tests
Increased liver function tests.

CAUTION
1. Report promptly any signs of acute intolerance syndrome. Stop drug.
2. Shake the rectal suspension thoroughly before administering.

Precautions for Use
By Infants and Children: Safety and effectiveness by those under 12 years of age not established.
By Those over 60 Years of Age: None.

▷ **Advisability of Use During Pregnancy**
Pregnancy Category: B. See Pregnancy Code at the back of this book.
Animal studies: No drug-induced birth defects found in rat or rabbit studies.
Human studies: Adequate studies of pregnant women are not available.
Use this drug only if clearly needed. Ask your physician for guidance.

Advisability of Use if Breast-Feeding
Presence of this drug in breast milk: Yes.
Avoid drug or refrain from nursing.

Habit-Forming Potential: None.

Effects of Overdosage: Headache, dizziness, nausea, vomiting, abdominal cramping.

Possible Effects of Long-Term Use: None reported.

Suggested Periodic Examinations While Taking This Drug (at physician's discretion)
Kidney function tests, urinalysis.

▷ **While Taking This Drug, Observe the Following**
Foods: Decreased mesalamine levels. Follow prescribed diet.
Beverages: No restrictions. May be taken with milk.
▷ *Alcohol:* No interactions expected.
Tobacco Smoking: No interactions expected.
▷ *Other Drugs:* No interactions expected.
▷ *Driving, Hazardous Activities:* No restrictions.
Aviation Note: The use of this drug *is probably not a disqualification* for piloting. Consult a designated Aviation Medical Examiner.
Exposure to Sun: No restrictions.

METAPROTERENOL (met a proh TER e nohl)

Other Name: Orciprenaline

Introduced: 1964 **Prescription:** USA: Yes; Canada: Yes **Available as Generic:** Yes **Class:** Antiasthmatic, bronchodilator **Controlled Drug:** USA: No; Canada: No

Brand Names: Alupent, Arm-a-Med, Dey-Dose, Dey-Lute, Metaprel, Prometa

Metaproterenol

BENEFITS versus RISKS	
Possible Benefits	*Possible Risks*
VERY EFFECTIVE RELIEF OF BRONCHOSPASM	Increased blood pressure Fine hand tremor Fast heart rate Irregular heart rhythm (with excessive use)

▷ **Principal Uses**
As a Single Drug Product: Uses currently included in FDA approved labeling: (1) Relieves acute bronchial asthma and reduces the frequency and severity of chronic, recurrent asthmatic attacks; (2) used to relieve reversible bronchospasm associated with chronic bronchitis and emphysema; (3) eases symptoms in obstructive bronchial disease.
Other (unlabeled) generally accepted uses: (1) Has been used in threatened abortion.

How This Drug Works: This drug acts to dilate those bronchial tubes that are in sustained constriction, thereby increasing the size of the airway and improving the ability to breathe.

Available Dosage Forms and Strengths
Powder for inhalation — 0.65 mg/inhalation
Solution for nebulizer — 0.4%, 0.6% and 5%
Syrup — 10 mg per 5-ml teaspoonful
Tablets — 10 mg, 20 mg

▷ **Usual Adult Dosage Range:** Inhaler: 2 or 3 inhalations/3 to 4 hours; do not exceed 12 inhalations/day. Hand nebulizer: 5 to 15 inhalations/4 hours; do not exceed 40 inhalations/day. Syrup and tablets: 20 mg/6 to 8 hours.
Note: Actual dosage and administration schedule must be determined by the physician for each patient individually.

Conditions Requiring Dosing Adjustments
Liver function: Specific guidelines for dosing adjustment in patients with liver compromise are not usually indicated.
Kidney function: Dosing changes are not indicated in kidney compromise.

▷ **Dosing Instructions:** May be taken on empty stomach or with food or milk. Tablets should not be crushed for administration. For aerosol and nebulizer, follow the written instructions carefully. Do not overuse.

Usual Duration of Use: According to individual requirements. Do not use beyond the time necessary to terminate episodes of asthma.

▷ **This Drug Should Not Be Taken If**
- you have had an allergic reaction to any dosage form of it previously.
- you currently have an irregular heart rhythm.
- you are taking, or have taken within the past 2 weeks, any monoamine oxidase (MAO) type A inhibitor drug (see Drug Classes).

▷ **Inform Your Physician Before Taking This Drug If**
- you are overly sensitive to other sympathetic stimulant drugs.
- you currently use epinephrine (Adrenalin, Primatene Mist, etc.) to relieve asthmatic breathing.

Metaproterenol

- you have any type of heart or circulatory disorder, especially high blood pressure or coronary heart disease.
- you have diabetes or an overactive thyroid gland (hyperthyroidism).
- you are taking any form of digitalis or any stimulant drug.

Possible Side-Effects (natural, expected and unavoidable drug actions)
Aerosol—dryness or irritation of mouth or throat, altered taste.
Tablet—nervousness, palpitation.

▷ **Possible Adverse Effects** (unusual, unexpected and infrequent reactions)
If any of the following develop, consult your physician promptly for guidance.
Mild Adverse Effects
Headache, dizziness, restlessness, insomnia, fine tremor of hands.
Rapid, pounding heartbeat; increased sweating; muscle cramps in arms and legs.
Nausea, heartburn, vomiting.
Serious Adverse Effects
Rapid or irregular heart rhythm, intensification of angina, increased blood pressure.
Hallucinations and psychosis (rare).
Paradoxical spasm of the bronchi (rare).

▷ **Possible Effects on Sexual Function:** None reported.

Natural Diseases or Disorders That May Be Activated By This Drug
Latent coronary artery disease, diabetes or high blood pressure.

Possible Effects on Laboratory Tests
Urine sugar tests: positive (unreliable results with Benedict's solution).

CAUTION

1. Combined use of this drug by aerosol inhalation with beclomethasone aerosol (Beclovent, Vanceril) may increase the risk of toxicity due to fluorocarbon propellants. Use this aerosol 20 to 30 minutes *before* beclomethasone aerosol as this will reduce the risk of toxicity and will enhance the penetration of beclomethasone.
2. *Avoid excessive use of aerosol inhalation.* Excessive or prolonged use of this drug by inhalation can reduce its effectiveness and cause serious heart rhythm disturbances, including cardiac arrest.
3. Do not combine this drug with epinephrine. These two drugs may be used alternately if an interval of 4 hours is allowed between doses.
4. If you do not respond to your usually effective dose, ask your doctor for help. Do not increase the size or frequency of the dose without your physician's approval.

Precautions for Use
By Infants and Children: Safety and effectiveness of the aerosol and nebulized solution not established for children under 12 years of age. Safety and effectiveness of the syrup and tablet not established for children under 6 years of age.
By Those over 60 Years of Age: Avoid excessive and continual use. If acute asthma is not relieved promptly, other drugs will have to be tried. Watch for nervousness, palpitations, irregular heart rhythm and muscle tremors. Use with extreme caution if you have hardening of the arteries, heart disease or high blood pressure.

▷ **Advisability of Use During Pregnancy**
  Pregnancy Category: C. See Pregnancy Code at the back of this book.
  Animal studies: Significant birth defects reported in rabbit studies.
  Human studies: Adequate studies of pregnant women are not available.
  Avoid use during first 3 months. Use during the last 6 months only if clearly needed.

Advisability of Use if Breast-Feeding
  Presence of this drug in breast milk: Unknown.
  Avoid drug or refrain from nursing.

Habit-Forming Potential: None.

Effects of Overdosage: Nervousness, palpitation, rapid heart rate, sweating, headache, tremor, vomiting, chest pain.

Possible Effects of Long-Term Use: Loss of effectiveness. See *CAUTION* category.

Suggested Periodic Examinations While Taking This Drug (at physician's discretion)
  Blood pressure measurements, evaluation of heart status.

▷ **While Taking This Drug, Observe the Following**
  Foods: No restrictions.
  Beverages: Avoid excessive use of caffeine-containing beverages: coffee, tea, cola, chocolate.
▷ *Alcohol:* No interactions expected.
  Tobacco Smoking: No interactions expected.
▷ *Other Drugs*
  Metaproterenol *taken concurrently* with
  • monoamine oxidase (MAO) type A inhibitor drugs may cause excessive increase in blood pressure and undesirable heart stimulation.
▷ *Driving, Hazardous Activities:* Usually no restrictions. Use caution if excessive nervousness or dizziness occurs.
  Aviation Note: The use of this drug *is a disqualification* for piloting. Consult a designated Aviation Medical Examiner.
  Exposure to Sun: No restrictions.
  Heavy Exercise or Exertion: Use caution. Excessive exercise can induce asthma in sensitive individuals.

METFORMIN (Met FOR min)

Other Names: None

Introduced: 1995 **Prescription:** USA: Yes; Canada: Yes **Available as Generic:** USA: No; Canada: No **Class:** Oral hypoglycemic agent, Biguanide
Controlled Drug: USA: No; Canada: No

Brand Names: Glucophage

Warning: Avoid excessive alcohol intake with this drug. Alcohol can cause lactic acidosis, a condition which metformin can also rarely cause. All oral hypoglycemic agents may carry the risk of increased cardiovascular death based on a 1975 study of tolbutamide and phenformin.

Metformin

BENEFITS versus RISKS	
Possible Benefits	*Possible Risks*
EFFECTIVE GLUCOSE CONTROL WITHOUT INSULIN INJECTIONS	LACTIC ACIDOSIS (RARE)
MAY BE USED CONCURRENTLY WITH A SULFONYLUREA	Possible anemia with long-term use
DOES NOT LEAD TO WEIGHT GAIN	
TAKEN BY MOUTH VERSUS INJECTION OF INSULIN	
Usually avoids excessive lowering of blood sugar	
Favorable effects on lipids	

▷ **Principal Uses**

As a Single Drug Product: Uses currently included in FDA approved labeling: (1) Used in combination with diet restrictions to treat noninsulin dependent diabetes; (2) can be combined with a sulfonylurea (see Drug Classes) in those patients who do not have an adequate response to diet restrictions plus a sulfonylurea.

Other (unlabeled) generally accepted uses: (1) May be used as single agent therapy to overcome insulin resistance.

How This Drug Works: This biguanide decreases sugar (glucose) production in the liver. It also increases sensitivity of the body to insulin.

Available Dosage Forms and Strengths
Tablets — 500 mg, 850 mg

▷ **Recommended Dosage Ranges (Actual dosage and administration schedule must be determined by the physician for each patient individually.)**

Infants and Children: Not approved for use in this population.

12 to 60 Years of Age: Dosing is started at 500 mg twice daily. It is best to take this medicine with the morning and evening meal. Typical effective dosages are 850 mg twice daily. Maximum dose is 850 mg three times daily.

Over 60 Years of Age: Lower doses are used. Some patients may have acceptable blood sugar control with as little as 500 mg daily. If this dose is used, it should be taken with the morning meal. The dose may be slowly increased as needed and tolerated.

Conditions Requiring Dosing Adjustments

Liver function: This drug should **not** be used in patients with liver compromise.

Kidney function: This drug should **not** be used in females with steady state creatinine levels greater than 1.4 or in males with steady state creatinine levels greater than 1.5.

▷ **Dosing Instructions:** This drug should be taken with the morning and evening meal if it has been prescribed on a twice daily basis.

Usual Duration of Use: Continual use on a regular schedule for a week is usually necessary to determine this drug's effectiveness in establishing tight glucose control. A month of continuous use will be needed before an effect on glycosylated hemoglobin (a measure of past success of glucose control) is seen. Long-term use (months to years) requires periodic evaluation of response and dosage adjustment. Consult your physician on a regular basis.

Possible Advantages of This Drug
Does not lead to weight gain.
Can be used (because of its mechanism of action) in combination with a sulfonylurea.
Can be used to overcome insulin resistance.
Does not cause excessive lowering of blood sugar (hypoglycemia) when used as monotherapy.

Currently a "Drug of Choice"
for treatment of hyperglycemia in the elderly.

▷ **This Drug Should Not Be Taken If**
- you have had an allergic reaction to any dosage form of it or related medicines previously.
- you have impaired kidneys (serum creatinine greater than 1.4 for females or 1.5 for males).
- you have liver disease.
- you are an alcoholic.
- you have a heart or lung insufficiency (increased lactic acidosis risk).
- you are going to have a radiology test that uses iodinated contrast media (ask your doctor).
- you have chronic metabolic acidosis or ketoacidosis.
- you are breast-feeding.

▷ **Inform Your Physician Before Taking This Drug If**
- you are planning to have surgery soon.
- you have a history of megaloblastic anemia.
- you have seen another physician and a diagnosis of ketoacidosis has been made.
- you are uncertain of how much metformin to take or how often to take it.

Possible Side-Effects (natural, expected and unavoidable drug actions)
Lactic acidosis (rare).

▷ **Possible Adverse Effects** (unusual, unexpected and infrequent reactions)
If any of the following develop, consult your physician promptly for guidance.
Mild Adverse Effects
Allergic Reactions: Rash.
Metallic taste (3%).
Nausea, vomiting or diarrhea.
Anorexia, headache, dizziness or tiredness.
Serious Adverse Effects
Allergic Reactions: Not reported.
Idiosyncratic Reactions: None reported.
Lactic acidosis (rare).
Lowered vitamin B12 levels and resultant anemia (megaloblastic).
Drug-induced porphyria.

Metformin

All oral hypoglycemic agents carry a label indicating that they may increase risk of cardiovascular death (based on a 1975 study of tolbutamide and phenformin).

▷ **Possible Effects on Sexual Function:** None reported.

Possible Delayed Adverse Effects: Low vitamin B12 levels and anemia (megaloblastic).

▷ **Adverse Effects That May Mimic Natural Diseases or Disorders**
Acidosis may mimic ketoacidosis, which is seen in diabetics.

Natural Diseases or Disorders That May Be Activated by This Drug
None reported.

Possible Effects on Laboratory Tests
Blood glucose: decreased.

CAUTION
1. This drug may cause lactic acidosis. Ask your doctor for signs or symptoms which may occur.
2. Drugs in this class (phenformin) or tolbutamide were reported to increase risk of cardiovascular death. While there is no data to support that effect for this medicine, patients should be closely followed.

Precautions for Use
By Infants and Children:
Safety and effectiveness for use by those under 18 years of age have not been established.

By Those over 60 Years of Age: Smaller starting doses (500 mg daily) are indicated. People in this age group tend to have an age-related decline in kidney function as well as a more compromised ability to tolerate lower blood sugar levels.

▷ **Advisability of Use During Pregnancy**
Pregnancy Category: B. See Pregnancy Code at the back of this book.
Animal studies: No birth defects in rats at two times the typical human dose.
Human studies: Information from adequate studies of pregnant women is not available. The manufacturer does not recommend the use of this drug in pregnancy. Insulin is still considered the drug of choice to control blood sugar in pregnancy.

Advisability of Use if Breast-Feeding
Presence of this drug in breast milk: Yes.
Avoid drug or refrain from nursing.

Habit-Forming Potential: None.

Effects of Overdosage: Nausea and vomiting, pulmonary edema, hemorrhage from the stomach, lactic acidosis, seizures, intractable lowering of the blood pressure, coma.

Possible Effects of Long-Term Use: Lowering of vitamin B12 and resultant anemia (megaloblastic).

Suggested Periodic Examinations While Taking This Drug (at physician's discretion)
Vitamin B12 levels, tests of kidney and liver function.

▷ **While Taking This Drug, Observe the Following**
  Foods: No restrictions.
  Nutritional Support: Diet as prescribed by your doctor.
  Beverages: No restrictions.
▷ *Alcohol:* Used with extreme caution. Alcohol worsens the effect of metformin on lactate. Avoid alcohol in excessive amounts.
  Tobacco Smoking: No interactions expected.
  Marijuana Smoking: May worsen dizziness.
▷ *Other Drugs*
  Metformin may *increase* the effects of
  • insulin in the sense that the lowering of blood sugar will be increased.
  Metformin *taken concurrently* with
  • ACE inhibitors (see Drug Classes) may exacerbate lowering of blood sugar to an undesirable extent.
  • beta blockers (see Drug Classes) may slow recovery from any hypoglycemia which occurs and can also block symptoms of low blood sugar.
  • itraconazole or other azole antifungal agents can result in severe lowering of the blood sugar.
  • thyroid hormones (see Drug Classes) can result in blunting of metformin's therapeutic effect.
  The following drugs may *increase* the effects of metformin
  • cimetidine and result in toxicity.
  • oral hypoglycemic agents (see Drug Classes). This effect may be used to therapeutic advantage.
▷ *Driving, Hazardous Activities:* This drug may cause drowsiness or dizziness. Restrict activities as necessary.
  Aviation Note: Diabetes **is a disqualification** for piloting. Consult a designated Aviation Medical Examiner.
  Exposure to Sun: Use caution. Some medicines which are similar can cause increased sensitivity to the sun.
  Heavy Exercise or Exertion: Heavy exercise will tend to use sugar up faster than usual. This drug will have an effect on lowering the blood sugar. Be alert to the symptoms of low blood sugar.
  Occurrence of Unrelated Illness: Infections or other illness may still require use of insulin to achieve acceptable blood sugar control.
  Discontinuation: Periodic physician evaluations of the continued benefit of this medicine are needed.

METHADONE (METH a dohn)

Introduced: 1948   **Prescription:** USA: Yes   **Available as Generic:** Yes   **Class:** Strong analgesic, opioids   **Controlled Drug:** USA: C-II*

Brand Name: Dolophine, Diskets

*See Schedules of Controlled Drugs at the back of this book.

Methadone

BENEFITS versus RISKS	
Possible Benefits	*Possible Risks*
EFFECTIVE RELIEF OF MODERATE TO SEVERE PAIN	POTENTIAL FOR HABIT FORMATION (DEPENDENCE)
SUBSTITUTION AND WITHDRAWAL IN HEROIN ADDICTION	Weakness, fainting Disorientation, hallucinations Interference with urination Constipation

▷ **Principal Uses**
As a Single Drug Product: Uses currently included in FDA approved labeling: (1) This potent analgesic is used by mouth or injection to relieve moderate to severe pain of any cause; (2) Used to provide an appropriate substitute for heroin or other narcotics in treatment programs for drug addiction. Other (unlabeled) generally accepted uses: (1) May have a role in neonatal drug withdrawal; (2) minor role in restless leg syndrome.

How This Drug Works: Depresses certain brain functions and blocks pain perception and calms the emotional response to pain. Relieves heroin withdrawal by long acting presence at receptors, and must itself be slowly withdrawn.

Available Dosage Forms and Strengths
    Concentrate — 10 mg per ml
    Injection — 10 mg per ml
    Oral solution — 5 mg, 10 mg per 5-ml teaspoonful (8% alcohol)
    Tablets — 5 mg, 10 mg
    Tablets, dispersible — 40 mg

▷ **Usual Adult Dosage Range:** Taken by mouth: 2.5 to 10 mg/3 to 4 hours as needed to relieve pain. The total daily dosage should not exceed 80 mg. (Dosage schedules for maintenance treatment during heroin withdrawal must be individualized.) **Note: Actual dosage and administration schedule must be determined by the physician for each patient individually.**

Conditions Requiring Dosing Adjustments
Liver function: This drug should be used with caution in patients with liver compromise, and consideration given to decreased dosages.
Kidney function: Patients with mild kidney failure should be given the usual dose every 6 hours. Patients with moderate to severe failure should be given the usual dose every 8 hours. Patients with severe failure should be given the usual dose every 8 to 12 hours.

▷ **Dosing Instructions:** The tablet may be crushed and taken with or following food to reduce stomach irritation or nausea. Concentrate must be diluted in 3 ounces (or more) of water before swallowing.

Usual Duration of Use: Continual use should not exceed 5 to 7 days without reassessment of need.

▷ **This Drug Should Not Be Taken If**
- you have had an allergic reaction to any dosage form of it previously.
- you are having an acute attack of asthma.

▷ **Inform Your Physician Before Taking This Drug If**
- you have a history of drug abuse or alcoholism.
- you have impaired liver or kidney function.
- you have a history of asthma or other chronic lung disease.
- you are taking any other drugs that have a sedative effect.
- you are taking, or have taken within the past 14 days, any monoamine oxidase (MAO) type A inhibitor drug (see Drug Class Section).
- you plan to have surgery under general anesthesia in the near future.

Possible Side-Effects (natural, expected and unavoidable drug actions)
Drowsiness, light-headedness, weakness, euphoria, dry mouth, urinary retention, constipation.

▷ **Possible Adverse Effects** (unusual, unexpected and infrequent reactions)
If any of the following develop, consult your physician promptly for guidance.

Mild Adverse Effects
Allergic Reactions: Skin rash, hives, itching.
Headache, dizziness, impaired concentration, sensation of drunkenness, confusion, depression, blurred or double vision.
Facial flushing, sweating, heart palpitation.
Nausea, vomiting.

Serious Adverse Effects
Drop in blood pressure, causing severe weakness and fainting.
Disorientation, hallucinations, unstable gait, tremor, muscle twitching.
Drug-induced porphyria.
Billiary tract spasm.
Liver toxicity (rare).
Respiratory depression.

▷ **Possible Effects on Sexual Function:** Decreased libido, impotence, delayed ejaculation, inhibited female orgasm, male infertility, loss of menstruation. (These effects do not occur with short-term use for pain relief; however, they are very common with long-term use and addiction.) Swelling and tenderness of the male breast tissue (gynecomastia).

▷ **Adverse Effects That May Mimic Natural Diseases or Disorders**
Paradoxical behavioral disturbances may suggest psychotic disorder.

Possible Effects on Laboratory Tests
Blood thyroid hormone levels: T_3 and T_4 levels increased; free T_4 level decreased.
Urine pregnancy tests: False positive results with Gravindex.
Urine screening tests for drug abuse: May be **positive**. (Test results depend upon amount of drug taken and testing method used.)

CAUTION
1. If you have asthma, chronic bronchitis or emphysema, the excessive use of this drug may cause significant respiratory difficulty, thickening of bronchial secretions and suppression of coughing.
2. The concurrent use of this drug with atropinelike drugs can increase the risk of urinary retention and reduced intestinal function.
3. Do not take this drug following acute head injury.

Methadone

Precautions for Use

By Infants and Children: Do not use this drug in infants under 1 year of age because of their vulnerability to life-threatening respiratory depression.

By Those over 60 Years of Age: Small starting doses and short-term use are indicated. May be increased risk of drowsiness, dizziness, unsteadiness, falling, urinary retention and constipation (often leading to fecal impaction).

▷ **Advisability of Use During Pregnancy**

Pregnancy Category: D if used in high doses or for prolonged amounts of time near the birth of the baby. See Pregnancy Code at the back of this book.

Animal studies: Significant birth defects reported in mice and hamster studies.

Human studies: Adequate studies of pregnant women are not available.

Ask your doctor for guidance.

Advisability of Use if Breast-Feeding

Presence of this drug in breast milk: Yes.

Avoid drug or refrain from nursing.

Habit-Forming Potential: This drug can cause psychological and physical dependence (see Glossary).

Effects of Overdosage: Marked drowsiness, confusion, tremors, convulsions, stupor leading to coma.

Possible Effects of Long-Term Use: Psychological and physical dependence, chronic constipation.

Suggested Periodic Examinations While Taking This Drug (at physician's discretion)

None.

▷ **While Taking This Drug, Observe the Following**

Foods: No restrictions.

Beverages: No restrictions. May be taken with milk.

▷ *Alcohol:* Opioid analgesics can intensify the intoxicating effects of alcohol, and alcohol can intensify the depressant effects of opioids on brain function, breathing and circulation. Alcohol is best avoided.

Tobacco Smoking: No interactions expected.

Marijuana Smoking: Increase in drowsiness and pain relief; impairment of mental and physical performance.

▷ *Other Drugs*

Methadone may *increase* the effects of
- other drugs with sedative effects, and cause excessive sedation.

Methadone *taken concurrently* with
- monoamine oxidase (MAO) type A inhibitor drugs (see Drug Classes) requires close observation for signs of nervous system toxicity.

The following drugs may *decrease* the effects of methadone
- phenytoin (Dilantin, etc.).
- rifampin (Rifadin, Rimactane, etc.).

▷ *Driving, Hazardous Activities:* This drug can impair mental alertness, judgment, reaction time and physical coordination. Avoid hazardous activities.

Aviation Note: The use of this drug *is a disqualification* for piloting. Consult a designated Aviation Medical Examiner.

Exposure to Sun: No restrictions.
Discontinuation: It is advisable to limit this drug to short-term use. If it is necessary to use it for extended periods of time, discontinuation should be gradual to minimize possible effects of withdrawal (stomach cramps, tearing eyes, nasal discharge, chills and tremors).

METHOTREXATE (meth oh TREX ayt)

Other Names: Amethopterin, MTX
Introduced: 1948   **Prescription:** USA: Yes; Canada: Yes   **Available as Generic:** Yes   **Class:** Anticancer drugs, antipsoriasis   **Controlled Drug:** USA: No; Canada: No
Brand Names: Abitrexate, Folex, Folex PFS, Mexate, Rheumatrex Dose Pack

BENEFITS versus RISKS	
Possible Benefits	*Possible Risks*
EFFECTIVE TREATMENT OF SOME CASES OF SEVERE DISABLING PSORIASIS	GASTROINTESTINAL ULCERATION AND BLEEDING
EFFECTIVE TREATMENT OF CERTAIN ADULT AND CHILDHOOD CANCERS	MOUTH AND THROAT ULCERATON
PREVENTION OF REJECTION OF BONE MARROW TRANSPLANTS	SEVERE BONE MARROW DEPRESSION
Helpful adjunctive therapy in severe, refractory rheumatoid arthritis and related disorders	DAMAGE TO LUNGS, LIVER OR KIDNEYS
	Loss of hair

▷ **Principal Uses**

As a Single Drug Product: Uses currently included in FDA approved labeling: (1) Combination therapy of acute lymphocytic leukemia; (2) combination therapy of various types of adult and childhood cancer; (3) severe and widespread forms of disabling psoriasis that have failed to respond to all standard treatment procedures; (4) various types of both adult and childhood cancer; (5) used to prevent rejection of transplanted bone marrow; (6) used in the treatment of connective tissue disorders such as rheumatoid arthritis and related conditions. Its use in rheumatoid arthritis is restricted to the treatment of selected adults with severe active disease that has failed to respond to conventional therapy.

Other (unlabeled) generally accepted uses: (1) Used in a variety of neoplastic syndromes in combination therapy; (2) may have a role in helping decrease steroid use in steroid-dependent asthma; (3) helps lessen neutropenia in Felty's syndrome.

How This Drug Works: By interfering with the normal utilization of folic acid in tissue cell reproduction, this drug retards abnormally rapid tissue growth (as in psoriasis and cancer).

Available Dosage Forms and Strengths

Injections — 2.5 mg per ml, 10 mg per ml and 25 mg per ml
Intrathecal cryodessicated powder — 20 mg, 50 mg, 100 mg

Injections (preservative-free) — 25 mg, 50 mg, 100 mg, 250 per ml
Tablets — 2.5 mg

▷ **Usual Adult Dosage Range**

For psoriasis (alternate schedules): (1) 10 to 50 mg once/week; (2) 2.5 to 5 mg/12 hours for 3 doses, or every 8 hours for 4 doses, once a week up to a maximum of 30 mg/week; (3) 2.5 mg/day for 5 days, followed by 2 days without drug, with gradual increase in dosage to a maximum of 6.25 mg/day.

For rheumatoid arthritis (alternate schedules): (1) single oral dose of 7.5 mg once weekly; (2) divided doses of 2.5 mg every 12 hours for 3 doses per week. Dosage may be increased gradually as needed and tolerated. Do not exceed a weekly dose of 20 mg.

Note: Actual dosage and administration schedule must be determined by the physician for each patient individually.

Conditions Requiring Dosing Adjustments

Liver function: It should be used with caution and in decreased dose in patients with liver compromise.

Kidney function: Methotrexate should be used as a result of a benefit to risk decision. Increased systemic adverse effects may occur if this medication is used in patients with compromised kidneys. This drug should **not** be given to patients with moderate to severe kidney failure (creatinine clearances less than 40 ml/min). In patients with mild to moderate kidney failure, 50% of the usual dose should be given in the usual dosing interval.

▷ **Dosing Instructions:** The tablet may be crushed and taken with food to reduce stomach irritation. Drink at least 2 to 3 quarts of liquids daily.

Usual Duration of Use: Use on a regular schedule for several weeks determines benefit in reducing the severity and extent of psoriasis. Response in rheumatoid arthritis usually begins after 3 to 6 weeks of treatment. When a favorable response has been achieved, the dosage should be reduced to the smallest amount that will maintain acceptable improvement. Long-term use (months to years) requires physician supervision.

▷ **This Drug Should Not Be Taken If**
- you have had an allergic reaction to it previously.
- you currently have, or have had a recent exposure to, either chicken pox or shingles (herpes zoster).
- you are pregnant or planning pregnancy in the near future, and you are taking this drug to treat psoriasis or rheumatoid arthritis.
- you have active liver disease, peptic ulcer, regional enteritis or ulcerative colitis.
- you are making little or no urine.
- you currently have a blood cell or bone marrow disorder.

▷ **Inform Your Physician Before Taking This Drug If**
- you have a chronic infection of any kind.
- you have impaired liver or kidney function.
- you have a history of bone marrow impairment of any kind, especially drug-induced bone marrow depression.
- you are dehydrated.
- you have a history of gout, peptic ulcer disease, regional enteritis or ulcerative colitis.

Possible Side-Effects (natural, expected and unavoidable drug actions)
The following are due to the pharmacological actions of this drug. **Report such developments to your physician promptly.**
Sores on the lips, in the mouth or throat; vomiting; intestinal cramping; diarrhea (may be bloody); painful urination; bloody urine.
Reduced resistance to infection, fatigue, weakness, fever, abnormal bleeding or bruising (bone marrow depression).

▷ **Possible Adverse Effects** (unusual, unexpected and infrequent reactions)
If any of the following develop, consult your physician promptly for guidance.
Mild Adverse Effects
Allergic Reactions: Skin rash, hives, itching.
Headache, drowsiness, blurred vision.
Loss of appetite, nausea, vomiting.
Loss of hair, loss of skin pigmentation, acne.
Serious Adverse Effects
Allergic Reactions: Drug-induced pneumonia: cough, chest pain, shortness of breath. Anaphylaxis.
Nervous system toxicity: speech disturbances, paralysis, seizures.
Liver toxicity with jaundice (see Glossary).
Kidney toxicity: reduced urine volume, kidney failure.
Colitis or toxic megacolon.
Immune suppression and subsequent infection with Pneumocystis carinii pneumonia.
Severe skin reactions (toxic epidermal necrolysis).
Chromosomal damage (from occupational exposure.

▷ **Possible Effects on Sexual Function:** Altered timing and pattern of menstruation.

Possible Delayed Adverse Effects: Some reports suggest that methotrexate therapy may contribute to the later development of secondary cancers. Other studies have not confirmed this.

Possible Effects on Laboratory Tests
Complete blood cell counts: decreased red cells, hemoglobin, white cells and platelets.
Blood uric acid level: increased.
Liver function tests: increased liver enzymes (ALT/GPT, AST/GOT and alkaline phosphatase), increased bilirubin.
Kidney function tests: increased blood urea nitrogen (BUN) level; increased urine creatinine content (kidney damage).
Fecal occult blood test: positive.
Sperm count: decreased.

CAUTION
1. This drug must be monitored carefully by a physician who is skilled in its proper administration. Request the Patient Package Insert that is available with this drug (Rheumatrex Dose Pack) and read it thoroughly.
2. Appropriate laboratory examinations, performed before and during the use of this drug, are mandatory.
3. Women with potential for pregnancy should have a pregnancy test

Methotrexate

before taking this drug and should use an effective form of contraception during its use and for 8 weeks following its discontinuation.
4. Live virus vaccines should be avoided during use of this drug. Live virus vaccines could actually produce infection rather than stimulate an immune response.

Precautions for Use
By Those over 60 Years of Age: Careful evaluation of kidney function should be made before starting treatment and during the entire course of therapy.

▷ **Advisability of Use During Pregnancy**
Pregnancy Category: X. See Pregnancy Code at the back of this book.
Animal studies: Skull and facial defects reported in mice.
Human studies: This drug is known to cause fetal deaths and birth defects. Its use during pregnancy to treat psoriasis or rheumatoid arthritis cannot be justified.

Advisability of Use if Breast-Feeding
Presence of this drug in breast milk: Yes.
Avoid drug or refrain from nursing.

Habit-Forming Potential: None.

Effects of Overdosage: The side-effects and adverse effects listed previously develop earlier and with greater severity.

Possible Effects of Long-Term Use: Liver compromise (fibrosis and cirrhosis) occurs in 3–5% of long-term users (35 to 49 months).

Suggested Periodic Examinations While Taking This Drug (at physician's discretion)
Complete blood cell counts, liver and kidney function tests, blood uric acid levels, chest X-ray examinations.

▷ **While Taking This Drug, Observe the Following**
Foods: Avoid highly seasoned foods that could be irritating. Between courses of treatment, eat liberally of the following foods: beef, chicken, lamb and pork liver, asparagus, navy beans, kale and spinach. Any food will reduce the peak methotrexate level obtained.
Beverages: No restrictions. This drug may be taken with milk.
▷ *Alcohol:* Avoid completely.
Tobacco Smoking: No interactions expected.
▷ *Other Drugs*
Methotrexate may *decrease* the effects of
- digoxin (Lanoxin).
- phenytoin (Dilantin).

The following drugs may *increase* the effects of methotrexate and enhance its toxicity
- aspirin and other salicylates.
- NSAIDs (see Drug Classes).
- probenecid (Benemid).

Methotrexate *taken concurrently* with
- Cholestyramine and other cholesterol lowering resins may result in decreased methotrexate effectiveness.
- cyclosporine (Sandimune) can result in increased toxicity from both drugs. The combination should be avoided.

- etretinate results in increased liver toxicity.
- pneumococcal or smallpox vaccine may result in decreased immune response to the vaccine.
- sulfa drugs such as sulfamethoxazole can result in increased hematologic toxicity.
- thiazide diuretics (see Drug Classes) may increase risk of myelosuppression.
- yellow fever vaccine can result in blunted response and benefit from the vaccine.

▷ *Driving, Hazardous Activities:* This drug may cause drowsiness, dizziness or blurred vision. Restrict activities as necessary.

Aviation Note: The use of this drug *is a disqualification* for piloting. Consult a designated Aviation Medical Examiner.

Exposure to Sun: Use caution. This drug can cause photosensitivity. Avoid ultraviolet lamps.

METHYCLOTHIAZIDE (METHY klo thigh a zyde)

Introduced: **Prescription:** USA: Yes; Canada: No **Available as Generic:** USA: Yes; Canada: Yes **Class:** Thiazide Diuretic **Controlled Drug:** Usa: No; Canada: No

Brand Names: ✢Duretic, Aquatensen, Enduron

BENEFITS versus RISKS	
Possible Benefits	*Possible Risks*
Effective, well-tolerated diuretic	Loss of blood potassium and magnesium
Enhances the effectiveness of other antihypertensives	Abnormal heart beats caused by loss of electrolytes
	Increased blood sugar, uric acid and calcium
	Rare blood cell disorders

Please see the combined thiazide diuretic profile for further information.

METHYLPHENIDATE (meth il FEN i dayt)

Introduced: 1956 **Prescription:** USA: Yes; Canada: Yes **Available as Generic:** USA: Yes; Canada: Yes **Class:** Stimulant, amphetaminelike drugs **Controlled Drug:** USA: C-II*; Canada:

Brand Names: ✢PMS-Methylphenidate, Ritalin, Ritalin-SR

*See Schedules of Controlled Drugs at the back of this book.

Methylphenidate

> **BENEFITS versus RISKS**
>
> *Possible Benefits*
> EFFECTIVE CONTROL OF NARCOLEPSY
> USEFUL AS ADJUNCTIVE TREATMENT IN THE ATTENTION-DEFICIT DISORDERS OF CHILDHOOD
> Useful in treatment of mild to moderate depression
> Useful in some cases of emotional withdrawal in the elderly
>
> *Possible Risks*
> POTENTIAL FOR SERIOUS PSYCHOLOGICAL DEPENDENCE
> SUPPRESSION OF GROWTH IN CHILDHOOD
> Abnormal behavior
> Rare blood cell disorders

▷ **Principal Uses**

As a Single Drug Product: Used primarily to treat (1) narcolepsy, recurrent spells of uncontrollable drowsiness and sleep; and (2) attention-deficit disorders of childhood, formerly known as the hyperactive child syndrome, minimal brain damage and minimal brain dysfunction.

Other (unlabeled) generally accepted uses: (1) Additional uses include the treatment of mild to moderate depression; (2) management of apathetic and withdrawal states in the elderly; (3) combination therapy of chronic pain, particularly cancer pain; (4) could have a role in helping autism.

How This Drug Works: This activates the brain stem, improves alertness and concentration, and increases learning ability and attention span.

Available Dosage Forms and Strengths

Tablets — 5 mg, 10 mg, 20 mg

Tablets, prolonged-action — 20 mg

▷ **Usual Adult Dosage Range:** 5 to 20 mg 2 or 3 times/day. **Note: Actual dosage and administration schedule must be determined by the physician for each patient individually.**

Conditions Requiring Dosing Adjustments

Liver function: Used with caution and in decreased dose in patients with liver compromise.

Kidney function: The kidney does not appear to to be involved in the elimination of this drug.

▷ **Dosing Instructions:** The regular tablet may be crushed and taken 30 to 45 minutes before meals. The prolonged-action tablet should be taken whole, not crushed.

Usual Duration of Use: Use on a regular schedule for 3 to 4 weeks determines effectiveness in controlling the symptoms of narcolepsy or improving the behavior of attention-deficit children. Long-term use (months to years) requires physician supervision and periodic evaluation.

▷ **This Drug Should Not Be Taken If**
- you have had an allergic reaction to it previously.
- you have glaucoma (inadequately treated).
- you are experiencing a period of severe anxiety, nervous tension or emotional depression.

▷ **Inform Your Physician Before Taking This Drug If**
- you have high blood pressure, angina or epilepsy.

Methylphenidate

- you are taking, or have taken within the past 14 days, any monoamine oxidase (MAO) type A inhibitor drug (see Drug Class Section).

Possible Side-Effects (natural, expected and unavoidable drug actions)
Nervousness, insomnia.

▷ **Possible Adverse Effects** (unusual, unexpected and infrequent reactions)
If any of the following develop, consult your physician promptly for guidance.
Mild Adverse Effects
Allergic Reactions: Skin rash, hives, drug fever, joint pains.
Headache, dizziness, rapid and forceful heart palpitation.
Reduced appetite, nausea, abdominal discomfort.
Stuttering and hallucinations.
Serious Adverse Effects
Allergic Reactions: Severe skin reactions, extensive bruising due to allergic destruction of blood platelets (see Glossary).
Porphyria (rare).
Liver toxicity (associated with intravenous abuse of the drug).
Muscle damage (rhabdomyolysis).
Idiosyncratic Reaction: Abnormal patterns of behavior.
Abnormally low red blood cell and white blood cell counts.
Growth suppression

▷ **Possible Effects on Sexual Function:** None reported.

Natural Diseases or Disorders That May Be Activated by This Drug
Latent epilepsy.

Possible Effects on Laboratory Tests
Blood platelet counts: occasionally decreased.
Prothrombin time: increased.
White and red blood cell counts: decreased.

CAUTION
1. Careful dosage adjustments on an individual basis are mandatory.
2. Paradoxical reactions (see Glossary) can occur, causing aggravation of initial symptoms for which this drug was prescribed.

Precautions for Use
By Infants and Children: Safety and effectiveness for those under 6 years of age not established. If this drug is not benefical in managing an attention deficit disorder after a trial of one month, it should be stopped. During long-term use, monitor the child for normal growth and development.
By Those over 60 Years of Age: Started with small doses. May be increased risk of nervousness, agitation, insomnia, high blood pressure, angina or disturbance of heart rhythm.

▷ **Advisability of Use During Pregnancy**
Pregnancy Category: B. See Pregnancy Code at the back of this book.
Animal studies: No birth defects found in mouse studies.
Human studies: Adequate studies of pregnant women are not available.
Use this drug only if clearly needed. Ask physician for guidance.

Advisability of Use if Breast-Feeding
Presence of this drug in breast milk: Unknown.
Avoid drug or refrain from nursing.

Habit-Forming Potential: This drug can produce tolerance and cause serious psychological dependence (see Glossary), a potentially dangerous characteristic of amphetaminelike drugs (see Drug Classes).

Effects of Overdosage: Headache, vomiting, agitation, tremors, muscle twitching, dry mouth, sweating, fever, confusion, hallucinations, seizures, coma.

Possible Effects of Long-Term Use: Suppression of growth (in weight and/or height) has been reported in children during long-term use of this drug.

Suggested Periodic Examinations While Taking This Drug (at physician's discretion)
Complete blood cell counts, blood pressure measurements.

▷ **While Taking This Drug, Observe the Following**
Foods: Avoid foods rich in tyramine (see Glossary); this drug in combination with tyramine may cause an excessive rise in blood pressure.
Beverages: Avoid beverages prepared from meat or meat extracts. This drug may be taken with milk.

▷ *Alcohol:* Avoid beer, Chianti wines and vermouth (may have high tyramine contents).
Tobacco Smoking: No interactions expected.

▷ *Other Drugs*
Methylphenidate may *increase* the effects of
- tricyclic antidepressants, and enhance their toxic effects (see Drug Classes).

Methylphenidate may *decrease* the effects of
- guanethidine (Ismelin), and impair its ability to lower blood pressure.

Methylphenidate *taken concurrently* with
- anticonvulsants may cause a significant change in the pattern of epileptic seizures; dosage adjustments may be necessary for proper control.
- monoamine oxidase (MAO) type A inhibitor drugs (see Drug Class Section) may cause a significant rise in blood pressure. Avoid the concurrent use of these drugs.
- morphine may be used to great therapeutic benefit to increase alertness, especially if high doses of morphine must be used.

▷ *Driving, Hazardous Activities:* This drug may cause dizziness or drowsiness. Restrict activities as necessary.
Aviation Note: The use of this drug *is a disqualification* for piloting. Consult a designated Aviation Medical Examiner.
Exposure to Sun: No restrictions.
Discontinuation: If it has been necessary to use this drug for an extended period of time, do not discontinue it abruptly. Careful supervision is necessary during withdrawal to prevent severe depression and erratic behavior.

METHYLPREDNISOLONE (meth il pred NIS oh lohn)

Introduced: 1957 **Prescription:** USA: Yes; Canada: Yes **Available as Generic:** USA: Yes; Canada: Yes **Class:** Cortisonelike drugs **Controlled Drug:** USA: No; Canada: No

Brand Names: A-Methapred, Depo-Medrol, Mar-Pred 40, Medrol, ◆Medrol Acne Lotion, Medrol Enpak, ◆Medrol Veriderm Cream, Meprolone, ◆Neo-Medrol Acne Lotion, ◆Neo-Medrol Veriderm, Solu-Medrol

Methylprednisolone

BENEFITS versus RISKS	
Possible Benefits	*Possible Risks*
EFFECTIVE RELIEF OF SYMPTOMS IN A WIDE VARIETY OF INFLAMMATORY AND ALLERGIC DISORDERS EFFECTIVE IMMUNO-SUPPRESSION in selected benign and malignant disorders	Short-term use (up to 10 days) is usually well tolerated Long-term use (exceeding 2 weeks) is associated with many adverse effects: ALTERED MOOD AND PERSONALITY CATARACTS, GLAUCOMA HYPERTENSION OSTEOPOROSIS ASEPTIC BONE NECROSIS INCREASED SUSCEPTIBILITY TO INFECTIONS (See Possible Adverse Effects and Possible Effects of Long-Term Use)

▷ **Principal Uses**

As a Single Drug Product: Uses currently included in FDA approved labeling: (1) Used in the treatment of a wide variety of allergic and inflammatory conditions. Used most commonly in the management of serious skin disorders, asthma, regional enteritis, multiple sclerosis, lupus erythematosus, ulcerative colitis and all types of major rheumatic disorders including bursitis, tendinitis and most forms of arthritis; (2) helps treat low platelet counts of unknown cause (idiopathic thrombocytopenic purpura).

Other (unlabeled) generally accepted uses: (1) Treatment of refractory anemia; (2) therapy of chronic obstrctive pulmonary disease; (3) combination treatment of acute nonlymphoblastic leukemia; (4) combination therapy of severe vomiting caused by chemotherapy; (5) helps prevent rejection of transplanted organs; (6) combination therapy of pneumocystis carinii pneumonia in AIDS patients; (7) helps treat bone cysts in children; (8) has a role in croup; (9) can help symptoms in Still's disease; (10) used by intramuscular injection to treat polymalgia rheumatica.

How This Drug Works: Anti-inflammatory effect is due to its ability to block normal defensive functions of certain white blood cells. Immunosuppressant effect is attributed to a reduced production of lymphocytes and antibodies.

Available Dosage Forms and Strengths
Ointment — 0.25% and 1%
Retention enema — 40 mg/bottle
Tablets — 2 mg, 4 mg, 8 mg, 16 mg, 24 mg, 32 mg

▷ **Usual Adult Dosage Range:** 4 to 48 mg daily as a single dose or in divided doses. **Note: Actual dosage and administration schedule must be determined by the physician for each patient individually.**

Conditions Requiring Dosing Adjustments

Liver function: Specific dosage adjustments in liver compromise are not defined. It is a rare cause of liver changes (hepatomegaly).

Kidney function: This drug can worsen existing kidney compromise. A benefit to risk decision must be made regarding the use of methylprednisolone in these patients.

▷ **Dosing Instructions:** The tablet may be crushed and taken with or following food to prevent stomach irritation, preferably in the morning.

Usual Duration of Use: For acute disorders: 4 to 10 days. For chronic disorders: according to individual requirements. Duration of use should not exceed the time necessary to obtain adequate symptomatic relief in acute self-limiting conditions, or the time required to stabilize a chronic condition and permit gradual withdrawal. Because of its intermediate duration of action, this drug is appropriate for alternate-day administration. Consult your physician on a regular basis.

▷ **This Drug Should Not Be Taken If**
- you have had an allergic reaction to any dosage form of it previously.
- you have active peptic ulcer disease.
- you have had recent bowel surgery where an anastamosis was performed.
- you have an active eye infection caused by the herpes simplex virus.
- you have active tuberculosis.

▷ **Inform Your Physician Before Taking This Drug If**
- you have had an adverse reaction to any cortisonelike drug in the past.
- you have a history of peptic ulcer disease, thrombophlebitis or tuberculosis.
- you have any of the following: diabetes, glaucoma, high blood pressure, deficient thyroid function or myasthenia gravis.
- you plan to have surgery of any kind in the near future.
- you have liver compromise.

Possible Side-Effects (natural, expected and unavoidable drug actions)
Increased appetite, weight gain, retention of salt and water, excretion of potassium, increased susceptibility to infection.

▷ **Possible Adverse Effects** (unusual, unexpected and infrequent reactions)
If any of the following develop, consult your physician promptly for guidance.

Mild Adverse Effects
Allergic Reaction: Skin rash.
Headache, dizziness, insomnia.
Acid indigestion, abdominal distension.
Muscle cramping, weakness and joint pain.
Acne, excessive growth of facial hair.

Serious Adverse Effects
Allergic Reactions: Anaphylaxis.
Mental and emotional disturbances of serious magnitude.
Reactivation of latent tuberculosis.
Development of peptic ulcer.
Hallucinations.
Seizures.
Toxic megacolon.
Liver or kidney compromise.
Blindness.
Muscle changes (myopathy).
Suppression of the adrenal gland.

Increased blood pressure.
Abnormal heart beats (arrythmias).
Development of inflammation of the pancreas.
Thrombophlebitis (inflammation of a vein with the formation of blood clot)—pain or tenderness in thigh or leg, with or without swelling of the foot, ankle or leg.
Pulmonary embolism (movement of a blood clot to the lung)—sudden shortness of breath, pain in the chest, coughing, bloody sputum.

▷ **Possible Effects on Sexual Function:** Altered timing and pattern of menstruation.

▷ **Adverse Effects That May Mimic Natural Diseases or Disorders**
Pattern of symptoms and signs resembling Cushing's syndrome.

Natural Diseases or Disorders That May Be Activated by This Drug
Latent diabetes, glaucoma, peptic ulcer disease, tuberculosis.

Possible Effects on Laboratory Tests
Blood amylase and lipase levels: increased (possible pancreatitis).
Glucose tolerance test (GTT): decreased.
Blood potassium level: decreased.
Blood testosterone level: decreased.

CAUTION
1. Best to carry an identification card that says you are taking this drug, if your course of treatment is to exceed 1 week.
2. Do not stop this drug abruptly after long-term treatment.
3. If vaccination against measles, rabies, smallpox or yellow fever is required, discontinue this drug 72 hours before vaccination and do not resume it for at least 14 days after vaccination.

Precautions for Use

By Infants and Children: Avoid prolonged use if possible. During long-term use, watch for suppression of normal growth. Intracranial pressure may increase. Long-term use may increase risk for adrenal gland deficiency during stress for as long as 18 months after the drug is stopped.

By Those over 60 Years of Age: Cortisonelike drugs should be used very sparingly after 60 and only when the disorder under treatment is unresponsive to adequate trials of unrelated drugs. Avoid prolonged use of this drug. Continual use (even in small doses) can increase the severity of diabetes, enhance fluid retention, raise blood pressure, weaken resistance to infection, induce stomach ulcer and accelerate the development of cataract and osteoporosis.

▷ **Advisability of Use During Pregnancy**
Pregnancy Category: C. See Pregnancy Code at the back of this book.
Animal studies: Birth defects reported in mice, rats and rabbits.
Human studies: Adequate studies of pregnant women are not available.
Avoid completely during the first 3 months. Limit use during the last 6 months as much as possible. If used, the infant should be examined for possible deficiency of adrenal gland function.

Advisability of Use if Breast-Feeding
Presence of this drug in breast milk: Yes.
Avoid drug or refrain from nursing.

Habit-Forming Potential: Use of this drug to suppress symptoms over an extended period of time may produce a state of functional dependence (see Glossary). In the treatment of asthma and rheumatoid arthritis, the dose should be kept as small as possible and withdrawal should be attempted after periods of reasonable improvement. Such procedures may reduce the degree of "steroid rebound"—the return of symptoms as the drug is withdrawn.

Effects of Overdosage: Fatigue, muscle weakness, stomach irritation, acid indigestion, excessive sweating, facial flushing, fluid retention, swelling of extremities, increased blood pressure.

Possible Effects of Long-Term Use: Increased blood sugar (possible diabetes), increased fat deposits on the trunk of the body ("buffalo hump"), rounding of the face ("moon face"), thinning and fragility of skin, loss of texture and strength of bones (osteoporosis, aseptic necrosis), cataracts, glaucoma, retarded growth and development in children.

Suggested Periodic Examinations While Taking This Drug (at physician's discretion)
Measurements of blood pressure, blood sugar and potassium levels.
Complete eye examinations at regular intervals.
Chest X-ray if history of tuberculosis.
Determination of the rate of development of the growing child to detect retardation of normal growth.

▷ **While Taking This Drug, Observe the Following**
Foods: No interactions expected. Ask physician regarding need to restrict salt intake or to eat potassium-rich foods. During long-term use of this drug, it is advisable to eat high-protein diet.
Nutritional Support: During long-term use, take a vitamin supplement. During wound repair, take a zinc supplement.
Beverages: No restrictions. Drink all forms of milk liberally.
▷ *Alcohol:* No interactions expected. Use caution if you are prone to peptic ulcer disease.
Tobacco Smoking: Nicotine increases the blood levels of naturally produced cortisone and related hormones. Heavy smoking may add to the expected actions of this drug and requires close observation for excessive effects.
Marijuana Smoking: May cause additional impairment of immunity.
▷ **Other Drugs**
Methylprednisolone may *decrease* the effects of
- insulin and require higher doses.
- isoniazid (INH, Niconyl, etc.).
- salicylates (aspirin, sodium salicylate, etc.).

Methylprednisolone *taken concurrently* with
- amphotericin B may result in additive potassium loss.
- carbamazepine (Tegretol) may result decreased methylprednisolone effectiveness.
- cyclosporine (Sandimmune) can result in increased steroid levels and cyclosporine toxicity.
- ketoconazole may increase blood levels of methylprednisolone and result in toxicity (abnormal heartbeats or psychiatric reactions).
- NSAIDs may cause increased risk of ulceration of the stomach or intestine.

- oral anticoagulants may either increase or decrease their effectiveness; consult physician regarding the need for prothrombin time testing and dosage adjustment.
- thiazide diuretics (see Drug Classes) can result in additive potassium loss.
- vaccines (such as flu or pneumococcal) may result in a blunting of the immune response to the vaccine.

The following drugs may *decrease* the effects of methylprednisolone
- antacids may reduce its absorption.
- barbiturates (Amytal, Butisol, phenobarbital, etc.).
- phenytoin (Dilantin, etc.).
- rifampin (Rifadin, Rimactane, etc.).

▷ *Driving, Hazardous Activities:* Usually no restrictions. Be alert to the rare occurrence of dizziness.

Aviation Note: The use of this drug *may be a disqualification* for piloting. Consult a designated Aviation Medical Examiner.

Exposure to Sun: No restrictions.

Occurrence of Unrelated Illness: This drug may decrease resistance to infection. Tell your doctor if you develop an infection of any kind. It may also reduce your body's ability to respond to stress of acute illness, injury or surgery. Keep your physician fully informed of any significant changes in your state of health.

Discontinuation: After extended use of this drug, do **not** stop it abruptly. Ask your doctor for help regarding gradual withdrawal. For a period of 2 years after discontinuing this drug, it is essential in the event of illness, injury or surgery that you inform attending medical personnel that you have used this drug. The period of impaired response to stress following the use of cortisonelike drugs may last for 1 to 2 years.

METHYSERGIDE (meth i SER jide)

Introduced: 1961 **Prescription:** USA: Yes; Canada: Yes **Available as Generic:** USA: No; Canada: No **Class:** Vascular headache preventive
Controlled Drug: USA: No; Canada: No

Brand Name: Sansert

BENEFITS versus RISKS	
Possible Benefits	*Possible Risks*
EFFECTIVE PREVENTION OF MIGRAINE AND CLUSTER HEADACHES	FIBROSIS (SCARRING) INSIDE CHEST AND ABDOMINAL CAVITIES, OF HEART AND LUNG TISSUES, ADJACENT TO MAJOR BLOOD VESSELS AND INTERNAL ORGANS (see Effects of Long-Term Use)
	Aggravation of hypertension, coronary artery disease and peripheral vascular disease

Methysergide

▷ **Principal Uses**

As a Single Drug Product: Uses currently included in FDA approved labeling: (1) Prevention of frequent and/or disabling vascular headaches (migraine and cluster neuralgia) that have not responded to other conventional treatment.

Other (unlabeled) generally accepted uses: May have a role in therapy of some strokes.

How This Drug Works: By blocking the inflammatory and vasoconstrictor effects of serotonin, this drug prevents blood vessel constriction that initiates vascular headaches.

Available Dosage Forms and Strengths
Tablets — 2 mg

▷ **Recommended Dosage Ranges** (Actual dosage and administration schedule must be determined by the physician for each patient individually.)

Infants and Children: Use not recommended.

12 to 60 Years of Age: 4 to 6 mg daily, in divided doses.

Over 60 Years of Age: 2 to 4 mg daily, in divided doses. Use very cautiously, with frequent monitoring for adverse effects.

Conditions Requiring Dosing Adjustments

Liver function: This drug should not be used in patients with liver compromise.

Kidney function: This drug should not be used in patients with renal compromise.

▷ **Dosing Instructions:** The tablet may be crushed and taken with food or milk to reduce stomach irritation. Limit continual (uninterrupted) use to 6 months; avoid drug completely for a period of 4 weeks between courses.

Usual Duration of Use: Use on a regular schedule for 3 weeks usually determines effectiveness in preventing recurrence of vascular headache. If significant benefit does not occur during this trial, this drug should be stopped. Long-term use (months to years) requires periodic physician evaluation.

▷ **This Drug Should Not Be Taken If**
- you have had an allergic reaction to it previously.
- you are pregnant.
- you currently have a severe infection.
- you have any of the following conditions:
    angina pectoris.
    Buerger's disease.
    chronic lung disease.
    connective tissue (collagen) disease.
    coronary artery disease.
    hardening of the arteries (arteriosclerosis).
    heart valve disease.
    high blood pressure (significant hypertension).
    kidney disease or significantly impaired kidney function.
    liver disease or significantly impaired liver function.
    active peptic ulcer disease.
    peripheral vascular disease.

phlebitis of any kind.
Raynaud's disease or phenomenon.

▷ **Inform Your Physician Before Taking This Drug If**
- you have had an adverse reaction to *any other form of ergot*.
- you have a history of peptic ulcer disease.

Possible Side-Effects (natural, expected and unavoidable drug actions)
Fluid retention, weight gain (in some individuals).

▷ **Possible Adverse Effects** (unusual, unexpected and infrequent reactions)
If any of the following develop, consult your physician promptly for guidance.

Mild Adverse Effects
Allergic Reactions: Skin rashes, flushing of the face, transient loss of scalp hair.
Dizziness, drowsiness, agitation, unsteadiness, altered vision.
Heartburn, nausea, vomiting, diarrhea.
Weight gain.
Transient muscle and joint pains.

Serious Adverse Effects
Idiosyncratic Reactions: Nightmares, hallucinations, acute mental disturbances.
Fibrosis (scar tissue formation) involving the chest and/or abdominal cavities, heart valves, lungs, kidneys, major blood vessels.
Spasm and narrowing of coronary and peripheral arteries: anginal chest pain; cold and painful extremities; leg cramps on walking.
Hemolytic anemia (see Glossary).
Abnormally low white blood cell counts.
Impaired circulation to the extremities (peripheral ischemia).
Heart attack (myocardial infarction) (very rare).

▷ **Possible Effects on Sexual Function:** Fibrosis of penile tissues.

▷ **Adverse Effects That May Mimic Natural Diseases or Disorders**
Swelling of the hands, lower legs, feet and ankles (peripheral edema) may suggest heart or kidney dysfunction.

Natural Diseases or Disorders That May Be Activated by This Drug
Latent coronary artery insufficiency (angina), Buerger's disease, Raynaud's disease, peptic ulcer disease.

Possible Effects on Laboratory Tests
Complete blood cell counts: decreased white cells (lymphocytes).
Stomach hydrochloric acid: increased.
Kidney function tests: increased blood urea nitrogen (BUN).

CAUTION
1. Continual use is limited to 6 months. Gradual reduction of dose is advised during the last 2 to 3 weeks of each course to prevent withdrawal headache rebound. Omit drug for a period of 4 to 6 weeks before resuming. This "drug-free" period is mandatory to reduce the risk of developing fibrosis of internal tissues.
2. Promptly report: fatigue, fever, chest pain, difficult breathing, stomach or flank pain, changes in pattern of urination.
3. This drug is useful only for the prevention of recurring vascular head-

aches; it is not recommended for the treatment of acute attacks of headache. It is ineffective and should not be used for tension headaches.

Precautions for Use
By Infants and Children: Use of this drug is not recommended.
By Those over 60 Years of Age: The age-related changes in blood vessels, circulatory functions and kidney function can make you more susceptible to the serious adverse effects of this drug. See the list of diseases and disorders above that are contraindications to the use this drug. Ask your doctor for help.

▷ **Advisability of Use During Pregnancy**
Pregnancy Category:
X. See Pregnancy Code at the back of this book.
Animal studies: No information available.
Human studies: Adequate studies of pregnant women are not available.
The manufacturer states that this drug is contraindicated during entire pregnancy.

Advisability of Use if Breast-Feeding
Presence of this drug in breast milk: Yes.
Avoid drug or refrain from nursing.

Habit-Forming Potential: None.

Effects of Overdosage: Nausea, vomiting, stomach pain, diarrhea, dizziness, excitement, cold hands and feet.

Possible Effects of Long-Term Use: Formation of scar tissue (fibrosis) inside chest cavity and/or abdominal cavity, on heart valves, in lung tissues, and surrounding major blood vessels and internal organs. This potentially dangerous reaction requires close and continual medical supervision while taking this drug.

Suggested Periodic Examinations While Taking This Drug (at physician's discretion)
Careful examination at regular intervals (6 to 12 months) for scar tissue formation or circulatory complications.
Complete blood cell counts.
Kidney function tests.

▷ **While Taking This Drug, Observe the Following**
Foods: No restrictions other than foods to which you are allergic. Some vascular headaches are due to food allergy.
Beverages: No restrictions.
▷ *Alcohol:* No interactions expected. Observe closely to determine if alcoholic beverages can initiate a migrainelike headache.
Tobacco Smoking: Avoid completely.
▷ *Other Drugs*
Methysergide *taken concurrently* with
- beta blocker drugs (see Drug Classes), may result in hazardous constriction of peripheral arteries; monitor the combined effects of these drugs on circulation in the extremities.

▷ *Driving, Hazardous Activities:* This drug may cause dizziness, drowsiness or impaired vision. Restrict activities as necessary.

Aviation Note: The use of this drug *is a disqualification* for piloting. Consult a designated Aviation Medical Examiner.

Exposure to Sun: No restrictions.

Exposure to Cold: Use caution. Cold environments may increase the occurrence of reduced circulation (blood flow) to the extremities.

Discontinuation: If this drug has been taken for an extended period of time, do not stop it abruptly. Gradual withdrawal (dosage reduction) over 2 to 3 weeks can prevent the development of rebound vascular headaches.

METOCLOPRAMIDE (met oh kloh PRA mide)

Introduced: 1973 **Prescription:** USA: Yes; Canada: Yes **Available as Generic:** Yes **Class:** Gastrointestinal stimulant, antivomiting agent **Controlled Drug:** USA: No; Canada: No

Brand Names: ✦Apo-Metoclop, ✦Clopra, ✦Emex, ✦Maxeran, Maxolon, Octamide, Reclomide, Reglan

BENEFITS versus RISKS	
Possible Benefits	*Possible Risks*
EFFECTIVE STOMACH STIMULANT FOR CORRECTING DELAYED EMPTYING	Sedation and fatigue (10%)
	Parkinson-like reactions (see Glossary)
Symptomatic relief in reflux esophagitis	Tardive dyskinesia (see Glossary), rare
Relief of nausea and vomiting associated with migraine headache	

▷ **Principal Uses**

As a Single Drug Product: Uses currently included in FDA approved labeling: (1) Helps stomach retention (gastroparesis) associated with diabetes; (2) acid reflux from the stomach into the esophagus (esophagitis); (3) the nausea and vomiting associated with migraine headaches; (4) the nausea and vomiting induced by anticancer drugs; (5) helps decrease the time needed to place a tube in the intestine; (6) used prior to cesarian section to decrease post-delivery nausea or vomiting.

Other (unlabeled) generally accepted uses: (1) Used as a preparatory drug in stomach hemorrhage; (2) may help gastrointestinal symptoms in anorexia nervosa; (3) eases drug-induced slowed functioning of the intestine (adynamic ileus); (4) decreases the frequency of accumulations of food in the stomach (bezoars); (5) can be of benefit in migraine attacks.

How This Drug Works: This drug inhibits relaxation of the stomach muscles and enhances the stimulation of the parasympathetic nervous system that is responsible for stomach muscle contractions. This action accelerates emptying of the stomach into the intestine.

Available Dosage Forms and Strengths

Injection — 5 mg per ml and 10 mg per ml

Syrup — 5 mg per 5-ml teaspoonful

Tablets — 5 mg, 10 mg

▷ **Usual Adult Dosage Range:** 10 to 15 mg 4 times/day. The total daily dose should not exceed 0.5 mg per kilogram of body weight. **Note: Actual** dosage and administration schedule must be determined by the physician for each patient individually.

Conditions Requiring Dosing Adjustments

Liver function: Specific dosage adjustments in liver compromise are not defined.

Kidney function: In patients with moderate kidney failure, 75% of the usual dose can be given at the usual dosing interval. In severe kidney failure, 50% of the usual dose can be given at the usual dosing interval. A benefit to risk decision must be made regarding the use of metoclopramide in these patients.

▷ **Dosing Instructions:** Take tablet or syrup 30 minutes before each meal and at bedtime. The tablet may be crushed for administration.

Usual Duration of Use: Use on a regular schedule for 5 to 7 days determines benefit in accelerating stomach emptying and relieving symptoms of heartburn, fullness and belching. Long-term use (months to years) requires physician supervision.

▷ **This Drug Should Not Be Taken If**
- you have had an allergic reaction to it previously.
- you have a seizure disorder of any kind.
- you have active gastrointestinal bleeding.
- you are taking or have taken within the last 14 days a MAO inhibitor (see Drug Classes).
- you are taking tricyclic antidepressants.
- you have a pheochromocytoma (adrenalin-producing tumor).

▷ **Inform Your Physician Before Taking This Drug If**
- you are allergic or overly sensitive to procaine or procainamide.
- you have impaired liver or kidney function.
- you have Parkinson's disease.
- you have epilepsy.
- you have high blood pressure.
- you have a history of depression.
- you are taking any atropinelike drugs, antipsychotic drugs or opioid analgesics (see Drug Classes Section).

Possible Side-Effects (natural, expected and unavoidable drug actions)

Drowsiness and lethargy (10%), breast tenderness and swelling, milk production.

▷ **Possible Adverse Effects** (unusual, unexpected and infrequent reactions)

If any of the following develop, consult your physician promptly for guidance.

Mild Adverse Effects

Allergic Reaction: Skin rash. Mild decreases in blood pressure.

Headache, dizziness, restlessness, depression, insomnia.

Dry mouth, nausea, diarrhea, constipation.

Urinary retention or incontinence.

Serious Adverse Effects

Idiosyncratic Reactions: Neuroleptic malignant syndrome (see Glossary), bronchospastic reactions in asthmatics.

Parkinson-like reactions (see Glossary).
Tardive dyskinesia (see Glossary).
Severe decrease in white blood cells (agranulocytosis) (very rare).
Abnormal heartbeats.
Severe increases in blood pressure (hypertensive crisis).
Tardive dyskinesia (rare).
Drug-induced porphyria.
Abnormal fixed positioning of the eyes (oculogyric crisis).

▷ **Possible Effects on Sexual Function**
Decreased libido (80%), impaired erection (60%), decreased sperm count.
Altered timing and pattern of menstruation.

Possible Effects on Laboratory Tests
Blood lithium level: increased.
Blood thyroid stimulating hormone (TSH) level: increased.

Precautions for Use
By Infants and Children: Watch for development of Parkinson-like reactions soon after starting therapy. Use of the smallest effective dose can minimize such reactions.
By Those over 60 Years of Age: Parkinson-like reactions and tardive dyskinesias are more likely to occur with the use of high doses over an extended period of time. The smallest effective dose should be identified and used only when clearly needed.

▷ **Advisability of Use During Pregnancy**
Pregnancy Category: B. See Pregnancy Code at the back of this book.
Animal studies: No birth defects found due to this drug.
Human studies: Adequate studies of pregnant women are not available.
Use this drug only if clearly needed.

Advisability of Use if Breast-Feeding
Presence of this drug in breast milk: Yes.
Avoid drug or refrain from nursing.

Habit-Forming Potential: None.

Effects of Overdosage: Marked drowsiness, confusion, muscle spasms, jerking movements of head and face, tremors, shuffling gait.

Possible Effects of Long-Term Use: Parkinson-like reactions may appear within several months of use. Tardive dyskinesias usually occur after a year of continual use; they may persist after this drug is discontinued.

Suggested Periodic Examinations While Taking This Drug (at physician's discretion)
During long-term use, observe for the development of fine, wormlike movements on the surface of the tongue; these may be the first indications of an emerging tardive dyskinesia.

▷ **While Taking This Drug, Observe the Following**
Foods: No restrictions.
Beverages: No restrictions. May be taken with milk.
▷ *Alcohol:* Use with extreme caution. Combined effects can result in excessive sedation and marked intoxication. Alcohol is best avoided.
Tobacco Smoking: No interactions expected.

▷ *Other Drugs*
  Metoclopramide may **decrease** the effects of
  • cimetidine (Tagamet).
  • digoxin (slow-dissolving dosage forms), and reduce its effectiveness.
  Metoclopramide **taken concurrently** with
  • major antipsychotic drugs (phenothiazines, thiothixenes, haloperidol, etc.) may increase the risk of developing Parkinson-like reactions.
  • cyclosporine (Sandimmune) may result in increased cyclosporine levels and toxicity.
  The following drugs may **decrease** the effects of metoclopramide
  • atropinelike drugs.
  • opioid analgesics (see Drug Classes).
▷ *Driving, Hazardous Activities:* This drug may cause drowsiness and dizziness. Restrict activities as necessary.
  Aviation Note: The use of this drug **may be a disqualification** for piloting. Consult a designated Aviation Medical Examiner.
  Exposure to Sun: No restrictions.

METOLAZONE (me TOHL a zohn)

Introduced: 1974 **Prescription:** USA: Yes; Canada: Yes **Available as Generic:** USA: No; Canada: No **Class:** Antihypertensive, diuretic, sulfonamides **Controlled Drug:** USA: No; Canada: No

Brand Names: Diulo, Microx, Mykrox, Zaroxolyn

BENEFITS versus RISKS	
Possible Benefits	*Possible Risks*
EFFECTIVE, WELL-TOLERATED DIURETIC	Loss of body potassium
POSSIBLY EFFECTIVE IN MILD HYPERTENSION	Increased blood sugar
	Increased blood uric acid
	Rare liver damage, jaundice
ENHANCES EFFECTIVENESS OF OTHER ANTIHYPERTENSIVES	Rare blood cell disorder: abnormally low white blood cell count

Please see thiazide diuretic profile for further information.

METOPROLOL (me TOH proh lohl)

Introduced: 1974 **Prescription:** USA: Yes; Canada: Yes **Available as Generic:** No **Class:** Antihypertensive, beta-adrenergic blocker **Controlled Drug:** USA: No; Canada: No

Brand Names: ✦Apo-Metoprolol, ✦Betaloc, ✦Co-Betaloc [CD], Lopressor, Lopressor Slow-release, Lopressor HCT [CD], Lopressor OROS, ✦Nu-Metop, ✦Novo-Metoprol, Toprol, Toprol XL

Metoprolol

BENEFITS versus RISKS	
Possible Benefits	*Possible Risks*
EFFECTIVE, WELL-TOLERATED ANTIHYPERTENSIVE in mild to moderate high blood pressure May help reduce death from heart attack (myocardial infarction)	CONGESTIVE HEART FAILURE in advanced heart disease Worsening of angina in coronary heart disease (abrupt withdrawal) Masking of low blood sugar (hypoglycemia) in drug-treated diabetes Provocation of asthma (with high doses)

▷ **Principal Uses**

As a Single Drug Product: Uses currently included in FDA approved labeling: (1) Treatment of mild to moderately severe high blood pressure. May be used alone or with other antihypertensive drugs, such as diuretics; (2) helps reduce the frequency and severity of angina; (3) Used to reduce the risk of recurrent heart attack.

Other (unlabeled) generally accepted uses: (1) May help reduce symptoms of pathology of the heart muscle (dilated cardiomyopathy); (2) can be a second line drug in treating panic attacks; (3) may decrease operative blood loss and perioperative arrhythmias in elective hysterectomy; (4) used to decrease pressure in the eye (intraocular pressure) in open angle glaucoma.

How This Drug Works: By blocking certain actions of the sympathetic nervous system, this drug
- reduces the rate, the contraction force and ejection pressure of the heart.
- reduces contraction of blood vessel walls, resulting in expansion and consequent lowering of blood pressure.
- prolongs the conduction time of nerve impulses through the heart, of benefit in the management of certain heart rhythm disorders.

Available Dosage Forms and Strengths
Injection — 1 mg per ml
Tablets — 50 mg, 100 mg
Tablets, prolonged-action — 50 mg, 100 mg, 200 mg

▷ **Usual Adult Dosage Range:** Initially, 50 mg twice daily (12 hours apart). The dose may be increased gradually at intervals of 7 to 10 days as needed and tolerated, up to 300 mg/day. For maintenance, 100 mg twice/day. The total daily dose should not exceed 450 mg. **Note: Actual dosage and administration schedule must be determined by the physician for each patient individually.**

Conditions Requiring Dosing Adjustments

Liver function: This drug should be used with caution in patients with liver compromise.

Kidney function: The kidneys are minimally involved in the elimination of this drug.

▷ **Dosing Instructions:** The regular tablet may be crushed and taken without regard to eating. Prolonged-action forms should be swallowed whole (not altered). Do not discontinue this drug abruptly.

Usual Duration of Use: Use on a regular schedule for 10 to 14 days determines effectiveness in lowering blood pressure. The long-term use of this drug (months to years) will be determined by your response to an overall treatment program (weight reduction, salt restriction, smoking cessation, etc.). Consult your physician on a regular basis.

Currently a "Drug of Choice"
for initiating treatment of hypertension with a single drug, especially for those subject to bronchial asthma or diabetes.

▷ **This Drug Should Not Be Taken If**
- you have had an allergic reaction to it previously.
- you have congestive heart failure.
- you have had a heart attack and your heart rate is less than 45 beats per minute.
- you have an abnormally slow heart rate or a serious form of heart block.
- you are taking, or have taken within the past 14 days, any monoamine oxidase (MAO) type A inhibitor drug (see Drug Class Section).

▷ **Inform Your Physician Before Taking This Drug If**
- you have had an adverse reaction to any beta blocker drug in the past (see Drug Classes).
- you have a history of serious heart disease.
- you have a history of hay fever (allergic rhinitis), asthma, chronic bronchitis or emphysema. People with bronchial asthma should generally not be given beta blockers. This drug is somewhat selective for the heart, and may be used in asthmatics with great caution.
- you have a history of overactive thyroid function (hyperthyroidism).
- you have a history of low blood sugar (hypoglycemia).
- you have impaired liver or kidney function.
- you have diabetes or myasthenia gravis.
- you currently take any form of digitalis, quinidine or reserpine, or any calcium blocker drug (see Drug Class Section).
- you have a history of poor circulation to the extremeties (peripheral vascular disease).
- you have a history of periodic cramps of your legs (intermittent claudication).
- you plan to have surgery under general anesthesia in the near future.

Possible Side-Effects (natural, expected and unavoidable drug actions)
Lethargy and fatigability (10%), cold extremities, slow heart rate (15%), light-headedness in upright position (see Orthostatic Hypotension in Glossary).

▷ **Possible Adverse Effects** (unusual, unexpected and infrequent reactions)
If any of the following develop, consult your physician promptly for guidance.
Mild Adverse Effects
Allergic Reactions: Skin rash, itching.
Worsening of psoriasis.

Headache, fatigue, dizziness (10%), insomnia, abnormal dreams.
Indigestion, nausea, vomiting, constipation, diarrhea.
Eye and joint pain.
Joint and muscle discomfort, fluid retention (edema).
Serious Adverse Effects
Mental depression (5%), anxiety.
Chest pain, shortness of breath, precipitation of congestive heart failure.
Induction of bronchial asthma (in asthmatic individuals).
Abnormally slow heartbeat (bradycardia).
Rebound hypertension (if the drug is abruptly stopped).
Hallucinations.
Precipitation of myasthenia gravis.
Carpal tunnel syndrome (rare).
Low or high blood sugar (hyper or hypoglycemia).
Liver compromise (hepatitis) (very rare).

▷ **Possible Effects on Sexual Function:** Decreased libido (4 times more common in men); impaired erection (less common with this drug than with most other beta blockers); Peyronie's disease (see Glossary).

Possible Effects on Laboratory Tests
Blood HDL cholesterol level: decreased.
Blood LDL cholesterol level: decreased.
Blood VLDL cholesterol level: increased.
Blood glucose level: increased.
Blood triglyceride levels: increased.

CAUTION
1. ***Do not stop this drug suddenly*** without the knowledge and help of your physician. Carry a note with you that says you take this drug.
2. Ask your doctor or pharmacist before using nasal decongestants usually present in over-the-counter cold preparations and nose drops. These can cause undesirable increases in blood pressure when used with beta blockers.
3. Report the development of any tendency to emotional depression.

Precautions for Use
By Infants and Children: Safety and effectiveness for use by those under 12 years of age have not been established. However, if this drug is used, observe for the development of low blood sugar (hypoglycemia) during periods of reduced food intake.

By Those over 60 Years of Age: Proceed **cautiously** with all antihypertensive drugs. Unacceptably high blood pressure should be reduced slowly, avoiding the risks associated with excessively low blood pressure. Therapy is started with small doses, and the blood pressure checked often. Sudden, rapid and excessive reduction of blood pressure can predispose to stroke or heart attack. Watch for dizziness, unsteadiness, tendency to fall, confusion, hallucinations, depression or urinary frequency.

▷ **Advisability of Use During Pregnancy**
Pregnancy Category: C. See Pregnancy Code at the back of this book.
Animal studies: No significant increase in birth defects due to this drug.
Human studies: Adequate studies of pregnant women are not available.
Use this drug only if clearly needed. Ask physician for guidance.

Advisability of Use if Breast-Feeding
Presence of this drug in breast milk: Yes, in large amounts.
Avoid drug or refrain from nursing.

Habit-Forming Potential: None.

Effects of Overdosage: Weakness, slow pulse, low blood pressure, fainting, cold and sweaty skin, congestive heart failure, possible coma and convulsions.

Possible Effects of Long-Term Use: Reduced heart reserve and eventual heart failure in susceptible individuals with advanced heart disease.

Suggested Periodic Examinations While Taking This Drug (at physician's discretion)
Measurements of blood pressure, evaluation of heart function.

▷ **While Taking This Drug, Observe the Following**

Foods: The peak drug concentrantion and therefore, the peak effect of this drug will increase if it is taken with food. Avoid excessive salt intake.

Beverages: No restrictions. May be taken with milk.

▷ *Alcohol:* Use with caution. Alcohol may exaggerate this drug's ability to lower the blood pressure and may increase its mild sedative effect.

Tobacco Smoking: Nicotine may reduce this drug's benefit in treating high blood pressure. Additionally, high doses of this drug may potentiate the constriction of the bronchial tubes caused by regular smoking.

▷ *Other Drugs*

Metoprolol may *increase* the effects of
- other antihypertensive drugs, and cause excessive lowering of the blood pressure. Dosage adjustments may be necessary.
- reserpine (Ser-Ap-Es, etc.), and cause sedation, depression, slowing of the heart rate and lowering of the blood pressure.
- verapamil (Calan, Isoptin), and cause excessive depression of heart function; monitor this combination closely.

Metoprolol *taken concurrently* with
- amiodarone may result in extremely slow heartbeat and cardiac arrest.
- clonidine (Catapres) requires close monitoring for rebound high blood pressure if clonidine is withdrawn while metoprolol is still being taken.
- fluoxetine (Prozac) may cause metoprolol toxicity.
- insulin requires close monitoring to avoid undetected hypoglycemia (see Glossary).
- lidocaine can lead to lidocaine toxicity (cardiac arrest).
- oral hypoglycemic agents (see Drug Classes) can result in prolonged hypoglycemia if it occurs.
- phenothiazines (see Drug Classes) can result in low blood pressure or toxicity due to the phenothiazine.
- quinidine can lead to abnormally slow heartbeat and shortness of breath.

The following drugs may *increase* the effects of metoprolol
- cimetidine (Tagamet).
- methimazole (Tapazole).
- MAO inhibitors (see Drug Classes).
- birth control pills (oral contraceptives).
- propylthiouracil (Propacil).

The following drugs may *decrease* the effects of metoprolol
- barbiturates (phenobarbital, etc.).
- indomethacin (Indocin), and possibly other "aspirin substitutes," or NSAIDs may impair metoprolol's antihypertensive effect.
- rifampin (Rifadin, Rimactane).

▷ *Driving, Hazardous Activities:* Use caution until the full extent of drowsiness, lethargy and blood pressure change has been determined.

Aviation Note: The use of this drug *is a disqualification* for piloting. Consult a designated Aviation Medical Examiner.

Exposure to Sun: No restrictions.

Exposure to Heat: Caution advised. Hot environments can lower the blood pressure and exaggerate the effects of this drug.

Exposure to Cold: Caution advised. Cold environments can increase circulatory deficiency in the extremities that may occur with this drug. The elderly should take precautions to prevent hypothermia (see Glossary).

Heavy Exercise or Exertion: It is advisable to avoid exertion that produces light-headedness, excessive fatigue or muscle cramping. The use of this drug may intensify the hypertensive response to isometric exercise.

Occurrence of Unrelated Illness: Fever can lower the blood pressure and require adjustment of dosage. Nausea or vomiting may interrupt the regular dosage schedule. Ask your doctor for help.

Discontinuation: It is advisable to avoid sudden discontinuation of this drug in all situations. If possible, gradual reduction of dose over a period of 1 to 2 weeks is recommended. Ask your physician for specific guidance.

METRONIDAZOLE (me troh NI da zohl)

Introduced: 1960   **Prescription:** USA: Yes; Canada: Yes   **Available as Generic:** Yes   **Class:** Anti-infective   **Controlled Drug:** USA: No; Canada: No

Brand Names: ◆Apo-Metronidazole, Femazole, Flagyl, Flagystatin, Lagyl, Metizol, MetroGel, Metro IV, Metryl, ◆Neo-Tric, ◆Novo-Nidazole, Protostat, SK Metronidazole, ◆Trikacide

BENEFITS versus RISKS	
Possible Benefits	*Possible Risks*
EFFECTIVE TREATMENT FOR TRICHOMONAS INFECTIONS, AMEBIC DYSENTERY AND GIARDIASIS	Superinfection with yeast organisms Peripheral neuropathy (see Glossary) Abnormally low white blood cell count (transient)
Effective treatment for some anaerobic bacterial infections	Colitis
Effective local treatment for rosacea	Aggravation of epilepsy

▷ **Principal Uses**

As a Single Drug Product: Uses currently included in FDA approved labeling: (1) Treats trichomonas infections of the vaginal canal and cervix and of the male urethra; (2) it is also used to treat amebic dysentery and liver abscess, giardia infections of the intestine and serious infections caused by certain strains of anaerobic bacteria; (3) treats gardnerella infections of the vagina; (4) treatment of rosacea with local application of a gel dosage form; (5) used in terapy of pseudomembranous colitis; (6) has a role in treating bed sores (decubitis ulcers); (7) can help prevent infection (prophylaxis) in gynecologic, appendectomy or colorectal surgery.

Other (unlabeled) generally accepted uses: (1) combination therapy with gentamicin in treating intraabdominal infections; (2) combination antibiotic treatment of duodenal ulcers caused by H. pylori; (3) can help treat infections caused by Giardia lamblia; (4) used to help heal the lesions in Crohn's disease.

How This Drug Works: By interacting with DNA, this drug destroys essential components (nucleus) that are needed for life and growth of infecting organisms.

Available Dosage Forms and Strengths
  Gel — 0.75%
  Injection — 500 mg per 100 ml
  Tablets — 250 mg, 500 mg

▷ **Usual Adult Dosage Range:** Varies with infection to be treated.

For trichomoniasis: One-day course—2 grams as a single dose; or 1 gram for 2 doses 12 hours apart. Seven-day course—250 mg 3 times/day for 7 consecutive days. (The 7-day course is preferred.)

For amebiasis: 500 to 750 mg 3 times/day for 5 to 10 consecutive days.

For giardiasis: 2 grams once/day for 3 days; or 250 to 500 mg 3 times/day for 5 to 7 days.

The total daily dosage should not exceed 4 grams (4000 mg).

Note: Actual dosage and administration schedule must be determined by the physician for each patient individually.

Conditions Requiring Dosing Adjustments

Liver function: The dose should be decreased by one third in mild to moderate liver compromise. It should not be used in severe liver compromise.

Kidney function: In severe kidney failure, 50% of the normal dose can be given at the usual dosing interval. A benefit to risk decision must be made regarding the use of metronidazole in these patients as there is a risk of systemic lupus erythematosus (SLE) from the metabolites of this drug.

▷ **Dosing Instructions:** The tablet may be crushed and taken with or following food to reduce stomach irritation.

Usual Duration of Use: Use on a regular schedule as outlined is needed to ensure effectiveness. Do not repeat the course of treatment without your physician's approval.

▷ **This Drug Should Not Be Taken If**
- you have had an allergic reaction to it or any the parabens contained in the gel form previously.
- you are pregnant.
- you currently have a bone marrow or blood cell disorder.
- you have any type of central nervous system disorder, including epilepsy.

▷ **Inform Your Physician Before Taking This Drug If**
- you have a history of any type of blood cell disorder, especially one induced by drugs.
- you have a history of seizures or peripheral neuropathy.

Metronidazole 641

- you have impaired liver or kidney function.
- you have a history of alcoholism.
- you are pregnant or breast-feeding.

Possible Side-Effects (natural, expected and unavoidable drug actions)
A sharp, metallic, unpleasant taste.
Dark discoloration of the urine (of no significance).
Superinfection (see Glossary) by yeast organisms in the mouth or vagina.

▷ **Possible Adverse Effects** (unusual, unexpected and infrequent reactions)
If any of the following develop, consult your physician promptly for guidance.

Mild Adverse Effects
Allergic Reactions: Skin rash, hives, flushing, itching.
Headache, dizziness, incoordination, unsteadiness, incontinence.
Discoloration of urine.
Loss of appetite, nausea, vomiting, abdominal cramps, diarrhea.
Irritation of mouth and tongue, possibly due to yeast infection.

Serious Adverse Effects
Idiosyncratic Reactions: Abnormal behavior, confusion, depression, Herxheimer reaction (sweating, diarrhea, vomiting, scalding urination, joint pain and itching).
Peripheral neuropathy (see Glossary).
Abnormally low white blood cell count (transient): fever, sore throat, infections.
Disulfiram (nausea, vomiting) type reaction if alcoholic beverages are consumed.
Seizures.
Drug-induced pneumonitis (rare).
Drug-induced porphyria (rare).
Pseudomembranous colitis.
Pancreatitis (rare).
Hemolytic-uremic syndrome (rare).

▷ **Possible Effects on Sexual Function:** Decreased libido; decreased vaginal secretions (difficult or painful intercourse).

Possible Delayed Adverse Effects: Studies have shown that this drug can cause cancer in mice and possibly in rats. There is no evidence to date that this drug causes cancer in man when used in the dosages specified earlier. Follow your physician's instructions exactly. Avoid unnecessary or prolonged use.

▷ **Adverse Effects That May Mimic Natural Diseases or Disorders**
Behavioral changes may suggest spontaneous psychosis.

Natural Diseases or Disorders That May Be Activated by This Drug
Latent yeast infections.

Possible Effects on Laboratory Tests
White blood cell counts: decreased.
Prothrombin time: increased.

CAUTION
1. Troublesome and persistent diarrhea can develop. If diarrhea persists for more than 24 hours, stop this drug and call your physician.

642   Metronidazole

2. Stop this drug immediately if you develop any signs of toxic effects on the brain or nervous system: Confusion, irritability, dizziness, incoordination, unsteady stance or gait, muscle jerking or twitching, numbness or weakness in the extremities.

Precautions for Use

By Infants and Children: Avoid use in those with a history of bone marrow or blood cell disorders.

By Those over 60 Years of Age: Natural changes in the skin may predispose to yeast infections in the genital and anal regions. Report the development of rashes and itching promptly.

▷ **Advisability of Use During Pregnancy**

Pregnancy Category: B. See Pregnancy Code at the back of this book.

Animal studies: No birth defects reported in rat studies. However, this drug is known to cause cancer in mice and possibly in rats.

Human studies: No increase in birth defects reported in 206 exposures to this drug during the first 3 months. However, information from adequate studies of pregnant women is not available.

The manufacturer advises against the use of this drug during the first 3 months. Use during the last 6 months is not advised unless it is absolutely essential to the mother's health.

Advisability of Use if Breast-Feeding

Presence of this drug in breast milk: Yes.

Avoid drug or refrain from nursing.

Habit-Forming Potential: None.

Effects of Overdosage: Weakness, stomach irritation, nausea, vomiting, confusion, disorientation.

Possible Effects of Long-Term Use: None reported. Avoid long-term use.

Suggested Periodic Examinations While Taking This Drug (at physician's discretion)

Complete blood cell counts.

▷ **While Taking This Drug, Observe the Following**

Foods: No restrictions.

Beverages: No restrictions. May be taken with milk.

▷ *Alcohol:* Use caution until combined effects have been determined. A disulfiramlike reaction has been reported (see Glossary).

Tobacco Smoking: No interactions expected.

▷ *Other Drugs*

Metronidazole may *increase* the effects of
- warfarin (Coumadin, etc.), and cause abnormal bleeding. The prothrombin time should be monitored closely, especially during the first 10 days of concurrent use.

Metronidazole *taken concurrently* with
- antacids may decrease absorption of metronidazole.
- birth control pills (oral contraceptives) may block the effectiveness of contraception and result in pregnancy.
- cholestyramine or other cholesterol lowering resins may decrease metronidazole absorption and lower its therapeutic effect.
- cotrimoxazole or other sulfa drugs may result in a disulfiram effect.

- cyclosporine (Sandimmune) can lead to cyclosporine toxicity.
- disulfiram (Antabuse) may cause severe emotional and behavioral disturbances.
- lithium can cause lithium toxicity.

▷ *Driving, Hazardous Activities:* This drug may cause dizziness or incoordination. Restrict activities as necessary.

Aviation Note: The use of this drug **may be a disqualification** for piloting. Consult a designated Aviation Medical Examiner.

Exposure to Sun: No restrictions.

MEXILETINE (mex IL e teen)

Introduced: 1973 **Prescription:** USA: Yes; Canada: Yes **Available as Generic:** No **Class:** Antiarrhythmic **Controlled Drug:** USA: No; Canada: No
Brand Name: Mexitil

BENEFITS versus RISKS	
Possible Benefits	*Possible Risks*
EFFECTIVE TREATMENT IN 30% OF SELECTED HEART RHYTHM DISORDERS	NARROW TREATMENT RANGE FREQUENT ADVERSE EFFECTS (up to 40% of users) WORSENING OF SOME ARRHYTHMIAS Rare seizures, liver injury and reduced white blood cell count

▷ **Principal Uses**
As a Single Drug Product: Uses currently included in FDA approved labeling: (1) Helps correct premature beats that arise in the ventricles (lower heart chambers) which are refractory to other agents.
Other (unlabeled) generally accepted uses: (1) May have a role in reducing symptoms in diabetic nerve damage (neuropathy); (2) has shown some benefit in combination therapy of Wolf-Parkinson-White syndrome.

How This Drug Works: By slowing the transmission of electrical impulses throughout the conduction system of the heart, this drug assists in restoring normal heart rate and rhythm in selected types of arrhythmia.

Available Dosage Forms and Strengths
Capsules — 150 mg, 200 mg, 250 mg

▷ **Usual Adult Dosage Range:** A loading dose of 400 to 600 mg is given, followed by 150 to 300 mg every 6 to 8 hours. Dose can be increased at intervals of 2 to 3 days, as needed and tolerated to a maximum total daily dose of 1200 mg. Measurement of drug blood levels is advised (when available) to determine the optimal dose and schedule. **Note: Actual dosage and administration schedule must be determined by the physician for each patient individually.**

Conditions Requiring Dosing Adjustments
Liver function: In liver compromise, the dose should be decreased by one fourth to one third. Blood levels should be obtained at prudent intervals.

Mexiletine

Kidney function: The dose should be decreased and blood levels obtained more frequently in patients with severe kidney failure.

▷ **Dosing Instructions:** The capsule may be opened and taken with food or antacid to reduce stomach irritation. Take at same times each day to obtain uniform results.

Usual Duration of Use: Use on a regular schedule for 1 to 2 weeks determines effectiveness in correcting or preventing responsive rhythm disorders. Long-term use requires physician supervision.

▷ **This Drug Should Not Be Taken If**
- you have had an allergic reaction to it previously.
- you have second-degree or third-degree heart block (determined by electrocardiogram), uncorrected by a pacemaker.

▷ **Inform Your Physician Before Taking This Drug If**
- you have had adverse reactions to other antiarrhythmic drugs in the past.
- you have a history of heart disease of any kind, especially "heart block" or heart failure.
- you have impaired liver function.
- you have Parkinson's disease.
- you are prone to low blood pressure.
- you have a seizure disorder of any kind.
- you take any form of digitalis, a potassium supplement or any diuretic drug that can cause potassium loss (ask physician).

Possible Side-Effects (natural, expected and unavoidable drug actions)
Nervousness (11%), light-headedness (10%).

▷ **Possible Adverse Effects** (unusual, unexpected and infrequent reactions)
If any of the following develop, consult your physician promptly for guidance.

Mild Adverse Effects

Allergic Reaction: Skin rash (4%).

Headache (7%), dizziness (26%), visual disturbance (7%), fatigue (3%), weakness (5%), tremor (13%).

Loss of appetite, indigestion, nausea (39%), vomiting, constipation (4%), diarrhea (5%), abdominal pain (1%).

Unpleasant taste.

Serious Adverse Effects

Idiosyncratic Reactions: Depression, confusion, amnesia, hallucinations, seizures (all rare).

Drug-induced heart rhythm disorders (1%), shortness of breath (5%), palpitations (7%), chest pain (7%), swelling of feet.

Congestive heart failure.

Urinary retention.

Liver damage with jaundice (see Glossary).

Abnormally low white blood cell and blood platelet counts (rare): Fever, sore throat, abnormal bleeding or bruising.

Systemic lupus erythematosus (rare).

▷ **Possible Effects on Sexual Function:** Decreased libido, impotence (rare).

▷ **Adverse Effects That May Mimic Natural Diseases or Disorders**
Liver toxicity may suggest viral hepatitis.

Mexiletine

Natural Diseases or Disorders That May Be Activated by This Drug
Latent epilepsy.

Possible Effects on Laboratory Tests
Blood white cell and platelet counts: decreased.
Liver function tests: increased liver enzymes (ALT/GPT, AST/GOT) increased in less than 1% of users.

CAUTION
1. Thorough evaluation of your heart function (including electrocardiograms) is necessary prior to using this drug.
2. Periodic evaluation of your heart function is needed to determine your response to this drug. Some individuals may experience worsening of their heart rhythm disorder and/or deterioration of heart function. Close monitoring of heart rate, rhythm and overall performance is essential.
3. Dosage must be adjusted carefully for each individual. Do not change your dosage without the knowledge and supervision of your physician.
4. Do not take any other antiarrhythmic drug while taking this drug unless you are directed to do so by your physician.
5. Carry a card of personal identification with the notation that you are taking this drug. Inform all attending medical personnel that you are taking this drug, especially if you require surgery of any kind.

Precautions for Use
By Infants and Children: Safety and effectiveness for those under 12 years of age not established. Initial use of this drug requires hospitalization and supervision by a qualified cardiologist.
By Those over 60 Years of Age: Reduced liver function may require reduction in dosage. Observe carefully for light-headedness, dizziness, unsteadiness and tendency to fall.

▷ **Advisability of Use During Pregnancy**
Pregnancy Category: C. See Pregnancy Code at the back of this book.
Animal studies: No birth defects reported in mice, rats or rabbits. However, an increased rate of fetal resorption was found.
Human studies: Adequate studies of pregnant women are not available.
Avoid during first 3 months. Use this drug only if clearly needed. Ask physician for guidance.

Advisability of Use if Breast-Feeding
Presence of this drug in breast milk: Yes.
Avoid drug or refrain from nursing.

Habit-Forming Potential: None.

Effects of Overdosage: Impaired urination, constipation, marked drop in blood pressure, abnormal heart rhythms, congestive heart failure, dizziness, incoordination, seizures.

Possible Effects of Long-Term Use: None reported.

Suggested Periodic Examinations While Taking This Drug (at physician's discretion)
Electrocardiograms, complete blood cell counts, liver function tests.

▷ **While Taking This Drug, Observe the Following**
Foods: No restrictions. Ask physician regarding need for salt restriction.
Beverages: No restrictions. May be taken with milk.

▷ *Alcohol:* Use caution. Alcohol can increase the blood-pressure-lowering effects of this drug.
Tobacco Smoking: Nicotine can cause irritability of the heart and reduce the effectiveness of this drug. Follow physician's advice regarding smoking.

▷ *Other Drugs*
Mexiletine may *increase* the effects of
- antihypertensive drugs, and cause excessive lowering of blood pressure.
- beta blocker drugs (see Drug Classes).
- theophylline (Theodur, others) leading to theophylline toxicity and seizures.

The following drugs may *decrease* the effects of mexiletine
- phenytoin (Dilantin, etc.).
- rifampin (Rifadin, Rimactane).

▷ *Driving, Hazardous Activities:* This drug may cause weakness, dizziness or blurred vision. Restrict activities as necessary.
Aviation Note: The use of this drug *may be a disqualification* for piloting. Consult a designated Aviation Medical Examiner.
Exposure to Sun: No restrictions.
Occurrence of Unrelated Illness: Vomiting, diarrhea or dehydration can affect this drug's action adversely. Report such developments promptly.
Discontinuation: This drug should not be stopped abruptly following long-term use. Ask your physician for guidance regarding gradual dose reduction.

MINOXIDIL (min OX i dil)

Introduced: 1972 **Prescription:** USA: Yes; Canada: Yes **Available as Generic:** Yes **Class:** Antihypertensive, hair growth stimulant **Controlled Drug:** USA: No; Canada: No
Brand Names: Loniten, Minodyl, Rogaine

BENEFITS versus RISKS	
Possible Benefits	*Possible Risks*
A POTENT, LONG-ACTING ANTIHYPERTENSIVE	EXCESSIVE BODY HAIR GROWTH (in 80% of users)
EFFECTIVE IN 75% OF CASES OF SEVERE HYPERTENSION	SALT AND WATER RETENTION
	Excessively rapid heart rate
EFFECTIVE IN ACCELERATED AND MALIGNANT HYPERTENSION	Aggravation of angina
	Local scalp irritation (topical use)
Moderately effective in treating male-pattern baldness	

▷ **Principal Uses**
As a Single Drug Product: Uses currently included in FDA approved labeling: (1) Treatment of severe high blood pressure that cannot be controlled by conventional therapy; (2) the treatment of female androgenic baldness or male-pattern baldness.
Other (unlabeled) generally accepted uses: (1) Supportive therapy in hair

transplants; (2) this drug has shown promising results in facilitating erection in patients with impotence caused by nerve dysfunction.

How This Drug Works: (1) Directly relaxes constricted muscles in the walls of small arteries, and permits expansion of the arteries and lowering of blood pressure. (2) The drug may act directly on the hair follicle, and also may increase the size of previously closed small blood vessels in the scalp (improve blood flow) and restore small hair follicles to normal size and activity.

Available Dosage Forms and Strengths
    Tablets — 2.5 mg, 10 mg
Topical solution — 2%

▷ **Usual Adult Dosage Range:** For hypertension: Initially, 5 mg/24 hours in one dose. Gradually increase dose to 10 mg, 20 mg, then 40 mg/24 hours, taken in 1 or 2 divided doses daily, as needed and tolerated. The usual maintenance dose is 10 to 40 mg/24 hours. The total daily dosage should not exceed 50 mg. For male-pattern baldness: Apply thinly 1 ml of topical solution to the balding area of the scalp twice daily. The total daily dosage should not exceed 2 ml. **Note: Actual dosage and administration schedule must be determined by the physician for each patient individually.**

Conditions Requiring Dosing Adjustments
Liver function: This drug is metabolized (90%) in the liver. It should be used with caution in patients with liver compromise.
Kidney function: In moderate kidney failure, the dose should be decreased empirically.

▷ **Dosing Instructions:** For hypertension: Tablets may be crushed and taken with or following food to prevent nausea. Take at the same time each day. For baldness: *The topical solution is for external, local use only; it is not to be swallowed.* Begin application at the center of the bald area; apply thinly to cover the entire area. The scalp and hair must be dry at the time of application. Follow instructions carefully.

Usual Duration of Use: Use on a regular schedule for 3 to 7 days usually determines effectiveness in controlling severe hypertension. Continual use of the topical solution for at least 4 months is necessary to determine its ability to promote hair growth. Long-term use (months to years) of both dosage forms requires physician supervision.

▷ **This Drug Should Not Be Taken If**
- you have had an allergic reaction to it previously.
- you are known to have a pheochromocytoma (an adrenalin-producing tumor).
- you have pulmonary hypertension due to mitral valve stenosis.
- you have had a heart attack.
- you have heart disease of any kind.

▷ **Inform Your Physician Before Taking This Drug If**
- you are pregnant or planning pregnancy.
- you have a history of coronary artery disease or impaired heart function.
- you have a history of stroke or impaired brain circulation.
- you have impaired liver or kidney function.

Possible Side-Effects (natural, expected and unavoidable drug actions)
Increased heart rate, fluid retention with weight gain (7%), excessive hair growth on face, arms, legs and back (80%).

▷ **Possible Adverse Effects** (unusual, unexpected and infrequent reactions)
If any of the following develop, consult your physician promptly for guidance.
Mild Adverse Effects
Allergic Reactions: Skin rash (less than 1%). Localized dermatitis at site of application of topical solution.
Headache, dizziness, fainting (1–2%).
Nausea, increased thirst.
Hair growth, and changes in hair color.
Weight gain.
Mild increase in liver enzymes.
Serious Adverse Effects
Allergic Reactions: Serious skin rash (Stevens-Johnson syndrome).
Idiosyncratic Reaction: Fluid formation around the heart (pericardial effusion) (3%).
Development of angina pectoris; development of high blood pressure in the lung circulation (pulmonary hypertension).
Systemic lupus erythematosus (rare).
Low white blood cells or platelets (rare).

▷ **Possible Effects on Sexual Function:** Male breast tenderness (gynecomastia) (less than 1%). Some data to support this drug balancing male ability to ejaculate and have a healthy sex drive may have been blunted by other drugs which treat high blood pressure.

Natural Diseases or Disorders That May Be Activated by This Drug
Latent coronary artery disease with symptomatic angina.

Possible Effects on Laboratory Tests
Blood HDL cholesterol level: increased.
Blood LDL cholesterol level: decreased.

CAUTION
1. Long-term use for hypertension usually requires the concurrent use of an effective diuretic to counteract salt and water retention.
2. The long-term use of this drug for hypertension may require concurrent use of a beta blocker drug to control excessive acceleration of the heart.
3. Best to avoid combining this drug and guanethidine; the combination can cause severe orthostatic hypotension (see Glossary).
4. Consult your physician regarding the advisability of using a "no salt added" diet.
5. Little of this drug is absorbed into the general circulation when the topical solution is applied to the scalp. However, some systemic effects have been reported. Inform your physician promptly if you experience any unusual symptoms while using the topical solution.

Precautions for Use
By Infants and Children: Dosage schedules should be determined by a qualified pediatrician. Monitor closely for salt and water retention.
By Those over 60 Years of Age: Treatment with small doses and a limit of total

daily dose to 75 mg is indicated. Headache, palpitation and rapid heart rate due to this drug are more common in this age group and can mimic acute anxiety states. Observe for dizziness, unsteadiness, fainting and falling.

▷ **Advisability of Use During Pregnancy**
Pregnancy Category: C. See Pregnancy Code at the back of this book.
Animal studies: No birth defects reported in rats or rabbits. However, studies did reveal decreased fertility and increased fetal deaths.
Human studies: Adequate studies of pregnant women are not available.
Avoid during the first 3 months. Use only if clearly needed during the last 6 months.

Advisability of Use if Breast-Feeding
Presence of this drug in breast milk: Yes.
Avoid drug or refrain from nursing.

Habit-Forming Potential: None.

Effects of Overdosage: Headache, dizziness, weakness, nausea, marked low blood pressure, weak and rapid pulse, loss of consciousness.

Possible Effects of Long-Term Use: Excessive growth of body hair occurs in 80% of users after 1 to 2 months of continual treatment for hypertension. Close to 100% of users will experience this effect after 1 year of continual treatment. This may be accompanied by darkening of the skin and coarsening of facial features.

Suggested Periodic Examinations While Taking This Drug (at physician's discretion)
Body weight measurement for insidious gain due to water retention.
Electrocardiographic and echocardiographic heart examinations.

▷ **While Taking This Drug, Observe the Following**
Foods: Avoid excessive salt and heavily salted foods.
Beverages: No restrictions. May be taken with milk.
▷ *Alcohol:* Use with extreme caution. Alcohol can exaggerate the blood-pressure-lowering effects of this drug.
Tobacco Smoking: Best avoided. Nicotine can contribute significantly to the development of angina in susceptible individuals.
▷ *Other Drugs*
Minoxidil may *increase* the effects of
- all other antihypertensive drugs; careful dosage adjustments are mandatory.

Minoxidil *taken concurrently* with
- guanethidine (Ismelin, Esimil) may cause severe orthostatic hypotension; avoid this combination.
- NSAIDs may blunt the therapeutic benefit of minoxidil.

▷ *Driving, Hazardous Activities:* This drug may cause dizziness and fatigue. Restrict activities as necessary.
Aviation Note: The use of this drug *is a disqualification* for piloting. Consult a designated Aviation Medical Examiner.
Exposure to Sun: No restrictions.
Discontinuation: This drug should not be stopped abruptly. If it is to be discontinued, consult your physician regarding gradual reduction in dosage and

appropriate replacement with other drugs for the management of hypertension. Following discontinuation of the topical solution, the pretreatment pattern of baldness may return within 3 to 4 months.

MISOPROSTOL (mi soh PROH stohl)

Introduced: 1987 **Prescription:** USA: Yes; Canada: Yes **Available as Generic:** USA: No; Canada: No **Class:** Stomach ulcer preventive, antiulcer
Controlled Drug: USA: No; Canada: No
Brand Name: Arthrotec, Cytotec

BENEFITS versus RISKS	
Possible Benefits	*Possible Risks*
EFFECTIVE PREVENTION OF STOMACH ULCERATION WHILE TAKING ANTI-INFLAMMATORY DRUGS (93% reduction of ulcer development)	ABORTION (11%)
	Diarrhea (14% to 40%), transient
	Neuropathy (rare)
Effective treatment of duodenal ulcer	

▷ **Principal Uses**

As a Single Drug Product: Uses currently included in FDA approved labeling: (1) Prevents development of stomach ulcers during long-term use of anti-inflammatory drugs as therapy for arthritis and related conditions.

Other (unlabeled) generally accepted uses: (1) Used (in Canada and other countries) for treatment of active duodenal ulcer unrelated to use of anti-inflammatory drugs; (2) has seen some use in inducing abortions; (3) used in combination with cyclosporine or prednisone to decrease transplanted organ rejection; (4) may have a benefit in helping ripen the cervix in preparation for a vaginal delivery.

How This Drug Works: This drug protects the lining of the stomach and duodenum and prevents ulceration due to anti-inflammatory drugs by: (1) replacing tissue prostaglandins that are depleted by anti-inflammatory drugs; (2) inhibiting the secretion of stomach acid; (3) increasing the local production of bicarbonate (to neutralize acids) and of mucus (to protect stomach and duodenal tissues). The combined effects prevent new ulcer formation and promote healing of existing ulcer(s).

Available Dosage Forms and Strengths
Tablets — 100 mcg and 200 mcg

Conditions Requiring Dosing Adjustments
Liver function: Specific dosage adjustments in liver compromise are not defined.
Kidney function: The dose of misoprostol should be decreased if it is used in patients with compromised kidneys, and is not well tolerated.

▷ **Usual Adult Dosage Range**
For prevention of stomach ulcer—100 to 200 mcg 4 times daily, taken concurrently during the use of any anti-inflammatory drug (see Antiarthritic/Anti-inflammatory Drug Classes).

For treatment of duodenal ulcer—200 mcg 4 times daily for 4 to 8 weeks.
Note: Actual dosage and administration schedule must be determined by the physician for each patient individually.

▷ **Dosing Instructions:** The tablet may be crushed and taken with each of 3 daily meals; take the last (fourth) dose of the day with food at bedtime.

Usual Duration of Use: For prevention of stomach ulcer, use is recommended for the entire period of anti-inflammatory drug use. For treatment of duodenal ulcer, continual use on a regular schedule for 4 weeks is recommended; if ulcer healing is not complete, a second course of 4 weeks is advised. Long-term use (months to years) requires periodic physician evaluation of response and dosage adjustment.

Possible Advantages of This Drug: Significantly more effective than histamine (H-2)-blocking drugs (cimetidine, famotidine, nizatidine, ranitidine) or sucralfate in preventing the development of stomach ulcers.

▷ **This Drug Should Not Be Taken If**
- you have had an allergic reaction to it previously.
- you are allergic to any type of prostaglandin.
- you are pregnant or breast-feeding.
- you are not able or willing to use effective contraception (oral contraceptives or intrauterine device) while taking this drug.

▷ **Inform Your Physician Before Taking This Drug If**
- you have a history of peptic ulcer disease or Crohn's disease.
- you have impaired kidney function.
- you have a seizure disorder.

Possible Side-Effects (natural, expected and unavoidable drug actions)
Diarrhea (14–40% of users), usually beginning after 13 days of use and subsiding spontaneously after 8 days.
Abortion (miscarriage) of pregnancy (11% of users); this is often incomplete and accompanied by serious uterine bleeding that may require hospitalization and urgent treatment.

▷ **Possible Adverse Effects** (unusual, unexpected and infrequent reactions)
If any of the following develop, consult your physician promptly for guidance.
Mild Adverse Effects
Allergic Reaction: Skin rash.
Headache (2.4%), dizziness.
Ringing in the ears.
Abdominal pain (12.8%), indigestion (2%), nausea (3.2%), vomiting (1.3%), flatulence (2.9%), constipation (1.1%).
Menstrual irregularity (0.3%), menstrual cramps (0.6%), heavy menstrual flow (0.5%), spotting between periods (0.7%).
Serious Adverse Effects
Allergic Reactions: None reported.
Postmenopausal vaginal bleeding; this may require further evaluation.
Anemia and low blood platelets (rare).
Bronchospasm (rare).
Neuropathy (rare).
Abortion (if taken while pregnant).

Misoprostol

▷ **Possible Effects on Sexual Function:** Reduced libido and impotence reported rarely, but causal relationship not established.

▷ **Natural Diseases or Disorders That May Be Activated by This Drug**
Latent epilepsy.

Possible Effects on Laboratory Tests
Mild increase in liver function enzymes.

▷ *CAUTION*
1. Do not take this drug if you are pregnant. It can cause abortion.
2. Do not make this drug available to others who may be pregnant or who may become pregnant.
3. If this drug is prescribed, it is advisable that you have a negative serum pregnancy test within 2 weeks before starting treatment.
4. Start taking this drug only on the second or third day of your next normal menstrual period.
5. Initiate effective contraceptive measures when you begin to take this drug. Discuss the use of oral contraceptives or intrauterine devices with your physician.
6. Should pregnancy occur while you are taking this drug, stop the drug immediately and inform your physician.

Precautions for Use
By Infants and Children: Safety and effectiveness for those under 18 years of age not established.
By Those over 60 Years of Age: This drug is usually well tolerated by this age group. However, some forms of prostaglandins can cause drops in blood pressure; watch for light-headedness or faintness that may indicate low blood pressure. Report any such development to your physician.

▷ **Advisability of Use During Pregnancy**
Pregnancy Category: X. See Pregnancy Code at the back of this book.
Animal studies: No birth defects due to this drug found in rat or rabbit studies.
Human studies: Information from studies of pregnant women confirms that this drug can cause abortion, sometimes incomplete; unpassed products of conception can cause life-threatening complications.
Avoid this drug completely.

Advisability of Use if Breast-Feeding
Presence of this drug in breast milk: Unknown.
Avoid drug or refrain from nursing.

Habit-Forming Potential: None.

Effects of Overdosage: Abdominal pain, diarrhea, fever, drowsiness, weakness, tremor, convulsions, difficult breathing.

Possible Effects of Long-Term Use: Unknown at this time.

Suggested Periodic Examinations While Taking This Drug (at physician's discretion)
Monitoring for accidental pregnancy.

▷ **While Taking This Drug, Observe the Following**
Foods: No restrictions.
Beverages: No restrictions. May be taken with milk.

▷ *Alcohol:* No interactions expected. However, alcohol can promote the development of stomach ulcer and reduce the effectiveness of this drug.
Tobacco Smoking: No interactions expected. However, nicotine is conducive to the development of stomach ulcer. Smoking should be avoided.
▷ *Other Drugs*
Misoprostol *taken concurrently* with
- antacids that contain magnesium may increase the risk of diarrhea; avoid this combination. Antacids in general may decrease misoprostol absorption and lessen therapeutic benefit.
- indomethacin and some other NSAIDs may relsult in decreased NSAID levels.

▷ *Driving, Hazardous Activities:* This drug may cause dizziness, light-headedness, stomach pain or diarrhea. Restrict activities as necessary.
Aviation Note: The use of this drug *may be a disqualification* for piloting. Consult a designated Aviation Medical Examiner.
Exposure to Sun: No restrictions.
Discontinuation: This drug should be taken as combination therapy while you are taking antiarthritic/anti-inflammatory drugs that can cause stomach ulceration. Call your doctor if you have reason to stop it prematurely.

MOLINDONE (moh LIN dohn)

Introduced: 1971 **Prescription:** USA: Yes **Available as Generic:** No **Class:** Strong tranquilizer, antipsychotic **Controlled Drug:** USA: No
Brand Name: Moban

BENEFITS versus RISKS	
Possible Benefits	*Possible Risks*
EFFECTIVE TREATMENT OF SOME CASES OF ACUTE AND CHRONIC SCHIZOPHRENIA	NARROW TREATMENT MARGIN SERIOUS TOXIC EFFECTS ON BRAIN:
May be effective in schizophrenia that has not responded to other drugs	PARKINSON-LIKE REACTIONS SEVERE RESTLESSNESS ABNORMAL INVOLUNTARY MOVEMENTS TARDIVE DYSKINESIAS (see Glossary) Liver toxicity, jaundice Atropinelike side-effects

▷ **Principal Uses**
As a Single Drug Product: Uses currently included in FDA approved labeling: (1) Helps manage acute and chronic schizophrenia to control thought disorder, disorientation, hallucinations, perceptual distortions and hostility; (2) May have a small role in helping relieve depression.
Other (unlabeled) generally accepted uses: (1) May be of help in children with conduct disorders.

Molindone

How This Drug Works: Acts on nerve transmitters (serotonin and dopamine) to restore the activity in the reticular activating system of the brain, and improve distorted patterns of thinking and behavior.

Available Dosage Forms and Strengths
  Concentrate — 20 mg per ml
  Tablets — 5 mg, 10 mg, 25 mg, 50 mg, 100 mg

▷ **Usual Adult Dosage Range:** Initially, 50 to 75 mg/day in 3 or 4 divided doses; dose may be increased gradually in 3 days to 100 mg/day as needed and tolerated. For maintenance: mild psychosis—5 to 15 mg, 3 or 4 times/day; moderate psychosis—10 to 25 mg, 3 or 4 times/day; severe psychosis—up to 225 mg/day, in 3 or 4 divided doses. The total daily dosage should not exceed 225 mg. **Note: Actual dosage and administration schedule must be determined by the physician for each patient individually.**

Conditions Requiring Dosing Adjustments
  Liver function: Specific dosage adjustments in liver compromise are not defined. It should be used with caution in patients with liver compromise as it is a rare cause of liver toxicity (hepatoxicity).
  Kidney function: The kidney is minimally (3%) involved in the elimination of molindone.

▷ **Dosing Instructions:** The tablet may be crushed and taken with food or milk to reduce stomach irritation. The liquid concentrate may be diluted with water, milk, fruit juice or carbonated beverages.

Usual Duration of Use: Use on a regular schedule for 3 to 6 weeks is usually necessary to determine this drug's effectiveness in controlling the features of schizophrenia. Long-term use (months to years) requires supervision and periodic evaluation by your physician. Consult your physician on a regular basis.

▷ **This Drug Should Not Be Taken If**
- you have had an allergic reaction to it previously.
- you have acute alcoholic intoxication.

▷ **Inform Your Physician Before Taking This Drug If**
- you are taking any drugs that have sedative effects.
- you use alcohol excessively.
- you have any type of seizure disorder.
- you are pregnant or are breast-feeding.
- you have a history of neuroleptic malignant syndrome.
- you have any type of glaucoma.
- you have Parkinson's disease or an enlarged prostate gland.
- you have impaired liver or kidney function.
- you have a history of breast cancer.

Possible Side-Effects (natural, expected and unavoidable drug actions)
  Drowsiness, dry mouth, nasal congestion, constipation, impaired urination. Parkinson-like reactions (see Glossary).

▷ **Possible Adverse Effects** (unusual, unexpected and infrequent reactions)
  If any of the following develop, consult your physician promptly for guidance.
  Mild Adverse Effects
  Allergic Reaction: Skin rash.

Headache, dizziness, blurred vision, lethargy, unsteadiness, insomnia, depression, euphoria, ringing in ears.
Rapid heartbeat, low blood pressure, fainting.
Loss of appetite, indigestion, nausea.
Temporary lowering or increase in white blood cells.

Serious Adverse Effects
Allergic Reactions: Liver reaction with jaundice (rare, questionable)
Idiosyncratic Reactions: Neuroleptic malignant syndrome (see Glossary).
Spasms of face and neck muscles, abnormal involuntary movements of extremities, severe restlessness.
Development of tardive dyskinesias (see Glossary).
Lowering of the blood pressure on standing (orthostatic hypotension).
Lowering of the seizure threshold.
Liver toxicity (rare).

▷ **Possible Effects on Sexual Function**
Increased libido; male breast enlargement and tenderness; painful and extended erections; female breast enlargement with milk formation.
Altered timing and pattern of menstruation.

▷ **Adverse Effects That May Mimic Natural Diseases or Disorders**
Parkinson-like reactions may be mistaken for naturally occurring Parkinson's disease.
Rare liver reaction may suggest viral hepatitis.

Possible Effects on Laboratory Tests
Liver function enzymes: increased.
Blood urea nitrogen: increased.

CAUTION
1. This drug may alter the pattern of epileptic seizures and require dosage adjustments of anticonvulsant drugs.
2. Obtain prompt evaluation of any change or disturbance of vision.
3. There is a very narrow margin between the effective therapeutic dose and the dose that can cause Parkinson-like reactions. Inform your physician promptly if suggestive symptoms develop.

Precautions for Use
By Infants and Children: Safety and effectiveness for those under 12 years of age not established.
By Those over 60 Years of Age: Start treatment with small doses. This drug can aggravate an existing prostatism (see Glossary). You may be more susceptible to the development of Parkinson-like reactions or tardive dyskinesia. Report any suggestive symptoms promptly.

▷ **Advisability of Use During Pregnancy**
Pregnancy Category: C. See Pregnancy Code at the back of this book.
Animal studies: No birth defects reported in mice, rats or rabbits.
Human studies: Adequate studies of pregnant women are not available.
Because of its inherent toxicity for brain tissue, avoid use during pregnancy if possible.

Advisability of Use if Breast-Feeding
Presence of this drug in breast milk: Unknown.
Avoid drug or refrain from nursing.

Habit-Forming Potential: None.

Effects of Overdosage: Marked drowsiness, weakness, tremor, agitation, impaired stance and gait, stupor progressing to coma, possible seizures.

Possible Effects of Long-Term Use: Development of tardive dyskinesias.

Suggested Periodic Examinations While Taking This Drug (at physician's discretion)
Complete blood cell counts, liver function tests.

▷ **While Taking This Drug, Observe the Following**
Foods: No restrictions.
Beverages: No restrictions. May be taken with milk.
▷ *Alcohol:* Avoid completely. Alcohol can increase the sedative action of this drug and enhance its depressant effects on brain function. Also, this drug can increase the intoxicating effects of alcohol.
Tobacco Smoking: No interactions expected.
▷ *Other Drugs*
Molindone may *increase* the effects of
- all drugs containing atropine or having atropinelike effects (see Drug Class Section).
- all drugs with sedative effects, and cause excessive sedation.

Molindone *taken concurrently* with
- antiepileptic drugs (anticonvulsants) may require close monitoring for changes in seizure patterns and need for dosage adjustments.

▷ *Driving, Hazardous Activities:* This drug may cause dizziness and drowsiness. Restrict activities as necessary.
Aviation Note: The use of this drug *is a disqualification* for piloting. Consult a designated Aviation Medical Examiner.
Exposure to Sun: No restrictions.
Exposure to Heat: Use caution and avoid excessive heat as much as possible. This drug may impair the regulation of body temperature and increase the risk of heat stroke.
Discontinuation: Do not stop taking this drug suddenly after long-term use. Ask your physician for guidance regarding gradual dosage reduction and withdrawal.

MORPHINE (MOR feen)

Other Name: MS (morphine sulfate)

Introduced: 1806   **Prescription:** USA: Yes; Canada: Yes   **Available as Generic:** Yes   **Class:** Strong analgesic, opioids   **Controlled Drug:** USA: C-II*; Canada: No

Brand Names: Astramorph, Astramorph PF, Duramorph, ✤Epimorph, Infumorph, ✤Morphine H.P., ✤Morphitec, ✤M.O.S., ✤M.O.S.-S.R., MS Contin, MSIR, OMS Concentrate, Oramorph SR, Paregoric, RMS Uniserts, Roxanol, Roxanol 100, Roxanol SR, ✤Statex

*See Schedules of Controlled Drugs at the back of this book.

Morphine

BENEFITS versus RISKS	
Possible Benefits	*Possible Risks*
EFFECTIVE RELIEF OF MODERATE TO SEVERE PAIN	POTENTIAL FOR HABIT FORMATION (DEPENDENCE)
	Respiratory depression
	Disorientation, hallucinations
	Interference with urination
	Constipation

▷ **Principal Uses**
As a Single Drug Product: Uses currently included in FDA approved labeling: Given by mouth, suppository or injection to relieve moderate to severe pain of: (1)Heart attack, cancer, operations, fluid on the lungs and other causes; (2) it is also used as an adjunct to anesthesia.
Other (unlabeled) generally accepted uses: (1) Therapy of pain in sickle cell crisis; (2) used in patient controlled analgesia pumps to fight pain.

How This Drug Works: Acting primarily as a depressant of certain brain functions, this drug suppresses the perception of pain and calms the emotional response to pain.

Available Dosage Forms and Strengths
Injection — 0.5 mg, 1 mg, 2 mg, 4 mg, 5 mg, 8 mg, 10 mg, 15 mg, 25 mg, 50 mg (all per ml)
Oral Solution — 20 mg per ml; 10 mg, 20 mg, 100 mg per 5-ml teaspoonful
Suppositories — 5 mg, 10 mg, 20 mg, 30 mg
Syrup — 1 mg, 5 mg, 10 mg, 20 mg, 50 mg (all per ml) Canada only
Tablets — 5 mg, 10 mg, 15 mg, 25 mg, 30 mg, 50 mg
Tablets, soluble — 10 mg, 15 mg, 30 mg
Tablets, sustained-release — 15 mg, 30 mg, 60 mg, 100 mg, 200 mg

▷ **Recommended Dosage Ranges** (Actual dosage and administration schedule must be determined by the physician for each patient individually.)
Infants and Children: 0.1 to 0.2 mg/kg of body weight every 4 hours, as needed. Single dose should not exceed 15 mg.
12 to 60 Years of Age: By injection—5 to 20 mg every 4 hours, as needed.
By mouth (regular solution, syrup and tablets)—10 to 30 mg every 4 hours, as needed.
By mouth (sustained-release forms)—30 mg every 8 to 12 hours, as needed.
By suppository—10 to 30 mg every 4 hours, as needed.
Over 60 Years of Age: Same as 12 to 60 years of age, using the lower end of the range initially; increase dose cautiously, as needed and tolerated.

Conditions Requiring Dosing Adjustments
Liver function: The dose and frequency **must** be adjusted (decreased) with liver compromise.
Kidney function: The dose and frequency should be adjusted in renal compromise.

Morphine

▷ **Dosing Instructions:** The regular tablet may be crushed and taken with or following food to reduce stomach irritation or nausea. The sustained-release tablet should be swallowed whole; do not break it in half, crush it or chew it. The oral liquid may be mixed with fruit juice to improve taste.

Usual Duration of Use: As required to control pain. For short-term, self-limiting conditions, continual use should not exceed 5 to 7 days without interruption and reassessment of need. For the long-term management of severe chronic pain, it is advisable to determine an optimal fixed-dosage schedule.

▷ **This Drug Should Not Be Taken If**
- you have had an allergic reaction to any dosage form of it previously.
- you are having an acute attack of asthma.
- you have acute respiratory depression.

▷ **Inform Your Physician Before Taking This Drug If**
- you are taking, or have taken within the past 14 days, any monoamine oxidase (MAO) type A inhibitor drug (see Drug Class Section).
- you are taking: atropinelike drugs, antihypertensives, metoclopramide (Reglan), zidovudine (AZT).
- you are taking any other drugs that have a sedative effect.
- you have a history of drug abuse or alcoholism.
- you have impaired liver or kidney function.
- you have prostate gland enlargement. (See **prostatism** in the Glossary.)
- you have a history of asthma, emphysema, epilepsy, gallbladder disease, or inflammatory bowel disease.
- you have a tendency toward constipation.
- you have a history of low blood pressure.
- you plan to have surgery under general anesthesia in the near future.

Possible Side-Effects (natural, expected and unavoidable drug actions)
  Drowsiness, light-headedness, weakness, euphoria, dry mouth, urinary retention, constipation.

▷ **Possible Adverse Effects** (unusual, unexpected and infrequent reactions)
  If any of the following develop, consult your physician promptly for guidance.
  Mild Adverse Effects
  Allergic Reactions: Skin rash, hives, itching (especially if the intravenous form is injected too quickly).
  Headache, dizziness, impaired concentration, sensation of drunkenness, confusion, depression, blurred or double vision.
  Miosis or pinpoint pupils.
  Facial flushing, sweating, heart palpitation.
  Nausea, vomiting.
  Spasm of the biliary tract.
  Urine retention.
  Serious Adverse Effects
  Allergic Reactions: Swelling of throat or vocal cords, spasm of larynx or bronchial tubes.
  Hallucinations, psychosis.
  Drop in blood pressure, causing severe weakness and fainting.

Disorientation, hallucinations, unstable gait, tremor, muscle twitching.
Drug-induced myasthenia gravis.
Respiratory depression.
Seizures.
Drug-induced porphyria (rare).

▷ **Possible Effects on Sexual Function:** Reduced libido and/or potency. Amenorrhea and disruption of ovulation.

▷ **Adverse Effects That May Mimic Natural Diseases or Disorders**
Paradoxical behavioral disturbances may suggest psychotic disorder.

Possible Effects on Laboratory Tests
Blood amylase and lipase levels: increased (natural side-effects).
Liver function tests: increased liver enzymes (ALT/GPT, AST/GOT and alkaline phosphatase), increased bilirubin.
Urine screening tests for drug abuse: May be **positive**. (Test results depend upon amount of drug taken and testing method used.)

CAUTION
1. If you have asthma, chronic bronchitis or emphysema, excessive use of this drug may cause significant respiratory difficulty, thickening of bronchial secretions and suppression of coughing.
2. Taking this drug with atropinelike drugs can increase the risk of urinary retention and reduced intestinal function.
3. Do not take this drug following acute head injury.

Precautions for Use
By Infants and Children: Used very cautiously in infants under 2 years of age because of vulnerability to life-threatening respiratory depression. Watch for any indication of paradoxical excitement in this age group.
By Those over 60 Years of Age: Small doses and short-term use indicated. There may be increased risk of drowsiness, dizziness, unsteadiness, falling, urinary retention and constipation (often leading to fecal impaction).

▷ **Advisability of Use During Pregnancy**
Pregnancy Category: C. See Pregnancy Code at the back of this book.
Animal studies: Significant skeletal birth defects reported in mouse and hamster studies.
Human studies: Adequate studies of pregnant women are not available. However, no significant increase in birth defects was found in 448 exposures to this drug.
Avoid during the first 3 months. Use sparingly and in small doses during the last 6 months only if clearly needed.

Advisability of Use if Breast-Feeding
Presence of this drug in breast milk: Yes.
Avoid drug or refrain from nursing.

Habit-Forming Potential: This drug can cause psychological and physical dependence (see Glossary).

Effects of Overdosage: Marked drowsiness, dizziness, confusion, restlessness, depressed breathing, tremors, convulsions, stupor progressing to coma.

Possible Effects of Long-Term Use: Psychological and physical dependence, chronic constipation.

Suggested Periodic Examinations While Taking This Drug (at physician's discretion)
 None.

▷ **While Taking This Drug, Observe the Following**
 Foods: No restrictions.
 Beverages: No restrictions. May be taken with milk.
▷ *Alcohol:* Alcohol is best avoided. Opioid analgesics can intensify the intoxicating effects of alcohol, and alcohol can intensify the depressant effects of opioids on brain function, breathing and circulation.
 Tobacco Smoking: No interactions expected.
 Marijuana Smoking: Increase in drowsiness and pain relief; impairment of mental and physical performance.
▷ *Other Drugs*
 Morphine may *increase* the effects of
 • other drugs with sedative effects.
 • antihypertensives, and cause excessive lowering of blood pressure.
 • atropinelike drugs, and increase the risk of constipation and urinary retention.
 Morphine may *decrease* the effects of
 • metoclopramide (Reglan).
 Morphine *taken concurrently* with
 • cimetidine (Tagamet) may result in morphine toxicity.
 • monoamine oxidase (MAO) type A inhibitor drugs (see Drug Classes) may cause the equivalent of an acute narcotic overdose: unconsciousness; severe depression of breathing, heart action and circulation. A variation of this reaction can be excitability, convulsions, high fever and rapid heart action.
 • phenothiazines (see Drug Class Section) may cause excessive and prolonged depression of brain functions, breathing and circulation.
 • zidovudine (AZT) may increase the toxicity of both drugs; avoid concurrent use.
▷ *Driving, Hazardous Activities:* This drug can impair mental alertness, judgment, reaction, time and physical coordination. Avoid hazardous activities.
 Aviation Note: The use of this drug *is a disqualification* for piloting. Consult a designated Aviation Medical Examiner.
 Exposure to Sun: No restrictions.
 Discontinuation: It is advisable to limit this drug to short-term use. Longer term use requires gradual tapering (decreasing) of doses to minimize possible effects of withdrawal: body aches, fever, sweating, nervousness, trembling, weakness, runny nose, sneezing, rapid heart rate, nausea, vomiting, stomach cramps, diarrhea.

MUPIROCIN (Myou PEER oh sin)

Introduced: 1987 **Prescription:** USA: Yes; Canada: Yes **Available as**
Generic: USA: No; Canada: No **Class:** Topical antibiotic **Controlled**
Drug: USA: No; Canada: No
Brand Names: Bactroban

BENEFITS versus RISKS

Possible Benefits | *Possible Risks*
EFFECTIVE TOPICAL TREATMENT OF STAPH AND STREP SKIN INFECTIONS | Skin irritation

---

▷ **Principal Uses**
   As a Single Drug Product: Uses currently included in FDA approved labeling: (1) Used to treat skin infections caused by Staphylococcal and Streptococcal infections such as ecthyma or impetigo.
   Other (unlabeled) generally accepted uses: (1) Used in burns where resistant Staphylococcus aureus is causing infection; (2) helps prevent opportunistic infections of venous access devices such as intravascular cannulas; (3) treats cellulitis caused by gram positive organisms; (4) has been used in some specific situations in skin surgery to prevent infections; (5) used in a newly available formulation to eradicate Staph Aureus from the interior of the noses of health care workers who have become carriers of this bacteria; (6) has recently been used to erradicate vaginal staph infections.

How This Drug Works: This drug binds to a specific enzyme (isoleucyl transfer-RNA synthetase) and stops susceptible bacteria from being able to make critical proteins.

Available Dosage Forms and Strengths
   Topical ointment — 2%
        — 20 mg per gram (Canada)

▷ **Recommended Dosage Ranges (Actual dosage and administration schedule must be determined by the physician for each patient individually.)**
   Infants and Children: Not indicated in infants.
      Children 5 to 15 years old have been given a thin coat of the 2% ointment applied to the infection site 3 times daily for three to five consecutive days.
   16 to 60 Years of Age: The 2% ointment has been applied 3 times daily for 5 to 14 days. Some more involved or extensive infections have been treated for longer periods. If the infection in question has not resolved after the initial course of the ointment, the site should be evaluated by a physician and systemic antibiotics or other treatment considered.
   Over 60 Years of Age: Same as 16 to 60 years of age.

Conditions Requiring Dosing Adjustments
   Liver function: This ointment is not usually systemically absorbed to an appreciable extent. If the ointment is applied to an extensive skin area, metabo-

lism of the active antibiotic does occur in the liver—yet there are no existing guidelines for dosage adjustments.

Kidney function: A substance in this formulation (polyethylene glycol) may be toxic to the kidneys if the ointment is applied over an extensive burn or wound area.

▷ **Dosing Instructions:** This medicine should be applied as a thin film or as described by your doctor. Call your doctor if the condition has not improved or worsens during the course of treatment. Do **not** combine this medicine with other ointments or treatments unless your doctor has prescribed this approach.

Usual Duration of Use: Continual use on a regular schedule for several days is usually necessary to determine this drug's effectiveness in treating skin infections. Long-term use (months to years) requires periodic physician evaluation. Consult your physician on a regular basis.

Possible Advantages of This Drug
Effective topical treatment of skin infections.

▷ **This Drug Should Not Be Taken If**
- you have had an allergic reaction to any dosage form of it previously.

▷ **Inform Your Physician Before Taking This Drug If**
- several days have passed since this medicine has been prescribed and there has been no change or worsening of the wound.
- pain at the site of the infection increases.
- you are uncertain of how much mupirocin to apply or how often to apply it.

Possible Side-Effects (natural, expected and unavoidable drug actions)
Irritation at the site of infection secondary to the polyethylene glycol component.

▷ **Possible Adverse Effects** (unusual, unexpected and infrequent reactions)
If any of the following develop, consult your physician promptly for guidance.

Mild Adverse Effects
Allergic Reactions: Skin rash and irritation at the infection site.
Soreness, stinging or pain at the infection site.

Serious Adverse Effects
Allergic Reactions: Not defined as the medicine is not appreciably absorbed.
If this medicine is applied to an extensive skin area, polyethylene glycol may be absorbed and cause kidney toxicity.

▷ **Possible Effects on Sexual Function:** Not reported.

Possible Delayed Adverse Effects: This medicine is indicated for short term use.

▷ **Adverse Effects That May Mimic Natural Diseases or Disorders**
None reported.

Natural Diseases or Disorders That May Be Activated by This Drug
None reported.

Possible Effects on Laboratory Tests
None reported.

CAUTION
1. Do not apply this medicine to an area of skin larger than that your doctor prescribed.

Precautions for Use
By Infants and Children:
Safety and effectiveness for use by those under 5 years of age have not been established.
By Those over 60 Years of Age: No special changes needed.

▷ **Advisability of Use During Pregnancy**
Pregnancy Category: B. See Pregnancy Code at the back of this book.
Animal studies: No fetal problems defined.
Human studies: Information from adequate studies of pregnant women is not available.

Advisability of Use if Breast-Feeding
Presence of this drug in breast milk: Unknown.
Avoid drug or refrain from nursing.

Habit-Forming Potential: None.

Effects of Overdosage: If this medicine is applied to an extensive area of skin, excessive amounts of polyethylene glycol may be absorbed and cause kidney toxicity.

Possible Effects of Long-Term Use: None defined.

Suggested Periodic Examinations While Taking This Drug (at physician's discretion)
None.

▷ **While Taking This Drug, Observe the Following**
Foods: No restrictions.
Beverages: No restrictions.
▷ *Alcohol:* No restrictions.
Tobacco Smoking: No interactions expected.
▷ *Other Drugs*
Mupirocin **taken concurrently** with
- other medications which are toxic to the kidneys may result in additive kidney toxicity if mupirocin is applied to a large area of skin.

Aviation Note: The use of this drug **does not appear to be a restriction** for piloting. Consult a designated Aviation Medical Examiner.
Exposure to Sun: No restrictions.

NABUMETONE (na BYU me tohn)

Introduced: 1984 **Prescription:** USA: Yes **Available as Generic:** No **Class:** Nonsteroidal anti-inflammatory drug (NSAID) **Controlled Drug:** USA: No

Brand Name: Relafen

BENEFITS versus RISKS	
Possible Benefits	**Possible Risks**
EFFECTIVE RELIEF OF MILD TO MODERATE PAIN AND INFLAMMATION ASSOCIATED WITH OSTEOARTHRITIS AND RHEUMATOID ARTHRITIS	Gastrointestinal ulceration (0.3–0.8%) Drug-induced hepatitis (less than 1%) Drug-induced kidney damage (less than 1%) Very rare lung fibrosis. Mild fluid retention (3–9%)

Please see the acetic acid nonsteroidal anti-inflammatory drug profile for further information.

NADOLOL (nay DOH lohl)

Introduced: 1976 **Prescription:** USA: Yes; Canada: Yes **Available as Generic:** No **Class:** Antianginal, antihypertensive, beta-adrenergic blocker **Controlled Drug:** USA: No; Canada: No
Brand Names: Corgard, Corzide [CD], ◆Apo-Nadol, Syn-Nadol

BENEFITS versus RISKS	
Possible Benefits	**Possible Risks**
EFFECTIVE, WELL-TOLERATED ANTIHYPERTENSIVE in mild to moderate high blood pressure EFFECTIVE ANTIANGINAL DRUG IN CLASSICAL CORONARY ARTERY DISEASE with moderate to severe angina	CONGESTIVE HEART FAILURE in advanced heart disease Provocation of asthma (in predisposed patients) Masking of hypoglycemia in drug-dependent diabetes Worsening of angina following abrupt withdrawal

▷ **Principal Uses**

As a Single Drug Product: Uses currently included in FDA approved labeling: (1) Treatment of moderately high blood pressure; (2) helps prevent attacks of effort-induced angina. (This drug is contraindicated in Prinzmetal's vasospastic angina.)

Other (unlabeled) generally accepted uses: (1) Helps prevent hemorrhage from bulging veins (esophageal varices) in cirrhosis; (2) may have an adjunctive role in helping prevent and reduce migraine severity; (3) may have a role in helping prevent death after a heart attack (myocardial infarction); (4) may help ease tremor in patients taking lithium; (5) helps decrease risk of ruptured blood vessels in the esophagus (esophageal varices) in patients with cirrhosis.

As a Combination Drug Product [CD]: This drug is available in combination with bendroflumethiazide, a mild diuretic antihypertensive drug. This combination product is more effective and more convenient for long-term use.

How This Drug Works: By blocking certain actions of the sympathetic nervous system, this drug
- reduces the rate and contraction force of the heart, lowering oxygen requirements of the heart muscle, reducing ejection pressure of the blood leaving the heart; consequently reducing the frequency of angina and lowering blood pressure.
- reduces the degree of contraction of blood vessel walls, resulting expansion and consequent lowering of blood pressure.
- prolongs conduction time of nerve impulses through the heart, of benefit in the management of certain heart rhythm disorders.

Available Dosage Forms and Strengths
Tablets — 20 mg, 40 mg, 80 mg, 120 mg, 160 mg

▷ **Usual Adult Dosage Range:** For hypertension: Initially, 40 mg daily in one dose; this may be increased gradually as needed and tolerated, up to 320 mg/24 hours. The usual maintenance dose is 80 to 320 mg/24 hours. The total daily dosage should not exceed 320 mg. For angina: Initially, 40 mg daily in one dose; increase gradually at intervals of 3 to 7 days up to 240 mg/24 hours. The usual maintenance dose is 80 to 240 mg/24 hours. The total daily dose should not exceed 240 mg. **Note: Actual dosage and administration schedule must be determined by the physician for each patient individually.**

Conditions Requiring Dosing Adjustments
Liver function: The liver is not significantly involved in the elimination of this medication.
Kidney function: In patients with moderate kidney failure, the usual dose should be given every 24 to 36 hours. In patients with severe kidney failure, the dose can be given every 40 to 60 hours.

▷ **Dosing Instructions:** The tablet may be crushed and taken without regard to eating. Do not stop this drug abruptly.

Usual Duration of Use: Use on a regular schedule for 10 to 14 days determines this drug's effectiveness in lowering blood pressure and preventing angina. The long-term use of this drug (months to years) will be determined by your response to an overall treatment program (weight reduction, salt restriction, smoking cessation, etc.). Consult your physician on a regular basis.

Possible Advantages of This Drug
Does not reduce blood flow to the kidney.
Can be used concurrently with other drugs that may reduce blood flow to the kidney (such as most anti-inflammatory aspirin substitutes).

▷ **This Drug Should Not Be Taken If**
- you have had an allergic reaction to it previously.
- you have congestive heart failure.
- you have an abnormally slow heart rate or a serious form of heart block.
- you are subject to bronchial asthma.
- you are presently experiencing seasonal hay fever.
- you are taking, or have taken within the past 14 days, any monoamine oxidase (MAO) type A inhibitor drug (see Drug Classes).

▷ **Inform Your Physician Before Taking This Drug If**
- you have had an adverse reaction to any beta blocker (see Drug Class Section).
- you have a history of serious heart disease.
- you have a history of hay fever (allergic rhinitis), asthma, chronic bronchitis or emphysema.
- you have a history of overactive thyroid function (hyperthyroidism).
- you have a history of low blood sugar (hypoglycemia).
- you have impaired liver or kidney function.
- you have diabetes or myasthenia gravis.
- you are pregnant or are breast-feeding.
- you have difficulty with blood circulation to the periphery (peripheral vascular disease).
- you are currently taking any form of digitalis, quinidine or reserpine, or any calcium blocker drug (see Drug Class Section).
- you plan to have surgery under general anesthesia in the near future.

Possible Side-Effects (natural, expected and unavoidable drug actions)
Lethargy and fatigability, cold extremities, slow heart rate, light-headedness in upright position (see Orthostatic Hypotension in Glossary).

▷ **Possible Adverse Effects** (unusual, unexpected and infrequent reactions)
If any of the following develop, consult your physician promptly for guidance.

Mild Adverse Effects
Allergic Reactions: Skin rash, itching, drug fever.
Headache, dizziness, insomnia, vivid dreaming, visual disturbances, ringing in ears, slurred speech, paresthesias.
Hair loss and sweating.
Indigestion, nausea, vomiting, diarrhea, abdominal pain.
Cough.
Increased blood potassium.
Numbness and tingling of extremities.

Serious Adverse Effects
Allergic Reaction: Facial swelling, anaphylaxis.
Chest pain, shortness of breath, precipitation of congestive heart failure.
Intensification of heart block.
Bronchospasm (rare).
Carpal tunnel syndrome (rare).
Induction of bronchial asthma (in asthmatic individuals).
Masking of warning indications of acute hypoglycemia in drug-treated diabetes.
Rare cause of pancreatitis.
Severe slowing of the heart (2%).
May precipitate cramping when walking (intermittent claudication).
Excessively low blood pressure.

▷ **Possible Effects on Sexual Function:** Decreased libido, impotence (4%), impaired erection (36%).

▷ **Adverse Effects That May Mimic Natural Diseases or Disorders**
Impaired circulation to the extremities may resemble Raynaud's phenomenon.

Natural Diseases or Disorders That May Be Activated by This Drug
Bronchial asthma, Prinzmetal's variant (vasospastic) angina, latent Raynaud's disease, myasthenia gravis (questionable).

Possible Effects on Laboratory Tests
Blood HDL cholesterol level: decreased.
Blood VLDL cholesterol level: increased.
Blood triglyceride levels: increased.

CAUTION
1. **Do not stop this drug suddenly** without the knowledge and help of your doctor. Carry a note on your person that you are taking this drug.
2. Ask your physician or pharmacist **before** using nasal decongestants usually present in over-the-counter cold preparations and nose drops. These can cause rapid blood pressure increases when combined with beta blocker drugs.
3. Report the development of any tendency to emotional depression.

Precautions for Use
By Infants and Children: Safety and effectiveness for those under 12 years of age not established. However, if this drug is used, observe for the development of low blood sugar (hypoglycemia) during periods of reduced food intake.

By Those over 60 Years of Age: Unacceptably high blood pressure should be reduced without creating the risks associated with excessively low blood pressure. Small doses, and frequent blood pressure checks needed. Sudden, rapid and excessive reduction of blood pressure can predispose to stroke or heart attack. Watch for dizziness, unsteadiness, tendency to fall, confusion, hallucinations, depression or urinary frequency.

▷ **Advisability of Use During Pregnancy**
Pregnancy Category: C. See Pregnancy Code at the back of this book.
Animal studies: No significant increase in birth defects due to this drug, but embryotoxicity reported in rabbits.
Human studies: Adequate studies of pregnant women are not available.
Avoid use during the first 3 months if possible. Use this drug only if clearly needed. Ask physician for guidance.

Advisability of Use if Breast-Feeding
Presence of this drug in breast milk: Yes, in large amounts.
Avoid drug or refrain from nursing.

Habit-Forming Potential: None.

Effects of Overdosage: Weakness, slow pulse, low blood pressure, fainting, cold and sweaty skin, congestive heart failure, possible coma and convulsions.

Possible Effects of Long-Term Use: Reduced heart reserve and eventual heart failure in susceptible individuals with advanced heart disease.

Suggested Periodic Examinations While Taking This Drug (at physician's discretion)
Measurements of blood pressure, evaluation of heart function.

▷ **While Taking This Drug, Observe the Following**
Foods: No restrictions. Avoid excessive salt intake.
Beverages: No restrictions. May be taken with milk.

▷ *Alcohol:* Use with caution. Alcohol may exaggerate this drug's ability to lower blood pressure and may increase its mild sedative effect.

Tobacco Smoking: Nicotine may reduce this drug's effectiveness in treating high blood pressure and angina. In addition, high doses of this drug may potentiate the constriction of the bronchial tubes caused by regular smoking.

▷ *Other Drugs*

Nadolol may **increase** the effects of
- other antihypertensive drugs, and cause excessive lowering of blood pressure. Dosage adjustments may be necessary.
- reserpine (Ser-Ap-Es, etc.), and cause sedation, depression, slowing of the heart rate and lowering of blood pressure.
- verapamil (Calan, Isoptin) or other calcium channel blockers (see Drug Classes), and cause excessive depression of heart function; monitor this combination closely.

Nadolol may **decrease** the effects of
- theophyllines (Aminophyllin, Theo-Dur, etc.), and reduce their effectiveness in treating asthma.

Nadolol **taken concurrently** with
- antacids containing aluminum can block absorption of this medicine and lessen therapeutic nadolol effects.
- amiodarone (Codarone) and cause severe slowing of the heart and potentially stop the heart (cardiac arrest).
- clonidine (Catapres) requires close monitoring for rebound high blood pressure if clonidine is withdrawn while nadolol is still being taken.
- epinephrine can cause serious hypertension, slowing of the heart and should anaphylaxis occur—epinephrine resistance.
- ergot derivatives (see Drug Class) can cause decreased blood flow to the extremities (peripheral ischemia).
- insulin requires close monitoring to avoid undetected hypoglycemia (see Glossary).
- lidocaine can lead to lidocaine toxicity (depressed heart function, cardiac arrest).
- oral hypoglycemic agents (see Drug Class) and cause slowed recovery from any hypoglycemia which may occur.

The following drugs may **decrease** the effects of nadolol
- indomethacin (Indocin), and possibly other "aspirin substitutes," or NSAIDs may impair nadolol's antihypertensive effect.

▷ *Driving, Hazardous Activities:* Use caution until the full extent of drowsiness, lethargy and blood pressure change has been determined.

Aviation Note: The use of this drug **is a disqualification** for piloting. Consult a designated Aviation Medical Examiner.

Exposure to Sun: No restrictions.

Exposure to Heat: Caution advised. Hot environments can lower the blood pressure and exaggerate the effects of this drug.

Exposure to Cold: Caution advised. Cold environments can enhance the circulatory deficiency in the extremities that may occur with this drug. The elderly should take precautions to prevent hypothermia (see Glossary).

Heavy Exercise or Exertion: It is advisable to avoid exertion that produces light-headedness, excessive fatigue or muscle cramping. The use of this drug may intensify the hypertensive response to isometric exercise.

Occurrence of Unrelated Illness: Fever that accompanies systemic infections can lower blood pressure and require dose decreases. Nausea or vomiting may interrupt the regular dosage schedule. Ask your physician for guidance.

Discontinuation: It is advisable to avoid sudden discontinuation of this drug in all situations. If possible, gradual reduction of dose over a period of 2 to 3 weeks is recommended. Ask your physician for specific guidance.

NAFARELIN (NAF a re lin)

Introduced: 1984 **Prescription:** USA: Yes **Available as Generic:** USA: No
Class: Gonadotropin-releasing hormone **Controlled Drug:** USA: No
Brand Name: Synarel

BENEFITS versus RISKS	
Possible Benefits	*Possible Risks*
VERY EFFECTIVE TREATMENT OF ENDOMETRIOSIS: Relief of symptoms (94%); reduction of lesions (86%)	Symptoms of estrogen deficiency (during treatment) Masculinizing effects (during treatment) Loss of bone density Lowering of the white blood cell count

▷ **Principal Uses**

As a Single Drug Product: Uses currently included in FDA approved labeling: (1) Treats endometriosis: reduction in the size and activity of endometrial implants within the pelvis; relief of pelvic pain associated with menstruation. (2) also used to treat precocious puberty due to excessive production of gonadotropic hormones.

Other (unlabeled) generally accepted uses: (1) Intranasal dosing helps control abnormal hair growth in women; (2) can be injected below the skin (subcutaneously) to help benign prostatic hyperplasia; (3) may be used before surgery to help decrease size of some tumors (myomas).

How This Drug Works: This drug stimulates the pituitary gland to secrete two additional hormones that regulate production of estrogen by the ovaries. Initially this drug causes an increase in the production of estrogen, but with continued use the high levels of estrogen suppress (via a feed-back mechanism) hormones that stimulate the ovary and thus estrogen production is significantly reduced. The implants of endometrium (from the lining of the uterus) that are attached to the pelvic wall are stimulated by the cyclic rise and fall of estrogen that accompanies menstruation. As a result of suppressing estrogen production, the displaced endometrial tissue (endometriosis) becomes dormant; the conditions responsible for premenstrual and menstrual pain are no longer active.

Nafarelin

Available Dosage Forms and Strengths
Nasal solution — 2 mg per ml (10 ml bottle)

▷ **Usual Adult Dosage Range:** 400 mcg daily. Spray 1 dose of 200 mcg into one nostril in the morning and 1 dose of 200 mcg into the other nostril in the evening, 12 hours apart. Begin treatment between days 2 and 4 of the menstrual cycle.

If regular menstruation persists after 2 months of treatment, the dose may be increased to 800 mcg daily: 1 spray into each nostril (a total of 2 sprays, 400 mcg) in the morning and again in the evening.

Note: Actual dosage and administration schedule must be determined by the physician for each patient individually.

Conditions Requiring Dosing Adjustments
Liver function: The liver plays a minor role in the elimination of this medication.
Kidney function: Specific guidelines are not available for dose. Decreases kidney compromise.

▷ **Dosing Instructions:** Carefully read and follow the patient instructions provided with this drug. The solution is to be sprayed directly into the nostrils; it is not to be swallowed. Time the start of therapy and daily dosing exactly as directed.

If you need to use a nasal decongestant (spray or drops), the decongestant should not be used for at least 30 minutes after dosing the nafarelin spray; earlier use could impair absorption of nafarelin.

Usual Duration of Use: Use on a regular schedule for 2 to 3 months usually determines effectiveness in relieving endometriosis symptoms. The standard course of treatment is limited to 6 months.

After 6 months of treatment, 60% of users are free of symptoms, 32% have mild symptoms, 7% have moderate symptoms and 1% will have severe symptoms. Six months after stopping this drug, of the 60% who obtain complete relief 50% will remain free of symptoms, 33% will have mild symptoms and 17% will have moderate symptoms.

If symptoms of endometriosis recur following a 6 month course of treatment and a repeat course is considered, it is advisable to measure bone density before retreatment is started.

Possible Advantages of This Drug
Causes fewer masculinizing effects than danazol.
Less tendency than danazol to increase blood cholesterol levels.
Unlike danazol, this drug does not cause abnormally low HDL cholesterol levels or abnormally high LDL cholesterol levels.

Currently a "Drug of Choice"
for the management of symptoms associated with endometriosis.

▷ **This Drug Should Not Be Taken If**
- you have had an allergic reaction to it previously.
- you are pregnant or breast-feeding.
- you have abnormal vaginal bleeding of unknown cause.

▷ **Inform Your Physician Before Taking This Drug If**
- you have used this drug, danazol or similar drugs previously.
- you are taking any type of estrogen, progesterone or oral contraceptive.

- you are planning pregnancy in the near future.
- you have a family history of osteoporosis.
- you use alcohol or tobacco regularly.
- you have a history of low white blood cells.
- you are using anticonvulsants or cortisonelike drugs.
- you are subject to allergic or infectious rhinitis and use nasal decongestants frequently.

Possible Side-Effects (natural, expected and unavoidable drug actions)

Effects due to reduced estrogen production: hot flashes (90%), headaches (19%), emotional lability (15%), insomnia (8%).

Masculinizing effects: acne (13%), muscle aches (10%), fluid retention (8%), increased skin oil (8%), weight gain (8%), excessive hair growth (2%).

▷ **Possible Adverse Effects** (unusual, unexpected and infrequent reactions)

If any of the following develop, consult your physician promptly for guidance.

Mild Adverse Effects

Allergic Reactions: Skin rash, hives (less than 1%).

Nasal irritation (10%).

Vaginal dryness (14–57%)

Depression (2%).

Serious Adverse Effects

Loss of vertebral bone density: at completion of 6 months of treatment, bone density decreases an average of 8.7% and bone mass decreases an average of 4.3%; partial recovery during the posttreatment period restores bone density loss to 4.9% and bone mass loss to 3.3%.

Lowering of the white blood cell count (12.5%).

Transient prostate enlargement.

Uterine bleeding.

▷ **Possible Effects on Sexual Function**

Decreased libido (22%), vaginal dryness (14–57%), reduced breast size (10%).

Impotence occurred in most men who had used this drug for prostate problems.

Galactorrhea.

Natural Diseases or Disorders That May Be Activated by This Drug

Worsening of or increased progression of osteoporosis.

Possible Effects on Laboratory Tests

Blood testosterone level: decreased in men with benign enlargement of prostate gland.

Blood progesterone: decreased to less than 4 ng/ml.

CAUTION

1. With continual use of this drug in proper dosage, menstruation will cease. If regular menstruation persists, call your doctor. Dosage adjustment may be necessary.
2. Use this drug consistently on a regular basis. Missed doses can result in breakthrough bleeding and ovulation.
3. It is advisable to avoid pregnancy during the course of treatment. Use

a nonhormonal method of birth control; do not use oral contraceptives. Inform your physician promptly if you think you may be pregnant.

4. If you need to use nasal decongestant sprays or drops, delay their use for at least 30 minutes after the intranasal spray of nafarelin.

Precautions for Use
By Infants and Children: Safety and effectiveness for those under 18 years of age not established.
By Those over 60 Years of Age: If used for prostatism, impotence is a common side effect. Depression (29%) and hot flashes (100%) were also reported.

▷ **Advisability of Use During Pregnancy**
Pregnancy Category:
X. See Pregnancy Code at the back of this book.
Animal studies: Major fetal abnormalities and increased fetal deaths due to this drug have been demonstrated in rat studies.
Human studies: Adequate studies of pregnant women are not available.
Avoid this drug during entire pregnancy.

Advisability of Use if Breast-Feeding
Presence of this drug in breast milk: Unknown.
Avoid drug or refrain from nursing.

Habit-Forming Potential: None.

Effects of Overdosage: No significant effects expected.

Possible Effects of Long-Term Use: Continual use should be limited to 6 months. If repeated courses of treatment are considered, determination of bone density and mass should be made to assess possible bone loss, predisposition to osteoporosis and possible therapy.

Suggested Periodic Examinations While Taking This Drug (at physician's discretion)
Blood cholesterol and triglyceride profiles.
Bone density and mass measurements.

▷ **While Taking This Drug, Observe the Following**
Foods: No restrictions.
Beverages: No restrictions.
▷ *Alcohol:* No interactions expected.
Tobacco Smoking: No interactions expected.
▷ *Other Drugs*
The following drugs will *decrease* the effects of nafarelin
- estrogens
- oral contraceptives
▷ *Driving, Hazardous Activities:* No restrictions.
Aviation Note:
The use of this drug **is not a disqualification** for piloting. Consult a designated Aviation Medical Examiner for confirmation.
Exposure to Sun: No restrictions.
Discontinuation: Normal ovarian function (ovulation, menstruation, etc.) is usually restored within 4 to 8 weeks after discontinuation of this drug.
Special Storage Instructions: Store in an upright position at room temperature. Protect from light.

NALTREXONE (Nail TREX own)

Introduced: 1995   **Prescription:** USA: Yes; Canada: Yes   **Available as Generic:** USA: No; Canada: No   **Class:** Antialcoholism, opioid antagonist
Controlled Drug: USA: No; Canada: No

Brand Names: Trexan, ReVia

Warning: This medication can cause liver damage if taken in excessive doses. If abdominal pain, white stools, yellowing of the eyes or skin occurs, call your doctor immediately.

BENEFITS versus RISKS	
Possible Benefits	*Possible Risks*
CONTROL OF CRAVING FOR ALCOHOL	LIVER DAMAGE IF EXCESSIVE DOSES TAKEN
PART OF AN EFFECTIVE COMBIATION APPROACH TO ALCOHOLISM	
ONCE DAILY DOSING	

▷ **Principal Uses**
  As a Single Drug Product: Uses currently included in FDA approved labeling: (1) Used as part of a comprehensive program to help alcohol dependence; (2) used to treat narcotic addiction.
  Other (unlabeled) generally accepted uses: (1) May help women with a specific type of cessation of menstruation (hypothalamic amenorrhea); (2) could have a role in treating Tourette's syndrome.

How This Drug Works: (1) In helping addiction to narcotics, this medicine acts as an antagonist to the effects of opioid medicines and blocks the effects or perceived benefit of the drug to the addicted patient.
  (2) The exact mechanism of action in alcohol addiction is unknown. It is thought that this drug interferes with the body's own opioids which may be released in response to drinking alcoholic beverages. If the effect of the body's own opioids (endogenous) is blocked, the craving for alcohol is thereby thought to be reduced.

Available Dosage Forms and Strengths
  Tablets — 50 mg

▷ **Recommended Dosage Ranges (Actual dosage and administration schedule must be determined by the physician for each patient individually.)**
  Infants and Children: Not indicated.
  18 to 60 Years of Age: 50 mg daily.
  Over 60 Years of Age: Same as 12 to 60 years of age.

Conditions Requiring Dosing Adjustments
  Liver function: This drug is extensively metabolized in the liver and is contraindicated in acute hepatitis or liver failure.
  Kidney function: Metabolites of this drug are removed via the kidneys, however, specific guidelines for dosing changes are not available.

▷ **Dosing Instructions:** If there is any question of opioid dependence, a narcan challenge test must be performed by the physician. Naltrexone is almost completely absorbed after oral dosing. This medicine may be taken with or without food.

Usual Duration of Use: Continual use on a regular schedule for 12 weeks is usually necessary to determine this drug's effectiveness in treating alcoholism. This drug should be a part of a comprehensive alcohol treatment program. Long-term use (months to years) requires periodic evaluation of response and dosage adjustment. Consult your physician on a regular basis.

Possible Advantages of This Drug
Actually decreases the craving for alcohol.

▷ **This Drug Should Not Be Taken If**
- you have had an allergic reaction to any dosage form of it previously.
- you have liver failure or acute hepatitis.
- you are in opioid withdrawal.
- you are physically dependent on narcotics.

▷ **Inform Your Physician Before Taking This Drug If**
- you have a history of viral hepatitis.
- you are planning surgery or a diagnostic procedure requiring anesthesia.
- you are uncertain of how much naltrexone to take or how often to take it.
- you take other prescription or non-prescription medicines which were not discussed with your doctor when naltrexone was prescribed.

Possible Side-Effects (natural, expected and unavoidable drug actions)
None.

▷ **Possible Adverse Effects** (unusual, unexpected and infrequent reactions)
If any of the following develop, consult your physician promptly for guidance.
Mild Adverse Effects
Allergic Reactions: Rash.
Oily skin, itching, hair loss.
Nose bleeds, muscle pain.
Weight loss, fatigue, nervousness.
Sleep disturbances.
Depression (5–7%).
Serious Adverse Effects
Allergic Reactions: None reported.
Idiosyncratic Reactions: None reported.
Liver toxicity.
Precipitation of acute withdrawal syndrome in patients dependent on narcotics.
Suicidal ideation (2%).
Abnormal platelet function (idiopathic thrombocytopenic purpura) (rare).

▷ **Possible Effects on Sexual Function:** Delayed ejaculation (less than 10%).

Possible Delayed Adverse Effects: None reported.

▷ **Adverse Effects That May Mimic Natural Diseases or Disorders**
Liver problems may mimic acute hepatitis.

Natural Diseases or Disorders That May Be Activated by This Drug
None.

Possible Effects on Laboratory Tests
Liver function tests: Increased.

CAUTION
1. The therapeutic dose and doses that can cause liver damage are fairly close. Make certain that you understand how much and how often to take this medicine.
2. Self administration of any narcotic drug may be fatal.

Precautions for Use
By Infants and Children:
Safety and effectiveness for use by those under 18 years of age have not been established.
By Those over 60 Years of Age: None.

▷ **Advisability of Use During Pregnancy**
Pregnancy Category: C. See Pregnancy Code at the back of this book.
Animal studies: This drug has been shown to be embryocidal in rats and rabbits at roughly 140 times the typical human dose.
Human studies: Information from adequate studies of pregnant women is not available. Ask your doctor for help with this benefit to risk decision.

Advisability of Use if Breast-Feeding
Presence of this drug in breast milk: Unknown.
Avoid drug or refrain from nursing.

Habit-Forming Potential: None.

Effects of Overdosage: Human subjects who received over 800 mg daily for a week showed no adverse effects.

Possible Effects of Long-Term Use: None defined.

Suggested Periodic Examinations While Taking This Drug (at physician's discretion)
Liver function tests.

▷ **While Taking This Drug, Observe the Following**
Foods: No restrictions.
Nutritional Support: Not indicated.
Beverages: No restrictions.
▷ *Alcohol:* Obviously not recommended.
Tobacco Smoking: No interactions expected.
Marijuana Smoking: Not to be attempted.
▷ *Other Drugs*
Naltrexone *taken concurrently* with
- narcotic medicines may result in a severe reaction.
- other drugs which are toxic to the liver may result in increased risk of liver toxicity.
- thioridazine may result in somnolence and lethargy.

▷ *Driving, Hazardous Activities:* This drug may cause fatigue. Restrict activities as necessary.
Aviation Note: Alcoholism **is a disqualification** for piloting. Consult a designated Aviation Medical Examiner.
Exposure to Sun: No restrictions.
Discontinuation: Do not stop this medicine without the knowledge of your doctor.

NAPROXEN (na PROX en)

Introduced: 1974 **Prescription:** USA: No (200mg) Yes (250mg); Canada: Yes **Available as Generic:** Yes **Class:** Mild analgesic, anti-inflammatory **Controlled Drug:** USA: No; Canada: No

Brand Names: Aleve (220 mg non-prescription), Anaprox, Anaprox DS, ✦Apo-Naproxen, Naprosyn, ✦Naxen, ✦Novo-Anaprox, ✦Nu-Naprox, ✦Synflex

BENEFITS versus RISKS	
Possible Benefits	*Possible Risks*
EFFECTIVE RELIEF OF MILD TO MODERATE PAIN AND INFLAMMATION	Gastrointestinal pain, ulceration, bleeding (rare)
	Drug-induced hepatitis with jaundice (rare)
	Rare kidney damage
	Mild fluid retention
	Rare reduced white blood cell counts
	Rare hemolytic anemia

Please see the propionic acid nonsteroidal anti-inflammatory drug profile for further information.

NEDOCROMIL (Na DOK ra mil)

Introduced: 1992 **Prescription:** USA: Yes; Canada: Yes **Available as Generic:** USA: No; Canada: No **Class:** Asthma Preventive **Controlled Drug:** USA: No; Canada: No

Brand Names: Tilade

BENEFITS versus RISKS	
Possible Benefits	*Possible Risks*
EFFECTIVE PREVENTION OF RECURRENT ASTHMA	Acute bronchospasm (rare)
Prevention of exercise induced asthma	Taste disorder

▷ **Principal Uses**

As a Single Drug Product: Uses currently included in FDA approved labeling: (1) Maintenance therapy of mild to moderate bronchial asthma; (2) has a steroid sparing effect which may allow reduction or even elimination of oral steroids.

Other (unlabeled) generally accepted uses: (1) May have a role in helping ease allergic rhinitis; (2) can help vernal conjunctivitis when instilled as an eye drop; (3) may help exercise induced asthma.

How This Drug Works: This drug inhibits the release of inflammatory chemical mediators such as histamine, prostaglandins and leukotrienes which cause bronchial constriction and inflammation seen in acute asthma.

Available Dosage Forms and Strengths
Inhaler — 16.2 gram canister
Solution for inhalation — 2 mg per actuation

▷ **Recommended Dosage Ranges (Actual dosage and administration schedule must be determined by the physician for each patient individually.)**
Infants and Children: Safety and efficacy not established.
12 to 60 Years of Age: Two inhalations four times daily to provide a total of 14 mg per day.
Over 60 Years of Age: Same as 12 to 60 years of age.

Conditions Requiring Dosing Adjustments
Liver function: Adjustments in dose in liver compromise are not defined.
Kidney function: Adjustments in dose in kidney compromise are not defined.

▷ **Dosing Instructions:** Follow the instructions on the leaflet provided in the medication box carefully. Nedocromil use must be continued, even when you are symptom-free.

Usual Duration of Use: Use on a regular schedule for a week usually determines effectiveness in helping prevent acute asthma. Long-term use (months to years) requires periodic phylsician evaluation of response and dosage adjustment.

Possible Advantages of This Drug
Usually well tolerated.
Rare serious adverse effects.

▷ **This Drug Should Not Be Taken If**
- you have had an allergic reaction to any dosage form of it previously.

▷ **Inform Your Physician Before Taking This Drug If**
- you have impaired kidney function.
- you have angina or a heart rhythm disorder.
- you are uncertain of how to take nedocromil, or how often to take it.

Possible Side-Effects (natural, expected and unavoidable drug actions)
Unpleasant taste (12%).
Mild throat irritation or hoarseness. This may be lessened by taking a few swallows of water after each inhalation.

▷ **Possible Adverse Effects** (unusual, unexpected and infrequent reactions)
If any of the following develop, consult your physician promptly for guidance.
Mild Adverse Effects
Allergic Reactions: Skin rash, hives.
Headache (4.8%), dizziness (1–2%).
Unpleasant taste (12%).
Nausea or vomiting (4 and 1.8% respectively).
Cough (less than 10%).
Serious Adverse Effects
Allergic Reactions: Anaphylactoid reaction, allergic pneumonitis (allergic reaction of the lung tissue).
Bronchospasm (5.4%)

▷ **Possible Effects on Sexual Function:** None reported.

Possible Delayed Adverse Effects: Pneumonitis (very rare).

Possible Effects on Laboratory Tests
Liver function tests: increased ALT.

CAUTION
1. This drug does **not** act as a bronchodilator and should not be used for immediate relief of acute asthma.
2. If use of this drug has allowed you to stop taking a cortisone-related drug, you may need to resume the cortisone-related drug if you are injured, have an infection or need surgery.
3. If severe asthma returns, contact your doctor promptly.
4. If you use a bronchodilator drug by inhalation, it is best to take it about five minutes before inhaling nedocromil.

Precautions for Use
By Infants and Children:
Safety and effectiveness for those under 12 years of age not established.
By Those over 60 Years of Age: This drug does not work in therapy of chronic bronchitis or emphysema.

▷ **Advisability of Use During Pregnancy**
Pregnancy Category: B. See Pregnancy Code at the back of this book.
Animal studies: Rat, mice and rabbit studies show no impairment of fertility or harm to the fetus.
Human studies: Adequate studies of pregnant women are not available.
Ask your doctor for guidance.

Advisability of Use if Breast-Feeding
Presence of this drug in breast milk: Unknown.
Avoid drug or refrain from nursing.

Habit-Forming Potential: None.

Effects of Overdosage: Head shaking, tremor and salivation were seen in dogs given high doses.

Suggested Periodic Examinations While Taking This Drug (at physician's discretion)
Sputum analysis and X-ray if pneumonitis suspected.
Liver function tests.

▷ **While Taking This Drug, Observe the Following**
Foods: No restrictions.
Beverages: Avoid all beverages to which you may be allergic.
▷ *Alcohol:* No interaction expected.
Tobacco Smoking: Follow your doctor's advice regarding smoking.
▷ *Other Drugs*
Nedocromil may make it possible to reduce the dose or frequency of use of cortisone-like drugs. Ask your doctor for guidance.
There are no known adverse drug interactions at present.
▷ *Driving, Hazardous Activities:* This drug may cause dizziness. Restrict activities as necessary.
Aviation Note: The use of this drug **may be a disqualification** for piloting. Consult a designated Aviation Medical Examiner.
Exposure to Sun: No restrictions.
Heavy Exercise or Exertion: This drug may enable you to partake in exercise. Ask your doctor for guidance.

Discontinuation: If this drug has made it possible to reduce or stop cortisone-like drugs, and you must stop nedocromil, you may have to resume the cortisone-like drug as well as other measures to control asthma.

NEFAZODONE (Na FAZ oh dohne)

Introduced: 1994   **Prescription:** USA: Yes; Canada: Yes   **Available as Generic:** USA: No; Canada: No   **Class:** phenylpiperidine antidepressant
Controlled Drug: USA: No; Canada: No
Brand Names: Serzone

BENEFITS versus RISKS	
Possible Benefits	*Possible Risks*
EFFECTIVE TREATMENT OF DEPRESSION	Dizziness
Fewer cardiovascular side effects than older agents	Mild blood pressure changes on standing
Minimal anticholinergic side effects	
Decreased sedation	

▷ **Principal Uses**
  As a Single Drug Product: Use currently included in FDA approved labeling: (1) Treatment of major depression.
   Other (unlabeled) generally accepted use: (1) May have a role in pain management.
  How This Drug Works: This antidepressant is unique in that it:
   1. Blocks the reuptake of a specific nerve transmitting chemical (5-HT).
   2. Acts as a 5-HT2 antagonist.
   Because of this unique mechanism of action, this drug has fewer cardiovascular and anticholinergic side effects than previously available agents.
  Available Dosage Forms and Strengths
   Tablets — 100 mg, 150 mg, 200 mg, 250 mg
▷ **Recommended Dosage Ranges (Actual dosage and administration schedule must be determined by the physician for each patient individually.)**
  Infants and Children: Not indicated.
  18 to 60 Years of Age: The starting dose for this medicine is 200 mg daily. This is given as 100 mg in the morning and 100 mg in the evening. The dose is increased as needed and tolerated in 100 mg increments with at least one week separating any dose increase. The maximum dose is 600 mg daily.
  Over 60 Years of Age: Dosing in this population starts with 100 mg daily in two divided doses. The medicine is then increased (however at a slower rate than in younger patients) as needed and tolerated.
  Conditions Requiring Dosing Adjustments
  Liver function: The dose should be decreased in patients with liver compromise.
  Kidney function: No specific dosing changes are presently identified.
▷ **Dosing Instructions:** Food delays the absorption and decreases total absorption, but this effect is not believed to be clinically significant.

Usual Duration of Use: Continual use on a regular schedule for four to five weeks is usually necessary to determine this drug's effectiveness in treating depression.

Long-term use (months to years) requires periodic evaluation of response and dosage adjustment. See your doctor regularly.

Possible Advantages of This Drug
Two different mechanisms of action.
Decreased side effects versus other available agents.

▷ **This Drug Should Not Be Taken If**
- you have had an allergic reaction to any dosage form of it previously.
- you are taking astemizole or terfenadine.
- you are taking a MAO inhibitor (see Drug Classes).

▷ **Inform Your Physician Before Taking This Drug If**
- you take a triazolobenzodiazepine such as triazolam or alprazolam.
- you have a history of seizure disorder.
- you have a history of heart disease.
- you are uncertain of how much nefazodone to take or how often to take it.
- you take other prescription or non-prescription medicines which were not discussed with your doctor when nefazodone was prescribed.

Possible Side-Effects (natural, expected and unavoidable drug actions)
Dry mouth and constipation.

▷ **Possible Adverse Effects** (unusual, unexpected and infrequent reactions)
If any of the following develop, consult your physician promptly for guidance.

Mild Adverse Effects
Allergic Reactions: Skin rash.
Dry mouth or blurred vision.
Nausea (23%), ringing in the ears (3%).
Headache, dizziness and tremor.
Insomnia (1.5%), confusion (8%) and agitation (1.2%).
Slowed heart rate.

Serious Adverse Effects
Allergic Reactions: Not defined.
Idiosyncratic Reactions: Not identified.
Lowered blood pressure on standing (postural hypotension).
Activation of mania (rare).
Seizures (rare).

▷ **Possible Effects on Sexual Function:** Impotence, absence of orgasm or abnormal ejaculation have all been rarely reported. Priapism has been reported with a structuraly similar drug.

Possible Delayed Adverse Effects: None reported.

▷ **Adverse Effects That May Mimic Natural Diseases or Disorders**
None reported.

Natural Diseases or Disorders That May Be Activated by This Drug
None reported.

Possible Effects on Laboratory Tests
Hematocrit: decreased.

Nefazodone

CAUTION
1. Risk of suicide is present in depressed patients. Small quantities of this medicine should be dispensed at a time when therapy is started. Appropriate suicide precautions should be taken.
2. This medicine **must not** be taken with MAO inhibitor. 14 days **must** elapse once a MAO inhibitor is stopped before nefazodone is started.

Precautions for Use
By Infants and Children:
Safety and effectiveness for use by those under 18 years of age have not been established.
By Those over 60 Years of Age: Lower starting doses and more gradual increases in dose are indicated.

▷ **Advisability of Use During Pregnancy**
Pregnancy Category: C. See Pregnancy Code at the back of this book.
Animal studies: Increased rat pup mortality was seen when doses five times the typical human dose were used.
Human studies: Information from adequate studies of pregnant women is not available. Ask your doctor for guidance.

Advisability of Use if Breast-Feeding
Presence of this drug in breast milk: Unknown.
Avoid drug or refrain from nursing.

Habit-Forming Potential: None defined at present.

Effects of Overdosage: Nausea, vomiting and somnolence.

Possible Effects of Long-Term Use: None reported.

Suggested Periodic Examinations While Taking This Drug (at physician's discretion)
Periodic checks of heart rate.

▷ **While Taking This Drug, Observe the Following**
Foods: No restrictions.
Beverages: No restrictions.
▷ *Alcohol:* This combination is not recommended.
Tobacco Smoking: No interactions expected.
Marijuana Smoking: Increased somnolence.
▷ *Other Drugs*
Nefazodone may *increase* the effects of
- alprazolam (Xanax).
- digoxin. Increased blood level checks are suggested.
- haloperidol (Haldol).
- triazolam (Halcion).

Nefazodone *taken concurrently* with
- astemizole (Hismanal) can cause serious heart toxicity.
- MAO inhibitors (see Drug Classes) may cause serious toxicity.
- terfenadine (seldane) may cause serious heart rhythm problems.

▷ *Driving, Hazardous Activities:* This drug may cause somnolence. Restrict activities as necessary.
Aviation Note: The use of this drug **is a disqualification** for piloting. Consult a designated Aviation Medical Examiner.

Exposure to Sun: Use caution, photosensitivity is possible.
Discontinuation: Do not stop this medication without discussing this with your doctor.

NEOSTIGMINE (nee oh STIG meen)

Introduced: 1931 **Prescription:** USA: Yes; Canada: Yes **Available as Generic:** USA: Yes; Canada: Yes **Class:** Antimyasthenic **Controlled Drug:** USA: No; Canada: No
Brand Name: Prostigmin, ✦PMS-Neostigmine, Viaderm-K.C.

BENEFITS versus RISKS	
Possible Benefits	*Possible Risks*
MODERATELY EFFECTIVE TREATMENT OF OCULAR AND MILD FORMS OF MYASTHENIA GRAVIS (symptomatic relief of muscle weakness)	Cholinergic crisis (overdose): Excessive salivation, nausea, vomiting, stomach cramps, diarrhea, shortness of breath (asthmalike wheezing), weakness.
Eases postoperative bowel slowing or block (paralytic ileus)	

▷ **Principal Uses**

As a Single Drug Product: Uses currently included in FDA approved labeling: (1) Treats ocular and milder forms of myasthenia gravis by providing temporary relief of muscle weakness and fatigability; (2) reverses depression of bowel function which may occur after surgery; (3) used to ease symptoms of bladder instability.

Other (unlabeled) generally accepted uses: (1) Used to reverse neuromuscular blockade caused by atracurium.

How This Drug Works: This drug inhibits cholinesterase, the enzyme that destroys acetylcholine. This results in higher levels of acetylcholine, the nerve transmitter that facilitates the stimulation of muscular activity. The net effects are increased muscle strength and endurance.

Available Dosage Forms and Strengths
Injection — 0.25, 0.5 and 1.0 mg per ml
Tablets — 15 mg

▷ **Usual Adult Dosage Range:** Initially: 15 mg/3 to 4 hours; adjust dosage as needed and tolerated. Maintenance: up to 300 mg/24 hours; the average dose is 75 to 150 mg/24 hours. **Note: Actual dosage and administration schedule must be determined by the physician for each patient individually.**

Conditions Requiring Dosing Adjustments
Liver function: Neostigmine should be used with caution in patients with compromised livers.
Kidney function: Half of a given dose of neostigmine is eliminated unchanged by the kidney, however, specific guidelines for decreasing doses are not available.

▷ **Dosing Instructions:** The tablet may be crushed and taken with food or milk to reduce the intensity of side-effects. Larger portions of the daily maintenance dosage should be timed according to the pattern of fatigue and weakness.

Usual Duration of Use: Use on a regular schedule (with dosage adjustment) for 10 to 14 days determines effectiveness in relieving the symptoms of myasthenia gravis. Long-term use (months to years) requires periodic physician evaluation.

▷ **This Drug Should Not Be Taken If**
- you have had an allergic reaction to it previously.
- you are known to be allergic to bromide compounds.
- you have an obstruction in your urinary tract or intestine.

▷ **Inform Your Physician Before Taking This Drug If**
- you have any type of seizure disorder.
- you are subject to heart rhythm disorders or bronchial asthma.
- you have recurrent urinary tract infections.
- you have prostatism (see Glossary).
- you plan to have surgery under general anesthesia in the near future.

Possible Side-Effects (natural, expected and unavoidable drug actions)
Small pupils, watering of eyes, slow pulse, excessive salivation, nausea, vomiting, stomach cramps, diarrhea, urge to urinate, increased sweating.

▷ **Possible Adverse Effects** (unusual, unexpected and infrequent reactions)
If any of the following develop, consult your physician promptly for guidance.
Mild Adverse Effects
Allergic Reaction: Skin rash.
Nervousness, anxiety, unsteadiness, muscle cramps or twitching.
Serious Adverse Effects
Confusion, slurred speech, seizures, difficult breathing (asthmatic wheezing).
Increased muscle weakness or paralysis.
Excessive vomiting or diarrhea may induce abnormally low blood potassium levels (hypokalemia). This will accentuate muscle weakness.
Abnormally slow heartbeat (bradycardia) (rare).
Drug-induced porphyria (rare).

▷ **Possible Effects on Sexual Function:** None reported.

▷ **Adverse Effects That May Mimic Natural Diseases or Disorders**
Seizures may suggest the possibility of epilepsy.

Natural Diseases or Disorders That May Be Activated by This Drug
Latent bronchial asthma.

Possible Effects on Laboratory Tests
None reported.

CAUTION
1. Certain drugs can block the action of this drug and reduce its effectiveness in treating myasthenia gravis. (See *Other Drugs* below.) Ask physician before starting any new drug, prescription or over-the-counter.
2. Dosing must be carefully individualized. Variations in response may occur from time to time. Because generalized muscle weakness is a major symptom of both myasthenia crisis (underdosage) and cholinergic crisis (overdosage), it may be difficult to recognize the correct cause.

As a rule, weakness that begins within 1 hour after taking this drug probably represents overdosage; weakness that begins 3 or more hours after taking this drug is probably due to underdosage. Observe these time relationships and inform your physician.
3. In long-term therapy, watch for development of resistance to the drug's therapeutic action (loss of effectiveness). Ask your doctor about the advisability of stopping this drug for a few days to see if responsiveness can be restored.

Precautions for Use
  By Infants and Children: Dosage and administration schedule must be modified if kidney function is severely impaired.
  By Those over 60 Years of Age: The natural decline of kidney function with aging may require smaller doses to prevent accumulation of this drug to toxic levels.

▷ **Advisability of Use During Pregnancy**
  Pregnancy Category: C. See Pregnancy Code at the back of this book.
    Animal studies: No information available.
    Human studies: Adequate studies of pregnant women are not available.
    There are no reports of birth defects due to the use of this drug during pregnancy. However, there are reports of significant muscular weakness in 20% of newborn infants whose mothers had taken this drug during pregnancy. Ask your physician for guidance.

Advisability of Use if Breast-Feeding
  Presence of this drug in breast milk: Probably not.
  Monitor nursing infant closely and discontinue drug or nursing if adverse effects develop.

Habit-Forming Potential: None.

Effects of Overdosage: Generalized muscular weakness, blurred vision, very small pupils, slow heart rate, difficult breathing (wheezing), excessive salivation, nausea, vomiting, stomach cramps, diarrhea, muscle cramps or twitching. This syndrome constitutes the cholinergic crisis.

Possible Effects of Long-Term Use: Development of tolerance (see Glossary) with loss of therapeutic benefit.

Suggested Periodic Examinations While Taking This Drug (at physician's discretion)
  Assessment of drug effectiveness and dosage schedule for best results.

▷ **While Taking This Drug, Observe the Following**
  Foods: No restrictions.
  Beverages: No restrictions. May be taken with milk.
▷ *Alcohol:* Use caution. Weakness and unsteadiness may be accentuated.
  Tobacco Smoking: No interactions expected.
▷ *Other Drugs*
  The following drugs may *decrease* the effects of neostigmine
  • atropine (belladonna).
  • clindamycin (Cleocin).
  • guanadrel (Hylorel).
  • guanethidine (Esimil, Ismelin).
  • procainamide (Procan SR, Pronestyl).

- quinidine (Cardioquin, Duraquin, etc.).
- quinine (Quinamm).

Neostigmine *taken concurrently* with
- edrophonium may cause cholinergic crisis in patients with myasthenic weakness.
- hydrocortisone can cause decreased neostigmine benefits.
- physostigmine can result in additive adverse effects.

▷ *Driving, Hazardous Activities:* This drug may cause blurred vision, confusion or generalized weakness. Restrict activities as necessary.

Aviation Note: The use of this drug *is a disqualification* for piloting. Consult a designated Aviation Medical Examiner.

Exposure to Sun: No restrictions.

Exposure to Heat: Use caution. This may cause excessive sweating and increased weakness.

Exposure to Environmental Chemicals: Avoid excessive exposure (inhalation, skin contamination) to the insecticides Baygon, Diazinon and Sevin. These can accentuate potential toxicity of this drug.

Discontinuation: Do not stop this drug abruptly without your doctor's knowledge and help.

NIACIN (NI a sin)

Other Names: Nicotinic acid, vitamin B-3

Introduced: 1937 **Prescription:** USA: Tablets and liquid—no; capsules—yes; Canada: No **Available as Generic:** USA: Yes; Canada: Yes **Class:** Anticholesterol, vasodilator, vitamins **Controlled Drug:** USA: No; Canada: No

Brand Names: ✦Antivert [CD], Niac, Niacels, Niacin TR, Niacor, Nia-bid, Nia-plus, Nicobid, Nico-400, Nicolar, Nicotinex, ✦Novoniacin, SK-Niacin, Slo-Niacin, Span-Niacin-150

BENEFITS versus RISKS	
Possible Benefits	*Possible Risks*
EFFECTIVE REDUCTION OF TOTAL CHOLESTEROL, LOW DENSITY CHOLESTEROL AND TRIGLYCERIDES IN TYPES II, III, IV AND V CHOLESTEROL DISORDERS (25% reduction of total cholesterol, 35% reduction of LDL cholesterol, and 20% elevation of HDL cholesterol, a beneficial effect)	Activation of peptic ulcer Drug-induced hepatitis Aggravation of diabetes or gout
Specific prevention and treatment of pellagra (niacin-deficiency disease)	

▷ **Principal Uses**

As a Single Drug Product: Uses currently included in FDA approved labeling: (1) Certain patterns of abnormally high blood levels of cholesterol and triglycerides; (2) pellagra, a niacin (vitamin B-3) deficiency disorder characterized by dementia, dermatitis and diarrhea; (3) therapy of Hartnup disease.

Other (unlabeled) generally accepted uses: (1) Therapy of certain types of vertigo and tinnitus (ringing in the ears); (2) may help decrease diarrhea in patients with cholera; (3) treatment of Chilblains.

As a Combination Drug Product [CD]: In Canada this drug is combined with meclizine to enhance its effectiveness in the treatment of motion sickness and vertigo.

How This Drug Works

It is thought that it may inhibit the initial production of triglycerides and impair the conversion of fatty tissue to cholesterol and triglycerides.

This drug corrects the specific deficiency of vitamin B-3 that is responsible for the symptoms of pellagra.

This drug causes direct dilation of peripheral blood vessels in the skin of the face and neck; for this reason it has been used to increase the blood flow to the inner ear in an attempt to relieve some types of vertigo and ringing in the ears. The effectiveness of this application is questionable.

Available Dosage Forms and Strengths

Capsules, prolonged-action — 125 mg, 250 mg, 300 mg, 400 mg, 500 mg
Oral solution — 50 mg per 5-ml teaspoonful
Tablets — 20 mg, 25 mg, 50 mg, 100 mg, 500 mg
Tablets, prolonged-action — 150 mg, 250 mg, 500 mg, 750 mg

▷ **Usual Adult Dosage Range**

For cholesterol disorders: Initially 100 mg 3 times daily. Dose may be increased in increments of 300 mg daily at intervals of 4 to 7 days as needed and tolerated. The usual maintenance dose is 1 to 2 grams 3 times daily. The total daily dosage should not exceed 6 grams.

For prevention of pellagra: 10 to 20 mg daily.

For treatment of pellagra: 50 mg 3 to 10 times daily.

Note: Actual dosage and administration schedule must be determined by the physician for each patient individually.

Conditions Requiring Dosing Adjustments

Liver function: This drug is metabolized in the liver and is contraindicated in liver disease.

Kidney function: Specific guidelines for adjustment of dosing are not available.

▷ **Dosing Instructions:** Take with or immediately following meals to prevent stomach irritation. Also take one-half of an adult's aspirin tablet or 1 children's aspirin tablet with each dose of niacin to prevent facial flushing and itching. Dosage should be increased very slowly over 2 to 3 months as needed. The prolonged-action form of niacin is preferable to improve tolerance. The regular tablet may be crushed for administration, but the prolonged-action capsules and tablets should not be altered.

Usual Duration of Use: Use on a regular schedule for 3 to 5 weeks determines benefit in reducing levels of cholesterol and triglycerides. Long-term use (months to years) requires periodic physician evaluation.

Currently a "Drug of Choice"
for initiating treatment of elevated LDL cholesterol and VLDL triglycerides.

▷ **This Drug Should Not Be Taken If**
- you have had an allergic reaction to it previously.
- you have active peptic ulcer disease or inflammatory bowel disease.
- you have active liver disease.

▷ **Inform Your Physician Before Taking This Drug If**
- you are prone to low blood pressure.
- you have a heart rhythm disorder of any kind.
- you have a history of peptic ulcer disease, inflammatory bowel disease, liver disease, jaundice or gallbladder disease.
- you have diabetes or gout.

Possible Side-Effects (natural, expected and unavoidable drug actions)
Flushing, itching, tingling and feeling of warmth usually in the face and neck. Sensitive individuals may experience orthostatic hypotension (see Glossary).

▷ **Possible Adverse Effects** (unusual, unexpected and infrequent reactions)
If any of the following develop, consult your physician promptly for guidance.

Mild Adverse Effects
Allergic Reactions: Skin rash, itching, hives.
Headache, dizziness, faintness, impaired vision.
Indigestion, nausea, vomiting, diarrhea.
Flushing and tingling.
Dryness of skin, grayish-black pigmentation of skin folds.

Serious Adverse Effects
Drug-induced hepatitis with jaundice (see Glossary): yellow eyes and skin, dark-colored urine, light-colored stools.
Worsening of diabetes and gout.
Development of heart rhythm disorders.
Myopathy.
Abnormal blood sugar.
Peptic ulcers.

▷ **Possible Effects on Sexual Function:** None reported.

▷ **Adverse Effects That May Mimic Natural Diseases or Disorders**
Liver reactions may suggest viral hepatitis.

Natural Diseases or Disorders That May Be Activated by This Drug
Latent diabetes, gout, inflammatory bowel disease or peptic ulcer.

Possible Effects on Laboratory Tests
Complete blood cell counts: decreased eosinophils and lymphocytes.
Blood total cholesterol, LDL cholesterol and triglyceride levels: decreased.
Blood HDL cholesterol level: increased.
Blood glucose level: increased.
Glucose tolerance test (GGT): decreased.
Blood uric acid level: increased.
Liver function tests: increased liver enzymes (ALT/GPT, AST/GOT and alkaline phosphatase), increased bilirubin.
Urine sugar tests: inaccurate test results with Benedict's solution.

Niacin

CAUTION
1. Large doses may cause increases in blood levels of sugar and uric acid. Diabetics or gout patients should monitor their status regularly.
2. Periodic measurements of blood cholesterol and triglyceride levels are essential for monitoring response and determining the need for changes in dosage or medication.
3. Recent reports indicate that the prolonged-action dosage forms of niacin may be more likely to cause liver damage than the rapidly absorbed (crystalline) forms. Ask your doctor which is the most appropriate dosage form and schedule for you.

Precautions for Use

By Infants and Children: Safety and effectiveness for use of large doses by those under 12 years of age have not been established.

By Those over 60 Years of Age: Observe for the possible development of low blood pressure (light-headedness, dizziness, faintness) and heart rhythm disorders.

▷ **Advisability of Use During Pregnancy**

Pregnancy Category: C. See Pregnancy Code at the back of this book.

Animal studies: Significant birth defects due to this drug were found in chicks.

Human studies: Adequate studies of pregnant women are not available.

Use this drug only if clearly needed. Avoid completely during the first 3 months.

Advisability of Use if Breast-Feeding

Presence of this drug in breast milk: Unknown.

Avoid drug or refrain from nursing.

Habit-Forming Potential: None.

Effects of Overdosage: Generalized flushing, nausea, vomiting, stomach cramps, diarrhea, weakness, fainting.

Possible Effects of Long-Term Use: Increased blood levels of sugar and uric acid; liver damage.

Suggested Periodic Examinations While Taking This Drug (at physician's discretion)

Measurements of blood levels of total cholesterol, HDL and LDL cholesterol fractions, triglycerides, sugar and uric acid.

Liver function tests.

▷ **While Taking This Drug, Observe the Following**

Foods: Follow the low-cholesterol diet prescribed by your physician.

Beverages: No restrictions. May be taken with milk.

▷ *Alcohol:* Use with caution. Alcohol used with large doses of this drug may cause excessive lowering of blood pressure.

Tobacco Smoking: No interactions expected.

▷ *Other Drugs*

Niacin may *increase* the effects of
- some antihypertensive drugs, and cause excessive lowering of blood pressure.

Niacin may *decrease* the effects of
- antidiabetic drugs (insulin and sulfonylureas), by raising the level of blood sugar.

- probenecid (Benemid) and sulfinpyrazone (Anturane), by raising the level of blood uric acid.

Niacin *taken concurrently* with
- lovastatin and other cholesterol lowering drugs may result in reversible muscle problems (myopathy or rhabdomyolysis).

▷ *Driving, Hazardous Activities:* This drug may cause dizziness and faintness. Restrict activities as necessary.

Aviation Note: The use of this drug *may be a disqualification* for piloting. Consult a designated Aviation Medical Examiner.

Exposure to Sun: No restrictions.

Discontinuation: Do not stop this drug without your physician's knowledge and guidance. Abrupt withdrawal may be followed by excessive increase in blood cholesterol and triglyceride levels.

NICARDIPINE (ni KAR de peen)

Introduced: 1984 **Prescription:** USA: Yes **Available as Generic:** USA: No **Class:** Antianginal, antihypertensive, calcium channel blocker **Controlled Drug:** USA: No

Brand Name: Cardene, Cardene SR

BENEFITS versus RISKS	
Possible Benefits	*Possible Risks*
EFFECTIVE PREVENTION OF CLASSICAL ANGINA-OF-EFFORT	Increase in angina upon starting treatment (7%)
EFFECTIVE TREATMENT OF HYPERTENSION	Water retention, ankle swelling (8%)

▷ **Principal Uses**

As a Single Drug Product: Uses currently included in FDA approved labeling: (1) Treats classical angina-of-effort (due to atherosclerotic disease of the coronary arteries) or angina caused by spasm of the coronary arteries; (2) mild to moderate hypertension.

Other (unlabeled) generally accepted uses: (1) Combination therapy in preventing recurrance of stroke; (2) may have a role in helping correct congestive heart failure; (3) can help refractory (not responding to nonsteroidal anti-inflammatory drugs) menstrual pain; (4) may help decrease the frequency and severity of migraine attacks; (5) can halt the progression of atherosclerosis; (6) lowers postoperative hypertension; (7) may prevent vessel spasm in some kinds of vascular surgery; (8) could have a role in some premature labor.

How This Drug Works: By blocking passage of calcium through certain cell walls (which is necessary for the function of nerve and muscle tissue), this drug inhibits the contraction of coronary arteries and peripheral arterioles. As a result of these effects, this drug
- promotes dilation of the coronary arteries (antianginal effect).
- reduces the degree of contraction of peripheral arterial walls, resulting in lowering of blood pressure. This further reduces the workload of the heart during exertion and helps prevent of angina.

Nicardipine

Available Dosage Forms and Strengths
    Capsules — 20 mg, 30 mg
    SR Capsules — 30 mg, 45 mg, 60mg

▷ **Usual Adult Dosage Range:** Initially 20 mg 3 times daily, 6 to 8 hours apart. Dose may be increased gradually at 3-day intervals (as needed and tolerated) up to 40 mg 3 times daily. The total daily dosage should not exceed 120 mg. **Note: Actual dosage and administration schedule must be determined by the physician for each patient individually.**

Conditions Requiring Dosing Adjustments
    Liver function: The dose should be started at 20 mg twice a day. If the dose must be increased, it should be slowly advanced and given twice a day.
    Kidney function: In patients with moderate kidney failure, the starting dose should be 20 mg twice daily. If the dose is increased, it should be titrated slowly, and the twice daily dosing interval retained. Nicardipine can cause urine retention, and should be used as a benefit to risk decision in patients with urine outflow problems.

▷ **Dosing Instructions:** May be taken with or following food to reduce stomach irritation. However, if taken after a high-fat meal, total absorption of this drug may be reduced by 20% to 30%. The capsule should be swallowed whole (not altered).

Usual Duration of Use: Use on a regular schedule for 2 to 4 weeks determines benefit in reducing the frequency and severity of angina or controlling hypertension. For long-term use (months to years), the smallest effective dose should be used. Physician supervision and periodic evaluation are essential.

Possible Advantages of This Drug
    Does not impair heart function or cause heart rhythm abnormalities.
    Can be used safely with beta blockers, digoxin, diuretics and nitrate.

▷ **This Drug Should Not Be Taken If**
- you have had an allergic reaction to it previously.
- you have advanced aortic stenosis.

▷ **Inform Your Physician Before Taking This Drug If**
- you have had an adverse reaction to any calcium blocker (see Drug Classes).
- you currently take any form of digitalis or a beta blocker drug (see Drug Class Section).
- you are taking any drugs that lower blood pressure.
- you are taking cimetidine (Tagamet) or cyclosporine (Sandimmune).
- you have a history of congestive heart failure, heart attack or stroke.
- you have a history of circulation impairment to the fingers.
- you have Duchenne muscular dystrophy.
- you are subject to disturbances of heart rhythm.
- you have impaired liver or kidney function.

Possible Side-Effects (natural, expected and unavoidable drug actions)
    Rapid heart rate (3.4%), swelling of the feet and ankles (8%), flushing and sensation of warmth (9.7%).

▷ **Possible Adverse Effects** (unusual, unexpected and infrequent reactions)
If any of the following develop, consult your physician promptly for guidance.
Mild Adverse Effects
Allergic Reaction: Skin rash (0.4%–1.2%).
Headache (6.4%–8.2%), dizziness (4%–6.9%), weakness (4.2%–5.8%), nervousness (0.6%), ringing in the ears (tinitis), blurred vision, confusion.
Palpitation (3.3%–4.1%), shortness of breath (0.6%).
Indigestion (0.8%–1.5%), nausea (1.9%–2.2%), vomiting (0.4%), constipation (0.6%).
Joint and muscle pain (1%).
Abnormal growth (hyperplasia) of the gums.
Serious Adverse Effects
Allergic Reactions: None reported.
Increased frequency or severity of angina on initiation of treatment or following an increase in dose (7%).
Difficult urination (rare).
Marked drop in blood pressure with fainting (0.8%).
Decreased white blood cell counts.

▷ **Possible Effects on Sexual Function:** Rare impotence (less than 1%).

▷ **Adverse Effects That May Mimic Natural Diseases or Disorders**
Flushing and warmth may resemble menopausal "hot flushes."

Possible Effects on Laboratory Tests
None reported.

CAUTION
1. If you are checking your own blood pressure, check it just before each dose and 1 to 2 hours after each dose to obtain an accurate picture of drug effect.
2. Be sure to tell all physicians and dentists you consult that you take this drug. Note the use of this drug on your card of personal identification.
3. You may use nitroglycerin and other nitrate drugs as needed to relieve acute episodes of angina pain. However, if you detect that your angina attacks are becoming more frequent or intense, call your doctor promptly.

Precautions for Use
By Infants and Children: Safety and effectiveness for those under 18 years of age not established.
By Those over 60 Years of Age: Usually well tolerated, however, watch for development of weakness, dizziness, fainting and falling. Take necessary precautions to prevent injury. Report promptly any changes in your pattern of thirst and urination.

▷ **Advisability of Use During Pregnancy**
Pregnancy Category: C. See Pregnancy Code at the back of this book.
Animal studies: Embryo and fetal toxicity reported in small animals, but no birth defects due to this drug.
Human studies: Adequate studies of pregnant women are not available.
Avoid this drug during the first 3 months. Use during the last 6 months only if clearly needed. Ask physician for guidance.

Nicardipine

Advisability of Use if Breast-Feeding
Presence of this drug in breast milk: Probably yes.
Avoid drug or refrain from nursing.

Habit-Forming Potential: None.

Effects of Overdosage: Weakness, light-headedness, fainting, fast pulse, low blood pressure, shortness of breath, flushed and warm skin, tremors.

Possible Effects of Long-Term Use: None reported.

Suggested Periodic Examinations While Taking This Drug (at physician's discretion)
Evaluations of heart function, including electrocardiograms; measurements of blood pressure in supine, sitting and standing positions.

▷ **While Taking This Drug, Observe the Following**

Foods: Food decreases the amount of this drug which is absorbed. It is also prudent to avoid excessive salt intake.

Beverages: No restrictions. May be taken with milk.

▷ *Alcohol:* Use with caution until combined effects have been determined. Alcohol may exaggerate the drop in blood pressure experienced by some individuals.

Tobacco Smoking: Nicotine may reduce the effectiveness of this drug. Follow your physician's advice regarding smoking.

Marijuana Smoking: Possible reduced effectiveness of this drug; mild to moderate increase in angina; possible changes in electrocardiogram, confusing interpretation.

▷ *Other Drugs*

Nicardipine may *increase* the effects of
- cyclosporine (Sandimmune), and cause kidney toxicity.

Nicardipine *taken concurrently* with
- amiodarone (Codarone) may result in cardiac arrest.
- beta blocker drugs or digitalis preparations (see Drug Classes Section) may affect heart rate and rhythm adversely. Careful monitoring by your physician is necessary if these drugs are taken concurrently.
- magnesium may cause worsening of neuromuscular blockade and further lowering of blood pressure.
- phenytoin (Dilantin) may result in phenytoin toxicity or decreased efficacy of Nicardipine.

The following drugs may *increase* the effects of nicardipine
- cimetidine (Tagamet).

▷ *Driving, Hazardous Activities:* Usually no restrictions. This drug may cause drowsiness or dizziness. Restrict activities as necessary.

Aviation Note: Coronary artery disease and hypertension **are disqualifications** for piloting. Consult a designated Aviation Medical Examiner.

Exposure to Sun: No restrictions.

Exposure to Heat: Caution advised. Hot environments can exaggerate the blood-pressure-lowering effects of this drug. Observe for light-headedness or weakness.

Heavy Exercise or Exertion: This drug may improve your ability to be more active without resulting angina pain. Use caution and avoid excessive exercise that could impair heart function in the absence of warning pain.

Discontinuation: Do not stop this drug abruptly. Ask your doctor about gradual withdrawal. Watch for possible development of rebound angina.

NICOTINE (NIK oh teen)

Introduced: 1992   **Prescription:** USA: Yes; Canada: Yes   **Available as Generic:** USA: No; Canada: No   **Class:** Smoking cessation adjunct
Controlled Drug: USA: No; Canada: No

Brand Names: Habitrol, Nicoderm, Nicorette, Nicorette DS, Nicotrol, ProStep

BENEFITS versus RISKS	
Possible Benefits	*Possible Risks*
EFFECTIVE REDUCTION OF NICOTINE CRAVING AND WITHDRAWAL EFFECTS when used adjunctively in smoking-cessation treatment programs	Aggravation of existing angina, heart rhythm disorders, hypertension, insulin-dependent diabetes, peptic ulcer and vascular diseases Increased risk of abortion (if used during pregnancy)

▷ **Principal Uses**

As a Single Drug Product: Uses currently included in FDA approved labeling: Nicotine chewing gum and nicotine transdermal systems are used adjunctively in behavior modification programs to assist cigarette smokers who wish to abstain from smoking.

Other (unlabeled) generally accepted uses: (1) Some early European data studying combination gum and patch use appears to show an increased success rate. The technique used the gum to halt "breakthrough" cigarette cravings. The thinking is that the craving resulted from an insufficient nicotine level provided by the patch, and that the gum provided a short term increase which stopped the craving; (2) may have a role in easing symptoms of ulcerative colitis.

How This Drug Works: By providing an alternate source of nicotine (for nicotine-dependent smokers), the appropriate use of these drug products can reduce nicotine craving and lessen smoking withdrawal effects such as irritability, nervousness, headache, fatigue, sleep disturbances, and drowsiness.

Available Dosage Forms and Strengths

Nicotine chewing gum tablets
 Nicotine (Nicorette—2 mg)
  (Nicorette DS—4 mg) — 2 mg (U.S., Canada)
   — 4 mg (U.S., Canada).
 Nicotine Transdermal Systems — 16-hour Systems (U.S. only): 5 mg, 10 mg, 15 mg
  — 24-hour Systems: 7 mg (U.S., Canada), 11 mg (U.S.), 14 mg (U.S., Canada), 21 mg (U.S., Canada) and 22 mg (U.S.)

How to Store

Store nicotine gum at room temperature and protect from light. Store nicotine patches at room temperature and be especially careful to avoid exposing the patches to temperatures greater than 86 degrees F (30 C). Do not store unpouched. Once opened, patches should be used promptly because they may lose their strength.

Nicotine

▷ **Recommended Dosage Ranges (Actual dosage and administration schedule must be determined by the physician for each patient individually.)**

Infants and Children: Avoid use completely in children. Avoid accidental exposure to patches.

12 to 60 Years of Age: For chewing gum tablets: Initially, 1 piece every hour while awake (10 to 12 pieces daily); supplement with 1 additional piece if and when needed to control urge to smoke. Total daily dosage should not exceed 30 pieces (60 mg).

For transdermal systems: Dosage depends upon patient characteristics and product used.

For those weighing 100 pounds or more, smoking 10 or more cigarettes daily, and *without* cardiovascular disease:

Using a 16-hour system (Nicotrol): Initially one 15 mg patch applied for 16 hours daily for 4 to 12 weeks. For those who have abstained from smoking, reduce dose to one 10 mg patch applied for 16 hours daily for the next 2 to 4 weeks; then to one 5 mg patch applied for 16 hours daily for the following 2 to 4 weeks.

Using a 24-hour system: Habitrol, Nicoderm—initially one 21 mg patch applied daily for 4 to 8 weeks. For those who have abstained from smoking, reduce dose to one 14 mg patch daily for the next 2 to 4 weeks; then to one 7 mg patch daily for the following 2 to 4 weeks. ProStep—initially one 22 mg patch applied daily for 4 to 8 weeks. For those who have abstained from smoking, reduce dose to one 11 mg patch daily for 2 to 4 weeks.

For those weighing less than 100 pounds, smoking less than 10 cigarettes daily, or *with* cardiovascular disease:

Using a 24-hour system (Habitrol, Nicoderm): Initially one 14 mg patch applied daily for 4 to 8 weeks. For those who have abstained from smoking, reduce dose to one 7 mg patch daily for the next 2 to 4 weeks. (ProStep): Initially one 11 mg patch applied daily for 4 to 8 weeks.

Over 60 Years of Age: Same as 12 to 60 years of age.

Conditions Requiring Dosing Adjustments

Liver function: Consideration must be given to decreasing the starting dose if the liver is conpromised.

Kidney function: Doses are decreased in severe kidney compromise.

▷ **Dosing Instructions:** Carefully follow the manufacturer's directions provided with each product.

For chewing gum: Limit use to one piece of gum at a time. This product is much harder than typical chewing gum. Chew each piece slowly and intermittently for 30 minutes. A tingling of your gum tissue or peppery taste usually indicates release of a sufficient amount of nicotine. Try to gradually reduce the number of pieces chewed each day by using it only when there is an urge to smoke. During participation in a smoking-cessation program, always have the gum available as a defense against smoking.

For transdermal systems: Apply a new patch at the same time each day. Do not alter the patch in any way. Apply the patch to the upper arm or body where the skin is clean, dry, and free of hair, oil, scars and irritation of any kind; alternate sites of application. Press the patch firmly in place for 10 seconds; ensure good contact throughout. Wash your hands when you have finished applying the patch. Replace patches that are dislodged by showering, bathing or swimming.

Usual Duration of Use: Use on a regular schedule for 2 to 3 months determines effectiveness in achieving lasting cessation of smoking. Nicotine chewing gum should not be used for more than 6 months; transdermal systems should not be used for more than 20 weeks. Long-term use requires periodic physician evaluation of response and dosage adjustment.

Possible Advantages of This Drug

Provides control and flexibility of gradual nicotine withdrawal for use in supervised smoking-cessation programs.

Currently a "Drug of Choice"

for those individuals who are motivated to stop smoking but find it difficult to withdraw abruptly.

▷ **This Drug Should Not Be Taken If**
- you have had an allergic reaction to any dosage form of it previously.
- you have severe, uncontrolled or a pattern of worsening angina (physician's discretion).
- you have uncontrolled, life-threatening heart rhythm disorders (physician's discretion).
- you have had a recent heart attack (physician's discretion).

▷ **Inform Your Physician Before Taking This Drug If**
- you have any form of angina (coronary heart disease).
- you have had a heart attack at any time.
- you are subject to heart rhythm disorders.
- you have insulin-dependent diabetes.
- you have hypertension (high blood pressure).
- you have hyperthyroidism (overactive thyroid function).
- you have a pheochromocytoma (adrenalin-producing tumor).
- you have a history of esophagitis or peptic ulcer disease.
- you have a history of Buerger's disease or Raynaud's disorder.
- you currently have any dental problems or skin disorders.
- you have a history of kidney or liver disease.
- you have already taken a 3 month course of the patch from another doctor.
- you think you are pregnant or plan to become pregnant.
- you are uncertain of how much or how often to take it.

Possible Side-Effects (natural, expected and unavoidable drug actions)

For chewing gum: Mouth or throat irritation; injury to teeth or dental repairs.

For transdermal systems: redness, itching or burning at site of application (mild and transient).

▷ **Possible Adverse Effects** (unusual, unexpected and infrequent reactions)

If any of the following develop, consult your physician promptly for guidance.

Mild Adverse Effects

Allergic Reactions: Skin rash, hives, itching, local or generalized swellings.

Headache, light-headedness, dizziness, drowsiness, irritability, nervousness, insomnia, joint pain, muscle aches, abnormal dreams.
Rapid heartbeat, palpitation, increased sweating.
Increased or decreased appetite, nausea, dry mouth, indigestion, constipation or diarrhea.

Serious Adverse Effects
Irregular heart rhythms, chest pain (angina), edema.
See Effects of Overdosage.
Stroke (rare).

▷ **Possible Effects on Sexual Function:** There is some data questioning an effect on sperm, but a distinct demonstration of an effect is lacking.

Natural Diseases or Disorders That May Be Activated by This Drug
Latent angina, atrial fibrillation, hypertension, peptic ulcer disease, temporomandibular joint (TMJ) disorder (by chewing gum).

Possible Effects on Laboratory Tests
Free fatty acids (FFA blood level): increased.
Blood glucose: increased.
Prothrombin time (INR): decreased.
Urine Screening Test for drug abuse: no effect.

CAUTION
1. For these drug products to be safe and effective, it is mandatory that all smoking be stopped immediately at the beginning of drug treatment.
2. Extended use of chewing gum may cause damage to mouth tissues and teeth, may loosen fillings and stick to dentures, and may initiate or aggravate temporomandibular joint dysfunction.
3. Smoking cessation and the use of these drug products can result in increased blood levels of insulin (in insulin-dependent diabetics); dosage reduction of insulin may be necessary to prevent hypoglycemic reactions.
4. If you are taking any of the following drugs, consult your physician regarding the need to reduce their dosage while participating in a smoking-cessation program: aminophylline, oxtriphylline, theophylline, beta blocker drugs, propoxyphene, oxazepam, prazosin, pentazocine, imipramine.
5. If you are taking any of the following drugs, consult your physician regarding the need to increase their dosage while participating in a smoking cessation program: isoproterenol, phynylephrine.
6. Used patches should be folded in half with the adhesive sides sealed together; place them in the orginal pouch or aluminum foil and dispose of them promptly; keep out of reach of children and animals.
7. Use of antacids such as Tums prior to chewing nicotine gum can increase the amount of nicotine absorbed from the gum.
8. Habitrol patches have only been shown to be effective when they are part of a complete smoking cessation program which includes counseling.

Precautions for Use
By Infants and Children:
Safety and effectiveness for those under 12 years of age not established.

By Those over 60 Years of Age: Because of the increased possibility of cardiovascular disorders in this age group, treatment is cautiously started. Watch closely for adverse effects.

▷ **Advisability of Use During Pregnancy**
Pregnancy Category: For nicotine chewing gum: X. For nicotine transdermal systems: D. See Pregnancy Code at the back of this book.
Animal studies: Impaired fertility found in mouse, rat and rabbit studies. Birth defects found in high-dose studies of mice.
Human studies: Adequate studies of pregnant women are not available. However, it is known that cigarette smoking during pregnancy may cause low birth weight, increased risk of abortion, and increased risk of newborn death.
The use of these drug products is not recommended during pregnancy.

Advisability of Use if Breast-Feeding
Presence of this drug in breast milk: Yes.
Avoid drug or refrain from nursing.

Habit-Forming Potential: The prolonged use of these drug products (beyond 3 months) may perpetuate the physical dependence of nicotine-dependent smokers.

Effects of Overdosage: Nausea, vomiting, increased salivation, stomach cramps, diarrhea, headache, dizziness, impaired vision and hearing, weakness, confusion, fainting, difficult breathing, seizures.

Possible Effects of Long-Term Use: Perpetuation of nicotine dependence.

Suggested Periodic Examinations While Taking This Drug (at physician's discretion)
Evaluation of patient's ability to abstain from smoking.
Evaluation of patient's blood pressure and heart function.

▷ **While Taking This Drug, Observe the Following**
Foods: No restrictions.
Beverages: No restrictions.
▷ *Alcohol:* May cause an increase in cardiovascular effects.
Tobacco Smoking: Avoid all forms of tobacco completely.
Marijuana Smoking: Avoid completely.
▷ *Other Drugs*
Nicotine may *increase* the effects of
- adenosine.
- niacin (flushing and dizziness).

The following drugs may *increase* the effects of nicotine
- antacids such as Tums used prior to chewing nicotine containing gum may increase the absorption of nicotine from the gum.
- cimetidine (Tagamet).
- lithium.
- ranitidine (Zantac).

Nicotine *taken concurrently* with
- niacin (Nicobid, others) can cause severe facial flushing.

▷ *Driving, Hazardous Activities:* This drug may cause dizziness or drowsiness. Restrict activities as necessary.

Aviation Note: The use of this drug **may be a disqualification** for piloting. Consult a designated Aviation Medical Examiner.

Exposure to Sun: No restrictions.

Exposure to Cold: Use caution until tolerance is determined. Cold environments may enhance the vasospastic action of nicotine.

Heavy Exercise or Exertion: Use caution in patients with angina, coronary artery disease or hypertension.

Discontinuation: As soon as a lasting cessation of smoking has been achieved, these drugs should be gradually reduced in dosage and then discontinued. Continual use of the chewing gum should not exceed 6 months; continual use of the transdermal systems should not exceed 20 weeks.

NIFEDIPINE (ni FED i peen)

Introduced: 1972 **Prescription:** USA: Yes; Canada: Yes **Available as Generic:** Yes **Class:** Antianginal, antihypertensive, calcium channel blocker **Controlled Drug:** USA: No; Canada: No

Brand Names: Adalat, Adalat CC, ✦Adalat P.A., ✦Adalat FT, ✦Apo-Nifed, ✦Gen-Nifedipine, ✦Novo-Nifedin, ✦Nu-Nifed, Procardia, Procardia XL

BENEFITS versus RISKS	
Possible Benefits	*Possible Risks*
EFFECTIVE PREVENTION OF BOTH MAJOR TYPES OF ANGINA	Rare increase in angina upon starting treatment
EFFECTIVE TREATMENT OF HYPERTENSION	Rare precipitation of congestive heart failure
	Rare anemia and low white blood cell counts
	Very rare drug-induced hepatitis
	Fainting (rare)

▷ **Principal Uses**

As a Single Drug Product: Uses currently included in FDA approved labeling: (1) Treats angina pectoris due to coronary artery spasm (Prinzmetal's variant angina) that occurs spontaneously and is not associated with exertion; and (2) classical angina-of-effort (due to atherosclerotic disease of the coronary arteries) in people who have not responded to or cannot tolerate the nitrates and beta blocker drugs customarily used to treat this disorder.

The sustained release tablets are used to treat mild to moderate hypertension.

Other (unlabeled) generally accepted uses: (1) Treatment of symptoms associated with Raynaud's phenomenon; (2) may stop the progression of atherosclerosis; (3) can have a role in congestive heart failure; (4) therapy of pulmonary hypertension; (5) helps decrease risk of heart attack after coronary artery bypass grafting; (6) could have a role in some neurologically based pain disorders; (7) may have a role in tardive dyskinesia; (8) can help urticaria of unknown cause; (9) therapy of achalasia or esophageal spasm; (10) helps intractable hiccups; (11)

Nifedipine

helps amaurosis fugax; (12) has a role in helping abnormal reactions to cold (chilblains).

How This Drug Works: By blocking passage of calcium through certain cell walls (which is necessary for the function of nerve and muscle tissue), this drug slows the spread of electrical activity through the heart and inhibits the contraction of coronary arteries and peripheral arterioles. As a result of these combined effects, this drug
- prevents spontaneous spasm of coronary arteries (Prinzmetal's angina).
- reduces the rate and contraction force of the heart during exertion, decreasing oxygen requirements of the heart muscle, and reducing the occurrence of effort-induced angina (classical angina pectoris).
- reduces the degree of contraction of peripheral arterial walls, resulting in their relaxation and consequent lowering of blood pressure. This further reduces the workload of the heart during exertion and helps prevent angina.

Available Dosage Forms and Strengths
Capsules — 5 mg (Canada), 10 mg (U.S. and Canada) and 20 mg (U.S.)
Tablets — 10 mg, 20 mg (Canada)
Tablets, extended-release — 10 mg, 20 mg (Canada), 30 mg, 60 mg, 90 mg (U.S.)
Tablets, sustained release — 30 mg, 60 mg, 90 mg

▷ **Recommended Dosage Ranges** (Actual dosage and administration schedule must be determined by the physician for each patient individually.)
Infants and Children: Dosage not established.
12 to 60 Years of Age: Initially, 10 mg 3 times daily. Dose may be increased gradually at 7- to 14-day intervals (as needed and tolerated) up to 30 mg 3 or 4 times/day. The usual maintenance dose is 10 to 20 mg 3 times/day. Maximum total daily dosage should not exceed 180 mg.
For hypertension: Initially a single 30-mg or 60-mg sustained release tablet taken once daily. Gradually increased as a single daily dose if needed.
Hypertensive crisis: 10 to 20 mg of nifedipine is given under the tongue.
Over 60 Years of Age: Same as 12 to 60 years of age.

Conditions Requiring Dosing Adjustments
Liver function: Specific dosage adjustments in liver compromise are not defined, and the dose should be empirically decreased. This drug is also a rare cause of liver toxicity (allergic hepatitis), and should be used with caution in patients with compromised livers. It is also a potential cause of portal hypertension, and should not be used in patients with portal hypertension.
Kidney function: In patients with compromised kidneys, nifedipine should be used as a benefit to risk decision as it can lead to kidney toxicity.

▷ **Dosing Instructions:** May be taken with or following food to reduce stomach irritation. The capsule should be swallowed whole (not altered). The sustained release tablet should be taken whole (not altered).

Usual Duration of Use: Use on a regular schedule for 2 to 4 weeks determines effectiveness in reducing the frequency and severity of angina and in controlling hypertension. For long-term use (months to years), the smallest effective dose should be used. Supervision and periodic physician evaluation are essential.

Possible Advantages of This Drug

The sustained release form of this drug permits effective once-a-day treatment for both angina and hypertension.

▷ **This Drug Should Not Be Taken If**
- you have had an allergic reaction to it previously.
- you have active liver disease.
- you have low blood pressure—systolic pressure below 90.
- you have significant narrowing or your aorta (aortic stenosis) ask your doctor.

▷ **Inform Your Physician Before Taking This Drug If**
- you have had an adverse response to any calcium blocker.
- you currently take any form of digitalis or a beta blocker drug (see Drug Class Section).
- you are taking any drugs that lower blood pressure.
- you have a history of congestive heart failure, heart attack or stroke.
- you are subject to disturbances of heart rhythm.
- you have impaired liver or kidney function.
- you have abnormal circulation to your fingers.
- you have diabetes or Duchenne muscular dystrophy.
- you have a history of drug-induced liver damage.

Possible Side-Effects (natural, expected and unavoidable drug actions)

Low blood pressure, rapid heart rate, swelling of the feet and ankles (7%), flushing and sensation of warmth (25%), sweating.

▷ **Possible Adverse Effects** (unusual, unexpected and infrequent reactions)

If any of the following develop, consult your physician promptly for guidance.

Mild Adverse Effects

Allergic Reactions: Skin rash, hives, itching, fever.

Headache (23%), dizziness (27%), weakness (12%), nervousness (7%), blurred vision, eye pain and swelling around the eyes.

Pedal edema (50%).

Depression (rare).

Abnormal growth of the gums.

Ringing in the ears (tinitis).

Sleep disturbances (2–7%).

Increased or decreased blood potassium.

Bedwetting (rare).

Palpitation (7%), shortness of breath, wheezing (6%), cough.

Heartburn (11%), nausea, taste disturbances, cramps, diarrhea (2%).

Tremors, muscle cramps (8%).

Serious Adverse Effects

Allergic Reaction: Drug-induced hepatitis (very rare), drug eruptions and erysipelaslike reactions and exfoliative dermatitis.

Idiosyncratic Reactions: Joint stiffness and inflammation.

Increased frequency or severity of angina on initiation of treatment or following an increase in dose.

Abnormal muscle movements (myoclonus) (rare).

Kidney toxicity (rare).
Pulmonary edema (rare).
Acute psychosis (very rare).
Worsening of circulation to the fingers.
Marked drop in blood pressure with fainting.
Low white blood cells, platelets and hemoglobin (rare).

▷ **Possible Effects on Sexual Function:** Altered timing and pattern of menstruation; excessive menstrual bleeding.
Tenderness and swelling of the male breast tissue (gynecomastia).

▷ **Adverse Effects That May Mimic Natural Diseases or Disorders**
An allergic rash and swelling of the legs may resemble erysipelas.
Drug-induced hepatitis may suggest viral hepatitis.

Possible Effects on Laboratory Tests
Bleeding time: increased.
Blood total cholesterol level: no effect in age group under 60 years old; decreased in those over 60 years old.
Blood HDL cholesterol level: no effect, or increased.
Blood LDL and VLDL cholesterol levels: no effect.
Blood triglyceride levels: no effect, or decreased.

CAUTION
1. Be sure to tell all health care providers you consult that you are taking this drug. Note the use of this drug on your card of personal identification.
2. You may use nitroglycerin and other nitrate drugs as needed to relieve acute episodes of angina pain. However, if you detect that your angina attacks are becoming more frequent or intense, call your doctor.

Precautions for Use
By Infants and Children: Safety and effectiveness for those under 12 years of age not established.
By Those over 60 Years of Age: You may be more susceptible to the development of weakness, dizziness, fainting and falling. Take necessary precautions to prevent injury. Report promptly any changes in your pattern of thirst and urination.

▷ **Advisability of Use During Pregnancy**
Pregnancy Category: C. See Pregnancy Code at the back of this book.
Animal studies: Embryo and fetal deaths reported in mice, rats and rabbits; birth defects reported in rats.
Human studies: Adequate studies of pregnant women are not available.
Avoid this drug during the first 3 months. Use during the last 6 months only if clearly needed. Ask physician for guidance.

Advisability of Use if Breast-Feeding
Presence of this drug in breast milk: Yes.
Avoid drug or refrain from nursing.

Habit-Forming Potential: None.

Effects of Overdosage: Weakness, light-headedness, fainting, fast pulse, low blood pressure, shortness of breath, flushed and warm skin, tremors.

Possible Effects of Long-Term Use: None reported.

Nifedipine

Suggested Periodic Examinations While Taking This Drug (at physician's discretion)

Evaluations of heart function, including electrocardiograms; measurements of blood pressure in supine, sitting and standing positions.

▷ **While Taking This Drug, Observe the Following**

Foods: Grapefruit juice may greatly increase the absorption (bioavailability) of nifedipine and result in an exaggerated therapeutic effect. It is also prudent to avoid excessive salt intake.

Beverages: No restrictions. May be taken with milk.

▷ *Alcohol:* Use with caution. Alcohol may exaggerate the drop in blood pressure experienced by some people.

Tobacco Smoking: Nicotine may reduce the effectiveness of this drug. Follow your physician's advice regarding smoking.

Marijuana Smoking: Possible reduced effectiveness of this drug; mild to moderate increase in angina; possible changes in electrocardiogram, confusing interpretation.

▷ *Other Drugs*

Nifedipine *taken concurrently* with
- amiodarone (Codarone) may cause the heart to stop.
- beta blocker drugs or digitalis preparations (see Drug Classes) may affect heart rate and rhythm adversely. Careful monitoring by your physician is necessary if these drugs are taken concurrently.
- cyclosporine (Sandimmune) can lead to nifedipine toxicity.
- diltiazem may lead to nifedipine toxicity.
- oral hypoglycemic agents (see Drug Classes) or insulin may result in loss of glucose control.
- magnesium can cause additive lowering of the blood pressure.
- phenytoin (Dilantin) can cause phenytoin toxicity.
- rifampin can decrease nifedipine effectiveness.
- theophylline can reduce the therapeutic benefit of nifedipine and may lead to theophylline toxicity as well.
- vincristine can cause vincristine toxicity.

The following drug may *increase* the effects of nifedipine
- cimetidine (Tagamet).
- quinidine can lead to nifedipine toxicity as well as decreased quinidine effectiveness.
- ranitidine (Zantac).

▷ *Driving, Hazardous Activities:* Usually no restrictions. This drug may cause drowsiness or dizziness. Restrict activities as necessary.

Aviation Note: Coronary artery disease *is a disqualification* for piloting. Consult a designated Aviation Medical Examiner.

Exposure to Sun: No restrictions.

Exposure to Heat: Caution advised. Hot environments can exaggerate the blood-pressure-lowering effects of this drug. Observe for light-headedness or weakness.

Heavy Exercise or Exertion: This drug may improve your ability to be more active without resulting angina pain. Use caution and avoid excessive exercise that could impair heart function in the absence of warning pain.

Discontinuation: Do not stop this drug abruptly. Consult your physician regarding gradual withdrawal. Observe for the possible development of rebound angina.

NITROFURANTOIN (ni troh fyur AN toin)

Introduced: 1953 **Prescription:** USA: Yes; Canada: Yes **Available as Generic:** Yes **Class:** Urinary anti-infective **Controlled Drug:** USA: No; Canada: No
Brand Names: ✦Apo-Nitrofurantoin, Furadantin, Furalan, Furan, Furanite, Furatoin, Macrodantin, Macrodantin MACPAC, ✦Nephronex, ✦Novofuran, Parfuran

BENEFITS versus RISKS	
Possible Benefits	*Possible Risks*
EFFECTIVE TREATMENT OF SOME URINARY TRACT INFECTIONS	ALLERGIC REACTIONS: Anaphylaxis Rashes, hives Repetitive asthma Lung inflammation Drug-induced hepatitis Peripheral neuropathy (see Glossary) Blood cell disorders: hemolytic anemia (see Glossary) Reduced white blood cell count Superinfections

▷ **Principal Uses**
 As a Single Drug Product: Use currently included in FDA approved labeling: (1) Because this drug is concentrated in the urine and attains low levels in the blood, its use is limited to the prevention or treatment of infections in the urinary tract.
 Other (unlabeled) generally accepted uses: (1) May be useful after transurethral resection of the prostate (TURP).
How This Drug Works: By interfering with some bacterial enzyme systems, this drug is bacteriostatic (growth retarding) in low to moderate concentrations and bactericidal (killing) in high concentrations.
Available Dosage Forms and Strengths
 Capsules — 25 mg, 50 mg, 100 mg
 Oral suspension — 25 mg per 5-ml teaspoonful
 Tablets — 50 mg, 100 mg
▷ **Usual Adult Dosage Range:** For treatment of active infections: 50 to 100 mg/6 hours. For prevention: 50 to 100 mg once/day at bedtime. The total daily dosage should not exceed 600 mg. **Note: Actual dosage and administration schedule must be determined by the physician for each patient individually.**
Conditions Requiring Dosing Adjustments
 Liver function: Specific dosage adjustments in liver compromise are not defined.

Nitrofurantoin

Kidney function: In patients with moderate kidney failure, the drug should **not** be used. It is capable of causing crystalluria, and patients who do use this drug should drink adequate quantities of water.

▷ **Dosing Instructions:** The tablet may be crushed and is best taken with or following food to facilitate absorption and reduce stomach irritation. This drug can stain the teeth yellow on contact.

Usual Duration of Use: Use on a regular schedule for 7 to 10 days determines effectiveness in curing urinary tract infections. Long-term use for prevention (months to years) requires physician supervision and periodic evaluation.

▷ **This Drug Should Not Be Taken If**
- you have had an allergic reaction to it previously.
- you have moderate to severely impaired kidney function.
- you have active liver disease.
- you have a prostate infection.
- you are in the last month of pregnancy.

▷ **Inform Your Physician Before Taking This Drug If**
- you are allergic to any nitrofuran drug.
- you have impaired liver or kidney function.
- you have a deficiency of glucose-6-phosphate dehydrogenase in your red blood cells.
- you have a history of peripheral neuropathy.
- you have a history of lung disease.
- you are nursing your baby.
- you have chronic anemia or diabetes.

Possible Side-Effects (natural, expected and unavoidable drug actions)
Superinfections (see Glossary) in the urinary tract.
Brown discoloration of the urine, of no significance.

▷ **Possible Adverse Effects** (unusual, unexpected and infrequent reactions)
If any of the following develop, consult your physician promptly for guidance.

Mild Adverse Effects
Allergic Reactions: Skin rashes, hives, localized swellings, itching, fever.
Headache, dizziness, drowsiness, burning and tearing of eyes, impaired color vision, muscle aching, loss of hair.
Tingling of the extremeties (paresthesias).
Loss of appetite, nausea, vomiting, diarrhea, abdominal cramping.

Serious Adverse Effects
Allergic Reactions: Anaphylaxis (see Glossary), interstitial pneumonitis (lung inflammation), asthma, hepatitis.
Idiosyncratic Reaction: Hemolytic anemia (see Glossary).
Peripheral neuropathy (see Glossary).
Blood cell disorders: reduced red and white blood cell counts.
Methemoglobinemia.
Trigeminal neuralgia (rare).
Change in acid base balance of the body (metabolic acidosis).
Drug-induced porphyria (rare).

Fever (rare).
Pancreatitis (rare).
Drug-induced inflammation of the parotid gland.
Crystalluria.
Systemic lupus erythematosus (also associated with erythema multiforme) (rare).

▷ **Possible Effects on Sexual Function:** Male infertility (rare).

▷ **Adverse Effects That May Mimic Natural Diseases or Disorders**
Allergic pneumonitis may suggest an infectious pneumonia.
Allergic hepatitis may suggest viral hepatitis.

Natural Diseases or Disorders That May Be Activated by This Drug
Latent asthma.

Possible Effects on Laboratory Tests
Complete blood cell counts: decreased red cells, hemoglobin, white cells and platelets; increased white cells and eosinophils (allergic reactions and drug-induced lung inflammation).
Blood amylase level: increased (pancreatic reaction).
Liver function tests: increased liver enzymes (ALT/GPT, AST/GOT and alkaline phosphatase), increased bilirubin.
Kidney function tests: increased blood creatinine and urea nitrogen (BUN) levels (kidney damage).
Urine sugar tests: false positive result with Benedict's solution.

CAUTION
Troublesome and persistent diarrhea can develop. If diarrhea persists for more than 24 hours, stop this drug and consult your physician.

Precautions for Use
By Infants and Children: This drug should not be used in infants under 1 month of age. Watch closely for the possible development of increased intracranial pressure.
By Those over 60 Years of Age: Dosage must be carefully individualized on the basis of kidney function. This age group is more susceptible to skin rashes, nausea, vomiting and constipation.

▷ **Advisability of Use During Pregnancy**
Pregnancy Category: C. See Pregnancy Code at the back of this book.
Animal studies: No information available.
Human studies: No significant increase in birth defects reported in 590 exposures. Adequate studies of pregnant women are not available.
Avoid use of drug during the last few weeks of pregnancy. Use otherwise only if clearly needed. Ask your physician for guidance.

Advisability of Use if Breast-Feeding
Presence of this drug in breast milk: Yes, in small amounts.
Avoid drug or refrain from nursing.

Habit-Forming Potential: None.

Effects of Overdosage: Nausea, vomiting, diarrhea.

Possible Effects of Long-Term Use: Allergic reactions in lungs or liver, peripheral neuropathy, superinfections within the urinary tract.

Suggested Periodic Examinations While Taking This Drug (at physician's discretion)
   Complete blood cell counts, liver function tests, X-ray examinations of lungs during long-term use.
▷ **While Taking This Drug, Observe the Following**
   Foods: No restrictions. Eat liberally of the following foods: beef, chicken, lamb and pork liver, asparagus, navy beans (good sources of folic acid).
   Beverages: No restrictions. May be taken with milk.
▷ *Alcohol:* Use with extreme caution. This drug, in combination with alcohol, may cause a disulfiramlike reaction (see Glossary) in sensitive individuals.
   Tobacco Smoking: No interactions expected.
▷ *Other Drugs*
   The following drugs may *decrease* the effects of nitrofurantoin
   • antacids that contain magnesium can prevent the absorption of nitrofurantoin and reduce its effectiveness.
   Nitrofurantoin **taken concurrently** with
   • birth control pills (oral contraceptives) may result in loss of contraception and pregnancy.
▷ *Driving, Hazardous Activities:* This drug may cause dizziness. Restrict activities as necessary.
   Aviation Note: The use of this drug **may be a disqualification** for piloting. Consult a designated Aviation Medical Examiner.
   Exposure to Sun: No restrictions.

NITROGLYCERIN (ni troh GLIS er in)

Introduced: 1847   **Prescription:** USA: Yes; Canada: No   **Available as Generic:** Yes   **Class:** Antianginal, nitrates   **Controlled Drug:** USA: No; Canada: No

Brand Names: Deponit, Minitran Transdermal Delivery System, Nitro-Bid, Nitrocap TD, Nitrocine Transdermal, Nitrocine Timecaps, Nitrodisc, Nitro-Dur, Nitro-Dur II, Nitrogard, ✦Nitrogard-SR, Nitroglyn, Nitrol, ✦Nitrol TSAR Kit, Nitrolin, Nitrolingual Spray, Nitrong, ✦Nitrong SR, Nitrospan, ✦Nitrostabilin, Nitrostat, Nitro Transdermal System, NTS Transdermal Patch, Transderm-Nitro, ✦Tridil

BENEFITS versus RISKS	
Possible Benefits	*Possible Risks*
EFFECTIVE RELIEF AND PREVENTION OF ANGINA	Orthostatic hypotension (see Glossary) with and without fainting
EFFECTIVE ADJUNCTIVE TREATMENT IN SELECTED CASES OF CONGESTIVE HEART FAILURE	Skin rash (rare)
	Altered hemoglobin with large doses (very rare)
	Low blood platelets (rare)

▷ **Principal Uses**
   As a Single Drug Product: Uses currently included in FDA approved labeling: (1) Treatment of symptomatic coronary artery disease. The rapid-action

forms are used to relieve acute attacks of anginal pain at their onset. The sustained-action forms are used to prevent the development of angina; (2) helps improve breathing dificulty caused by heart failure (left ventricle); (3) intravenous nitroglycerin is used in surgery to control blood pressure; (4) helps relieve congestive heart failure after heart attacks.

Other (unlabeled) generally accepted uses: (1) May help ease spasms of the Sphincter of Oddi; (2) topical use may help in impotence; (3) can help reduce the extent of heart damage if given following a heart attack (myocardial infarction); (4) helps relax cocaine-constricted heart arteries; (5) eases the pain of peripheral neuropathy; may be of help in easing esophageal problems (achalasia); (6) when the anal sphincter does not work correctly, this drug can help reduce the muscle pressure and ease constipation; (7) nitroglycerin in combination with vasopressin may be of use in stopping bleeding esophageal varices; (8) can help loss of vision that has been caused by a clot in the retinal artery; (9) if ergot medications (see Drug Class) have shut down circulation to the extremeties, nitroglycerin can open up the circulation; (10) used to delay contractions in order to rotate an abnormally positioned fetus.

How This Drug Works: By direct action on the muscles in blood vessel walls, this drug relaxes and dilates both arteries and veins. Its beneficial effects in angina are due to two mechanisms of action: (1) dilation of narrowed coronary arteries; (2) dilation of veins in the general circulation, with consequent reduction of the volume and pressure of blood entering the heart. The net effects are improved blood supply to the heart muscle and reduced work load for the heart. Both actions reduce the frequency and severity of angina.

Available Dosage Forms and Strengths
Canisters, translingual spray — 13.8 grams (200 doses), 0.4 mg per metered dose
Capsules, prolonged-action — 2.5 mg, 2.6 mg, 6.5 mg, 9 mg
Ointment — 2%
Tablets, buccal — 1 mg, 2 mg, 3 mg
Tablets, prolonged-action — 2.6 mg, 6.5 mg, 9 mg
Tablets, sublingual — 0.15 mg, 0.3 mg, 0.4 mg, 0.6 mg
Transdermal systems — 2.5 mg, 5 mg, 7.5 mg, 10 mg, 15 mg (all per 24 hours)

▷ **Usual Adult Dosage Range:** According to dosage form:
Sublingual spray—1 metered spray (0.4 mg) under tongue/3 to 5 minutes, up to 3 doses within 15 minutes, to relieve acute angina. To prevent angina, 1 spray taken 5 to 10 minutes before exertion.
Sublingual tablets—0.15 to 0.6 mg dissolved under tongue at 5-minute intervals to relieve acute angina.
Prolonged-action tablets—1.3 to 6.5 mg at 8- to 12-hour intervals to prevent angina.
Prolonged-action capsules—2.5 to 9 mg at 8- to 12-hour intervals to prevent angina.
Ointment—2.5 to 5 cm (1 to 2 inches, 15 to 30 mg) applied in a thin, even layer of uniform size to hairless skin at 3- to 4-hour intervals to prevent angina.

Buccal tablets—1 to 2 mg/4 to 5 hours placed between cheek and gum.
Transdermal patches—5-sq.-cm to 30-sq.-cm patch applied to hairless skin once/24 hours to prevent angina.
Note: Actual dosage and administration schedule must be determined by the physician for each patient individually.

Conditions Requiring Dosing Adjustments
Liver function: Specific dosage adjustments in liver compromise are not defined.
Kidney function: Specific guidelines for dosing changes are not available. This drug can discolor urine.

▷ **Dosing Instructions:** Dosage forms to be swallowed are best taken when stomach is empty (1 hour before or 2 hours after eating) to obtain maximal blood levels. Tablets should not be crushed for administration. Capsules may be opened, but the contents should not be crushed or chewed before swallowing.

Usual Duration of Use: Use on a regular schedule for 3 to 5 days is often needed to determine effectiveness in preventing and relieving acute anginal attacks. Individual dosage adjustments will be necessary for optimal results. Long-term use (months to years) requires physician supervision.

▷ **This Drug Should Not Be Taken If**
- you have had an allergic reaction to it previously.
- you are severely anemic.
- you have had recent head trauma.
- you have hyperthyroidism.
- you have increased intraocular pressure.
- you have abnormal growth of the heart muscle in response to vascular disease (hypertrophic cardiomyopathy).
- you have closed-angle glaucoma (inadequately treated).

▷ **Inform Your Physician Before Taking This Drug If**
- you have had an unfavorable response to other nitrate drugs in the past.
- you have low blood pressure.
- you have any form of glaucoma.
- you have had recent bleeding in your head.

Possible Side-Effects (natural, expected and unavoidable drug actions)
Flushing of face, headaches (50%), orthostatic hypotension (see Glossary), rapid heart rate, palpitation.

▷ **Possible Adverse Effects** (unusual, unexpected and infrequent reactions)
If any of the following develop, consult your physician promptly for guidance.
Mild Adverse Effects
Allergic Reaction: Skin rash.
Throbbing headaches (may be severe and persistent), dizziness, fainting.
Nausea, vomiting, taste disorders.
Serious Adverse Effects
Allergic Reactions: Severe skin reactions with peeling.
Idiosyncratic Reaction: Methemoglobinemia (very rare).
Abnormally slow heart beat (bradycardia) (rare).
Low blood supply to the head (transient ischemic attacks).
Increased intracranial pressure.

▷ **Possible Effects on Sexual Function**
  Correction of impotence (1 report following sublingual use).
  The preventive use of nitroglycerin prior to sexual activity has been recommended to eliminate or reduce the risk of angina. Consult your physician for guidance.

▷ **Adverse Effects That May Mimic Natural Diseases or Disorders**
  Hypotensive spells (sudden drops in blood pressure) due to this drug may be mistaken for late-onset epilepsy.

Possible Effects on Laboratory Tests
  Blood platelet count: decreased.

CAUTION
  1. This drug can provoke migraine headaches in susceptible individuals.
  2. Patients with impaired brain circulation (cerebral arteriosclerosis) have increased risk of transient ischemic attacks—periods of temporary speech impairment, paralysis, numbness, etc.
  3. Tolerance to long-acting forms of nitrates will happen in most patients after 24 hours of continuous use. A nitrate free interval of 10 hours usually restores effectiveness.
  4. Many over-the-counter (OTC) drug products for allergies, colds and coughs contain drugs that may counteract the desired effects of this drug. Ask your physician or pharmacist for help before using any such medications.

Precautions for Use
  By Infants and Children: Limited usefulness and experience in this age group. Dosage schedules not established.
  By Those over 60 Years of Age: Begin treatment with small doses and increase dose cautiously as needed and tolerated. You may be more susceptible to the development of flushing, throbbing headache, dizziness, "blackout" spells, fainting and falling.

▷ **Advisability of Use During Pregnancy**
  Pregnancy Category: C. See Pregnancy Code at the back of this book.
  Animal studies: No information available.
  Human studies: Adequate studies of pregnant women are not available.
  Use this drug only if clearly needed. Ask physician for guidance.

Advisability of Use if Breast-Feeding
  Presence of this drug in breast milk: Unknown.
  Watch nursing infant closely and discontinue drug or nursing if adverse effects develop.

Habit-Forming Potential: None.

Effects of Overdosage: Throbbing headache, dizziness, marked flushing, nausea, vomiting, abdominal cramps, confusion, delirium, paralysis, seizures, circulatory collapse.

Possible Effects of Long-Term Use: The development of tolerance (see Glossary) and the temporary loss of effectiveness.

Suggested Periodic Examinations While Taking This Drug (at physician's discretion)
  Measurements of blood pressure and internal eye pressures.
  Evaluation of hemoglobin.

▷ **While Taking This Drug, Observe the Following**
   Foods: No restrictions.
   Beverages: No restrictions. May be taken with milk.
▷ *Alcohol:* Avoid alcohol completely. This combination may result in severe lowering of the blood pressure. There is a potential for collapse of the circulation and pumping effectiveness of the heart.
   Tobacco Smoking: Nicotine can reduce the effectiveness of this drug. Follow your physician's advice regarding smoking.
   Marijuana Smoking: Possible reduced effectiveness of this drug; mild to moderate increase in angina; possible changes in the electrocardiogram, confusing interpretation.
▷ *Other Drugs*
   Nitroglycerin **taken concurrently** with
   - antihypertensive drugs may cause excessive lowering of blood pressure. Careful dosage adjustments may be necessary.
   - dihydroergotamine or similar ergot medicines (see drug Classes) may result in ergotamine toxicity.
   - heparin can result in decreased therapeutic benefit of heparin.
   The following drugs may *increase* the effects of nitroglycerin
   - aspirin, in analgesic doses (500 mg or more).
▷ *Driving, Hazardous Activities:* Usually no restrictions. This drug may cause dizziness or faintness. Restrict activities as necessary.
   Aviation Note: Coronary artery disease **is a disqualification** for piloting. Consult a designated Aviation Medical Examiner.
   Exposure to Sun: No restrictions.
   Exposure to Heat: Hot environments can cause significant lowering of blood pressure.
   Exposure to Cold: Cold environments can increase the need for this drug and limit its effectiveness.
   Heavy Exercise or Exertion: This drug can increase your tolerance for exercise. Use good judgment regarding excessive exertion in the absence of anginal pain.
   Discontinuation: Do not stop this drug abruptly after long-term use. It is advisable to reduce the dose (of the prolonged-action dosage forms) gradually over a period of to 6 weeks. Observe for rebound angina.
   Special Storage Instructions: For sublingual tablets, to prevent loss of strength
   - keep tablets in the original glass container.
   - do not transfer tablets to a plastic or metallic container (such as a pillbox).
   - do not place absorbent cotton, paper (such as the prescription label), or other material inside the container.
   - do not store other drugs in the same container.
   - close the container tightly immediately after each use.
   - store at room temperature.

NIZATIDINE (ni ZA te deen)

Introduced: 1986 **Prescription:** USA: Yes **Available as Generic:** No **Class:** Antiulcer, H-2 receptor blocker **Controlled Drug:** USA: No
Brand Name: Axid

BENEFITS versus RISKS

Possible Benefits	Possible Risks
EFFECTIVE TREATMENT OF PEPTIC ULCER DISEASE: relief of symptoms, acceleration of healing and prevention of recurrence in many cases CONTROL OF HYPERSECRETORY STOMACH DISORDERS Beneficial in treatment of reflux esophagitis	Drug-induced liver damage (rare) Abnormally low blood platelet count (rare)

Please see the histamine (H2) blocking drug profile for more information.

NORFLOXACIN (nor FLOX a sin)

Introduced: 1986 **Prescription:** USA: Yes; Canada: Yes **Available as Generic:** USA: No; Canada: No **Class:** Anti-infectives **Controlled Drug:** USA: No; Canada: No

Brand Name: Noroxin, Chibroxin

Warning: Some physicians are using the name "Norflox" to identify this drug when issuing orders (for inpatients) or prescriptions (for outpatients). Norflox is not an accepted name for this drug in any setting for any reason. This coinage of an abbreviated name has resulted in serious medication errors—the dispensing of Norflex, the generic drug orphenadrine, a skeletal muscle relaxant. Ask your pharmacist to verify that you are getting the right drug—an anti-infective.

Warning: Reports are being made for some drugs in this class which find tendon rupture as a rare adverse effect. Ask your doctor about limits on strenuous exercise while you are taking this medicine. A rare idiosyncratic reaction has also been reported which presents as mental confusion and disorientation. Use of this medicine after head trauma may be a risk factor. If you have suffered a fall, ask your doctor if a medicine in a different antibiotic class should be substituted. If you are taking this drug and notice a change in your thinking, call your doctor.

BENEFITS versus RISKS

Possible Benefits	Possible Risks
Effective treatment of urinary tract infections Effective treatment of bacterial gastroenteritis and gonorrhea	Infrequent nausea, indigestion Rare impairment of vision Rare seizure and neurological compromise

Norfloxacin

▷ **Principal Uses**

As a Single Drug Product: Uses currently included in FDA approved labeling: (1) Treat urinary tract infections (in adults) caused by a wide variety of bacteria sensitive to the action of this drug (including gonorrhea); (2) also used as an ophthalmic solution to treat eye infections and conjunctivitis. Other (unlabeled) generally accepted uses: (1) Used in a variety of infections where it is effective against the bacteria usually causing the problem such as prostatitis, certain pneumonias and Salmonella; (2) used in gastroenteritis caused by certain bacteria, to prevent traveler's diarrhea.

How This Drug Works: By inhibiting essential enzyme systems of bacterial nucleic acids (DNA), this drug prevents bacterial reproduction (with low doses) and destroys bacteria (with higher doses).

Available Dosage Forms and Strengths
Tablets — 400 mg
Ophthalmic Solution — 3 mg per ml

▷ **Usual Adult Dosage Range:** Uncomplicated urinary tract infections—400 mg/ 12 hours for 3 days. Complicated urinary tract infections—400 mg/12 hours for 10 to 21 days. Total daily dosage should not exceed 800 mg. **Note: Actual dosage and administration schedule must be determined by the physician for each patient individually.**

Conditions Requiring Dosing Adjustments

Liver function: Norfloxacin should be used with caution in patients with compromised livers, and blood levels and liver function tests obtained.

Kidney function: In patients with moderate to severe kidney compromise, the dose should be decreased to 400 mg daily. Since norfloxacin is a rare cause of crystalluria, patients taking the drug should drink adequate quantities of water.

▷ **Dosing Instructions:** Preferably taken with a full glass of water 1 hour before or 2 hours after eating. Avoid antacids for 2 hours after taking this drug. The tablet may be crushed for administration. Take the full course prescribed.

Usual Duration of Use: Continual use on a regular schedule for 3 to 21 days (depending upon the nature of the infection) is usually necessary to determine this drug's effectiveness in eradicating the infection.

▷ **This Drug Should Not Be Taken If**
- you have had an allergic reaction to any dosage form of it previously.
- you are pregnant or breast-feeding.
- it is prescribed for a child under 18 years of age.

▷ **Inform Your Physician Before Taking This Drug If**
- you are allergic to cinoxacin (Cinobac) or nalidixic acid (NegGram).
- you have a history of psychosis.
- you have a history of intracranial pressure elevation (ask your doctor).
- you have a seizure disorder.
- you have impaired liver or kidney function.

Possible Side-Effects (natural, expected and unavoidable drug actions)
None reported.

▷ **Possible Adverse Effects** (unusual, unexpected and infrequent reactions)
If any of the following develop, consult your physician promptly for guidance.

Mild Adverse Effects
   Allergic Reactions: Skin rash (0.4%), hives (0.1%), localized swelling, itching (0.1%).
   Headache (1.6%), dizziness (1.2%), mental depression (4 reports), seizures (3 reports).
   Drowsiness, mood alterations, nervousness, insomnia, hallucinations (all less than 1%).
   Lowering of blood glucose.
   Visual disturbances: blurred or double vision, altered color vision, increased sensitivity to light (all less than 0.1%).
   Dry mouth, decreased appetite (0.1%), nausea (2%), indigestion (0.3%), vomiting, (0.2%), diarrhea (0.2%).
   Swollen or painful tendons and joints (0.1%).
Serious Adverse Effects
   Allergic Reactions: Exfoliative dermatitis (1 report), anaphylactic reaction (see Glossary).
   One medication of this class has had instances of severe neurological compromise reported with use of the drug. Stop the medication immediately and call your doctor if you experience confusion, trouble speaking or disorientation once taking this drug.
   One medicine belonging to this class has been associated with tendon rupture. Ask your doctor for guidance regarding exercise or activity while you are taking this drug.
   Lowering of neutrophilic white blood cells.
   Seizures (rare).
   Formation of crystals of the drug in the urine.
   Worsening of myasthenia gravis.

▷ **Possible Effects on Sexual Function:** Vaginitis with discharge has been reported.

Natural Diseases or Disorders That May Be Activated by This Drug
   Latent epilepsy.

Possible Effects on Laboratory Tests
   Red and white blood cell counts: rarely decreased.
   Liver function tests: rarely increased liver enzymes (ALT/GPT, AST/GOT).
   Kidney function tests: rarely increased blood creatinine and urea nitrogen (BUN) levels.
   Blood sugar: decreased.

CAUTION
   1. Crystal formation in the kidney can occur (especially with high doses or prolonged use). This can be prevented by drinking large amounts of water, up to 2 quarts/24 hours.
   2. This drug may decrease saliva formation and predispose to formation of dental cavities or gum disease. Consult your dentist if mouth dryness persists.

Precautions for Use
   By Infants and Children: Safety for use by those who have not attained complete bone growth not established. This drug can impair normal bone growth and development in test animals. Avoid its use in children until they are 18.

By Those over 60 Years of Age: Impaired kidney function requires dosage reduction. Consult your physician.

▷ **Advisability of Use During Pregnancy**
Pregnancy Category: C. See Pregnancy Code at the back of this book.
Animal studies: Mouse, rat, rabbit and monkey studies reveal no birth defects due to this drug. However, this drug can cause impaired bone development in immature dogs.
Human studies: Adequate studies of pregnant women are not available.
This drug should be avoided during entire pregnancy.

Advisability of Use if Breast-Feeding
Presence of this drug in breast milk: Unknown.
Avoid drug or refrain from nursing.

Habit-Forming Potential: None.

Effects of Overdosage: Nausea, vomiting, diarrhea, seizures.

Possible Effects of Long-Term Use: Crystal formation in kidneys with high doses and inadequate fluid intake.

Suggested Periodic Examinations While Taking This Drug (at physician's discretion)
Liver function tests, urine analysis.

▷ **While Taking This Drug, Observe the Following**
Foods: Avoid taking this drug after eating dairy foods. Take this drug one hour before or two hours after eating dairy foods such as milk or cottage cheese.
Beverages: No restrictions.
▷ *Alcohol:* No interactions expected.
Tobacco Smoking: No interactions expected.
▷ *Other Drugs*
Norfloxacin **taken concurrently** with
- Nitrofurantoin (Macrodantin, etc.) may antagonize the antibacterial action of norfloxacin in the urinary tract. Avoid this combination.
- cyclosporine (Sandimmune) may cause toxic effects on the kidney.
- iron salts will decrease the therapeutic benefits of norfloxacin.
- sucralfate (Carafate) will decrease absorption of norfloxacin.
- theophylline will lead to theophylline toxicity over time.
- warfarin will lead to increased risk of bleeding.
- zinc will decrease norfloxacin effectiveness.

The following drug may *increase* the effects of norfloxacin
- probenecid (Benemid).

The following drugs may *decrease* the effects of norfloxacin
- antacids may reduce its absorption.

▷ *Driving, Hazardous Activities:* This drug may cause dizziness or impaired vision. Restrict activities as necessary.
Aviation Note: The use of this drug **may be a disqualification** for piloting. Consult a designated Aviation Medical Examiner.
Exposure to Sun: Sunglasses advised if eyes are overly sensitive to bright light.
Discontinuation: If you experience no adverse effects from this drug, take the full course prescribed for maximal results. Consult your physician when to stop taking this medication.

NORTRIPTYLINE (nor TRIP ti leen)

Introduced: 1963 **Prescription:** USA: Yes; Canada: Yes **Available as Generic:** USA: Yes; Canada: No **Class:** Antidepressant **Controlled Drug:** USA: No; Canada: No

Brand Names: Aventyl, Pamelor

BENEFITS versus RISKS	
Possible Benefits	*Possible Risks*
EFFECTIVE RELIEF OF ENDOGENOUS DEPRESSION Possibly beneficial in other depressive disorders Possibly beneficial in the management of some types of chronic, severe pain	ADVERSE BEHAVIORAL EFFECTS: confusion, disorientation, hallucinations, delusions CONVERSION OF DEPRESSION TO MANIA in manic-depressive disorders Aggravation of schizophrenia Irregular heart rhythms Rare blood cell abnormalities

▷ **Principal Uses**

As a Single Drug Product

Uses currently included in FDA approved labeling (1) Relieves symptoms associated with spontaneous (endogenous) depression. This drug should be used only when a diagnosis of a true, primary depression of significant degree has been established. It should not be used to treat the symptoms of mild and transient (reactive) depression that may be associated with many life situations in the absence of a bona fide affective illness.

Other (unlabeled) generally accepted uses: (1) Used in conjunction with other drugs to manage chronic, severe pain associated with such conditions as cancer, migraine headache, severe arthritis, peripheral neuropathy, AIDS, etc.; (2) helps decrease the frequency of bedwetting; (3) may have a role in helping severe PMS; (4) can help attention deficit hyperactivity disorder (ADHD).

How This Drug Works: It is thought that this drug relieves depression by slowly restoring to normal levels certain constituents of brain tissue (norepinephrine and serotonin) that transmit nerve impulses.

Available Dosage Forms and Strengths

Capsules — 10 mg, 25 mg, 50 mg, 75 mg
Oral solution — 10 mg per 5-ml teaspoonful (alcohol 4%)

▷ **Usual Adult Dosage Range:** Initially 25 mg 3 or 4 times daily. Dose may be increased cautiously as needed and tolerated by 10 to 25 mg daily at intervals of 1 week. Usual maintenance dose is 50 to 100 mg/24 hours. Total dose should not exceed 150 mg/24 hours. When the optimal requirement is determined, it may be taken at bedtime as one dose. **Note: Actual dosage and administration schedule must be determined by the physician for each patient individually.**

Conditions Requiring Dosing Adjustments

Liver function: Specific dosage adjustments in liver compromise are not defined, however, the patient should be closely followed, and levels obtained. This drug is also a rare cause of hepatoxicity, and should be used with caution in patients with compromised livers.

Kidney function: Specific dosing changes in renal compromise are not usually needed. Nortriptaline can cause a decrease in urine outflow, and should be used as a benefit to risk decision in patients with urine outflow problems.

▷ **Dosing Instructions:** The capsule may be opened and may be taken without regard to meals.

Usual Duration of Use: Some benefit may be apparent within 1 to 2 weeks, but adequate response may require continual use for 3 months or longer. Long-term use should not exceed 6 months without physician evaluation regarding the need for continuation of the drug.

Possible Advantages of This Drug
Causes less daytime sedation.
Causes fewer atropinelike side-effects.
Causes orthostatic hypotension infrequently (see Glossary).

▷ **This Drug Should Not Be Taken If**
- you have had an allergic reaction to it previously.
- you are taking or have taken within the past 14 days any monoamine oxidase (MAO) type A inhibitor drug (see Drug Classes).
- you are recovering from a recent heart attack.
- you have narrow-angle glaucoma.

▷ **Inform Your Physician Before Taking This Drug If**
- you are allergic or sensitive to any other tricyclic antidepressant (see Drug Class Section).
- you have a history of: diabetes, epilepsy, glaucoma, heart disease, prostate gland enlargement or overactive thyroid function.
- you plan to have surgery under general anesthesia in the near future.
- you have a history of bone marrow suppression.
- you have a history of low blood pressure.

Possible Side-Effects (natural, expected and unavoidable drug actions)
Light-headedness, drowsiness, blurred vision, dry mouth, constipation, impaired urination (see Prostatism in Glossary).

▷ **Possible Adverse Effects** (unusual, unexpected and infrequent reactions)
If any of the following develop, consult your physician promptly for guidance.

Mild Adverse Effects
Allergic Reactions: Skin rash, hives, swelling of face or tongue, drug fever (see Glossary).
Headache, dizziness, memory problems, weakness, fainting, unsteady gait, tremors, blurred vision, hearing toxicity.
Peculiar taste, weight gain, cavities (dental caries), irritation of tongue or mouth, nausea, indigestion.
Fluctuation of blood sugar levels.

Serious Adverse Effects
Allergic Reactions: Hepatitis, with or without jaundice (see Glossary).
Confusion, disorientation, hallucinations, delusions.
Aggravation of paranoid psychoses and schizophrenia; seizures.
Heart palpitation and irregular rhythm.

Bone marrow depression (see Glossary)—fatigue, weakness, fever, sore throat, abnormal bleeding or bruising.
Drug-induced porphyria (rare).
Excessive urination leading to sodium loss.
Peripheral neuritis (see Glossary)—numbness, tingling, pain, loss of strength in arms and legs.
Parkinson-like disorders (see Glossary)—usually mild and infrequent; more likely to occur in the elderly.

▷ **Possible Effects on Sexual Function:** Decreased libido, increased libido (antidepressant effect), male impotence, inhibited female orgasm, male and female breast enlargement, milk production, swelling of testicles.

▷ **Adverse Effects That May Mimic Natural Diseases or Disorders**
Liver toxicity may suggest viral hepatitis.

Natural Diseases or Disorders That May Be Activated by This Drug
Latent diabetes, epilepsy, glaucoma, prostatism.

Possible Effects on Laboratory Tests
White blood cell and platelet counts: decreased.
Blood glucose levels: increased and decreased (fluctuations).
Liver function tests: increased liver enzymes (ALT/GPT, AST/GOT and alkaline phosphatase), increased bilirubin.

CAUTION
1. Dose must be individualized. Report for follow-up evaluation and laboratory tests as directed by your physician.
2. It is advisable to withhold this drug if electroconvulsive therapy (ECT, "shock" treatment) is to be used to treat your depression.

Precautions for Use

By Infants and Children: Safety and effectiveness for those under 6 years of age not established.

By Those over 60 Years of Age: Usual dosage is 30 to 50 mg daily in divided doses. During the first 2 weeks of treatment, watch for confusion, agitation, forgetfulness, delusions disorientation and hallucinations. Reduction of dosage or discontinuation may be necessary. Unsteadiness may predispose to falling and injury. This drug can increase the degree of impaired urination associated with prostate gland enlargement (prostatism).

▷ **Advisability of Use During Pregnancy**

Pregnancy Category: D. See Pregnancy Code at the back of this book.
Animal studies: Results are inconclusive.
Human studies: No defects reported in 21 exposures to amitriptyline, a closely related drug. Adequate studies of pregnant women are not available for this drug.
Avoid use of drug during first 3 months. Use during last 6 months only if clearly needed. Ask your physician for guidance.

Advisability of Use if Breast-Feeding
Presence of this drug in breast milk: Yes, in small amounts.
Monitor nursing infant closely and discontinue drug or nursing if adverse effects develop: excessive drowsiness and failure to feed.

Habit-Forming Potential: Psychological or physical dependence is rare and unexpected.

718   Nortriptyline

Effects of Overdosage: Confusion, hallucinations, marked drowsiness, heart palpitations, dilated pupils, tremors, stupor, deep sleep, coma, convulsions.

Suggested Periodic Examinations While Taking This Drug (at physician's discretion)
Complete blood cell counts, liver function tests, serial blood pressure readings and electrocardiograms.

▷ **While Taking This Drug, Observe the Following**
Foods: No restrictions. This drug may increase the appetite and cause excessive weight gain.
Beverages: No restrictions. May be taken with milk.

▷ *Alcohol:* Avoid completely. This drug can markedly increase the intoxicating effects of alcohol and accentuate its depressant action on brain function.
Tobacco Smoking: May hasten the elimination of this drug. Higher doses may be necessary.

▷ *Other Drugs*
Nortriptyline may *increase* the effects of
- atropinelike drugs (see Drug Class Section).
- dicoumarol, and increase the risk of bleeding.
- epinephrine (Adrenalin).
- phenytoin (Dilantin) by increasing blood levels.
- warfarin (Coumadin).

Nortriptyline may *decrease* the effects of
- clonidine (Catapres).
- ephedrine (Primatene tablets).
- guanethidine (Ismelin).

Nortriptyline *taken concurrently* with
- activated charcoal will decrease and almost block absorption (useful in overdose situations).
- disulfiram (Antabuse) may cause acute dementia: confusion, disorientation, hallucinations.
- fluconazole (Diflucan) may result in large increases in nortriptyline levels and result in toxic reactions.
- monoamine oxidase (MAO) inhibitor drugs may cause high fever, delirium and convulsions (see Drug Class Section).
- norepinephrine can cause a serious increase in blood pressure, abnormal heart rhythmns and fast heart rate. Avoid the combination.
- phenothiazines (see Drug Class) can result in increased phenothiazine levels and toxicity as well as additive anticholinergic problems.
- thyroid preparations may impair heart rhythm and function. Ask physician for guidance regarding adjustment of thyroid dose.

The following drugs may *increase* the effects of nortriptyline
- cimetidine (Tagamet), and cause nortriptyline toxicity.
- fluoxetine (Prozac).
- quinidine (Quinaglute, etc,), and cause nortriptyline toxicity.

The following drugs may *decrease* the effects of nortriptyline
- barbiturates (see Drug Classes), and reduce its effectiveness.
- carbamazepine (Tegretol).
- conjugated estrogens.

▷ *Driving, Hazardous Activities:* This drug may impair mental alertness, judgment, physical coordination and reaction time. Avoid hazardous activities.

Aviation Note: The use of this drug *is a disqualification* for piloting. Consult a designated Aviation Medical Examiner.

Exposure to Sun: Use caution. This drug may cause photosensitivity (see Glossary).

Exposure to Heat: This drug can inhibit sweating and impair the body's adaptation to hot environments, increasing the risk of heat stroke. Avoid saunas.

Exposure to Cold: The elderly should use caution and avoid conditions conducive to hypothermia (see Glossary).

Discontinuation: Best to slowly discontinue this drug. Abrupt withdrawal after long-term use can cause headache, malaise and nausea.

OFLOXACIN (oh FLOX a sin)

Introduced: 1984 **Prescription:** USA: Yes **Available as Generic:** USA: No **Class:** Anti-infective **Controlled Drug:** USA: No
Brand Name: Floxin, Ocuflox

Warning: Reports are being made for some drugs in this class which find tendon rupture as a rare adverse effect. Ask your doctor about limits on strenuous exercise while you are taking this medicine. A rare idiosyncratic reaction has also been reported which presents as mental confusion and disorientation. Use of this medicine after head trauma may be a risk factor. If you have suffered a fall, ask your doctor if a medicine in a different antibiotic class should be substituted. If you are taking this drug and notice a change in your thinking, call your doctor.

BENEFITS versus RISKS	
Possible Benefits	*Possible Risks*
HIGHLY EFFECTIVE TREATMENT FOR INFECTIONS OF THE LOWER RESPIRATORY TRACT, URINARY TRACT, SKIN AND SKIN STRUCTURES, due to susceptible organisms EFFECTIVE TREATMENT FOR SOME SEXUALLY TRANSMITTED DISEASES Effective treatment for some infections of the prostate gland	Rare but serious allergic reactions Rare seizures and hallucinations Dizziness (1–5%) Nausea (3–10%), diarrhea (1–4%)

▷ **Principal Uses**

As a Single Drug Product: Uses currently included in FDA approved labeling: (1) Treats responsive infections (in adults) of: (1) the lower respiratory tract (lungs and bronchial tubes); (2) the urinary tract (kidneys, bladder, urethra and prostate gland); (3) skin and related tissues; (4) certain sexually transmitted diseases: gonorrheal and chlamydial infections of the urethra and cervix; (5) infections of the eye.

Other (unlabeled) generally accepted uses: (1) May have a role in combination therapy of leprosy; (2) used to treat traveler's diarrhea; (3) treats bone infections in combination with surgery.

How This Drug Works: By interfering with the bacterial enzyme DNA gyrase (required for DNA synthesis and cell reproduction), this drug arrests bacterial growth (in low concentrations) and destroys bacteria (in high concentrations).

Available Dosage Forms and Strengths
>   Tablets — 200 mg, 300 mg, 400 mg
> Ophthalmic solution — 3 mg per ml

▷ **Usual Adult Dosage Range:** 200 mg to 400 mg/12 hours, depending upon the nature and severity of the infection. The total daily dosage should not exceed 800 mg. **Note: Actual dosage and administration schedule must be determined by the physician for each patient individually.**

Conditions Requiring Dosing Adjustments
Liver function: Dosage adjustments do not appear to be needed.
Kidney function: In patients with moderate kidney failure, the usual dose can be given every 24 hours. In patients with severe failure, one half the usual dose should be given every 24 hours.

▷ **Dosing Instructions:** Do not take with food. The tablet may be crushed and is preferably taken 1 hour before or 2 hours after eating. Drink fluids liberally during the entire course of treatment. Avoid antacids containing aluminum or magnesium and supplements containing iron or zinc for 2 hours before and after dosing.

Usual Duration of Use: Use on a regular schedule for up to 10 days determines effectiveness in eradicating the infection. The drug should be continued for at least 2 days after all indications of infection have disappeared. Prostate gland infections may require continual treatment for 6 weeks. Long-term use requires periodic physician evaluation of response.

Possible Advantages of This Drug
Very broad spectrum of antibacterial activity.
Capable of establishing effective drug levels throughout the prostate gland.
Effective one-dose treatment for uncomplicated gonorrheal infection of the urethra.
No significant effect on kidney function.
No reports of serious drug-induced colitis.

▷ **This Drug Should Not Be Taken If**
- you have had an allergic reaction to it previously.
- you are pregnant or breast-feeding.
- you have a seizure disorder that is not adequately controlled.
- it is prescribed for a person under 18 years of age (as it may cause arthropathies-joint problems, as well as defects in cartilage).

▷ **Inform Your Physician Before Taking This Drug If**
- you are allergic to cinoxacin (Cinobac), nalidixic acid (NegGram), ciprofloxacin (Cipro) or norfloxacin (Noroxin).
- you have a history of a seizure disorder or a circulatory disorder of the brain.
- you have a history of psychosis or intracranial pressure elevation.

- you have impaired liver or kidney function.
- you are taking any form of probenecid or theophylline.

Possible Side-Effects (natural, expected and unavoidable drug actions)
Superinfections: vaginitis (1–3%). (See Superinfection in the Glossary.)

▷ **Possible Adverse Effects** (unusual, unexpected and infrequent reactions)
If any of the following develop, consult your physician promptly for guidance.

Mild Adverse Effects
Allergic Reactions: Rash (1–3%), itching (1–3%), fever (1–3%).
Headache (1–9%), dizziness (1–5%), weakness (1–3%), drowsiness (1–3%), nervousness (1–3%), joint and muscle pain (less than 1%), insomnia (3–7%), visual disturbances (1–3%).
Decreased appetite (1–3%), altered taste (1–3%), dry mouth (1–3%), nausea (3–10%), vomiting (1–3%), indigestion (1%), diarrhea (1–4%).

Serious Adverse Effects
Allergic Reactions: Anaphylactoid reactions (see Glossary).
Idiosyncratic Reactions: Rare aphasia may be idiosyncratic.
Central nervous system stimulation: restlessness, tremor, confusion, hallucinations, seizures (all very rare).
Intracranial hypertension (rare).
Drug-induced hepatitis (rare).

▷ **Possible Effects on Sexual Function:** Painful menstruation, excessive menstrual bleeding.

▷ **Natural Diseases or Disorders That May Be Activated by This Drug**
Latent epilepsy.

Possible Effects on Laboratory Tests
Complete blood cell counts: rarely decreased lymphocytes; rarely increased eosinophils.
Liver function tests: rarely increased liver enzymes (ALT/GPT, AST/GOT).
Blood creatinine level: rarely increased.
Blood glucose levels: rare fluctuations.

CAUTION
1. Crystal formation in the kidney may occur with high doses and prolonged use. This can be prevented by drinking large amounts of water, up to 2 quarts/24 hours.
2. Drugs of this class may decrease the formation of saliva and predispose to the development of dental cavities or gum disease. Consult your dentist if dry mouth persists.
3. Very rare case reports of aphasia, disorientation and confusion has occurred. Stop the drug and call your doctor immediately if this occurs.

Precautions for Use
By Infants and Children: Safety and effectiveness for those under 18 years of age not established. Avoid the use of this drug completely. It can impair normal bone growth and development in immature animals.
By Those over 60 Years of Age: Impaired kidney function will require dosage reduction.
If you are taking theophylline concurrently with this drug, observe closely for possible theophylline accumulation and toxicity.

Ofloxacin

▷ **Advisability of Use During Pregnancy**
Pregnancy Category: C. See Pregnancy Code at the back of this book.
Animal studies: Mild skeletal defects due to this drug were found in rat studies; toxic effects on the fetus were shown in rat and rabbit studies. This drug can impair normal bone development in immature dogs.
Human studies: Adequate studies of pregnant women are not available. However, the potential for adverse effects on fetal bone development contraindicates the use of this drug during entire pregnancy.

Advisability of Use if Breast-Feeding
Presence of this drug in breast milk: Yes.
Avoid drug or refrain from nursing.

Habit-Forming Potential: None.

Effects of Overdosage: Nausea, vomiting, diarrhea, confusion, hallucinations, seizures.

Possible Effects of Long-Term Use: Superinfections (see Glossary).

Suggested Periodic Examinations While Taking This Drug (at physician's discretion)
Liver function tests, urine analysis.

▷ **While Taking This Drug, Observe the Following**
Foods: No restrictions.
Beverages: No restrictions. May be taken with milk.
▷ *Alcohol:* No interactions expected.
Tobacco Smoking: No interactions expected.
▷ *Other Drugs*
Ofloxacin may *increase* the effects of
- theophylline, and cause theophylline toxicity.
- warfarin (Coumadin) and lead to bleeding.

The following drug may *increase* the effects of ofloxacin
- probenecid (Benemid).

The following drugs may *decrease* the effects of ofloxacin
- antacids containing aluminum or magnesium can reduce the absorption of ofloxacin and lessen its effectiveness.
- iron salts.
- sucralfate (Carafate).
- zinc salts.

▷ *Driving, Hazardous Activities:* This drug may cause drowsiness, dizziness and impaired vision. Restrict activities as necessary.
Aviation Note: The use of this drug **may be a disqualification** for piloting. Consult a designated Aviation Medical Examiner.
Exposure to Sun: This drug may rarely cause photosensitivity (see Glossary).
Discontinuation: If you experience no adverse effects from this drug, take the full course prescribed for best results.

OLSALAZINE (ohl SAL a zeen)

Introduced: 1987 **Prescription:** USA: Yes; Canada: Yes **Available as Generic:** USA: No; Canada: No **Class:** Bowel anti-inflammatory **Controlled Drug:** USA: No; Canada: No

Brand Name: Dipentum

BENEFITS versus RISKS
Possible Benefits   *Possible Risks*
EFFECTIVE SUPPRESSION OF INFLAMMATORY BOWEL DISEASE   RARE BONE MARROW DEPRESSION (see Glossary) Rare drug-induced hepatitis Occasional aggravation of ulcerative colitis

▷ **Principal Uses**
　As a Single Drug Product: Uses currently included in FDA approved labeling: Used to maintain remission of chronic ulcerative colitis and proctitis.
　Other (unlabeled) generally accepted uses: Has a role in treatment of active ulcerative colitis.

How This Drug Works: This drug suppresses the formation of prostaglandins (and related compounds), tissue substances that induce inflammation, tissue destruction and diarrhea—the main features of ulcerative colitis and proctitis.

Available Dosage Forms and Strengths
　　Capsules — 250 mg
　Tablet (in Canada only) — 500 mg

▷ **Recommended Dosage Ranges** (Actual dosage and administration schedule must be determined by the physician for each patient individually.)
　Infants and Children: Dosage not established.
　12 to 60 Years of Age: 500 mg twice daily, morning and evening.
　Over 60 Years of Age: Same as 12 to 60 years of age.

Conditions Requiring Dosing Adjustments
　Liver function: Dosage adjustments do not appear to be needed in liver compromise. This drug is also a rare cause of hepatoxicity (granulomatous hepatitis), and should be used with caution in patients with compromised livers.
　Kidney function: Some of the metabolites of olsalazine are eliminated by the kidneys. There is potential for kidney damage by one of these compounds, and the drug should be used as a benefit to risk in patients with compromised kidneys.

▷ **Dosing Instructions:** The capsule may be opened and taken with food, preferably with breakfast and dinner.

Usual Duration of Use: Use on a regular schedule for 1 to 3 weeks determines effectiveness in controlling the symptoms of ulcerative colitis. Long-term use (months to years) requires physician supervision.

Olsalazine

Possible Advantages of This Drug
Does not inhibit sperm production or cause infertility.

▷ **This Drug Should Not Be Taken If**
- you have had an allergic reaction to it previously.
- you have severely impaired kidney function.
- you are allergic to aspirin.

▷ **Inform Your Physician Before Taking This Drug If**
- you are allergic to aspirin (or other salicylates), mesalamine or sulfasalazine.
- you are allergic by nature: history of hay fever, asthma, hives, eczema.
- you have impaired kidney function.
- you have severe liver disease.
- you are currently taking sulfasalazine (Azulfidine).

Possible Side-Effects (natural, expected and unavoidable drug actions)
None.

▷ **Possible Adverse Effects** (unusual, unexpected and infrequent reactions)
If any of the following develop, consult your physician promptly for guidance.

Mild Adverse Effects
Allergic Reactions: Skin rash (2.3%), itching (1.3%).
Headache (5%), drowsiness (1.8%), depression (1.5%), dizziness (1%).
Loss of appetite (1.3%), indigestion (4%), nausea (5%), vomiting (1%), stomach pain (10%), diarrhea (11%).
Paresthesias (rare).
Blurred vision (rare).
Joint aches and pains (4%).

Serious Adverse Effects
Allergic Reactions: Dermatitis, hair loss (rare).
Rare bone marrow depression (see Glossary): fatigue, weakness, fever, sore throat, abnormal bleeding or bruising.
Rare drug-induced hepatitis (see Glossary).
Rare pancreatitis.
Rare kidney damage.
Pericarditis (rare).
Spasm of the bronchi of the lung (rare).

▷ **Possible Effects on Sexual Function:** Rare impotence, excessive menstrual flow.

Possible Effects on Laboratory Tests
Complete blood cell counts: decreased red cells, hemoglobin, white cells and platelets; increased eosinophils.
Liver function tests: increased liver enzymes (ALT/GPT, AST/GOT and alkaline phosphatase), increased bilirubin.
Urinalysis: red blood cells and protein present.

CAUTION
1. Report promptly any signs of infection or unusual bleeding or bruising.
2. Report promptly any indications of active or intensified ulcerative colitis: abdominal cramping, bloody diarrhea, fever.

Precautions for Use
By Infants and Children: Safety and effectiveness for those under 12 years of age not established.
By Those over 60 Years of Age: None.

▷ **Advisability of Use During Pregnancy**
Pregnancy Category: C. See Pregnancy Code at the back of this book.
Animal studies: Rat studies reveal toxic effects on the fetus, retarded bone development, and impaired development of internal organs.
Human studies: Adequate studies of pregnant women are not available.
Use this drug only if clearly needed. Ask your physician for guidance.

Advisability of Use if Breast-Feeding
Presence of this drug in breast milk: Unknown.
Avoid drug or refrain from nursing.

Habit-Forming Potential: None.

Effects of Overdosage: Headache, dizziness, nausea, vomiting, abdominal cramping.

Possible Effects of Long-Term Use: Bone marrow depression (impaired production of blood cells).

Suggested Periodic Examinations While Taking This Drug (at physician's discretion)
Complete blood cell counts.
Liver function tests.
Kidney function tests, urinalysis.

▷ **While Taking This Drug, Observe the Following**
Foods: No restrictions. Follow prescribed diet.
Beverages: No restrictions. May be taken with milk.
▷ *Alcohol:* No interactions expected.
Tobacco Smoking: No interactions expected.
▷ *Other Drugs:* No interactions expected.
▷ *Driving, Hazardous Activities:* This drug may cause drowsiness or dizziness. Restrict activities as necessary.
Aviation Note: The use of this drug **may be a disqualification** for piloting. Consult a designated Aviation Medical Examiner.
Exposure to Sun: Use caution. This drug can cause photosensitization (see Glossary).

OMEPRAZOLE (oh ME pra zohl)

Introduced: 1986 **Prescription:** USA: Yes; Canada: Yes **Available as Generic:** USA: No; Canada: No **Class:** Antiulcer, gastric acid inhibitor
Controlled Drug: USA: No; Canada: No

Brand Name: Prilosec, ✦Losec

Omeprazole

BENEFITS versus RISKS	
Possible Benefits	*Possible Risks*
VERY EFFECTIVE TREATMENT OF CONDITIONS ASSOCIATED WITH EXCESSIVE PRODUCTION OF GASTRIC ACID: Zollinger-Ellison syndrome, mastocytosis, endocrine adenoma VERY EFFECTIVE TREATMENT OF REFLUX ESOPHAGITIS VERY EFFECTIVE TREATMENT OF GASTRIC AND DUODENAL ULCERS	Rare aplastic anemia (see Glossary) Rare liver failure

▷ **Principal Uses**

As a Single Drug Product: Uses currently included in FDA approved labeling: (1) Inhibits stomach acid formation in: acute and chronic gastritis, reflux esophagitis, Zollinger-Ellison syndrome, mastocytosis, endocrine adenomas and active duodenal ulcer; (2) recently approved for long-term use in erosive esophagitis.

Other (unlabeled) generally accepted uses: (1) Used to help gastric ulcers; (2) combination therapy with clarithramycin in patients with positive Helicobacter pylori cultures; (3) may have a role in severe bleeding of the stomach (hemorrhagic gastritis).

How This Drug Works: Inhibits a specific enzyme system (proton pump H/K ATPase) in the stomach lining, stopping production of stomach acid and thereby (1) eliminates a principal cause of the condition under treatment, and (2) creates an environment conducive to healing.

Available Dosage Forms and Strengths

Capsules, delayed-release — 20 mg

▷ **Usual Adult Dosage Range:** Reflux esophagitis: 20 mg to 40 mg once daily for 4 to 8 weeks.

Excessive stomach acid conditions: 60 mg once daily for as long as necessary.

Gastric and duodenal ulcer: 20 mg to 40 mg once daily for 4 to 8 weeks.

In extreme conditions, doses of 120 mg three times a day have been used.

Note: Actual dosage and administration schedule must be determined by the physician for each patient individually.

Conditions Requiring Dosing Adjustments

Liver function: Dosing adjustments are not defined, however, patients should be monitored closely.

Kidney function: Dosage adjustments do not appear to be needed.

▷ **Dosing Instructions:** Take immediately before eating, preferably the morning meal. The capsule should be swallowed whole without opening; the contents should not be crushed or chewed. This drug may be taken concurrently with antacids if they are needed to relieve stomach pain.

Usual Duration of Use: Use on a regular schedule for 2 to 3 weeks determines benefit in suppressing stomach acid production. Long-term use (months to years) requires periodic physician evaluation of response.

Omeprazole

Possible Advantages of This Drug
Effectively inhibits acid secretion at all times: basal conditions (stomach empty and at rest) and following food, alcohol, smoking or other stimulants.
Is more effective than H-2 receptor blocking drugs in treating severe reflux esophagitis and refractory duodenal ulcer.

Currently a "Drug of Choice"
for the short-term treatment of severe reflux esophagitis and for the long-term treatment of Zollinger-Ellison syndrome and erosive esophagitis.

▷ **This Drug Should Not Be Taken If**
- you have had an allergic reaction to it previously.
- you have a currently active bone marrow or blood cell disorder.

▷ **Inform Your Physician Before Taking This Drug If**
- you have a history of liver disease or impaired liver function.
- you have a history of any type of bone marrow or blood cell disorder, especially one that is drug-induced.
- you are currently taking any anticoagulant medication, diazepam (Valium) or phenytoin (Dilantin, etc.).

Possible Side-Effects (natural, expected and unavoidable drug actions)
None reported.

▷ **Possible Adverse Effects** (unusual, unexpected and infrequent reactions)
If any of the following develop, consult your physician promptly for guidance.

Mild Adverse Effects
Allergic Reactions: Skin rash (1.5%), itching.
Headache (6.9%), dizziness (1.5%), muscle pain or ringing in the ears (1%), drowsiness, paresthesias, weakness (1.1%).
Indigestion (2.4%), nausea (2.2%), vomiting (1.5%), diarrhea (3%), constipation (1.1%).

Serious Adverse Effects
Allergic Reactions: rare allergic kidney damage (interstitial nephritis).
Rare bone marrow depression (see Glossary): fatigue, weakness, fever, sore throat, infections, abnormal bleeding or bruising.
Rare liver damage with jaundice (see Glossary).
Rare urinary tract infection: painful urination, cloudy or bloody urine.
Rare chest pain or angina.
Rare half-facial pain.
Yeast infection (Candida) of the esophagus.
Rare kidney inflammation (interstitial nephritis).

Possible Effects on Sexual Function
Drug-induced male breast enlargement and tenderness (gynecomastia) has been rarely reported.

▷ **Adverse Effects That May Mimic Natural Diseases or Disorders**
Persistent infection or bruising may reflect bone marrow depression; blood counts advisable.
Liver reactions may suggest viral hepatitis.

728 Omeprazole

Possible Effects on Laboratory Tests
Complete blood cell counts: decreased red cells, hemoglobin, white cells and platelets.
Blood glucose level: decreased.
Liver function tests: increased liver enzymes (ALT/GPT, AST/GOT and alkaline phosphatase), increased bilirubin.

CAUTION
1. Follow your physician's instructions exactly regarding the length of time you take this drug. Do not extend its use without his guidance.
2. Report promptly any indications of infection.
3. Inform your physician if you plan to take any other medications (prescription or over-the-counter) while taking omeprazole.
4. While this drug effectively treats ulcers, it does not preclude the possibility of cancer of the stomach.

Precautions for Use
By Infants and Children: Safety and effectiveness for those under 12 years of age not established.
By Those over 60 Years of Age: Slower elimination of this drug makes it possible to achieve satisfactory response with smaller doses; this reduces the risk of adverse effects. Limit the daily dose to 20 mg if possible.

▷ Advisability of Use During Pregnancy
Pregnancy Category: C. See Pregnancy Code at the back of this book.
Animal studies: No drug-induced birth defects found in rats; drug-induced embryo and fetal toxicity were demonstrated in rats and rabbits.
Human studies: Adequate studies of pregnant women are not available.
Avoid use if possible. Use only if clearly necessary and for the shortest possible time.

Advisability of Use if Breast-Feeding
Presence of this drug in breast milk: Unknown.
Avoid drug or refrain from nursing.

Habit-Forming Potential: None.

Effects of Overdosage:
Possible drowsiness, dizziness, lethargy, abdominal pain, nausea.

Possible Effects of Long-Term Use:
Some long-term (2 year) studies in rats revealed the development of drug-induced carcinoid tumors in the stomach. To date, long-term use of this drug (more than 5 years) in humans has not revealed any drug-induced tumor potential. Pending more studies of long-term human use, it is advisable to limit the use of this drug to the shortest duration possible.

Suggested Periodic Examinations While Taking This Drug (at physician's discretion)
Complete blood cell counts.

▷ While Taking This Drug, Observe the Following
Foods: No restrictions.
Beverages: No restrictions. May be taken with milk.
▷ *Alcohol:* No interactions expected. However, alcohol is best avoided; it stimulates the secretion of stomach acid.

Tobacco Smoking: No interactions expected. However, smoking is best avoided; it may stimulate the secretion of stomach acid.

▷ *Other Drugs*
Omeprazole may *increase* the effects of
- anticoagulants (warfarin, etc.) and increase the risk of bleeding.
- cyclosporine by increasing the level (decreased levels also reported).
- diazepam (Valium) and cause excessive sedation.
- digoxin and lead to toxicity.
- phenytoin (Dilantin, etc.) and cause phenytoin toxicity.

Omeprazole may *decrease* the effects of
- ampicillin.
- amoxicillin.
- iron preparations.
- ketoconazole (Nizoral).

▷ *Driving, Hazardous Activities:* This drug may cause drowsiness and dizziness. Limit activities as necessary.

Aviation Note: The use of this drug **may be a disqualification** for piloting. Consult a designated Aviation Medical Examiner.

Exposure to Sun: No restrictions.

Discontinuation: The duration of use will vary according to the condition under treatment and individual patient response. Premature discontinuation could result in incomplete healing or prompt recurrence of symptoms.

ONDANSETRON (On DAN sa tron)

Introduced: 1993 **Prescription:** USA: Yes; Canada: Yes **Available as Generic:** USA: No; Canada: No **Class:** Antiemetic, 5HT3 antagonist
Controlled Drug: USA: No; Canada: No
Brand Name: Zofran

BENEFITS versus RISKS	
Possible Benefits	*Possible Risks*
EFFECTIVE ORAL TREATMENT AND RELIEF OR PREVENTION OF SEVERE VOMITING WHICH CAN OCCUR AFTER SOME TYPES OF CHEMOTHERAPY OR RADIATION TREATMENTS	Bronchospasm (rare) Grand mal seizures (rare) Rare liver toxicity Rare heart rate and rhythm changes Rare low potassium

▷ **Principal Uses**
As a Single Drug Product: Uses currently included in FDA approved labeling: (1) Prevention of nausea and vomiting associated with initial and repeat courses of chemotherapy; (2) Treatment or prevention of postoperative nausea and vomiting.

Other (unlabeled) generally accepted uses: (1) Prevention or treatment of emesis (vomiting) caused by radiation therapy; (2) may have a role in treating schizophrenia.

How This Drug Works: Ondansetron antagonizes 5HT3 receptors. It appears to block vomiting by blocking serotonin (a chemical causing vomiting) at 5HT3 receptors.

Ondansetron

Available Dosage Forms and Strengths
    Tablets — 4 mg
            — 8 mg
    Intravenous — 2 mg per ml

How To Store
    Keep at room temperature. Avoid exposing this medicine to extreme humidity.

▷ **Recommended Dosage Ranges** (Actual dosage and administration schedule must be determined by the physician for each patient individually.)
    Infants and Children: Little information is available regarding use in those less than four years old.
    4 to 12 Years of Age: One four mg tablet given three times by mouth daily. The method and frequency is the same as for adults.
    12 to 60 Years of Age: One 8 mg tablet given three times a day. The first dose should be given 30 minutes before the start of the emetogenic chemotherapy. Subsequent doses should be given 4 hours and 8 hours after the first dose.
    Over 60 Years of Age: Same as 12 to 60 years of age.

Conditions Requiring Dosing Adjustments
    Liver function: Maximum dose in people with severe liver failure is 8 mg per day.
    Kidney function: Studies have not been conducted in patients with impaired kidneys. Decision to use ondansetron in these patients must be made by your physician. Only 10% of the drug is removed unchanged by the kidneys.

▷ **Dosing Instructions:** May be taken on an empty stomach.
    Usual Duration of Use: Since chemotherapy can cause vomiting long after it has been given, continual use on a regular schedule for 3 days is usually necessary.

Possible Advantages of This Drug
    Effective oral prevention of severe vomiting caused by some kinds of chemotherapy which have been poorly controlled by earlier agents.

Currently a "Drug of Choice"
    for control of vomiting secondary to emetogenic (likely to cause vomiting) cancer chemotherapy.

▷ **This Drug Should Not Be Taken If**
- you have had an allergic reaction to any dosage form of it previously.

▷ **Inform Your Physician Before Taking This Drug If**
- you have a history of liver disease.
- you have a history of kidney disease.
- you have a history of alcoholism.
- you are unsure of how much to take or how often to take ondansetron.

Possible Side-Effects (natural, expected and unavoidable drug actions)
    Constipation, sedation.

▷ **Possible Adverse Effects** (unusual, unexpected and infrequent reactions)
    If any of the following develop, consult your physician promptly for guidance.

Mild Adverse Effects
　Allergic Reactions: Skin rash (1%).
　Headache (up to 40%), sedation (6–10%), dizziness and lightheadedness (5%), constipation (3–11%), diarrhea (7%), dry mouth (5%).
Serious Adverse Effects
　Allergic Reactions: Anaphylaxis (rare).
　Rare: Extrapyramidal reactions (abnormal body movements), seizures, angina, tachycardia, arrhythmias, bronchospasm, liver failure, hypokalemia (low potassium).

▷ **Possible Effects on Sexual Function:** None reported.

Possible Delayed Adverse Effects: None reported.

▷ **Adverse Effects That May Mimic Natural Diseases or Disorders**
　Changes in liver enzymes may mimic hepatitis; however, specific antibodies will not be present. Bronchospasm may mimic asthma.

Natural Diseases or Disorders That May Be Activated by This Drug
　Epilepsy, asthma.

Possible Effects on Laboratory Tests
　Liver function tests: Transient increases in SGPT, SGOT and bilirubin.

CAUTION
　1. Even though you do not feel an urge to vomit, continue ondansetron for the prescribed length of therapy. The vomit causing effect of cancer chemotherapy or radiation therapy continues after the medicine or radiation has been given.

Precautions for Use
By Infants and Children:
　Safety and effectiveness for those under 3 years of age not established.
By Those over 60 Years of Age: Same as for general adult population.

▷ **Advisability of Use During Pregnancy**
Pregnancy Category: B. See Pregnancy Code at the back of this book.
　Animal studies: Ondansetron and its metabolites pass into the milk. No adverse effects on gestation, postnatal development or reproductive performance has been observed in rats.
　Human studies: Adequate studies of pregnant women are not available. Ask your physician for guidance.

Advisability of Use if Breast-Feeding
　Presence of this drug in breast milk: This medicine is excreted in the milk of rats; however, human data is not available. Caution should be used if this medicine is to be used in nursing mothers.

Habit-Forming Potential: None.

Effects of Overdosage: Doses 10 times greater than recommended have not resulted in illness.

Possible Effects of Long-Term Use: Not indicated for long term use.

Suggested Periodic Examinations While Taking This Drug (at physician's discretion)
　Observe for vomiting occurrence and frequency.

▷ **While Taking This Drug, Observe the Following**
Foods: No restrictions.
Beverages: No restrictions.
▷ *Alcohol:* Additive sedation and potential additive urge to vomit if alcohol is taken in large doses. Alcohol abuse which has led to liver problems may limit the the total dose which can be given.
Tobacco Smoking: No direct clinical documenting restrictions.
Marijuana Smoking: May induce additive sedation and provide additive antiemetic effects.
▷ *Other Drugs*
The following drugs may *increase* the effects of ondansetron
- allopurinol (Zyloprim).
- cimetidine (Tamamet).
- disulfiram (Antabuse).
- fluconazole (Diflucan).
- isoniazid (Nydrazid).
- macrolide antibiotics (erythromycin, azithromycin and clarithromycin).
- metronidazole (Flagyl).
- monoamine oxidase inhibitor antidepressants (MAO inhibitors—Nardil).

The following drugs may *decrease* the effects of ondansetron
- barbiturates.
- carbamazepine (Tegretol).
- phenylbutazone (Butazolidin, Azolid).
- phenytoin (Dilantin).
- rifampin (Rifadin) and rifabutin (Mycobutin).
- tolbutamide (Orinase).

▷ *Driving, Hazardous Activities:* This drug may cause drowsiness and dizziness. Restrict activities as necessary.
Aviation Note: The use of this drug **may be a disqualification** for piloting. Consult a designated Aviation Medical Examiner.
Exposure to Sun: No restrictions.
Discontinuation: Ondansetron may be stopped after you've completed the prescribed course (usually 3 days) of therapy.

ORAL CONTRACEPTIVES (or al kon tra SEP tivs)

Other Names: Estrogens/progestins, OCs, Birth control pills

Introduced: 1956   **Prescription:** USA: Yes; Canada: Yes   **Available as Generic:** USA: Yes, in some forms; Canada: No   **Class:** Female sex hormones   **Controlled Drug:** USA: No; Canada: No

Brand Names: Brevicon, Demulen, Desogen, Enovid, Genora, Jenest 28, Levlen, Loestrin, Lo/Ovral, Micronor*, ◆Minestrin 1/20, Mini-Ovral, Modicon, NEE, Nelova, Nelova 1/50 M, Nelova 10/11, Norcept-E 1/35, Nordette, Norethin 1/35E, Norethin 1/50M, Norinyl, Norlestrin, Nor-Q.D.*, Ortho Cyclen, Ortho Tri-Cyclen, Ortho-Novum, Ovcon, Ovral, Ovrette*, ◆Synphasic, Tri-Levlen, Tri-Norinyl, Triphasil, Triquilar, Zovia

*"Mini-Pill" type, contains progestin only.

Oral Contraceptives

BENEFITS versus RISKS	
Possible Benefits	*Possible Risks*
HIGHLY EFFECTIVE FOR CONTRACEPTIVE PROTECTION	SERIOUS, LIFE-THREATENING THROMBOEMBOLIC DISORDERS in susceptible individuals
Moderately effective as adjunctive treatment in management of excessive menses and endometriosis	Hypertension
	Fluid retention
	Intensification of migrainelike headaches
	Intensification of fibrocystic breast changes
	Accelerated growth of uterine fibroid tumors
	Drug-induced hepatitis with jaundice
	Benign liver tumors (rare)

▷ **Principal Uses**

As a Single Drug Product: Uses currently included in FDA approved labeling: (1) Prevention of conception. The "Mini-Pill" contains only one component—a progestin. This has been shown to be slightly less effective than the combination of estrogen and progestin in preventing pregnancy; (2) used in cases where women do not make enough hormones (female hypogonadism); (3) helps decrease excessive blood flow at menstruation (menorrhagia).

Other (unlabeled) generally accepted uses: (1) May be of benefit in abnormal hair growth in women (hirsutism); (2) has a protective effect against osteoporosis.

As a Combination Drug Product [CD]:

Uses currently included in FDA approved labeling: (1) Most oral contraceptives consist of a combination of an estrogen and a progestin. These products are the most effective form of medicinal contraception available; (2) they are sometimes used to treat menstrual irregularity, excessively heavy menstrual flow and endometriosis.

Other (unlabeled) generally accepted uses: (1) Gestodene has been reported to inhibit certain breast cancer cell lines. Clinical studies are needed; (2) may have a protective effect against osteoporosis; triphasic oral contraceptives can help in the prevention or treatment of menopause symptoms.

How This Drug Works: When estrogen and progestin are taken in sufficient dosage and on a regular basis, the blood and tissue levels of these hormones increase to resemble those that occur during pregnancy. This results in suppression of the two pituitary gland hormones that normally cause ovulation (the formation and release of an egg by the ovary). In addition, these drugs may (1) alter the cervical mucus so that it resists the passage of sperm, and (2) alter the lining of the uterus so that it resists implantation of the egg (if ovulation occurs).

Available Dosage Forms and Strengths

Tablets — several combinations of synthetic estrogens and progestins in varying strengths; see the package label of the brand prescribed.

Oral Contraceptives

▷ **Usual Adult Dosage Range:** Initiate treatment with the first tablet on the fifth day after the onset of menstruation. Follow with 1 tablet daily (taken at the same time each day) for 21 consecutive days. Resume treatment on the eighth day following the last tablet taken during the preceding cycle. The schedule is to take the drug daily for 3 weeks and to omit it for 1 week. For the Mini-Pill (progestin only), initiate treatment on the first day of menstruation and take 1 tablet daily, every day, throughout the year (no interruption). **Note: Actual dosage and administration schedule must be determined by the physician for each patient individually.**

Conditions Requiring Dosing Adjustments
Liver function: These agents are contraindicated in liver disease.
Kidney function: Oral contraceptives are not significantly eliminated by the kidneys.

▷ **Dosing Instructions:** The tablets may be crushed and taken with or after food to reduce stomach irritation. To ensure regular (every day) use and uniform blood levels, it is best to take the tablet at the same time daily.

Usual Duration of Use: According to individual needs and circumstances. Long-term use (months to years) requires physician supervision and evaluation every 6 months.

▷ **This Drug Should Not Be Taken If**
- you have had an allergic reaction to any dosage form of it.
- you have a history of thrombophlebitis, embolism, heart attack or stroke.
- you have breast cancer.
- you have active liver disease, seriously impaired liver function or a history of liver tumor.
- you are a heavy smoker.
- you have diabetes and have developed circulatory disease.
- you have high blood pressure.
- you have not had any periods (amenorrhea).
- you have abnormal and unexplained vaginal bleeding.
- you have sickle cell disease.
- you are pregnant.

▷ **Inform Your Physician Before Taking This Drug If**
- you have had an adverse reaction to any oral contraceptive.
- you have a history of cancer of the breast or reproductive organs.
- you have any of the following conditions: fibrocystic breast changes, fibroid tumors of the uterus, endometriosis, migrainelike headaches, epilepsy, asthma, epilepsy, elevated lipids, prolapse of the mitral valve of the heart, heart disease, high blood pressure, gallbladder disease, diabetes or porphyria.
- you smoke tobacco on a regular basis.
- you plan to have surgery in the near future.

Possible Side-Effects (natural, expected and unavoidable drug actions)
Fluid retention, weight gain, "breakthrough" bleeding (spotting in middle of menstrual cycle), altered menstrual pattern, lack of menstruation (during and following cessation of drug), increased susceptibility to yeast infection of the genital tissues.

▷ **Possible Adverse Effects** (unusual, unexpected and infrequent reactions)
If any of the following develop, consult your physician promptly for guidance.

Mild Adverse Effects
Allergic Reactions: Skin rash, hives, itching.
Headache, nervous tension, irritability, accentuation of migraine headaches.
Nausea, vomiting, bloating, diarrhea.
Tannish pigmentation of the face.
Reduced tolerance to contact lenses.
Impaired color vision: blue tinge to objects, blue halo around lights.

Serious Adverse Effects
Allergic Reactions: Erythema multiforme and nodosum (skin reactions), loss of scalp hair.
Idiosyncratic Reactions: Joint and muscle pains.
Emotional depression, rise in blood pressure (in some people).
Eye changes: optic neuritis, retinal thrombosis, altered curvature of the cornea, cataracts.
Gallbladder disease, benign liver tumors, jaundice, rise in blood sugar.
Erosion of uterine cervix, enlargement of uterine fibroid tumors, cystitislike syndrome.
Abnormal glucose tolerance leading to high blood glucose (hyperglycemia).
Thrombophlebitis (inflammation of a vein with formation of blood clot)—pain or tenderness in thigh or leg, with or without swelling of foot or leg.
Drug-induced porphyria (rare).
Retinopathy (rare).
Pulmonary embolism (movement of blood clot to lung)—sudden shortness of breath, pain in chest, coughing, bloody sputum.
Stroke (blood clot in brain)—headaches, blackout, sudden weakness or paralysis of any part of the body, severe dizziness, altered vision, slurred speech, inability to speak.
Heart attack (blood clot in coronary artery)—sudden pain in chest, neck, jaw or arm; weakness; sweating; nausea.
Mesenteric thrombosis—blood clot in abdominal artery.

▷ **Possible Effects on Sexual Function**
Decreased libido (14–50%).
Altered character of menstruation; midcycle spotting.
Breast enlargement and tenderness with milk production.
Absent menstruation and infertility (temporary) after discontinuation of drug.

Possible Delayed Adverse Effects: Estrogens taken during pregnancy can predispose the female child to the later development of cancer of the vagina or cervix following puberty.

▷ **Adverse Effects That May Mimic Natural Diseases or Disorders**
Liver reactions may suggest viral hepatitis.

Natural Diseases or Disorders That May Be Activated by This Drug
Latent hypertension, diabetes mellitus, acute intermittent porphyria, lupus erythematosuslike syndrome.

Oral Contraceptives

Possible Effects on Laboratory Tests
Blood lupus erythematosus (LE) cells: positive.
Blood clotting time: decreased.
Blood prothrombin time: decreased.
Blood amylase and lipase levels: increased (very rare pancreatitis).
Blood total cholesterol, HDL cholesterol, LDL and VLDL cholesterol levels: usually no effects; some variability depending upon estrogen and progestin content of preparation used.
Blood triglyceride levels: no effect to increased, depending upon estrogen and progestin content of preparation used.
Blood glucose level: increased.
Blood thyroid stimulating hormone (TSH) level: no effect.
Blood thyroid hormone levels: T_3 and T_4 increased; free T_4 either no effect or decreased.
Liver function tests: increased liver enzymes (ALT/GPT, AST/GOT and alkaline phosphatase), increased bilirubin.

CAUTION

1. Serious adverse effects due to these drugs are a very low risk. However, any unusual development should be reported and evaluated promptly.
2. Studies indicate that women over 30 years of age who smoke and use oral contraceptives are at significantly greater risk of having a serious cardiovascular event than are nonusers.
3. The risk of thromboembolism increases with the amount of estrogen in the product and with the age of the user. Low-estrogen combinations are advised.
4. It is advisable to discontinue these drugs 1 month prior to elective surgery to reduce the risk of postsurgical thromboembolism.
5. Investigate promptly any alteration or disturbance of vision that occurs during the use of these drugs.
6. Investigate promptly the nature of recurrent, persistent or severe headaches that develop while taking these drugs.
7. Observe for significant change of mood. Discontinue this drug if depression develops.
8. Certain commonly used drugs may reduce the effectiveness of oral contraceptives. Some of these are listed in the category of *Other Drugs*.
9. Diarrhea lasting more than a few hours (and occurring during the days the drug is taken) can prevent adequate absorption of these drugs and impair their effectiveness as contraceptives.
10. If 2 consecutive menstrual periods are missed, consult your physician regarding the advisability of performing a pregnancy test. Do not continue to use these drugs until your pregnancy status is determined.
11. Many antibiotics may decrease the effectiveness of birth control pills (oral contraceptives). If your doctor prescribes an antibiotic, ask if a different method of birth control is needed.

▷ **Advisability of Use During Pregnancy**
Pregnancy Category: X. See Pregnancy Code at the back of this book.
Animal studies: Genital defects reported in mice and guinea pigs; cleft palate reported in rodents.
Human studies: Information from studies of pregnant women indicates that

estrogens can masculinize the female fetus. In addition, limb defects and heart malformations have been reported.

It is now known that estrogens taken during pregnancy can predispose the female child to the development of cancer of the vagina or cervix following puberty.

Avoid these drugs completely during entire pregnancy.

Advisability of Use if Breast-Feeding

Presence of these drugs in breast milk: Yes, in minute amounts.

These drugs may suppress milk formation if started early following delivery.

Breast-feeding is considered to be safe during the use of oral contraceptives.

Habit-Forming Potential: None.

Effects of Overdosage: Headache, drowsiness, nausea, vomiting, fluid retention, abnormal vaginal bleeding, breast enlargement and discomfort.

Possible Effects of Long-Term Use: High blood pressure, gallbladder disease with stones, accelerated growth of uterine fibroid tumors, absent menstruation and impaired fertility after discontinuation of drug.

Suggested Periodic Examinations While Taking This Drug (at physician's discretion)

Regular (every 6 months) evaluation of the breasts and pelvic organs, including Pap smears. Liver function tests as indicated.

▷ **While Taking This Drug, Observe the Following**

Foods: Avoid excessive use of salt if fluid retention occurs.

Beverages: No restrictions. May be taken with milk.

▷ *Alcohol:* No interactions expected.

Tobacco Smoking: Studies indicate that heavy smoking (15 or more cigarettes daily) in association with the use of oral contraceptives significantly increases the risk of heart attack (coronary thrombosis). Heavy smoking should be considered a contraindication to the use of oral contraceptives.

▷ *Other Drugs*

Oral contraceptives may *increase* the effects of
- some benzodiazepines, and cause excessive sedation.
- cyclosporine (Sandimmune) and cause toxicity.
- metoprolol (Lopressor), and cause excessive beta blocker effects.
- prednisolone and prednisone, and cause excessive cortisonelike effects.
- theophyllines, and increase the risk of toxic effects.

Oral contraceptives *taken concurrently* with
- antibiotics can seriously impair effectiveness and allow pregnancy to occur.
- antidiabetic drugs may cause unpredictable fluctuations of blood sugar.
- tricyclic antidepressants (Elavil, Sinequan, etc.) may enhance their adverse effects and reduce their antidepressant effectiveness.
- troleandomycin (TAO) may increase occurance of liver toxicity and jaundice.
- warfarin (Coumadin) may cause unpredictable alterations of prothrombin activity.

The following drugs may *decrease* the effects of oral contraceptives (and impair their effectiveness)

- barbiturates (phenobarbital, etc.; see Drug Class Section).
- carbamazepine (Tegretol).
- griseofulvin (Fulvicin, etc.).
- penicillins (ampicillin, penicillin V).
- phenytoin (Dilantin).
- primidone (Mysoline).
- rifampin (Rifadin, Rimactane).
- tetracyclines (see Drug Classes).

▷ *Driving, Hazardous Activities:* Usually no restrictions. Consult your physician for assessment of individual risk and for guidance regarding specific restrictions.

Aviation Note: Usually no restrictions. However, watch for the rare occurrence of disturbed vision and to restrict activities accordingly. Consult a designated Aviation Medical Examiner.

Exposure to Sun: Use caution. These drugs can cause photosensitivity (see Glossary).

Discontinuation: Do not stop this drug if "breakthrough" bleeding occurs. If spotting or bleeding continues, consult your physician. A preparation with a higher estrogen content may be required. Remember: Omitting this drug for only 1 day may allow pregnancy to occur. It is advisable to avoid pregnancy for 3 to 6 months after discontinuing these drugs; aborted fetuses from women who became pregnant within 6 months after discontinuation reveal significantly increased chromosome abnormalities.

OXAPROZIN (OX a proh zin)

Introduced: 1992 **Prescription:** USA: Yes **Available as Generic:** USA: No **Class:** NSAID, mild analgesic **Controlled Drug:** USA: No
Brand Names: Daypro

BENEFITS versus RISKS	
Possible Benefits	*Possible Risks*
EFFECTIVE RELIEF OF MILD TO MODERATE PAIN AND INFLAMMATION ONCE DAILY DOSING	Gastrointestinal pain, ulceration and bleeding (rare) Rare kidney toxicity Rare fluid retention

Please refer to the propionic acid nonsteroidal antiinflammatory drug profile for further information.

OXICAMS
(Nonsteroidal antiinflammatory drug)

Piroxicam (peer OX i kam)

Introduced: 1978 **Prescription:** USA: Yes; Canada: Yes **Available as Generic:** Yes **Class:** Mild analgesic, anti-inflammatory **Controlled Drug:** USA: No; Canada: No
Brand Names: ◆Apo-Piroxicam, Feldene, ◆Novo-Pirocam, ◆Nu-Pirox

BENEFITS versus RISKS	
Possible Benefits	*Possible Risks*
EFFECTIVE RELIEF OF MILD TO MODERATE PAIN AND INFLAMMATION	Gastrointestinal pain, ulceration, bleeding. Drug-induced hepatitis (rare) Rare kidney damage Mild fluid retention Reduced white blood cell and platelet counts

▷ **Principal Uses**

As a Single Drug Product: Uses currently included in FDA approved labeling: (1) Relieves mild to moderately severe pain and inflammation associated with (1) rheumatoid arthritis, (2) osteoarthritis.

Other (unlabeled) generally accepted uses: (1) Treats the morning and evening pain associated with ankylosing spondylitis; (2) helps relieve the pain and inflammation of acute gout; (3) used to treat terminal cancer pain in combination with doxepin; (4) may have a role in easing temporal arteritis.

How This Drug Works: This drug suppresses the formation of prostaglandins (and related compounds), chemicals involved in the production of inflammation and pain.

Available Dosage Forms and Strengths

Capsules — 10 mg, 20 mg
Rectal Suppository — 10 mg, 20 mg

▷ **Usual Adult Dosage Range:** As antiarthritic: 10 mg twice daily, 12 hours apart; or 20 mg once daily. The total daily dosage should not exceed 40 mg, and then for no more than 5 days. **Note: Actual dosage and administration schedule must be determined by the physician for each patient individually.**

Conditions Requiring Dosing Adjustments

Liver function: This drug should be used with caution in patients with liver compromise, and the dose should be empirically decreased.

Kidney function: Piroxicam should be used with caution in renal compromise and kidney function followed closely.

▷ **Dosing Instructions:** Take with or following food to prevent stomach irritation. Take with a full glass of water and remain upright (do not lie down) for 30 minutes. The capsule may be opened for administration.

Usual Duration of Use: Use on a regular schedule for 2 weeks usually determines effectiveness in relieving the discomfort of arthritis. Long-term use (months to years) requires physician supervision and periodic evaluation.

▷ **This Drug Should Not Be Taken If**
- you have had an allergic reaction to it previously.
- you are subject to asthma or nasal polyps caused by aspirin.
- you have active peptic ulcer disease or any form of gastrointestinal bleeding.
- you have a bleeding disorder or a blood cell disorder.

- you have active liver disease.
- you have severe impairment of kidney function.

▷ **Inform Your Physician Before Taking This Drug If**
- you are allergic to aspirin or to other aspirin substitutes.
- you have a history of peptic ulcer disease, regional enteritis or ulcerative colitis.
- you have a history of any type of bleeding disorder.
- you have impaired liver or kidney function.
- you have high blood pressure or a history of heart failure.
- you are taking any of the following: acetaminophen, aspirin or other aspirin substitutes, anticoagulants, oral antidiabetic drugs.
- you plan to have surgery of any type in the near future.

Possible Side-Effects (natural, expected and unavoidable drug actions)
Fluid retention (weight gain), prolongation of bleeding time.

▷ **Possible Adverse Effects** (unusual, unexpected and infrequent reactions)
If any of the following develop, consult your physician promptly for guidance.

Mild Adverse Effects
Allergic Reactions: Skin rash, itching, spontaneous bruising.
Headache, dizziness, hair loss, altered or blurred vision, ringing in the ears, drowsiness, fatigue, paresthesias, inability to concentrate.
Indigestion, nausea, vomiting, abdominal pain, breast pain, diarrhea.

Serious Adverse Effects
Active peptic ulcer, stomach or intestinal bleeding.
Drug-induced liver damage.
Serious skin damage (toxic epidermal necrolysis).
Pancreatitis (rare).
Kidney damage with painful urination, bloody urine, reduced urine formation.
Rare bone marrow depression (see Glossary): fatigue, weakness, fever, sore throat, abnormal bleeding or bruising.
Blood clotting problems.
Increased blood potassium.
Decreased sodium (following abnormal urine excretion) (rare).

▷ **Possible Effects on Sexual Function:** None reported.

Possible Delayed Adverse Effects: Mild anemia due to "silent" blood loss from the stomach.

▷ **Adverse Effects That May Mimic Natural Diseases or Disorders**
Liver reaction may suggest viral hepatitis.

Natural Diseases or Disorders That May Be Activated by This Drug
Peptic ulcer disease, ulcerative colitis.

Possible Effects on Laboratory Tests
Red blood cell count and hemoglobin level: decreased.
Bleeding time: increased.
Blood uric acid level: increased.
Liver function tests: increased liver enzymes (ALT/GPT, AST/GOT and alkaline phosphatase), increased bilirubin.

Kidney function tests: blood creatinine and urea nitrogen (BUN) levels increased; urine analysis positive for red blood cells, casts and increased protein content (kidney damage).

Fecal occult blood test: positive.

CAUTION
1. The smallest effective dose should always be used.
2. This drug may hide early signs of infection. Tell your doctor if you think you are developing an infection.

Precautions for Use

By Infants and Children: Indications and dose recommendations for those under 12 years of age not established.

By Those over 60 Years of Age: Small doses are advisable until tolerance is determined. Observe for any indications of liver or kidney toxicity, fluid retention, dizziness, confusion, impaired memory, stomach bleeding or constipation.

▷ **Advisability of Use During Pregnancy**

Pregnancy Category: B. Category D in the last three months of pregnancy. See Pregnancy Code at the back of this book.

Animal studies: No birth defects reported due to this drug.

Human studies: Adequate studies of pregnant women are not available.

The manufacturer does not recommend the use of this drug during pregnancy.

Advisability of Use if Breast-Feeding

Presence of this drug in breast milk: Yes.

Avoid drug or refrain from nursing.

Habit-Forming Potential: None.

Effects of Overdosage: Possible drowsiness, dizziness, ringing in the ears, nausea, vomiting, indigestion.

Possible Effects of Long-Term Use: Development of anemia due to "silent" bleeding from the gastrointestinal tract.

Suggested Periodic Examinations While Taking This Drug (at physician's discretion)

Complete blood cell counts, liver and kidney function tests.

Complete eye examinations if vision is altered in any way.

Hearing examinations if ringing in the ears or hearing loss develops.

▷ **While Taking This Drug, Observe the Following**

Foods: No restrictions.

Beverages: No restrictions. May be taken with milk.

▷ *Alcohol:* Use with caution. Both alcohol and piroxicam can irritate the stomach lining, and can increase the risk of stomach ulceration and/or bleeding.

Tobacco Smoking: No interactions expected.

▷ *Other Drugs*

Piroxicam may *increase* the effects of
- acetaminophen (Tylenol, etc.), and increase the risk of kidney damage; avoid prolonged use of this combination.
- anticoagulants (Coumadin, etc.), and increase the risk of bleeding; monitor prothrombin time, adjust dose accordingly.

Piroxicam *taken concurrently* with the following drugs may increase the risk of bleeding; avoid these combinations:
- aspirin.
- antihypertensives will blunt their therapeutic benefit.
- beta blockers (atenolol and others) can decrease the effectiveness of the beta blocker.
- dipyridamole (Persantine).
- indomethacin (Indocin).
- lithium can lead to lithium toxicity.
- sulfinpyrazone (Anturane).
- valproic acid (Depakene).

▷ *Driving, Hazardous Activities:* This drug may cause drowsiness or dizziness. Restrict activities as necessary.

Aviation Note: The use of this drug **may be a disqualification** for piloting. Consult a designated Aviation Medical Examiner.

Exposure to Sun: This drug may cause photosensitivity (see Glossary). Use caution.

OXTRIPHYLLINE (ox TRY fi lin)

Other Names: choline theophyllinate, theophylline cholinate

Introduced: 1965 **Prescription:** USA: Yes; Canada: Yes **Available as Generic:** Yes **Class:** Antiasthmatic, bronchodilator, xanthines **Controlled Drug:** USA: No; Canada: No

Brand Names: ✦Apo-Oxtriphylline, Choledyl, Choledyl Delayed-release, Choledyl SA, ✦Novotriphyl

BENEFITS versus RISKS	
Possible Benefits	*Possible Risks*
EFFECTIVE PREVENTION AND RELIEF OF ACUTE BRONCHIAL ASTHMA	NARROW TREATMENT RANGE FREQUENT STOMACH DISTRESS Gastrointestinal bleeding
MODERATELY EFFECTIVE CONTROL OF CHRONIC, RECURRENT BRONCHIAL ASTHMA	Central nervous system toxicity, seizures Heart rhythm disturbances
Moderately effective symptomatic relief in chronic bronchitis and emphysema	

▷ **Principal Uses**

As a Single Drug Product: Uses currently included in FDA approved labeling: (1) Used primarily to relieve the shortness of breath and wheezing characteristic of acute bronchial asthma, and to prevent the recurrence of asthmatic episodes; (2) It is also useful in relieving the asthmaticlike symptoms that are associated with some types of chronic bronchitis and emphysema.

Other (unlabeled) generally accepted uses: Please see the theophylline profile.

As a Combination Drug Product [CD]: This drug is available in combination with guaifenesin to provide an expectorant effect that thins the mucus secretions in the bronchial tubes.

How This Drug Works: This drug yields 64% free theophylline, the active medicinal component. By inhibiting the enzyme phosphodiesterase, this drug produces an increase in the tissue chemical cyclic AMP. This causes relaxation of the muscles in the bronchial tubes and blood vessels of the lung, resulting in relief of bronchospasm, expanded lung capacity and improved lung circulation.

Available Dosage Forms and Strengths

Oral solution — 100 mg per 5-ml teaspoonful (20% alcohol)
Syrup — 50 mg per 5-ml teaspoonful
Tablets — 100 mg, 200 mg (U.S., Canada) and 300 mg (Canada)
Tablets, delayed-release — 100 mg, 200 mg
Tablets, extended-release — 400 mg, 600 mg

▷ **Recommended Dosage Ranges** (Actual dosage and administration schedule must be determined by the physician for each patient individually.)

Note: All doses of oxtriphylline are to be calculated as theophylline-equivalents; all dosages cited below are for theophylline.

Infants and Children: For acute attack of asthma (not currently taking theophylline)—loading dose of 5 to 6 mg/kg of body weight.

For acute attack while currently taking theophylline—a single dose of 2.5 mg/kg of body weight, if no indications of theophylline toxicity. Monitor blood levels of theophylline.

For maintenance during acute attack—dosage is based on age:

Up to 6 months of age—0.07 for each week of age + 1.7 = the mg/kg of body weight, given every 8 hours.

6 months to 1 year of age—0.05 for each week of age + 1.25 = the mg/kg of body weight, given every 6 hours.

1 to 9 years of age—5 mg/kg of body weight, every 6 hours.

9 to 12 years of age—4 mg/kg of body weight, every 6 hours.

12 to 16 years of age—3 mg/kg of body weight, every 6 hours.

For chronic treatment to prevent recurrence of asthma—dosage is based on age:

Initially 16 mg/kg of body weight, in 3 or 4 divided doses at 6 to 8 hour intervals, up to a maximum of 400 mg daily. Increase dose as needed and tolerated by increments of 25% every 2 to 3 days. Limit total daily dosage as follows:

Up to 1 year of age—0.3 for each week of age + 8.0 = the mg/kg of body weight, per day.

1 to 9 years of age—22 mg/kg of body weight, per day.

9 to 12 years of age—20 mg/kg of body weight, per day.

12 to 16 years of age—18 mg/kg of body weight, per day.

16 years of age and over—13 mg/kg of body weight or 900 mg per day, whichever is less.

Note: It is advisable to measure blood levels of theophylline periodically during chronic therapy. The delayed-release tablets of oxtriphylline should not be used in children up to 6 years of age. The extended-release tablets of oxtriphylline should not be used in children up to 12 years of age.

16 to 60 Years of Age: For acute attack of asthma (not currently taking theophylline)—loading dose of 5 to 6 mg/kg of body weight.

For acute attack while currently taking theophylline—a single dose of 2.5 mg/kg of body weight, if no indications of theophylline toxicity. Monitor blood levels of theophylline.

For maintenance during acute attack—for nonsmokers: 3 mg/kg of body weight, every 8 hours; for smokers: 4 mg/kg of body weight, every 6 hours.

For chronic treatment to prevent recurrence of asthma—Initially 6 to 8 mg/kg of body weight, in 3 or 4 divided doses at 6 to 8 hour intervals, up to a maximum of 400 mg daily. Increase dose as needed and tolerated by increments of 25% every 2 to 3 days. The total daily dosage should not exceed 13 mg/kg of body weight or 900 mg, whichever is less.

Over 60 Years of Age: For acute attack—same as 16 to 60 years of age.

For maintenance during acute attack—2 mg/kg of body weight, every 8 hours.

Conditions Requiring Dosing Adjustments

Liver function: The dose **must** be lowered, and blood levels obtained frequently.

Kidney function: Blood drug levels should be closely followed in severe kidney failure.

▷ **Dosing Instructions:** The regular tablets may be crushed and taken with or following food to reduce stomach irritation. The delayed-release and extended-release tablets should be swallowed whole and not altered. Do not refrigerate any liquid dosage forms of this drug.

Usual Duration of Use: Use on a regular schedule for 48 to 72 hours determines this drug's effectiveness in controlling breathing problems associated with bronchial asthma and chronic lung disease. Long-term use (months to years) requires physician supervision and periodic evaluation.

▷ **This Drug Should Not Be Taken If**
- you have had an allergic reaction to oxtriphylline, aminophylline, dyphylline or theophylline.
- you have active peptic ulcer disease.
- you have an uncontrolled seizure disorder.

▷ **Inform Your Physician Before Taking This Drug If**
- you have had an unfavorable reaction to any xanthine drug (see Drug Class Section).
- you have a seizure disorder of any kind.
- you have a history of peptic ulcer disease.
- you have impaired liver or kidney function.
- you have hypertension, heart disease or any type of heart rhythm disorder.

Possible Side-Effects (natural, expected and unavoidable drug actions)
Nervousness, insomnia, rapid heart rate, increased urine volume.

▷ **Possible Adverse Effects** (unusual, unexpected and infrequent reactions)
If any of the following develop, consult your physician promptly for guidance.

Mild Adverse Effects
  Allergic Reactions: Skin rash, hives.
  Headache, dizziness, irritability, tremor, fatigue, weakness.
  Loss of appetite, nausea, vomiting, abdominal pain, diarrhea, excessive thirst.
  Flushing of face.

Serious Adverse Effects
  Idiosyncratic Reactions: Marked anxiety, confusion, behavioral disturbances.
  Central nervous system toxicity: muscle twitching, seizures.
  Heart rhythm abnormalities, rapid breathing, low blood pressure.
  Gastrointestinal bleeding.

▷ **Possible Effects on Sexual Function:** None reported.

Natural Diseases or Disorders That May Be Activated by This Drug
  Latent peptic ulcer disease.

Possible Effects on Laboratory Tests
  Blood uric acid level: increased.
  Fecal occult blood test: positive (large doses may cause stomach bleeding).

CAUTION
1. This drug should not be taken concurrently with other antiasthmatic drugs unless you are directed to do so by your physician. Serious overdosage could result.
2. It has been reported that influenza vaccine may delay the elimination of this drug and cause accumulation to toxic levels.

Precautions for Use
By Infants and Children: Do not exceed recommended doses. Observe for indications of toxicity: irritability, agitation, tremors, lethargy, fever, vomiting, rapid heart rate and breathing, seizures. Monitor blood levels of drug during long-term use.

By Those over 60 Years of Age: Small starting doses are indicated. There may be increased risk of stomach irritation, nausea, vomiting or diarrhea. When used concurrently with coffee (caffeine) or with nasal decongestants, this drug may cause excessive stimulation and a hyperactivity syndrome.

▷ **Advisability of Use During Pregnancy**
Pregnancy Category: C. See Pregnancy Code at the back of this book.
  Animal studies: Significant birth defects due to this drug reported in mice.
  Human studies: Adequate studies of pregnant women are not available. No increase in birth defects reported in 394 exposures to theophylline.
  Avoid this drug during the first 3 months. Use it otherwise only if clearly needed. Ask your physician for guidance.

Advisability of Use if Breast-Feeding
  Presence of this drug in breast milk: Yes.
  Avoid drug or refrain from nursing.

Habit-Forming Potential: None.

Effects of Overdosage: Nausea, vomiting, restlessness, irritability, confusion, delirium, seizures, high fever, weak pulse, coma.

Possible Effects of Long-Term Use: Gastrointestinal irritation.

Oxtriphylline

Suggested Periodic Examinations While Taking This Drug (at physician's discretion)
Measurement of blood theophylline levels, especially with high dosage or long-term use. (See Therapeutic Drug Monitoring in Section One.)

▷ **While Taking This Drug, Observe the Following**
Foods: No restrictions.
Beverages: Avoid excessive use of caffeine-containing beverages: coffee, tea, cola; this combination could cause nervousness and insomnia.
▷ *Alcohol:* No interactions expected. May have additive effect on stomach irritation.
Tobacco Smoking: May hasten the elimination of this drug and reduce its effectiveness. Higher doses may be necessary to maintain a therapeutic blood level.

▷ *Other Drugs*
Oxtriphylline may *decrease* the effects of
- lithium (Lithane, Lithobid, etc.), and reduce its effectiveness.

Oxtriphylline *taken concurrently* with
- halothane (anesthesia) may cause heart rhythm abnormalities.
- phenytoin (Dilantin) may cause decreased effects of both drugs. Monitor blood levels and adjust dosages as appropriate.

The following drugs may *increase* the effects of oxtriphylline
- allopurinol (Lopurin, Zyloprim).
- cimetidine (Tagamet).
- ciprofloxacin (Cipro).
- disulfiram (Antabuse).
- erythromycin (E-Mycin, Erythrocin, etc.).
- mexiletine (Mexitil).
- norfloxacin (Noroxin).
- oral contraceptives.
- ranitidine (Zantac).
- ticlopidine (Ticlid).
- troleandomycin (TAO).

The following drugs may *decrease* the effects of oxtriphylline
- barbiturates (phenobarbital, etc.).
- beta blocker drugs (see Drug Classes).
- carbamazepine (Tegretol).
- primidone (Mysoline).
- rifampin (Rifadin, Rimactane, etc.).

▷ *Driving, Hazardous Activities:* This drug may cause dizziness. Restrict activities as necessary.
Aviation Note: The use of this drug *may be a disqualification* for piloting. Consult a designated Aviation Medical Examiner.
Exposure to Sun: No restrictions.
Occurrence of Unrelated Illness: Acute viral respiratory infections can delay the elimination of this drug significantly. Observe closely for indications of toxicity and the need to reduce dosage or lengthen the dosage interval.
Discontinuation: Avoid prolonged and unnecessary use of this drug. When you have achieved an asthma-free state, withdraw this drug gradually over several days.

OXYCODONE (ox ee KOH dohn)

Introduced: 1950 **Prescription:** USA: Yes; Canada: Yes **Available as Generic:** USA: Yes; Canada: No **Class:** Analgesic, narcotic **Controlled Drug:** USA: C-II*; Canada: No

Brand Names: ◆Endocet [CD], ◆Endodan [CD], ◆Oxycocet [CD], ◆Oxycodan [CD], Percocet [CD], ◆Percocet-Demi [CD], Percodan [CD], Percodan-Demi [CD], Roxicodone, Roxiprin [CD], SK-Oxycodone, ◆Supeudol, Tylox [CD]

BENEFITS versus RISKS	
Possible Benefits	*Possible Risks*
EFFECTIVE RELIEF OF MODERATE TO SEVERE PAIN	POTENTIAL FOR HABIT FORMATION (DEPENDENCE)
	Sedative effects
	Mild allergic reactions (infrequent)
	Nausea, constipation

▷ **Principal Uses**

As a Single Drug Product: Uses currently included in FDA approved labeling: (1) Used in tablet and suppository form (Canada) to relieve moderate to severe pain.

Other (unlabeled) generally accepted uses: None.

As a Combination Drug Product [CD]: Oxycodone is available in combinations with acetaminophen and with aspirin. These milder pain relievers are added to enhance the analgesic effect and to reduce fever when present.

How This Drug Works: Acting primarily as a depressant of certain brain functions, this drug suppresses pain perception and calms the emotional response to pain.

Available Dosage Forms and Strengths
  Solution — 5 mg per 5-ml teaspoonful
  Suppositories — 10 mg, 20 mg (Canada)
    Tablets — 5 mg, 10 mg (Canada)
    Tablets — 2.44 mg, 4.88 mg (in combination drugs)

▷ **Usual Adult Dosage Range:** 5 mg/3 to 6 hours. Current pain theory says that pain medicines should be scheduled; for example, given every 4 hours. The outdated as needed method tended to result in less than optimal therapy. May be increased to 10 mg/4 hours if needed for severe pain. The total daily dosage should not exceed 60 mg. **Note: Actual dosage and administration schedule must be determined by the physician for each patient individually.**

Conditions Requiring Dosing Adjustments

Liver function: Dosage adjustments should be empirically made in liver failure.

Kidney function: Dosage adjustment does not appear to be needed.

▷ **Dosing Instructions:** The tablet may be crushed and taken with or following food to reduce stomach irritation or nausea.

*See Schedules of Controlled Drugs at the back of this book.

Oxycodone

    Usual Duration of Use: As required to control pain. Continual use should not exceed 5 to 7 days without interruption and reassessment of need.

▷ **This Drug Should Not Be Taken If**
- you have had an allergic reaction to any dosage form of it previously.
- you are having an acute attack of asthma.
- patients allergic to aspirin should **not** be given Percodan.

▷ **Inform Your Physician Before Taking This Drug If**
- you have had an unfavorable reaction to any narcotic drug in the past.
- you have had a head injury with increased pressure (intracranial) in the head.
- you have a history of drug abuse or alcoholism.
- you have chronic lung disease with impaired breathing.
- you have impaired liver or kidney function.
- you have gallbladder disease, a seizure disorder or an underactive thyroid gland.
- you have difficulty emptying the urinary bladder.
- you are taking any other drugs that have a sedative effect.
- you plan to have surgery under general anesthesia in the near future.

Possible Side-Effects (natural, expected and unavoidable drug actions)
Drowsiness, light-headedness, dry mouth, urinary retention, constipation.

▷ **Possible Adverse Effects** (unusual, unexpected and infrequent reactions)
    If any of the following develop, consult your physician promptly for guidance.
    Mild Adverse Effects
    Allergic Reactions: Skin rash, hives, itching.
    Idiosyncratic Reactions: Skin rash and itching when combined with dairy products (milk or cheese).
    Dizziness, impaired concentration, sensation of drunkenness, confusion, depression, blurred or double vision.
    Nausea, vomiting.
    Serious Adverse Effects
    Impaired breathing: use with caution in chronic lung disease.
    Abnormal body movements (if the drug is abruptly stopped).

▷ **Possible Effects on Sexual Function:** Blunted sexual responses.

Possible Effects on Laboratory Tests
    Urine screening tests for drug abuse: *initial* test result may be falsely **positive**; *confirmatory* test result will be **negative**. (Test results depend upon amount of drug taken and testing method used.)

CAUTION
1. If you have asthma, chronic bronchitis or emphysema, the excessive use of this drug may cause significant respiratory difficulty, thickening of bronchial secretions and suppression of coughing.
2. The concurrent use of this drug with atropinelike drugs can increase the risk of urinary retention and reduced intestinal function.
3. Do not take this drug following acute head injury.

Precautions for Use
    By Infants and Children: Do not use this drug in children under 2 years of age because of their vulnerability to life-threatening respiratory depression.

By Those over 60 Years of Age: Small starting doses and short-term therapy are indicated. There may be increased susceptibility to the development of drowsiness, dizziness, unsteadiness, falling, urinary retention and constipation (often leading to fecal impaction).

▷ **Advisability of Use During Pregnancy**
Pregnancy Category: C. See Pregnancy Code at the back of this book.
Animal studies: No information available.
Human studies: Adequate studies of pregnant women are not available. Oxycodone taken repeatedly during the last few weeks before delivery may cause withdrawal symptoms in the newborn infant.
Use this drug only if clearly needed and in small, infrequent doses.

Advisability of Use if Breast-Feeding
Presence of this drug in breast milk: Unknown.
Avoid drug or refrain from nursing.

Habit-Forming Potential: Psychological and/or physical dependence can develop with use of large doses for an extended period of time.

Effects of Overdosage: Drowsiness, restlessness, agitation, nausea, vomiting, dry mouth, vertigo, weakness, lethargy, stupor, coma, seizures.

Possible Effects of Long-Term Use: Psychological and physical dependence, chronic constipation.

Suggested Periodic Examinations While Taking This Drug (at physician's discretion)
None.

▷ **While Taking This Drug, Observe the Following**
Foods: No restrictions.
Beverages: No restrictions. May be taken with milk.
▷ *Alcohol:* Oxycodone can intensify the intoxicating effects of alcohol, and alcohol can intensify the depressant effects of oxycodone on brain function, breathing and circulation. Combined use is best avoided.
Tobacco Smoking: No interactions expected.
Marijuana Smoking: Increase in drowsiness and pain relief; impairment of mental and physical performance.
▷ *Other Drugs*
Oxycodone may *increase* the effects of
 • other drugs with sedative effects.
 • atropinelike drugs, and increase the risk of constipation and urinary retention.
▷ *Driving, Hazardous Activities:* This drug can impair mental alertness, judgment, reaction time and physical coordination. Avoid hazardous activities accordingly.
Aviation Note: The use of this drug *is a disqualification* for piloting. Consult a designated Aviation Medical Examiner.
Exposure to Sun: No restrictions.
Discontinuation: It is advisable to limit this drug to short-term use. If it is necessary to use it for extended periods of time, discontinuation should be gradual to minimize possible effects of withdrawal.

PAROXETINE (pa ROCKS a teen)

Introduced: 1993 **Prescription:** USA: Yes; Canada: Yes **Available as Generic:** USA: No; Canada: No **Class:** **Controlled Drug:** USA: No; Canada: No
Brand Names: Paxil

BENEFITS versus RISKS	
Possible Benefits	*Possible Risks*
EFFECTIVE CONTROL OF DEPRESSION	Withdrawal symptoms
	Abnormal ejaculation in males
Better adverse effect profile than tricyclic antidepressants	

▷ **Principal Uses**
　As a Single Drug Product: Uses currently included in FDA approved labeling: (1) Treatment of depression.
　Other (unlabeled) generally accepted uses: (1) Can have a role in diabetic nerve pain (neuropathy).
How This Drug Works: This phenylpiperidine antidepressant inhibits the uptake of a chemical important in mood (serotonin). When more of this chemical is available in the brain, a positive impact on thinking is often realized.
Available Dosage Forms and Strengths
　Capsules — 20 mg, 30 mg
▷ **Recommended Dosage Ranges (Actual dosage and administration schedule must be determined by the physician for each patient individually.)**
　Infants and Children: Not indicated.
　18 to 60 Years of Age: The usual starting dose is 20 mg, given in the morning. The dose can then be increased as needed and tolerated in 10 mg intervals to a maximum of 50 mg daily.
　Over 60 Years of Age: The starting dose in this population is 10 mg daily. The maximum dose is 40 mg daily.
Conditions Requiring Dosing Adjustments
　Liver function: Starting dose is 10 mg and the maximum dose is 40 mg daily. Drug levels may be needed.
　Kidney function: The starting dose and maximum dose are the same as those used in patients with liver compromise.
▷ **Dosing Instructions:** The absorption of this medicine is not changed by food.
Usual Duration of Use: Continual use on a regular schedule for 14 days is usually necessary to determine this drug's effectiveness in treating depression. Long-term use (months to years) requires periodic evaluation of response and dosage adjustment. Consult your physician on a regular basis.
Possible Advantages of This Drug
　Fewer side effects than tricyclic antidepressants.
▷ **This Drug Should Not Be Taken If**
- you have had an allergic reaction to any dosage form of it previously.
- you are currently taking, or have taken within the last 14 days a MAO inhibitor (see Drug Classes) medication.

Paroxetine

▷ **Inform Your Physician Before Taking This Drug If**
- you are pregnant or are breast feeding.
- you have a history of mania.
- you have a history of seizures.
- you take diuretics or typically drink little water.
- you have a history of liver or kidney disease.
- you take other prescription or non-prescription medicines which were not discussed with your doctor when paroxetine was prescribed.

Possible Side-Effects (natural, expected and unavoidable drug actions)
Lowered blood pressure and fainting upon standing (postural hypotension).

▷ **Possible Adverse Effects** (unusual, unexpected and infrequent reactions)
If any of the following develop, consult your physician promptly for guidance.

Mild Adverse Effects
Allergic Reactions: Skin rash and itching.
Palpitations (2.9%).
Loss of appetite, taste disorders (2.4%) or constipation (13%).
Tingling of the hands (paresthesias) (3.8%).
Sweating (12%).
Nervousness (5.2%) insomnia (14%), sedation (23%).
Dizziness (up to 12%), blurred vision (5%).

Serious Adverse Effects
Allergic Reactions: Not reported.
Idiosyncratic Reactions: None reported.
Abnormal movements or positioning of the mouth or face.
Seizures (rare).

▷ **Possible Effects on Sexual Function:** Galactorrhea. Abnormal ejaculation (12.9%), inability to achieve orgasm (10%), impotence or sexual dysfunction (10%).

Possible Delayed Adverse Effects: None reported.

▷ **Adverse Effects That May Mimic Natural Diseases or Disorders**
Increased liver enzymes may mimic early hepatitis.

Natural Diseases or Disorders That May Be Activated by This Drug
None reported.

Possible Effects on Laboratory Tests
Liver function tests: increased.

CAUTION
1. Take this medicine as prescribed and do not stop taking it without discussing discontinuation with your doctor.

Precautions for Use
By Infants and Children: Safety and effectiveness for use by those under 18 years of age have not been established.
By Those over 60 Years of Age: Lower starting and maximum doses are indicated.

▷ **Advisability of Use During Pregnancy**
Pregnancy Category: B. See Pregnancy Code at the back of this book.
Animal studies: Reproduction studies in rabbits or rats using doses of up to 10 times the typical human dose have not revealed any fetal changes.

752 Paroxetine

Human studies: Information from adequate studies of pregnant women is not available.
Ask your doctor for guidance.

Advisability of Use if Breast-Feeding
Presence of this drug in breast milk: Yes, in small amounts.
Ask your doctor for guidance.

Habit-Forming Potential: None, however a withdrawal syndrome characterized by dizziness, confusion, sweating and tremor has been described.

Effects of Overdosage: Confusion, heart rhythm changes, seizures.

Possible Effects of Long-Term Use: Not defined.

Suggested Periodic Examinations While Taking This Drug (at physician's discretion)
Liver function tests.

▷ **While Taking This Drug, Observe the Following**
Foods: No restrictions.
Nutritional Support: Not indicated.
Beverages: No restrictions.
▷ *Alcohol:* Alcohol does not have any documented negative effects on this medicine.
Tobacco Smoking: No interactions expected.
Marijuana Smoking: Additive sedation.
▷ *Other Drugs*
Paroxetine may *increase* the effects of
- desipramine.

Paroxetine *taken concurrently* with
- MAO inhibitors (see Drug Classes) may result in a fatal serotonin syndrome. Do **not** combine these medicines.
- warfarin (Coumadin) may result in bleeding.

The following drugs may *increase* the effects of paroxetine
- cimetidine (Tagamet).

▷ *Driving, Hazardous Activities:* This drug may frequently cause sedation. Restrict activities as necessary.
Aviation Note: The use of this drug **is a disqualification** for piloting. Consult a designated Aviation Medical Examiner.
Exposure to Sun: No specific restrictions.
Exposure to Heat: This medicine can cause excessive sweating. If you work or are frequently in a hot environment, be careful to replace enough fluids to avoid dehydration.
Heavy Exercise or Exertion: Since this medicine may cause excessive sweating, be careful to replace lost fluids.
Occurrence of Unrelated Illness: Illnesses which cause fevers may be worsened in their ability to cause dehydration.
Discontinuation: Do not stop this medicine without first talking with your doctor.

PENBUTOLOL (pen BYU toh lohl)

Introduced: 1976 **Prescription:** USA: Yes **Available as Generic:** No **Class:** Antihypertensive, beta-adrenergic blocker **Controlled Drug:** USA: No
Brand Name: Levatol

BENEFITS versus RISKS	
Possible Benefits	*Possible Risks*
EFFECTIVE, WELL-TOLERATED ANTIHYPERTENSIVE in mild to moderate high blood pressure	CONGESTIVE HEART FAILURE in advanced heart disease
Worsening of angina in coronary heart disease (abrupt withdrawal)
Masking of low blood sugar (hypoglycemia) in drug-treated diabetes
Provocation of asthma

▷ **Principal Uses**

As a Single Drug Product: Uses currently included in FDA approved labeling: (1) Treatment of mild to moderately severe high blood pressure. May be used alone or concurrently with other antihypertensive drugs, such as diuretics.

Other (unlabeled) generally accepted uses: (1) May help curb aggressive behavior; (2) can help decrease the frequency and severity of angina attacks; (3) may help decrease death from heart attack (myocardial infarction); (4) can have a supportive role in panic attacks.

How This Drug Works: By blocking certain actions of the sympathetic nervous system, this drug
- reduces the rate and contraction force of the heart, thus lowering the ejection pressure of the blood leaving the heart.
- reduces the degree of contraction of blood vessel walls, resulting in their expansion and consequent lowering of blood pressure.

Available Dosage Forms and Strengths
Tablets — 20 mg

▷ **Usual Adult Dosage Range:** Initially 20 mg once daily. The dose may be increased gradually by 10 mg/day at intervals of 2 weeks as needed and tolerated up to 80 mg/day. For maintenance, 20 to 40 mg once daily is usually adequate. The total daily dose should not exceed 80 mg. **Note: Actual dosage and administration schedule must be determined by the physician for each patient individually.**

Conditions Requiring Dosing Adjustments
Liver function: Dosage adjustments should be considered in mild to moderate liver disease, however, specific guidelines are not available.
Kidney function: Penbutolol elimination does not significantly involve the kidneys.

▷ **Dosing Instructions:** The tablet may be crushed and taken without regard to eating. Do not stop this drug abruptly.

Penbutolol

Usual Duration of Use: Use on a regular schedule for up to 2 weeks determines the full effect in lowering blood pressure. Long-term use of this drug (months to years) will be determined by the course of your blood pressure over time and your response to an overall treatment program (weight reduction, salt restriction, smoking cessation, etc.).

Possible Advantages of This Drug
Adequate control of blood pressure with a single daily dose.
Causes less slowing of the heart rate than most other beta blocker drugs.

Currently a "Drug of Choice"
for initiating treatment of hypertension with a single drug.

▷ **This Drug Should Not Be Taken If**
- you have had an allergic reaction to it previously.
- you have congestive heart failure.
- you have an abnormally slow heart rate or a serious form of heart block.
- you have abnormal growth of the left side of the heart (left ventricular hypertrophy).
- you are subject to bronchial asthma.

▷ **Inform Your Physician Before Taking This Drug If**
- you have had an adverse reaction to any beta blocker (see Drug Class Section).
- you have a history of serious heart disease.
- you are a diabetic.
- you have a history of hay fever (allergic rhinitis), asthma, chronic bronchitis or emphysema.
- you have a history of overactive thyroid function (hyperthyroidism).
- you have a history of low blood sugar (hypoglycemia).
- you have impaired liver or kidney function.
- you have diabetes or myasthenia gravis.
- you have impaired circulation in the extremities (Raynaud's disorder, claudication pains in legs).
- you take any form of digitalis, quinidine or reserpine, or any calcium blocker drug (see Drug Classes).
- you plan to have surgery under general anesthesia in the near future.

Possible Side-Effects (natural, expected and unavoidable drug actions)
Lethargy and fatigability, cold extremities, slow heart rate, light-headedness in upright position (see Orthostatic Hypotension in Glossary).

▷ **Possible Adverse Effects** (unusual, unexpected and infrequent reactions)
If any of the following develop, consult your physician promptly for guidance.
Mild Adverse Effects
Allergic Reactions: Skin rash, itching, reversible hair loss.
Headache, dizziness, blurred vision, insomnia, abnormal dreams.
Indigestion, nausea, vomiting, constipation, diarrhea.
Joint and muscle discomfort.
Serious Adverse Effects
Allergic Reactions: Anaphylactoid reaction (see Glossary).
Mental depression, anxiety, disorientation, short-term memory loss, hallucinations.

Carpal tunnel syndrome (rare).
High blood sugar.
Worsening of circulatory problems in those with preexisting conditions such as Raynaud's phenomenon.
Bronchospasm (1–2%).
Chest pain, shortness of breath, precipitation of congestive heart failure.
Rebound hypertension (if abruptly stopped).
Induction of bronchial asthma (in asthmatic individuals).
Aggravation of myasthenia gravis.
Abnormally low white blood cell and platelet counts: fever, sore throat, abnormal bleeding or bruising.

▷ **Possible Effects on Sexual Function:** Decreased libido and impotence, rare but more common with higher doses; Peyronie's disease (see Glossary).

▷ **Adverse Effects That May Mimic Natural Diseases or Disorders**
Reduced blood flow to extremities may resemble Raynaud's phenomenon (see Glossary).

Natural Diseases or Disorders That May Be Activated by This Drug
Raynaud's disease, intermittent claudication, myasthenia gravis.

Possible Effects on Laboratory Tests
White blood cell and platelet counts: decreased.
Uric acid: increased.
Blood sugar: increased.

CAUTION
1. *Do not stop this drug suddenly* without the knowledge and help of your doctor. Carry a notation on your person that you are taking this drug.
2. Ask your physician or pharmacist before using nasal decongestants usually present in over-the-counter cold preparations and nose drops. These can cause sudden increases in blood pressure when taken with beta blockers.
3. Report the development of any tendency to emotional depression.

Precautions for Use
By Infants and Children: Safety and effectiveness for those under 12 years of age not established. However, if this drug is used, observe for the development of low blood sugar (hypoglycemia) during periods of reduced food intake.

By Those over 60 Years of Age: Unacceptably high blood pressure should be reduced without creating the risks associated with excessively low blood pressure. Small starting doses and frequent blood pressure checks are needed. Sudden, rapid and excessive reduction of blood pressure can predispose to stroke or heart attack. Observe for dizziness, unsteadiness, tendency to fall, confusion, hallucinations, depression or urinary frequency.

▷ **Advisability of Use During Pregnancy**
Pregnancy Category: C. See Pregnancy Code at the back of this book.
Animal studies: No birth defects due to this drug found in rat or rabbit studies.

756 Penbutolol

Human studies: Adequate studies of pregnant women are not available. Use this drug only if clearly needed. Ask physician for guidance.

Advisability of Use if Breast-Feeding
Presence of this drug in breast milk: Unknown.
Avoid drug or refrain from nursing.

Habit-Forming Potential: None.

Effects of Overdosage: Weakness, slow pulse, low blood pressure, fainting, cold and sweaty skin, congestive heart failure, possible coma and convulsions.

Possible Effects of Long-Term Use: Reduced heart reserve and eventual heart failure in susceptible individuals with advanced heart disease.

Suggested Periodic Examinations While Taking This Drug (at physician's discretion)
Measurements of blood pressure, evaluation of heart function.
Complete blood cell counts.

▷ **While Taking This Drug, Observe the Following**
Foods: No restrictions. Avoid excessive salt intake.
Beverages: No restrictions. May be taken with milk.

▷ *Alcohol:* Alcohol may exaggerate this drug's ability to lower the blood pressure and may increase its mild sedative effect.
Tobacco Smoking: Nicotine may reduce this drug's benefit in treating high blood pressure. In addition, high doses of this drug may worsen constriction of the bronchial tubes caused by regular smoking.

▷ *Other Drugs*
Penbutolol may *increase* the effects of
- other antihypertensive drugs, and cause excessive lowering of the blood pressure. Dosage adjustments may be necessary.
- reserpine (Ser-Ap-Es, etc.), and cause sedation, depression, slowing of the heart rate and lowering of the blood pressure. This combination is best avoided.
- verapamil (Calan, Isoptin), and cause excessive depression of heart function; monitor this combination closely.

Pebutolol may *decrease* the effects of
- epinephrine resulting in decreased benefit when used to correct allergic reactions. Slow heartbeat and elevated blood pressure may also occur.

Penbutolol *taken concurrently* with
- clonidine (Catapres) requires close monitoring for rebound high blood pressure if clonidine is withdrawn while penbutolol is still being taken.
- insulin or oral hypoglycemic agents requires close monitoring to avoid undetected hypoglycemia (see Glossary).
- amiodarone (Codarone) may cause slow heartbeat and arrest. Combination is best avoided.

The following drugs may *increase* the effects of penbutolol
- methimazole (Tapazole).
- birth control pills (oral contraceptives).
- propylthiouracil (Propacil).

The following drugs may *decrease* the effects of penbutolol
- barbiturates (phenobarbital, etc.).

- indomethacin (Indocin), and possibly other "aspirin substitutes," or NSAIDs may impair penbutolol's antihypertensive effect.
- rifampin (Rifadin, Rimactane).

▷ *Driving, Hazardous Activities:* Use caution until the full extent of fatigue, dizziness and blood pressure change have been determined.

Aviation Note: The use of this drug *is a disqualification* for piloting. Consult a designated Aviation Medical Examiner.

Exposure to Sun: No restrictions.

Exposure to Heat: Hot environments can lower the blood pressure and exaggerate the effects of this drug.

Exposure to Cold: Cold environments can worsen the circulatory deficiency in the extremities that may occur with this drug. The elderly should take precautions to prevent hypothermia (see Glossary).

Heavy Exercise or Exertion: It is advisable to avoid exertion that produces light-headedness, excessive fatigue or muscle cramping. The use of this drug may intensify the hypertensive response to isometric exercise.

Occurrence of Unrelated Illness: Fever can lower the blood pressure and require adjustment of dosage. Nausea or vomiting may interrupt the regular dosage schedule. Ask your physician for guidance.

Discontinuation: It is advisable to avoid sudden discontinuation of this drug in all situations. If possible, gradual reduction of dose over a period of 2 to 3 weeks is recommended. Ask your physician for specific guidance.

PENICILLAMINE (pen i SIL a meen)

Introduced: 1963　**Prescription:** USA: Yes; Canada: Yes　**Available as Generic:** USA: No; Canada: No　**Class:** Chelating agent, antirheumatic
Controlled Drug: USA: No; Canada: No
Brand Names: Cuprimine, Depen

BENEFITS versus RISKS	
Possible Benefits	*Possible Risks*
EFFECTIVE TREATMENT OF WILSON'S DISEASE (COPPER TOXICITY)	SEVERE ALLERGIC REACTIONS BONE MARROW DEPRESSION (see Glossary)
Partially effective treatment of rheumatoid arthritis	Drug-induced damage of lungs, liver, pancreas and kidneys
Effective treatment of cystinuria and cystine kidney stones	
Partially effective treatment of poisoning due to heavy metals: iron, lead, mercury and zinc.	

▷ **Principal Uses**

As a Single Drug Product: Uses currently included in FDA approved labeling: Treatment of (1) Wilson's disease (copper toxicity of brain, cornea, liver and kidneys); (2) severe rheumatoid arthritis that has failed to respond to less hazardous conventional treatment; also helps rheumatoid arthritis which presents with interstitial lung disease; (3) cystinuria and cystine stone formation (excessive amounts of cystine in the urine).

Other (unlabeled) generally accepted uses: (1) Treatment of heavy metal poisoning, especially that due to lead and mercury; (2) may be of benefit in increasing survival in scleroderma; (3) eases the progression of systemic sclerosis.

How This Drug Works: In Wilson's disease and heavy metal poisoning—this drug chelates (bonds tightly to) copper, iron, lead, mercury and zinc (in body tissues) to form soluble compounds that are readily extracted and excreted in the urine.

In rheumatoid arthritis—this drug favorably modifies the abnormal immune reactions within joint structures that cause inflammation, swelling, pain and tissue destruction.

In cystinuria—this drug combines with cystine to form a compound that is readily excreted in the urine. The reduction of cystine concentrations prevents the formation of cystine stones in the urinary tract.

Available Dosage Forms and Strengths
  Capsules — 125 mg, 250 mg
  Tablets — 250 mg

▷ **Recommended Dosage Ranges** (Actual dosage and administration schedule must be determined by the physician for each patient individually.)

Infants and Children: For Wilson's disease: From 6 months to 12 years of age—20 mg/kg of body weight daily, in 4 divided doses.

For rheumatoid arthritis: Initially 3 mg/kg of body weight (up to 250 mg) daily, in 2 divided doses, for 3 months; then 6 mg/kg of body weight (up to 500 mg) daily, in 2 divided doses, for 3 months; as needed and tolerated, gradually increase dose to a maximum of 10 mg/kg of body weight daily, in 3 to 4 divided doses.

For cystinuria: 30 mg/kg of body weight daily, in 4 divided doses.

For lead poisoning: 25 to 40 mg/kg of body weight daily, in 2 to 3 divided doses.

12 to 60 Years of Age: For Wilson's disease: 250 mg 4 times daily.

For rheumatoid arthritis: Initially 125 or 250 mg once daily as a single dose; increase dose gradually, as needed and tolerated, by 125 or 250 mg daily at intervals of 2 to 3 months. The total daily dose should not exceed 1000 mg for small individuals, 1500 mg for large individuals.

For cystinuria and cystine stones: 500 mg 4 times daily.

For heavy metal poisoning: 500 mg to 1500 mg daily for 1 to 2 months.

Over 60 Years of Age: Initially 125 mg daily; gradually increase dose, as needed and tolerated, by 125 mg daily at intervals of 2 to 3 months. The total daily dose should not exceed 750 mg.

Conditions Requiring Dosing Adjustments

Liver function: Dosage adjustments do not appear to be needed. This drug is a rare cause of liver toxicity, and should be used with caution in patients with compromised livers.

Kidney function: In patients with moderate kidney failure, the drug should **not** be given. It is also a cause of kidney problems (nephropathy and renal failure), and should be used as a benefit to risk decision in patients with compromised kidneys.

▷ **Dosing Instructions:** Take this drug on an empty stomach, 1 hour before or 2 hours after eating. The capsule may be opened and the tablet may be crushed for administration.

Usual Duration of Use: Use on a regular schedule for 2 to 3 months determines benefit in relieving the symptoms of Wilson's disease or rheumatoid arthritis. Long-term use (months to years) requires periodic physician evaluation.

▷ **This Drug Should Not Be Taken If**
- you have had an allergic reaction to it previously.
- you are pregnant and using this drug to treat rheumatoid arthritis or cystinuria.
- you currently have a bone marrow or blood cell disorder.
- you are currently taking drugs for malaria, gold therapy or other cytotoxic drugs.
- you have active liver disease.

▷ **Inform Your Physician Before Taking This Drug If**
- you are allergic to any type of penicillin.
- you have a history of drug-induced bone marrow depression.
- you have a history of myasthenia gravis, pancreatitis, peptic ulcer disease or systemic lupus erythematosus.
- you have impaired liver or kidney function.
- you are planning pregnancy.
- you are taking any type of gold or immune-suppressant drugs.
- you are planning surgery or dental procedures in the near future.

Possible Side-Effects (natural, expected and unavoidable drug actions)
Deficiency of pyridoxine (vitamin B_6): optic neuritis (eye pain, blurred vision); peripheral neuritis (pain, numbness, tingling in extremities).

▷ **Possible Adverse Effects** (unusual, unexpected and infrequent reactions)
If any of the following develop, consult your physician promptly for guidance.

Mild Adverse Effects
Allergic Reactions: Skin rash, hives, itching.
Blurred vision.
Ringing or buzzing in ears.
Loss of appetite, mouth sores, altered taste, nausea, vomiting, stomach pain, diarrhea.

Serious Adverse Effects
Allergic Reactions: Severe dermatitis, fever, joint pain, swollen lymph glands.
Bone marrow depression (see Glossary).
Very rare leukemia (one case of acute lymphoblastic).
Bronchiolitis (cough, wheezing, shortness of breath).
Lung toxicity (pulmonary bleeding, Goodpasture's syndrome or alveolitis).
Abnormal muscle quivering (fasciculation).
Hepatitis with jaundice (see Glossary).
Pancreatitis (fever, severe stomach pain, nausea, vomiting).
Peptic ulcer, stomach or duodenum.
Drug-induced porphyria.
Kidney damage (cloudy/bloody urine, swelling of face, legs, feet).
Myasthenia gravis syndrome (extreme muscle weakness, difficulty breathing, chewing, swallowing, talking; double vision).
Systemic lupus erythematosus (SLE) syndrome (skin rash, skin blisters, fever, fatigue, chest pain, joint pain).

▷ **Possible Effects on Sexual Function:** Swelling and tenderness of male breast tissue.

Possible Delayed Adverse Effects: None reported.

▷ **Adverse Effects That May Mimic Natural Diseases or Disorders**
Drug-induced hepatitis may suggest viral hepatitis.
Myasthenia gravis syndrome.
Systemic lupus erythematosus (SLE) syndrome.

Natural Diseases or Disorders That May Be Activated by This Drug
Peptic ulcer, hemolytic anemia.

Possible Effects on Laboratory Tests
Complete blood cell counts: decreased red cells, hemoglobin, white cells and platelets; increased eosinophils.
Blood LE cells: positive.
Liver function tests: increased liver enzymes (ALT/GPT, AST/GOT and alkaline phosphatase), increased bilirubin.
Kidney function tests: increased blood urea nitrogen (BUN) and creatinine levels; increased urine protein content.
Partial Thromboplastin time (PTT): Decreased.
Urine copper: increased.

CAUTION
1. Ask your doctor about the advisability of taking pyridoxine (vitamin B_6) to prevent optic neuritis and peripheral neuritis. The recommended amount is 25 mg daily.
2. Comply fully with your physician's request for periodic laboratory tests: blood counts, liver and kidney function tests.
3. Report promptly any indications of bone marrow depression: unusual fatigue or weakness, fever or sore throat, abnormal bleeding or bruising.
4. Do not interrupt your regular, continual dosing of this drug; even brief periods of interruption may cause significant allergic reactions following resumption of treatment. If dosing is interrupted for any reason, it should be resumed with small doses and gradually increased until the previous full dosage is restored.
5. If you are to have surgery, reduce the dose of this drug to 250 mg daily until your wound is fully healed. This drug can impair or delay wound healing.

Precautions for Use
By Infants and Children: Safety and effectiveness for those under 6 months of age not established.
By Those over 60 Years of Age: May have increased levels of bone marrow depression while using this drug. Report promptly any indication of unusual fatigability, infection, bruising or bleeding.

▷ **Advisability of Use During Pregnancy**
Pregnancy Category: D. See Pregnancy Code at the back of this book.
Animal studies: Rat studies reveal drug-induced cleft palates and skeletal defects.
Human studies: Adequate studies of pregnant women are not available. Birth defects have been reported in infants born to mothers with rheumatoid arthritis or cystinuria who took this drug during pregnancy.

If you have rheumatoid arthritis, do not use this drug. If you have cystinuria, avoid this drug if possible. If you have Wilson's disease, limit the daily dose to 1000 mg; if cesarean section is planned, limit the daily dose to 250 mg during the last 6 weeks of pregnancy and following delivery until wound healing is complete.

Advisability of Use if Breast-Feeding
Presence of this drug in breast milk: Unknown.
Avoid drug or refrain from nursing.

Habit-Forming Potential: None.

Effects of Overdosage: Nausea, vomiting, diarrhea, stomach pain.

Possible Effects of Long-Term Use: Increased risk of bone marrow depression, liver or kidney damage.

Suggested Periodic Examinations While Taking This Drug (at physician's discretion)
Complete blood cell counts every 2 weeks during the first 6 months of treatment; then monthly thereafter.
Urinalysis every 2 weeks during the first 6 months of treatment; then monthly thereafter.
Liver and kidney function tests every 6 months during the first 18 months of treatment.

▷ **While Taking This Drug, Observe the Following**
Foods: Follow the diet prescribed by your physician.
Nutritional Support: Recommended daily supplement of pyridoxine (vitamin B_6)—25 mg.
Beverages: Do not take this drug with milk.
▷ *Alcohol:* No interactions expected.
Tobacco Smoking: No interactions expected.
▷ *Other Drugs*
Penicillamine may *decrease* the effects of
- digoxin (Lanoxin).

The following drugs may *increase* the effects of penicillamine
- chloroquine (Aralen).
- indomethacin (Indocin) and perhaps other NSAIDs.

The following drugs may *decrease* the effects of penicillamine
- all antacids containing aluminum and/or magnesium.
- iron preparations.
- probenecid (Benemid).
- sucralfate (Carafate).

Penicillamine *taken concurrently with*
- birth control pills (oral contraceptives) can result in breast swelling and tenderness.
- gold (Auranofin) may result in increased bone marrow depression and rashes.
- heparin may result in decreased therapeutic benefit.

▷ *Driving, Hazardous Activities:* No restrictions.
Aviation Note: The use of this drug *may be a disqualification* for piloting. Consult a designated Aviation Medical Examiner.

Exposure to Sun: No restrictions.
Discontinuation: To be determined by your physician. Do not stop this drug without your physician's knowledge and guidance.

PENICILLIN V (pen i SIL in VEE)

Introduced: 1953   **Prescription:** USA: Yes; Canada: Yes   **Available as Generic:** USA: Yes; Canada: Yes   **Class:** Antibiotic, penicillins   **Controlled Drug:** USA: No; Canada: No

Brand Names: ◆Apo-Pen-VK, Beepen VK, Betapen-VK, Ledercillin VK, ◆Nadopen-V, ◆Novopen-VK, ◆Nu-Pen-VK, Penapar VK, Pen-V, ◆Pen-Vee, Pen-Vee K, ◆PVF, ◆PVF K, Robicillin VK, SK-Penicillin VK, Uticillin VK, V-Cillin K, ◆VC-K 500, Veetids

BENEFITS versus RISKS	
Possible Benefits	*Possible Risks*
EFFECTIVE TREATMENT OF INFECTIONS due to susceptible microorganisms	ALLERGIC REACTIONS, mild to severe Superinfections (yeast) Drug-induced colitis

▷ **Principal Uses**
   As a Single Drug Product: Uses currently included in FDA approved labeling: (1) Used to treat responsive infections of the upper and lower respiratory tract, the middle ear and the skin; (2) Helps prevent rheumatic fever and bacterial endocarditis in people with valvular heart disease.
   Other (unlabeled) generally accepted uses: (1) Combination therapy of animal bite wounds; (2) treatment of stage one Lyme disease in children; (3) therapy of Lyme disease involving the central nervous system.

How This Drug Works: This drug destroys susceptible infecting bacteria by interfering with their ability to produce new protective cell walls as they multiply and grow.

Available Dosage Forms and Strengths
   Oral solution — 125 mg, 250 mg per 5-ml teaspoonful
   Tablets — 125 mg, 250 mg, 500 mg

▷ **Usual Adult Dosage Range:** Dosage is based upon sensitivity testing of the bacteria causing the infection, the severity of the infection and response of the patient. Depending upon the specific infection, the dosage range is 125 to 500 mg/6 to 8 hours. For the prevention of bacterial endocarditis: 2 grams (2000 mg) taken 1 hour before the procedure, followed by 1 gram 6 hours later. The total daily dosage should not exceed 7 grams (7000 mg).
   Note: Actual dosage and administration schedule must be determined by the physician for each patient individually.

Conditions Requiring Dosing Adjustments
   Liver function: Dosage adjustments do not appear to be needed.
   Kidney function: In patients with renal compromise, no more than 250 mg should be given every 6 hours.

▷ **Dosing Instructions:** The tablet may be crushed and taken on an empty stomach or with food or milk. Absorption may be slightly faster if taken when stomach is empty.

Usual Duration of Use: For all streptococcal infections—not less than 10 consecutive days (without interruption) to reduce the possibility of developing rheumatic fever or glomerulonephritis. For all other infections—as long as necessary to eradicate the infection.

▷ **This Drug Should Not Be Taken If**
- you have had an allergic reaction to any dosage form of it previously.
- you are certain you are allergic to *any* form of penicillin.

▷ **Inform Your Physician Before Taking This Drug If**
- you suspect you may be allergic to penicillin or you have a history of a previous "reaction" of any type to penicillin.
- you are allergic to any cephalosporin antibiotic (Ancef, Anspor, Ceclor, Ceporan, Ceporex, Kafocin, Keflex, Keflin, Kefzol, Loridine, Ultracef, Velosef; see Drug Classes).
- you are allergic by nature (hay fever, asthma, hives, eczema).

Possible Side-Effects (natural, expected and unavoidable drug actions)
Superinfections (see Glossary), often due to yeast organisms.

▷ **Possible Adverse Effects** (unusual, unexpected and infrequent reactions)
If any of the following develop, consult your physician promptly for guidance.

Mild Adverse Effects
Allergic Reactions: Skin rashes, hives, itching.
Irritations of mouth and tongue, "black tongue," nausea, vomiting, mild diarrhea, dizziness (rare).

Serious Adverse Effects
Allergic Reactions: Anaphylactic reaction (see Glossary), severe skin reactions, drug fever, swollen painful joints, sore throat, abnormal bleeding or bruising.
Severe skin reactions (Stevens-Johnson syndrome, bullous pemphigoid).
Drug-induced colitis.
Rare hemolytic anemia.
Drug-induced periarteritis nodosa (rare).
Rare drug-induced meningitis.
Drug-induced porphyria.
Abnormal liver function.

▷ **Possible Effects on Sexual Function:** None reported.

Possible Effects on Laboratory Tests
Complete blood counts: decreased red cells, hemoglobin, white cells and platelets; increased eosinophils (allergic reaction).
Prothrombin time: occasionally increased.
Liver function tests: increased aspartate aminotransferase (AST/GOT) and bilirubin.

CAUTION
1. Take the exact dose and the full course prescribed.
2. If this drug must be used concurrently with antibiotics like erythromycin or tetracycline, give the penicillin first.

Precautions for Use
By Infants and Children: Observe the allergic child closely for evidence of a developing allergy to penicillin. This drug may cause diarrhea, which sometimes necessitates discontinuation.

764   Penicillin V

By Those over 60 Years of Age: Natural changes in the skin may predispose to prolonged itching reactions in the genital and anal regions. Report such reactions promptly.

▷ **Advisability of Use During Pregnancy**
Pregnancy Category: B. See Pregnancy Code at the back of this book.
Animal studies: Birth defects of the limbs reported in mice. (Not confirmed in other studies.)
Human studies: Adequate studies of pregnant women indicate no increased risk of birth defects in 3546 pregnancies exposed to penicillin derivatives.
This drug is considered safe for use during any period of pregnancy.

Advisability of Use if Breast-Feeding
Presence of this drug in breast milk: Yes.
The nursing infant may be sensitized to penicillin and be at risk for developing diarrhea or yeast infections.
Avoid drug if possible or refrain from nursing.

Habit-Forming Potential: None.

Effects of Overdosage: Possible nausea, vomiting and/or diarrhea.

Possible Effects of Long-Term Use: Superinfections, often due to yeast organisms.

Suggested Periodic Examinations While Taking This Drug (at physician's discretion)
Complete blood cell counts, kidney function tests.

▷ **While Taking This Drug, Observe the Following**
Foods: No restrictions.
Beverages: No restrictions. May be taken with milk.
▷ *Alcohol:* No interactions expected.
Tobacco Smoking: No interactions expected.
▷ *Other Drugs*
Penicillin V may *decrease* the effects of
- birth control pills (oral contraceptives), and impair their effectiveness in preventing pregnancy.

The following drugs may *decrease* the effects of penicillin V
- antacids may reduce the absorption of penicillin V.
- chloramphenicol (Chloromycetin).
- erythromycin (Erythrocin, E-Mycin, etc.).
- tetracyclines (Achromycin, Declomycin, Minocin, etc.). (See Drug Class Section.)

▷ *Driving, Hazardous Activities:* Usually no restrictions. Be alert to the rare occurrence of dizziness and/or nausea, and restrict activities accordingly.
Aviation Note: The use of this drug *may be a disqualification* for piloting. Consult a designated Aviation Medical Examiner.
Exposure to Sun: No restrictions.
Special Storage Instructions: Oral solutions should be refrigerated.
Observe the Following Expiration Times: Do not take the oral solution of this drug if older than 7 days when kept at room temperature or 14 days when kept refrigerated.

PENTAMIDINE (pent AM i deen)

Introduced: 1985　**Prescription:** USA: Yes; Canada: Yes　**Available as Generic:** USA: No; Canada: No　**Class:** Anti-infective, antiprotozoal
Controlled Drug: USA: No; Canada: No
Brand Names: NebuPent, ♦Pentacarinat, ♦Pneumopent

BENEFITS versus RISKS	
Possible Benefits	*Possible Risks*
PREVENTION AND TREATMENT OF PNEUMOCYSTIS CARINII PNEUMONIA (AIDS-RELATED)	Kidney damage Liver damage (8.7%) Low white blood cells (2.8%) Rare pancreatitis Rare hypoglycemia (see Glossary) Cough and bronchospasm

▷ **Principal Uses**
As a Single Drug Product: Uses currently included in FDA approved labeling: (1) Prevention (by inhalation of aerosol) of AIDS-related Pneumocystis carinii pneumonia; (2) treatment of pneumocystis carinii pneumonia.
Other (unlabeled) generally accepted uses: (1) Treatment of mild Pneumocystis carinii pneumonia; (2) therapy of the parasite causing leishmaniasis.

How This Drug Works: This drug may interfere with RNA and DNA formation and inhibit the production of essential proteins. It interferes with sugar use in parasites.

Available Dosage Forms and Strengths
Powder for inhalation solution — Vials of 60 mg (Canada) and 300 mg (United States and Canada)

▷ **Recommended Dosage Ranges** (Actual dosage and administration schedule must be determined by the physician for each patient individually.)
Infants and Children: Dosage not established.
12 to 60 Years of Age: For prevention—(1) oral inhalation of 300 mg of NebuPent or Pentacarinat every 4 weeks, or 150 mg every 2 weeks; or (2) oral inhalation of 60 mg of Pneumopent every 24 to 72 hours for a total of 5 doses over a 2 week period; then 60 mg every 2 weeks.
For treatment—oral inhalation of 600 mg of NebuPent or Pentacarinat daily for 21 days.
Over 60 Years of Age: Same as 12 to 60 years of age.

Conditions Requiring Dosing Adjustments
Liver function: The role of the liver in the elimination of this medication has not been fully characterized. This drug is a rare cause of hepatotoxicity, and should be used with caution in patients with compromised livers.
Kidney function: Used with caution in kidney failure, however, the kidney is minimally involved in the elimination of this drug.

▷ **Dosing Instructions:** Oral inhalation of NebuPent and Pentacarinat for prevention should be continued over a period of 30 to 45 minutes; for treatment, over a period of 25 to 30 minutes.

Pentamidine

Oral inhalation of Pneumopent for prevention should be continued over a period of 15 minutes.

For optimal distribution of pentamidine in the lungs, oral inhalation should be administered to patients in a supine or recumbent position.

Oral inhalations of pentamidine should be administered in a well ventilated room.

If a bronchodilator inhaler is used to prevent bronchospasm and coughing, administer this 5 to 10 minutes before inhalation of pentamidine.

Usual Duration of Use: Use on a regular schedule for 3 to 4 months determines effectiveness in preventing development of Pneumocystis carinii pneumonia in HIV-infected individuals. Continual use for 3 to 4 weeks is needed to evaluate its effectiveness in controlling active pneumonia. Long-term use (months to years) requires periodic physician evaluation of response.

Possible Advantages of This Drug
Usually well tolerated, with mild and minimal adverse effects. Drug of choice for pneumocystis prevention is Septra.

▷ **This Drug Should Not Be Taken If**
- you have had an allergic reaction to any form of it previously.
- you have uncontrolled bronchial asthma.

▷ **Inform Your Physician Before Taking This Drug If**
- you have a history of bronchial asthma.
- you have a history of pancreatitis.
- you are a diabetic.
- you have a history of abnormal heartbeats (arrhythmias).
- your liver or kidney function is compromised.
- you have very low blood pressure.
- you smoke tobacco regularly.

Possible Side-Effects (natural, expected and unavoidable drug actions)
Unpleasant, metallic taste.

▷ **Possible Adverse Effects** (unusual, unexpected and infrequent reactions)
If any of the following develop, consult your physician promptly for guidance.

Mild Adverse Effects
Allergic Reactions: Skin rash.
Throat discomfort, coughing, wheezing, chest congestion.
Lowering of blood pressure, fast heart rate.
Lowered blood sugar (6–40%).

Serious Adverse Effects
Kidney or liver damage.
Severe skin damage (toxic epidermal necrolysis, Stevens-Johnson syndrome) (rare).
Low blood calcium or magnesium (rare).
Rare hypoglycemia (see Glossary).
Rare pancreatitis.
Low blood platelets, hemoglobin and white blood cells.
Abnormal heart rhythm (torsade de pointes or ventricular changes).
Hallucinations.

▷ **Possible Effects on Sexual Function:** None reported.

Natural Diseases or Disorders That May Be Activated by This Drug
Bronchial asthma.

Possible Effects on Laboratory Tests
Blood glucose levels: decreased or increased.
Blood urea nitrogen (BUN) and creatinine: increased.
Complete blood count: white blood cells, hemoglobin and platelets decreased.
Liver function tests: increased SGOT, SGPT and CPK.
Blood calcium or magnesium: decreased.

CAUTION
1. Cigarette smokers and asthmatics are more likely to experience acute coughing and wheezing when using inhalation pentamidine.
2. Inhalation bronchodilators (such as pirbuterol or terbutaline), if used to prevent bronchospasm, should be given 5 to 10 minutes before inhalation of pentamidine.

Precautions for Use
By Infants and Children: Pentamidine is an alternative to cotrimoxazole to prevent Pneumocystis carinii pneumonia in children with HIV who are over 5 years old. Recommended schedule is 300 mg every 4 weeks inhaled by nebulizer. Prophylaxis is started when the CD4 count in a 5-year-old is less than 500.
By Those over 60 Years of Age: No information available.

▷ **Advisability of Use During Pregnancy**
Pregnancy Category:
C. See Pregnancy Code at the back of this book.
Animal studies: None performed using inhalation pentamidine.
Human studies: Adequate studies of pregnant women are not available.
Use this drug only if clearly needed. Ask your physician for guidance.

Advisability of Use if Breast-Feeding
Presence of this drug in breast milk: Unknown.
Monitor nursing infant closely and discontinue drug or nursing if adverse effects develop.

Habit-Forming Potential: None.

Effects of Overdosage: Throat irritation, coughing, bronchospasm.

Possible Effects of Long-Term Use: Pancreatitis.

Suggested Periodic Examinations While Taking This Drug (at physician's discretion)
Blood urea nitrogen (BUN), liver function tests, blood glucose, complete blood count (CBC) and blood pressure should be followed.

▷ **While Taking This Drug, Observe the Following**
Foods: No restrictions, however, your doctor may order supplemental folic acid.
Beverages: No restrictions.
▷ *Alcohol:* No interactions expected.
Tobacco Smoking: Avoid completely. Continued smoking may provoke coughing and bronchospasm.

▷ **Other Drugs**
Pentamidine *taken concurrently* with
- amphotericin B may result in increased risk of kidney toxicity.
- cotrimoxazole can result in antagonism of therapeutic effect of both drugs.
- foscarnet may cause very low blood calcium or magnesium levels.

▷ *Driving, Hazardous Activities:* No restrictions.

Aviation Note: The use of this drug *may be a disqualification* for piloting. Consult a designated Aviation Medical Examiner.

Exposure to Sun: No restrictions.

Discontinuation: To be determined by your physician.

PENTAZOCINE (pen TAZ oh seen)

Introduced: 1967   **Prescription:** USA: Yes; Canada: Yes   **Available as Generic:** USA: No; Canada: No   **Class:** Analgesic, narcotic   **Controlled Drug:** USA: C-IV*; Canada: No

Brand Names: Talacen [CD], Talwin, Talwin Compound [CD], ✦Talwin Compound-50 [CD], Talwin Nx [CD]

BENEFITS versus RISKS	
Possible Benefits	*Possible Risks*
EFFECTIVE RELIEF OF MODERATE TO SEVERE PAIN	POTENTIAL FOR HABIT FORMATION (DEPENDENCE) Respiratory depression Sedative effects Mental and behavioral disturbances Low blood pressure, fainting Nausea, constipation

▷ **Principal Uses**

As a Single Drug Product: Uses currently included in FDA approved labeling: (1) Relieves acute or chronic pain of moderate to severe degree from any cause.

Other (unlabeled) generally accepted uses: None.

As a Combination Drug Product [CD]: Pentazocine is available in combinations with acetaminophen and with aspirin. These milder pain relievers are added to enhance the analgesic effect and to reduce fever when present. In the United States the tablet form of pentazocine also contains naloxone (Talwin Nx), a narcotic antagonist that renders the drug ineffective if abused.

How This Drug Works: Acting primarily as a depressant of certain brain functions, this drug suppresses the perception of pain and calms the emotional response to pain.

Available Dosage Forms and Strengths
Injection — 30 mg per ml
Tablets — 50 mg (Canada)
Tablets — 50 mg with 0.5 mg of naloxone (USA)

*See Schedules of Controlled Drugs at the back of this book.

Pentazocine

▷ **Usual Adult Dosage Range:** 50 mg/3 to 4 hours as needed. May be increased to 100 mg/4 hours if needed for severe pain. The total daily dosage should not exceed 600 mg. **Note: Actual dosage and administration schedule must be determined by the physician for each patient individually.**

Conditions Requiring Dosing Adjustments
Liver function: Doses should be decreased or the time between doses lengthened.
Kidney function: For moderate to severe kidney failure, the dose should be reduced by 25–50%.

▷ **Dosing Instructions:** The tablet may be crushed and taken with or following food to reduce stomach irritation or nausea.

Usual Duration of Use: As required to control pain. Continual use should not exceed 5 to 7 days without interruption and reassessment of need.

▷ **This Drug Should Not Be Taken If**
- you have had an allergic reaction to any dosage form of it previously.
- you are having an acute attack of asthma.
- you have increased intracranial pressure or brain damage.

▷ **Inform Your Physician Before Taking This Drug If**
- you have had an unfavorable reaction to any narcotic drug in the past.
- you have a history of drug abuse or alcoholism.
- you have chronic lung disease with impaired breathing.
- you have impaired liver or kidney function.
- you have gallbladder disease, a seizure disorder or an underactive thyroid gland.
- you have difficulty emptying the urinary bladder.
- you are taking any other drugs that have a sedative effect.
- you plan to have surgery under general anesthesia in the near future.

Possible Side-Effects (natural, expected and unavoidable drug actions)
Drowsiness, light-headedness, weakness, urinary retention, constipation.

▷ **Possible Adverse Effects** (unusual, unexpected and infrequent reactions)
If any of the following develop, consult your physician promptly for guidance.
Mild Adverse Effects
Allergic Reactions: Skin rash, hives, itching, swelling of face.
Headache, dizziness, impaired concentration, sensation of drunkenness, blurred or double vision, flushing, sweating.
Increased or decreased blood pressure.
Drug fever (rare).
Nausea, vomiting, indigestion, diarrhea.
Serious Adverse Effects
Marked drop in blood pressure, possible fainting.
Impaired breathing: Use with caution in chronic lung disease.
Mental and behavioral disturbances, hallucinations, psychosis, tremor.
Drug-induced seizure (rare).
Drug-induced porphyria (rare).
Toxic epidermal necrolysis (rare).
Fibrous muscle replacement (rare).
Rare kidney problems.

Fixed positioning of the eyes (oculogyric crisis) (rare).
Bone marrow depression (see Glossary) of a mild and reversible nature (rare).
Aggravation of prostatism (see Glossary).

▷ **Possible Effects on Sexual Function:** Blunting of sexual response.

Natural Diseases or Disorders That May Be Activated by This Drug
Porphyria (see Glossary).

Possible Effects on Laboratory Tests
White blood cell count: rarely decreased.
Blood amylase and lipase levels: increased (natural side-effects).

CAUTION
1. The use of this drug with atropinelike drugs may increase the risk of urinary retention and reduced intestinal function.
2. Do not take this drug following acute head injury.

Precautions for Use
By Infants and Children: Safety and effectiveness for those under 12 years of age not established.
By Those over 60 Years of Age: Use small doses initially and increase dosage as needed and tolerated. Limit use to short-term treatment only. There may be increased susceptibility to development of drowsiness, dizziness, unsteadiness, falling, urinary retention and constipation.

▷ **Advisability of Use During Pregnancy**
Pregnancy Category: C (B or D in high dose or extended use). See Pregnancy Code at the back of this book.
Animal studies: Significant birth defects reported in hamsters.
Human studies: Adequate studies of pregnant women are not available. Pentazocine taken repeatedly during the last few weeks before delivery may cause withdrawal symptoms in the newborn infant.
Avoid this drug during the first 3 months. Use only if clearly needed and in small, infrequent doses during the last 6 months.

Advisability of Use if Breast-Feeding
Presence of this drug in breast milk: Expected.
Avoid drug or refrain from nursing.

Habit-Forming Potential: Psychological and/or physical dependence can develop with use of large doses for an extended period of time.

Effects of Overdosage: Anxiety, disturbed thoughts, hallucinations, progressive drowsiness, stupor, depressed breathing.

Possible Effects of Long-Term Use: Psychological and physical dependence, chronic constipation.

Suggested Periodic Examinations While Taking This Drug (at physician's discretion)
Complete blood cell counts, if used for an extended period of time.

▷ **While Taking This Drug, Observe the Following**
Foods: No restrictions.
Beverages: No restrictions. May be taken with milk.
▷ *Alcohol:* Pentazocine can intensify the intoxicating effects of alcohol, and

alcohol can intensify the depressant effects of pentazocine on brain function, breathing and circulation. Best to avoid combination.
Tobacco Smoking: Heavy smoking may reduce the effectiveness of pentazocine and make larger doses necessary.
Marijuana Smoking: Increase in drowsiness and pain relief; impairment of mental and physical performance.

▷ *Other Drugs*
Pentazocine may **increase** the effects of
- other drugs with sedative effects.
- atropinelike drugs, and increase the risk of constipation and urinary retention.
- cyclosporine (Sandimmune) and cause toxicity.
- MAO inhibitors (see Drug Classes) may result in muscle rigidity.

▷ *Driving, Hazardous Activities:* This drug can impair mental alertness, judgment, reaction time and physical coordination. Avoid hazardous activities accordingly.
Aviation Note: The use of this drug **is a disqualification** for piloting. Consult a designated Aviation Medical Examiner.
Exposure to Sun: No restrictions.
Discontinuation: It is advisable to limit this drug to short-term use. If it is necessary to use it for extended periods of time, discontinuation should be gradual to minimize possible effects of withdrawal.

PENTOXIFYLLINE (pen tox I fi leen)

Other Name: Oxpentifylline
Introduced: 1972 **Prescription:** USA: Yes; Canada: Yes **Available as Generic:** No **Class:** Blood flow agent, xanthines **Controlled Drug:** USA: No; Canada: No
Brand Name: Trental

BENEFITS versus RISKS	
Possible Benefits	*Possible Risks*
IMPROVED BLOOD FLOW IN PERIPHERAL ARTERIAL DISEASE	Reduced blood pressure, angina, abnormal heart rhythms
REDUCTION OF INTERMITTENT CLAUDICATION PAIN	Rare low blood counts and aplastic anemia
	Indigestion, nausea, vomiting
	Dizziness, flushing

▷ **Principal Uses**
As a Single Drug Product: Uses currently included in FDA approved labeling: (1) Adjunctive treatment in the management of peripheral obstructive arterial disease to improve arterial blood flow and reduce the frequency and severity of muscle pain due to intermittent claudication.
Other (unlabeled) generally accepted uses: (1) Decreases hemodialysis shunt clots (thrombosis); (2) may have a role in treating impotence which is caused by blood vessel problems (vascular impotence); (3) can increase the motility of sperm; (4) helps decrease interleukin 6 and tumor necrosis

factor in patients with cerebral malaria; (5) has had variable results in AIDS patients in attempting to halt weight loss which may be caused by tumor necrosis factor; (6) may ease skin tightening in some cases; (7) has been used to relieve symptoms of septic shock; (8) has been used to help heal refractory ulcers in diabetics; (9) can help decrease insulin requirements in diabetics.

How This Drug Works: Improves blood flow and increases oxygen supply to working muscles by way of three mechanisms: (1) reduction of blood viscosity due to decreased levels of fibrinogen in the blood; (2) increased flexibility of the red blood cells (carrying oxygen) due to an increase in cyclic AMP (enzyme) within red blood cells; this permits easier passage through the small blood vessels of the microcirculation; and (3) prevention of red blood cell and platelet aggregation.

Inhibits interleukin-6 and tumor necrosis factor.

Available Dosage Forms and Strengths
Tablets, prolonged-action — 400 mg

▷ **Usual Adult Dosage Range:** 400 mg 3 times/day. If adverse nervous system or gastrointestinal effects occur, reduce the dose to 400 mg twice/day. **Note: Actual dosage and administration schedule must be determined by the physician for each patient individually.**

Conditions Requiring Dosing Adjustments
Liver function: Dosing changes do not appear to be needed in liver compromise.
Kidney function: The dose should be empirically decreased in patients with compromised kidneys.

▷ **Dosing Instructions:** Take with or following food to reduce stomach irritation. Swallow the tablet whole without breaking, crushing or chewing.

Usual Duration of Use: Use on a regular schedule for 2 to 4 weeks determines effectiveness in preventing or delaying the pains of intermittent claudication associated with walking. Treatment for a minimum of 3 months is recommended to determine full effectiveness. Long-term use (months to years) requires physician supervision and periodic evaluation.

Possible Advantages of This Drug
Reduces blood viscosity and thereby improves blood flow through small vessels.
Increases supply of oxygen to working muscles.

Currently a "Drug of Choice"
for treating peripheral arterial disease and reducing the frequency and severity of intermittent claudication pain.

▷ **This Drug Should Not Be Taken If**
- you have had an allergic reaction to it previously.

▷ **Inform Your Physician Before Taking This Drug If**
- you are allergic to other xanthine drugs: caffeine, theophylline, theobromine.
- you have impaired kidney function.
- you have low blood pressure, impaired brain circulation or coronary artery disease.
- you are a diabetic.

- you smoke tobacco.
- you are taking any antihypertensive drugs.

Possible Side-Effects (natural, expected and unavoidable drug actions)
Usually none with recommended doses.

▷ **Possible Adverse Effects** (unusual, unexpected and infrequent reactions)
If any of the following develop, consult your physician promptly for guidance.

Mild Adverse Effects
Allergic Reaction: Skin rash.
Headache (1.2%), blurred vision and scotoma (less than 1%), dizziness (1.9%), tremor.
May worsen glucose control in diabetics.
Nose bleeds (rare).
Indigestion (2.8%), nausea (2.2%), vomiting (1.2%).

Serious Adverse Effects
Development of angina or heart rhythm disorders in the presence of coronary artery disease.
Liver toxicity (rare).
Rare low platelets, white blood cells or all cells.
Rare auditory hallucinations.
Retinal bleeding (rare).

▷ **Possible Effects on Sexual Function**
May help reverse impotence caused by circulatory problems.

Possible Effects on Laboratory Tests
Complete blood cell counts: rarely decreased red cells, hemoglobin, white cells and platelets.

CAUTION
Use this drug with caution in the presence of impaired circulation within the brain (cerebral arteriosclerosis) or coronary artery disease. If any related symptoms develop, consult your physician for prompt evaluation.

Precautions for Use
By Infants and Children: Safety and effectiveness for those under 18 years of age not established. Use by this age group is not anticipated.
By Those over 60 Years of Age: You may be more susceptible to the adverse effects listed. Observe closely for any indications of dizziness or chest pain and report these promptly.

▷ **Advisability of Use During Pregnancy**
Pregnancy Category: C. See Pregnancy Code at the back of this book.
Animal studies: Increased fetal resorptions reported in rats, but no birth defects found in rats or rabbits.
Human studies: Adequate studies of pregnant women are not available.
Avoid use during the first 3 months. Use otherwise only if clearly needed.

Advisability of Use if Breast-Feeding
Presence of this drug in breast milk: Yes.
Avoid drug or refrain from nursing.

Habit-Forming Potential: None.

Effects of Overdosage: Drowsiness, flushing, faintness, excitement, seizures.

Possible Effects of Long-Term Use: None reported.

774　Pergolide

Suggested Periodic Examinations While Taking This Drug (at physician's discretion)
Blood pressure measurements, evaluation of heart status.

▷ **While Taking This Drug, Observe the Following**
Foods: No restrictions.
Beverages: No restrictions. May be taken with milk.
▷ *Alcohol:* Alcohol may increase the blood-pressure-lowering effect of this drug.
Tobacco Smoking: Nicotine constricts arteries and will impair the effectiveness of this drug significantly. Avoid all use of tobacco.
▷ Other Drugs
Pentoxifylline may *increase* the effects of
- antihypertensive drugs, and cause excessive lowering of blood pressure.
- warfarin (Coumadin, etc.), and increase the possibility of unwanted bleeding; monitor prothrombin times as appropriate.

Pentoxifylline *taken concurrently* with
- cimetidine (Tagamet), nizatidine, famotidine and ranitidine may result in pentoxifylline toxicity (increases drug absorption).
- theophylline may result in theophylline toxicity.

▷ *Driving, Hazardous Activities:* This drug may cause drowsiness or dizziness. Restrict activities as necessary.
Aviation Note: The use of this drug *may be a disqualification* for piloting. Consult a designated Aviation Medical Examiner.
Exposure to Sun: No restrictions.

PERGOLIDE (PER go lide)

Introduced: 1980　**Prescription:** USA: Yes　**Available as Generic:** USA: No　**Class:** Antiparkinsonism, dopamine agonist, ergot derivative
Controlled Drug: USA: No
Brand Name: Permax

BENEFITS versus RISKS	
Possible Benefits	*Possible Risks*
ADDITIVE RELIEF OF SYMPTOMS OF PARKINSON'S DISEASE when used concurrently with levodopa/carbidopa (Sinemet) PERMITS A 5–30% REDUCTION IN SINEMET DOSAGE	ABNORMAL INVOLUNTARY MOVEMENTS (62%) HALLUCINATIONS (14%) INITIAL FALL IN BLOOD PRESSURE/ORTHOSTATIC HYPOTENSION (10%) Premature heart contractions (ventricular)

▷ **Principal Uses**
As a Single Drug Product: Uses currently included in FDA approved labeling: (1) As an adjunct to levodopa/carbidopa treatment of Parkinson's disease for people who experience intolerable abnormal movements (dyskinesia) and/or increasing "on-off" episodes due to levodopa. The addition of pergolide (1) permits reduction of the daily dose of levodopa with consequent lessening of dyskinesia and erratic drug response, and (2) provides additional relief of parkinsonian symptoms.

Other (unlabeled) generally accepted uses: (1) May have a role in helping reduce drug craving in cocaine withdrawal; (2) helps in some conditions where excess prolactin is made.

How This Drug Works: By directly stimulating part of the brain (dopamine receptor sites in the corpus striatum), this drug helps to compensate for the deficiency of dopamine that is responsible for the rigidity, tremor and sluggish movement characteristic of Parkinson's disease.

Available Dosage Forms and Strengths
Tablets — 0.05 mg, 0.25 mg, 1 mg

▷ **Usual Adult Dosage Range**
Initially 0.05 mg daily for the first 2 days; gradually increase the daily dose by 0.1 mg or 0.15 mg every third day over the next 12 days. If needed and tolerated, the daily dose may be increased further by 0.25 mg every third day until an optimal respose is achieved. The total daily dosage should be divided into 3 equal portions and given at 6 to 8 hour intervals. The usual maintenance dose is 3 mg/24 hours; do not exceed 5 mg/24 hours.

During the gradual introduction of pergolide, the concurrent dose of levodopa/carbidopa (Sinemet) may be cautiously decreased in accord with your physician's instructions.

Note: Actual dosage and administration schedule must be determined by the physician for each patient individually.

Conditions Requiring Dosing Adjustments
Liver function: Specific guidelines for dosing adjustments in liver compromise are not available. It should be used with caution.
Kidney function: Consideration should be given to empiric decreases in dosage.

▷ **Dosing Instructions:** The tablet may be crushed and taken with food or milk to reduce stomach irritation.

Usual Duration of Use: Use on a regular schedule for 4 to 6 weeks determines effectiveness in controlling the symptoms of Parkinson's disease and permitting reduction of levodopa/carbidopa dosage. Long-term use (months to years) requires periodic physician evaluation of response.

Possible Advantages of This Drug: It may provide a more effective and uniform control of parkinsonian symptoms and a reduction of some adverse effects of long-term levodopa therapy.

▷ **This Drug Should Not Be Taken If**
- you have had an allergic reaction to it previously.
- you have had a serious adverse effect from any ergot preparation.
- you have severe coronary artery disease or peripheral vascular disease.

▷ **Inform Your Physician Before Taking This Drug If**
- you have constitutionally low blood pressure.
- you are pregnant or breast-feeding.
- you are taking any antihypertensive drugs or antipsychotic drugs (see Drug Classes).
- you have any degree of coronary artery disease, especially angina or a history of heart attack.
- you have any type of heart rhythm disorder.

- you have impaired liver or kidney function.
- you have a seizure disorder.

Possible Side-Effects (natural, expected and unavoidable drug actions)
Weakness (4.2%), chest pain—possibly anginal (3.7%), peripheral edema (7.4%), orthostatic hypotension (see Glossary) (10%).

▷ **Possible Adverse Effects** (unusual, unexpected and infrequent reactions)
If any of the following develop, consult your physician promptly for guidance.

Mild Adverse Effects
Allergic Reactions: Skin rash (3.2%), facial swelling (1.1%).
Headache (5.3%), dizziness (19%), hallucinations (14%), confusion (11%), drowsiness (10%), insomnia (8%), anxiety (6%), double vision (2%).
Nasal congestion (12%), shortness of breath (5%), palpitation (2%), fainting (2%).
Altered taste (1.6%), loss of appetite (4.8%), dry mouth (3.7%), indigestion (6.4%), nausea (24%), vomiting (2.7%), constipation (10%), diarrhea (6.4%).

Serious Adverse Effects
Allergic Reactions: None reported.
Idiosyncratic Reactions: "Flu-like" symptoms (3%).
Abnormal involuntary movements (dyskinesia) (62%), psychotic behavior (2%).
Abnormal heartbeats (ventricular arrhythmias).
Paranoid delusions (up to 18%).

▷ **Possible Effects on Sexual Function:** Infrequent reports of altered libido (both increased and decreased), impotence, breast pain, priapism (see Glossary).

▷ **Adverse Effects That May Mimic Natural Diseases or Disorders**
Effects on mental function and behavior may resemble psychotic disorders.

▷ **Natural Diseases or Disorders That May Be Activated by This Drug**
Coronary artery disease with anginal syndrome, heart rhythm disorders, Raynaud's syndrome (see Glossary), seizure disorders.

Possible Effects on Laboratory Tests
Blood prolactin level: decreased (marked reduction).

CAUTION
1. May cause abnormal movements (dyskinesias) and intensify existing dyskinesias. Watch carefully for the development of tremors, twitching or abnormal, involuntary movements of any kind. Report these promptly.
2. Low starting doses help prevent the possibility of excessive drop in blood pressure. See dosage routine outlined above.
3. Inform your physician promptly if you become pregnant or plan pregnancy. This drug has been reported (rarely) to cause abortion and birth defects.

Precautions for Use
By Infants and Children: This drug is not utilized by this age group.
By Those over 60 Years of Age: Small initial doses are mandatory. Watch closely for any tendency to light-headedness or faintness, especially on

arising from a lying or sitting position. You may be more susceptible to the development of impaired thinking, confusion, agitation, nightmares or hallucinations.

▷ **Advisability of Use During Pregnancy**
Pregnancy Category: B. See Pregnancy Code at the back of this book.
Animal studies: No birth defects due to this drug were found in mouse or rabbit studies.
Human studies: Adequate studies of pregnant women are not available. However, there are four reports of birth defects associated with the use of this drug and infrequent reports of abortion. Causal relationships have not been established, but prudence advises against the use of this drug during pregnancy. Consult your physician for guidance.

Advisability of Use if Breast-Feeding
Presence of this drug in breast milk: Unknown.
Avoid drug or refrain from nursing.

Habit-Forming Potential: None.

Effects of Overdosage: Nausea, vomiting, palpitations, low blood pressure, agitation, severe involuntary movements, hallucinations, seizures.

Possible Effects of Long-Term Use: Increased risk of developing dyskinesias.

Suggested Periodic Examinations While Taking This Drug (at physician's discretion)
Regular evaluation of drug response, heart function and blood pressure status.

▷ **While Taking This Drug, Observe the Following**
Foods: No restrictions.
Beverages: No restrictions. May be taken with milk.
▷ *Alcohol:* Alcohol can exaggerate the blood-pressure-lowering and sedative effects of this drug.
Tobacco Smoking: No interactions expected.
▷ *Other Drugs*
Pergolide *taken concurrently* with
- antihypertensive drugs (and other drugs that can lower blood pressure) requires careful monitoring for excessive drops in pressure. Dosage adjustments may be necessary.

The following drugs may *decrease* the effects of pergolide and diminish its effectiveness
- chlorprothixene (Taractan).
- haloperidol (Haldol).
- metoclopramide (Reglan).
- phenothiazines (see Drug Class Section).
- thiothixene (Navane).

▷ *Driving, Hazardous Activities:* This drug may cause dizziness, drowsiness, impaired coordination or fainting. Restrict activities as necessary.
Aviation Note: The use of this drug *is a disqualification* for piloting. Consult a designated Aviation Medical Examiner.
Exposure to Sun: No restrictions.
Exposure to Heat: Use caution until the combined effects have been determined. Hot environments can cause lowering of blood pressure.

Discontinuation: Do not stop this drug abruptly. Sudden withdrawal can cause confusion, paranoid thinking and severe hallucinations. Consult your physician regarding a schedule for gradual withdrawal.

PERPHENAZINE (per FEN a zeen)

Introduced: 1957 **Prescription:** USA: Yes; Canada: Yes **Available as Generic:** USA: Yes; Canada: Yes **Class:** Strong tranquilizer, phenothiazines **Controlled Drug:** USA: No; Canada: No

Brand Names: ◆Apo-Perphenazine, ◆PMS-Perphenazine, ◆Elavil Plus [CD], Etrafon [CD], Etrafon-A [CD], Etrafon Forte [CD], ◆Phenazine, ◆PMS-Levazine, Triavil [CD], Trilafon

BENEFITS versus RISKS	
Possible Benefits	*Possible Risks*
EFFECTIVE CONTROL OF ACUTE MENTAL DISORDERS	SERIOUS TOXIC EFFECTS ON BRAIN with long-term use
Beneficial effects on thinking, mood and behavior	Liver damage with jaundice (infrequent)
Relief of anxiety and tension	Rare blood cell disorders: hemolytic anemia, abnormally low white blood cell and platelet counts
Moderately effective control of nausea and vomiting	

▷ **Principal Uses**

As a Single Drug Product: Uses currently included in FDA approved labeling: (1) Used to treat acute and chronic psychotic disorders such as agitated depression, schizophrenia and similar states of mental dysfunction; (2) It may be used as a tranquilizer to help agitated and disruptive behavior in the absence of true psychosis; (3) sometimes used to treat severe nausea and vomiting.

Other (unlabeled) generally accepted uses: (1) Can ease tremors caused by tricyclic antidepressants.

As a Combination Drug Product [CD]: Available combined with amitriptyline, an effective antidepressant. In some cases of severe agitated depression, the combination of a specific antipsychotic drug and a specific antidepressant drug will be more effective than either drug used alone.

How This Drug Works: By inhibiting dopamine, this drug acts to correct an imbalance of nerve impulse transmissions thought to be responsible for mental disorders.

Available Dosage Forms and Strengths
Concentrate — 16 mg per 5-ml teaspoonful
Injection — 5 mg per ml
Tablets — 2 mg, 4 mg, 8 mg, 16 mg
Tablets, prolonged-action — 8 mg

▷ **Usual Adult Dosage Range:** Initially 2 to 16 mg 2 to 4 times daily. Dose may be increased by 4 mg at 3- to 4-day intervals as needed and tolerated. Usual dosage range is 8 to 24 mg daily. The total daily dosage should not exceed 64 mg. **Note: Actual dosage and administration schedule must be determined by the physician for each patient individually.**

Perphenazine 779

Conditions Requiring Dosing Adjustments
Liver function: The dose should be empirically decreased in patients with liver compromise. Perphenazine is contraindicated in patients with moderare to severe liver compromise.
Kidney function: The kidney is minimally involved in the elimination of this drug.

▷ **Dosing Instructions:** May be taken with or following meals to reduce stomach irritation. The regular tablets may be crushed for administration; the prolonged-action tablets should be taken whole, not broken, crushed or chewed.

Usual Duration of Use: Use on a regular schedule for several weeks determines this drug's effectiveness in controlling psychotic disorders. If it is not significantly beneficial within 6 weeks, it should be stopped. Long-term use (months to years) requires periodic physician evaluation of response, and consideration of continued need.

▷ **This Drug Should Not Be Taken If**
- you are allergic to any of the drugs bearing the brand names listed.
- you have active liver disease.
- you have brain damage in the subcortical area.
- you have cancer of the breast.
- you have a current blood cell or bone marrow disorder.

▷ **Inform Your Physician Before Taking This Drug If**
- you are allergic or abnormally sensitive to any phenothiazine (see Drug Classes).
- you have impaired liver or kidney function.
- you have any type of seizure disorder.
- you have diabetes, glaucoma or heart disease.
- you have a history of lupus erythematosus.
- you have an allergy to sulfites.
- you are taking any drug with sedative effects.
- you plan to have surgery under general or spinal anesthesia soon.

Possible Side-Effects (natural, expected and unavoidable drug actions)
Drowsiness (usually during the first 2 weeks), orthostatic hypotension (see Glossary), blurred vision, dry mouth, nasal congestion, constipation, impaired urination.
Pink or purple coloration of urine, of no significance.

▷ **Possible Adverse Effects** (unusual, unexpected and infrequent reactions)
If any of the following develop, consult your physician promptly for guidance.
Mild Adverse Effects
Allergic Reactions: Skin rash, hives, low-grade fever.
Lowering of body temperature, especially in the elderly. (See Hypothermia in Glossary).
Increased appetite and weight gain.
Dizziness, weakness, agitation, insomnia, impaired day and night vision.
Chronic constipation, fecal impaction.
Serious Adverse Effects
Allergic Reactions: Hepatitis with jaundice (see Glossary), severe skin reactions, anaphylactic reaction (see Glossary).

Idiosyncratic Reactions: Neuroleptic malignant syndrome (see Glossary).
Depression, disorientation, seizures, deposits in cornea, lens and retina.
Rapid heart rate, heart rhythm disorders.
Blood cell disorders: hemolytic anemia, reduced white blood cell and blood platelet counts.
Drug-induced porphyria.
Nervous system reactions: Parkinson-like disorders (see Glossary), severe restlessness, muscle spasms involving the face and neck, tardive dyskinesia (see Glossary).

▷ **Possible Effects on Sexual Function**
Altered timing and pattern of menstruation.
Female breast enlargement with milk production.
Male breast enlargement and tenderness.
Painful and extended duration of erection.
Inhibited ejaculation.
False positive pregnancy test results.

▷ **Adverse Effects That May Mimic Natural Diseases or Disorders**
Nervous system reactions may suggest true Parkinson's disease.
Liver reactions may suggest viral hepatitis.
Reactions resembling systemic lupus erythematosus can occur.

Natural Diseases or Disorders That May Be Activated by This Drug
Latent epilepsy, glaucoma, diabetes mellitus, prostatism (see Glossary).

Possible Effects on Laboratory Tests
White blood cell counts: decreased.
Blood bilirubin level: increased (jaundice—see Glossary).
Blood glucose level: increased.
Glucose tolerance test (GTT): decreased in 35% of those taking this drug.

CAUTION

1. Many over-the-counter medications (see OTC Drugs in Glossary) for allergies, colds and coughs contain drugs that can interact unfavorably with this drug. Ask your physician or pharmacist for help **before** using any such medications.
2. Antacids that contain aluminum and/or magnesium can prevent the absorption of this drug and reduce its effectiveness.
3. Obtain prompt evaluation of any change or disturbance of vision.

Precautions for Use

By Infants and Children: Use of this drug is not recommended in children under 12 years of age. Do not use this drug in the presence of symptoms suggestive of Reye syndrome (see Glossary). Children with acute infectious diseases (flulike infections, chicken pox, measles, etc.) are more prone to develop spasms of the face, back and extremities if this drug is used to control nausea or vomiting.

By Those over 60 Years of Age: Small starting doses are advisable. Increased susceptibility to development of drowsiness, lethargy, constipation, lowering of body temperature (hypothermia) and orthostatic hypotension (see Glossary). This drug can enhance existing prostatism (see Glossary). You may also be more susceptible to the development of Parkinson-like reactions and/or tardive dyskinesia (see discussion of these terms in Glossary). These reactions must be recognized early since they may become unresponsive to treatment and irreversible.

▷ **Advisability of Use During Pregnancy**
Pregnancy Category: C. See Pregnancy Code at the back of this book.
Animal studies: Cleft palate reported in mouse and rat studies.
Human studies: No increase in birth defects reported in 166 exposures. Information from adequate studies of pregnant women is not available.
Avoid drug during the first 3 months; avoid during the last month because of possible effects on the newborn infant.

Advisability of Use if Breast-Feeding
Presence of this drug in breast milk: Yes, in minute amounts.
Monitor nursing infant closely and discontinue drug or nursing if adverse effects develop.

Habit-Forming Potential: None.

Effects of Overdosage: Marked drowsiness, weakness, tremor, agitation, unsteadiness, deep sleep, coma, convulsions.

Possible Effects of Long-Term Use: Opacities in the cornea or lens of the eye, pigmentation of the retina.
Tardive dyskinesia (see Glossary).

Suggested Periodic Examinations While Taking This Drug (at physician's discretion)
Complete blood cell counts, especially between the fourth and tenth weeks of treatment.
Liver function tests, electrocardiograms.
Complete eye examinations—eye structures and vision.
Careful inspection of the tongue for early evidence of fine, involuntary, wavelike movements that could indicate the beginning of tardive dyskinesia.

▷ **While Taking This Drug, Observe the Following**
Foods: No restrictions.
Nutritional Support: A riboflavin (vitamin B-2) supplement should be taken with long-term use.
Beverages: No restrictions. May be taken with milk.
▷ *Alcohol:* Avoid completely. Alcohol can increase the sedative action of phenothiazines and accentuate their depressant effects on brain function and blood pressure. Phenothiazines can increase the intoxicating effects of alcohol.
Tobacco Smoking: Possible reduction of drowsiness from drug.
Marijuana Smoking: Moderate increase in drowsiness; accentuation of orthostatic hypotension; increased risk of precipitating latent psychoses, confusing the interpretation of mental status and drug responses.

▷ *Other Drugs*
Perphenazine may *increase* the effects of
- all sedative drugs, especially meperidine (Demerol), and cause excessive sedation.
- all atropinelike drugs, and cause nervous system toxicity.

Perphenazine may *decrease* the effects of
- guanethidine (Ismelin, Esimil), and reduce its effectiveness in lowering blood pressure.
- oral hypoglycemic drugs and cause loss of glucose control.

Perphenazine *taken concurrently* with
- lithium (Lithobid, Lithotabs) may impair the effectiveness of lithium and cause nervous system toxicity.

The following drugs may *decrease* the effects of perphenazine
- antacids containing aluminum and/or magnesium.
- barbiturates (see Drug Class Section).
- benztropine (Cogentin).
- disulfiram (Antabuse).
- trihexyphenidyl (Artane).

▷ *Driving, Hazardous Activities:* This drug can impair mental alertness, judgment and physical coordination. Avoid hazardous activities.

Aviation Note: The use of this drug *is a disqualification* for piloting. Consult a designated Aviation Medical Examiner.

Exposure to Sun: Use caution. Some phenothiazines can cause photosensitivity (see Glossary).

Exposure to Heat: Use caution and avoid excessive heat as much as possible. This drug may impair the regulation of body temperature and increase the risk of heat stroke.

Exposure to Cold: Use caution and dress warmly. This drug can increase the risk of hypothermia in the elderly.

Discontinuation: After a period of long-term use, do not stop this drug suddenly. Gradual withdrawal over 2 to 3 weeks under physician supervision is recommended. Do not discontinue this drug without your physician's knowledge and approval. The relapse rate of schizophrenia after discontinuation is 50–60%.

PHENELZINE (FEN el zeen)

Introduced: 1961 **Prescription:** USA: Yes; Canada: Yes **Available as Generic:** No **Class:** Antidepressant, MAO type A inhibitor **Controlled Drug:** USA: No; Canada: No

Brand Name: Nardil

BENEFITS versus RISKS	
Possible Benefits	*Possible Risks*
EFFECTIVE RELIEF OF REACTIVE, NEUROTIC, ATYPICAL DEPRESSIONS with associated anxiety or phobia Beneficial in some depressions that are not responsive to other treatments	DANGEROUS INTERACTIONS WITH MANY DRUGS AND FOODS CONDUCIVE TO HYPERTENSIVE CRISIS DISORDERED HEART RATE AND RHYTHM Drug-induced hepatitis (rare) Mental changes: agitation, confusion, impaired memory, hypomania

▷ **Principal Uses**
  As a Single Drug Product: Uses currently included in FDA approved labeling: (1) Used to treat severe situational (reactive or neurotic) depression, atypical depression, and (though less effective) severe endogenous depression. Because of the supervision required during its use and its potential for serious adverse effects, this drug is usually reserved to treat depressions that have not responded satisfactorily to other antidepressant therapy.
  Other (unlabeled) generally accepted uses: (1) Helps control binge eating in bulimia; (2) may be useful in treating chronic headache patients who also suffer from depression or anxiety; (3) a long term study found phenelzine beneficial in treating social phobia; (4) rare use in intractable narcolepsy; (5) may be of benefit in posttraumatic stress disorder.

How This Drug Works: By blocking an enzyme (monoamine oxidase type A) in brain tissue, this drug produces an increase of nerve impulse transmitters that maintain normal mood and emotional stability.

Available Dosage Forms and Strengths
  Tablets — 15 mg

▷ **Usual Adult Dosage Range:** Initially, 15 mg 3 times/day; increase rapidly up to 60 mg/day, as needed and tolerated, until improvement is apparent. For maintenance, reduce dose gradually over several weeks to the smallest dose that will maintain improvement; this may be as low as 15 mg daily or every other day. The total daily dosage should not exceed 90 mg. **Note: Actual dose and dosing schedule must be individually determined by the physician.**

Conditions Requiring Dosing Adjustments
  Liver function: Phenelzine is contraindicated in patients with increased liver function tests or history of liver compromise.
  Kidney function: No specific dosing changes are indicated in renal compromise.

▷ **Dosing Instructions:** The tablet may be crushed and taken on an empty stomach or with food. Do not take this drug in the late evening; it can interfere with sleep.

Usual Duration of Use: Use on a regular schedule for 3 to 4 weeks usually determines effectiveness in relieving depression. Once the optimal maintenance dose has been determined, it may be continued indefinitely. Long-term use (months to years) requires physician supervision.

▷ **This Drug Should Not Be Taken If**
  - you have had an allergic reaction to it previously.
  - you have advanced heart disease.
  - you have active liver disease or impaired liver function.
  - you have an adrenalin-producing tumor (pheochromocytoma).
  - you are taking any of the following drugs: another MAO type A inhibitor, a tricyclic antidepressant, carbamazepine (see Drug Classes).

▷ **Inform Your Physician Before Taking This Drug If**
  - you have high blood pressure.
  - you have had a stroke, or you have impaired circulation to the brain.
  - you have coronary heart disease.

- you have frequent or severe headaches.
- you have diabetes, epilepsy, schizophrenia or an overactive thyroid gland (hyperthyroidism).
- you are pregnant or are breast-feeding.
- you have impaired kidney function.
- you plan to have surgery under general or spinal anesthesia in the near future.

Possible Side-Effects (natural, expected and unavoidable drug actions)
Insomnia if taken in the evening.
Orthostatic hypotension (see Glossary).
Fluid retention (swelling of feet and ankles).

▷ **Possible Adverse Effects** (unusual, unexpected and infrequent reactions)
If any of the following develop, consult your physician promptly for guidance.
Mild Adverse Effects
Allergic Reaction: Skin rash.
Headache, dizziness, drowsiness, weakness, agitation, confusion, impaired memory, tremors, muscle twitching, blurred vision, impaired red-green color vision.
Dry mouth, increased appetite, indigestion, constipation.
Serious Adverse Effects
Drug-induced hepatitis with jaundice (see Glossary).
Hypertensive crisis: rapid and extreme rise in blood pressure, severe throbbing headache, palpitation, nausea, vomiting, sweating, risk of brain hemorrhage.
Peripheral neuropathy.
Seizures (rare).
Drug-induced porphyria.
Neuroleptic malignant syndrome (rare).
Unusual excitement or nervousness.
Disturbances of heart rate and rhythm.
Low white blood cell count.

▷ **Possible Effects on Sexual Function**
Decreased libido (30% of males, 28% of females).
Impaired erection (50%); inhibited ejaculation (60%).
Inhibited orgasm (30% of males, 35% of females).

▷ **Adverse Effects That May Mimic Natural Diseases or Disorders**
Drug-induced hepatitis may suggest viral hepatitis.

Natural Diseases or Disorders That May Be Activated by This Drug
Latent epilepsy, schizophrenia.
This drug may convert depression into the manic phase of a manic-depressive disorder.

Possible Effects on Laboratory Tests
White blood cell counts: decreased.
Blood glucose level: increased.
Liver function tests: increased liver enzymes (ALT/GPT and AST/GOT), increased bilirubin.
Systemic lupus erythematosus cells: positive.

CAUTION
1. The lowest effective dose should be identified and not exceeded.
2. The development of a severe headache or palpitation may indicate a dangerous elevation of blood pressure. Stop this drug immediately and call your doctor.
3. This drug may suppress anginal pain that would normally serve as a warning of excessive demand on the heart.
4. May increase the possibility of hypoglycemic reactions if used concurrently with insulin or oral antidiabetic drugs (sulfonylureas; see Drug Class Section). It may also delay recovery from hypoglycemia.
5. This drug can alter the threshold for convulsions in anyone with epilepsy or a seizure disorder. Dose decreases of anticonvulsant drugs may be needed.
6. This drug should be discontinued 2 weeks before elective surgery under general or spinal anesthesia. Consult your surgeon or anesthesiologist.
7. Many over-the-counter drug products contain ingredients that can cause serious interactions if taken with this drug. Avoid use of: cold and sinus medications, nasal decongestants, hay fever preparations, asthma inhalants, appetite and weight control products, "pep" pills. Ask your physician or pharmacist about their safe use with this drug.
8. It is advisable to carry a card of personal identification with the notation that you are taking this drug. Notify all medical personnel that may attend you that you are taking this drug.

Precautions for Use
By Infants and Children: Safety and effectiveness for those under 16 years of age not established.

By Those over 60 Years of Age: This drug is not recommended for use by anyone over 60. However, if poor response to other treatment justifies consideration of a trial of this drug, it should not be used in patients with high blood pressure, hardening of the arteries, impaired circulation within the brain, or coronary artery disease. This drug will intensify existing prostatism (see Glossary). Fluid retention is more prominent in this age group.

▷ Advisability of Use During Pregnancy
Pregnancy Category: C. See Pregnancy Code at the back of this book.
Animal studies: No information available.
Human studies: Adequate studies of pregnant women are not available. Birth defects have been reported with the use of this drug.
Avoid this drug completely if possible. Ask your physician for guidance.

Advisability of Use if Breast-Feeding
Presence of this drug in breast milk: Probably yes.
Avoid drug or refrain from nursing.

Habit-Forming Potential: None.

Effects of Overdosage: Overstimulation, agitation, anxiety, restlessness, insomnia, confusion, delirium, hallucinations, seizures, high fever, circulatory collapse, coma.

Possible Effects of Long-Term Use: The conversion of mental depression into a state of hypomania: excessive mental and physical activity, excitement, agitation, loud and rapid talking, delusional thinking.

Suggested Periodic Examinations While Taking This Drug (at physician's discretion)
Blood pressure measurements in lying, sitting and standing positions.
Complete blood cell counts, liver function tests.

▷ **While Taking This Drug, Observe the Following**

Foods: ***All tyramine-rich foods should be avoided completely.*** See Tyramine in the Glossary for a compete list of foods and beverages to avoid while taking this drug. A pyridoxine deficiency may develop and require supplementation (symptoms of peripheral neuropathy would result if this vitamin is not replaced).

Beverages: Limit coffee, tea and cola beverages to one serving daily. See Tyramine in the Glossary.

▷ *Alcohol:* Alcohol can increase the depressant effects of this drug on brain function.

Tobacco Smoking: No interactions expected.

▷ *Other Drugs*

Phenelzine may *increase* the effects of
- amphetamine and related drugs.
- appetite suppressants.
- all drugs with stimulant effects on the nervous system, and cause excessive rise in blood pressure.
- all drugs with sedative effects, and cause excessive sedation.
- insulin.
- sulfonylureas (see Drug Classes) or other oral hypoglycemic agents.

Phenelzine *taken concurrently* with
- antihistamines can worsen the anticholinergic side effects of antihistamines.
- carbamazepine (Tegretol) may cause severe toxic reactions.
- dextromethorphan (non-prescription cough medicine with a "DM") and cause severe toxic reactions.
- dopamine (Intropin) may cause severe toxic reactions.
- levodopa (Dopar, Sinemet) may cause a dangerous rise in blood pressure.
- meperidine (Demerol) may cause high fever, seizures and coma.
- methyldopa (Aldomet) may cause a dangerous rise in blood pressure.
- methylphenidate (Ritalin) may cause severe headache, weakness and numbness in the extremities.
- nadolol (Corgard) and metoprolol (Lopressor) or other beta blockers (see Drug Classes) may result in significant decreases in heart rate.
- phenothiazines or other antipsychotics may cause exaggeration of the central nervous system and depression of breathing effects.
- tryptophan (L-Tryptophan) can cause toxic reactions.
- tricyclic antidepressants may cause severe toxic reactions including high fever, delirium, tremor, seizures and coma.

Note: Consult your physician before taking *any other drugs* while taking phenelzine.

▷ *Driving, Hazardous Activities:* This drug may cause dizziness, drowsiness and blurred vision. Restrict activities as necessary.

Aviation Note: The use of this drug ***is a disqualification*** for piloting. Consult a designated Aviation Medical Examiner.

Exposure to Sun: No restrictions.

Occurrence of Unrelated Illness: Because of the very serious and life-threatening interactions that can occur between this drug and many others, you **must** tell each physician and dentist you consult that you are taking this drug.

Discontinuation: If this drug is not effective after 4 weeks of continual use, it should be stopped. If it is effective, continue to take it in proper dosage until advised to stop. Do not stop it abruptly. If another antidepressant is to be tried, a drug-free waiting period of 14 days must pass between stopping this drug and starting the new one. Avoid tyramine-rich foods and other interacting drugs during this 14-day period.

PHENOBARBITAL (fee noh BAR bi tawl)

Other Name: Phenobarbitone

Introduced: 1912 **Prescription:** USA: Yes; Canada: Yes **Available as Generic:** Yes **Class:** Sedative, anticonvulsant, barbiturates **Controlled Drug:** USA: C-IV*; Canada: C

Brand Names: Aminodrox-Forte, Antispasmodic[CD], Azpan, Barbidonna [CD], Barbidonna Elixir [CD], Barbita, Belap, Belladenal [CD], Belladenal-S [CD], ✦Belladenal Spacetabs [CD], ✦Bellergal [CD], Bellergal-S [CD], ✦Bellergal Spacetabs [CD], Bronchotabs [CD], Bronkolixir [CD], ✦Cafergot-PB, Chardonna-2 [CD], Daricon PB, ✦Diclophen [CD], Dilantin w/Phenobarbital [CD], Donphen, Donna-Sed, Donnatal [CD], Eskabarb, Eskaphen B [CD], ✦Gardenal, Hybephen [CD], Hypnaldyne [CD], Kinesed [CD], Luminal, Mudrane GG Elixir & Tablets [CD], Mudrane Tablets [CD], ✦Neuro-Spasex [CD], ✦Neuro-Trasentin [CD], ✦Neuro-Trasentin Forte [CD], Phedral [CD], ✦Phenaphen Capsules [CD], ✦Phenaphen No. 2, 3, 4 [CD], Phenergan w/Codeine [CD], Quadrinal [CD], Relaxadron, SBP [CD], Scodonnar [CD], Sedacord, SK-Phenobarbital, Solfoton, Spasquid [CD], Spazcaps, Tedral Preparations [CD], T.E.P. [CD], Thalfed [CD], Theocord [CD], Theolixer, Vitaphen

BENEFITS versus RISKS	
Possible Benefits	*Possible Risks*
EFFECTIVE CONTROL OF TONIC-CLONIC SEIZURES AND ALL TYPES OF PARTIAL SEIZURES	POTENTIAL FOR DEPENDENCE LIFE-THREATENING TOXICITY WITH OVERDOSAGE
EFFECTIVE CONTROL OF FEBRILE SEIZURES OF CHILDHOOD	Drug-induced hepatitis Rare drug induced decreased kidney function
Effective relief of anxiety and nervous tension	Rare blood cell disorders: abnormally low red cell, white cell and platelet counts

*See Schedules of Controlled Drugs at the back of this book.

Phenobarbital

▷ **Principal Uses**

As a Single Drug Product: Uses currently included in FDA approved lableing: (1) Used as a mild sedative; (2) as an anticonvulsant to control grand mal epilepsy and all types of partial seizures. It is also used to control febrile seizures of childhood.

Other (unlabeled) generally accepted uses: (1) May be helpful in detoxification of sedative-hypnotic addiction; (2) can help control seizures found in cerebral malaria; (3) eases neonatal seizures; (4) may have a role in pain syndromes.

As a Combination Drug Product [CD]: This drug is available in many combinations with derivatives of belladonna, an antispasmodic commonly used to treat functional disorders of the gastrointestinal tract. It is also available in combination with bronchodilators for the treatment of asthma, and with ergotamine for the treatment of headaches.

How This Drug Works: By impeding the transfer of sodium and potassium across cell membranes, this drug selectively blocks the transmission of nerve impulses. This could serve to produce a sedative effect and to suppress the spread of nerve impulses that are responsible for epileptic seizures.

Available Dosage Forms and Strengths

Capsules — 16 mg
 Elixir — 15 mg, 20 mg per 5-ml teaspoonful
 Tablets — 8 mg, 16 mg, 32 mg, 65 mg, 100 mg

▷ **Usual Adult Dosage Range:** As sedative—15 to 30 mg 2 to 4 times/day. As hypnotic—100 to 200 mg at bedtime. As anticonvulsant—120 to 250 mg given as a single dose at bedtime. Dose is used to keep blood levels from 15 to 40 mcg/ml. **Note: Actual dose and dosing schedule must be determined by the physician for each patient individually.**

Conditions Requiring Dosing Adjustments

Liver function: It should be used with caution, in decreased doses and blood levels obtained more frequently in patients with liver compromise.

Kidney function: This drug should be used with caution and in decreased dose in patients with compromised kidneys. Blood levels should be obtained at prudent intervals.

▷ **Dosing Instructions:** Regular tablets may be crushed and capsules opened and taken with or after food to reduce stomach irritation. Prolonged-action dosage forms should be swallowed whole without alteration.

Usual Duration of Use: Use on a regular schedule for 3 to 5 days determines effectiveness in relieving anxiety and tension, and for 4 to 6 weeks to determine its ability to control seizures. If used to treat anxiety-tension states, its use should not exceed 4 weeks without reappraisal of continued need. Long-term use for seizure control (months to years) requires physician supervision and periodic evaluation.

▷ **This Drug Should Not Be Taken If**
- you have had an allergic reaction to it previously.
- you have severe liver impairment.
- you are subject to acute intermittent porphyria (see Glossary).
- you have respiratory disease that makes it difficult to breathe.

▷ **Inform Your Physician Before Taking This Drug If**
- you are allergic or overly sensitive to any barbiturate (see Drug Class Section).
- you are pregnant or planning pregnancy.
- you have a history of alcohol or drug abuse.
- you are taking any drugs with sedative effects.
- you have any type of seizure disorder.
- you have myasthenia gravis.
- you have impaired liver, kidney or thyroid gland function.
- you plan to have surgery under general anesthesia in the near future.

Possible Side-Effects (natural, expected and unavoidable drug actions)
Drowsiness, impaired concentration, mental and physical sluggishness.

▷ **Possible Adverse Effects** (unusual, unexpected and infrequent reactions)
If any of the following develop, consult your physician promptly for guidance.

Mild Adverse Effects
Allergic Reactions: Skin rashes, hives, localized swellings of face, drug fever (see Glossary).
Dizziness, unsteadiness, impaired vision, double vision.
Nausea, vomiting, diarrhea.
Abnormal growth of the gums.
Shoulder-hand syndrome: pain and stiffness in the shoulder, pain and swelling in the hand.

Serious Adverse Effects
Allergic Reactions: Drug-induced hepatitis with jaundice (see Glossary), severe skin disorders (Stevens-Johnson syndrome or toxic epidermal necrolysis).
Osteoporosis (possible with long term use).
Idiosyncratic Reactions: Paradoxical excitement and delirium (instead of sedation).
Drug-induced myasthenia gravis.
Respiratory depression.
Mental depression, abnormal involuntary movements.
Blood cell disorders: deficiencies of all blood cell types causing fatigue, weakness, fever, sore throat, abnormal bleeding or bruising.
Blood clotting disorders in neonates.
Kidney disease (rare).
Optic neuropathy (rare).
Drug-induced seizures.
Low blood calcium.

▷ **Possible Effects on Sexual Function**
Decreased libido and/or impotence (16%).
Decreased effectiveness of oral contraceptives taken concurrently (71%).

▷ **Adverse Effects That May Mimic Natural Diseases or Disorders**
Liver reactions may suggest viral hepatitis.

Natural Diseases or Disorders That May Be Activated by This Drug
Acute intermittent and/or cutaneous porphyria, systemic lupus erythematosus.

Possible Effects on Laboratory Tests
>   Complete blood cell counts: decreased red cells, hemoglobin, white cells and platelets.
>   Blood lupus erythematosus (LE) cells: positive.
>   Prothrombin time: decreased (when taken concurrently with warfarin).
>   Blood calcium level: decreased (with long-term use).
>   Blood thyroxine (T_4) level: decreased.
>   Liver function tests: increased liver enzymes (ALT/GPT, AST/GOT and alkaline phosphatase), increased bilirubin.
>   Urine sugar tests: no effect with TesTape; false low results with Clinistix and Diastix.
>   Urine screening tests for drug abuse: may be **positive**. (Test results depend upon amount of drug taken and testing method used.)

CAUTION
>   1. Accurate diagnosis and classification of the seizure pattern are essential for correct selection of the most appropriate drug for therapy.
>   2. Emotional stress or physical trauma (including surgery) may require increased anticonvulsant dosage to control seizures.
>   3. Prolonged-action dosage forms of this drug are not appropriate for the treatment of seizures and should not be used.

Precautions for Use
>   *By Infants and Children:* This drug should not be given to the hyperkinetic child. Observe for possible paradoxical stimulation and hyperactivity; this can occur in 10% to 40% of children. Changes associated with puberty characteristically slow the metabolism of this drug and permit its gradual accumulation. Blood levels of this drug in young adolescents should be monitored every 3 months to detect rising concentrations and early toxicity.
>   *By Those over 60 Years of Age:* It is advisable to avoid all barbiturates in the elderly. If use of this drug is attempted, small starting doses are indicated. Watch for confusion, delirium, agitation and excitement. Do not use this drug concurrently with other drugs for mental disorders. This drug is conducive to the development of hypothermia (see Glossary).

▷ **Advisability of Use During Pregnancy**
>   *Pregnancy Category:* D. See Pregnancy Code at the back of this book.
>   Animal studies: Conflicting reports of cleft palate and skeletal defects in mouse, rat and rabbit studies.
>   Human studies: Information from studies of pregnant women indicates no increase in birth defects in 8037 exposures to this drug. However, it is reported that barbiturates can cause fetal damage when taken during pregnancy.
>   Avoid use of drug during entire pregnancy if possible. If it is clearly needed to control seizures, the mother should receive vitamin K prior to delivery and the infant should receive it at birth.

Advisability of Use if Breast-Feeding
>   Presence of this drug in breast milk: Yes, in small amounts.
>   Monitor nursing infant closely and discontinue drug or nursing if adverse effects develop.

Habit-Forming Potential: Psychological and physical dependence can occur with prolonged use of excessive doses—300 to 700 mg/day for 1 to 2 months. Dependence is not likely to occur with usual sedative or anticonvulsant doses.

Effects of Overdosage: Behavior similar to alcoholic intoxication—confusion, slurred speech, physical incoordination, staggering gait, drowsiness, stupor leading to coma.

Possible Effects of Long-Term Use: Psychological and/or physical dependence; syndrome of chronic intoxication—headache, depression, impaired vision, dizziness, slurred speech, incoordination. Megaloblastic anemia due to folic acid deficiency. Rickets or osteomalacia due to deficiencies of vitamin D and calcium.

Suggested Periodic Examinations While Taking This Drug (at physician's discretion)
When used to control seizures, blood phenobarbital levels are needed.
Time to sample blood for phenobarbital level: Just before next dose.
Recommended therapeutic range: For adults—15–40 mcg/ml; for children—15–30 mcg/ml.
Complete blood cell counts, liver function tests.
During long-term use: blood levels of folic acid, vitamin B-12, calcium and phosphorus; densitometry (DEXA) studies for demineralization of bone.

▷ **While Taking This Drug, Observe the Following**
Foods: No restrictions. Eat liberally of foods rich in folic acid—fortified breakfast cereals, liver, legumes, green leafy vegetables.
Beverages: No restrictions. May be taken with milk or fruit juices.
▷ *Alcohol:* Avoid completely. Alcohol can increase greatly the sedative and depressant actions of this drug on brain functions.
Tobacco Smoking: May enhance the sedative effects of this drug and increase drowsiness.
Marijuana Smoking: Increased drowsiness, unsteadiness; significantly impaired mental and physical performance.
▷ *Other Drugs*
Phenobarbital may *increase* the effects of
- all other drugs with sedative effects, and cause excessive sedation.

Phenobarbital may *decrease* the effects of
- anticoagulants (Coumadin, etc.), and require dosage adjustments.
- certain beta blockers (Inderal, Lopressor), and reduce their effectiveness.
- cortisonelike drugs.
- cyclosporine (Sandimmune).
- diltiazem.
- disopyramide.
- doxycycline (Vibramycin).
- griseofulvin (Fulvicin, etc.).
- metoprolol.
- oral contraceptives, and reduce their effectiveness in preventing pregnancy.
- quinidine (Quinaglute, etc.), and reduce its effectiveness.
- theophyllines (Aminophyllin, Theo-Dur, etc.), and reduce their antiasthmatic effectiveness.
- tricyclic antidepressants.
- verapamil (Calan) and reduce its effectiveness.
- warfarin and increase risk of clots.

Phenobarbital *taken concurrently* with
- colestipol and other cholesterol lowering resins may bind phenobarbital and limit absorption.
- influenza vaccine may cause phenobarbital toxicity.
- itraconazole may decrease the anti-fungal effect of itraconazole.
- phenytoin (Dilantin) may alter phenytoin blood levels: a high phenobarbital level will increase the phenytoin level; a low phenobarbital level will decrease the phenytoin level. Periodic determination of blood levels of both drugs is advised.
- primidone (Mysoline) may lead to phenobarbital toxicity.

The following drugs may *increase* the effects of phenobarbital
- valproic acid (Depakene).

▷ *Driving, Hazardous Activities:* This drug may cause drowsiness and may impair mental alertness, judgment, physical coordination and reaction time. Restrict activities as necessary.

Aviation Note: The use of this drug *is a disqualification* for piloting. Consult a designated Aviation Medical Examiner.

Exposure to Sun: Use caution. This drug may cause photosensitivity.

Exposure to Cold: Observe the elderly for possible hypothermia (see Glossary) while taking this drug.

Discontinuation: If used as an anticonvulsant, this drug must not be stopped abruptly. Sudden withdrawal can precipitate status epilepticus (repetitive seizures). Gradual reduction in dosage should be made over a period of 3 months. Total drug withdrawal may be attempted after a period of 3 to 5 years without a seizure. However, seizures are likely to recur in 40% of adults and in 20–30% of children.

PHENYTOIN (FEN i toh in)

Other Name: Diphenylhydantoin

Introduced: 1938   **Prescription:** USA: Yes; Canada: Yes   **Available as Generic:** USA: Yes; Canada: Yes   **Class:** Anticonvulsant, hydantoins
Controlled Drug: USA: No; Canada: No

Brand Names: Dilantin, Dilantin w/Phenobarbital [CD], Di-Phen, Diphenylan, ✦Mebroin [CD]

BENEFITS versus RISKS	
Possible Benefits	*Possible Risks*
EFFECTIVE CONTROL OF TONIC-CLONIC (GRAND MAL), PSYCHOMOTOR (TEMPORAL LOBE), MYOCLONIC AND FOCAL SEIZURES IN 80% OF USERS	VERY NARROW TREATMENT MARGIN POSSIBLE BIRTH DEFECTS Overgrowth of gums Excessive hair growth Rare blood cell disorders: impaired production of all blood cells Drug-induced hepatitis Drug-induced nephritis

▷ **Principal Uses**

As a Single Drug Product: Uses currently included in FDA approved labeling: (1) As an antiepileptic drug to control grand mal, psychomotor, myoclonic and focal seizures. It can also be used to control seizures following brain surgery.

Other (unlabeled) generally accepted uses: (1) Used to initiate treatment of trigeminal neuralgia; it is sometimes effective in relieving the severe facial pain of this disorder; (2) used in chronic pain syndromes; (3) may have a role (as an applied powder) in helping heal wounds.

As a Combination Drug Product [CD]: This drug is available in combination with phenobarbital, another effective anticonvulsant. Some seizure disorders require the combined actions of these two drugs for effective control.

How This Drug Works: By promoting the loss of sodium from nerve fibers, this drug lowers and stabilizes their excitability and thereby inhibits the repetitious spread of electrical impulses along nerve pathways. This action may prevent seizures altogether, or it may reduce their frequency and severity.

Available Dosage Forms and Strengths
Capsules (extended) — 30 mg, 100 mg
Capsules (prompt) — 30 mg, 100 mg
Injection — 50 mg per ml
Oral suspension — 30 mg, 125 mg per 5-ml teaspoonful
Tablets, chewable — 50 mg

▷ **Usual Adult Dosage Range:** Initially, 100 mg 3 times/day. Dose may be increased cautiously by 100 mg/week as needed and tolerated. Once the optimal maintenance dose has been identified, the total daily dose may be taken as a single dose every 24 hours if Dilantin capsules are used. No other formulation is approved for once-a-day use. The total daily dosage should not exceed 600 mg. **Note: Actual dosage and administration schedule must be determined by the physician for each patient individually.**

Conditions Requiring Dosing Adjustments

Liver function: The maintenance dose should be decreased based on blood levels.

Kidney function: The dose or dosing interval must be decreased in moderate kidney failure.

▷ **Dosing Instructions:** May be taken with or after food to reduce stomach irritation. The capsule may be opened and the tablet may be crushed for administration.

Usual Duration of Use: Use on a regular schedule for 2 to 3 weeks usually determines benefit in reducing frequency and severity of seizures. Optimal control will require careful dosage adjustments over a period of several months. Long-term use (months to years) requires ongoing physician supervision.

▷ **This Drug Should Not Be Taken If**
- you have had an allergic reaction to this drug or to other hydantoin drugs previously.
- you have sinus bradycardia or serious heart block.

▷ **Inform Your Physician Before Taking This Drug If**
- you are taking any other drugs at this time.
- you have a history of liver disease or impaired liver function.
- you have low blood pressure, diabetes or any type of heart disease.
- you are pregnant or are planning pregnancy.
- you plan to have surgery under general anesthesia in the near future.

Possible Side-Effects (natural, expected and unavoidable drug actions)
Mild fatigue, sluggishness and drowsiness (in sensitive individuals).
Pink to red to brown coloration of urine (of no significance).

▷ **Possible Adverse Effects** (unusual, unexpected and infrequent reactions)
If any of the following develop, consult your physician promptly for guidance.

Mild Adverse Effects
Allergic Reactions: Skin rashes (5–10%), hives, drug fever (see Glossary).
Headache, dizziness, nervousness, insomnia, muscle twitching.
Nausea, vomiting, constipation.
Bedwetting.
Abnormal eye movements.
Low blood calcium and elevated blood sugar.
Overgrowth of gum tissues (most common in children).
Excessive growth of body hair (most common in young girls).

Serious Adverse Effects
Allergic Reactions: Drug-induced hepatitis, with or without jaundice (see Glossary). Drug-induced nephritis, with acute kidney failure. Severe skin reactions (TEN, Stevens-Johnson or erythema multiforme). Myocarditis, generalized enlargement of lymph glands (pseudolymphoma).
Idiosyncratic Reaction: Hemolytic anemia (see Glossary).
Acute psychotic episodes (rare).
Blood clotting disorders in infants of mothers maintained on phenytoin (rare).
Bone marrow depression (see Glossary): fatigue, weakness, fever, sore throat, abnormal bleeding or bruising.
Drug-induced periarteritis nodosa.
Drug-induced seizures.
Drug-induced low thyroid function.
Drug-induced myasthenia gravis.
Abnormal IgA (increased risk of respiratory infections).
Peripheral neuropathy.
Drug-induced porphyria.
Serious heart rhythm problems (with rapid intravenous use).
Mental confusion, unsteadiness, double vision, jerky eye movements, slurred speech.
Myopathy (rare).
Joint pain and swelling.
Elevated blood sugar, due to inhibition of insulin release.

▷ **Possible Effects on Sexual Function**
Decreased libido and/or impotence (11%).
Peyronie's disease (see Glossary).
Decreased effectiveness of oral contraceptives taken concurrently (24%).

▷ **Adverse Effects That May Mimic Natural Diseases or Disorders**
Drug-induced hepatitis may suggest viral hepatitis.
Skin reactions may resemble lupus erythematosus.

Natural Diseases or Disorders That May Be Activated by This Drug
Latent diabetes, porphyria, systemic lupus erythematosus.

Possible Effects on Laboratory Tests
Complete blood cell counts: decreased red cells, hemoglobin, white cells and platelets; increased eosinophils (allergic reaction).
Blood lupus erythematosus (LE) cells: positive.
Prothrombin time: increased (when taken concurrently with warfarin).
Blood calcium level: decreased.
Blood total cholesterol, LDL and VLDL cholesterol levels: no effects.
Blood HDL cholesterol level: increased.
Blood triglyceride levels: no effect.
Blood glucose level: increased.
Blood thyroid hormone levels: T_3, T_4 and free T_4 increased.
Liver function tests: increased liver enzymes (ALT/GPT, AST/GOT and alkaline phosphatase), increased bilirubin.

CAUTION
1. Some brand name capsules of this drug have a significantly longer duration of action than generic name capsules of the same strength. To assure a correct dosing schedule, it is necessary to distinguish between "prompt" action and "extended" action capsules. Do not substitute one for the other without your physician's knowledge and guidance.
2. When used for the treatment of epilepsy, ***this drug must not be stopped abruptly.***
3. Periodic measurements of blood levels of this drug are essential in determining appropriate dosage. (See Therapeutic Drug Monitoring Section.)
4. Regularity of drug use is essential for successful management of seizure disorders. Take this drug at the same time each day.
5. Shake the suspension form of this drug thoroughly before measuring the dose. Use a standard measuring device to assure that the dose is based upon a 5-ml teaspoon.
6. Side-effects and mild adverse effects are usually most apparent during the first several days of treatment, and often subside with continued use.
7. It may be necessary to take folic acid to prevent anemia while taking this drug. Consult your physician regarding this.
8. It is advisable to carry a card of personal identification with a notation that you are taking this drug.

Precautions for Use
By Infants and Children: Elimination of this drug varies widely with age. Periodic measurement of blood levels is essential for all ages. Some children will require more than one dose daily for good control. Observe for early indications of drug toxicity: jerky eye movements, unsteadiness in stance and gait, slurred speech, abnormal involuntary movements of the extremities and odd behavior.

By Those over 60 Years of Age: You may be more sensitive to all of the actions of this drug and require smaller doses. Observe closely for any indications of early toxicity: drowsiness, fatigue, confusion, unsteadiness, disturbances of vision, slurred speech, muscle twitching.

▷ **Advisability of Use During Pregnancy**
Pregnancy Category: D. See Pregnancy Code at the back of this book.
Animal studies: Cleft lip and palate, skeletal and visceral defects in mice; skeletal and visceral defects in rats.
Human studies: Available information is conflicting. Some studies suggest a small but significant increase in the occurrence of birth defects associated with the use of phenytoin during pregnancy. The incidence of birth defects in children of epileptics not taking anticonvulsant drugs is 3.2%; the incidence with the use of anticonvulsant drugs during pregnancy increases to 6.4%. The "fetal hydantoin syndrome" in the newborn infant exposed to phenytoin during pregnancy consists of birth defects of the skull, face and limbs, deficient growth and development, and subnormal intelligence and performance. Other effects on the infant include reduction in blood clotting factors that predispose it to severe bruising and hemorrhage.
Discuss with your physician the advantages and possible disadvantages of using this drug during pregnancy. It is advisable to use the smallest maintenance dose that will control seizures. In addition, you should be given vitamin K during the last month of pregnancy to prevent a deficiency of blood clotting factors in the fetus.

Advisability of Use if Breast-Feeding
Presence of this drug in breast milk: Yes, in trace amounts.
Monitor nursing infant closely and discontinue drug or nursing if adverse effects develop.

Habit-Forming Potential: None.

Effects of Overdosage: Drowsiness, jerky eye movements, hand tremor, unsteadiness, slurred speech, hallucinations, delusions, nausea, vomiting, stupor progressing to coma.

Possible Effects of Long-Term Use: Low blood calcium resulting in rickets or osteomalacia; megaloblastic anemia; peripheral neuropathy (see Glossary); schizophreniclike psychosis. Lymphosarcoma, malignant lymphoma and leukemia have been associated with long-term use; a cause-and-effect relationship (see Glossary) has not been established.

Suggested Periodic Examinations While Taking This Drug (at physician's discretion)
Monitoring of blood phenytoin levels to guide dosage.
Time to sample blood for phenytoin level: Just before next dose.
Recommended therapeutic range: 10 to 20 ng/ml.
Complete blood cell counts, liver function tests.
Measurements of the following blood levels: glucose, calcium, phosphorus, folic acid, vitamin B-12.
Skeletal X-ray studies for demineralization of bone.

▷ **While Taking This Drug, Observe the Following**
Foods: No restrictions.
Nutritional Support: Supplements of folic acid, calcium, vitamin D and vitamin K may be necessary.

Beverages: No restrictions. May be taken with milk.
▷ *Alcohol:* Use extreme caution. Alcohol (in large quantities or with continual use) may reduce this drug's effectiveness in preventing seizures.
Tobacco Smoking: No interactions expected.
▷ *Other Drugs*
   Phenytoin may ***decrease*** the effects of
   - acetaminophen.
   - conjugated estrogens.
   - cortisonelike drugs (see Drug Class Section).
   - cyclosporine.
   - disopyramide.
   - doxycycline (Vibramycin, etc.).
   - itraconazole.
   - levodopa (Larodopa, Sinemet).
   - levothyroxine.
   - meperidine.
   - methadone (Dolophine).
   - mexiletine (Mexitil).
   - miconazole.
   - oral contraceptives (birth control pills).
   - oral hypoglycemic agents (see Drug Class).
   - quinidine (Quinaglute, etc.).

   Phenytoin ***taken concurrently*** with
   - oral anticoagulants (Coumadin, etc.) can either increase or decrease the anticoagulant effect; monitor this combination very closely with serial prothrombin testing.
   - carbamazepine (Tegretol) may result in increased or decreased levels of phenytoin.
   - chlordiazepoxide (and perhaps other benzodiazepines) may increase or decrease pheyntoin levels. Levels should be obtained more frequently if these drugs are combined.
   - ciprofloxacin (Cipro) may increase or decrease phenytoin levels.
   - dopamine will result in very low blood pressure.
   - primidone (Mysoline) may alter primidone actions and enhance its toxicity.
   - theophyllines (Aminophyllin, Theo-Dur, etc.) may cause a decrease in the effectiveness of both drugs.
   - warfarin (Coumadin) may result in an initial increased risk of bleeding and a subsequent decrease in anticoagulation.

   The following drugs may ***increase*** the effects of phenytoin
   - amiodarone (Codarone).
   - chloramphenicol (Chloromycetin).
   - chlorpheniramine.
   - cimetidine (Tagamet).
   - cotrimoxazole.
   - diltiazem.
   - disulfiram (Antabuse).
   - felbamate.
   - fluconazole (Diflucan).
   - fluoxetine (Prozac).

- ibuprofen and perhaps other NSAIDs.
- isoniazid (INH, Niconyl, etc.).
- nifedipine.
- phenacemide (Phenurone).
- sulfonamides (see Drug Class Section).
- tricyclic antidepressants (see drug Classes).
- trimethoprim (Proloprim, Trimpex).
- valproic acid (Depakene).

The following drugs may *decrease* the effects of phenytoin
- bleomycin.
- carmustine.
- cisplatin.
- diazoxide.
- folic acid.
- methotrexate.
- rifampin.
- vinblastine.

▷ *Driving, Hazardous Activities:* This drug may impair mental alertness, vision and coordination. Restrict activities as necessary.

Aviation Note: The use of this drug *is a disqualification* for piloting. Consult a designated Aviation Medical Examiner.

Exposure to Sun: Use caution. This drug may cause photosensitivity (see Glossary).

Occurrence of Unrelated Illness: Intercurrent infections may slow the elimination of this drug and increase the risk of toxicity due to higher blood levels.

*Discontinuation: **This drug must not be discontinued abruptly.*** Sudden withdrawal can precipitate severe and repeated seizures. If this drug is to be discontinued, gradual reduction in dosage should be made over a period of 3 months. Total drug withdrawal may be attempted after a period of 3 to 4 years without a seizure. However, seizures are likely to recur in 40% of adults and in 20–30% of children.

PILOCARPINE (pi loh KAR peen)

Introduced: 1875 **Prescription:** USA: Yes; Canada: No **Available as Generic:** Yes **Class:** Antiglaucoma **Controlled Drug:** USA: No; Canada: No

Brand Names: Adsorbocarpine, Almocarpine, Akarpine, E-Pilo Preparations [CD], I-Pilopine, Isopto Carpine, ✦Minims, ✦Miocarpine, Ocusert Pilo-20, -40, PE Preparations [CD], Pilagan, Pilocar, ✦Pilopine HS, Piloptic-1,-2, Pilosyst 20/40, Salagen, ✦Spersacarpine

BENEFITS versus RISKS	
Possible Benefits	*Possible Risks*
EFFECTIVE REDUCTION OF INTERNAL EYE PRESSURE FOR CONTROL OF ACUTE AND CHRONIC GLAUCOMA	Mild side-effects with systemic absorption Minor eye discomfort Altered vision

Pilocarpine

▷ **Principal Uses**

As a Single Drug Product: Uses currently included in FDA approved labeling: (1) Used exclusively for the management of all types of glaucoma. Selection of the appropriate dosage form and strength must be carefully individualized.

Other (unlabeled) generally accepted uses: (1) Treatment of Adie's syndrome; (2) can help in situations where the salivary glands fail to work.

As a Combination Drug Product [CD]: This drug is combined with epinephrine (in eye drop solutions) to utilize the actions of both drugs in lowering internal eye pressure. The opposite effects of these two drugs on the size of the pupil (pilocarpine constricts, epinephrine dilates) provides a balance that prevents excessive constriction or dilation.

How This Drug Works: By directly stimulating constriction of the pupil, this drug enlarges the outflow canal in the anterior chamber of the eye and promotes the drainage of excess fluid (aqueous humor), thus lowering the internal eye pressure.

Available Dosage Forms and Strengths

Eye drop solutions — 0.25%, 0.5%, 1%, 2%, 3%, 4%, 5%, 6%, 8% and 10%
Gel — 4%
Ocuserts — 20 mcg and 40 mcg
Tablet — 5 mg

▷ **Usual Adult Dosage Range:** For chronic glaucoma—eye drop solutions: 1 drop of a 0.5% to 4% solution 4 times/day. Eye gel: apply 0.5 inch strip of gel into the eye once daily at bedtime. Ocusert: insert one into affected eye and replace every 7 days with a new one. **Note: Actual dose and dosing schedule must be determined by the physician for each patient individually.**

Conditions Requiring Dosing Adjustments

Liver function: The specific elimination of this drug is unclear.
Kidney function: The elimination of this drug has yet to be defined.

▷ **Dosing Instructions:** To avoid excessive absorption into the body, press finger against inner corner of the eye (to close off the tear duct) during and for 2 minutes following instillation of the eye drop. Place the gel and the Ocusert in the eye at bedtime.

Usual Duration of Use: Use on a regular schedule for 1 to 2 weeks usually determines this drug's effectiveness in controlling internal eye pressure. Long-term use (months to years) requires physician supervision.

▷ **This Drug Should Not Be Taken If**
- you have had an allergic reaction to it previously.
- you have active bronchial asthma.

▷ **Inform Your Physician Before Taking This Drug If**
- you have a history of bronchial asthma.
- you have a history of acute iritis.
- you have significant heart disease.
- you have chronic obstructive pulmonary disease.
- you have gallstones.

Possible Side-Effects (natural, expected and unavoidable drug actions)

Temporary impairment of vision, usually lasting 2 to 3 hours following instillation of drops.

Pilocarpine

▷ **Possible Adverse Effects** (unusual, unexpected and infrequent reactions)
   If any of the following develop, consult your physician promptly for guidance.
   Mild Adverse Effects
      Allergic Reactions: Itching of the eyes, eyelid itching and/or swelling.
      Headache, heart palpitation, tremors.
      Sweating.
   Serious Adverse Effects
      Provocation of acute asthma in susceptible individuals.
      Atrioventricular block (abnormal heart conduction).
      Retinal detachment (rare).

▷ **Possible Effects on Sexual Function:** None reported.

Possible Effects on Laboratory Tests
   Red blood cell and white blood cell counts: increased.

Precautions for Use
   By Those over 60 Years of Age: Maintain personal cleanliness to prevent eye infections. Report promptly any indication of possible infection involving the eyes.

▷ **Advisability of Use During Pregnancy**
   Pregnancy Category: C. See Pregnancy Code at the back of this book.
      Animal studies: Significant birth defects due to this drug reported in rats.
      Human studies: Adequate studies of pregnant women are not available.
      Limit use to the smallest effective dose. Minimize systemic absorption (see Dosing Instructions).

Advisability of Use if Breast-Feeding
   Presence of this drug in breast milk: May be present in small amounts.
   Monitor nursing infant closely and discontinue drug or nursing if adverse effects develop.

Habit-Forming Potential: None.

Effects of Overdosage: Flushing of face, increased flow of saliva, sweating. If solution is swallowed: nausea, vomiting, diarrhea, profuse sweating, rapid pulse, difficult breathing, loss of consciousness.

Possible Effects of Long-Term Use: Development of tolerance (see Glossary), temporary loss of effectiveness.

Suggested Periodic Examinations While Taking This Drug (at physician's discretion)
   Measurement of internal eye pressure on a regular basis.
   Examination of eyes for development of cataracts.

▷ **While Taking This Drug, Observe the Following**
   Foods: No restrictions.
   Beverages: No restrictions.
▷   *Alcohol:* Use caution. If this drug is absorbed, it may prolong the effect of alcohol on the brain.
   Tobacco Smoking: No interactions expected.
   Marijuana Smoking: Sustained additional decrease in internal eye pressure.
▷ *Other Drugs*
   The following drugs may ***decrease*** the effects of pilocarpine
   • atropine and drugs with atropinelike actions (see Drug Classes).

Pilocarpine *taken concurrently* with
- epinephrine will result in increased myopia.
- timolol can produce additive effects in treating glaucoma.

▷ *Driving, Hazardous Activities:* This drug may impair your ability to focus your vision properly. Restrict activities as necessary.

Aviation Note: The use of this drug *may be a disqualification* for piloting. Consult a designated Aviation Medical Examiner.

Exposure to Sun: No restrictions.

Discontinuation: Do not stop regular use of this drug without consulting your physician. Periodic discontinuation and temporary substitution of another drug may be necessary to preserve its effectiveness in treating glaucoma.

PINDOLOL (PIN doh lohl)

Introduced: 1972   **Prescription:** USA: Yes; Canada: Yes   **Available as Generic:** Yes   **Class:** Antihypertensive, beta-adrenergic blocker   **Controlled Drug:** USA: No; Canada: No

Brand Names: ✦Apo-Pindol, ✦Novo-Pindol, ✦Nu-Pindol, ✦Syn-Pindolol, ✦Viskazide [CD], Visken

BENEFITS versus RISKS	
Possible Benefits	*Possible Risks*
EFFECTIVE, WELL-TOLERATED ANTIHYPERTENSIVE in mild to moderate high blood pressure	CONGESTIVE HEART FAILURE in advanced heart disease Worsening of angina in coronary heart disease (abrupt withdrawal) Masking of low blood sugar (hypoglycemia) in drug-treated diabetes Provocation of asthma (with high doses)

▷ **Principal Uses**

As a Single Drug Product: Uses currently included in FDA approved labeling: (1) The treatment of mild to moderate high blood pressure. May be used alone or concurrently with other antihypertensive drugs, such as diuretics.

Other (unlabeled) generally accepted uses: (1) May be of benefit in helping control aggressive behavior; (2) can help prevent migraine headaches; (3) combination therapy with dogoxin may be effective in limiting some abnormal heart rhythmns (atrial fibrillation); (4) can be of benefit in some kinds of anxiety; (5) decreases sympathetic output in hyperthyroidism.

As a Combination Drug Product [CD]: This drug is available in combination with hydrochlorothiazide (in Canada). The addition of a thiazide diuretic to this beta blocker drug enhances its effectiveness as an antihypertensive.

How This Drug Works: By blocking certain actions of the sympathetic nervous system, this drug
- reduces the rate and contraction force of the heart, thus lowering the ejection pressure of the blood leaving the heart.

Pindolol

- reduces the degree of contraction of blood vessel walls, resulting in their relaxation and consequent lowering of blood pressure.

Available Dosage Forms and Strengths
Tablets — 5 mg, 10 mg, 15 mg (Canada)

▷ **Usual Adult Dosage Range:** Initially, 5 mg twice daily (12 hours apart). The dose may be increased gradually by 10 mg/day at intervals of 2 to 3 weeks as needed and tolerated up to 60 mg/day. For maintenance, 5 to 10 mg 2 or 3 times/day. The total daily dose should not exceed 60 mg. **Note: Actual dosage and administration schedule must be determined by the physician for each patient individually.**

Conditions Requiring Dosing Adjustments
Liver function: The dose should be empirically decreased in patients with severe liver compromise and in those with combined liver and kidney compromise.
Kidney function: The dose should be decreased if urine output is significatly decreased.

▷ **Dosing Instructions:** The tablet may be crushed and taken without regard to eating. Do not stop this drug abruptly.

Usual Duration of Use: Use on a regular schedule for 2 to 3 weeks usually determines effectiveness in lowering blood pressure. The long-term use of this drug (months to years) will be determined by the course of your blood pressure over time and your response to an overall treatment program (weight reduction, salt restriction, smoking cessation, etc.). Consult your physician on a regular basis.

Possible Advantages of This Drug: Causes less slowing of the heart rate than most other beta blocker drugs.

Currently a "Drug of Choice"
for initiating treatment of hypertension with a single drug.

▷ **This Drug Should Not Be Taken If**
- you have bronchial asthma.
- you have had an allergic reaction to it previously.
- you have congestive heart failure.
- you have an abnormally slow heart rate or a serious form of heart block.
- you are taking, or have taken within the past 14 days, any monoamine oxidase (MAO) type A inhibitor drug (see Drug Classes).

▷ **Inform Your Physician Before Taking This Drug If**
- you have had an adverse reaction to any beta blocker in the past (see Drug Classes).
- you have a history of serious heart disease.
- you have a history of hay fever (allergic rhinitis), asthma, chronic bronchitis or emphysema.
- you have a history of overactive thyroid function (hyperthyroidism).
- you have a history of low blood sugar (hypoglycemia) or diabetes.
- you have impaired liver or kidney function.
- you have diabetes or myasthenia gravis.
- you currently take any form of digitalis, quinidine or reserpine, or any calcium blocker drug (see Drug Class Section).
- you plan to have surgery under general anesthesia in the near future.

Possible Side-Effects (natural, expected and unavoidable drug actions)
   Lethargy and fatigability (15%), cold extremities, slow heart rate, light-headedness in upright position (see Orthostatic Hypotension in Glossary).

▷ **Possible Adverse Effects** (unusual, unexpected and infrequent reactions)
   If any of the following develop, consult your physician promptly for guidance.
   Mild Adverse Effects
   Allergic Reactions: Skin rash, itching.
   Headache (5%), dizziness (17%), insomnia (19%), abnormal dreams, fainting.
   Indigestion, nausea (7%), vomiting, constipation, diarrhea.
   Joint and muscle discomfort (11%), fluid retention (edema) (11%).
   Serious Adverse Effects
   Mental depression, anxiety.
   Chest pain, shortness of breath, precipitation of congestive heart failure.
   Induction of bronchial asthma (in asthmatic individuals).
   Abnormally slow heart beat.
   Congestive heart failure (2%).
   Drug-induced systemic lupus erythematosus (rare).
   Drug-induced myasthenia gravis.
   Depression.
   Low blood glucose.

▷ **Possible Effects on Sexual Function:** Decreased libido, impaired erection (rare).

Possible Effects on Laboratory Tests
   Blood lupus erythematosus (LE) cells: positive (one case of drug-induced LE).
   Blood total cholesterol level: decreased (with long-term use).
   Blood HDL cholesterol level: increased.
   Blood LDL and VLDL cholesterol levels: no effects.
   Blood triglyceride levels: no effects.
   Glucose tolerance test (GTT): decreased.
   Liver function tests: slightly increased liver enzymes (ALT/GPT and AST/GOT) in 7% of drug users.

CAUTION
   1. ***Do not stop this drug suddenly*** without the knowledge and help of your doctor. Carry a notation on your person that you are taking this drug.
   2. Ask your doctor or pharmacist before using nasal decongestants usually present in over-the-counter cold preparations and nose drops. These can cause sudden increases in blood pressure when taken concurrently with beta blocker drugs.
   3. Report the development of any tendency to emotional depression.

Precautions for Use
   By Infants and Children: Safety and effectiveness for those under 12 years of age not established. However, if this drug is used, observe for the development of low blood sugar (hypoglycemia) during periods of reduced food intake.
   By Those over 60 Years of Age: Unacceptably high blood pressure should be

reduced without creating the risks associated with excessively low blood pressure. Small starting doses, and frequent blood pressure checks are indicated. Sudden, rapid and excessive reduction of blood pressure can predispose to stroke or heart attack. Watch for dizziness, unsteadiness, tendency to fall, confusion, hallucinations, depression or urinary frequency.

▷ **Advisability of Use During Pregnancy**
Pregnancy Category: B. See Pregnancy Code at the back of this book.
Animal studies: No significant increase in birth defects due to this drug.
Human studies: Adequate studies of pregnant women are not available.
Use this drug only if clearly needed. Ask physician for guidance.

Advisability of Use if Breast-Feeding
Presence of this drug in breast milk: Yes.
Avoid drug or refrain from nursing.

Habit-Forming Potential: None.

Effects of Overdosage: Weakness, slow pulse, low blood pressure, fainting, cold and sweaty skin, congestive heart failure, possible coma and convulsions.

Possible Effects of Long-Term Use: Reduced heart reserve and eventual heart failure in susceptible individuals with advanced heart disease.

Suggested Periodic Examinations While Taking This Drug (at physician's discretion)
Measurements of blood pressure, evaluation of heart function.

▷ **While Taking This Drug, Observe the Following**
Foods: No restrictions. Avoid excessive salt intake.
Beverages: No restrictions. May be taken with milk.
▷ *Alcohol:* Use with caution. Alcohol may exaggerate this drug's ability to lower the blood pressure and may increase its mild sedative effect.
Tobacco Smoking: Nicotine may reduce this drug's effectiveness in treating high blood pressure. In addition, high doses of this drug may worsen constriction of the bronchial tubes caused by regular smoking.

▷ *Other Drugs*
Pindolol may *increase* the effects of
- other antihypertensive drugs, and cause excessive lowering of the blood pressure. Dosage adjustments may be necessary.
- reserpine (Ser-Ap-Es, etc.), and cause sedation, depression, slowing of the heart rate and lowering of the blood pressure.
- verapamil (Calan, Isoptin), and cause excessive depression of heart function; monitor this combination closely.

Pindolol *taken concurrently* with
- clonidine (Catapres) requires close monitoring for rebound high blood pressure if clonidine is withdrawn while pindolol is still being taken.
- insulin requires close monitoring to avoid undetected hypoglycemia (see Glossary).
- oral hypoglycemic agents (see Drug Classes) can result in slowed recovery from low blood sugar.

The following drugs may *increase* the effects of pindolol
- cimetidine (Tagamet).
- methimazole (Tapazole).

- oral contraceptives.
- propylthiouracil (Propacil).

The following drugs may *decrease* the effects of pindolol
- barbiturates (phenobarbital, etc.).
- indomethacin (Indocin), and possibly other "aspirin substitutes," or NSAIDs may impair pindolol's antihypertensive effect.
- rifampin (Rifadin, Rimactane).
- theophylline.

▷ *Driving, Hazardous Activities:* Use caution until the full extent of fatigue, dizziness and blood pressure change have been determined.

Aviation Note: The use of this drug *is a disqualification* for piloting. Consult a designated Aviation Medical Examiner.

Exposure to Sun: No restrictions.

Exposure to Heat: Caution advised. Hot environments can lower the blood pressure and exaggerate the effects of this drug.

Exposure to Cold: Caution advised. Cold environments can enhance the circulatory deficiency in the extremities that may occur with this drug. The elderly should take precautions to prevent hypothermia (see Glossary).

Heavy Exercise or Exertion: It is advisable to avoid exertion that produces light-headedness, excessive fatigue or muscle cramping. The use of this drug may intensify the hypertensive response to isometric exercise.

Occurrence of Unrelated Illness: Fever can lower the blood pressure and require adjustment of dosage. Nausea or vomiting may interrupt regular doses. Ask your doctor for help.

Discontinuation: It is advisable to avoid sudden discontinuation of this drug in all situations. If possible, gradual reduction of dose over a period of 2 to 3 weeks is recommended. Ask your physician for specific guidance.

PIRBUTEROL (peer BYU ter ohl)

Introduced: 1983 **Prescription:** USA: Yes **Available as Generic:** No **Class:** Antiasthmatic, bronchodilator **Controlled Drug:** USA: No
Brand Name: Maxair

BENEFITS versus RISKS	
Possible Benefits	*Possible Risks*
VERY EFFECTIVE RELIEF OF BRONCHOSPASM	Increased blood pressure Nervousness Fine hand tremor Irregular heart rhythm (with excessive use)

▷ **Principal Uses**

As a Single Drug Product: Uses curently included in FDA approved labeling: (1) relieves acute attacks of bronchial asthma; (2) reduces the frequency and severity of chronic, recurrent asthmatic attacks (prevention); (3) relieves reversible bronchospasm associated with chronic bronchitis, bronchiectasis and emphysema.

Other (unlabeled) generally accepted uses: May help high blood potassium seen in kidney failure.

Pirbuterol

How This Drug Works: By increasing the production of cyclic AMP, this drug relaxes constricted bronchial muscles to relieve asthmatic wheezing.

Available Dosage Forms and Strengths
Aerosol — 200 mcg per actuation (in canisters of 300 inhalations)

▷ **Usual Adult Dosage Range:** Inhaler—1 to 2 inhalations (200 to 400 mcg) every 4 to 6 hours. **Do not exceed** 12 inhalations (2400 mcg)/24 hours. **Note: Actual dosage and administration schedule must be determined by the physician for each patient individually.**

Conditions Requiring Dosing Adjustments
Liver function: It should be used with caution in patients with liver compromise who use it frequently. Guidelines for dosage adjustments are not available.
Kidney function: The kidneys do not appear to play a role in the elimination of this drug.

▷ **Dosing Instructions:** Carefully follow the "Patient's Instructions for Use" provided with the inhaler. Do not overuse.

Usual Duration of Use: According to individual requirements. Do not use beyond the time necessary to terminate episodes of asthma.

Possible Advantages of This Drug
Has a more rapid onset of action and a longer duration of effect than most other drugs of this class.

▷ **This Drug Should Not Be Taken If**
- you have had an allergic reaction to it previously.
- you currently have an irregular heart rhythm.
- you are taking, or have taken within the past 2 weeks, any monoamine oxidase (MAO) type A inhibitor drug (see Drug Classes).

▷ **Inform Your Physician Before Taking This Drug If**
- you have any type of heart or circulatory disorder, especially high blood pressure, coronary heart disease or heart rhythm abnormality.
- you have diabetes or hyperthyroidism.
- you have any type of seizure disorder.
- you are taking any form of digitalis or any stimulant drug.

Possible Side-Effects (natural, expected and unavoidable drug actions)
Aerosol—dryness or irritation of mouth or throat, altered taste.

▷ **Possible Adverse Effects** (unusual, unexpected and infrequent reactions)
If any of the following develop, consult your physician promptly for guidance.
Mild Adverse Effects
Allergic Reactions: Skin rash, itching (less than 1%).
Headache (2%), dizziness (1.2%), nervousness (6.9%), fine tremor of hands (6%).
Palpitations (1.7%), rapid heart rate (1.2%), chest pain (1.3%), cough (1.2%).
Nausea (1.7%), diarrhea (1.3%), taste disorders (rare).
Serious Adverse Effects
Irregular heart rhythm, increased blood pressure.

▷ **Possible Effects on Sexual Function:** None reported.

Natural Diseases or Disorders That May Be Activated By This Drug
Latent coronary artery disease, diabetes, epilepsy or high blood pressure.

Possible Effects on Laboratory Tests
None reported.

CAUTION
1. Combined use of this drug by inhalation with beclomethasone aerosol (Beclovent, Vanceril) may increase the risk of toxicity due to fluorocarbon propellants. Advisable to use pirbuterol aerosol 20 to 30 minutes **before** beclomethasone aerosol. This will reduce the risk of toxicity and help beclomethasone reach the lung.
2. Excessive or prolonged use of this drug by inhalation can reduce its effectiveness and cause serious heart rhythm disturbances, including cardiac arrest.

Precautions for Use
By Infants and Children: Safety and effectiveness of use in children under 12 years of age have not been established.
By Those over 60 Years of Age: Avoid excessive and continual use. If acute asthma is not relieved promptly, other drugs will have to be tried. Observe for the development of nervousness, palpitations, irregular heart rhythm and muscle tremors.

▷ **Advisability of Use During Pregnancy**
Pregnancy Category: C. See Pregnancy Code at the back of this book.
  Animal studies: High-dose studies in rabbits revealed abortion and increased fetal deaths. Studies in rats and rabbits found no drug associated birth defects.
  Human studies: Adequate studies of pregnant women are not available.
  Avoid use during first 3 months if possible.

Advisability of Use if Breast-Feeding
Presence of this drug in breast milk: Unknown.
Avoid drug or refrain from nursing.

Habit-Forming Potential: None.

Effects of Overdosage: Nervousness, palpitation, rapid heart rate, sweating, headache, tremor, vomiting, chest pain.

Possible Effects of Long-Term Use: Loss of effectiveness.

Suggested Periodic Examinations While Taking This Drug (at physician's discretion)
Blood pressure measurements, evaluation of heart status.

▷ **While Taking This Drug, Observe the Following**
Foods: No restrictions.
Beverages: Avoid excessive use of caffeine-containing beverages—coffee, tea, cola, chocolate.
▷ *Alcohol:* No interactions expected.
Tobacco Smoking: No interactions expected.
▷ *Other Drugs*
  Pirbuterol **taken concurrently** with
  • monoamine oxidase (MAO) type A inhibitor drugs may cause excessive increase in blood pressure and undesirable heart stimulation.

▷ *Driving, Hazardous Activities:* Use caution if excessive nervousness or dizziness occurs.
Aviation Note: The use of this drug ***is a disqualification*** for piloting. Consult a designated Aviation Medical Examiner.
Exposure to Sun: No restrictions.
Heavy Exercise or Exertion: Use caution. Excessive exercise can induce asthma in sensitive individuals.

PIROXICAM (peer OX i kam)

Introduced: 1978 **Prescription:** USA: Yes; Canada: Yes **Available as Generic:** Yes **Class:** Mild analgesic, anti-inflammatory **Controlled Drug:** USA: No; Canada: No
Brand Names: ✦Apo-Piroxicam, Feldene, ✦Novopirocam, Nu-Pirox

BENEFITS versus RISKS	
Possible Benefits	*Possible Risks*
EFFECTIVE RELIEF OF MILD TO MODERATE PAIN AND INFLAMMATION	Gastrointestinal pain, ulceration, bleeding. Drug-induced hepatitis (rare) Rare kidney damage Mild fluid retention Reduced white blood cell and platelet counts

Please see the oxicam nonsteroidal anti-inflammatory drug profile for further information.

PRAVASTATIN (pra vah STA tin)

Introduced: 1986 **Prescription:** USA: Yes; Canada: Yes **Available as Generic:** USA: No; Canada: No **Class:** Cholesterol reducer **Controlled Drug:** USA: No; Canada: No
Brand Name: Pravachol

BENEFITS versus RISKS	
Possible Benefits	*Possible Risks*
EFFECTIVE REDUCTION OF TOTAL BLOOD CHOLESTEROL AND LDL CHOLESTEROL	Drug-induced hepatitis (without jaundice) 1.3% Drug-induced myositis (muscle inflammation) 0.6%

▷ **Principal Uses**
As a Single Drug Product: Uses currently included in FDA approved labeling: Treatment of abnormally high total blood cholesterol levels (in individuals with Types IIa and IIb hypercholesterolemia) due to increased fractions of low-density lipoprotein (LDL) cholesterol. It is used in conjunction with a cholesterol-lowering diet. It should not be used until an

adequate trial of nondrug methods for lowering cholesterol has proved to be ineffective.

Other (unlabeled) generally accepted uses: Familial hypercholesterolemia.

How This Drug Works: This drug blocks the liver enzyme that starts production of cholesterol. Its principal action is the reduction of low-density lipoproteins (LDL), the fraction of total blood cholesterol that is thought to increase the risk of coronary heart disease. This drug may also increase the level of high-density lipoproteins (HDL), the cholesterol fraction that is thought to reduce the risk of heart disease.

Available Dosage Forms and Strengths
Tablets — 10 mg, 20 mg (Canada) and 20 mg (United States).

▷ **Recommended Dosage Ranges** (Actual dosage and administration schedule must be determined by the physician for each patient individually.)
Infants and Children: Under 2 years of age—do not use this drug.
2 to 18 years of age—dosage not established.
18 to 60 Years of Age: Initially 10 to 40 mg daily (depending upon cholesterol level), taken at bedtime. Maintenance dosage is 10 to 20 mg daily; adjust as needed and tolerated at intervals of 4 weeks.
Over 60 Years of Age: Same as 18 to 60 years of age.

Conditions Requiring Dosing Adjustments
Liver function: This drug should be used with caution in patients with liver compromise, and the starting dose decreased to 10 mg per day. Pravastatin is contraindicated in acute liver disease.
Kidney function: Patients with significant renal compromise can be given a starting dose of 10 mg per day. Pravastatin should be used with caution in renal compromise.

▷ **Dosing Instructions:** The tablet may be crushed and can be taken without regard to eating. Preferably taken at bedtime. (The highest rates of cholesterol production occur between midnight and 5 A.M.).

Usual Duration of Use: Use on a regular schedule for 4 to 6 weeks usually determines effectiveness in reducing blood levels of total and LDL cholesterol. Long-term use (months to years) requires periodic physician evaluation.

Possible Advantages of This Drug: Recent studies indicate that drugs of this class (HMG-CoA reductase inhibitors) are more effective and better tolerated than other drugs currently available for reducing total and LDL cholesterol. Its long-term effects are yet to be determined. See Cholesterol Disorders in Section Two.

▷ **This Drug Should Not Be Taken If**
- you have had an allergic reaction to it previously.
- you have active liver disease.
- you are pregnant or breast-feeding.

▷ **Inform Your Physician Before Taking This Drug If**
- you have previously taken any other drugs in this class: lovastatin (Mevacor), simvastatin (Zocor).
- you have a history of liver disease or impaired liver function.
- you are not using any method of birth control, or you are planning pregnancy.

- you regularly consume substantial amounts of alcohol.
- you have kidney disease.
- you have cataracts or impaired vision.
- you have any type of chronic muscular disorder.
- you plan to have major surgery in the near future.

Possible Side-Effects (natural, expected and unavoidable drug actions)
Development of abnormal liver function tests without associated symptoms.

▷ **Possible Adverse Effects** (unusual, unexpected and infrequent reactions)
If any of the following develop, consult your physician promptly for guidance.

Mild Adverse Effects
Allergic Reactions: Skin rash, itching (1.3%).
Headache (1.7%), dizziness (1.0%).
Flu-like syndrome.
Indigestion (2.0%), stomach pain (2.0%), nausea (2.9%), excessive gas (2.7%), constipation (2.4%), diarrhea (2.0%).
Muscle cramps and/or pain (1.4%).

Serious Adverse Effects
Marked and persistent abnormal liver function tests with focal hepatitis (without jaundice) occurred in 1.3%.
Acute myositis (muscle pain and tenderness) occurred in 0.6% during long-term use.
Low white blood cells (Leukopenia) (rare).

▷ **Possible Effects on Sexual Function:** None reported.

Possible Delayed Adverse Effects: None reported to date.

Natural Diseases or Disorders That May Be Activated by This Drug
Latent liver disease.

Possible Effects on Laboratory Tests
Blood alanine aminotransferase (ALT) enzyme level: increased (with higher doses of drug).
Blood total cholesterol, LDL cholesterol and triglyceride levels: decreased.
Blood HDL cholesterol level: increased.

CAUTION
1. If pregnancy occurs while taking this drug, discontinue it immediately and consult your physician.
2. Report promptly any development of muscle pain or tenderness, especially if accompanied by fever or malaise.
3. Report promptly the development of altered or impaired vision so that appropriate evaluation can be made.

Precautions for Use
By Infants and Children: Safety and effectiveness for those under 18 years of age not established.
By Those over 60 Years of Age: Inform your physician regarding any personal or family history of cataracts. Comply with all recommendations regarding periodic eye examinations. Report promptly any alterations in vision.

▷ **Advisability of Use During Pregnancy**
Pregnancy Category: X. See Pregnancy Code at the back of this book.
Animal studies: Mouse and rat studies reveal skeletal birth defects due to a closely related drug of this class.

Human studies: Adequate studies of pregnant women are not available. This drug should be avoided during entire pregnancy.

Advisability of Use if Breast-Feeding
Presence of this drug in breast milk: Yes, in small amounts.
Avoid drug or refrain from nursing.

Habit-Forming Potential: None.

Effects of Overdosage: Increased indigestion, stomach distress, nausea, diarrhea.

Possible Effects of Long-Term Use: Abnormal liver function with focal hepatitis.

Suggested Periodic Examinations While Taking This Drug (at physician's discretion)
Blood cholesterol studies: total cholesterol, HDL and LDL fractions.
Liver function tests before treatment, every 6 weeks during the first 3 months of use, every 8 weeks for the rest of the first year, and at 6-month intervals thereafter.
Complete eye examination at beginning of treatment and at any time that significant change in vision occurs. Ask your physician for guidance.

▷ **While Taking This Drug, Observe the Following**
  Foods: Follow a standard low-cholesterol diet.
  Beverages: No restrictions. May be taken with milk.
▷ *Alcohol:* No interactions expected. Use sparingly.
  Tobacco Smoking: No interactions expected.
▷ *Other Drugs*
  Pravastatin *taken concurrently* with
  • cyclosporine (Sandimmune) increases the risk for myopathy.
  • gemfibrozil (Lopid) may alter the absorption and excretion of pravastatin; these drugs should not be taken concurrently.
  • warfarin (Coumadin) can increase the risk of bleeding.
  The following drug may *decrease* the effects of pravastatin
  • cholestyramine (Questran), may reduce absorption of pravastatin; take pravastatin 1 hour before or 4 hours after cholestyramine.
▷ *Driving, Hazardous Activities:* This drug may cause dizziness. Restrict activities as necessary.
  Aviation Note: The use of this drug *may be a disqualification* for piloting. Consult a designated Aviation Medical Examiner.
  Exposure to Sun: No restrictions.
  Discontinuation: Do not stop this drug without your doctor's knowledge and help. There may be a significant increase in blood cholesterol levels following discontinuation of this drug.

PRAZOSIN (PRA zoh sin)

Introduced: 1970 **Prescription:** USA: Yes; Canada: Yes **Available as Generic:** Yes **Class:** Antihypertensive **Controlled Drug:** USA: No; Canada: No

Brand Names: ✦Apo-Prazo, Minipress, Minizide [CD], ✦Novo-Prazin, ✦Nu-Prazo

Prazosin

BENEFITS versus RISKS	
Possible Benefits	*Possible Risks*
EFFECTIVE INITIAL THERAPY FOR MILD TO MODERATE HYPERTENSION	"First dose" drop in blood pressure with fainting (0.15%)
EFFECTIVE ANTIHYPERTENSIVE IN CASES OF MODERATE TO SEVERE HYPERTENSION	Cause of paroxysmal tachycardia (5.3%)
EFFECTIVE CONTROL OF HYPERTENSION IN PHEOCHROMOCYTOMA	
Effective in presence of impaired kidney function	

▷ **Principal Uses**
  As a Single Drug Product: Uses currently included in FDA approved labeling: (1) Used to start treatment in mild to moderate hypertension. Also used in conjunction with other drugs, to treat moderate to severe hypertension.
  Other (unlabeled) generally accepted uses: (1) Combination therapy of congestive heart failure; (2) helps control high blood pressure in a rare tumor (pheochromocytoma); (3) may have an adjunctive role in controlling urine outflow problems caused by prostatic obstruction; (4) may help relieve the symptoms of Raynaud's phenomenon; (5) can ease symptoms of angina.
  As a Combination Drug Product [CD]: This drug is available in combination with polythiazide, a diuretic of the thiazide class of drugs. By utilizing two different methods of drug action, this combination product is more effective and more convenient for long-term use.

How This Drug Works: By blocking certain actions of the sympathetic nervous system, this drug causes direct relaxation and expansion of blood vessel walls, thus lowering the pressure of the blood within the vessels.

Available Dosage Forms and Strengths
  Capsules — 1 mg, 2 mg, 5 mg

▷ **Usual Adult Dosage Range:** Initiate treatment with a "test dose" of 1 mg to determine the patient's response within the first 2 hours. If tolerated satisfactorily, dose is increased cautiously up to 15 mg/24 hours in 2 or 3 divided doses. The total daily dosage should not exceed 20 mg. **Note: Actual dose and dosing schedule must be determined by the physician for each patient individually.**

Conditions Requiring Dosing Adjustments
  Liver function: It should be used with caution and in lower doses in patients with liver compromise. The drug is 97% protein bound.
  Kidney function: Patients with kidney failure may have adequate response to smaller doses.

▷ **Dosing Instructions:** May be taken without regard to food. The capsule may be opened for administration.

Usual Duration of Use: Use on a regular schedule for 4 to 6 weeks usually determines effectiveness in controlling hypertension. Long-term use (months to years) requires supervision and periodic physician evaluation.

Possible Advantages of This Drug
Effective initial treatment of hypertension.
Does not alter blood cholesterol, potassium or sugar levels.

▷ **This Drug Should Not Be Taken If**
- you have had an allergic reaction to it previously.
- you are experiencing mental depression.
- you have angina (active coronary artery disease) and you are not taking a beta-blocking drug. (Consult your physician.)

▷ **Inform Your Physician Before Taking This Drug If**
- you have experienced orthostatic hypotension (see Glossary) when using other antihypertensive drugs.
- you have a history of mental depression.
- you have impaired circulation to the brain, or a history of stroke.
- you have coronary artery disease.
- you have active liver disease or impaired liver function.
- you plan to have surgery under general anesthesia in the near future.

Possible Side-Effects (natural, expected and unavoidable drug actions)
Orthostatic hypotension, drowsiness (7%), salt and water retention, dry mouth, nasal congestion, constipation.

▷ **Possible Adverse Effects** (unusual, unexpected and infrequent reactions)
If any of the following develop, consult your physician promptly for guidance.
Mild Adverse Effects
Allergic Reactions: Skin rash, itching.
Headache (7.8%), dizziness (10.3%), fatigue (6.9%), weakness (6.5%), nervousness, sweating, numbness and tingling, blurred vision, reddened eyes, ringing in the ears.
Edema.
Nose bleeds (less than 4%).
Palpitation (5.3%), rapid heart rate, shortness of breath.
Nausea (4.9%), vomiting, diarrhea, abdominal pain, constipation.
Urinary frequency and incontinence.
Serious Adverse Effects
Mental depression, sleep disturbance.
Paroxysmal tachycardia (heart rates of 120 to 160).

▷ **Possible Effects on Sexual Function**
Decreased libido (14%); impotence (less than 1%).
Retrograde ejaculation. Priapism (see Glossary).

Natural Diseases or Disorders That May Be Activated by This Drug
Latent coronary artery insufficiency.

Possible Effects on Laboratory Tests
Blood total cholesterol level: no effect in some; decreased in others.
Blood HDL cholesterol level: no effect in some; increased in others.
Blood LDL cholesterol level: no effect.
Blood VLDL cholesterol level: no effect in some; decreased in others.
Blood triglyceride levels: no effect in some; decreased in others.
Blood glucose level: increased.
Glucose tolerance test (GTT): decreased.

Blood thyroid stimulating hormone (TSH) level: increased.
Blood thyroxine (T_4) level: increased.

CAUTION
1. Observe for the possible "first dose" response of precipitous drop in blood pressure, with or without fainting; this usually occurs within 30 to 90 minutes. Limit initial doses to 1 mg taken at bedtime for the first 3 days; remain supine after taking these trial doses.

Precautions for Use
By Infants and Children: Safety and effectiveness for use by those under 12 years of age have not been established.

By Those over 60 Years of Age: Begin treatment with no more than 1 mg/day for the first 3 days. Subsequent increases in dose must be very gradual and carefully supervised by your physician. The occurrence of orthostatic hypotension can cause unexpected falls and injury; sit or lie down promptly if you feel light-headed or dizzy. Report any indications of dizziness or chest pain promptly.

▷ **Advisability of Use During Pregnancy**
Pregnancy Category: C. See Pregnancy Code at the back of this book.
Animal studies: No birth defects found.
Human studies: Adequate studies of pregnant women are not available.
Use this drug only if clearly needed. Ask your physician for guidance.

Advisability of Use if Breast-Feeding
Presence of this drug in breast milk: Yes, in small amounts.
Monitor nursing infant closely and discontinue drug or nursing if adverse effects develop.

Habit-Forming Potential: None.

Effects of Overdosage: Orthostatic hypotension, headache, generalized flushing, rapid heart rate, extreme weakness, irregular heart rhythm, circulatory collapse.

Possible Effects of Long-Term Use: None reported.

Suggested Periodic Examinations While Taking This Drug (at physician's discretion)
Measurements of blood pressure in lying, sitting and standing positions.
Measurements of body weight to detect fluid retention.

▷ **While Taking This Drug, Observe the Following**
Foods: No restrictions. Avoid excessive salt intake.
Beverages: No restrictions. May be taken with milk.

▷ *Alcohol:* Use with extreme caution. Alcohol can exaggerate the blood-pressure-lowering actions of this drug and cause excessive reduction.
Tobacco Smoking: Nicotine can worsen this drug's ability to intensify coronary insufficiency in susceptible individuals. All forms of tobacco should be avoided.

▷ *Other Drugs*
The following drugs may *increase* the effects of prazosin
- beta-adrenergic-blocking drugs (see Drug Classes); severity and duration of the "first dose" hypotensive response may be increased.
- verapamil (Calan) may increase the blood level of prazosin and require dose reduction.

Prazocin *taken concurrently* with
- NSAIDs (see Drug Classes).

▷ *Driving, Hazardous Activities:* This drug may cause dizziness or drowsiness. Restrict activities as necessary.

Aviation Note: The use of this drug *is a disqualification* for piloting. Consult a designated Aviation Medical Examiner.

Exposure to Sun: No restrictions.

Exposure to Cold: Use caution until combined effect has been determined. Cold environments may increase this drug's ability to cause coronary insufficiency (angina) in susceptible individuals.

Heavy Exercise or Exertion: Excessive exertion can augment this drug's ability to induce angina.

Discontinuation: If you are taking this drug as part of your treatment program for congestive heart failure, do not stop it abruptly. Ask your physician for guidance.

PREDNISOLONE (pred NIS oh lohn)

Introduced: 1955 **Prescription:** USA: Yes; Canada: Yes **Available as Generic:** USA: Yes; Canada: Yes **Class:** Cortisonelike drugs **Controlled Drug:** USA: No; Canada: No

Brand Names: ✦Ak-Cide [CD], A & D with prednisolone [CD], ✦Ak-Pred, ✦Ak-Tate, Blephamide, Cortalone, Delta-Cortef, Duapred, Econopred Ophthalmic, Fernisolone-P, Hydelta-TBA, Hydeltrasol, ✦Inflamase, ✦Inflamase Forte, Isopto Cetapred [CD], Key-Pred, Meticortelone, Menti-Derm, Metimyd [CD], Metreton, ✦Minims Prednisolone, Niscort, Nor-Pred, ✦Nova-Pred, ✦Novoprednisolone, Ophtho-Tate, Optimyd [CD], Otobione [CD], Pediapred, Pediaject, Predcor, ✦Pred Forte, Pred-G [CD], ✦Pred Mild, Prelone, PSP-IV, Savacort, Sterane, TBA Pred, ✦Vasocidin [CD]

BENEFITS versus RISKS	
Possible Benefits	*Possible Risks*
EFFECTIVE RELIEF OF SYMPTOMS IN A WIDE VARIETY OF INFLAMMATORY AND ALLERGIC DISORDERS	Short-term use (up to 10 days) is usually well tolerated
EFFECTIVE IMMUNO-SUPPRESSION in selected benign and malignant disorders	Long-term use (exceeding 2 weeks) is associated with many possible adverse effects:
Prevention of rejection in organ transplantation	ALTERED MOOD AND PERSONALITY
	CATARACTS, GLAUCOMA
	HYPERTENSION
	OSTEOPOROSIS
	ASEPTIC BONE NECROSIS
	INCREASED SUSCEPTIBILITY TO INFECTIONS
	(See Possible Adverse Effects and Possible Effects of Long-Term Use below)

Prednisolone

▷ **Principal Uses**

As a Single Drug Product: Uses currently included in FDA approved labeling: (1) Used in the treatment of a wide variety of allergic and inflammatory conditions. It is used most commonly in the management of serious skin disorders, asthma, regional enteritis, ulcerative colitis and all types of major rheumatic disorders including bursitis, tendinitis, most forms of arthritis and inflammatory eye conditions; (2) used as part of combination therapy in lymphoma; (3) used in some kinds of adrenal insufficiencies; (4) used to help tuberculosis patients who also have inflammation around the heart without fluid buildup; (5) eases symptoms in ulcerative colitis.

Other (unlabeled) generally accepted uses: (1) Used as part of combination therapy in acute leukemias (lymphoblastic, lymphocytic and myelogenous); (2) may have a role in combination therapy of breast cancer; (3) can help relieve the muscle pain of familial Mediterranean Fever; (4) part of a combination therapy in treating abnormal liver tumors (hemangiomas); (5) Can help subfertile men decrease seminal antibodies and become fertile; (6) helps people who have drug-induced lowering of white blood cells recover; (7) treats anaphylactic reactions of unknown cause; (8) treats thrombocytopenic purpura of unknown cause; (9) eases symptoms in myasthenia gravis; (10) can help reflex sympathetic dystrophy.

How This Drug Works: Not fully established. It is thought that this drug's anti-inflammatory effect is due to its ability to inhibit the normal defensive functions of certain white blood cells. Its immunosuppressant effect is attributed to a reduced production of lymphocytes and antibodies.

Available Dosage Forms and Strengths
Eye ointment — 0.6%
Eye suspension — 1%
Syrup — 15 mg per 5-ml teaspoonful
Tablets — 5 mg

▷ **Usual Adult Dosage Range:** 5 to 60 mg daily as a single dose or in divided doses. The total daily dosage should not exceed 250 mg. **Note: Actual dosage and administration schedule must be determined by the physician for each patient individually.**

Conditions Requiring Dosing Adjustments

Liver function: Dosing adjustments do not appear to be needed in liver compromise.

Kidney function: Dosing adjustments in renal compromise do not appear to be needed. This drug can cause proteinuria, and may be a benefit to risk use in patients with kidney compromise (nephropathy) which causes them to lose protein.

▷ **Dosing Instructions:** The tablet may be crushed and taken with or following food to prevent stomach irritation, preferably in the morning.

Usual Duration of Use: For acute disorders: 4 to 10 days. For chronic disorders: according to individual requirements. The duration of use should not exceed the time needed to obtain adequate symptomatic relief in acute self-limiting conditions; or the time required to stabilize a chronic condition and permit gradual withdrawal. Because of its intermediate duration of action, this drug is appropriate for alternate day administration. Consult your physician on a regular basis.

Note: The information categories provided in this Profile are appropriate for prednisolone. For specific information that is normally found in those categories that have been omitted from this Profile, the reader is referred to the Drug Profile of Prednisone which follows. Prednisolone is a derivative of Prednisone; all significant actions and effects are shared by both drugs.

PREDNISONE (PRED ni sohn)

Introduced: 1955   **Prescription:** USA: Yes; Canada: Yes   **Available as Generic:** USA: Yes; Canada: Yes   **Class:** Cortisonelike drugs   **Controlled Drug:** USA: No; Canada: No

Brand Names: ✦Apo-Prednisone, Deltasone, Liquid Pred, Meticorten, ✦Metreton [CD], ✦Novoprednisone, Orasone, Panasol-S, Paracort, Prednicen-M, SK-Prednisone, Sterapred, ✦Winpred

BENEFITS versus RISKS	
Possible Benefits	*Possible Risks*
EFFECTIVE RELIEF OF SYMPTOMS IN A WIDE VARIETY OF INFLAMMATORY AND ALLERGIC DISORDERS EFFECTIVE IMMUNOSUPPRESSION in selected benign and malignant disorders Prevention of rejection in organ transplantation	Short-term use (up to 10 days) is usually well tolerated Long-term use (exceeding 2 weeks) is associated with many possible adverse effects: ALTERED MOOD AND PERSONALITY CATARACTS, GLAUCOMA HYPERTENSION OSTEOPOROSIS ASEPTIC BONE NECROSIS INCREASED SUSCEPTIBILITY TO INFECTIONS (See Possible Adverse Effects and Possible Effects of Long-Term Use below)

▷ **Principal Uses**

As a Single Drug Product: Uses currently included in FDA approved labeling: Treats a wide variety of allergic and inflammatory conditions. It is used most commonly in the management of serious skin disorders, asthma, gout, lupus erythematosus, regional enteritis, ulcerative colitis, nephrotic syndrome and all types of major rheumatic disorders including bursitis, tendinitis and most forms of arthritis; (2) used as part of combination therapy of lymphoma; (3) helps address adrenal insufficiency.

Other (unlabeled) generally accepted uses: (1) Used in combination therapy of acute (lymphoblastic, lymphocytic and myelogenous) leukemias; (2) combination therapy of breast cancer; (3) may be helpful in therapy of familial mediterranean fever; (4) used with other medications to treat liver tumors (hemangiomas); (5) may help subfertile men decrease seminal antibodies and become fertile; (6) helps prevent early lung deterioration in children with AIDS; (7) eases symptoms in alcoholics who have hepatitis and encephalopathy; (8) used in some chronic pain syndromes.

How This Drug Works: It is thought that this drug's anti-inflammatory effect is due to its ability to inhibit the normal defensive functions of certain white blood cells. Its immunosuppressant effect is attributed to a reduced production of lymphocytes and antibodies.

Available Dosage Forms and Strengths
    Oral solution — 5 mg per 5-ml teaspoonful
        Syrup — 5 mg per 5-ml teaspoonful (alcohol 5%)
        Tablets — 1 mg, 2.5 mg, 5 mg, 10 mg, 20 mg, 25 mg, 50 mg

▷ **Usual Adult Dosage Range:** 5 to 60 mg daily as a single dose or in divided doses. The total daily dosage should not exceed 250 mg. **Note: Actual dosage and administration schedule must be determined by the physician for each patient individually.**

Conditions Requiring Dosing Adjustments
  Liver function: Dosing adjustments do not appear to be needed in liver compromise.
  Kidney function: Dosing adjustments in renal compromise do not appear to be needed. This drug is a possible cause of proteinuria. Its use is a benefit to risk decision in patients who have protein losing renal compromise (nephropathy).

▷ **Dosing Instructions:** The tablet may be crushed and taken with or following food to prevent stomach irritation, preferably in the morning.

Usual Duration of Use: For acute disorders: 4 to 10 days. For chronic disorders: according to individual requirements. The duration of use should not exceed the time necessary to obtain adequate symptomatic relief in acute self-limiting conditions; or the time required to stabilize a chronic condition and permit gradual withdrawal. Because of its intermediate duration of action, this drug is appropriate for alternate day administration. Consult your physician on a regular basis.

▷ **This Drug Should Not Be Taken If**
- you have had an allergic reaction to any dosage form of it previously.
- you have active peptic ulcer disease.
- you have an active herpes simplex virus eye infection.
- you have active tuberculosis.
- you have a systemic fungal infection.

▷ **Inform Your Physician Before Taking This Drug If**
- you have had an adverse reaction to any cortisonelike drug.
- you have a history of peptic ulcer disease, thrombophlebitis or tuberculosis.
- you have: diabetes, kidney failure, glaucoma, high blood pressure, deficient thyroid function or myasthenia gravis.
- you have osteoporosis.
- you plan to have surgery of any kind in the near future.

Possible Side-Effects (natural, expected and unavoidable drug actions)
  Increased appetite, weight gain, retention of salt and water, excretion of potassium, increased susceptibility to infection.

▷ **Possible Adverse Effects** (unusual, unexpected and infrequent reactions)
If any of the following develop, consult your physician promptly for guidance.
Mild Adverse Effects
Allergic Reaction: Skin rash.
Headache, dizziness, insomnia.
Acid indigestion, abdominal distention.
Patchy blue areas on the great toe (blue toe syndrome).
Muscle cramping and weakness.
Elevated intracranial pressure (pseudotumor cerebri).
Acne, excessive growth of facial hair.
Serious Adverse Effects
Mental and emotional disturbances of serious magnitude.
Reactivation of latent tuberculosis.
Development of peptic ulcer.
Increased blood pressure.
Development of inflammation of the pancreas.
Thrombophlebitis (inflammation of a vein with the formation of blood clot)—pain or tenderness in thigh or leg, with or without swelling of the foot, ankle or leg.
Seizures (rare).
Increased intraocular (in the eye) pressure.
Kaposi's sarcoma (rare).
Necrosis of bone.
Superinfections.
Increased blood sugar.
Drug-induced porphyria.
Pulmonary embolism (movement of a blood clot to the lung)—sudden shortness of breath, pain in the chest, coughing, bloody sputum.
Low blood platelets (rare).

▷ **Possible Effects on Sexual Function**
Altered timing and pattern of menstruation.
Correction of male infertility when due to autoantibodies that suppress sperm activity.

▷ **Adverse Effects That May Mimic Natural Diseases or Disorders**
Pattern of symptoms and signs resembling Cushing's syndrome.

Natural Diseases or Disorders That May Be Activated by This Drug
Latent diabetes, glaucoma, peptic ulcer disease, tuberculosis.

Possible Effects on Laboratory Tests
Complete blood cell counts: decreased eosinophils, lymphocytes and platelets.
Blood amylase level: increased (possible pancreatitis).
Blood total cholesterol and HDL cholesterol levels: increased.
Blood LDL cholesterol level: no effect.
Blood triglyceride levels: no significant effect.
Blood glucose level: increased.
Glucose tolerance test (GTT): decreased.
Blood potassium level: decreased.
Blood testosterone level: decreased.

Prednisone

Blood thyroid hormone (T_3): decreased.
Blood uric acid level: increased.
Urine sugar tests: no effect with TesTape; false low result with Clinistix and Diastix.
Fecal occult blood test: positive (if gastrointestinal bleeding).

CAUTION
1. If therapy is to exceed one week, it is advisable to carry a card of personal identification with a notation that you are taking this drug.
2. Do not stop this drug abruptly after long-term use.
3. If vaccination against measles, rabies, smallpox or yellow fever is required, discontinue this drug 72 hours before vaccination and do not resume it for at least 14 days after vaccination.

Precautions for Use
By Infants and Children: Avoid prolonged use if possible. During long-term use, observe for suppression of normal growth and the possibility of increased intracranial pressure. Following long-term use, the child may be at risk for adrenal gland deficiency during stress for as long as 18 months after cessation of this drug.

By Those over 60 Years of Age: Cortisonelike drugs should only be used when the disorder under treatment is unresponsive to adequate trials of unrelated drugs. Avoid the prolonged use of this drug. Continual use (even in small doses) can increase severity of diabetes, enhance fluid retention, raise blood pressure, weaken resistance to infection, induce stomach ulcer and accelerate development of cataract and osteoporosis.

▷ **Advisability of Use During Pregnancy**
Pregnancy Category: B or C. See Pregnancy Code at the back of this book.
Animal studies: Birth defects reported in mice, rats and rabbits.
Human studies: Adequate studies of pregnant women are not available.
Avoid completely during the first 3 months. Limit use during the last 6 months as much as possible. If used, examine infant for possible deficiency of adrenal gland function.

Advisability of Use if Breast-Feeding
Presence of this drug in breast milk: Yes.
Avoid drug or refrain from nursing.

Habit-Forming Potential: Long-term use of this drug may produce a state of functional dependence (see Glossary). In therapy of asthma and rheumatoid arthritis, it is advisable to keep the dose as small as possible and to attempt drug withdrawal after periods of reasonable improvement. Such procedures may reduce the degree of "steroid rebound"—the return of symptoms as the drug is withdrawn.

Effects of Overdosage: Fatigue, muscle weakness, stomach irritation, acid indigestion, excessive sweating, facial flushing, fluid retention, swelling of extremities, increased blood pressure.

Possible Effects of Long-Term Use: Increased blood sugar (possible diabetes), increased fat deposits on the trunk of the body ("buffalo hump"), rounding of the face ("moon face"), thinning and fragility of skin, loss of texture and strength of bones (osteoporosis, aseptic necrosis), cataracts, glaucoma, retarded growth and development in children.

Suggested Periodic Examinations While Taking This Drug (at physician's discretion)
    Measurements of blood pressure, blood sugar and potassium levels.
    Complete eye examinations at regular intervals.
    Chest X-ray if history of tuberculosis.
    Determination of the rate of development of the growing child to detect retardation of normal growth.

▷ **While Taking This Drug, Observe the Following**
    Foods: No interactions expected. Ask physician regarding need to restrict salt intake or to eat potassium-rich foods. During long-term use of this drug, it is advisable to eat a high-protein diet.
    Nutritional Support: During long-term use, take a vitamin D supplement. During wound repair, take a zinc supplement. Potassium loss may need to be replaced.
    Beverages: No restrictions. Drink all forms of milk liberally.
▷   *Alcohol:* No interactions expected. Use caution if you are prone to peptic ulcers.
    Tobacco Smoking: Nicotine increases the blood levels of naturally produced cortisone and related hormones. Heavy smoking may add to the expected actions of this drug and requires close observation for excessive effects.
    Marijuana Smoking: May cause additional impairment of immunity.
▷   *Other Drugs*
    Prednisone may ***decrease*** the effects of
- isoniazid (INH, Niconyl, etc.).
- salicylates (aspirin, sodium salicylate, etc.).

Prednisone ***taken concurrently*** with
- amphotericin B may result in additive potassium loss.
- birth control pills (oral contraceptives) will prolong the prednisone effect.
- cyclosporine (Sandimmune) can cause increased cyclosporine levels and increased prednisone levels. Dose decreases may be needed for both drugs.
- foscarnet may result in additive potassium loss.
- ketoconazole will lessen the therapeutic benefit of ketoconazole.
- NSAIDs may result in additive stomach and intestinal irritation.
- oral hypoglycemic agents (see Drug Class) or insulin may result in loss of glucose control.
- oral anticoagulants may either increase or decrease their effectiveness; consult physician regarding the need for prothrombin time testing and dosage adjustment.
- pneumococcal or smallpox vaccine will blunt the response to the vaccine.
- thiazide diuretics (see drug class) or loop diuretics may result in additive potassium loss.

The following drugs may ***decrease*** the effects of prednisone
- antacids may reduce its absorption.
- barbiturates (Amytal, Butisol, phenobarbital, etc.).
- carbamazepine (Tegretol).
- phenytoin (Dilantin, etc.).
- primidone (Mysoline).
- rifampin (Rifadin, Rimactane, etc.).

▷ *Driving, Hazardous Activities:* Usually no restrictions. Be alert to the rare occurrence of dizziness.

Aviation Note: The use of this drug **may be a disqualification** for piloting. Consult a designated Aviation Medical Examiner.

Exposure to Sun: No restrictions.

Occurrence of Unrelated Illness: This drug may decrease natural resistance to infection. Tell your doctor if you develop an infection of any kind. It may also reduce your body's ability to respond to the stress of acute illness, injury or surgery. Keep your doctor informed of any significant changes in your state of health.

Discontinuation: After long-term use, do not stop it abruptly. Ask physician for guidance regarding gradual withdrawal. For a period of 2 years after discontinuing this drug, it is essential in the event of illness, injury or surgery that you tell attending medical personnel that you have used this drug in the past. The period of impaired response to stress following the use of cortisonelike drugs may last for 1 to 2 years.

PRIMAQUINE (PRIM a kween)

Introduced: 1955   Prescription: USA: Yes; Canada: Yes   Available as Generic: USA: Yes; Canada: Yes   Class: Anti-infective, antiprotozoal
Controlled Drug: USA: No; Canada: No
Brand Names: None in United States or Canada

BENEFITS versus RISKS	
Possible Benefits	*Possible Risks*
EFFECTIVE PREVENTION AND TREATMENT OF CERTAIN TYPES OF MALARIA	HEMOLYTIC ANEMIA (see Glossary)
EFFECTIVE ADJUNCTIVE TREATMENT OF PNEUMOCYSTIS CARINII PNEUMONIA	Methemoglobinemia Rare decreased white blood cell counts

▷ **Principal Uses**

As a Single Drug Product: Uses currently included in FDA approved labeling: Prevention of malaria caused by P. vivax and P. falciparum.

Other (unlabeled) generally accepted uses: Treatment (in combination with clindamycin) of AIDS-related Pneumocystis carinii pneumonia. This combined drug therapy is used in patients who are unresponsive or intolerant to standard treatment.

How This Drug Works: It is thought that by altering DNA, this drug inhibits development of certain protozoal organisms in blood and body tissues, thus producing cures and preventing relapses.

Available Dosage Forms and Strengths
Tablets — 26.3 mg (15 mg base)

▷ **Recommended Dosage Ranges** (Actual dosage and administration schedule must be determined by the physician for each patient individually.)

Infants and Children: 680 mcg (390 mcg base)/kg of body weight, once daily for 14 days.

12 to 60 Years of Age: For malaria—26.3 mg (15 mg base), once daily for 14 days.
For Pneumocystis carinii pneumonia—15 to 30 mg base, once daily for 21 days.
Over 60 Years of Age: Same as 12 to 60 years of age.

Conditions Requiring Dosing Adjustments
Liver function: No specific guidelines for dose decreases in liver compromise are available.
Kidney function: Specific guidelines for dosage adjustment in patients with compromised kidneys have not been developed.

▷ **Dosing Instructions:** Take with food or antacids to reduce stomach irritation. Swallow the tablet whole. Take the full course prescribed.

Usual Duration of Use: Use on a regular schedule for 2 to 3 weeks usually determines effectiveness in controlling protozoal infections. Long-term use requires periodic physician evaluation of response and dosage adjustment.

▷ **This Drug Should Not Be Taken If**
- you have had an allergic reaction to it previously.
- you are pregnant.
- you are currently taking quinacrine (Atabrine).
- you are acutely ill with lupus erythematosus or rheumatoid arthritis.

▷ **Inform Your Physician Before Taking This Drug If**
- you are allergic to iodoquinol (Floraquin).
- you have a personal or family history of hemolytic anemia.
- you have glucose-6-phosphate dehydrogenase (G6PD) deficiency of your red blood cells.
- you have nicotinamide adenine dinucleotide methemoglobin (NADH) reductase deficiency.
- you are currently taking other drugs that can cause hemolytic anemia. (Ask your doctor.)
- you are planning pregnancy.

Possible Side-Effects (natural, expected and unavoidable drug actions)
None.

▷ **Possible Adverse Effects** (unusual, unexpected and infrequent reactions)
If any of the following develop, consult your physician promptly for guidance.
Mild Adverse Effects
Allergic Reactions: Itching.
Headache, confusion, depression, visual disturbances.
Nausea, vomiting, stomach pain.
Serious Adverse Effects
Idiosyncratic Reactions: Hemolytic anemia (see Glossary), more common in those with G6PD deficiency; methemoglobin formation, more common in those with NADH methemoglobin reductase deficiency.
Abnormally low white blood cell counts (fever, sore throat, infections).
Possible increase of blood pressure; heart rhythm disturbances.
Drug-induced methemoglobinemia.

▷ **Possible Effects on Sexual Function:** None reported.

Possible Delayed Adverse Effects: None reported.

Possible Effects on Laboratory Tests
   Complete blood cell counts: decreased red cells, hemoblogin and white cells.
   Methemoglobin: increased.
CAUTION
   1. Not to be taken during acute malaria; it may induce hemolysis.
   2. Avoid concurrent use of other drugs that may cause hemolysis.
Precautions for Use
   By Infants and Children: No specific information available.
   By Those over 60 Years of Age: No specific information available.
▷ **Advisability of Use During Pregnancy**
   Pregnancy Category:
   C. See Pregnancy Code at the back of this book.
   Animal studies: No information available.
   Human studies: Adequate studies of pregnant women are not available.
   This drug is not recommended for use during pregnancy because it may cause hemolysis in a fetus deficient in G6PD.
Advisability of Use if Breast-Feeding
   Presence of this drug in breast milk: Unknown.
   Avoid drug or refrain from nursing.
Habit-Forming Potential: None.
Effects of Overdosage: Nausea, vomiting, stomach cramps.
Possible Effects of Long-Term Use: None reported.
Suggested Periodic Examinations While Taking This Drug (at physician's discretion)
   Complete blood cell counts.
▷ **While Taking This Drug, Observe the Following**
   Foods: No restrictions.
   Beverages: No restrictions.
▷ *Alcohol:* No interactions expected.
   Tobacco Smoking: No interactions expected.
▷ *Other Drugs*
   Primaquine **taken concurrently** with
   • aurothioglucose may increase hematological toxicity of primaquine.
   • quinacrine (Atabrine) may increase primaquine's toxicity. Avoid the concurrent use of these drugs.
▷ *Driving, Hazardous Activities:* This drug may cause confusion and visual disturbances. Restrict activities as necessary.
   Aviation Note: The use of this drug **may be a disqualification** for piloting. Consult a designated Aviation Medical Examiner.
   Exposure to Sun: No restrictions.
   Discontinuation: To be determined by your physician.

PRIMIDONE (PRI mi dohn)

Introduced: 1953 **Prescription:** USA: Yes; Canada: Yes **Available as Generic:** USA: Yes; Canada: Yes **Class:** Anticonvulsant **Controlled Drug:** USA: No; Canada: No
Brand Names: ✦Apo-Primidone, Myidone, Mysoline, ✦PMS-Primidone

BENEFITS versus RISKS	
Possible Benefits	*Possible Risks*

EFFECTIVE CONTROL OF TONIC-CLONIC (GRAND MAL) AND ALL TYPES OF PARTIAL SEIZURES	Allergic skin reactions
	Rare blood cell disorders:
	  megaloblastic anemia, deficient
	  white blood cells and platelets

▷ **Principal Uses**

As a Single Drug Product: Uses currently included in FDA approved labeling: (1) This drug is used exclusively to control generalized grand mal seizures and all types of partial seizures. It can be used to supplement the anticonvulsant action of phenytoin.

Other (unlabeled) generally accepted uses: (1) May have a minor role in helping in therapy of orthostatic tremor; (2) can help ringing in the ears.

How This Drug Works: Reduces and stabilizes the excitability of nerve fibers and inhibits the repetitious spread of electrical impulses along nerve pathways. This action may prevent seizures altogether, or it may reduce their frequency and severity. (Part of this drug's action is attributable to phenobarbital, one of its conversion products in the body.)

Available Dosage Forms and Strengths
  Oral suspensions — 250 mg per 5-ml teaspoonful
  Tablets — 50 mg, 250 mg

▷ **Usual Adult Dosage Range:** Initially, 100 mg/24 hours as a single dose at bedtime for 3 days; 100 to 125 mg twice a day for days 4 through 6, 100 to 125 mg three times a day for days 7 through 9, and an ongoing (maintenance) dose of 250 mg 3 times/day, 6 to 8 hours apart. Total daily dosage should not exceed 2000 mg. **Note: Actual dosage and administration schedule must be determined by the physician for each patient individually.**

Conditions Requiring Dosing Adjustments

Liver function: The dose **must** be decreased, and blood levels obtained more frequently in patients with liver compromise.

Kidney function: In patients with mild to moderate kidney failure, the usual dose can be given every eight hours. Patients with moderate to severe kidney failure can be given the usual dose every 8–12 hours. Patients with severe kidney failure should be given the usual dose every 12–24 hours. Primidone should be used with caution in renal compromise as it can be a cause of crystalluria.

▷ **Dosing Instructions:** The tablet may be crushed and taken with or following food to reduce stomach irritation. Shake the suspension well before measuring the dose.

Usual Duration of Use: Use on a regular schedule for 2 to 4 weeks usually determines effectiveness in reducing the frequency and severity of seizures. Long-term use (months to years) requires physician supervision.

▷ **This Drug Should Not Be Taken If**
  • you have had an allergic reaction to it previously.
  • you are allergic to phenobarbital.
  • you have a history of porphyria.

▷ **Inform Your Physician Before Taking This Drug If**
- you have had an allergic or idiosyncratic reaction to any barbiturate drug in the past.
- you have a family history of intermittent porphyria.
- you have impaired liver, kidney or thyroid gland function.
- you have asthma, emphysema or myasthenia gravis.
- you are pregnant or planning pregnancy.
- you plan to have surgery under general anesthesia in the near future.

Possible Side-Effects (natural, expected and unavoidable drug actions)
Drowsiness, impaired concentration, mental and physical sluggishness.

▷ **Possible Adverse Effects** (unusual, unexpected and infrequent reactions)
If any of the following develop, consult your physician promptly for guidance.

Mild Adverse Effects
Allergic Reactions: Skin rashes, hives, localized swellings. "Hangover" effect, dizziness, unsteadiness, impaired vision, double vision, fatigue, emotional disturbances.
Low blood pressure, faintness.
Shoulder pain, joint pain.
Nausea, vomiting, thirst, increased urine volume.

Serious Adverse Effects
Allergic Reaction: Swelling of lymph glands.
Idiosyncratic Reactions: Paradoxical anxiety, seizures, agitation, restlessness, rage.
Visual hallucinations.
Drug-induced porphyria.
Drug-induced systemic lupus erythematosus.
Drug-induced low thyroid gland function (hypothyroidism).
Blood cell disorders: megaloblastic anemia due to folic acid depletion; deficient production of white blood cells and blood platelets.
Auditory hallucinations (rare).

▷ **Possible Effects on Sexual Function**
Decreased libido and/or impotence (22%).
Decreased effectiveness of oral contraceptives taken concurrently.

▷ **Adverse Effects That May Mimic Natural Diseases or Disorders**
Allergic swelling of lymph glands may suggest a naturally occurring lymphoma.

Natural Diseases or Disorders That May Be Activated by This Drug
Acute intermittent and/or cutaneous porphyria (see Glossary).
Systemic lupus erythematosus.

Possible Effects on Laboratory Tests
Complete blood cell counts: decreased red cells, hemoglobin, white cells and platelets; increased eosinophils.
Blood lupus erythematosus (LE) cells: positive.
Prothrombin time: decreased (when taken concurrently with warfarin).
Urine screening tests for drug abuse: may be **positive** for phenobarbital (a normal derivative of this drug). (Test results depend upon amount of drug taken and testing method used.)

CAUTION
1. This drug must not be stopped abruptly.
2. The wide variation of this drug's action from person to person requires careful individualization of dosage schedules.
3. Regularity of drug use is essential for the successful management of seizure disorders. Take your medication at the same time each day.
4. Side-effects and mild adverse effects are usually most apparent during the first several weeks of treatment and often subside with continued use.
5. It may be necessary to take folic acid to prevent anemia while taking this drug. Consult your physician.
6. It is advisable to carry a card of personal identification with a notation that you are taking this drug.

Precautions for Use
By Infants and Children: This drug should be used with caution in the hyperkinetic (overactive) child. Observe for possible paradoxical hyperactivity. Changes associated with puberty characteristically slow the metabolism of phenobarbital and permit its gradual accumulation. Measurements of blood levels in young adolescents can detect rising concentrations of this drug that could lead to toxicity. (See Therapeutic Drug Monitoring in Section One.)

By Those over 60 Years of Age: It is advisable to avoid all barbiturates in the elderly. If use of this drug is attempted, small starting doses are indicated. Watch for confusion, delirium, agitation or paradoxical excitement. This drug may be conducive to hypothermia (see Glossary).

▷ **Advisability of Use During Pregnancy**
Pregnancy Category: D. See Pregnancy Code at the back of this book.
Animal studies: Birth defects due to this drug reported in mice.
Human studies: Adequate studies of pregnant women are not available. However, recent reports suggest a possible association between the use of this drug during the first 3 months of pregnancy and the development of birth defects in the fetus. Discuss with your physician the advantages and possible disadvantages of using this drug during pregnancy. If it is used, determine the smallest maintenance dose that will prevent seizures.

The newborn infants of mothers who take this drug during pregnancy may develop abnormal bleeding or bruising due to the deficiency of certain blood clotting factors in the blood. Consult your physician regarding the need to take vitamin K during the last month of pregnancy.

Advisability of Use if Breast-Feeding
Presence of this drug in breast milk: Yes.
Monitor nursing infant closely and discontinue drug or nursing if adverse effects develop.

Habit-Forming Potential: None.

Effects of Overdosage: Drowsiness, jerky eye movements, blurred vision, staggering gait, incoordination, slurred speech, stupor progressing to coma.

Possible Effects of Long-Term Use: Enlargement of lymph glands; enlargement of thyroid gland. Megaloblastic anemia due to folic acid deficiency. Reduced blood levels of calcium and phosphorus, leading to rickets in children and loss of bone texture (osteomalacia) in adults.

Suggested Periodic Examinations While Taking This Drug (at physician's discretion)
Complete blood cell counts. Measurements of blood levels of calcium and phosphorus. Evaluation of lymph and thyroid glands. Skeletal X-ray examinations for bone demineralization during long-term use.

▷ **While Taking This Drug, Observe the Following**
Foods: No restrictions.
Nutritional Support: Consult your physician regarding the need for supplements of calcium, vitamin D, folic acid and vitamin K.
Beverages: No restrictions. May be taken with milk or fruit juice.
▷ *Alcohol:* Avoid completely. Alcohol can increase greatly the sedative and depressant effects of this drug on brain function.
Tobacco Smoking: May enhance the sedative effects of this drug and increase drowsiness.
▷ *Other Drugs*
Note: 15% of primidone is converted to phenobarbital in the body. See the Drug Profile of Phenobarbital for possible interactions with other drugs.
▷ *Driving, Hazardous Activities:* This drug may cause drowsiness and dizziness; it can also impair mental alertness, vision and physical coordination. Restrict activities as necessary.
Aviation Note: The use of this drug **is a disqualification** for piloting. Consult a designated Aviation Medical Examiner.
Exposure to Sun: No restrictions.
Occurrence of Unrelated Illness: Notify your physician of any illness or injury that prevents the use of this drug according to your regular dosage schedule.
Discontinuation: Do not stop this drug without your physician's knowledge and approval. Sudden withdrawal of any anticonvulsant drug can cause severe and repeated seizures.

PROBENECID (proh BEN e sid)

Introduced: 1951 **Prescription:** USA: Yes; Canada: No **Available as Generic:** USA: Yes; Canada: No **Class:** Antigout **Controlled Drug:** USA: No; Canada: No

Brand Names: ◆Ampicin PRB [CD], Benemid, ◆Benuryl, Colabid [CD], Col-Benemid [CD], Polycillin-PRB [CD], Probalan, Probampacin [CD], Proben-C [CD], ◆Pro-Biosan 500 Kit [CD], SK-Probenecid

BENEFITS versus RISKS	
Possible Benefits	*Possible Risks*
EFFECTIVE LONG-TERM PREVENTION OF ACUTE ATTACKS OF GOUT	Formation of uric acid kidney stones
Useful adjunct to penicillin therapy (to achieve high blood and tissue levels of penicillin)	Bone marrow depression (aplastic anemia) (rare)
	Drug-induced liver and kidney damage (both rare)

Probenecid

▷ **Principal Uses**

As a Single Drug Product: Uses currently included in FDA approved labeling: (1) Used in helping maintain penicillin levels in therapy of gonorrhea; (2) helps decrease elevated uric acid levels caused by thiazide diuretics; (3) helps prevent gout.

Other (unlabeled) generally accepted uses: (1) May have a role in preventing kidney toxicity in cisplatin chemotherapy; (2) adjunctive use in maintaining effective antibiotic levels in treatment of syphilis; (3) helps decrease uric acid in gout patients.

As a Combination Drug Product [CD]: This drug is available in combination with colchicine, a drug often used for the treatment of acute gout. Each drug works in a different way; when used in combination they provide both relief of the acute gout and some measure of protection from recurrence of acute attacks.

How This Drug Works: Works in the kidney (tubular systems) to increase uric acid excretion in the urine, this drug reduces the levels of uric acid in the blood and body tissues. It also works in the kidney to decrease the amount of penicillin excreted in the urine, and prolongs the presence of penicillin in the blood and helps achieve higher concentrations in body tissues.

Available Dosage Forms and Strengths
Tablets — 500 mg

▷ **Usual Adult Dosage Range:** Antigout: Initially, 250 mg twice/day for 1 week; then 500 mg twice/day. Adjunct to penicillin therapy: 500 mg 4 times/day. **Note: Actual dosage and administration schedule must be determined by the physician for each patient individually.**

Conditions Requiring Dosing Adjustments

Liver function: Specific guidelines for dosage adjustment in liver compromise are not available. It should be used with caution.

Kidney function: Patients with moderate kidney failure should **not** be given this drug as the effectiveness is questionable.

▷ **Dosing Instructions:** The tablet may be crushed and taken with or following food to reduce stomach irritation. Drink 2.5 to 3 quarts of liquids daily.

Usual Duration of Use: Use on a regular schedule for several months usually determines effectiveness in preventing acute attacks of gout. Long-term use (months to years) requires supervision and periodic evaluation by your physician.

▷ **This Drug Should Not Be Taken If**
- you have had an allergic reaction to it previously.
- you have active liver disease.
- you have acute kidney failure.
- you have an active blood cell or bone marrow disorder.
- you are experiencing an attack of acute gout at the present time.

▷ **Inform Your Physician Before Taking This Drug If**
- you have a history of kidney disease or kidney stones.
- you have a history of liver disease or impaired liver function.
- you have a history of peptic ulcer disease.
- you have a history of a blood cell or bone marrow disorder.
- you are taking any drug product that contains aspirin or aspirinlike drugs.

Possible Side-Effects (natural, expected and unavoidable drug actions)
   Development of kidney stones (composed of uric acid); this is preventable. Consult your physician regarding the use of sodium bicarbonate (or other urine alkalizer) to prevent stone formation.

▷ **Possible Adverse Effects** (unusual, unexpected and infrequent reactions)
   If any of the following develop, consult your physician promptly for guidance.
   Mild Adverse Effects
   Allergic Reactions: Skin rash, itching, drug fever (see Glossary).
   Headache, dizziness, flushing of face.
   Reduced appetite, sore gums, nausea, vomiting.
   Serious Adverse Effects
   Allergic Reaction: Anaphylactic reaction (see Glossary).
   Idiosyncratic Reaction: Hemolytic anemia (see Glossary).
   Bone marrow depression (see Glossary): fatigue, weakness, fever, sore throat, abnormal bleeding or bruising.
   Drug-induced liver damage with jaundice (see Glossary).
   Drug-induced porphyria.
   Fluid in the retina (retinal edema) (rare).
   Drug-induced kidney damage: marked fluid retention, reduced urine formation.

▷ **Possible Effects on Sexual Function:** None reported.

▷ **Adverse Effects That May Mimic Natural Diseases or Disorders**
   Liver reactions may suggest viral hepatitis.
   Kidney reactions may suggest nephrosis.

Possible Effects on Laboratory Tests
   Complete blood cell counts: decreased red cells, hemoglobin, white cells and platelets.
   Prothrombin time: increased (when taken concurrently with warfarin).
   Blood glucose level: decreased.
   Blood urea nitrogen (BUN) level: increased (kidney damage).
   Blood uric acid level: decreased.
   Liver function tests: increased liver enzymes (ALT/GPT, AST/GOT and alkaline phosphatase), increased bilirubin.
   Urine sugar tests: false positive with Benedict's solution and Clinitest.

CAUTION
1. This drug should not be started until 2 to 3 weeks after an acute attack of gout has subsided.
2. This drug may increase the frequency of acute attacks of gout during the first few months of treatment. Concurrent use of colchicine is advised to prevent acute attacks.
3. Aspirin (and aspirin-containing drug products) can reduce the effectiveness of this drug. Use acetaminophen or a nonaspirin analgesic for pain relief as needed.

Precautions for Use
   By Infants and Children: Safety and effectiveness for those under 2 years of age not established.
   By Those over 60 Years of Age: The natural decline in kidney function that occurs after 60 may require adjustment of your dosage. You may be more

susceptible to the serious adverse effects of this drug. Report any unusual symptoms promptly for evaluation.

▷ **Advisability of Use During Pregnancy**
Pregnancy Category: B. See Pregnancy Code at the back of this book.
Animal studies: No information available.
Human studies: Adequate studies of pregnant women are not available.
This drug has been used during pregnancy with no reports of birth defects or adverse effects on the fetus. Ask your physician for guidance.

Advisability of Use if Breast-Feeding
Presence of this drug in breast milk: Unknown.
Avoid drug or refrain from nursing.

Habit-Forming Potential: None.

Effects of Overdosage: Stomach irritation, nausea, vomiting, nervous agitation, delirium, seizures, coma.

Possible Effects of Long-Term Use: Formation of kidney stones. Kidney damage in sensitive individuals.

Suggested Periodic Examinations While Taking This Drug (at physician's discretion)
Complete blood cell counts, measurements of blood uric acid, liver and kidney function tests.

▷ **While Taking This Drug, Observe the Following**
Foods: Follow physician's advice regarding the need for a low-purine diet.
Beverages: A large intake of coffee, tea or cola beverages may reduce the effectiveness of treatment.

▷ *Alcohol:* No interactions expected. However, large amounts of alcohol can raise the blood uric acid level and reduce the effectiveness of treatment.
Tobacco Smoking: No interactions expected.

▷ *Other Drugs*
Probenecid may *increase* the effects of
- acyclovir (Zovirax) and result in toxicity unless doses are reduced.
- clofibrate (Atromid S).
- dyphylline (Neothylline).
- ketoprofen and perhaps other NSAIDs.
- methotrexate (Mexate), and increase its toxicity.
- midazolam (Versed) and increase the CNS depression.
- oral hypoglycemic agents (see Drug Class).
- thiopental (Pentothal), and prolong its anesthetic effect.
- zidovudine (Retrovir) and increase toxicity risk.

Probenecid *taken concurrently* with
- penicillins may cause a threefold to fivefold increase in penicillin blood levels, greatly increasing the effectiveness of each penicillin dose.
- cephalosporins may cause a doubling of antibiotic levels. Caution must be used to avoid toxicity.
- dapsone may cause up to a 50% increased dapsone level and result in toxicity unless dapsone doses are decreased.

The following drugs may *decrease* the effects of probenecid
- aspirin and other salicylates may reduce its effectiveness in promoting the excretion of uric acid.
- bismuth subsalicylate (Pepto-Bismol).

▷ *Driving, Hazardous Activities:* This drug may cause dizziness. Restrict activities as necessary.
  Aviation Note: The use of this drug **may be a disqualification** for piloting. Consult a designated Aviation Medical Examiner.
  Exposure to Sun: No restrictions.
  Discontinuation: Do not stop this drug without consulting your physician.

PROBUCOL (PROH byu kohl)

Introduced: 1971 **Prescription:** USA: Yes; Canada: Yes **Available as Generic:** USA: No; Canada: No **Class:** Anticholesterol **Controlled Drug:** USA: No; Canada: No

Brand Name: Lorelco

BENEFITS versus RISKS	
Possible Benefits	*Possible Risks*
EFFECTIVE REDUCTION OF TOTAL CHOLESTEROL AND LOW DENSITY CHOLESTEROL IN TYPE IIa CHOLESTEROL DISORDERS	CONCURRENT REDUCTION OF HIGH DENSITY (HDL) CHOLESTEROL (This is thought to be undesirable in the prevention and treatment of atherosclerosis.) Abnormal heart rhythms (ventricular fibrillation, Torsade De Pointes) Low blood platelets

▷ **Principal Uses**
  As a Single Drug Product: Uses currently included in FDA approved labeling: (1) Used for the reduction of abnormally high blood levels of cholesterol (type IIa) that have not responded to adequate control of diet, weight, diabetes and hypothyroidism.
  Other (unlabeled) generally accepted uses: None.

How This Drug Works: This drug may inhibit the absorption of dietary cholesterol, may inhibit the early stages of cholesterol production in the liver and may increase the rate of LDL cholesterol destruction and elimination.

Available Dosage Forms and Strengths
  Tablets — 250 mg, 500 mg

▷ **Usual Adult Dosage Range:** 250 mg to 500 mg twice daily. **Note: Actual dosage and administration schedule must be determined by the physician for each patient individually.**

Conditions Requiring Dosing Adjustments
  Liver function: It should be used with caution in patients with compromised biliary tracts.
  Kidney function: The kidney is minimally invloved in the elimination of this drug.

▷ **Dosing Instructions:** The tablet may be crushed and taken with the morning and evening meals.

Usual Duration of Use: Use on a regular schedule for 3 to 6 months usually determines effectiveness in lowering cholesterol blood levels. Long-term use (months to years) requires periodic physician evaluation of response.

▷ **This Drug Should Not Be Taken If**
- you have had an allergic reaction to it previously.
- you have had a heart attack (myocardial infarction) recently.
- you have serious heart arrhythmias.

▷ **Inform Your Physician Before Taking This Drug If**
- you are pregnant.
- you have a history of heart disease, heart rhythm disorder or abnormal electrocardiogram.
- you have low blood potassium or magnesium.
- you have impaired liver function or gallstones.

Possible Side-Effects (natural, expected and unavoidable drug actions)
None.

▷ **Possible Adverse Effects** (unusual, unexpected and infrequent reactions)
If any of the following develop, consult your physician promptly for guidance.

Mild Adverse Effects
Allergic Reactions: Rash, itching, swelling (angioedema) of face, mouth, hands or feet.
Blurred vision.
Ringing in the ears.
Urination at night.
Headache, dizziness, numbness or tingling in extremities (paresthesias).
Indigestion, excessive gas, abdominal discomfort, nausea, vomiting, diarrhea.

Serious Adverse Effects
Idiosyncratic Reactions: Dizziness, fainting, chest pain, heart palpitations.
Altered electrocardiogram.
Nodular goiter.
Peripheral neuritis (rare).
Ventricular heart arrhythmias.

▷ **Possible Effects on Sexual Function**
Altered timing and pattern of menstruation.
Impotence (rare).

Possible Effects on Laboratory Tests
Blood eosinophil count: increased (allergic reaction).
Blood total cholesterol, HDL and LDL cholesterol levels: decreased.
Blood triglyceride levels: decreased.
Blood uric acid level: increased (in women only).

CAUTION
1. Report promptly the development of chest pain, heart palpitations, dizziness or faintness.
2. Periodic measurements of blood cholesterol and triglycerides are essential to monitoring your response to treatment and determining the need for changes in dosage or medication.

834 Probucol

Precautions for Use
- *By Infants and Children:* Safety and effectiveness for those under 12 years of age not established.
- *By Those over 60 Years of Age:* It is advisable to have an electrocardiogram before starting this drug and at intervals of 6 months until it is determined that there is no drug-induced alteration of heart function.

▷ **Advisability of Use During Pregnancy**
Pregnancy Category: B. See Pregnancy Code at the back of this book.
- Animal studies: No drug-induced birth defects found in rodents.
- Human studies: Adequate studies of pregnant women are not available.
- Use this drug only if clearly needed. Because of the long persistence of this drug in body tissues, it is recommended that the drug be discontinued and that birth control be used for 6 months before attempting to establish pregnancy.
- The manufacturer does not recommend the use of this drug during pregnancy.

Advisability of Use if Breast-Feeding
- Presence of this drug in breast milk: Unknown.
- Avoid drug or refrain from nursing.

Habit-Forming Potential: None.

Effects of Overdosage: Abdominal distress, nausea, vomiting, diarrhea.

Possible Effects of Long-Term Use: Decrease in high density (HDL) cholesterol blood levels; increase in triglyceride blood levels.

Suggested Periodic Examinations While Taking This Drug (at physician's discretion)
- Measurements of blood levels of total cholesterol, HDL and LDL cholesterol fractions and triglycerides.
- Electrocardiograms (selectively).

▷ **While Taking This Drug, Observe the Following**
- *Foods:* Follow the low-cholesterol diet prescribed by your physician.
- *Beverages:* No restrictions.
▷ - *Alcohol:* No interactions expected.
- *Tobacco Smoking:* No interactions expected.
▷ - *Other Drugs*
   Probucol may *decrease* the effects of
   - chenodiol (Chenix), and impair its benefit in the therapy of gallstones.

   Probucol *taken concurrently* with
   - clofibrate (Atromid-S) can cause a serious lowering of HDL-cholesterol without gain in decreasing LDL-cholesterol.
▷ - *Driving, Hazardous Activities:* This drug may cause dizziness or faintness in sensitive individuals. Restrict activities as necessary.
- *Aviation Note:* The use of this drug *is usually not a disqualification* for piloting. Consult a designated Aviation Medical Examiner.
- *Exposure to Sun:* No restrictions.
- *Discontinuation:* Do not stop this drug without your physician's knowledge and guidance. Abrupt withdrawal may be followed by prompt and excessive increase in blood cholesterol levels.

PROCAINAMIDE (proh kayn A mide)

Introduced: 1950 **Prescription:** USA: Yes; Canada: Yes **Available as**
Generic: USA: Yes; Canada: No **Class:** Antiarrhythmic **Controlled**
Drug: USA: No; Canada: No
Brand Names: ♦Apo-Procainamide, Procamide SR, Procan SR, Promine, Pronestyl, Pronestyl-SR, Rhythmin

BENEFITS versus RISKS	
Possible Benefits	*Possible Risks*
EFFECTIVE TREATMENT OF SELECTED HEART RHYTHM DISORDERS	NARROW TREATMENT RANGE INDUCTION OF SYSTEMIC LUPUS ERYTHEMATOSUS SYNDROME in 20% of long-term users Provocation of abnormal heart rhythms Blood cell disorders: insufficient white blood cells and platelets

▷ **Principal Uses**

As a Single Drug Product: Uses currently included in FDA approved labeling: (1) Used to abolish and prevent the recurrence of premature beats arising in the ventricles (lower chambers) of the heart.

Other (unlabeled) generally accepted uses: (1) Used to treat and prevent atrial fibrillation, atrial flutter and abnormally rapid heart rates (tachycardia) that originate in the atria or the ventricles; (2) helps treat myotonia and improve breathing in myotonic dystrophy.

How This Drug Works: By slowing the activity of the pacemaker and delaying the transmission of electrical impulses through the conduction system and muscle of the heart, this drug assists in restoring normal heart rate and rhythm.

Available Dosage Forms and Strengths
  Capsules — 250 mg, 375 mg, 500 mg
  Injections — 100 mg per ml and 500 mg per ml
  Tablets — 250 mg, 375 mg, 500 mg
Tablets, prolonged-action — 250 mg, 500 mg, 750 mg, 1000 mg

▷ **Usual Adult Dosage Range:** Dose varies according to indication for use. Premature atrial or ventricular contractions: 250 to 500 mg/3 hours. Paroxysmal atrial tachycardia: initially, 1250 mg, followed in 1 hour by 750 mg; then 500 to 1000 mg/2 hours as needed and tolerated. Atrial fibrillation and flutter: the heart should be digitalized first; then initiate procainamide with 1250 mg, followed in 1 hour by 750 mg; follow with 500 to 1000 mg/2 hours as needed and tolerated. For maintenance: 500 to 1000 mg/4 to 6 hours. The total daily dosage should not exceed 6000 mg. **Note:** Actual dosage and administration schedule must be determined by the physician for each patient individually.

Conditions Requiring Dosing Adjustments

Liver function: This drug should be used with caution in patients with liver compromise, and blood levels appropriately obtained. It should be used as a benefit to risk in patients with compromised livers as it may be more likely to cause liver problems in this patient population.

Kidney function: Patients with moderate to severe kidney failure can be given the usual doses every 6–12 hours. Patients with severe kidney failure can be given the usual dose every 8–24 hours. The drug should be used with caution in renal compromise, and appropriate blood levels obtained.

▷ **Dosing Instructions:** Preferably taken on an empty stomach, 1 hour before or 2 hours after eating. However, it may be taken with or following food to reduce stomach irritation. The regular capsules may be opened and the regular tablets may be crushed for administration; however, the prolonged-action tablets should be swallowed whole without alteration.

Usual Duration of Use: Use on a regular schedule for 24 to 48 hours usually determines effectiveness in correcting or preventing responsive rhythm disorders. Long-term use requires supervision and periodic evaluation by your physician.

▷ **This Drug Should Not Be Taken If**
- you have had an allergic reaction to it previously.
- you have second-degree or third-degree heart block (determined by electrocardiogram).
- you have myasthenia gravis.

▷ **Inform Your Physician Before Taking This Drug If**
- you are allergic to procaine (Novocaine) or to other local anesthetics of the "-caine" drug class, such as those commonly used for glaucoma testing and for dental procedures.
- you have had any adverse reactions to other antiarrhythmic drugs.
- you have a history of heart disease of any kind, especially "heart block."
- you have a history of low blood pressure.
- you have a history of lupus erythematosus.
- you have a history of abnormally low blood platelet counts.
- you have impaired liver or kidney function.
- you have myasthenia gravis.
- you have an enlarged prostate gland.
- you are taking any form of digitalis or any diuretic drug that can cause excessive loss of body potassium (ask physician).
- you plan to have surgery under general anesthesia in the near future.

Possible Side-Effects (natural, expected and unavoidable drug actions)
Drop in blood pressure in susceptible individuals.

▷ **Possible Adverse Effects** (unusual, unexpected and infrequent reactions)
If any of the following develop, consult your physician promptly for guidance.

Mild Adverse Effects
Allergic Reactions: Skin rash, hives, itching, drug fever (see Glossary).
Weakness, light-headedness.
Loss of appetite, bitter taste, indigestion, nausea, vomiting, diarrhea.

Serious Adverse Effects
Allergic Reactions: Systemic lupus erythematosuslike syndrome: fever, skin eruptions, joint and muscle pains, pleurisy. (This is reported to occur in

at least 20% of users.) Idiosyncratic Reactions: Mental depression, hallucinations, psychotic behavior, hemolytic anemia (see Glossary).
Severe drop in blood pressure, fainting.
Drug-induced pancreatitis.
Drug-induced liver toxicity.
Myopathy.
Pericardial effusions.
Asthmalike breathing difficulties.
Induction of new heart rhythm disturbances.
Inability to empty urinary bladder, prostatism (see Glossary).
Peripheral neuropathy.
Blood cell disorders: abnormally low white blood cell count, causing fever, sore throat, infections; abnormally low blood platelet count, causing abnormal bleeding or bruising.

▷ **Possible Effects on Sexual Function:** None reported.

▷ **Adverse Effects That May Mimic Natural Diseases or Disorders**
Rare liver reaction may suggest viral hepatitis.

Natural Diseases or Disorders That May Be Activated by This Drug
Systemic lupus erythematosus, myasthenia gravis.

Possible Effects on Laboratory Tests
Complete blood cell counts: decreased red cells, hemoglobin, white cells and platelets; increased eosinophils.
Blood lupus erythematosus (LE) cells: positive.
Blood antinuclear antibodies (ANA): positive (in 50–80% of those using drug after 3 to 6 months).
Liver function tests: increased liver enzymes (ALT/GPT, AST/GOT and alkaline phosphatase), increased bilirubin.
Urine screening tests for drug abuse: *initial* test result may be falsely **positive**; *confirmatory* test result will be **negative**. (Test results depend upon amount of drug taken and testing method used.)

CAUTION

1. Thorough evaluation of your heart function (including electrocardiograms) is necessary prior to using this drug.
2. Periodic evaluation of your heart function is necessary to determine your response to this drug. Some individuals may experience worsening of their heart rhythm disorder and/or deterioration of heart function. Close monitoring of heart rate, rhythm and overall performance is essential.
3. Dosage must be adjusted carefully for each individual. Do not change your dosage without the knowledge and supervision of your physician.
4. Do not take any other antiarrhythmic drug while taking this drug unless directed to do so by your physician.

Precautions for Use
By Infants and Children: Blood cell counts should be monitored for loss of white blood cells.
By Those over 60 Years of Age: Reduced kidney function may require reduction in dosage. Observe carefully for light-headedness, dizziness, unsteadiness and tendency to fall.

Procainamide

▷ **Advisability of Use During Pregnancy**
   Pregnancy Category: C. See Pregnancy Code at the back of this book.
   Animal studies: No information available.
   Human studies: Adequate studies of pregnant women are not available.
   Use this drug only if clearly needed.

Advisability of Use if Breast-Feeding
   Presence of this drug in breast milk: Yes.
   Avoid drug or refrain from nursing.

Habit-Forming Potential: None.

Effects of Overdosage: Loss of appetite, nausea, vomiting, weakness, faintness, irregular heart rhythm, stupor, circulatory collapse, heart arrest.

Possible Effects of Long-Term Use: Lupus erythematosuslike syndrome (see above).

Suggested Periodic Examinations While Taking This Drug (at physician's discretion)
   Complete blood cell counts.
   Blood tests for the development of lupus erythematosus (LE) cells and antinuclear antibodies.
   Electrocardiograms to monitor the full effect of this drug on the mechanisms that influence heart rate and rhythm.

▷ **While Taking This Drug, Observe the Following**
   Foods: No restrictions.
   Beverages: Avoid excessive intake of coffee, tea and cola beverages. Avoid iced drinks. May be taken with milk.
▷ *Alcohol:* Use caution. Alcohol can increase the blood-pressure-lowering effects of this drug.
   Tobacco Smoking: Nicotine can cause irritability of the heart and reduce the effectiveness of this drug. Follow physician's advice regarding smoking.
▷ *Other Drugs*
   Procainamide may *increase* the effects of
   • antihypertensive drugs, and cause excessive lowering of blood pressure.
   The following drugs may *increase* the effects of procainamide
   • amiodirone (Codarone).
   • cimetidine (Tagamet).
   • quinidine (Quinaglute).
   • propranolol (Inderal).
   • ranitidine (Zantac).
   • trimethoprim (Proloprim, Bactrim).
▷ *Driving, Hazardous Activities:* This drug may cause dizziness or weakness. Restrict activities as necessary.
   Aviation Note: The use of this drug **may be a disqualification** for piloting. Consult a designated Aviation Medical Examiner.
   Exposure to Sun: No restrictions.
   Exposure to Heat: Use caution. Hot environments are conducive to lower blood pressure.
   Occurrence of Unrelated Illness: Vomiting, diarrhea or dehydration can affect this drug's action adversely. Report such developments promptly.
   Discontinuation: This drug should not be stopped abruptly after long-term use. Ask your physician for guidance regarding gradual dose reduction.

PROCHLORPERAZINE (proh klor PER a zeen)

Introduced: 1956 **Prescription:** USA: Yes; Canada: Yes **Available as Generic:** USA: Yes; Canada: Yes **Class:** Strong tranquilizer, antiemetic, phenothiazines **Controlled Drug:** USA: No; Canada: No
Brand Names: ◆Combid [CD], Compazine, Eskatrol, ◆PMS-prochlorperazine, Pro-Iso, ◆Stemetil, Ultrazine [CD]

BENEFITS versus RISKS	
Possible Benefits	*Possible Risks*
EFFECTIVE CONTROL OF ACUTE MENTAL DISORDERS in the majority of patients: beneficial effects on thinking, mood and behavior EFFECTIVE CONTROL OF NAUSEA AND VOMITING Relief of anxiety and nervous tension	SERIOUS TOXIC EFFECTS ON BRAIN with long-term use Liver damage with jaundice (infrequent) Rare blood cell disorders: abnormally low white cell and platelet counts

▷ **Principal Uses**

As a Single Drug Product: Uses currently included in FDA approved labeling: (1) Relieves severe nausea and vomiting; (2) sometimes used to treat schizophrenia; (3) helps prevent motion sickness.

Other (unlabeled) generally accepted uses: (1) Sometimes used to increase the effects of anesthesia; (2) may be of use in Meniere's disease.

How This Drug Works: By inhibiting the action of dopamine, this drug acts to correct an imbalance of nerve impulse transmissions that is thought to be responsible for certain mental disorders. By blocking the action of dopamine in the chemoreceptor trigger zone of the brain, this drug prevents stimulation of the vomiting center.

Available Dosage Forms and Strengths
Capsules, prolonged-action — 10 mg, 15 mg, 30 mg
Injection — 5 mg per ml
Suppositories — 2.5 mg, 5 mg, 25 mg
Syrup — 5 mg per 5-ml teaspoonful
Tablets — 5 mg, 10 mg, 25 mg

▷ **Usual Adult Dosage Range:** Initially, 5 mg/6 to 8 hours. If needed and tolerated, dose may be increased by 5 mg at intervals of 3 to 4 days. Usual range is 35 to 60 mg/24 hours. The total daily dosage should not exceed 150 mg.
Note: Actual dose and dosing schedule must be determined by the physician for each patient individually.

Conditions Requiring Dosing Adjustments
Liver function: This drug should be used with caution in patients with liver compromise. Specific guidelines for dosage adjustment are not available.
Kidney function: Specific guidelines for adjustment of dosages are not available.

▷ **Dosing Instructions:** The tablets may be crushed and taken with or following food to reduce stomach irritation. Prolonged-action capsules should be swallowed whole without alteration.

Duration of Use: Use on a regular schedule for 12 to 24 hours usually determines effectiveness in controlling nausea and vomiting. If used for severe anxiety-tension states or acute psychotic behavior, a trial of several weeks is usually necessary to determine effectiveness. If not significantly beneficial within 6 weeks, it should be stopped. Consult your physician on a regular basis.

▷ **This Drug Should Not Be Taken If**
- you have had an allergic reaction to it previously.
- you have active liver disease.
- you have extremely low blood pressure.
- you have cancer of the breast.
- you have a current blood cell or bone marrow disorder.

▷ **Inform Your Physician Before Taking This Drug If**
- you are allergic or abnormally sensitive to any phenothiazine drug (see Drug Class Section).
- you have impaired liver or kidney function.
- you have any type of seizure disorder.
- you have bone marrow depression or history of blood diseases.
- you have diabetes, glaucoma or heart disease.
- you have prostate trouble (prostatic hypertrophy).
- you have a history of lupus erythematosus.
- you are taking any drug with sedative effects.
- you plan to have surgery under general or spinal anesthesia in the near future.

Possible Side-Effects (natural, expected and unavoidable drug actions)

Drowsiness (usually during the first 2 weeks), orthostatic hypotension (see Glossary), blurred vision, dry mouth, nasal congestion, constipation, impaired urination.

Pink or purple coloration of urine, of no significance.

▷ **Possible Adverse Effects** (unusual, unexpected and infrequent reactions)

If any of the following develop, consult your physician promptly for guidance.

Mild Adverse Effects

Allergic Reactions: Skin rash, hives, low-grade fever.

Lowering of body temperature, especially in the elderly. (See Hypothermia in Glossary.)

Increased appetite and weight gain.

Increased blood pressure.

Dizziness, weakness, agitation, insomnia, impaired day and night vision.

Chronic constipation, fecal impaction, incontinence.

Serious Adverse Effects

Allergic Reactions: Hepatitis with jaundice (see Glossary), usually between second and fourth week; high fever; asthma; anaphylactic reaction (see Glossary).

Idiosyncratic Reactions: Toxic dermatitis, Stevens-Johnson syndrome. Neuroleptic malignant syndrome (see Glossary).

Liver toxicity (rare).

Abnormal eye positioning (oculogyric crisis).

Depression, disorientation, seizures.

Disturbances of heart rhythm, rapid heart rate.
Bone marrow depression (see Glossary): fever, sore throat, abnormal bleeding or bruising.
Drug-induced porphyria.
Parkinson-like disorders (see Glossary); muscle spasms of face, jaw, neck, back, extremities; extreme restlessness; slowed movements, muscle rigidity, tremors; tardive dyskinesias (see Glossary).

▷ **Possible Effects on Sexual Function**
Altered timing and pattern of menstruation.
Female breast enlargement with milk production.
Male breast enlargement and tenderness.
Inhibited ejaculation; priapism (see Glossary).
Causes false positive pregnancy test result.

▷ **Adverse Effects That May Mimic Natural Diseases or Disorders**
Nervous system reactions may suggest Parkinson's disease.
Liver reactions may suggest viral hepatitis.
Reactions resembling systemic lupus erythematosus can occur.

Natural Diseases or Disorders That May Be Activated by This Drug
Latent epilepsy, glaucoma, diabetes mellitus, prostatism (see Glossary).

Possible Effects on Laboratory Tests
White blood cell count: decreased.
Liver function tests: increased liver enzymes (ALT/GPT, AST/GOT and alkaline phosphatase), increased bilirubin.

CAUTION
1. Many over-the-counter medications (see OTC Drugs in Glossary) for allergies, colds and coughs contain drugs that can interact unfavorably with this drug. Ask your doctor or pharmacist for help before using any such medications.
2. Antacids that contain aluminum and/or magnesium can prevent the absorption of this drug and reduce its effectiveness.
3. Obtain prompt evaluation of any change or disturbance of vision.

Precautions for Use
By Infants and Children: Do not use this drug in infants under 2 years of age, or in children of any age with symptoms suggestive of Reye syndrome (see Glossary). Children with acute illnesses ("flulike" infections, measles, chicken pox, etc.) are very susceptible to adverse effects when this drug is given to control nausea and vomiting.

By Those over 60 Years of Age: Small starting doses are advisable. You may be more susceptible to drowsiness, lethargy, constipation, lowering of body temperature (hypothermia) and orthostatic hypotension (see Glossary). This drug can worsen existing prostatism (see Glossary). You may also be more susceptible to the development of Parkinson-like reactions and/or tardive dyskinesia (see discussion of these terms in Glossary). These reactions must be recognized early since they may become unresponsive to treatment and irreversible.

▷ **Advisability of Use During Pregnancy**
Pregnancy Category: C. See Pregnancy Code at the back of this book.
Animal studies: Cleft palate reported in mouse and rat studies.

Human studies: No increase in birth defects reported in 2023 exposures. Information from adequate studies of pregnant women is not available.

Limit use to small and infrequent doses. Avoid drug during the last month because of possible effects on the newborn infant.

Advisability of Use if Breast-Feeding
Presence of this drug in breast milk: Yes, in small amounts.
Monitor nursing infant closely and discontinue drug or nursing if adverse effects develop.

Habit-Forming Potential: None, but has been used in combination with pentazocine as a heroin substitute by drug abusers.

Effects of Overdosage: Marked drowsiness, weakness, tremor, agitation, unsteadiness, deep sleep, coma, convulsions.

Possible Effects of Long-Term Use: Tardive dyskinesias. Eye changes: opacities in cornea or lens, retinal pigmentation.

Suggested Periodic Examinations While Taking This Drug (at physician's discretion)
Complete blood cell counts, especially between the fourth and tenth weeks of treatment.
Liver function tests, electrocardiograms.
Complete eye examinations—eye structures and vision.
Careful inspection of the tongue for early evidence of fine, involuntary, wavelike movements that could indicate the beginning of tardive dyskinesia.

▷ **While Taking This Drug, Observe the Following**
Foods: No restrictions.
Nutritional Support: A riboflavin (vitamin B-2) supplement should be taken with long-term use.
Beverages: No restrictions. May be taken with milk.

▷ *Alcohol:* Avoid completely. Alcohol can increase the sedative action of phenothiazines and accentuate their depressant effects on brain function and blood pressure. Phenothiazines can increase the intoxicating effects of alcohol.

Tobacco Smoking: Possible reduction of drowsiness from drug.
Marijuana Smoking: Moderate increase in drowsiness; accentuation of orthostatic hypotension; increased risk of precipitating latent psychoses, confusing the interpretation of mental status and drug responses.

▷ *Other Drugs*
Prochlorperazine may *increase* the effects of
- all sedative drugs, especially meperidine (Demerol), and cause excessive sedation.
- all atropinelike drugs, and cause nervous system toxicity.

Prochlorperazine may *decrease* the effects of
- guanethidine (Ismelin, Esimil), and reduce its effectiveness in lowering blood pressure.

Prochlorperazine *taken concurrently* with
- oral hypoglycemic agents may blunt their therapeutic benefit.

- MAO inhibitors (see Drug Classes) may result in increased risk of abnormal body movements (extrapyramidal reactions).
- propranolol (Inderal) may cause increased effects of both drugs; monitor drug effects closely and adjust dosages as necessary.

The following drugs may *decrease* the effects of prochlorperazine
- antacids containing aluminum and/or magnesium.
- benztropine (Cogentin).
- trihexyphenidyl (Artane).

▷ *Driving, Hazardous Activities:* This drug can impair mental alertness, judgment and physical coordination. Avoid hazardous activities.

Aviation Note: The use of this drug *is a disqualification* for piloting. Consult a designated Aviation Medical Examiner.

Exposure to Sun: Use caution until sensitivity has been determined. Some phenothiazines can cause photosensitivity (see Glossary).

Exposure to Heat: Use caution and avoid excessive heat as much as possible. This drug may impair the regulation of body temperature and increase the risk of heat stroke.

Exposure to Cold: Use caution and dress warmly. This drug can increase the risk of hypothermia in the elderly.

Discontinuation: After long-term use, do not stop this drug suddenly. Gradual withdrawal over 2 to 3 weeks under physician supervision is recommended.

PROPIONIC ACIDS
(Nonsteroidal anti-inflammatory drugs)

Ibuprofen (i BYU proh fen)   **Fenoprofen** (FEN oh proh fen)   **Flurbiprofen** (Flur BI proh fen)   **Ketoprofen** (Kee toh PROH fen)   **Naproxen** (Na PROX in)   **Oxaprozin** (OX a proh zin)

Introduced: 1974, 1976, 1977, 1973, 1974, 1992   **Prescription:** USA: Varies; Canada: Yes   **Available as Generic:** Yes: ibuprofen, fenoprofen, flurbiprofen, ketoprofen and naproxen   **Class:** NSAID, Mild analgesic, anti-inflammatory   **Controlled Drug:** USA: No; Canada: No

Brand Names: Ibuprofen: , Aches-N-Pain, Actiprofen, Advil, ✦Amersol, ✦Apo-Ibuprofen, Bayer Select, Children's Advil, Children's Motrin, CoAdvil [CD], Dimetapp Sinus [CD], Dristan Sinus, Genpril, Guildprofen, Haltran, Ibuprohm, Ibu-Tab, Medipren, Medi-Profen, Midol IB, Motrin, Motrin IB, ✦Novo-Profen, Nuprin, PediaProfen, Rufen, Superior Pain Medicine, Supreme Pain Medicine, Fenoprofen:, Nalfon, Flurbiprofen:, Ansaid, ✦Apo-Flurbiprofen, ✦Froben, Ocufen, Ketoprofen:, ✦Apo-Keto, ✦Apo-Keto E, Orudis, Orudis SR, Oruvail, Oruvail ER, ✦Oruvail SR, ✦Rhodis , ✦Rhodis EC, ✦Rhodis EC suppository, Naproxen:, Aleve, Anaprox, Anaprox DS, ✦Apo-Naproxen, Naprosyn, ✦Naxen, ✦Novo-Naprox, ✦Nu-Naprox, ✦Synflex, Oxaprozin:, Daypro

Propionic Acids

BENEFITS versus RISKS	
Possible Benefits	*Possible Risks*
EFFECTIVE RELIEF OF MILD TO MODERATE PAIN AND INFLAMMATION	Gastrointestinal pain, ulceration, bleeding (rare) Rare kidney damage Rare fluid retention Rare bone marrow depression (except oxaprozin) Rare liver toxicity (naproxen, ketoprofen and flurbiprofen)

▷ **Principal Uses**

As a Single Drug Product: Uses currently included in FDA approved labeling: (1) All of the 6 agents in this class treat rheumatoid and osteoarthritis; (2) naproxen has the longest list of indications and is useful in: bursitis, gout, dysmenorrhea, pain, juvenile rheumatoid arthritis and tendonitis; (3) fenoprofen is the only agent approved to treat tennis elbow.

Other (unlabeled) generally accepted uses: (1) naproxen has been used to treat migraine and colds caused by rhinoviruses; (2) oxaprozin is useful in gout and tendonitis; (3) ketoprofen may have a role in temporal arteritis; (4) flurbiprofen has some support for therapy of periodontal disease and miosis inhibition; (5) fenoprofen has been used successfully in therapy of migraine; (6) ibuprofen treats interleukin 2 toxicity, chronic urticaria and can decrease IUD associated bleeding. All of the agents have been used for a variety of pains and fever.

How These Drugs Work: It is thought that these drugs reduces the tissue concentrations of prostaglandins (and related compounds), chemicals involved in the production of inflammation and pain.

Available Dosage Forms and Strengths

Ibuprofen:
  Caplets — 200 mg
  Oral suspension — 100 mg per 5-ml teaspoonful
    Tablets — 200 mg, 300 mg, 400 mg, 600 mg, 800 mg

Fenoprofen:
  Capsules — 200 mg, 300 mg
    Tablets — 600 mg

Flurbiprofen:
    Tablets — 50 mg (Canada) and 100 mg

Ketoprofen:
  Capsules — 50 mg, 75 mg, 100 mg, 150 mg
  Suppositories — 100 mg (in Canada)
  Enteric tablets — 50 mg (in Canada)

Naproxen:
  Oral suspension — 125 mg per 5 ml teaspoonful
    Tablets — 250 mg, 275 mg, 375 mg, 500 mg, 550 mg

Oxaprozin:
    Caplet — 600 mg

▷ **Usual Adult Dosage Range:** Ibuprofen: 200 to 800 mg 3 or 4 times/day. Total daily dosage should not exceed 3200 mg.

Fenoprofen: 300 to 600 mg three or four times daily. Daily maximum is 3200 mg.

Flurbiprofen: 100 to 200 mg daily in 2 to 4 divided doses. The lowest effective dose should be used. Daily maximum is 300 mg.

Ketoprofen: 75 mg three times daily or 50 mg four times daily. Usual daily dose is 150 to 300 mg divided into 3 or 4 doses. Daily maximum is 300 mg.

Naproxen: Gout: 750 mg initially, then 250 mg every 8 hours until attack is relieved. Arthritis: 250, 375 or 500 mg twice daily 12 hours apart.

Menstrual pain: 500 mg initially, then 250 mg every 6 to 8 hours as needed.

Oxaprozin: 1200 mg as a single daily dose in the morning. Daily maximum is 1800 mg.

Note: Actual dose and dosing schedule must be determined by the physician for each patient individually.

Conditions Requiring Dosing Adjustments

Liver function: All of these drugs are metabolized in the liver and are used with caution, and consideration is given to lower doses in patients with liver compromise.

Kidney function: These drugs share the risks common to most nonsteroidal anti-inflammatory drugs (NSAIDs). Some patients with kidney compromise are dependent on prostaglandins for kidney function. A benefit to risk decision must be made regarding the use of NSAIDS in these patients.

▷ **Dosing Instructions:** Take either on an empty stomach or with food or milk to prevent stomach irritation. Take with a full glass of water and remain upright (do not lie down) for 30 minutes. The tablets may be crushed and the capsules opened for administration except for ketoprofen tablets which should not be crushed or altered.

Usual Duration of Use: Use on a regular schedule for 1 to 2 weeks usually determines effectiveness. Peak oxaprozin effect may take 6 weeks. Long-term use requires supervision and periodic evaluation by the physician.

▷ **These Drugs Should Not Be Taken If**
- you have had an allergic reaction to them previously.
- you are subject to asthma or nasal polyps caused by aspirin.
- you have active peptic ulcer disease or any form of gastrointestinal bleeding.
- you have active liver disease (naproxen, ketoprofen and flurbiprofen).
- you have a bleeding disorder or a blood cell disorder.
- you have severe impairment of kidney function.

▷ **Inform Your Physician Before Taking These Drugs If**
- you are allergic to aspirin or to other aspirin substitutes.
- you have a history of peptic ulcer disease or any type of bleeding disorder.
- you have impaired liver or kidney function.
- you have high blood pressure or a history of heart failure.
- you are taking any of the following: acetaminophen, aspirin or other aspirin substitutes or anticoagulants.

Possible Side-Effects (natural, expected and unavoidable drug actions)
Fluid retention (weight gain); pink, red, purple or rust coloration of urine (ibuprofen only). Ringing in the ears.

▷ **Possible Adverse Effects** (unusual, unexpected and infrequent reactions)
  If any of the following develop, consult your physician promptly for guidance.
  Mild Adverse Effects
    Allergic Reactions: Skin rash, hives, itching.
    Headache, dizziness, altered or blurred vision, ringing in the ears, depression.
    Mouth sores, indigestion, nausea, vomiting, constipation, diarrhea.
  Serious Adverse Effects
    Allergic Reactions: Anaphylaxis (see Glossary), severe skin reactions.
    Idiosyncratic Reactions: Ibuprofen-drug-induced meningitis with fever and coma.
    Active peptic ulcer, with or without bleeding.
    Liver damage with jaundice (see Glossary).
    Kidney damage with painful urination, bloody urine, reduced urine formation.
    Rare bone marrow depression (see Glossary)—fatigue, weakness, fever, sore throat, abnormal bleeding or bruising.

▷ **Possible Effects on Sexual Function**
  Altered timing and pattern of menstruation (ibuprofen, ketoprofen and naproxen), and excessive menstrual bleeding (ibuprofen and ketoprofen); Male breast enlargement and tenderness (ibuprofen). Naproxen may rarely inhibit ejaculation. Ketoprofen may rarely decrease libido.

Possible Delayed Adverse Effects: Mild anemia due to "silent" blood loss from the stomach (less than that caused by aspirin).

▷ **Adverse Effects That May Mimic Natural Diseases or Disorders**
  Liver reaction may suggest viral hepatitis.

Natural Diseases or Disorders That May Be Activated by These Drugs
  Peptic ulcer disease, ulcerative colitis.

Possible Effects on Laboratory Tests
  Complete blood cell counts: decreased red cells, hemoglobin, white cells and platelets.
  Blood cholesterol level: increased.
  Blood lithium level: increased.
  Blood uric acid level: increased.
  Liver function tests: increased liver enzymes (ALT/GPT, AST/GOT and alkaline phosphatase), increased bilirubin.
  Kidney function tests: increased blood creatinine and urea nitrogen (BUN) levels.
  Fecal occult blood test: positive.

CAUTION
  1. Dosage should always be limited to the smallest amount that produces reasonable improvement.
  2. These drugs may mask early indications of infection. Inform your physician if you think you are developing an infection of any kind.

Precautions for Use
  By Infants and Children: Safety and effectiveness for those under 12 years of age not established.

By Those over 60 Years of Age: Small doses are advisable until tolerance is determined. Watch for signs of liver or kidney toxicity, fluid retention, dizziness, confusion, impaired memory, stomach bleeding or constipation.

▷ **Advisability of Use During Pregnancy**
Pregnancy Category: B for ibuprofen, fenoprofen, flurbiprofen, ketoprofen and naproxen. C for oxaprozin. See Pregnancy Code at the back of this book.
Animal studies: No birth defects reported in rats or rabbits.
Human studies: Adequate studies of pregnant women are not available.
Avoid these drugs during the last 3 months. Use during the first 6 months only if clearly needed. Ask physician for guidance.

Advisability of Use if Breast-Feeding
Presence of this drug in breast milk: Yes.
Avoid drug or refrain from nursing.

Habit-Forming Potential: None.

Effects of Overdosage: Drowsiness, dizziness, ringing in the ears, nausea, vomiting, diarrhea, confusion, unsteadiness, stupor progressing to coma.

Possible Effects of Long-Term Use: Fluid retention.

Suggested Periodic Examinations While Taking These Drugs (at physician's discretion)
Complete blood cell counts, liver and kidney function tests, complete eye examinations if vision is altered in any way.

▷ **While Taking These Drugs, Observe the Following**
Foods: No restrictions.
Beverages: No restrictions. May be taken with milk.
▷ *Alcohol:* Use with caution. The irritant action of alcohol on the stomach lining, added to the irritant action of these drugs, can increase the risk of stomach ulceration and/or bleeding.
Tobacco Smoking: No interactions expected.
▷ *Other Drugs*
These medicines may *increase* the effects of
- acetaminophen (Tylenol, etc.), and increase the risk of kidney damage; avoid prolonged use of this combination.
- anticoagulants (Coumadin, etc.), and increase the risk of bleeding; monitor prothrombin time, adjust dose accordingly.
- lithium (Lithobid, others) by causing toxic lithium levels.
- methotrexate (Mexate, others) and result in major methotrexate toxicity with possible anemia, hemorhage and blood infections.

These medicines may *decrease* the effects of
- diuretics such as hydrochlorothiazide (Esidrix) and furosemide (Lasix).
- beta blockers such as carteolol (Cartrol).

These medicines *taken concurrently* with the following drugs may increase the risk of bleeding; avoid these combinations:
- aspirin.
- dipyridamole (Persantine).
- indomethacin (Indocin).

- sulfinpyrazone (Anturane).
- valproic acid (Depakene).

▷ *Driving, Hazardous Activities:* These drugs may cause drowsiness or dizziness. Restrict activities as necessary.

Aviation Note: The use of these drugs **may be a disqualification** for piloting. Consult a designated Aviation Medical Examiner.

Exposure to Sun: Use caution until sensitivity is determined. Ibuprofen, ketoprofen, flurbiprofen and naproxen cause photosensitivity (see Glossary).

PROPRANOLOL (proh PRAN oh lohl)

Introduced: 1966   **Prescription:** USA: Yes; Canada: Yes   **Available as Generic:** Yes   **Class:** Antianginal, antiarrhythmic, antihypertensive, migraine preventive, beta-adrenergic blocker   **Controlled Drug:** USA: No; Canada: No

Brand Names: ◆Apo-Propranolol, ◆Detensol, Inderal, Inderal-LA, Inderide [CD], Inderide LA [CD], Ipran, ◆Novo-Pranol, ◆PMS Propranolol

BENEFITS versus RISKS	
Possible Benefits	*Possible Risks*
EFFECTIVE, WELL-TOLERATED AS: ANTIANGINAL DRUG in effort-induced angina; ANTIARRHYTHMIC DRUG in certain heart rhythm disorders; ANTIHYPERTENSIVE DRUG in mild to moderate hypertension EFFECTIVE PREVENTION OF MIGRAINE HEADACHES Effective adjunct in the prevention of recurrent heart attack (myocardial infarction) Effective adjunct in the management of pheochromocytoma	CONGESTIVE HEART FAILURE in advanced heart disease Worsening of angina in coronary heart disease (if drug is abruptly withdrawn) Masking of low blood sugar (hypoglycemia) in drug-treated diabetes Provocation of asthma Rare depression Rare blood cell disorders: low white cell and platelet counts

▷ **Principal Uses**

As a Single Drug Product: Uses currently included in FDA approved labeling: (1) Used to treat several serious cardiovascular disorders: classical effort-induced angina, certain types of heart rhythm disturbance and high blood pressure. It is also beneficial in preventing the recurrence of heart attacks (myocardial infarction); (2) In addition, it is used to reduce the frequency and severity of migraine headaches.

Other (unlabeled) generally accepted uses: (1) Control of physical signs of anxiety and nervous tension (as in stage fright); (2) helps control familial tremors and symptoms seen with markedly overactive thyroid function (thyrotoxicosis); (3) decreases abnormal abdominal fluid accumulation (ascites) in people with cirrhosis of the liver; (4) may have a role in combination therapy with metronidazole in resistant giardia infections; (5) helps control headaches caused by cyclosporine (Sandimmune); (6) may be useful in certain kinds of pain, especially after amputations; (7)

Propranolol

can help control panic attacks; (8) useful in helping decrease bleeding in patients with esophageal varices and liver cirrhosis; (9) helps fight giardiasis (a parasitic infection) that is resistant to metronidazole treatment.

As a Combination Drug Product [CD]: This drug is available in combination with hydrochlorothiazide for the treatment of hypertension. This combination product includes two drugs with different mechanisms of action; it is intended to provide greater effectiveness and convenience for long-term use.

How This Drug Works: By blocking certain actions of the sympathetic nervous system, this drug
- reduces rate and contraction force of the heart, lowering the ejection pressure of the blood leaving the heart and reducing the oxygen requirement for heart function.
- reduces the degree of contraction of blood vessel walls, resulting in their expansion and consequent lowering of blood pressure.
- prolongs the conduction time of nerve impulses through the heart, of benefit in the management of certain heart rhythm disorders.

Available Dosage Forms and Strengths
Capsules, prolonged-action — 60 mg, 80 mg, 120 mg, 160 mg
Concentrate — 80 mg/ml
Injection — 1 mg per ml
Oral solution — 4 mg/ml and 8 mg/ml
Tablets — 10 mg, 20 mg, 40 mg, 60 mg, 80 mg, 90 mg

▷ **Usual Adult Dosage Range:** Varies with indication.
Antianginal: Initially, 10 mg 3 or 4 times/day; increase dose gradually every 3 to 7 days as needed and tolerated. The total daily dosage should not exceed 400 mg.
Antiarrhythmic: 10 to 30 mg 3 or 4 times/day as needed and tolerated.
Antihypertensive: Initially, 40 mg twice/day; increase dose gradually as needed and tolerated. The total daily dosage should not exceed 640 mg.
Migraine headache prevention: Initially, 20 mg 4 times/day; increase dose gradually as needed and tolerated. The total daily dosage should not exceed 480 mg.
Note: Actual dosage and administration schedule must be determined by the physician for each patient individually.

Conditions Requiring Dosing Adjustments
Liver function: This drug should be used with caution in patients with liver compromise, however, specific guidelines for adjustment of dosages are not available.
Kidney function: Used with caution in people with combined kidney and liver compromise.

▷ **Dosing Instructions:** Preferably taken 1 hour before eating to maximize absorption. The tablet may be crushed for administration; to prevent harmless possible numbing effect, mix with soft food and swallow promptly. The prolonged-action capsules should be swallowed whole without alteration. Do not stop this drug abruptly.

Usual Duration of Use: Use on a regular schedule for 10 to 14 days usually determines effectiveness in preventing angina, controlling heart rhythm disorders and lowering blood pressure. Maximal effectiveness may require continual use for 6 to 8 weeks. The long-term use of this drug (months to years) will be determined by the course of your symptoms over time and your response to the overall treatment program (weight reduction, salt restriction, smoking cessation, etc.). Consult your physician on a regular basis.

▷ **This Drug Should Not Be Taken If**
- you have bronchial asthma
- you have had an allergic reaction to it previously.
- you have Prinzmetal's variant angina (coronary artery spasm).
- you have congestive heart failure.
- you have Raynaud's disease.
- you have an abnormally slow heart rate or a serious form of heart block.
- you are taking, or have taken within the past 14 days, any monoamine oxidase (MAO) type A inhibitor drug (see Drug Classes).

▷ **Inform Your Physician Before Taking This Drug If**
- you have had an adverse reaction to any beta blocker drug in the past (see Drug Classes).
- you have a history of serious heart disease.
- you have a history of hay fever (allergic rhinitis), asthma, chronic bronchitis or emphysema.
- you have a history of overactive thyroid function (hyperthyroidism).
- you have a history of low blood sugar (hypoglycemia).
- you have impaired liver or kidney function.
- you are allergic to bee stings.
- you have diabetes or myasthenia gravis.
- you are currently taking any form of digitalis, quinidine or reserpine, or any calcium blocker drug (see Drug Classes).
- you plan to have surgery under general anesthesia in the near future.

Possible Side-Effects (natural, expected and unavoidable drug actions)
Lethargy and fatigability, cold extremities, slow heart rate, light-headedness in upright position (see orthostatic hypotension in Glossary).

▷ **Possible Adverse Effects** (unusual, unexpected and infrequent reactions)
If any of the following develop, consult your physician promptly for guidance.
Mild Adverse Effects
Allergic Reactions: Skin rash, temporary loss of hair, drug fever (see Glossary).
Joint pain.
Headache, dizziness, insomnia, vivid dreams.
Indigestion, taste disorder, nausea, vomiting, diarrhea.
Weight gain.
Serious Adverse Effects
Allergic Reactions: Anaphylaxis.
Idiosyncratic Reactions: Acute behavioral disturbances: disorientation, confusion, hallucinations, amnesia. Paradoxical hypertension.
Mental depression, anxiety.
Chest pain, shortness of breath, precipitation of congestive heart failure.
Peripheral neuropathy (rare).

Hyperthyroidism (rare).
Drug-induced systemic lupus erythematosus.
Drug-induced myasthenia gravis.
Drug-induced porphyria (rare).
Kidney problems (interstitial nephritis) (rare).
Induction of bronchial asthma (in asthmatic individuals).
May precipitate problems walking (intermittent claudication).
Rare blood cell disorders: abnormally low white blood cell count, causing fever and sore throat; abnormally low blood platelet count, causing abnormal bleeding or bruising.
Carpal tunnel syndrome (rare).

▷ **Possible Effects on Sexual Function**
Decreased libido; impaired erection (28%); impotence (15%).
This drug has been found to have the highest incidence of libido reduction and erectile impairment of all beta blocker drugs.
Male infertility (inhibited sperm motility); Peyronie's disease (see Glossary).

▷ **Adverse Effects That May Mimic Natural Diseases or Disorders**
Reduced blood flow to extremities may resemble Raynaud's phenomenon (see Glossary).

Natural Diseases or Disorders That May Be Activated by This Drug
Prinzmetal's variant angina, Raynaud's disease, intermittent claudication, myasthenia gravis (questionable).

Possible Effects on Laboratory Tests
White blood cell count: occasionally decreased.
Blood platelet count: increased or decreased.
Bleeding time: increased.
Blood total cholesterol level: no effect in some; increased in others.
Blood HDL cholesterol level: no effect in some; decreased in others.
Blood LDL cholesterol level: no effect in some; increased and decreased in others.
Blood VLDL cholesterol level: no effect in some; increased in others.
Blood triglyceride levels: no effect in some; increased in others.
Blood glucose level: no effect in some; increased and decreased in others.
Glucose tolerance test (GTT): decreased.
Blood thyroid hormone levels: T_3—no effect in some, decreased in others; T_4—increased; free T_4—increased.
Blood uric acid level: no effect in some; increased in others.
Liver function tests: increased liver enzymes (ALT/GPT, AST/GOT and alkaline phosphatase); effects probably not due to liver damage.

CAUTION
1. ***Do not stop this drug suddenly*** without the knowledge and help of your doctor. Carry a notation on your person that you are taking this drug.
2. Ask your physician or pharmacist before using nasal decongestants usually present in over-the-counter cold preparations and nose drops. These can cause sudden increases in blood pressure when taken concurrently with beta blocker drugs.
3. Report the development of any tendency to emotional depression.

852   Propranolol

Precautions for Use

By Infants and Children: Safety and effectiveness for those under 12 years of age not established. However, if this drug is used, observe for the development of low blood sugar (hypoglycemia) during periods of reduced food intake.

By Those over 60 Years of Age: Unacceptably high blood pressure should be reduced without creating the risks associated with excessively low blood pressure. Therapy is started with small doses, and blood pressure checked frequently. Sudden, rapid and excessive reduction of blood pressure can predispose to stroke or heart attack. Observe for dizziness, unsteadiness, tendency to fall, confusion, hallucinations, depression or urinary frequency.

▷ **Advisability of Use During Pregnancy**

Pregnancy Category: C. See Pregnancy Code at the back of this book.

Animal studies: No significant increase in birth defects due to this drug. Some toxic effects on embryo reported.

Human studies: Adequate studies of pregnant women are not available.

Avoid use of drug during the first 3 months if possible. Use this drug only if clearly needed. Ask your physician for guidance.

Advisability of Use if Breast-Feeding

Presence of this drug in breast milk: Yes.

Monitor nursing infant closely and discontinue drug or nursing if adverse effects develop.

Habit-Forming Potential: None.

Effects of Overdosage: Weakness, slow pulse, low blood pressure, fainting, cold and sweaty skin, congestive heart failure, possible coma and convulsions.

Possible Effects of Long-Term Use: Reduced heart reserve and eventual heart failure in susceptible patients with advanced heart disease.

Suggested Periodic Examinations While Taking This Drug (at physician's discretion)

Complete blood cell counts.

Measurements of blood pressure, evaluation of heart function.

▷ **While Taking This Drug, Observe the Following**

Foods: No restrictions. Avoid excessive salt intake.

Beverages: No restrictions. May be taken with milk.

▷ *Alcohol:* Use with caution. Alcohol may exaggerate this drug's ability to lower the blood pressure and may increase its mild sedative effect.

Tobacco Smoking: Nicotine may reduce this drug's effectiveness in treating angina, heart rhythm disorders and high blood pressure. Smoking increases the rate of elimination of this drug and decreases its blood levels, especially in younger individuals. In addition, high doses of this drug may worsen the constriction of the bronchial tubes caused by regular smoking.

▷ *Other Drugs*

Propranolol may *increase* the effects of
- other antihypertensive drugs, and cause excessive lowering of blood pressure. Dosage adjustments may be necessary.
- lidocaine (Xylocaine, etc.).

- reserpine (Ser-Ap-Es, etc.), and cause sedation, depression, slowing of the heart rate and lowering of the blood pressure.
- verapamil (Calan, Isoptin), and cause excessive depression of heart function; monitor this combination closely.
- warfarin (Coumadin) and increase bleeding risk.

Propranolol may *decrease* the effects of
- albuterol.
- theophyllines (Aminophyllin, Theo-Dur, etc.), and reduce their antiasthmatic effectiveness.

Propranolol *taken concurrently* with
- amiodarone (Codaraone) may result in abnormal heart rhythms and low pulse. These agents should not be combined.
- clonidine (Catapres) requires close monitoring for rebound high blood pressure if clonidine is withdrawn while propranolol is still being taken.
- digoxin can result in severe slowing of the heart (bradycardia).
- epinephrine (Adrenalin, etc.) may cause marked rise in blood pressure and slowing of the heart rate.
- insulin requires close monitoring to avoid undetected hypoglycemia (see Glossary).
- oral hypoglycemic agents (see Drug Class) and cause slow recovery from any low blood sugar which may occur.
- quinidine can increase adverse effects without increased therapeutic benefits.
- X-ray contrast media such as diatrizoate results in up to an eight fold increased risk of severe allergic (aphylactoid) drug reactions.

The following drugs may *increase* the effects of propranolol
- chlorpromazine (Thorazine, etc.).
- cimetidine (Tagamet).
- diltiazem (Cardizem).
- disopyramide (Norpace).
- furosemide or other diuretics.
- methimazole (Tapazole).
- nicardipine (Cardene).
- propylthiouracil (Propacil).

The following drugs may *decrease* the effects of propranolol
- antacids.
- barbiturates (phenobarbital, etc.).
- indomethacin (Indocin), and possibly other "aspirin substitutes" or NSAIDs may impair propranolol's antihypertensive effect.
- rifampin (Rifadin, Rimactane).

▷ *Driving, Hazardous Activities:* Use caution until the full extent of drowsiness, lethargy and blood pressure change have been determined.

Aviation Note: The use of this drug *may be a disqualification* for piloting. Consult a designated Aviation Medical Examiner.

Exposure to Sun: No restrictions.

Exposure to Heat: Caution advised. Hot environments can lower blood pressure and exaggerate the effects of this drug.

Exposure to Cold: Caution advised. Cold environments can enhance the circulatory deficiency in the extremities that may occur with this drug. The elderly should take precautions to prevent hypothermia (see Glossary).

Heavy Exercise or Exertion: It is advisable to avoid exertion that produces light-headedness, excessive fatigue or muscle cramping. The use of this drug may intensify the hypertensive response to isometric exercise.

Occurrence of Unrelated Illness: Fever can lower blood pressure and require adjustment of dosage. Nausea or vomiting may interrupt the regular dosage schedule. Ask your physician for guidance.

Discontinuation: It is advisable to avoid sudden discontinuation of this drug in all situations; this is especially true in the presence of coronary artery disease. If possible, gradual reduction of dose over a period of 2 to 3 weeks is recommended. Ask your physician for specific guidance.

PROTRIPTYLINE (proh TRIP ti leen)

Introduced: 1966 **Prescription:** USA: Yes; Canada: Yes **Available as Generic:** USA: No; Canada: No **Class:** Antidepressant **Controlled Drug:** USA: No; Canada: No

Brand Names: ♦Triptil, Vivactil

BENEFITS versus RISKS

Possible Benefits	*Possible Risks*
EFFECTIVE RELIEF OF MAJOR ENDOGENOUS DEPRESSIONS	ADVERSE BEHAVIORAL EFFECTS: confusion, disorientation, hallucinations, delusions
Possibly beneficial in other depressive disorders	CONVERSION OF DEPRESSION TO MANIA in manic-depressive disorders
Possibly beneficial in the management of attention deficit disorder	Aggravation of schizophrenia
Possibly beneficial in the management of narcolepsy/cataplexy syndrome	Irregular heart rhythms Rare blood cell abnormalities

▷ **Principal Uses**

As a Single Drug Product: Uses currently included in FDA approved labeling: (1) Relieves symptoms associated with major spontaneous (endogenous) depression, depressed bipolar disorder and mixed bipolar disorder.

Other (unlabeled) generally accepted uses: (1) Treatment of sleep disorders such as apnea, hypersomnia and impaired morning arousal, (2) may have a role in treating glaucoma.

How This Drug Works: It is thought that this drug relieves depression by slowly restoring to normal levels certain constituents of brain tissue (norepinephrine and serotonin) that transmit nerve impulses.

Available Dosage Forms and Strengths
Tablets — 5 mg, 10 mg

▷ **Recommended Dosage Ranges** (Actual dosage and administration schedule must be determined by the physician for each patient individually.)

Infants and Children: Dosage not established.

12 to 60 Years of Age: Initially 5 to 10 mg, 3 or 4 times daily. Increase dose cautiously as needed and tolerated by 5 mg daily at intervals of 1 week.

The usual maintenance dose is 15 to 40 mg/24 hours, divided into 3 or 4 doses. The total daily dose should not exceed 60 mg.

Over 60 Years of Age: Initially 5 mg, 2 or 3 times daily to evaluate tolerance. Increase dose cautiously as needed and tolerated by 5 mg daily at intervals of 1 week. Doses above 20 mg daily require careful monitoring of heart function and blood pressure. The total daily dose should not exceed 40 mg.

Conditions Requiring Dosing Adjustments

Liver function: The dose should be empirically decreased, and blood levels obtained at appropriate intervals. Protriptyline is a rare cause of hepatotoxicity.

Kidney function: The kidney plays a minor role in the elimination of this drug.

▷ **Dosing Instructions:** The tablet may be crushed and taken without regard to meals.

For those individuals who experience a stimulating effect from this drug: (1) Necessary dosage increases should be made in the morning; (2) The last daily dose should be taken in the afternoon (3 to 4 P.M.) to avoid insomnia and disturbed dreaming.

Usual Duration of Use: Some benefit may be apparent within 1 to 2 weeks, but adequate response may require continual use for 3 months or longer. Long-term use should not exceed 6 months without evaluation regarding the need for continuation of the drug. Consult your physician on a regular basis.

Possible Advantages of This Drug

Causes less daytime sedation.

Causes orthostatic hypotension less frequently (see Glossary).

▷ **This Drug Should Not Be Taken If**
- you have had an allergic reaction to it previously.
- you are taking or have taken within the past 14 days any monoamine oxidase (MAO) type A inhibitor drug (see Drug Classes).
- you are recovering from a recent heart attack.
- you have narrow-angle glaucoma.

▷ **Inform Your Physician Before Taking This Drug If**
- you are allergic or sensitive to any other tricyclic antidepressant (see Drug Classes).
- you have a history of any of the following: diabetes, epilepsy, glaucoma, heart disease, prostate gland enlargement or overactive thyroid function.
- you have a history of psychosis.
- you work outside, particularly in hot weather.
- you plan to have surgery under general anesthesia in the near future.

Possible Side-Effects (natural, expected and unavoidable drug actions)

Light-headedness, blurred vision, dry mouth, constipation, impaired urination (see Prostatism in Glossary).

▷ **Possible Adverse Effects** (unusual, unexpected and infrequent reactions)

If any of the following develop, consult your physician promptly for guidance.

Mild Adverse Effects

Allergic Reactions: Skin rash, hives, swelling of face or tongue, drug fever (see Glossary).

Cavities (dental caries).
Blurred vision.
Ringing in the ears.
Headache, dizziness, weakness, fainting, unsteady gait, tremors.
Peculiar taste, irritation of tongue or mouth, nausea, indigestion.
Fluctuation of blood sugar levels.

Serious Adverse Effects
Allergic Reactions: Hepatitis, with or without jaundice (see Glossary).
Confusion, disorientation, hallucinations, delusions.
Aggravation of paranoid psychoses and schizophrenia; seizures.
Heart palpitation and irregular rhythm.
Bone marrow depression (see Glossary)—fatigue, weakness, fever, sore throat, abnormal bleeding or bruising.
Severe lowering of blood pressure on standing (orthostatic hypotension).
Peripheral neuritis (see Glossary)—numbness, tingling, pain, loss of strength in arms and legs.
Parkinson-like disorders (see Glossary)—usually mild and infrequent; more likely to occur in the elderly.

▷ **Possible Effects on Sexual Function:** Decreased libido, increased libido (antidepressant effect), male impotence, inhibited female orgasm, male and female breast enlargement, milk production, swelling of testicles.

▷ **Adverse Effects That May Mimic Natural Diseases or Disorders**
Liver toxicity may suggest viral hepatitis.

Natural Diseases or Disorders That May Be Activated by This Drug
Latent diabetes, epilepsy, glaucoma, prostatism.

Possible Effects on Laboratory Tests
White blood cell and platelet counts: decreased.
Blood glucose levels: increased and decreased (fluctuations).
Liver function tests: increased liver enzymes (ALT/GPT, AST/GOT and alkaline phosphatase), increased bilirubin.

CAUTION
1. Dosage must be adjusted for each person individually. Report for follow-up evaluation and laboratory tests as directed by your physician.
2. It is advisable to withhold this drug if electroconvulsive therapy (ECT, "shock" treatment) is to be used to treat your depression.

Precautions for Use
By Infants and Children: Safety and effectiveness for those under 6 years of age not established. This drug may be used to relieve symptoms of attention deficit disorder, with or without hyperactivity, in selected children over 6 years of age.
By Those over 60 Years of Age: Usual dosage is 15 to 30 mg daily in divided doses. During the first 2 weeks of treatment, observe for the development of confusion, agitation, forgetfulness, disorientation, delusions and hallucinations. Reduction of dosage or discontinuation may be necessary. Unsteadiness may predispose to falling and injury. This drug can increase the degree of impaired urination associated with prostate gland enlargement (prostatism).

▷ **Advisability of Use During Pregnancy**
Pregnancy Category: C. See Pregnancy Code at the back of this book.
Animal studies: No birth defects found in mouse, rat and rabbit studies.
Human studies: No defects reported in 21 exposures to amitriptyline, a closely related drug. Adequate studies of pregnant women are not available.
Avoid use of drug during first 3 months. Use during last 6 months only if clearly needed. Ask your physician for guidance.

Advisability of Use if Breast-Feeding
Presence of this drug in breast milk: Yes, in small amounts.
Monitor nursing infant closely and discontinue drug or nursing if adverse effects develop: excessive drowsiness and failure to feed.

Habit-Forming Potential: Psychological or physical dependence is rare and unexpected.

Effects of Overdosage: Confusion, hallucinations, marked drowsiness, heart palpitations, dilated pupils, tremors, stupor, deep sleep, coma, convulsions.

Suggested Periodic Examinations While Taking This Drug (at physician's discretion)
Complete blood cell counts, liver function tests, serial blood pressure readings and electrocardiograms.

▷ **While Taking This Drug, Observe the Following**
Foods: No restrictions. This drug may increase the appetite and cause excessive weight gain.
Beverages: No restrictions. May be taken with milk.
▷ *Alcohol:* Avoid completely. This drug can markedly increase the intoxicating effects of alcohol and accentuate its depressant action on brain function.
Tobacco Smoking: May hasten the elimination of this drug. Higher doses may be necessary.

▷ *Other Drugs*
Protriptyline may *increase* the effects of
- atropinelike drugs (see Drug Class Section).
- dicoumarol, and increase the risk of bleeding.
- epinephrine (Adrenalin).
- norepinephrine.
- phenytoin (Dilantin) and lead to toxicity.
- pseudoephedrine and cause high blood pressure and arrhythmias.

Protriptyline may *decrease* the effects of
- clonidine (Catapres), and cause loss of blood pressure control; do not use these drugs concurrently.
- guanethidine (Ismelin).

Protriptyline *taken concurrently* with
- disulfiram (Antabuse) may cause acute dementia: confusion, disorientation, hallucinations.
- monoamine oxidase (MAO) inhibitor drugs may cause high fever, delirium and convulsions (see Drug Classes).
- thyroid preparations may impair heart rhythm and function. Ask physician for guidance regarding adjustment of thyroid dose.

- warfarin (Coumadin) may result in prolonged anticoagulation. Increased INR testing (prothrombin times) is needed.

The following drugs may *increase* the effects of protriptyline
- cimetidine (Tagamet).
- estrogens (Premarin).
- fluoxetine (Prozac).
- lithium (Lithobid, etc.).
- methylphenidate (Ritalin).
- oral contraceptives.
- quinidine.
- ranitidine (Zantac).

The following drugs may *decrease* the effects of protriptyline
- barbiturates (see Drug Classes), and reduce its effectiveness.

▷ *Driving, Hazardous Activities:* This drug may impair mental alertness, judgment, physical coordination and reaction time. Avoid hazardous activities.

Aviation Note: The use of this drug *is a disqualification* for piloting. Consult a designated Aviation Medical Examiner.

Exposure to Sun: Use caution. This drug may cause photosensitivity (see Glossary).

Exposure to Heat: This drug can inhibit sweating and impair the body's adaptation to hot environments, increasing the risk of heat stroke. Avoid saunas.

Exposure to Cold: The elderly should use caution and avoid conditions conducive to hypothermia (see Glossary).

Discontinuation: It is advisable to discontinue this drug gradually. Abrupt withdrawal after long-term use can cause headache, malaise and nausea.

PYRAZINAMIDE (peer a ZIN a mide)

Introduced: 1968 Prescription: USA: Yes; Canada: Yes Available as Generic: USA: Yes; Canada: No Class: Anti-infective, antitubercular
Controlled Drug: USA: No; Canada: No
Brand Names: ◆PMS Pyrazinamide, ◆Tebrazid

BENEFITS versus RISKS	
Possible Benefits	*Possible Risks*
EFFECTIVE ADJUNCTIVE TREATMENT OF TUBERCULOSIS	DRUG-INDUCED HEPATITIS (0.3%) Activation of gouty arthritis Activation of porphyria Rare decreased platelets and hemoglobin

▷ **Principal Uses**

As a Single Drug Product: Uses currently included in FDA approved labeling: (1) Treatment of active tuberculosis, in combination with other antitubercular drugs

Other (unlabeled) generally accepted uses: (1) Combination therapy of mycobacterium xenopi infections; (2) combination therapy of resistant tuberculosis.

Pyrazinamide

How This Drug Works: This drug is ideal for killing tuberculosis organisms which are in acid environments such as in some kinds of white blood (macrophages) cells.

Available Dosage Forms and Strengths
Tablets — 500 mg

▷ **Recommended Dosage Ranges** (Actual dosage and administration schedule must be determined by the physician for each patient individually.)

Infants and Children: 7.5 to 15 mg/kg of body weight, twice daily; or 15 to 30 mg/kg of body weight, once daily.
Total daily dosage should not exceed 1.5 grams.

12 to 60 Years of Age: For tuberculosis without HIV infection—5 to 8.75 mg/kg of body weight, every 6 hours; or 6.7 to 11.7 mg/kg of body weight, every 8 hours.
For tuberculosis with HIV infection—20 to 30 mg/kg of body weight, daily for the first 2 months; or 50 to 70 mg/kg of body weight, twice a week.
Total daily dosage should not exceed 3 grams.

Over 60 Years of Age: Same as 12 to 60 years of age.

Conditions Requiring Dosing Adjustments
Liver function: It should be used with caution and in decreased doses in patients with liver compromise. Contraindicated in patients with severe liver dysfunction.

Kidney function: In patients with end stage renal failure, the dose **must** be adjusted to 12 to 20 mg/kg/day. Patients should be closely monitored.

▷ **Dosing Instructions:** The tablet may be crushed and taken with or following food to reduce stomach irritation. Take the full course prescribed. This drug should be taken concurrently with other antitubercular drugs to prevent the development of drug-resistant strains of tuberculosis bacteria.

Usual Duration of Use: Use on a regular schedule for 2 months usually determines effectiveness in contolling active tuberculosis. Long-term use of antitubercular drugs (6 months to 2 years) requires periodic physician evaluation.

Possible Advantages of This Drug
May reduce the period of drug treatment from 9 to 6 months in responsive infections.

▷ **This Drug Should Not Be Taken If**
- you have had an allergic reaction to it previously.
- you have permanent liver damage with impaired function.
- you have active gout.
- you have active peptic ulcer disease.

▷ **Inform Your Physician Before Taking This Drug If**
- you have had an allergic reaction to: ethionamide, isoniazid, niacin (nicotinic acid).
- you have a history of liver disease.
- you have a history of peptic ulcer or porphyria.
- you tried to take medicines for tuberculosis before, but did not complete the prescribed therapy.
- you have gout or diabetes.
- you have impaired kidney function.

Pyrazinamide

Possible Side-Effects (natural, expected and unavoidable drug actions)
Increased blood uric acid levels.

▷ **Possible Adverse Effects** (unusual, unexpected and infrequent reactions)
If any of the following develop, consult your physician promptly for guidance.

Mild Adverse Effects
Allergic Reactions: Skin rash, itching, fever.
Loss of appetite, nausea, vomiting.
Increased uric acid.
Joint pain.

Serious Adverse Effects
Idiosyncratic Reactions: rare sideroblastic anemia.
Decreased blood platelets (rare).
Seizures (rare).
Pellegra.
Drug-induced porphyria.
Kidney problems (interstitial nephritis).
Drug-induced hepatitis, with and without jaundice (see Glossary).
Gouty arthritis, due to increased blood uric acid levels.

▷ **Possible Effects on Sexual Function:** None reported.

▷ **Adverse Effects That May Mimic Natural Diseases or Disorders**
Drug-induced hepatitis may suggest viral hepatitis.

Natural Diseases or Disorders That May Be Activated by This Drug
Gout, peptic ulcer, porphyria.

Possible Effects on Laboratory Tests
Complete blood cell counts: decreased red cells, hemoglobin and platelets.
Prothrombin time: increased.
Blood uric acid level: increased.
Liver function tests: increased liver enzymes (ALT/GPT, AST/GOT and alkaline phosphatase), increased bilirubin.
Urine ketone tests: false positive test result with Acetest and Ketostix.

CAUTION
1. When this drug is used alone, tuberculosis bacteria rapidly develop resistance to it. To be effective, this drug must be used in combination with other effective antitubercular drugs, such as isoniazid and rifampin.
2. This drug may interfere with control of diabetes.

Precautions for Use
By Infants and Children: Safety and effectiveness for those under 12 years of age not established. The rare occurrence of drug-related seizure has been reported in a 2 year old child.
By Those over 60 Years of Age: No specific information available.

▷ **Advisability of Use During Pregnancy**
Pregnancy Category:
C. See Pregnancy Code at the back of this book.
Animal studies: No information available.
Human studies: Adequate studies of pregnant women are not available.
Use this drug only if clearly needed. Ask your physician for guidance.

Advisability of Use if Breast-Feeding
Presence of this drug in breast milk: Yes.
Avoid drug or refrain from nursing.

Habit-Forming Potential: None.

Effects of Overdosage: Nausea, vomiting, malaise.

Possible Effects of Long-Term Use: Liver damage.

Suggested Periodic Examinations While Taking This Drug (at physician's discretion)
Complete blood cell counts.
Liver function tests.
Uric acid blood levels.

▷ **While Taking This Drug, Observe the Following**
Foods: No restrictions.
Beverages: No restrictions. May be taken with milk.
▷ *Alcohol:* Use sparingly to minimize liver toxicity.
Tobacco Smoking: No interactions expected.
▷ *Other Drugs*
Pyrazinamide may *decrease* the effects of
- allopurinol (Zyloprim).
- BCG vaccine.
- cyclosporine (Sandimmune).
- probenecid (Benemid).
- sulfinpyrazone (Anturane).

▷ *Driving, Hazardous Activities:* No restrictions.
Aviation Note: The use of this drug is probably ***not a disqualification*** for piloting. Consult a designated Aviation Medical Examiner.
Exposure to Sun: Use caution. This drug may cause photosensitivity (see Glossary).
Discontinuation: If tolerated, this drug is usually taken for a minimum of 2 months. Do not stop it without your physician's knowledge and guidance.

PYRIDOSTIGMINE (peer id oh STIG meen)

Introduced: 1962 **Prescription:** USA: Yes; Canada: No **Available as Generic:** USA: No; Canada: No **Class:** Antimyasthenic **Controlled Drug:** USA: No; Canada: No

Brand Names: ✦Anaplex SR, Mestinon, Mestinon-SR, Mestinon Timespan, Regonol

BENEFITS versus RISKS	
Possible Benefits	*Possible Risks*
MODERATELY EFFECTIVE TREATMENT OF OCULAR AND MILD FORMS OF MYASTHENIA GRAVIS (symptomatic relief of muscle weakness)	Cholinergic crisis (overdose): excessive salivation, nausea, vomiting, stomach cramps, diarrhea, shortness of breath (asthmalike wheezing), excessive weakness

Pyridostigmine

▷ **Principal Uses**

As a Single Drug Product: Uses currently included in FDA approved labeling: (1) Used primarily to treat the ocular and milder forms of myasthenia gravis by providing temporary relief of muscle weakness and fatigability. It is most useful in long-term treatment when there is little or no difficulty in swallowing; (2) used to reverse muscle relaxants.

Other (unlabeled) generally accepted uses: (1) Used as part of combination therapy in chronic pain; (2) may help in combination therapy of Huntington's chorea and Lambert-Eaton syndrome; (3) adjunctive use with scopolamine to prevent side effects of scopolamine in treating motion sickness; (4) used in war zones to treat the effects of nerve gas; (5) may have a role in treating nonepidemic parotitis.

How This Drug Works: This drug inhibits cholinesterase, the enzyme that destroys acetylcholine. This results in higher levels of acetylcholine, the nerve transmitter that facilitates the stimulation of muscular activity. The net effects are increased muscle strength and endurance.

Available Dosage Forms and Strengths

Syrup — 60 mg per 5-ml teaspoonful (5% alcohol)
Tablets — 60 mg
Tablets, prolonged-action — 180 mg

▷ **Usual Adult Dosage Range:** Initially: 60 to 120 mg/3 to 4 hours; adjust dosage as needed and tolerated. Maintenance: 60 to 1500 mg/24 hours; the average dose is 600 mg/24 hours. Prolonged-action tablets: 180 to 540 mg once or twice a day, at least 6 hours apart. **Note: Actual dosage and administration schedule must be determined by the physician for each patient individually.**

Conditions Requiring Dosing Adjustments

Liver function: No dosing changes are defined in liver compromise.

Kidney function: This drug is primarily eliminated in the urine, however, specific guidelines for dosage adjustments in renal compromise are not available.

▷ **Dosing Instructions:** Take with food or milk to reduce the intensity of side-effects. Larger portions of the daily maintenance dosage should be timed according to the pattern of fatigue and weakness. The syrup will permit a finer adjustment of dosage. The regular tablet may be crushed for administration. The prolonged-action tablet should be taken whole (not altered).

Usual Duration of Use: Use on a regular schedule (with dosage adjustment) for 10 to 14 days usually determines effectiveness in relieving the symptoms of myasthenia gravis. Long-term use (months to years) requires periodic physician evaluation.

▷ **This Drug Should Not Be Taken If**
- you are known to be allergic to bromide compounds.
- you have a urinary obstruction or mechanical intestinal obstruction.

▷ **Inform Your Physician Before Taking This Drug If**
- you are subject to heart rhythm disorders or bronchial asthma.
- you are sensitive to bromides.
- you have recurrent urinary tract infections.

- you have prostatism (see Glossary).
- you plan to have surgery under general anesthesia in the near future.

Possible Side-Effects (natural, expected and unavoidable drug actions)
Small pupils, watering of eyes, slow pulse, excessive salivation, nausea, vomiting, stomach cramps, diarrhea, urge to urinate, increased sweating.

▷ **Possible Adverse Effects** (unusual, unexpected and infrequent reactions)
If any of the following develop, consult your physician promptly for guidance.
Mild Adverse Effects
Allergic Reaction: Skin rash.
Nervousness, anxiety, unsteadiness, muscle cramps or twitching.
Loss of scalp hair, sweating.
Change in the pupil of the eye (miosis).
Serious Adverse Effects
Confusion, slurred speech, seizures, difficult breathing (asthmatic wheezing).
Increased muscle weakness or paralysis.
Psychosis (rare).
Excessive vomiting or diarrhea may induce abnormally low blood potassium levels (hypokalemia). This will accentuate muscle weakness.

▷ **Possible Effects on Sexual Function:** None reported.

▷ **Adverse Effects That May Mimic Natural Diseases or Disorders**
Seizures may suggest the possibility of epilepsy.

Natural Diseases or Disorders That May Be Activated by This Drug
Latent bronchial asthma.

Possible Effects on Laboratory Tests
None reported.

CAUTION
1. Some drugs block the action of this drug and reduce its effectiveness in treating myasthenia gravis. (See *Other Drugs* below.) Ask your doctor before starting any new drug, prescription or over-the-counter.
2. Dosing must be carefully individualized. Variations in response may occur from time to time. Because generalized muscle weakness is a major symptom of both myasthenia crisis (underdosage) and cholinergic crisis (overdosage), it may be difficult to recognize the correct cause. As a rule, weakness that begins within 1 hour after taking this drug probably represents overdosage; weakness that begins 3 or more hours after taking this drug is probably due to underdosage. Observe these time relationships and inform your physician.
3. During long-term use of this drug, watch for development of resistance to the drug's therapeutic action (loss of effectiveness). Ask your doctor if the drug should be stopped for a few days to see if responsiveness can be restored.

Precautions for Use
By Infants and Children: The syrup form of this drug permits greater precision of dosage adjustment and ease of administration in this age group.
By Those over 60 Years of Age: The natural decline of kidney function with

aging may require smaller doses to prevent accumulation of this drug to toxic levels.

▷ **Advisability of Use During Pregnancy**
Pregnancy Category: C. See Pregnancy Code at the back of this book.
Animal studies: No information available.
Human studies: Adequate studies of pregnant women are not available.
There are no reports of birth defects due to the use of this drug during pregnancy. However, there are reports of significant muscular weakness in newborn infants whose mothers had taken this drug during pregnancy. Ask your physician for guidance.

Advisability of Use if Breast-Feeding
Presence of this drug in breast milk: Probably not.
Monitor nursing infant closely and discontinue drug or nursing if adverse effects develop.

Habit-Forming Potential: None.

Effects of Overdosage: Generalized muscular weakness, blurred vision, very small pupils, slow heart rate, difficult breathing (wheezing), excessive salivation, nausea, vomiting, stomach cramps, diarrhea, muscle cramps or twitching. This syndrome constitutes the cholinergic crisis.

Possible Effects of Long-Term Use: Development of tolerance (see Glossary) with loss of therapeutic effectiveness.

Suggested Periodic Examinations While Taking This Drug (at physician's discretion)
Assessment of drug effectiveness and dosage schedule for optimal therapeutic results.

▷ **While Taking This Drug, Observe the Following**
Foods: No restrictions.
Beverages: No restrictions. May be taken with milk.
▷ *Alcohol:* Use caution until the combined effects are determined. Weakness and unsteadiness may be accentuated.
Tobacco Smoking: No interactions expected.
▷ *Other Drugs*
The following drugs may *decrease* the effects of pyridostigmine
- atropine (belladonna).
- clindamycin (Cleocin).
- guanadrel (Hylorel).
- guanethidine (Esimil, Ismelin).
- procainamide (Procan SR, Pronestyl).
- quinidine (Cardioquin, Duraquin, etc.).
- quinine (Quinamm).
- steroids.
▷ *Driving, Hazardous Activities:* This drug may cause blurred vision, confusion or generalized weakness. Restrict activities as necessary.
Aviation Note: The use of this drug *is a disqualification* for piloting. Consult a designated Aviation Medical Examiner.
Exposure to Sun: No restrictions.
Exposure to Heat: Use caution. This may cause excessive sweating and increased weakness.

Exposure to Environmental Chemicals: Avoid excessive exposure (inhalation, skin contamination) to the insecticides Baygon, Diazinon and Sevin. These can worsen potential drug toxicity.

Discontinuation: Do not stop this drug abruptly without your doctor's knowledge and guidance.

PYRIMETHAMINE (peer i METH a meen)

Introduced: 1968 **Prescription:** USA: Yes; Canada: Yes **Available as Generic:** USA: No; Canada: No **Class:** Anti-infective, antiprotozoal
Controlled Drug: USA: No; Canada: No
Brand Names: Daraprim, Fansidar [CD]

BENEFITS versus RISKS	
Possible Benefits	*Possible Risks*
EFFECTIVE PREVENTION AND TREATMENT OF CERTAIN TYPES OF MALARIA	BONE MARROW DEPRESSION, APLASTIC ANEMIA (see Glossary) Serious skin reactions
Effective treatment of AIDS-related isosporiasis diarrhea	
Effective adjunctive treatment of AIDS-related toxoplasmosis	

▷ **Principal Uses**

As a Single Drug Product: Uses currently included in FDA approved labeling: (1) Prevention of chloroquine-resistant P. falciparum malaria, when taken with sulfadoxine; (2) Treatment of chloroquine-resistant P. falciparum malaria, when taken together with sulfadoxine and quinine; (3) therapy of toxoplasmosis.

Other (unlabeled) generally accepted uses: (1) Treatment of isosporiasis diarrhea in those with AIDS or ARC; (2) treatment of toxoplasmosis in those with AIDS; (3) prevention of pneumocystis carinii (PCP) pneumonia in HIV positive patients.

As a Combination Drug Product [CD]: This drug is combined with sulfadoxine in a single tablet and marketed with the brand name Fansidar. This combined dosage form is the one most commonly used to treat the conditions cited above.

How This Drug Works: Pyrimethamine: Interferes with protozoal nucleic acid and protein production by inhibiting essential enzyme systems.

Sulfadoxine: Interferes with the production of bacterial purines and DNA by inhibiting essential enzyme systems.

Available Dosage Forms and Strengths

Tablets — 25 mg of pyrimethamine and 500 mg of sulfadoxine (combined)

▷ **Recommended Dosage Ranges** (Actual dosage and administration schedule must be determined by the physician for each patient individually.)

Infants and Children: For treatment of malaria:

Up to 2 months of age—do not use these drugs.

2 months of age or over—1.25 mg of pyrimethamine/kg of body weight and 25 mg of sulfadoxine/kg of body weight, given as a single dose on the third day of quinine treatment.

For prevention of malaria:
Up to 2 months of age—do not use these drugs.
2 months to 4 years of age—¼ tablet once every 7 days; or ½ tablet once every 14 days.
4 to 8 years of age—½ tablet once every 7 days; or 1 tablet every 14 days.
9 to 14 years of age—¾ tablet once every 7 days; or 1½ tablets every 14 days.

14 to 60 Years of Age: For treatment of malaria: 3 tablets as a single dose on the third day of quinine treatment.

For prevention of malaria: 1 tablet once every 7 days; or 2 tablets once every 14 days.

For treatment of isosporiasis: 50 to 75 mg of pyrimethamine daily, as needed to control or eliminate infection.

For prevention of isosporiasis: 1 tablet of Fansidar once every 7 days. HIV-infected individuals will require long-term preventive treatment.

For treatment of toxoplasmosis: Usual dose is 2 mg/kg daily divided into two daily doses for 3 days, then 1 mg/kg/day every 2 or 3 days for four weeks.

Note: Sulfadiazine is the sulfa drug of choice to use in combination with pyrimethamine for treating AIDS-related cerebral toxoplasmosis. See the Drug Profile of sulfadiazine for detailed information.

For prevention of toxoplasmosis: Maintenance treatment following initial control of infection consists of pyrimethamine 25 mg per day, sulfadiazine 4 grams per day, and folinic acid 10 mg per day; this combination of 3 drugs is given for life.

Over 60 Years of Age: Same as 14 to 60 years of age.

Conditions Requiring Dosing Adjustments
Liver function: This drug should be used with caution in patients with liver compromise.
Kidney function: Pyrimethamine should be used with caution in renal compromise.

▷ **Dosing Instructions:** The regular tablet may be crushed and taken with food if necessary to reduce stomach irritation; take with a full glass of water. Take on a regular schedule.

For prevention of malaria—start 1 to 2 weeks before entering malarious area; continue on a regular schedule while in the area; continue for 4 weeks after leaving the area.

Usual Duration of Use: Use on a regular schedule for 4 to 6 weeks usually determines effectiveness in controlling malaria or toxoplasmosis. Long-term use in the management of AIDS (months to years) requires periodic physician evaluation.

Currently a "Drug of Choice"
for the treatment of AIDS-related cerebral toxoplasmosis (used together with sulfadiazine and folinic acid).

▷ **This Drug Should Not Be Taken If**
- you have had an allergic reaction to it previously.
- you are pregnant or breast-feeding.
- you have an active bone marrow or blood cell disorder.
- you have active liver disease.

Pyrimethamine

▷ **Inform Your Physician Before Taking This Drug If**
- (for sulfadoxine, Fansidar) you are allergic to sulfa drugs, furosemide, thiazide diuretics, oral antidiabetic drugs, or acetazolamide.
- you have a history of drug-induced bone marrow depression.
- you have porphyria or a seizure disorder.
- you have impaired liver or kidney function.
- you are planning pregnancy.
- you have a folate deficiency (ask your doctor).
- you are taking any other drugs currently.

Possible Side-Effects (natural, expected and unavoidable drug actions)
Folic acid deficiency: painful, burning tongue; loss of taste; megaloblastic anemia.

▷ **Possible Adverse Effects** (unusual, unexpected and infrequent reactions)
If any of the following develop, consult your physician promptly for guidance.
Mild Adverse Effects
Allergic Reactions: Skin rash, fever.
Headache, drowsiness, fatigue, nervousness.
Loss of appetite, nausea, vomiting, diarrhea.
Serious Adverse Effects
Allergic Reactions: Severe skin reactions (such as Stevens-Johnson syndrome).
Bone marrow depression, aplastic anemia (see Glossary): weakness, fatigue, fever, sore throat, abnormal bleeding or bruising.
Drug-induced hepatitis with jaundice (see Glossary): yellow eyes and skin, light-colored stools, dark urine.
Drug-induced porphyria.

▷ **Possible Effects on Sexual Function:** None reported.

▷ **Adverse Effects That May Mimic Natural Diseases or Disorders**
Liver reactions may suggest viral hepatitis.

Natural Diseases or Disorders That May Be Activated by This Drug
Latent epilepsy (pyrimethamine) and porphyria (sulfadoxine).

Possible Effects on Laboratory Tests
Complete blood cell counts: decreased red cells, hemoglobin, white cells and platelets.
Liver function tests: increased liver enzymes (ALT/GPT, AST/GOT and alkaline phosphatase), increased bilirubin.

CAUTION
1. Stop taking this drug immediately if a skin rash or itching develops.
2. Women of child-bearing age should use an effective means of contraception while taking this drug.
3. Folinic acid (not folic acid) should be taken routinely while taking pyrimethamine to prevent adverse effects on blood cell production.

Precautions for Use
By Infants and Children: Safety and effectiveness for those under 2 months of age not established.
By Those over 60 Years of Age: No information available.

Pyrimethamine

▷ **Advisability of Use During Pregnancy**
  Pregnancy Category: C. See Pregnancy Code at the back of this book.
  Animal studies: Rat studies reveal drug-induced birth defects.
  Human studies: Adequate studies of pregnant women are not available.
  This drug should be avoided during entire pregnancy because of its potential for harm to the fetus; it is a folic acid antagonist.
Advisability of Use if Breast-Feeding
  Presence of this drug in breast milk: Yes.
  Avoid drug or refrain from nursing.
Habit-Forming Potential: None.
Effects of Overdosage: Nausea, vomiting, unsteadiness, tremors, seizures, respiratory failure.
Possible Effects of Long-Term Use: Bone marrow depression (see Glossary).
Suggested Periodic Examinations While Taking This Drug (at physician's discretion)
  Complete blood cell counts.
  Liver function tests.

▷ **While Taking This Drug, Observe the Following**
  Foods: No restrictions.
  Nutritional Support: Folinic acid, 5 to 10 mg daily; if treating AIDS, 10 to 20 mg daily. (Do not use folic acid.)
  Beverages: No restrictions. Increase liquid intake to ensure 3 pints of urine output daily.
▷ *Alcohol:* No interactions expected.
  Tobacco Smoking: No interactions expected.
▷ *Other Drugs*
  Pyrimethamine may *increase* the effects of
  • chlorpromazine (Thorazine).
  The following drug may *decrease* the effects of pyrimethamine
  • folic acid.
  Pyrimethamine *taken concurrently* with
  • aurothioglucose may result in increased risk of blood cell problems.
  • cotrimoxazole increases risk of anemia (megaloblastic).
  • quinine will result in increased free (active) quinine.
▷ *Driving, Hazardous Activities:* This drug may cause fatigue and drowsiness. Restrict activities as necessary.
  Aviation Note: The use of this drug ***is a disqualification*** for piloting. Consult a designated Aviation Medical Examiner.
  Exposure to Sun: Use caution. This drug may cause photosensitivity (see Glossary).
  Discontinuation: To be determined by your physician.

QUAZEPAM (KWAH zee pam)

Introduced: 1982 **Prescription:** USA: Yes **Available as Generic:** USA: No **Class:** Hypnotic, benzodiazepines **Controlled Drug:** USA: C-IV*

Brand Name: Doral, Dormalin

BENEFITS versus RISKS

Possible Benefits	*Possible Risks*
EFFECTIVE HYPNOTIC during 4 weeks of continual use	Habit-forming potential with long-term use
NO SUPPRESSION OF REM (RAPID EYE MOVEMENT) SLEEP	Minor impairment of mental functions ("hangover" effect)
NO REM SLEEP REBOUND after discontinuation	
Wide margin of safety with therapeutic doses	

▷ **Principal Uses**

As a Single Drug Product: Uses currently included in FDA approved labeling: (1) Short-term treatment of insomnia consisting of difficulty in falling asleep, frequent nighttime awakenings, and/or early morning awakenings; (2) preoperative use (given the night before surgery) as a hypnotic. Other (unlabeled) generally accepted uses: None.

How This Drug Works: This drug selectively affects the benzodiazepine receptors in the brain (BZ-1 receptors) that are associated primarily with sleep mechanisms. Other benzodiazepine hypnotics affect both BZ-1 and BZ-2 receptors, the latter being associated with awareness, memory and judgment; this could account for the "morning-after" impairment of memory and mental functioning caused by shorter acting benzodiazepine hypnotics (notably triazolam and temazepam), but not by quazepam.

Available Dosage Forms and Strengths
Tablets — 7.5 mg, 15 mg

▷ **Recommended Dosage Ranges** (Actual dosage and administration schedule must be determined by the physician for each patient individually.)

Infants and Children: Up to 18 years of age—use not recommended.

18 to 60 Years of Age: Initially 15 mg at bedtime; on the third night, decrease to 7.5 mg, evaluate effectiveness; adjust further dosage as needed and tolerated.

Over 60 Years of Age: Same as 18 to 60 years of age. Usual maintenance dose is 7.5 mg, once daily at bedtime; use higher doses with caution.

Conditions Requiring Dosing Adjustments

Liver function: The dose **must** be decreased in patients with liver compromise.
Kidney function: Quazepam should be used with caution in renal compromise.

▷ **Dosing Instructions:** The tablet may be crushed and taken on an empty stomach or with food or milk. Do not stop this drug abruptly if taken for more than 4 weeks.

---

*See Schedules of Controlled Drugs at the back of this book.

Quazepam

Usual Duration of Use: Use for 3 nights usually determines this drug's effectiveness in relieving insomnia. If possible, this drug should be used for periods of 3 to 5 nights intermittently, repeated as needed with appropriate dosage adjustment. Avoid uninterrupted and prolonged use. The duration of use should not exceed 2 weeks without reappraisal of continued need.

Possible Advantages of This Drug
Effective the first night of use.
Maintains effectiveness on continual use for 4 weeks.
No effects on rapid-eye-movement (REM) sleep.
Minimal "hangover" effect on day after use.
Less likely to cause "next-morning" amnesia, cognitive impairment or mental dysfunction.
No daytime anxiety (drug-withdrawal effect).
No rebound insomnia when drug is discontinued.
No blood cell or liver toxicity.

▷ **This Drug Should Not Be Taken If**
- you have had an allergic reaction to it previously.
- you are pregnant.
- you have sleep apnea (periods where breathing stops while you sleep).
- you have acute narrow-angle glaucoma.

▷ **Inform Your Physician Before Taking This Drug If**
- you are allergic to any benzodiazepine (see Drug Classes).
- you have a history of alcoholism or drug abuse.
- you are planning pregnancy.
- you have impaired liver or kidney function.
- you have a history of serious depression or mental disorder.
- you are taking other drugs with sedative effects.
- you have: asthma, emphysema, epilepsy, myasthenia gravis.

Possible Side-Effects (natural, expected and unavoidable drug actions)
Mild "hangover" effects on arising: drowsiness, lethargy (12%).

▷ **Possible Adverse Effects** (unusual, unexpected and infrequent reactions)
If any of the following develop, consult your physician promptly for guidance.
Mild Adverse Effects
Allergic Reactions: Skin rash, itching (less than 1%).
Headache (4.5%), dizziness (1.5%), fatigue (1.9%), unsteadiness, blurred vision (less than 1%).
Dry mouth, nausea, vomiting, indigestion, constipation, diarrhea (all less than 1%).
Problems in moving and coordination (ataxia).
Serious Adverse Effects
Idiosyncratic Reactions: Nervousness, talkativeness, irritability, apprehension, euphoria, excitement, hallucinations. (Rare paradoxical reactions that may occur with any benzodiazepine.)
Withdrawal symptoms.

▷ **Possible Effects on Sexual Function:** Decreased libido, impotence (rare and questionable).

Possible Effects on Laboratory Tests
Urine screening tests for drug abuse: may be **positive**. (Test results depend upon amount of drug taken and testing method used.)

CAUTION
1. Do not stop taking this drug abruptly if it has been taken continually for more than 4 weeks.
2. Some over-the-counter drug products that contain antihistamines (allergy and cold preparations, sleep aids) can cause excessive sedation.
3. Regular nightly use of any hypnotic drug should be avoided.
4. This drug is changed by the liver into long-acting forms that can persist in the body for 24 hours or more. With continual use of this drug daily, these active drug forms may accumulate and produce increasing sedation. If you experience a "hangover" effect, avoid hazardous activities (driving, etc.) and the use of alcohol.

Precautions for Use

By Infants and Children: Safety and effectiveness for those under 18 years of age not established.

By Those over 60 Years of Age: It is advisable to use smaller doses at longer intervals. Watch for lethargy, indifference, fatigue, weakness, unsteadiness, disturbing dreams, nightmares and paradoxical reactions of excitement, agitation, anger, hostility and rage.

Because this is a long-acting benzodiazepine, it may cause residual sluggishness and unsteadiness with increased risk of falling during the day following bedtime use. This drug may also increase the number of periods of sleep apnea in this age group.

▷ **Advisability of Use During Pregnancy**

Pregnancy Category: X. See Pregnancy Code at the back of this book.
Animal studies: No significant birth defects reported in mouse and rabbit studies.
Human studies: Adequate studies of pregnant women are not available.
Several studies indicate an increased risk of birth defects if drugs of this class (benzodiazepines) are used during the first 3 months.
Frequent use in late pregnancy can cause the "floppy infant" syndrome in the newborn: weakness, lethargy, unresponsiveness, depressed breathing, low body temperature.
Avoid use during entire pregnancy.

Advisability of Use if Breast-Feeding
Presence of this drug in breast milk: Yes.
Avoid drug or refrain from nursing.

Habit-Forming Potential: This drug can produce psychological and/or physical dependence (see Glossary) if used in large doses for an extended period of time. Avoid continual use.

Effects of Overdosage: Marked drowsiness, weakness, feeling of drunkenness, staggering gait, tremor, stupor progressing to deep sleep or coma.

Possible Effects of Long-Term Use: Psychological and/or physical dependence.

Suggested Periodic Examinations While Taking This Drug (at physician's discretion)
None.

Quinacrine

▷ **While Taking This Drug, Observe the Following**
Foods: No restrictions.
Beverages: Avoid excessive intake of caffeine-containing beverages (coffee, tea, cola) within 4 hours of taking this drug. May be taken with milk.
▷ *Alcohol:* It is advisable to avoid alcohol completely—throughout the day and night—if it is necessary to drive or to engage in any hazardous activity.
Tobacco Smoking: Heavy smoking may reduce the hypnotic action of this drug.
Marijuana Smoking: Increased sedation and significant impairment of intellectual and physical performance.
▷ *Other Drugs*
Quazepam may *increase* the effects of
- digoxin (Lanoxin), and cause digoxin toxicity.
- phenytoin (Dilantin), and cause phenytoin toxicity.

Quazepam may *decrease* the effects of
- levodopa (Sinemet, etc.), and reduce its effectiveness in treating Parkinson's disease.

The following drugs may *increase* the effects of quazepam
- cimetidine (Tagamet).
- disulfiram (Antabuse).
- isoniazid (INH, Rifamate, etc.).
- oral contraceptives.
- valproic acid (Depakene).

The following drugs may *decrease* the effects of quazepam
- rifampin (Rimactane, etc.).
- theophylline (aminophylline, Theo-Dur, etc.).

▷ *Driving, Hazardous Activities:* This drug may impair mental alertness, judgment, physical coordination and reaction time. Avoid hazardous activities accordingly.
Aviation Note: The use of this drug ***is a disqualification*** for piloting. Consult a designated Aviation Medical Examiner.
Exposure to Sun: No restrictions.
Exposure to Heat: Use caution until the effect of excessive perspiration is determined. Because of reduced urine volume, this drug may accumulate in the body and produce effects of overdosage.
Discontinuation: Do **not** stop this drug abruptly if this drug has been taken for over 4 weeks without interruption. Dosage should be tapered gradually to prevent a withdrawal syndrome that could include depression, confusion, hallucinations, tremor, seizures, muscle cramping, sweating and vomiting.

QUINACRINE (KWIN a kreen)

Other Name: Mepacrine

Introduced: 1967   **Prescription:** USA: Yes; Canada: No   **Available as Generic:** USA: No; Canada: No   **Class:** Antiprotozoal, lupus suppressant
Controlled Drug: USA: No; Canada: No
Brand Name: Atabrine

Quinacrine

BENEFITS versus RISKS	
Possible Benefits	*Possible Risks*
HIGHLY EFFECTIVE TREATMENT FOR GIARDIASIS Effective treatment for mild to moderate discoid lupus erythematosus	Infrequent adverse behavioral effects: irritability, mood changes, hallucinations, psychotic thinking Yellow discoloration of skin Rare hepatitis Rare corneal and retinal changes, hepatitis, aplastic anemia with high-dose and/or long-term use

▷ **Principal Uses**

As a Single Drug Product: Uses currently included in FDA approved labeling: (1) Treats giardiasis (eradicate Giardia lamblia that are infecting the small intestine); (2) treats tapeworm infections; (3) can be used in preventing or treating malaria, however resistant forms are now present.

Other (unlabeled) generally accepted uses: (1) May have a role in helping asthma patients; (2) can be helpful in decreasing effects of lupus erythematosus; (3) has been used in treating malignant lung (pleural) effusions; (4) used to cause sterilization in women.

How This Drug Works: As an antiprotozoal, this drug inhibits DNA and RNA and prevents reproduction of infecting organisms. As a lupus suppressant, it is thought that this drug impairs the activities of nucleoproteins that are responsible for inflammatory autoimmune reactions.

Available Dosage Forms and Strengths
Tablets — 100 mg

▷ **Usual Adult Dosage Range:** For giardiasis: 100 mg 3 times a day for 5 to 7 days. For discoid lupus: 50 mg to 100 mg daily for several months.

Note: Actual dosage and administration schedule must be determined by the physician for each patient individually.

Conditions Requiring Dosing Adjustments

Liver function: It should be used with caution in combination with other liver toxic drugs.

Kidney function: It should be used with caution and in decreased dose in renal compromise. Quinacrine can discolor the urine.

▷ **Dosing Instructions:** The tablet may be crushed and taken after meals with a full glass of water, tea or fruit juice. The bitter taste can be disguised by mixing with jam, jelly, honey or chocolate syrup. Take the full course prescribed.

Usual Duration of Use: Use on a regular schedule for 5 to 7 days usually determines effectiveness in curing giardiasis. Continual use on a regular schedule for up to 6 months is usually required to realize benefit in controlling the skin lesions of lupus. Long-term use (months to years) requires periodic physician evaluation.

Currently a "Drug of Choice"
for treating symptomatic giardiasis (Giardia lamblia infection).

Quinacrine

▷ **This Drug Should Not Be Taken If**
- you have had an allergic reaction to it previously.
- you have active liver disease.
- you have active bone marrow disease or a blood cell disorder.
- you have porphyria.
- you have psoriasis.

▷ **Inform Your Physician Before Taking This Drug If**
- you are pregnant, planning pregnancy, or breast-feeding.
- you have a history of liver disease or impaired liver function.
- you have a history of bone marrow depression or blood cell disorder, especially drug-induced.
- you have a history of mental disorder (psychosis).
- you have a history of seizure disorder.
- you have any type of eye disorder or impaired vision.
- you have a history of alcohol abuse.
- you have a G6PD deficiency (ask your doctor).
- you have a history of porphyria or psoriasis.
- you are currently taking primaquine.

Possible Side-Effects (natural, expected and unavoidable drug actions)
Yellow discoloration of skin, eyes and urine (of no significance).
Blue-black discoloration of palate and nails with long-term use (of no significance).

▷ **Possible Adverse Effects** (unusual, unexpected and infrequent reactions)
If any of the following develop, consult your physician promptly for guidance.

Mild Adverse Effects
Allergic Reactions: Skin rashes, itching, peeling.
Headache, dizziness, nightmares.
Visual halos or blurred vision.
Loss of appetite, nausea, vomiting, stomach pain or cramping, diarrhea.
Low-grade fever, loss of scalp hair, joint and muscle aches.

Serious Adverse Effects
Allergic Reactions: Chronic dermatitis, exfoliative dermatitis.
Idiosyncratic Reactions: Heart rhythm disturbances; hemolytic anemia in those with glucose-6-phosphate dehydrogenase deficient red blood cells.
Acute behavioral reactions: excitement, agitation, hallucinations, nightmares, psychosis ("Mepacrine madness").
Seizures (rare).
Liver toxicity (rare).
Ear toxicity (ototoxicity).
Corneal swelling and deposits, impaired vision, retinopathy.
Bone marrow depression (see Glossary): fatigue, weakness, fever, sore throat, abnormal bruising or bleeding.

▷ **Possible Effects on Sexual Function:** None reported.

Possible Delayed Adverse Effects: Aplastic anemia (see Glossary) and retinal damage are rare occurrences after discontinuation of this drug.

▷ **Adverse Effects That May Mimic Natural Diseases or Disorders**
Yellow discoloration of skin and eyes may suggest jaundice.
Acute behavioral reactions may suggest unrelated neuropsychiatric disorder.

Natural Diseases or Disorders That May Be Activated by This Drug
Porphyria, psoriasis.

Possible Effects on Laboratory Tests
Complete blood cell counts: decreased red cells, hemoglobin, white cells and platelets; increased eosinophils (allergic reaction).

Liver function tests: increased liver enzymes (ALT/GPT, AST/GOT and alkaline phosphatase), increased bilirubin.

Thrombin: increased activity.

CAUTION
1. Following therapy for giardia infection, 3 separate stool examinations taken 3 to 5 days apart, beginning 3 to 4 weeks after completion of medication should be obtained. If these examinations are negative (indicating a cure), any persistent symptoms may be a lactose intolerance induced by the infection. This may persist for several weeks.
2. During the long-term use of this drug for the treatment of lupus, report promptly any changes in vision that occur so appropriate evaluation can be made.
3. May increase thrombin, FPA and antithrombin three activity when used to treat lung effusions (fluid buildup) in cancer. Watch for abnormal bleeding.

Precautions for Use
By Infants and Children: This drug is not well tolerated by this age group. Dosage schedules and treatment monitoring should be supervised by a qualified pediatrician.

By Those over 60 Years of Age: Adverse behavioral reactions are more likely to occur in this age group. Observe closely for nervous irritability, mood changes, sleep disturbances, or other signs of toxic mental effects. Report these promptly.

▷ ## Advisability of Use During Pregnancy
Pregnancy Category: C. See Pregnancy Code at the back of this book.

Animal studies: Rat studies reveal increased fetal deaths but no birth defects.

Human studies: Adequate studies of pregnant women are not available. Hydrocephalus and absent kidney formation has been reported; possibly attributable to the use of this drug during pregnancy.

If possible, this drug should be avoided during the entire pregnancy.

Advisability of Use if Breast-Feeding
Presence of this drug in breast milk: Yes.

Avoid drug or refrain from nursing.

Habit-Forming Potential: None.

Effects of Overdosage:
Seizures, low blood pressure, heart rhythm abnormalities, circulatory collapse.

Possible Effects of Long-Term Use:
Yellow discoloration of skin, eyes and urine.

Blue-black discoloration of palate and nails.

Chronic dermatitis.

Retinal pigmentation and damage with impaired vision.

Drug-induced hepatitis.

Suggested Periodic Examinations While Taking This Drug (at physician's discretion)

Complete blood cell counts, liver function tests.

Complete eye examinations *before* start of long-term drug use and every 3 to 6 months during use.

▷ **While Taking This Drug, Observe the Following**

Foods: No restrictions.

Beverages: No restrictions. May be taken with milk.

▷ *Alcohol:* Use caution. This combination may cause a mild disulfiramlike reaction (see Glossary).

Tobacco Smoking: No interactions expected.

▷ *Other Drugs*

Quinacrine may *increase* the effects of
- primaquine and increase its toxic potential.
- aurothioglucose and cause increased risk of blood problems (dyscrasias).

▷ *Driving, Hazardous Activities:*

This drug may cause dizziness. Restrict activities as necessary.

Aviation Note:

The use of this drug **may be a disqualification** for piloting. Consult a designated Aviation Medical Examiner.

Exposure to Sun: No restrictions.

Discontinuation: During the long-term use of this drug for lupus, if no significant benefit is apparent after 6 months, this drug should be stopped.

QUINAPRIL (KWIN a pril)

Introduced: 1984 **Prescription:** USA: Yes **Available as Generic:** No **Class:** Antihypertensive, ACE inhibitor **Controlled Drug:** USA: No
Brand Name: Accupril

BENEFITS versus RISKS	
Possible Benefits	*Possible Risks*
EFFECTIVE CONTROL OF MILD TO MODERATE HIGH BLOOD PRESSURE	Headache (5.6%), dizziness (3.9%), fatigue (2.6%) Low blood pressure (0.4%) Low white blood cell counts (0.4%) Allergic swelling of face, tongue, throat, vocal cords (0.1%)

▷ **Principal Uses**

As a Single Drug Product: Uses currently included in FDA approved labeling: (1) Treats mild to moderate high blood pressure, either alone or combined with a thiazide diuretic; (2) treats symptoms of congestive heart failure.

Other (unlabeled) generally accepted uses: (1) Improves survival in patients with congestive heart failure.

How This Drug Works: By blocking certain enzyme systems (angiotensin-converting enzyme, ACE) that influence arterial function, this drug helps relax arterial walls and lowers resistance to blood flow that causes high blood pressure. This, in turn, reduces the work load of the heart and improves its performance.

Available Dosage Forms and Strengths
Tablets — 5 mg, 10 mg, 20 mg, 40 mg

▷ **Recommended Dosage Ranges** (Actual dosage and administration schedule must be determined by the physician for each patient individually.)
Infants and Children: Dosage not established.
12 to 60 Years of Age: Initially 10 mg once daily for those not taking a diuretic; 5 mg once daily for those taking a diuretic. Usual maintenance dose is 20 to 40 mg/day taken in a single dose. If once-a-day dosing does not give stable control of blood pressure over a 24 hour period, divide the dose equally into morning and evening doses. The total daily dosage should not exceed 80 mg.
Over 60 Years of Age: Same as 12 to 60 years of age, if kidney function is normal. If kidney function is significantly impaired, reduce dose by 50%. The total daily dose should not exceed 40 mg.

Conditions Requiring Dosing Adjustments
Liver function: Decreases in dose are not needed.
Kidney function: Patients with mild kidney failure can be given 10 mg daily. Those with moderate kidney failure should be given 5 mg daily. In severe kidney failure, 2.5 mg per day may be given.

▷ **Dosing Instructions:** The tablet may be crushed and taken on an empty stomach or with food, at same time each day.

Usual Duration of Use: Use on a regular schedule for 2 to 3 weeks usually determines effectiveness in controlling high blood pressure. The proper treatment of high blood pressure usually requires the long-term use of effective medications. Consult your physician on a regular basis.

Possible Advantages of This Drug
Usually controls blood pressure effectively with one daily dose.
Relatively low incidence of adverse effects.
No adverse influence on asthma, cholesterol blood levels or diabetes.
Sudden withdrawal does not result in a rapid increase in blood pressure.

▷ **This Drug Should Not Be Taken If**
- you have had an allergic reaction to it previously.
- you are pregnant (last 6 months).
- you currently have a blood cell or bone marrow disorder.
- you have an abnormally high level of blood potassium.

▷ **Inform Your Physician Before Taking This Drug If**
- you have had an allergic reaction (or other adverse effect) on using any other ACE inhibitor drug (see Drug Classes).
- you are planning pregnancy.
- you have a history of kidney disease or impaired kidney function.
- you have severe liver disease.
- you are immunosuppressed or are taking an immunosuppresant medicine.
- you are taking potassium supplements or have an elevated blood potassium.
- you have a low white blood cell count.

Quinapril

- you have scleroderma or systemic lupus erythematosus.
- you have cerebral artery disease.
- you have any form of heart disease.
- you are taking any of the following drugs: other antihypertensives, diuretics, nitrates or potassium supplements.
- you plan to have surgery under general anesthesia in the near future.

Possible Side-Effects (natural, expected and unavoidable drug actions)
  Dizziness (3.9%), orthostatic hypotension (0.5%) (see Glossary), fainting (0.4%), increased blood potassium level (2%).

▷ **Possible Adverse Effects** (unusual, unexpected and infrequent reactions)
  If any of the following develop, consult your physician promptly for guidance.

Mild Adverse Effects
  Allergic Reactions: Skin rash, itching (less than 1%).
  Headache (5.6%), fatigue (2.6%), drowsiness (0.5%), numbness and tingling (less than 1%), weakness (less than 1%).
  Taste disorders (rare).
  Cough (2%), chest pain, muscle pain (up to 5%), palpitation (less than 1.0%).
  Indigestion, nausea/vomiting (1.4%), constipation (less than 1%).

Serious Adverse Effects
  Allergic Reactions: Swelling (angioedema) of face, tongue and/or vocal cords (0.1%); can be life-threatening.
  Impairment of kidney function (2.0%).
  Blood cell problems have occurred with other ACE inhibitors, and caution should be used here.
  Low blood pressure and fainting.
  Increased blood potassium.

▷ **Possible Effects on Sexual Function:** None reported.

Possible Effects on Laboratory Tests
  Complete blood cell counts: decreased white cells and platelets.
  Blood potassium level: increased.
  Liver function tests: increased liver enzymes (ALT/GPT, AST/GOT and alkaline phosphatase).
  Kidney function tests: increased blood urea nitrogen (BUN) and creatinine.

CAUTION
1. Ask your doctor if other antihypertensive drugs (especially diuretics) should be stopped for 1 week before starting this drug.
2. **Inform your physician immediately if you become pregnant.** This drug should not be taken beyond the first 3 months of pregnancy.
3. **Report promptly** any indications of infection (fever, sore throat), and any indications of water retention (weight gain, puffiness, swollen feet or ankles).
4. Do not use a salt substitute without your physician's knowledge and approval. (Many salt substitutes contain potassium.)
5. Blood cell counts and urine analyses should be checked **before** starting this drug.

Precautions for Use

By Infants and Children: Safety and effectiveness for those in this age group not established.

By Those over 60 Years of Age: Small starting doses are indicated. Sudden and excessive lowering of blood pressure can predispose to stroke or heart attack in those with impaired brain circulation or coronary artery heart disease.

▷ **Advisability of Use During Pregnancy**

Pregnancy Category: C during the first three months (trimester). D in the last six months of pregnancy. See Pregnancy Codes at the back of this book.

Animal studies: No information available.

Human studies: The use of ACE inhibitor drugs during the last 6 months of pregnancy is known to possibly cause very serious injury and possible death to the fetus; skull and limb malformations, lung defects, and kidney failure have been reported in over 50 cases worldwide.

Avoid this drug completely during the last 6 months. During the first 3 months of pregnancy, use this drug only if clearly needed. Ask your physician for guidance.

Advisability of Use if Breast-Feeding

Presence of this drug in breast milk: Unknown.

Avoid drug or refrain from nursing.

Habit-Forming Potential: None.

Effects of Overdosage: Excessive drop in blood pressure, light-headedness, dizziness, fainting.

Possible Effects of Long-Term Use: Gradual increase in blood potassium level.

Suggested Periodic Examinations While Taking This Drug (at physician's discretion)

Before starting drug: Complete blood cell counts; urine analysis with measurement of protein content; blood potassium level.

During use of drug: Blood cell counts; measurements of blood potassium.

▷ **While Taking This Drug, Observe the Following**

Foods: Consult physician regarding salt intake.

Nutritional Support:

Do not take potassium supplements unless directed by your physician.

Beverages: No restrictions. May be taken with milk.

▷ *Alcohol:* Use caution until combined effect has been determined. Alcohol may enhance the blood-pressure-lowering effect of this drug.

Tobacco Smoking: No interactions expected.

▷ **Other Drugs**

Quinapril *taken concurrently* with
- cyclosporine (Sandimmune) may cause increased kidey toxicity.
- furosemide (Lasix) or bemetanide (Bumex) may cause decreased blood pressure on standing (postural hypotension).
- lithium can cause increased lithium blood levels and toxicity; monitor lithium blood levels and adjust dosage as necessary.
- potassium preparations (K-Lyte, Slow-K, etc.) may cause increased blood levels of potassium with risk of serious heart rhythm disturbances.

- potassium-sparing diuretics: amiloride (Moduretic), spironolactone (Aldactazide), triamterene (Dyazide) may cause increased blood levels of potassium with risk of serious heart rhythm disturbances.
- tetracycline can reduce the absorption of tetracycline by 29–37%.

▷ *Driving, Hazardous Activities:* Usually no restrictions. Be aware of possible drops in blood pressure with resultant dizziness or faintness.

Aviation Note: The use of this drug **may be a disqualification** for piloting. Consult a designated Aviation Medical Examiner.

Exposure to Sun: Caution advised. A similar drug of this class can cause photosensitivity.

Exposure to Heat: Caution advised. Avoid excessive perspiring with resultant loss of body water and drop in blood pressure.

Occurrence of Unrelated Illness: Report promptly any disorder that causes nausea, vomiting or diarrhea. Fluid and chemical imbalances must be corrected as soon as possible.

Discontinuation: This drug may be stopped abruptly without causing a sudden increase in blood pressure. However, you should consult your physician regarding withdrawal of this drug for any reason.

QUINIDINE (KWIN i deen)

Introduced: 1918 **Prescription:** USA: Yes; Canada: No **Available as Generic:** Yes **Class:** Antiarrhythmic **Controlled Drug:** USA: No; Canada: No

Brand Names: ◆Apo-Quinidine, ◆Biquin Durules, Cardioquin, Cin-Quin, Duraquin, ◆Natisedine, ◆Novoquinidine, Quinaglute Dura-Tabs, ◆Quinate, Quinidex Extentabs, ◆Quinobarb [CD]*, Quinora, Quin-Release, SK-Quinidine sulfate

BENEFITS versus RISKS	
Possible Benefits	*Possible Risks*
EFFECTIVE TREATMENT OF SELECTED HEART RHYTHM DISORDERS	NARROW TREATMENT RANGE FREQUENT ADVERSE EFFECTS NUMEROUS ALLERGIC AND IDIOSYNCRATIC REACTIONS Dose-related toxicity Provocation of abnormal heart rhythms Abnormally low blood platelet count (rare) Hemolytic anemia (rare) Kidney and liver toxicity (rare)

▷ **Principal Uses**

As a Single Drug Product: Uses currently included in FDA approved labeling: (1) Helps control the following types of abnormal heart rhythm: atrial fibrillation and flutter, paroxysmal atrial tachycardia, paroxysmal ven-

---

*Quinobarb contains phenylethylbarbiturate, a sedative of the barbiturate class.

tricular tachycardia, premature atrial and ventricular contractions; (2) intravenous treatment of malaria in people who can not take medicine by mouth.

Other (unlabeled) generally accepted uses: None.

As a Combination Drug Product [CD]: (1) This drug is available (in Canada) in combination with a barbiturate, a mild sedative that is added to allay the anxiety and nervous tension that often accompany heart rhythm disorders.

How This Drug Works: By slowing the activity of the pacemaker and delaying transmission of electrical impulses through the conduction system and muscle of the heart, this drug assists in restoring normal heart rate and rhythm.

Available Dosage Forms and Strengths
Capsules — 200 mg, 300 mg
Injections — 80 mg, 200 mg per ml
Tablets — 100 mg, 200 mg, 275 mg, 300 mg
Tablets, prolonged-action — 300 mg, 324 mg, 330 mg

▷ **Usual Adult Dosage Range:** Test dose: 200 mg, then observe for 2 hours for evidence of idiosyncrasy.

Dose varies with indication—

Premature atrial or ventricular contractions: 200 to 300 mg 3 or 4 times/day.

Paroxysmal atrial tachycardia: 400 to 600 mg/2 to 3 hours until paroxysm is terminated.

Atrial flutter: digitalize first; then individualize dosage schedule as appropriate.

Atrial fibrillation: digitalize first; then try 200 mg/2 to 3 hours for 5 to 8 doses; increase dose daily until normal rhythm is restored or toxic effects develop.

Maintenance schedule: 200 to 300 mg 3 or 4 times/day. The total daily dosage should not exceed 4000 mg.

Note: Actual dosage and administration schedule must be determined by the physician for each patient individually.

Conditions Requiring Dosing Adjustments

Liver function: This drug is extensively metabolized in the liver. Blood levels should be obtained to guide dosing.

Kidney function: Blood levels should be obtained, and used to guide dosing. Quinidine should be used with caution in renal compromise.

▷ **Dosing Instructions:** Preferably taken on an empty stomach to achieve high blood levels rapidly. However, it may be taken with or following food to reduce stomach irritation. The regular tablets may be crushed and the capsules opened for administration. The prolonged-action forms should be swallowed whole without alteration.

Usual Duration of Use: Use on a regular schedule for 2 to 4 days usually determines effectiveness in correcting or preventing responsive abnormal rhythms. Long-term use (months to years) requires physician supervision and periodic evaluation.

Quinidine

▷ **This Drug Should Not Be Taken If**
- you have had an allergic or idiosyncratic reaction to it previously.
- you currently have an acute infection of any kind.
- you have taken too much digoxin (digoxin toxicity).
- you have myasthenia gravis.
- you have abnormal heart rhythms caused by an escape mechanism (ask your specialist).

▷ **Inform Your Physician Before Taking This Drug If**
- you have coronary artery disease or myasthenia gravis.
- you have a history of hyperthyroidism.
- you usually have a very low blood pressure.
- you have had a deficiency of blood platelets in the past from any cause.
- you are now taking, or have taken recently, any digitalis preparation (digitoxin, digoxin, etc.).
- you plan to have surgery under general anesthesia in the near future.
- you have acute rheumatic fever or subacute bacterial endocarditis (SBE).

Possible Side-Effects (natural, expected and unavoidable drug actions)
Drop in blood pressure, may be marked in some patients.

▷ **Possible Adverse Effects** (unusual, unexpected and infrequent reactions)
If any of the following develop, consult your physician promptly for guidance.

Mild Adverse Effects
Allergic Reactions: Skin rash, hives, itching, drug fever (rare).
Dose-related toxicity (cinchonism): blurred vision, ringing in the ears, loss of hearing, dizziness.
Joint pain.
Irritation of the esophagus (esophagitis).
Nausea, vomiting, diarrhea (20% to 30% of users).

Serious Adverse Effects
Allergic Reactions: Severe skin reactions, hemolytic anemia (see Glossary), joint and muscle pains, anaphylactic reaction (see Glossary), reduced blood platelet count, drug-induced hepatitis (see Glossary).
Idiosyncratic Reactions: Skin rash, rapid heart rate, acute delirium and combative behavior, difficult breathing.
Psychosis (rare).
Drug-induced myasthenia gravis (rare).
Swelling of the lymph glands in the inguinal area (lymphadenopathy).
Kidney toxicity (rare).
Systemic lupus erythematosus (SLE) (rare).
Carpal tunnel syndrome (very rare).
Very low blood pressure, fainting (syncope).
Heart conduction abnormalities.
Optic neuritis, impaired vision.
Abnormally low white blood cell count: fever, sore throat, infections.

▷ **Possible Effects on Sexual Function:** None reported.

▷ **Adverse Effects That May Mimic Natural Diseases or Disorders**
Drug-induced hepatitis may suggest viral hepatitis.

Natural Diseases or Disorders That May Be Activated by This Drug
Systemic lupus erythematosus, myasthenia gravis, psoriasis (in sensitive individuals).

Possible Effects on Laboratory Tests
Complete blood cell counts: decreased red cells, hemoglobin, white cells and platelets; increased eosinophils (allergic reaction); marked increase of white blood cells in association with "quinidine fever" (very rare).
Antinuclear antibodies (ANA): positive.
Prothrombin time: increased (when taken concurrently with warfarin).
Liver function tests: increased liver enzymes (ALT/GPT, AST/GOT and alkaline phosphatase), increased bilirubin.

CAUTION
1. Wide variation in response from person to person. Dosage adjustments must be based upon individual reaction. Notify your physician of any events that you suspect may be drug related.
2. It is advisable to carry a card of personal identification that includes a notation that you are taking this drug.

Precautions for Use
By Infants and Children: A test for drug idiosyncrasy should be made before starting treatment with this drug. If there is no beneficial response after 3 days of adequate dosage, this drug should be discontinued.

By Those over 60 Years of Age: Small doses are mandatory until your individual response has been determined. Observe for the development of light-headedness, dizziness, weakness or sense of impending faint. Use caution to prevent falls.

▷ Advisability of Use During Pregnancy
Pregnancy Category: C. See Pregnancy Code at the back of this book.
Animal studies: No information available.
Human studies: Adequate studies of pregnant women are not available. No birth defects have been reported following use of this drug during pregnancy.
Use this drug only if clearly needed.

Advisability of Use if Breast-Feeding
Presence of this drug in breast milk: Yes.
Avoid drug or refrain from nursing.

Habit-Forming Potential: None.

Effects of Overdosage:
Nausea, vomiting, ringing in the ears, headache, jerky eye movements, double vision, altered color vision, confusion, delirium, hot skin, seizures, coma.

Possible Effects of Long-Term Use: None reported.

Suggested Periodic Examinations While Taking This Drug (at physician's discretion)
Complete blood cell counts, electrocardiograms.

▷ While Taking This Drug, Observe the Following
Foods: No restrictions.
Beverages: No restrictions. May be taken with milk.
▷   *Alcohol:* Use caution. Alcohol may enhance the blood-pressure-lowering effects of this drug.

▷ *Tobacco Smoking:* Nicotine can increase irritability of the heart and aggravate rhythm disorders. Avoid all forms of tobacco.

▷ *Other Drugs*
Quinidine may *increase* the effects of
- anticoagulants (Coumadin, etc.), and increase the risk of bleeding.
- digitoxin and digoxin (Lanoxin), and cause digitalis toxicity.
- disopyramide (Norpace).
- tricyclic antidepressants (doxepin).
- warfarin (Coumadin) and result in bleeding.

The following drugs may *increase* the effects of quinidine
- amiodarone (Codarone).
- cimetidine (Tagamet).
- ketoconazole.
- verapamil.

The following drugs may *decrease* the effects of quinidine
- barbiturates (phenobarbital, etc.).
- phenytoin (Dilantin).
- rifampin (Rifadin, Rimactane).

▷ *Driving, Hazardous Activities:* This drug may cause dizziness and alter vision. Restrict activities as necessary.

Aviation Note: The use of this drug *may be a disqualification* for piloting. Consult a designated Aviation Medical Examiner.

Exposure to Sun: Use caution. This drug may cause photosensitivity (See Glossary).

RAMIPRIL (ra MI pril)

Introduced: 1985   **Prescription:** USA: Yes   **Available as Generic:** No   **Class:** Antihypertensive, ACE inhibitor   **Controlled Drug:** USA: No   **Brand Name:** Altace

BENEFITS versus RISKS	
Possible Benefits	*Possible Risks*
EFFECTIVE CONTROL OF MILD TO SEVERE HIGH BLOOD PRESSURE	Headache (5.4%), dizziness (2.2%), fatigue (2.0%)
	Low blood pressure (0.5%)
	Allergic swelling of face, tongue or vocal cords (angioedema) (0.3%)

▷ **Principal Uses**
As a Single Drug Product
Uses currently included in FDA approved labeling: (1) Treats all degrees of high blood pressure, alone or concurrently with thiazide-type diuretics. Mild to moderate high blood pressure usually responds to low doses; severe high blood pressure may require higher doses, with greater risk of serious adverse effects; (2) helps decrease the size of the left ventricle and control blood pressure in people with left ventricular hypertrophy; (3) helps control blood pressure caused by abnormalities (stenosis) in the renal artery.

Other (unlabeled) generally accepted uses: (1) Helps improve survival in patients with congestive heart failure.

How This Drug Works: By blocking enzyme systems that influence arterial function, this drug helps relax arterial walls and lower resistance to blood flow that causes high blood pressure. This, in turn, reduces the work load of the heart and improves its performance.

Available Dosage Forms and Strengths
Capsules — 1.25 mg, 2.5 mg, 5 mg, 10 mg

▷ **Usual Adult Dosage Range:** Initially 2.5 mg once daily for 2 to 4 weeks. Usual maintenance dose is 2.5 to 20 mg/day in a single dose or in 2 divided doses.

If taking diuretics: Either discontinue the diuretic for 3 days before initiating this drug, or begin treatment with 1.25 mg of this drug.

Total daily dose should not exceed 5 mg if kidney function is significantly impaired. **Note: Actual dosage and administration schedule must be determined by the physician for each patient individually.**

Conditions Requiring Dosing Adjustments
Liver function: Patients should be followed closely if they have compromised livers.
Kidney function: Patients with moderate kidney failure or creatinine values of greater than 2.5, a dose of 1.25 mg of ramipril can be used daily.

▷ **Dosing Instructions:** Take on an empty stomach or with food, at same time each day. The capsule may be opened for administration.

Usual Duration of Use: Use on a regular schedule for 2 to 4 weeks usually determines effectiveness in controlling high blood pressure. The proper treatment of high blood pressure usually requires the long-term use of effective medications. Consult your physician on a regular basis.

▷ **This Drug Should Not Be Taken If**
- you have had an allergic reaction to it previously.
- you are pregnant (last 6 months).
- you have a history of angioedema (a serious allergic reaction) from any cause.
- you have active liver disease.
- you have an abnormally high level of blood potassium.

▷ **Inform Your Physician Before Taking This Drug If**
- you have had an unfavorable reaction to angiotensin-converting enzyme (ACE) inhibitor drugs previously: captopril (Capoten), enalapril (Vasotec), lisinopril (Prinivil, Zestril), others (see Drug Classes).
- you are pregnant (first 3 months), planning pregnancy, or breast-feeding.
- you have impaired liver or kidney function.
- you have scleroderma or systemic lupus erythematosus.
- you have any form of heart disease.
- you have diabetes.
- you take: other antihypertensives, diuretics, nitrates or potassium supplements.
- you have abnormal kidney circulation (ask your doctor).
- you take immunosuppressant therapy or have an autoimmune disease.

- you have an abormally elevated blood potassium level or take a potassium sparing diuretic.
- you have a condition which causes increased temperature.
- you have had low white blood cell counts.
- you plan to have surgery under general anesthesia in the near future.

Possible Side-Effects (natural, expected and unavoidable drug actions)
Dizziness (2.2%), light-headedness (0.5%).

▷ **Possible Adverse Effects** (unusual, unexpected and infrequent reactions)
If any of the following develop, consult your physician promptly for guidance.

Mild Adverse Effects
Allergic Reactions: Skin rash, itching.
Headache (5.4%), fatigue (2%), drowsiness, nervousness, numbness and tingling, insomnia.
Cough.
Chest pain, palpitation, drug-induced cough (12%).
Indigestion, stomach pain, nausea (1.1%), vomiting, diarrhea.
Excessive sweating, joint and muscle aches.

Serious Adverse Effects
Allergic Reactions: Swelling (angioedema) of face, tongue and/or vocal cords: can be life threatening (0.3%).
Profound lowering of the blood pressure.
Increased blood potassium.
Abnormally decreased blood sodium.

▷ **Possible Effects on Sexual Function:** Rare report of impotence (0.4%).

Possible Effects on Laboratory Tests
Complete blood cell counts: decreased red cells and hemoglobin (0.4% using this drug alone; 1.5% using this drug and a diuretic); decreased white cells, increased eosinophils (both rare).
Blood potassium level: increased (1%).
Liver function tests: increased liver enzymes (ALT/GPT, AST/GOT and alkaline phosphatase), increased bilirubin.
Kidney function tests: increased blood urea nitrogen (BUN) (0.5% using this drug alone; 3% using this drug and a diuretic); increased creatinine (1.2% using this drug alone; 1.5% using this drug and a diuretic).
Increased erythrocyte sedientation rate.

CAUTION
1. Ask your doctor if other antihypertensive drugs (especially diuretics) should be stopped for 1 week before starting this drug.
2. **Report promptly** any indications of infection (fever, sore throat), and any indications of water retention (weight gain, puffiness, swollen feet or ankles).
3. Do not use a salt substitute without your physician's knowledge and approval. (Many salt substitutes contain potassium.)
4. It is advisable to obtain blood cell counts and urine analyses **before** starting this drug.

5. **Notify your physician immediately if pregnancy occurs.** This drug should not be taken beyond the first 3 months of pregnancy.

Precautions for Use
By Infants and Children: Safety and effectiveness for use by those in this age group have not been established.
By Those over 60 Years of Age: Small doses are advisable until tolerance has been determined. Sudden and excessive lowering of blood pressure can predispose to stroke or heart attack in those with impaired brain circulation or coronary artery heart disease.

▷ **Advisability of Use During Pregnancy**
Pregnancy Category: D. See Pregnancy Code at the back of this book.
Animal studies: Fetal kidney defects found in rat studies; retarded growth found in mouse studies.
Human studies: Adequate studies of pregnant women are not available. However, drugs of this class taken during the last 6 months of pregnancy have been reported to cause serious fetal defects: skull and facial malformations, limb deformities, lung defects and kidney failure (over 50 cases reported worldwide).
Avoid this drug completely during the last 6 months. During the first 3 months of pregnancy, use this drug only if clearly needed. Ask your physician for guidance.

Advisability of Use if Breast-Feeding
Presence of this drug in breast milk: Yes.
Avoid drug or refrain from nursing.

Habit-Forming Potential: None.

Effects of Overdosage: Excessive drop in blood pressure—light-headedness, dizziness, fainting.

Possible Effects of Long-Term Use: Gradual increase in blood potassium level.

Suggested Periodic Examinations While Taking This Drug (at physician's discretion)
Before starting drug: Complete blood cell counts; urine analysis with measurement of protein content; blood potassium level.
During use of drug: Blood cell counts; measurements of blood potassium.

▷ **While Taking This Drug, Observe the Following**
Foods: Consult physician regarding salt intake.
Nutritional Support: **Do not take** potassium supplements unless directed by your physician.
Beverages: No restrictions. May be taken with milk.
▷ *Alcohol:* Use caution until combined effect has been determined. Alcohol may enhance the blood-pressure-lowering effect of this drug.
Tobacco Smoking: No interactions expected.
▷ *Other Drugs*
Ramipril *taken concurrently* with
- aspirin or other NSAIDs may blunt the blood pressure lowering response.
- lithium (Lithane, Lithotab, etc.) may cause increased blood lithium levels and symptoms of lithium toxicity. Monitor lithium levels closely.

- potassium preparations (K-Lyte, Slow-K, etc.) may cause increased blood levels of potassium with risk of serious heart rhythm disturbances.
- potassium-sparing diuretics: amiloride (Moduretic), spironolactone (Aldactazide), triamterene (Dyazide) may cause increased blood levels of potassium with risk of serious heart rhythm disturbances.
- cyclosporine (Sandimmune) may pose increased risk of kidney toxicity.
- loop diuretics such as furosemide (Lasix) or bumetanide (Bumex) may cause severe postural hypotension (see Glossary).

▷ *Driving, Hazardous Activities:* Usually no restrictions. Be aware of possible drops in blood pressure with resultant dizziness or faintness.

Aviation Note: The use of this drug **may be a disqualification** for piloting. Consult a designated Aviation Medical Examiner.

Exposure to Sun: Caution advised. A similar drug of this class can cause photosensitivity.

Exposure to Heat: Caution advised. Avoid excessive perspiring with resultant loss of body water and drop in blood pressure.

Occurrence of Unrelated Illness: Nausea, vomiting or diarrhea may cause fluid and chemical imbalances that must be corrected as soon as possible.

RANITIDINE (ra NI te deen)

Introduced: 1981   **Prescription:** USA: Yes; Canada: Yes   **Available as Generic:** Yes   **Class:** Antiulcer, H-2 receptor blocker   **Controlled Drug:** USA: No; Canada: No

Brand Name: Zantac, ◆Zantac-C, ◆Apo-Ranitidine, ◆Novo-Ranitidine, ◆Nu-Ranit

Warning: The brand names Zantac and Xanax are similar and can be mistaken for each other; this can lead to serious medication errors. These names represent very different drugs. Zantac is the generic drug ranitidine; it is used to treat peptic ulcer disease. Xanax is the generic drug alprazolam; it is a mild tranquilizer. Verify that you are taking the correct drug.

BENEFITS versus RISKS	
Possible Benefits	*Possible Risks*
EFFECTIVE TREATMENT OF PEPTIC ULCER DISEASE: relief of symptoms, acceleration of healing, prevention of recurrence	Drug-induced hepatitis (rare)
	Confusion (in severely ill elderly patients)
CONTROL OF HYPERSECRETORY STOMACH DISORDERS	Rare blood cell disorders
	Rare pancreatitis
Beneficial in treatment of reflux esophagitis	Rare liver toxicity

Author's note: Two of the four available H2 receptor blocking drugs are now available without prescription. It is expected that the remaining two H2s will pursue and achieve nonprescription status.

Please see the new histamine (H2) blocking drug profile for further information.

RIFABUTIN (RIF a byou tin)

Introduced: 1993 **Prescription:** USA: Yes; Canada: Not available
Available as Generic: USA: No; Canada: No **Class:** antimycobacterial agent (antitubercular) **Controlled Drug:** USA: No; Canada: Not available
Brand Name: Mycobutin

Warning: Rifabutin prophylaxis must not be given to people with active tuberculosis.

BENEFITS versus RISKS	
Possible Benefits	*Possible Risks*
PREVENTION OF DISSEMINATED MYCOBACTERIUM AVIUM COMPLEX (MAC) IN PEOPLE WITH ADVANCED HIV INFECTION.	NEUTROPENIA (2%) Rare low white blood cell counts (leukopenia) Rare low platelet counts (thrombocytopenia)

▷ **Principal Uses**
As a Single Drug Product: Uses currently included in FDA approved labeling: (1) Prevention of disseminated Mycobacterium avium complex (MAC) in patients with advanced HIV infection; (2) combination treatment of MAI infection.
Other (unlabeled) generally accepted use: (1) Some clinical trial use in pneumocystis carinii pneumonia.

How This Drug Works: Rifabutin inhibits DNA-dependant RNA polymerase (an enzyme critical to cells that are dividing) in E. coli. The exact mechanism of action of rifabutin in Mycobacterium avium or Mycobacterium intracellulare is not known.

Available Dosage Forms and Strengths
Rifabutin (Mycobutin) capsules — 150mg

How To Store
Keep at room temperature and avoid exposure to excessive humidity.

▷ **Recommended Dosage Ranges (Actual dosage and administration schedule must be determined by the physician for each patient individually.)**
Infants and Children: Safety and effectiveness of rifabutin in MAC prophylaxis has not clearly been established. Safety data comes from a trial of 22 children who were HIV positive:
Infants one year of age—18.5mg/kg/day.
Children 2–10 years—8.6mg/kg/day.
Adolescents 14 years—4.0mg/kg/day.
14 to 60 Years of Age: 300 mg once a day. People who are prone to nausea and vomiting may take 150 mg 2 times a day with food.
Over 60 Years of Age: Same as 12 to 60 years of age.

Conditions Requiring Dosing Adjustments
Liver function: At present, clear adjustments of dose in hepatic compromise are not defined, but the drug should be used with caution.
Kidney function: Elimination of rifabutin may actually be increased in people with compromised kidneys, yet the clinical effect is as yet unknown.

▷ **Dosing Instructions:** May be taken with food if you are prone to nausea and vomiting. May be mixed with foods such as applesauce for use in children.

Usual Duration of Use: Use on a regular schedule indefinitely is usually needed to assure this drug's effectiveness in prophylaxis of disseminated MAC. Long-term use (months to years) requires periodic physician evaluation of response.

If rifabutin is being used as a part of combination therapy of a Mycobacterium avium intracellularae infection, the ideal duration of treatment has not been identified, but treatment is usually ongoing.

Possible Advantages of This Drug
Oral treatment of very resistant organisms.

Currently a "Drug of Choice"
for prophylaxis (prevention) of disseminated MAC.

▷ **This Drug Should Not Be Taken If**
- you have had an allergic reaction to any dosage form of it previously.
- you have active tuberculosis (combination therapy with several medications is indicated).

▷ **Inform Your Physician Before Taking This Drug If**
- you are pregnant or plan to become pregnant.
- you are taking an oral contraceptive (a nonhormonal alternative method is advised).
- you have a history of blood disorders.
- you are taking an anticoagulant such as coumadin.
- you take other prescription or non-prescription medicines which were not discussed with your doctor when this medicine was prescribed.
- you are uncertain of how much to take or how often to take rifabutin.

Possible Side-Effects (natural, expected and unavoidable drug actions)
This medication may color saliva, urine, feces, sputum, perspiration, tears, and skin a brown-orange color. Soft contact lenses may become permanently stained by rifabutin or its metabolites.

Emergence of resistant Mycobacterium tuberculosis.

▷ **Possible Adverse Effects** (unusual, unexpected and infrequent reactions)
If any of the following develop, consult your physician promptly for guidance.

Mild Adverse Effects
Allergic Reactions: Skin rash, fever.
Change in taste perceptions, headache, loss of appetite, gastrointestinal upset, nausea, vomiting, and diarrhea, muscle aches, joint pains and a flu-like syndrome.
Taste disorders.

Serious Adverse Effects
Very rare confusion and aphasia and seizures, chest pain with dyspnea (trouble breathing), nonspecific T wave changes (a change in the way the heart beats), neutropenia-2%, rare leukopenia, anemia, thrombocytopenia and hepatitis.

▷ **Possible Effects on Sexual Function:** Potential alteration of pattern and timing of menstruation.
Decreased effectiveness of oral contraceptives taken together with this drug.

▷ **Adverse Effects That May Mimic Natural Diseases or Disorders**
Liver reactions similar to viral hepatitis.

Possible Effects on Laboratory Tests
Complete blood cell counts: neutropenia (decreases in a specific kind of white blood cells), thrombocytopenia (decreased platelets), anemia, leukopenia (decreased white blood cells).
Coagulation (clotting tests), decreased prothrombin time (when taken at the same time as coumadin).
Liver enzymes (alk phos, SGOT and SGPT) can be increased.

CAUTION
1. The effectiveness of oral contraceptives may be decreased.
2. May hasten the development of resistant Mycobacterium tuberculosis if used as monotherapy (as a single drug).
3. Urine, feces, saliva, sputum, sweat, tears and skin may be colored brown-orange with rifabutin and some of its metabolites. Soft contact lenses may be permanently stained.

Precautions for Use
By Infants and Children:
Safety and effectiveness for use in children has not been established.
By Those over 60 Years of Age: Specific precautions have not yet been developed, however since the drug is similar to rifampin, those over 60 may be more sensitive to the adverse effects of rifabutin.

▷ **Advisability of Use During Pregnancy**
Pregnancy Category: B. See Pregnancy Code at the back of this book.
Animal studies: At doses equal to 8 times the usual human dose, rifabutin caused an increase in skeletal variants in rats. Doses of 16 times the usual human dose caused maternotoxicity and fetal skeletal anomalies in rabbits.
Human studies: Adequate studies of pregnant women are not available.
Ask your physician for guidance.

Advisability of Use if Breast-Feeding
Presence of this drug in breast milk: It is not known whether rifabutin is excreted in breast milk.
A decision should be made to avoid drug or refrain from nursing.

Habit-Forming Potential: None.

Effects of Overdosage: No information is currently available on overdosage in humans.

Suggested Periodic Examinations While Taking This Drug (at physician's discretion)
This medication may cause neutropenia and thrombocytopenia, therefore, white blood cell counts and platelet counts should be checked. Liver function tests should also be obtained periodically.

▷ **While Taking This Drug, Observe the Following**
Foods: No restrictions.
Beverages: No restrictions.
▷ *Alcohol:* Potential exists for additive liver toxicity. It is best to avoid alcohol.

892   Rifampin

Tobacco Smoking: No interactions expected.

Marijuana Smoking: May be an additive cause of rashes and seizures in people with existing seizure disorders. Avoid marijuana completely.

▷ *Other Drugs*

Rifabutin may *decrease* the effects of
- antianxiety agents such as diazepam.
- anticoagulants such as coumadin.
- anticonvulsant drugs such as phenytoin.
- barbiturates.
- BCG live attenuated vaccine.
- beta blockers such as metopralol, propranolol.
- chloramphenicol.
- clofibrate.
- cortisonelike drugs (see Drug Class Section).
- cyclosporine.
- dapsone.
- digitalis preparations.
- disopyramide.
- ketoconazole.
- mexilitine.
- narcotics such as methadone.
- oral contraceptives.
- oral hypoglycemic agents (sulfonylureas such as tolbutamide).
- quinidine.
- theophylline.
- verapamil.
- zidovudine (the therapeutic effect will be lessened by a decreased drug level).

Rifabutin *taken concurrently* with
- anticoagulants such as coumadin will result in a decreased anticoagulant effect (the protime will decrease).
- fluconazole may result in increased rifabutin concentrations.

▷ *Driving, Hazardous Activities:* This drug may rarely be associated with confusion and seizures. Restrict activities as necessary.

Aviation Note: The use of this drug *may be a disqualification* for piloting. Consult a designated Aviation Medical Examiner.

Exposure to Sun: No restrictions.

Discontinuation: Do not stop or interrupt taking this medication without asking your doctor.

RIFAMPIN (RIF am pin)

Other Name: Rifampicin

Introduced: 1967   **Prescription:** USA: Yes; Canada: Yes   **Available as Generic:** No   **Class:** Antibiotic, rifamycins   **Controlled Drug:** USA: No; Canada: No

Brand Names: Rifadin, Rifadin IV, Rifamate [CD], Rimactane, Rimactane/INH Dual Pack [CD], ◆Rofact

BENEFITS versus RISKS	
Possible Benefits	**Possible Risks**
EFFECTIVE TREATMENT OF TUBERCULOSIS in combination with other drugs EFFECTIVE PREVENTION OF MENINGITIS by the elimination of meningococcus from the throat of carriers	DRUG-INDUCED HEPATITIS DRUG-INDUCED NEPHRITIS Flulike syndrome Rare blood cell disorder: abnormally low blood platelet count Rare coagulation defects Rare porphyria Rare colitis (pseudomembranous)

▷ **Principal Uses**

As a Single Drug Product: Uses currently included in FDA aproved labeling: (1) Treats active tuberculosis. It is usually given concurrently with other antitubercular drugs to enhance its effectiveness. It is also used to eliminate the meningitis germ (meningococcus) from the throats of healthy carriers so it cannot be spread to others; (2) treats tuberculosis in coal workers with good outcomes when combined with other antibucular drugs; (3) used to prevent tuberculosis in people exposed to patients with active disease.

Other (unlabeled) generally accepted uses: (1) Second line agent in combination with doxycycline in treatment of brucellosis; (2) has a place in preventing Haemophilus influenzae infections in people exposed to patients with active disease; (3) combination therapy of lepromatous leprosy; (4) used in combination with cotrimoxazole to eliminate methicillin resistant staphylococcus aureus (MRSA) from people who carry the bacteria.

As a Combination Drug Product [CD]: This drug is available in combination with isoniazid, another antitubercular drug that delays the development of drug-resistant strains of the tuberculosis germ.

How This Drug Works: This drug prevents the growth and multiplication of susceptible tuberculosis organisms by blocking specific enzyme systems that are involved in the formation of essential proteins.

Available Dosage Forms and Strengths
Capsules — 150 mg, 300 mg

▷ **Usual Adult Dosage Range:** For tuberculosis: 600 mg once/day. For meningococcus carriers: 600 mg once/day for 4 days. The total daily dosage should not exceed 600 mg. **Note: Actual dosage and administration schedule must be determined by the physician for each patient individually.**

Conditions Requiring Dosing Adjustments
Liver function: This drug can cause liver damage, and patients should be followed closely. In severe failure, the dose should be limited to 6 to 8 mg per kg twice a week.
Kidney function: Specific guidelines for dosing adjustments are not available.

▷ **Dosing Instructions:** Preferably taken with 8 ounces of water on an empty stomach (1 hour before or 2 hours after eating). However, it may be taken with food if necessary to reduce stomach irritation. The capsule may be opened and the contents mixed with applesauce or jelly for administration.

Usual Duration of Use: Use on a regular schedule for several months usually determines effectiveness in promoting recovery from tuberculosis. Long-term use (possibly 1 to 2 years) requires ongoing physician supervision and periodic evaluation.

▷ **This Drug Should Not Be Taken If**
- you have had an allergic reaction to it previously.
- you have active liver disease.

▷ **Inform Your Physician Before Taking This Drug If**
- you are pregnant.
- you have a history of liver disease or impaired liver function.
- you consume alcohol daily.
- you are taking an oral contraceptive. (An alternate method of contraception is advised.)
- you are taking an anticoagulant.

Possible Side-Effects (natural, expected and unavoidable drug actions)
Red, orange or brown discoloration of tears, sweat, saliva, sputum, urine or stool. Yellow discoloration of the skin (not jaundice). Note: In the absence of symptoms indicating illness, any discoloration is a harmless drug effect and does not indicate toxicity.
Possible fungal superinfections (see Glossary).

▷ **Possible Adverse Effects** (unusual, unexpected and infrequent reactions)
If any of the following develop, consult your physician promptly for guidance.
Mild Adverse Effects
Allergic Reactions: Skin rash, hives, itching, drug fever (see Glossary).
Headache, drowsiness, dizziness, blurred vision, impaired hearing, vague numbness and tingling.
Joint and muscle pain.
Loss of appetite, heartburn, nausea, vomiting, abdominal cramps, diarrhea.
Serious Adverse Effects
Skin problems (Stevens-Johnson syndrome).
Flulike syndrome: fever, chills, headache, dizziness, musculoskeletal pain, difficult breathing.
Drug-induced liver damage, with or without jaundice.
Drug-induced kidney damage: impaired urine production, bloody or cloudy urine.
Drug-induced porphyria.
Excessively low blood platelet count: abnormal bleeding or bruising.
Blood clotting problems (disseminated intravascular coagulopathy (rare).
Hemolytic anemia (rare).
Suppression of the adrenal gland (rare).
Pseudomembranous colitis (rare).
Gallstones (rare).
Pancreatitis (rare).

▷ **Possible Effects on Sexual Function**
    Altered timing and pattern of menstruation.
    Decreased effectiveness of oral contraceptives taken concurrently.
▷ **Adverse Effects That May Mimic Natural Diseases or Disorders**
    Liver reactions may suggest viral hepatitis.
    Kidney reactions may suggest an infectious nephritis.

Possible Effects on Laboratory Tests
    Complete blood cell counts: decreased red cells, hemoglobin, white cells and platelets; increased eosinophils (allergic reaction).
    Prothrombin time: increased (when taken concurrently with warfarin).
    Liver function tests: increased liver enzymes (ALT/GPT, AST/GOT and alkaline phosphatase), increased bilirubin.

CAUTION
1. This drug may permanently discolor soft contact lenses.
2. This drug may reduce the effectiveness of oral contraceptives; unplanned pregnancy could occur; an alternate method of contraception is advised.
3. When this drug is used alone in the treatment of tuberculosis, resistance can develop rapidly. This drug should only be used in conjunction with other antitubercular drugs.
4. To ensure the best possible response to treatment, take the full course of medication prescribed; this may be for several months or years.

Precautions for Use
    By Infants and Children: Monitor closely for possible liver toxicity or deficiency of blood platelets.
    By Those over 60 Years of Age: Natural changes in body composition and function make you more susceptible to the adverse effects of this drug. Report promptly any indications of possible drug toxicity.
▷ **Advisability of Use During Pregnancy**
    Pregnancy Category: C. See Pregnancy Code at the back of this book.
    Animal studies: Cleft palate and spinal defects reported in rodent studies.
    Human studies: Adequate studies of pregnant women are not available.
    If possible, avoid use of drug during the first 3 months.

Advisability of Use if Breast-Feeding
    Presence of this drug in breast milk: Yes.
    Avoid drug or refrain from nursing.

Habit-Forming Potential: None.

Effects of Overdosage: Nausea, vomiting, drowsiness, unconsciousness, severe liver damage, jaundice.

Possible Effects of Long-Term Use: Superinfections, fungal overgrowth of mouth or tongue.

Suggested Periodic Examinations While Taking This Drug (at physician's discretion)
    Complete blood cell counts, liver and kidney function tests.
    Hearing acuity tests if hearing loss is suspected.
▷ **While Taking This Drug, Observe the Following**
    Foods: No restrictions.
    Beverages: No restrictions.

▷ *Alcohol:* It is best to avoid alcohol completely to reduce the risk of liver toxicity.
Tobacco Smoking: No interactions expected.
▷ *Other Drugs*
Rifampin may **decrease** the effects of
- anticoagulants (Coumadin, etc.), and reduce their effectiveness.
- BCG vaccine.
- beta blockers: metoprolol, propranolol.
- cortisonelike drugs (see Drug Class Section).
- cyclosporine.
- dapsone.
- digitoxin, digoxin.
- disopyramide.
- enalapril.
- fluconazole.
- itraconazole.
- ketoconazole.
- methadone (Dolophine).
- mexiletine (Mexitil).
- nifedipine.
- oral contraceptives.
- oral hypoglycemic agents (se Drug Class).
- phenytoin (Dilantin).
- progestins.
- quinidine.
- sulfonylureas: chlorpropamide, tolbutamide.
- theophyllines (Aminophyllin, Theo-Dur, etc.).
- verapamil.
- warfarin.

The following drugs may **decrease** the effects of rifampin
- aminosalicylic acid (PAS), and reduce its antitubercular effectiveness.

▷ *Driving, Hazardous Activities:* This drug may cause dizziness, drowsiness, impaired vision and impaired hearing. Restrict activities as necessary.
Aviation Note: The use of this drug **may be a disqualification** for piloting. Consult a designated Aviation Medical Examiner.
Exposure to Sun: No restrictions.
Discontinuation: It is advisable not to interrupt or stop this drug without consulting your physician. Intermittent administration can increase the possibility of developing allergic reactions.

RISPERIDONE (Ris pair i doan)

Introduced: December 1993 **Prescription:** USA: Yes; Canada: Yes
Available as Generic: USA: No; Canada: No **Class:** Antipsychotic agent
Controlled Drug: USA: No; Canada: No

Brand Names: Risperdal

BENEFITS versus RISKS	
Possible Benefits	*Possible Risks*
TREATMENT OF SCHIZOPHRENIA REFRACTORY TO OTHER AGENTS	Change in heart function (prolonged QT interval—Rare).
DECREASED SIDE EFFECTS COMPARED TO OTHER AVAILABLE DRUGS	Involuntary movement disorder (tardive dyskinesia—Rare) Neuroleptic malignant syndrome (see Glossary—Rare)

▷ **Principal Uses**

As a Single Drug Product: Uses currently included in FDA approved labeling: (1) Short-term (6 to 9 weeks) treatment of chronic schizophrenia.

Other (unlabeled) generally accepted uses: (1) Treatment of acute schizophrenia; (2) treatment of aggression; (3) treatment of Tourette's syndrome; (4) can have a role in helping behavioral problems in people with mental retardation.

How This Drug Works: This medication acts to balance two nerve transmitters (dopamine and serotonin) and by doing so, helps restore more normal thinking and mood.

Available Dosage Forms and Strengths
Tablets — 1 mg, 2 mg, 3 mg, 4 mg

▷ **Recommended Dosage Ranges (Actual dosage and administration schedule must be determined by the physician for each patient individually.)**

Infants and Children: Safety and efficacy for those less than 18 years of age are not established.

18 to 60 Years of Age: Usual starting dose is 1 mg taken twice daily. Dosage may be increased as needed and tolerated by 1 mg on the second and third day for a total of 3 mg twice daily by the third day. If further dose changes are needed, they should be made at 1 week intervals. Doses greater than 6 mg per day are not recommended.

Over 60 Years of Age: Therapy is started with 0.5 mg twice daily. The dose is increased if needed and tolerated by 0.5 mg twice daily. Doses greater than 1.5 mg daily are achieved by small increases made at one week intervals. Careful attention must be paid to blood pressure and development of adverse effects.

Conditions Requiring Dosing Adjustments

Liver function: The starting dose must be decreased and adjusted as for those over 60 years old.

Kidney function: The starting dose must be decreased and adjusted as for those over 60 years old.

▷ **Dosing Instructions:** The tablet may be crushed, and medication effect is not changed by food.

Usual Duration of Use: Use on a regular schedule for 1 to 2 weeks usually determines effectiveness in helping control chronic schizophrenia. If long-term use is attempted, the lowest effective dose should be used. Periodic physician evaluation of response and dosage adjustment is required.

Risperidone

Possible Advantages of This Drug
Treatment of schizophrenia refractory to other therapy.

▷ **This Drug Should Not Be Taken If**
- you have had an allergic reaction to any dosage form of it previously.
- you have had neuroleptic malignant syndrome (ask your doctor).

▷ **Inform Your Physician Before Taking This Drug If**
- you have a history of breast cancer.
- you have liver or kidney compromise.
- you are pregnant or plan to become pregnant.
- you have had tardive dyskinesia in the past.
- you have a history of heart rhythm disturbances.
- you are uncertain of your risperidone dose or how often to take it.

Possible Side-Effects (natural, expected and unavoidable drug actions)
Increased prolactin levels may result in male and female breast tenderness and swelling.

▷ **Possible Adverse Effects** (unusual, unexpected and infrequent reactions)
If any of the following develop, consult your physician promptly for guidance.

Mild Adverse Effects
Allergic Reactions: skin rash.
Somnolence (3% to 41% of high dose patients).
Difficulty in concentrating/fatigue (1%).
Increased dreaming (1%).
Weight gain (18%).
Constipation.
Orthostatic hypotension (see Glossary—rare).
Increased urination (1%).

Serious Adverse Effects
Allergic Reactions: Anaphylactoid reactions.
Abnormal heart function (prolonged QT interval—rare).
Tardive dyskinesia (see Glossary—rare).
Neuroleptic malignant syndrome (rare).
Low sodium (1%).
Rare seizures (0.3%).
Low platelets (rare).
Abnormal liver function (rare).

▷ **Possible Effects on Sexual Function:** Diminshed sexual desire (1%). Delayed or absent orgasm (1%). Erectile dysfunction including priapism (1%), male or female breast tenderness or swelling (1%). Dry vagina or menstrual changes (menorrhagia—1%). Ejaculation failure (0.1–1%).

Possible Delayed Adverse Effects: Swelling and tenderness of male and female breast tissue.

Natural Diseases or Disorders That May Be Activated by This Drug
Some human cancers depend on prolactin for growth, and since risperidone increases prolactin, it should be used with caution in people with previously diagnosed breast cancer.

Possible Effects on Laboratory Tests
Liver function tests: increased SGPT, SGOT and LDH.

Complete blood counts: decreased platelets, white blood cells and hemoglobin.
Prolactin: increased.

CAUTION
1. Should be used with great caution, if at all in patients with cancer.
2. Call your doctor promptly if you have an increased tendency to infection or abnormal bleeding or bruising while taking this drug.
3. Used with great caution, if at all in patients with seizure history.

Precautions for Use
By Infants and Children:
Safety and effectiveness for those under 18 years of age not established.
By Those over 60 Years of Age: A lower starting dose and slow increases are indicated. Great care should be taken in those with heart disease. You may be more likely to experience postural hypotension (see Glossary) and problems with motor skills. Those with prostate problems may have increased risk of urine retention.

▷ **Advisability of Use During Pregnancy**
Pregnancy Category: C. See Pregnancy Code at the back of this book.
Animal studies: Increased rat pup death during the first few days of lactation.
Human studies: Adequate studies of pregnant women are not available. One case report of lack of formation of the corpus callosum of the brain in a fetus exposed to this drug while in the uterus.
Ask your doctor for guidance.

Advisability of Use if Breast-Feeding
Presence of this drug in breast milk: Yes.
Avoid drug or refrain from nursing.

Habit-Forming Potential: None.

Effects of Overdosage: Drowsiness, hypotension, tachycardia, low sodium and potsssium, ECG changes (prolonged QT interval), and seizure.

Suggested Periodic Examinations While Taking This Drug (at physician's discretion)
Liver function tests.
Electrolytes (sodium, and potassium).
ECG.
Prolactin level.

▷ **While Taking This Drug, Observe the Following**
Foods: No restrictions.
Beverages: No restrictions.
▷ *Alcohol:* Patients should avoid alcohol while taking risperidone.
Tobacco Smoking: No interactions expected.
Marijuana Smoking: Increased somnolence.
▷ *Other Drugs*
Risperidone may *decrease* the effects of
- levodopa (Sinemet, others).

Risperidone *taken concurrently* with
- cabramazepine (Tegretol) will decrease the drug level and perhaps the therapeutic effect of risperidone.

The following drugs may *increase* the effects of risperidone
- clozapine (Clozaril).

▷ *Driving, Hazardous Activities:* This drug may cause drowsiness and difficulty concentrating. Restrict activities as necessary.

Aviation Note: The use of this drug *is a disqualification* for piloting. Consult a designated Aviation Medical Examiner.

Exposure to Sun: Use caution. May cause photosensitivity.

Discontinuation: Consult your doctor before stopping this medication.

SALMETEROL (Sal ME ter all)

Introduced: February, 1994 **Prescription:** USA: Yes; Canada: Not available in Canada **Available as Generic:** USA: No **Class:** Sympathomimetic agent **Controlled Drug:** USA: No
Brand Names: Serevent

BENEFITS versus RISKS	
Possible Benefits	*Possible Risks*
LONG ACTING RELIEF OF BRONCHIAL ASTHMA PREVENTION OF NOCTURNAL ASTHMA SYMPTOMS	Rapid heart rate (tachycardia)

▷ **Principal Uses**
As a Single Drug Product: Uses currently included in FDA approved labeling: (1) Treatment and prevention of bronchospasm in asthma; (2) prevention of nocturnal asthma; (3) prevention of exercised induced bronchospasm. Other (unlabeled) generally accepted uses: (1) None at present.

How This Drug Works: This drug acts at specific sites (beta-2) in the lung and result in opening of the airways (bronchodilation), decreased airway reactivity and increased movement of mucous. It also appears to block release of chemicals from certain (mast) cells which worsen asthma.

Available Dosage Forms and Strengths
Inhaler — 13 gram canister which gives 25 mcg of salmeterol per use.

▷ **Recommended Dosage Ranges (Actual dosage and administration schedule must be determined by the physician for each patient individually.)**
Infants and Children: Safety and efficacy in those less than 12 years of age not established.
12 to 60 Years of Age: For prevention of asthma: Two inhalations (42 mcg) twice daily in the morning and evening. Doses should be given 12 hours apart.
For prevention of exercised induced asthma: Two inhalations at least 30 to 60 minutes **before** exercise. Additional doses of salmeterol should **not** be given for 12 hours.
Over 60 Years of Age: Same as 12 to 60 years of age.

Conditions Requiring Dosing Adjustments
Liver function: Used with caution as the drug may accumulate in liver failure.
Kidney function: Salmeterol has not been studied in kidney failure patients.

▷ **Dosing Instructions:** Follow written instructions on the inhaler closely. Has not been studied for use with a spacer or similar device. Should be shaken well before using.

Usual Duration of Use: Use on a regular schedule for 4 to 6 weeks usually determines effectiveness in preventing asthma attacks. Long-term use (months to years) requires periodic physician evaluation of response and dosage adjustment.

Possible Advantages of This Drug
Longer acting beta-two agent than medications previously available.

▷ **This Drug Should Not Be Taken If**
- you have had an allergic reaction to any dosage form of it previously.
- you currently have an irregular heart rhythm.
- you are taking, or have taken within the past 2 weeks, any monoamine oxidase (MAO) type A inhibitor.

▷ **Inform Your Physician Before Taking This Drug If**
- your breathing does not improve after administration of this drug.
- you have a overactive thyroid (hyperthyroidism).
- you have diabetes.
- you have abnormally high blood pressure.
- you are uncertain of how much salmeterol to take or how often to take it.

Possible Side-Effects (natural, expected and unavoidable drug actions)
Dryness or irritation of the mouth or throat, altered taste. Nervousness or palpitations.
Tachyphylaxis.

▷ **Possible Adverse Effects** (unusual, unexpected and infrequent reactions)
If any of the following develop, consult your physician promptly for guidance.
Mild Adverse Effects
Allergic Reactions: Skin rash and urticaria.
Rhinitis and laryngitis.
Nervousness and fatigue.
Headache, tremor and nervousness.
Serious Adverse Effects
Allergic Reactions: Not defined.
Rapid heart rate (tachycardia) and palpitations.
Paradoxical bronchospasm.
Respiratory arrest (rare).

▷ **Possible Effects on Sexual Function:** Dysmenorrhea.

Possible Delayed Adverse Effects: Not defined at present.

▷ **Adverse Effects That May Mimic Natural Diseases or Disorders**
Rapid heart rate may mimic heart disease.
Bronchospasm may mimic asthma.

Natural Diseases or Disorders That May Be Activated by This Drug
Latent coronary artery disease. Diabetes or high blood pressure.

Possible Effects on Laboratory Tests
Blood cholesterol profile: may be increased.
Blood glucose level: increased.

Salmeterol

CAUTION
1. Use of this drug by inhalation with beclomethasone aerosol (Beclovent, Vanceril) may increase the risk of fluorocarbon propellant toxicity. Use salmeterol aerosol 20 to 30 minutes **before** beclomethasone aerosol to reduce toxicity and enhance penetration of beclomethasone into the lungs.
2. Serious heart rhythm problems or cardiac arrest can result from excessive and prolonged use.
3. Call your doctor if you begin to have symptoms more frequently than usual, or if you begin to increase your use of the immediate bronchodilator which was prescribed for you.

Precautions for Use
  By Infants and Children:
    Safety and effectiveness for those under 12 years of age not established.
  By Those over 60 Years of Age: Avoid increased use. If asthma is not controlled as it has been in the past, call your doctor.

▷ **Advisability of Use During Pregnancy**
  Pregnancy Category: C. See Pregnancy Code at the back of this book.
    Animal studies: Rabbit studies have revealed cleft palate, limb and paw flexures and delayed bone formation.
    Human studies: Adequate studies of pregnant women are not available.
    Ask your doctor for guidance.

Advisability of Use if Breast-Feeding
  Presence of this drug in breast milk: Yes, but extent not defined.
  Avoid drug or refrain from nursing.

Habit-Forming Potential: None.

Effects of Overdosage: Exaggeration of pharmacologic effects: tachycardia and/or arrhythmia, muscle cramps, cardiac arrest and death.

Suggested Periodic Examinations While Taking This Drug (at physician's discretion)
  Blood pressure checks, evaluations of heart (cardiac) status.

▷ **While Taking This Drug, Observe the Following**
  Foods: No restrictions.
  Beverages:
    Avoid excessive caffeine as in coffee, tea, cola and chocolate.
▷ *Alcohol:* No interactions expected.
  Tobacco Smoking: No interactions expected.
    Salmeterol **taken concurrently** with
    • monoamine oxidase (MAO) type A inhibitor drugs can cause extreme increases in blood pressure and heart stimulation.
    The following drugs may *increase* the effects of salmeterol
    • tricyclic antidepressants.
    • methylzanthines such as caffeine or theophylline.
▷ *Driving, Hazardous Activities:* This drug may cause nervousness or dizziness. Restrict activities as necessary.
  Aviation Note: The use of this drug ***is a disqualification*** for piloting. Consult a designated Aviation Medical Examiner.

Exposure to Sun: No restrictions.
Heavy Exercise or Exertion: Use caution. May stress protective effects of this drug.

SELEGILINE (se LEDGE i leen)

Other Name: Deprenyl
Introduced: 1981 **Prescription:** USA: Yes **Available as Generic:** USA: No **Class:** Antiparkinsonism, monoamine oxidase (MAO) type B inhibitor **Controlled Drug:** USA: No
Brand Name: Eldepryl

BENEFITS versus RISKS

Possible Benefits
EFFECTIVE INITIAL TREATMENT OF PARKINSON'S DISEASE when started at the onset of symptoms
ADDITIVE RELIEF OF SYMPTOMS OF PARKINSON'S DISEASE when used concurrently with levodopa/carbidopa (Sinemet)
PERMITS UP TO 30% REDUCTION IN SINEMET DOSAGE

Possible Risks
ABNORMAL INVOLUNTARY MOVEMENTS (12%)
HALLUCINATIONS (5.4%)
INITIAL FALL IN BLOOD PRESSURE/ORTHOSTATIC HYPOTENSION (1.8%)

▷ **Principal Uses**

As a Single Drug Product: Uses currently included in FDA approved labeling: (1) Used to start drug treatment of very early Parkinson's disease (soon after onset of symptoms), thus delaying the use of levodopa/carbidopa. It is also used as an adjunct to levodopa/carbidopa treatment of Parkinson's disease for those individuals who experience intolerable abnormal movements (dyskinesia) and/or increasing "on-off" episodes due to loss of effectiveness of levodopa. The addition of selegiline (1) permits reduction of the daily dose of levodopa (by 25% to 30%) with consequent lessening of dyskinesia and erratic drug response, and (2) provides additional relief of parkinsonian symptoms.

Other (unlabeled) generally accepted uses: (1) Some improvement in Alzheimer's disease in patients treated with this drug.

How This Drug Works: By (1) inhibiting monoamine oxidase type B, the enzyme that inactivates dopamine in the brain, and by (2) slowing the restorage of released dopamine at nerve terminals, this drug helps to correct the deficiency of dopamine that is responsible for the rigidity, tremor and sluggish movement characteristic of Parkinson's disease.

Available Dosage Forms and Strengths
Tablets — 5 mg

▷ **Usual Adult Dosage Range**

5 mg once or twice daily. The usual maintenance dose is 5 mg after breakfast and 5 mg after lunch. A total daily dose of 10 mg is adequate to achieve

Selegiline

optimal benefit from this drug. Higher doses do not result in further improvement and are not advised.

During the gradual introduction of selegiline, the concurrent dose of levodopa/carbidopa (Sinemet) may be cautiously decreased in accord with your physician's instructions. Concurrent Sinemet dosage should be reduced by 10% to 20% when selegiline is started. **Note: Actual dosage and administration schedule must be determined by the physician for each patient individually.**

Conditions Requiring Dosing Adjustments

Liver function: This drug is extensively metabolized in the liver. Patients with liver compromise should be followed closely.

Kidney function: The kidney does not have a major role in the elimination of this medication. It can cause prostatic hypertrophy, and should be used with caution in patients with urine outflow problems.

▷ **Dosing Instructions:** The tablet may be crushed and taken with food or milk to reduce stomach irritation.

Usual Duration of Use: Use on a regular schedule for 4 to 6 weeks usually determines effectiveness in controlling the symptoms of Parkinson's disease and permitting reduction of levodopa/carbidopa dosage. Long-term use (months to years) requires periodic physician evaluation of response and dosage adjustment.

Possible Advantages of This Drug

It may provide a more effective and uniform control of parkinsonian symptoms and a significant reduction of some adverse effects associated with long-term levodopa therapy. Fifty to 60% of users show improvement.

It does not lose its effectiveness with long-term use.

It does not require avoidance of foods containing tyramine, as is necessary with monoamine oxidase (MAO) type A inhibitors.

It causes no life-threatening or irreversible adverse effects.

▷ **This Drug Should Not Be Taken If**
- you have had an allergic reaction to it previously.
- you have Huntington's disease, hereditary (essential) tremor or tardive dyskinesia (see Glossary).
- you are pregnant or breast-feeding.
- you take meperidine (Demerol).

▷ **Inform Your Physician Before Taking This Drug If**
- you have constitutionally low blood pressure.
- you have peptic ulcer disease.
- you have a history of heart rhythm disorder.
- you are taking any antihypertensive drugs or antipsychotic drugs (see Drug Classes).

Possible Side-Effects (natural, expected and unavoidable drug actions)

Weakness (0.3%), orthostatic hypotension (see Glossary) (1.8%), dry mouth (2%), insomnia (1.5%).

▷ **Possible Adverse Effects** (unusual, unexpected and infrequent reactions)

If any of the following develop, consult your physician promptly for guidance.

Mild Adverse Effects
    Headache (2%), dizziness (2.2%), blurred vision (rare), agitation (2.5%).
    Palpitations (0.2%), fainting (0.1%).
    Altered taste (0.1%), nausea and vomiting (7%), stomach pain (4%).
    Sleep disorders.

Serious Adverse Effects
    Dyskinesias: abnormal involuntary movements (12%).
    Confusion and hallucinations (5.4%), depression (0.4%), psychosis (0.2%), vivid dreams (2%).
    Aggravation of peptic ulcer (0.2%), gastrointestinal bleeding (0.2%).
    Growth of the prostate (rare).

▷ **Possible Effects on Sexual Function:** Transient decreases in penile sensation and anorgasmia have rarely been reported if doses exceed 10 mg per day. Increased libido may occur.

▷ **Adverse Effects That May Mimic Natural Diseases or Disorders**
    Effects on mental function and behavior may resemble psychotic disorders.

▷ **Natural Diseases or Disorders That May Be Activated by This Drug**
    Peptic ulcer disease.

Possible Effects on Laboratory Tests
    None reported.

CAUTION
1. This drug can initiate dyskinesias and can intensify existing dyskinesias. Watch carefully for the development of tremors, twitching or abnormal, involuntary movements of any kind. Report these promptly.
2. This drug potentiates the effects of levodopa. When this drug is added to current levodopa treatment, adverse effects of levodopa may develop or be intensified. The dose of levodopa must be reduced by 10% to 20% when treatment with selegiline begins.
3. Tell your doctor promptly if you become pregnant or plan pregnancy. The manufacturer does not recommend the use of this drug during pregnancy.

Precautions for Use
  By Infants and Children: This drug is not utilized by this age group.
  By Those over 60 Years of Age: This drug is well tolerated by the elderly. Observe closely for any tendency to light-headedness or faintness, especially on arising from a lying or sitting position.

▷ **Advisability of Use During Pregnancy**
  Pregnancy Category: C. See Pregnancy Code at the back of this book.
  Animal studies: No birth defects due to this drug were found in rat studies.
  Human studies: Adequate studies of pregnant women are not available. The manufacturer advises that this drug should not be taken during pregnancy.

Advisability of Use if Breast-Feeding
  Presence of this drug in breast milk: Unknown.
  Avoid drug or refrain from nursing.

Habit-Forming Potential: None.

Selegiline

Effects of Overdosage: Nausea, vomiting, palpitations, low blood pressure, agitation, severe involuntary movements, hallucinations.

Possible Effects of Long-Term Use: None reported.

Suggested Periodic Examinations While Taking This Drug (at physician's discretion)

Regular evaluation of drug response, heart function and blood pressure status.

▷ **While Taking This Drug, Observe the Following**

Foods: Caution should be used regarding tyramine containing foods, although the reaction with this drug may not be as severe as that seen with other MAO inhibitors.

Beverages: No restrictions. May be taken with milk.

▷ *Alcohol:* Use caution until the combined effects have been determined. Alcohol may exaggerate the blood-pressure-lowering and sedative effects of this drug.

Tobacco Smoking: No interactions expected.

▷ *Other Drugs*

Selegiline *taken concurrently* with
- amphetamine (dexedrine) can cause a severe increase in blood pressure.
- antidepressants such as amitriptyline (Elavil) may cause neurotoxic reactions such as seizures.
- antihypertensive drugs (and other drugs that can lower blood pressure) requires careful monitoring for excessive drops in pressure. Dosage adjustments may be necessary.
- fluoxetine (Prozac) may cause serotonin toxicity syndrome.
- lithium may increase risk of the serotonin toxicity syndrome.
- meperidine (Demerol) may cause a life-threatening reaction of unknown cause; avoid this combination.
- oral hypoglycemic agents (see Drug Classes) may cause very low blood sugars.
- tryptophan may cause a fatal serotonin syndrome.

The following drugs may *decrease* the effects of selegiline and diminish its effectiveness
- chlorprothixene (Taractan).
- haloperidol (Haldol).
- metoclopramide (Reglan).
- phenothiazines (see Drug Classes).
- reserpine (Ser-Ap-Es, etc.), in high doses.
- thiothixene (Navane).

▷ *Driving, Hazardous Activities:* This drug may cause dizziness, drowsiness, impaired coordination or fainting. Restrict activities as necessary.

Aviation Note: The use of this drug *is a disqualification* for piloting. Consult a designated Aviation Medical Examiner.

Exposure to Sun: No restrictions.

Exposure to Heat: Use caution until the combined effects have been determined. Hot environments can cause lowering of blood pressure.

Discontinuation: Do not stop this drug abruptly. Sudden withdrawal can cause prompt increase in parkinsonian symptoms and deterioration of control. Consult your physician regarding a schedule for gradual withdrawal and concurrent adjustment of Sinemet or other appropriate drugs.

SERTRALINE (SER tra leen)

Introduced: 1986 **Prescription:** USA: Yes **Available as Generic:** USA: No **Class:** Antidepressant **Controlled Drug:** USA: No
Brand Name: Zoloft

BENEFITS versus RISKS	
Possible Benefits	*Possible Risks*
EFFECTIVE TREATMENT OF MAJOR DEPRESSIVE DISORDERS	Frequent confusion
	Male sexual dysfunction (16%)
Possibly effective in relieving the symptoms of obsessive-compulsive disorder	Conversion of depression to mania in manic-depressive disorders (0.4%)
	Rare chest pain and heart attack
	Seizures (less than 0.1%)

▷ **Principal Uses**
  As a Single Drug Product: Uses currently included in FDA approved labeling: (1) Treats major forms of depression that have not responded well to other therapies. This drug should be used only when a diagnosis of a true, primary depression of significant degree has been established.
  Other (unlabeled) generally accepted uses: (1) May have a role in treating obesity. Rat studies have shown a decrease in eating that depends on the dose that is taken. Studies in humans are being conducted; (2) treatment of obsessive-compulsive disorder.
  How This Drug Works: This drug relieves depression by slowly restoring to normal levels a specific constituent of brain tissue (serotonin) that transmits nerve impulses.

Available Dosage Forms and Strengths
  Tablets — 50 mg, 100 mg

▷ **Recommended Dosage Ranges** (Actual dosage and administration schedule must be determined by the physician for each patient individually.)
  Infants and Children: Dosage not established.
  12 to 60 Years of Age: Initially 50 mg once daily, taken in the morning or evening. Increase dose gradually, as needed and tolerated, in increments of 50 mg at intervals of 1 week. The total daily dosage should not exceed 200 mg.
  Over 60 Years of Age: Same as 12 to 60 years of age. Adjust dosage as appropriate for impaired liver or kidney function.

Conditions Requiring Dosing Adjustments
  Liver function: This drug is a rare cause of liver damage. Patients should be followed closely.
  Kidney function: The role of the kidneys in the elimination of this drug is unknown.

▷ **Dosing Instructions:** The tablet may be crushed and is best taken with food to enhance absorption, but may be taken at any time with or without food.
  Usual Duration of Use: Use on a regular schedule for 4 to 8 weeks usually determines (1) this drug's effectiveness in relieving depression; (2) the pattern of both favorable and unfavorable drug effects. Long-term use

(months to years) requires periodic physician evaluation of response and dosage adjustment.

Possible Advantages of This Drug
Does not cause weight gain, a common side-effect of tricyclic antidepressants.
Less likely to cause dry mouth, constipation, urinary retention, orthostatic hypotension (see Glossary) and heart rhythm disturbances than tricyclic antidepressants.
Does not cause Parkinson-like reactions.

▷ **This Drug Should Not Be Taken If**
- you have had an allergic reaction to it previously.
- you are currently taking or have taken within the past 14 days any monoamine oxidase (MAO) type A inhibitor drug (see Drug Classes Section).

▷ **Inform Your Physician Before Taking This Drug If**
- you have experienced any adverse effects from antidepressant drugs.
- you have impaired liver or kidney function.
- you have Parkinson's disease.
- you have had a recent heart attack.
- you have a seizure disorder.
- you are pregnant or plan pregnancy while taking this drug.

Possible Side-Effects (natural, expected and unavoidable drug actions)
Decreased appetite (2.8%), weight loss (average 1 to 2 pounds).

▷ **Possible Adverse Effects** (unusual, unexpected and infrequent reactions)
If any of the following develop, consult your physician promptly for guidance.

Mild Adverse Effects
Allergic Reactions: Skin rash (2%), itching.
Headache (20%), nervousness (3%), insomnia (16%), drowsiness (13%), fatigue (10%), tremor (10%), dizziness (11%), impaired concentration (1.3%), abnormal vision (4%), numbness and tingling (2%), confusion (1%), hallucinations (rare).
Chest pain and increased blood pressure (rare).
Paresthesias (rare).
Dry mouth (16%), altered taste (1.2%), indigestion (6%), nausea (26%), vomiting (3.8%), diarrhea (17%), tongue ulceration (rare).

Serious Adverse Effects
Allergic Reactions: Dermatitis (various forms, rare).
Drug-induced seizures (less than 0.1%).
Hemorrhage into the anterior chamber of the eye.
Low blood sugar.
Bronchospasm (occasional).

▷ **Possible Effects on Sexual Function:** Male sexual dysfunction: delayed ejaculation (15.5%); female sexual dysfunction: inhibited orgasm (1.7%).
Swelling and tenderness of male and female breast tissue.

Natural Diseases or Disorders That May Be Activated by This Drug
Latent epilepsy.

Possible Effects on Laboratory Tests
Blood total cholesterol and triglyceride levels: increased.

Blood uric acid levels: decreased.
Liver function tests: increased liver enzymes (ALT/GPT, AST/GOT and alkaline phosphatase).

CAUTION
1. If any type of skin reaction develops (rash, hives, etc.), discontinue this drug and inform your physician promptly.
2. If dryness of the mouth develops and persists for more than 2 weeks, consult your dentist for guidance.
3. Ask your doctor or pharmacist before taking any other prescription or over-the-counter drug while taking this drug.
4. If you are advised to take any monoamine oxidase (MAO) type A inhibitor drug (see Drug Classes), allow an interval of 5 weeks after discontinuing this drug before starting the MAO inhibitor.
5. It is advisable to withhold this drug if electroconvulsive therapy (ECT, "shock" treatment) is to be used to treat your depression.

Precautions for Use
By Infants and Children: Safety and effectiveness for those under 12 years of age not established.
By Those over 60 Years of Age: The lowest effective dose should be used for maintenance treatment and adjusted as needed for reduced kidney function.

▷ **Advisability of Use During Pregnancy**
Pregnancy Category: B. See Pregnancy Code at the back of this book.
Animal studies: Delayed bone development due to this drug found in rat and rabbit studies.
Human studies: Adequate studies of pregnant women are not available.
Use this drug only if clearly needed. Ask your physician for guidance.

Advisability of Use if Breast-Feeding
Presence of this drug in breast milk: Unknown.
Avoid drug or refrain from nursing.

Habit-Forming Potential: None.

Effects of Overdosage: Agitation, restlessness, excitement, nausea, vomiting, seizures.

Possible Effects of Long-Term Use: None reported.

Suggested Periodic Examinations While Taking This Drug (at physician's discretion)
None.

▷ **While Taking This Drug, Observe the Following**
Foods: May increase peak blood level.
Beverages: No restrictions. May be taken with milk.
▷ *Alcohol:* Avoid completely.
Tobacco Smoking: No interactions expected.
▷ *Other Drugs*
Sertraline may *increase* the effects of
- diazepam (Valium).
- tolbutamide (Orinase).
- warfarin (Coumadin) and related oral anticoagulants.

Sertraline *taken concurrently* with
- antidiabetic drugs (insulin, oral hypoglycemics) may increase the risk of hypoglycemic reactions; monitor blood and urine sugar levels carefully.
- monoamine oxidase (MAO) type A inhibitor drugs may cause confusion, agitation, high fever, seizures and dangerous elevations of blood pressure. Avoid the concurrent use of these drugs.

▷ *Driving, Hazardous Activities:* This drug may cause drowsiness, dizziness, impaired judgment and altered vision. Restrict activities as necessary.

Aviation Note: The use of this drug *is a disqualification* for piloting. Consult a designated Aviation Medical Examiner.

Exposure to Sun: Use caution. This drug may (rarely) cause photosensitivity (see Glossary).

Discontinuation: The slow elimination of this drug from the body makes it unlikely that any withdrawal effects will result from abrupt discontinuation. However, call your doctor if you plan to stop this drug for any reason.

SIMVASTATIN (sim vah STA tin)

Introduced: 1986 **Prescription:** USA: Yes; Canada: Yes **Available as Generic:** USA: No; Canada: No **Class:** Cholesterol reducer **Controlled Drug:** USA: No; Canada: No
Brand Name: Zocor

BENEFITS versus RISKS	
Possible Benefits	*Possible Risks*
EFFECTIVE REDUCTION OF TOTAL BLOOD CHOLESTEROL AND LDL CHOLESTEROL in selected individuals	Drug-induced hepatitis (without jaundice) 1.0% Drug-induced myositis (muscle inflammation) rare

▷ **Principal Uses**

As a Single Drug Product: Uses currently included in FDA approved labeling: (1) Used in patients with elevated cholesterol to reduce death from heart disease (42% in one study) and decrease the number of nonfatal heart attacks; (2) Treatment of abnormally high total blood cholesterol levels (in individuals with Types IIa and IIb hypercholesterolemia) due to increased fractions of low-density lipoprotein (LDL) cholesterol. It is used in conjunction with a cholesterol-lowering diet. It should not be used until an adequate trial of nondrug methods for lowering cholesterol has proved to be ineffective.

Other (unlabeled) generally accepted uses: (1) Stops the progression of clogging arteries (atherosclerotic progression) in people with that disorder; (2) may help reduce lipid disorders that occur in kidney (nephrotic syndrome) problems; (3) can have a role as part of combination therapy in preventing gallstones.

How This Drug Works: This drug blocks the liver enzyme that starts production of cholesterol. It reduces low-density lipoproteins (LDL), the fraction of total blood cholesterol that is thought to increase the risk of coronary heart disease. This drug may also increase the level of high-density lipoproteins (HDL), the cholesterol fraction that reduces the risk of heart disease.

Available Dosage Forms and Strengths
Tablets — 5 mg, 10 mg, 20 mg, 40 mg

▷ **Recommended Dosage Ranges** (Actual dosage and administration schedule must be determined by the physician for each patient individually.)
Infants and Children: Under 2 years of age—do not use this drug.
2 to 20 years of age—dosage not established.
20 to 60 Years of Age: Initially 10 mg daily if LDL cholesterol is over 190 mg/dL, taken at bedtime. Increase dose as needed and tolerated by increments of 5 to 10 mg at intervals of 4 weeks. The total daily dose should not exceed 40 mg.
Over 60 Years of Age:
Initially 5 mg daily. Increase dose as needed and tolerated by increments of 5 mg at intervals of 4 weeks. The total daily dose should not exceed 20 mg.

Conditions Requiring Dosing Adjustments
Liver function: This drug achieves a high concentration in the liver, and is subsequently eliminated in the bile. It can be a rare cause of liver damage, and patients should be followed closely.
Kidney function: In severe kidney failure, the dose should be started at 5 mg, and the patient closely followed.

▷ **Dosing Instructions:** The tablet may be crushed and taken without regard to eating. Preferably taken at bedtime. (The highest rates of cholesterol production occur between midnight and 5 A.M.)

Usual Duration of Use: Use on a regular schedule for 4 to 6 weeks usually determines effectiveness in reducing blood levels of total and LDL cholesterol. Long-term use (months to years) requires periodic physician evaluation of response and dosage adjustment. Consult your physician on a regular basis.

Possible Advantages of This Drug: Recent studies indicate that drugs of this class (HMG-CoA reductase inhibitors) are more effective and better tolerated than other drugs currently available for reducing total and LDL cholesterol. Its long-term effects are yet to be determined.

▷ **This Drug Should Not Be Taken If**
- you have had an allergic reaction to it previously.
- you have active liver disease.
- you are pregnant or breast-feeding.

▷ **Inform Your Physician Before Taking This Drug If**
- you have previously taken any other drugs in this class: lovastatin (Mevacor), pravastatin (Pravachol).
- you have a history of liver disease or impaired liver function.
- you are not using any method of birth control, or you are planning pregnancy.
- you regularly consume substantial amounts of alcohol.
- you have cataracts or impaired vision.
- you have any type of chronic muscular disorder.
- you plan to have major surgery in the near future.

912 Simvastatin

Possible Side-Effects (natural, expected and unavoidable drug actions)
Development of abnormal liver function tests without associated symptoms.

▷ **Possible Adverse Effects** (unusual, unexpected and infrequent reactions)
If any of the following develop, consult your physician promptly for guidance.

Mild Adverse Effects
Headache (3.5%).
Indigestion (1.1%), nausea (1.3%), excessive gas (1.9%), constipation (2.3%), diarrhea (1.9%).
Lowering of the blood pressure.
Insomnia (occasional).

Serious Adverse Effects
Marked and persistent abnormal liver function tests with focal hepatitis (without jaundice) occurred in 1.0%.
Acute myositis (muscle pain and tenderness) occurred rarely during long-term use.
Lichen planus skin rash (rare).

▷ **Possible Effects on Sexual Function:** None reported.

Possible Delayed Adverse Effects: None reported to date.

Natural Diseases or Disorders That May Be Activated by This Drug
Latent liver disease.

Possible Effects on Laboratory Tests
Blood alanine aminotransferase (ALT) enzyme level: increased (with higher doses of drug).
Blood total cholesterol, LDL cholesterol and triglyceride levels: decreased.
Blood HDL cholesterol level: increased.

CAUTION
1. If pregnancy occurs while taking this drug, stop it immediately and consult your physician.
2. Report promptly any development of muscle pain or tenderness, especially if accompanied by fever or weakness (malaise).
3. Report promptly the development of altered or impaired vision so that appropriate evaluation can be made.

Precautions for Use
By Infants and Children: Safety and effectiveness for those under 20 years of age not established.
By Those over 60 Years of Age: Inform your physician regarding any personal or family history of cataracts. Comply with all recommendations regarding periodic eye examinations. Report promptly any alterations in vision.

▷ **Advisability of Use During Pregnancy**
Pregnancy Category: X. See Pregnancy Code at the back of this book.
Animal studies: Mouse and rat studies reveal skeletal birth defects due to a closely related drug of this class.
Human studies: Adequate studies of pregnant women are not available.
This drug should be avoided during entire pregnancy.

Advisability of Use if Breast-Feeding
Presence of this drug in breast milk: Unknown.
Avoid drug or refrain from nursing.

Habit-Forming Potential: None.

Effects of Overdosage: Increased indigestion, stomach distress, nausea, diarrhea.

Possible Effects of Long-Term Use: Abnormal liver function with focal hepatitis.

Suggested Periodic Examinations While Taking This Drug (at physician's discretion)
Blood cholesterol studies: total cholesterol, HDL and LDL fractions.
Liver function tests before treatment, every 6 weeks during the first 3 months of use, every 8 weeks for the rest of the first year, and at 6-month intervals thereafter.
Complete eye examination at beginning of treatment and at any time that significant change in vision occurs. Ask your physician for guidance.

▷ **While Taking This Drug, Observe the Following**
Foods: Follow a standard low-cholesterol diet.
Beverages: No restrictions. May be taken with milk.
▷ *Alcohol:* No interactions expected. Use sparingly.
Tobacco Smoking: No interactions expected.
▷ *Other Drugs*
Simvastatin may *increase* the effects of
- digoxin (Lanoxin).
- warfarin (Coumadin); monitor INR (prothrombin times).

Simvastatin *taken concurrently* with
- clofibrate or other fibrate compounds may result in increased risk of serious muscle toxicity.
- gemfibrozil (Lopid) may alter the absorption and excretion of simvastatin; these drugs should not be taken concurrently.
- cyclosporine (Sandimmune) can result in kidney failure and myopathy.

The following drug may *decrease* the effects of simvastatin
- cholestyramine (Questran), may reduce absorption of simvastatin; take simvastatin 1 hour before or 4 hours after cholestyramine.

▷ *Driving, Hazardous Activities:* No restrictions.
Aviation Note: No restrictions.
Exposure to Sun: No restrictions.
Discontinuation: Do not stop this drug without your physician's knowledge and guidance. There may be significant increase in blood cholesterol levels following discontinuation of this drug.

SPIRONOLACTONE (speer on oh LAK tohn)

Introduced: 1959 **Prescription:** USA: Yes; Canada: Yes **Available as Generic:** USA: Yes **Class:** Diuretic **Controlled Drug:** USA: No; Canada: No

Brand Names: Alatone, Aldactazide [CD], Aldactone, ✦Apo-Spirozide, ✦Novospiroton, ✦Novospirozine [CD], ✦Sincomen, Spironazide

Spironolactone

BENEFITS versus RISKS

Possible Benefits	*Possible Risks*
EFFECTIVE PREVENTION OF POTASSIUM LOSS when used adjunctively with other diuretics	ABNORMALLY HIGH BLOOD POTASSIUM LEVEL with excessive use
EFFECTIVE DIURETIC IN REFRACTORY CASES OF FLUID RETENTION when used adjunctively with other diuretics	Enlargement of male breast tissue Masculinization effects in women: excessive hair growth, deepening of the voice
	Rare hepatitis

▷ **Principal Uses**

As a Single Drug Product: Uses currently included in FDA approved labeling: (1) Used to manage congestive heart failure and disorders of the liver and kidney that are accompanied by excessive fluid retention (edema); (2) it is also used in conjunction with other measures to treat high blood pressure. It is used primarily in situations where it is advisable to prevent loss of potassium from the body; (3) used to decrease fluid in patients who have failed glucocorticoid treatment and have nephrotic syndrome.

Other (unlabeled) generally accepted uses: (1) May have an adjunctive role in treating acne; (2) can help treat lung problems (bronchopulmonary dysplasia) and slow the disease process; (3) can help precocious puberty in females; (4) eases fluid buildup in premenstrual syndrome.

As a Combination Drug Product [CD]: This drug is available in combination with hydrochlorothiazide, a different kind of diuretic that promotes the loss of potassium from the body. Spironolactone is used in this combination to counteract the potassium-wasting effect of the thiazide diuretic.

How This Drug Works: By inhibiting the action of aldosterone (an adrenal gland hormone), this drug prevents the reabsorption of sodium and the excretion of potassium by the kidney. Thus the drug promotes the excretion of sodium (and water with it) and the retention of potassium.

Available Dosage Forms and Strengths
Tablets — 25 mg, 50 mg, 100 mg

▷ **Usual Adult Dosage Range:** Initially, 25 to 100 mg/day for 5 days. The dose is then adjusted according to individual response. The usual maintenance dose is 50 to 200 mg/day, divided into 2 to 4 doses. The total daily dosage should not exceed 400 mg. **Note: Actual dosage and administration schedule must be determined by the physician for each patient individually.**

Conditions Requiring Dosing Adjustments

Liver function: This drug can be a rare cause of liver damage, and patients should be followed closely.

Kidney function: In patients with mild kidney failure, the drug can be given every 12 hours in the usual dose. In moderate kidney failure, spironolactone can be given every 12 to 24 hours in the usual dose. In severe kidney failure, this drug should **not** be given. Spironolactone is contraindicated in acute renal failure and in severe chronic renal compromise.

▷ **Dosing Instructions:** The tablet may be crushed and taken with or following meals to promote absorption of the drug and to reduce stomach irritation.

Usual Duration of Use: Use on a regular schedule for 5 to 10 days usually determines effectiveness in clearing edema, and for 2 to 3 weeks to determine its effect on hypertension. Long-term use (months to years) requires physician supervision and periodic evaluation.

▷ **This Drug Should Not Be Taken If**
- you have had an allergic reaction to it previously.
- you have severely impaired liver or kidney function.
- your creatinine is greater than 2.5 mg/dl.

▷ **Inform Your Physician Before Taking This Drug If**
- you have a history of liver or kidney disease.
- you have diabetes.
- you take: an anticoagulant, antihypertensives, a digitalis preparation, another diuretic, lithium or a potassium preparation.
- you plan to have surgery under general anesthesia in the near future.

Possible Side-Effects (natural, expected and unavoidable drug actions)
Abnormally high blood potassium levels (42%), abnormally low blood sodium levels (12%), dehydration (17%).

▷ **Possible Adverse Effects** (unusual, unexpected and infrequent reactions)
If any of the following develop, consult your physician promptly for guidance.

Mild Adverse Effects

Allergic Reactions: Skin rash, hives, itching, drug fever (see Glossary).

Headache, dizziness, unsteadiness, weakness, drowsiness, lethargy, confusion.

Dry mouth, nausea, vomiting, diarrhea.

Serious Adverse Effects

Allergic Reaction: Abnormally low blood platelet count (rare).

Symptomatic potassium excess: confusion, numbness and tingling in lips and extremities, fatigue, weakness, shortness of breath, slow heart rate, low blood pressure.

Masculine pattern of hair growth and deepening of the voice in women.

Stomach ulceration with bleeding (rare).

Possible association with decreased white blood cell counts.

Disruption in the acid base balance of the body (hyperchloremic metabolic acidosis.

Hepatitis (rare).

Systemic lupus erythematosus like syndrome (rare).

Thinning of the bones (rare).

▷ **Possible Effects on Sexual Function**

Decreased libido (close to 100%); impaired erection or impotence (30%).

Male breast enlargement and tenderness (close to 100% with high doses).

Female breast enlargement (100% with high doses); altered timing and pattern of menstruation; postmenopausal bleeding.

Decreased vaginal secretion.

Possible Effects on Laboratory Tests

White blood cell count: decreased (one report only).

Blood platelet count: decreased.

Prothrombin time: decreased.

Blood potassium level: increased.
Blood uric acid level: no effect in some; increased and decreased in others.

CAUTION
1. Do not take potassium supplements or increase your intake of potassium-rich foods while taking this drug.
2. Do not stop this drug abruptly unless abnormally high blood levels of potassium develop.
3. Ordinary doses of aspirin (600 mg) may reverse the diuretic effect of this drug. Observe response to this drug combination.
4. Avoid the excessive use of salt substitutes that contain potassium; these are a potential cause of potassium excess.

Precautions for Use
By Infants and Children: Limit the continual use of this drug in children to 1 month. Observe closely for indications of potassium accumulation.

By Those over 60 Years of Age: The natural decline in kidney function may predispose to potassium retention in the body. Watch for indications of potassium excess: slow heart rate, irregular heart rhythms, low blood pressure, confusion, drowsiness. The excessive use of diuretics can cause harmful loss of body water (dehydration), increased viscosity of the blood and an increased tendency of the blood to clot, predisposing to stroke, heart attack or thrombophlebitis.

▷ **Advisability of Use During Pregnancy**
Pregnancy Category: B. See Pregnancy Code at the back of this book.
Animal studies: This drug causes feminization of male rat fetuses.
Human studies: Adequate studies of pregnant women are not available.
This drug should not be used during pregnancy unless a very serious complication of pregnancy occurs for which this drug is significantly beneficial.

Advisability of Use if Breast-Feeding
Presence of this drug in breast milk: A metabolic end product (canrenone) is present.
Avoid drug or refrain from nursing.

Habit-Forming Potential: None.

Effects of Overdosage: Thirst, drowsiness, fatigue, weakness, nausea, vomiting, confusion, irregular heart rhythm, low blood pressure.

Possible Effects of Long-Term Use: Potassium accumulation to abnormally high blood levels. Male breast enlargement.

Suggested Periodic Examinations While Taking This Drug (at physician's discretion)
Measurements of blood sodium, potassium and chloride levels.
Kidney function tests.

▷ **While Taking This Drug, Observe the Following**
Foods: No restrictions. Avoid excessive restriction of salt.
Beverages: No restrictions. May be taken with milk.
▷ *Alcohol:* Use with caution. Alcohol may enhance the drowsiness and the blood-pressure-lowering effect of this drug.
Tobacco Smoking: No interactions expected.

▷ *Other Drugs*
Spironolactone may *increase* the effects of
- digoxin (Lanoxin).

Spironolactone may *decrease* the effects of
- anticoagulants (Coumadin, etc.).

Spironolactone *taken concurrently* with
- captopril (Capoten) or other ACE inhibitors (see Drug Classes) may cause excessively high blood potassium levels.
- cyclosporine (Sandimmune) may result in very elevated potassium levels.
- digitoxin (Crystodigin) may cause either increased or decreased digitoxin effects (unpredictable).
- lithium may cause accumulation of lithium to toxic levels.
- potassium preparations may cause excessively high blood potassium levels.

The following drugs may *decrease* the effects of spironolactone
- aspirin or other NSAIDs may reduce its diuretic effectiveness.

▷ *Driving, Hazardous Activities:* This drug may cause dizziness and drowsiness. Restrict activities as necessary.

Aviation Note: The use of this drug *may be a disqualification* for piloting. Consult a designated Aviation Medical Examiner.

Exposure to Sun: No restrictions.

Discontinuation: With high dosage or prolonged use, it is advisable to withdraw this drug gradually. Ask your physician for guidance.

STAVUDINE (STAV you dine)

Other Names: d4T
Introduced: June 1994 **Prescription:** USA: Yes; Canada: Yes **Available as Generic:** USA: No; Canada: No **Class:** Antiretroviral **Controlled Drug:** USA:No
Brand Name: Zerit

BENEFITS versus RISKS	
Possible Benefits	*Possible Risks*
INCREASED CD4 COUNTS IN ADULTS WITH ADVANCED HIV THERAPEUTIC OPTION FOR THOSE INTOLERANT OF AZT OR DIDANOSINE	PERIPHERAL NEUROPATHY Rare pancreatitis (1%)

▷ **Principal Uses**
As a Single Drug Product: Uses currently included in FDA approved labeling: (1) Treatment of advanced HIV in adults who have failed or are intolerant of AZT or didanosine.

Other (unlabeled) generally accepted uses: (1) The drug has been used in a small number of children; (2) approval pending for initial use in HIV positive patients; (3) combination therapy may offer a durable increase in CD4 count and decrease in viral load.

How This Drug Works: This drug inhibits HIV reproduction (replication) by: (1) Inhibiting an HIV enzyme (reverse transcriptase) which blocks the

Stavudine

ability of the virus to make nuclear material; (2) by inhibiting an enzyme (DNA polymerase gamma and beta) which blocks the ability to make DNA in the mitochondria.

Available Dosage Forms and Strengths
Capsules — 15 mg, 20 mg, 30 mg, 40 mg

▷ **Recommended Dosage Ranges (Actual dosage and administration schedule must be determined by the physician for each patient individually.)**
Infants and Children: Safety and efficacy not established.
18 to 60 Years of Age: Patients who weigh 60 kg (132 pounds) or more should be given 40 mg twice daily. Patients who weigh less than 60 kg should be given 30 mg twice daily.
In those who have had to stop this medicine because of peripheral neuropathy (with complete resolution of symptoms):
20 mg twice daily for patients who weigh 60 kg or more.
15 mg twice daily for those who weigh less than 60 kg.
Over 65 Years of Age: This drug has **not** been studied in those over 65.

Conditions Requiring Dosing Adjustments
Liver function: Liver involvement in elimination has not been studied in humans.
Kidney function: Patients with mild kidney compromise (creatinine clearance greater than 50 ml/min) failure may be given the usual weight-adjusted dose for adults. Those with mild to moderate kidney failure (creatinine clearance 26 to 50) should be given one half of the usual weight adjusted dose every 12 hours.
Those with severe kidney compromise (creatining clearance 10 to 25 ml/min) should be given one half the usual weight-adjusted dose every 24 hours.

▷ **Dosing Instructions:** This drug may be taken without regard to food.

Usual Duration of Use: Use on a regular schedule for several months usually determines effectiveness in slowing AIDS progression and increasing CD4 counts. Long-term use (months to years) requires periodic physician evaluation of response and dosage adjustment. The response as measured by increased CD4 count and decreased viral burden has been durable over several years in many patients.

Possible Advantages of This Drug
More favorable side-effect profile than other nucleoside analogs.
Increased CD4 count over time (may not be sustained).
Favorable profile for combination therapy.

▷ **This Drug Should Not Be Taken If**
- you have had an allergic reaction to any dosage form of it previously.

▷ **Inform Your Physician Before Taking This Drug If**
- you have had peripheral neuropathy caused by other drugs before.
- you have kidney or liver compromise.
- you have had pancreatitis.
- you have viatmin B12 deficiency or folic acid deficiency.
- you are uncertain of how much stavudine to take or how often to take it.

▷ **Possible Adverse Effects** (unusual, unexpected and infrequent reactions)
If any of the following develop, consult your physician promptly for guidance.

Mild Adverse Effects
   Allergic Reactions: Skin rash.
   Nausea and vomiting (4%).
   Abdominal pain (4%).
Serious Adverse Effects
   Allergic Reactions: Anaphylactoid rections (rare).
   Peripheral neuropathy (15–21%).
   Pancreatitis (1%).
   Liver toxicity (rare).
   Low white blood cell and platelet counts (rare).

▷ **Possible Effects on Sexual Function:** Rare impotence.

Possible Delayed Adverse Effects: Unknown.

▷ **Adverse Effects That May Mimic Natural Diseases or Disorders**
   Increased liver function tests may mimic hepatitis.

Possible Effects on Laboratory Tests
   Liver function tests: increased.
   Amylase: increased.
   Complete blood counts: decreased platelets and white blood cells.

CAUTION
   1. Stavudine has **not** been shown to decrease the risk of giving (transmission) of HIV to others through sexual contact or blood contamination.
   2. Promptly report the development of stomach pain and vomiting; this could indicate pancreatitis.
   3. Report developement of pain, numbness, tingling or burning in the hands or feet as this may be peripheral neuropathy.

Precautions for Use
   By Infants and Children:
   Safety and effectiveness for those under 18 years of age not established.
   By Those over 65 Years of Age: The drug has not been studied in this age group.

▷ **Advisability of Use During Pregnancy**
   Pregnancy Category: C. See Pregnancy Code at the back of this book.
      Animal studies: Clinical doses in rats have not revealed teratogenicity, however, doses of 399 times those used in humans have resulted in skeletal problems. Increased early rat death has also occurred at 399 times the human dose.
      Human studies: Adequate studies of pregnant women are not available.
      Ask your doctor for guidance.

Advisability of Use if Breast-Feeding
   Presence of this drug in breast milk: Yes.
   Refrain from nursing if you are taking this drug.

Habit-Forming Potential: None.

Effects of Overdosage: Adults treated with 12 to 24 times the recommended daily dose revealed no acute toxicity.

Possible Effects of Long-Term Use: Peripheral neuropathy and hepatic toxicity.

Suggested Periodic Examinations While Taking This Drug (at physician's discretion)
   Liver function tests, amylase and complete blood counts.
   CD4 or viral load measurement.

▷ **While Taking This Drug, Observe the Following**
  Foods: No restrictions.
  Beverages: No restrictions.
▷ *Alcohol:* No interactions expected.
  Tobacco Smoking: No interactions expected.
▷ *Other Drugs*
  Stavudine may *increase* the effects of
  • didanosine (Videx) at specific drug concentration ratios.
  • zidovudine (AZT) at specific drug concentration ratios.
  Stavudine may *decrease* the effects of
  • didanosine (Videx) at specific drug concentration ratios.
  • zidovudine (AZT) at specific drug concentration ratios (may only be a phosphorylated intermediate and not of clinical significance).
▷ *Driving, Hazardous Activities:* This drug may cause dizziness. Restrict activities as necessary.
  Aviation Note: The use of this drug **may be a disqualification** for piloting. Consult a designated Aviation Medical Examiner.
  Exposure to Sun: No restrictions.
  Discontinuation: Do not stop this drug without your doctor's knowledge and guidance.

STRONTIUM-89 (Stron TEE UM)

Introduced: June 1993 **Prescription:** USA: Yes; Canada: Yes **Available as Generic:** USA: No; Canada: No **Class:** Systemic Radionuclide
Controlled Drug: USA: No; Canada: No
Brand Names: Metastron

BENEFITS versus RISKS	
Possible Benefits	*Possible Risks*
EFFECTIVE RELIEF OF PRIMARY OR METASTATIC BONE CANCER PAIN	BONE MARROW TOXICITY (decreased white blood cells and platelets)
	Transient increase in bone pain

▷ **Principal Uses**
  As a Single Drug Product: Uses currently included in FDA approved labeling:
    (1) Used to treat primary or metastatic bone cancer pain.
  Other (unlabeled) generally accepted uses: None at present.
How This Drug Works: This radiopharmaceutical is selectively taken up by areas of bone cancer. Once it accumulates in cancerous areas, it emits radiation directly at the site of the cancer.
Available Dosage Forms and Strengths
  Injection — 10.9 to 22.6 mg of strontium in a total of 1 ml of water.
▷ **Recommended Dosage Ranges (Actual dosage and administration schedule must be determined by the physician for each patient individually.)**
  Infants and Children: Safety and efficacy for those less than 18 years old not established.

18 to 60 Years of Age: A dose of 4 mCi (148 MBq) is given intravenously over 1 to 2 minutes. The dose may also be calculated using 40 to 60 mcCI/kg. The dose may be repeated at 90 day intervals, if needed.

Over 60 Years of Age: Same as 18 to 60 years of age.

Conditions Requiring Dosing Adjustments

Liver function: Dosing changes in liver compromise do not appear to be needed.

Kidney function: This agent is primarily removed by the kidneys, however, decreases in doses are not presently defined.

▷ **Dosing Instructions:** You may eat and drink as you normally would. During the first week after injection, Strontium-89 will be present in the blood and the urine. A normal toilet should be used in preference to a urinal.

Usual Duration of Use: Use of previously prescribed pain medicine will be expected for 7 to 20 days after the injection. A maximum of 20 days after injection has been needed to determine peak effectiveness in controlling bone cancer pain. The dose may be repeated (if blood tests are acceptable) 90 days after the prior dose was given. Consult your physician on a regular basis.

Possible Advantages of This Drug

Effective control of bone cancer pain without the risks or compromise of narcotics.

▷ **This Drug Should Not Be Taken If**
- you have had an allergic reaction to any dosage form of it previously.
- you have cancer which does **not** involve the bone.

▷ **Inform Your Physician Before Taking This Drug If**
- you have a history of low platelets or white blood cell counts.
- you take other drugs which may lower white cells or platelets.

Possible Side-Effects (natural, expected and unavoidable drug actions)

May cause a calcium-like flushing when it is injected.

May cause a transient (up to 72 hours) increase in bone pain.

▷ **Possible Adverse Effects** (unusual, unexpected and infrequent reactions)

If any of the following develop, consult your physician promptly for guidance.

Mild Adverse Effects

Allergic Reactions: Chills and fever.

Mild calcium-like flushing on injection.

Transient (up to 72 hours) increase in bone pain.

Serious Adverse Effects

Allergic Reactions: None defined.

Bone marrow toxicity: Low white blood cell counts and low platelets.

Very rare bacterial infection of the blood (septicemia) following drug-induced decreases in white blood cells.

▷ **Possible Effects on Sexual Function:** None reported.

Possible Delayed Adverse Effects: Lowering of white blood cells (recovery in up to six months) and blood platelets (lowest count 12 to 16 weeks after therapy).

Natural Diseases or Disorders That May Be Activated by This Drug

Aplastic anemia.

Strontium-89

Possible Effects on Laboratory Tests
White blood cell counts: decreased.
Platelet counts: decreased.

CAUTION
1. Promptly report any signs of infection (lethargy, temperature, sore throat).
2. It may take up to 20 days for this agent to work. Narcotics will need to be continued.
3. Your blood and urine will contain radioactive Strontium for 7 days after injection. Ask your doctor for help on appropriate disposal.
4. This drug is a potential carcinogen.
5. Promptly report any abnormal bleeding or bruising.

Precautions for Use
By Infants and Children:
Safety and effectiveness for those under 18 years of age not established.
By Those over 60 Years of Age: Specific changes not presently needed.

▷ Advisability of Use During Pregnancy
Pregnancy Category: D. See Pregnancy Code at the back of this book.
Animal studies: Adequate studies evaluating potential to cause birth defects have not been performed.
Human studies: Adequate studies of pregnant women are not available.
This drug may cause fetal harm. Ask your doctor for advice.

Advisability of Use if Breast-Feeding
Presence of this drug in breast milk: This drug acts like calcium and is expected to be present in breast milk.
Avoid drug or refrain from nursing.

Habit-Forming Potential: None.

Effects of Overdosage:
May result in acute radiation syndrome with initial nausea and vomiting followed by depressed white cells, platelets and tendency to infections. Careful dosage calculations are indicated as this drug emits beta radiation.

Possible Effects of Long-Term Use:
Not indicated for long-term use.

Suggested Periodic Examinations While Taking This Drug (at physician's discretion)
Complete blood counts should be tested once every other week during therapy.

▷ While Taking This Drug, Observe the Following
Foods: No restrictions.
Beverages: No restrictions.
▷ *Alcohol:* No interactions expected.
Tobacco Smoking: No interactions expected.
Marijuana Smoking: No interactions expected.
▷ *Other Drugs*
Strontium-89 **taken concurrently** with
- medications which lower white blood cells or platelets may result in severe decreases.

▷ *Driving, Hazardous Activities:* This drug may cause a transient increase in bone pain. Restrict activities as necessary.

Aviation Note: The use of this drug **may be a disqualification** for piloting. Consult a designated Aviation Medical Examiner.
Exposure to Sun: No restrictions.
Discontinuation: Dosing may be repeated if blood counts are acceptable.

SUCRALFATE (soo KRAL fayt)

Introduced: 1978 **Prescription:** USA: Yes; Canada: Yes **Available as Generic:** No **Class:** Antiulcer **Controlled Drug:** USA: No; Canada: No
Brand Names: Carafate, ◆Sulcrate

BENEFITS versus RISKS	
Possible Benefits	*Possible Risks*
EFFECTIVE TREATMENT IN DUODENAL ULCER DISEASE	Constipation
	Skin rash, hives, itching
No serious adverse effects	Rare aluminum toxicity in kidney compromise
No significant drug interactions	

▷ **Principal Uses**

As a Single Drug Product: Uses currently included in FDA approved labeling: (1) Treats and prevents recurrance of duodenal ulcer disease in adults and children. It is effective when used alone, but may be used in with antacids for pain relief.

Other (unlabeled) generally accepted uses: (1) May be useful in treating gastric ulcers in people who can not tolerate other treatment; (2) can reduce the frequency of diarrhea caused by radiation therapy; (3) may have a role as a douche in promoting healing of vaginal ulcerations that are resistant to other measures; (4) can ease the pain and spasms associated with tonsillectomy.

How This Drug Works: This drug promotes ulcer healing in several ways: (1) formation of a protective coating over the ulcer and ulcer margins, preventing further damage; (2) Inhibition of the digestive action of pepsin; (3) the stimulation of active healing (tissue repair).

Available Dosage Forms and Strengths
  Tablets — 0.5 gram and 1 gram
  Suspension — 1 gram per 10 ml

▷ **Usual Adult Dosage Range:** 1 gram 4 times/day. **Note: Actual dosage and administration schedule must be determined by the physician for each patient individually.**

Conditions Requiring Dosing Adjustments
Liver function: Sucralfate is not absorbed.
Kidney function: Sucralfate is not absorbed.

▷ **Ced Dosing Instructions:** Take with water on an empty stomach at least 1 hour before or 2 hours after each meal and at bedtime. Swallow the tablets whole; do not alter or chew. Take the full course prescribed.

Usual Duration of Use: Use on a regular schedule for 6 to 8 weeks is usually needed for peak effect in promoting the healing of ulcers. Use beyond 8 weeks must be determined by your physician.

Sucralfate

▷ **This Drug Should Not Be Taken If**
- you have had an allergic reaction to it previously.

▷ **Inform Your Physician Before Taking This Drug If**
- you have chronic constipation.
- you are taking any other drugs at this time.

Possible Side-Effects (natural, expected and unavoidable drug actions)
Constipation (2.2%).

▷ **Possible Adverse Effects** (unusual, unexpected and infrequent reactions)
If any of the following develop, consult your physician promptly for guidance.

Mild Adverse Effects
Allergic Reactions: Skin rash, hives, itching.
Dizziness, light-headedness, drowsiness.
Dry mouth, indigestion, nausea, cramping, diarrhea.

Serious Adverse Effects
Increased risk of aluminum toxicity (seizures, jerks and encephalopathy) with patients in end stage kidney failure.

▷ **Possible Effects on Sexual Function:** None reported.

Possible Effects on Laboratory Tests
None reported.

CAUTION
1. If antacids are needed to relieve ulcer pain, do not take them within half an hour before or 2 hours after the dose of sucralfate.
2. This drug may impair the absorption of other drugs if they are taken close together. It is advisable to avoid taking any other drugs within 2 hours of taking sucralfate. This applies especially to cimetidine (Tagamet), phenytoin (Dilantin) and tetracyclines.

▷ **Advisability of Use During Pregnancy**
Pregnancy Category: B. See Pregnancy Code at the back of this book.
Animal studies: No birth defects reported in mouse, rat and rabbit studies.
Human studies: Adequate studies of pregnant women are not available.
It should be used only if clearly needed. Ask your physician for guidance.

Advisability of Use if Breast-Feeding
Presence of this drug in breast milk: Unknown.
Watch nursing infant closely and stop drug or nursing if adverse effects develop.

Habit-Forming Potential: None.

Effects of Overdosage: Nausea, stomach cramping, possible diarrhea.

Possible Effects of Long-Term Use: Deficiencies of vitamins A, D, E and K due to impaired absorption from the intestine.

Suggested Periodic Examinations While Taking This Drug (at physician's discretion)
None required.

▷ **While Taking This Drug, Observe the Following**
Foods: No restrictions. Follow diet prescribed by your physician.
Beverages: No restrictions. This drug is preferably taken with water.
▷ *Alcohol:* No interactions with drug expected. However, alcohol is best avoided because of its irritant effect on the stomach.

Tobacco Smoking: Nicotine can delay ulcer healing and reduce the effectiveness of this drug. Avoid all forms of tobacco.
▷ *Other Drugs*
Sucralfate may *decrease* the effects of
- cimetidine (Tagamet).
- ciprofloxacin (Cipro).
- digoxin (Lanoxin).
- enoxacin (Penetrex).
- fleroxacin.
- ketoconazole.
- lomefloxacin (Maxaquin).
- norfloxacin (Noroxin).
- ofloxacin (Floxin).
- phenytoin (Dilantin, etc.).
- quinidine.
- temafloxacin.
- tetracycline (Achromycin, Tetracyn, etc.).
- warfarin (Coumadin, etc.), and reduce its anticoagulant effect.

▷ *Driving, Hazardous Activities:* This drug may cause dizziness or drowsiness. Restrict activities as necessary.
Aviation Note: The use of this drug *may be a disqualification* for piloting. Consult a designated Aviation Medical Examiner.
Exposure to Sun: No restrictions.

SULFADIAZINE (sul fa DI a zeen)

Introduced: 1945 **Prescription:** USA: Yes; Canada: Yes **Available as Generic:** USA: Yes; Canada: No **Class:** Anti-infective, sulfonamide
Controlled Drug: USA: No; Canada: No

Brand Names: ◆Coptin [CD], Microsulfon, ◆Ovoquinol, SSD, Trisem [CD], Trisoralen [CD]

BENEFITS versus RISKS	
Possible Benefits	*Possible Risks*
EFFECTIVE TREATMENT OF INFECTIONS DUE TO SUSCEPTIBLE MICROORGANISMS	BONE MARROW DEPRESSION (see Glossary)
	DRUG-INDUCED HEPATITIS (see Glossary)
Effective treatment of AIDS-related paracoccidioidomycosis	SEVERE ALLERGIC REACTIONS
Effective adjunctive treatment of AIDS-related toxoplasmosis	Drug-induced kidney damage
Effective adjunctive treatment of certain types of malaria	

▷ **Principal Uses**
As a Single Drug Product: Uses currently included in FDA approved labeling: (1) Used alone to treat urinary tract infections.
Other (unlabeled) generally accepted uses: (1) Treats the following infec-

tions: chancroid, inclusion conjunctivitis, meningococcal meningitis, nocardiosis, recurrent rheumatic fever prevention, trachoma; (2) adjunctive use with other anti-infectives to treat certain types of malaria, H. influenzae meningitis, acute otitis media; (3) used with pyrimethamine to treat AIDS-related cerebral toxoplasmosis and pneumocystis carinii pneumonia.

As a Combination Drug Product [CD]: Combined with trimethoprim (Canada) to treat acute, chronic and recurrent urinary tract infections caused by susceptible organisms.

How This Drug Works: This drug prevents the growth and multiplication of susceptible organisms by interfering with their formation of folic acid, an essential element in the synthesis of RNA and DNA.

Available Dosage Forms and Strengths
Tablets — 500 mg
Vaginal Cream

▷ **Recommended Dosage Ranges** (Actual dosage and administration schedule must be determined by the physician for each patient individually.)

Infants and Children: Up to 2 months of age—use not recommended.
2 months of age and over—initially 75 mg/kg of body weight; then 37.5 mg/kg every 6 hours, or 25 mg/kg every 4 hours.
The total daily dose should not exceed 6 grams.

12 to 60 Years of Age: Initially 2 to 4 grams; then 1 gram every 4 to 6 hours. The total daily dose should not exceed 6 grams.
For treatment of AIDS-related cerebral toxoplasmosis—sulfadiazine 4 to 8 grams daily, pyrimethamine 25 to 100 mg daily, and folinic acid 10 to 20 mg daily.

Over 60 Years of Age: Same as 12 to 60 years of age.

Conditions Requiring Dosing Adjustments

Liver function: This drug can be a rare cause of liver damage, and patients should be followed closely. Specific guidelines for adjustment of dosing in liver compromise are not available.

Kidney function: It should be used with caution in renal compromise as it can cause crystalluria.

▷ **Dosing Instructions:** The tablet may be crushed and taken without regard to meals. If necessary, take with or following food to reduce stomach irritation. Take with a full glass of water. Increase liquid intake to ensure urine output of 3 pints daily.

Usual Duration of Use: Use on a regular schedule for 5 to 10 days usually determines effectiveness in controlling responsive infections. When treating AIDS-related infections, it is usually necessary to maintain regular drug therapy for 4 to 6 weeks to evaluate effectiveness. Maintenance long-term treatment is continued indefinitely. This requires periodic evaluation of response and dosage adjustment. Consult your physician on a regular basis.

Possible Advantages of This Drug
This is a short-acting sulfa drug, preferable to long-acting sulfa compounds which have a greater potential for adverse effects.

Currently a "Drug of Choice"
for treating AIDS-related cerebral toxoplasmosis, in combination with pyrimethamine and folinic acid.

▷ **This Drug Should Not Be Taken If**
- you have had an allergic reaction to it or any other sulfa drug.
- you are in the ninth month of pregnancy.
- you have an active blood cell or bone marrow disorder.
- you have active liver disease.

▷ **Inform Your Physician Before Taking This Drug If**
- you are allergic to acetazolamide, furosemide, oral antidiabetic drugs, or thiazide diuretics (see Drug Classes).
- you are allergic by nature: hayfever, asthma, hives or eczema.
- you have a history of drug-induced bone marrow depression.
- you have a history of drug-induced liver damage.
- you have glucose-6-phosphate dehydrogenase (G6PD) deficiency of your red blood cells.
- you have porphyria (see Glossary).
- you have impaired liver or kidney function.
- you are currently taking any other drugs.

Possible Side-Effects (natural, expected and unavoidable drug actions)
Reddish-brown discoloration of urine, of no significance.
Superinfections (see Glossary).

▷ **Possible Adverse Effects** (unusual, unexpected and infrequent reactions)
If any of the following develop, consult your physician promptly for guidance.
Mild Adverse Effects
Allergic Reactions: Skin rashes, hives, itching, swelling of face, redness of eyes, fever.
Headache, dizziness, impaired balance, ringing in ears, numbness and tingling in extremities.
Reduced appetite, mouth irritation, nausea, vomiting, stomach pain, diarrhea.

Serious Adverse Effects
Allergic Reactions: Anaphylactic reaction (see Glossary). Severe skin and joint reactions.
Idiosyncratic Reactions: Hemolytic anemia (see Glossary).
Bone marrow depression (see Glossary): fatigue, weakness, fever, sore throat, abnormal bleeding or bruising.
Encephalopathy (rare).
Drug-induced hepatitis, with or without jaundice (see Glossary): yellow skin and eyes, light-colored stools, dark urine.
Drug-induced kidney damage: painful urination, blood in urine.
Thyroid gland enlargement (goiter); impaired thyroid function.

▷ **Possible Effects on Sexual Function:** None reported.

▷ **Adverse Effects That May Mimic Natural Diseases or Disorders**
Drug-induced hepatitis may suggest viral hepatitis.
Thyroid gland enlargement may suggest unrelated goiter.

Natural Diseases or Disorders That May Be Activated by This Drug
Latent porphyria, hemolytic anemia.

Possible Effects on Laboratory Tests
Complete blood cell counts: decreased red cells, hemoglobin, white cells and platelets.
Liver function tests: increased liver enzymes (ALT/GPT, AST/GOT and alkaline phosphatase), increased bilirubin.
Kidney function tests: red blood cells and protein in urine; increased blood urea nitrogen (BUN) and creatinine.
Urine sugar tests: false positive test results with Benedict's reagent and Clinitest, but not with Clinistix or Tes-Tape.

CAUTION
1. If a skin rash develops, consult your physician immediately.
2. Avoid this drug during the last month of pregnancy.
3. The long-term use of this drug may reduce the effectiveness of oral contraceptives and result in breakthrough bleeding or pregnancy.

Precautions for Use
By Infants and Children: This drug should not be used by those under 2 months of age; it can cause severe jaundice and brain damage in the newborn infant.
By Those over 60 Years of Age: You are at increased risk for serious adverse effects: severe skin reactions, bone marrow depression, significant deficiency of blood platelets with resultant bruising or bleeding. Use this drug cautiously, in small doses and for short periods of time unless you are treating an AIDS-related infection.

▷ **Advisability of Use During Pregnancy**
Pregnancy Category:
B in the first or second three months, D if given near the birth of the baby. See Pregnancy Code at the back of this book.
Animal studies: Mouse and rat studies revealed cleft palates attributed to this drug.
Human studies: Adequate studies of pregnant women are not available.
Use this drug only if clearly needed during the first 8 months of pregnancy. Avoid it completely during the last month of pregnancy. Ask your physician for guidance.

Advisability of Use if Breast-Feeding
Presence of this drug in breast milk: Yes.
Avoid drug or refrain from nursing.

Habit-Forming Potential: None.

Effects of Overdosage: Nausea, vomiting, stomach pain, diarrhea, bloody urine, reduced urine formation.

Possible Effects of Long-Term Use: Bone marrow depression; thyroid gland enlargement, with or without reduced thyroid function; superinfections.

Suggested Periodic Examinations While Taking This Drug (at physician's discretion)
Complete blood cell counts, weekly for the first 8 weeks.
Liver and kidney function tests.

▷ **While Taking This Drug, Observe the Following**
   Foods: No restrictions.
   Nutritional Support: Folinic acid, 10 to 20 mg daily. *After* (not during) treatment with this drug, ask your physician for guidance regarding the need for supplemental vitamin C to correct any deficiency due to therapy.
   Beverages: No restrictions. May be taken with milk. Increase liquid intake to ensure a daily urine volume of 3 pints.
▷ *Alcohol:* Use with caution. Sulfonamide drugs may increase the intoxicating effects of alcohol.
   Tobacco Smoking: No interactions expected.
▷ *Other Drugs*
   Sulfadiazine may *increase* the effects of
   • oral anticoagulants (see Drug Classes). Monitor prothrombin times; adjust dosage as needed to prevent unwanted bleeding.
   • oral antidiabetic drugs (see Drug Classes). Adjust dosage as needed to prevent hypoglycemia (see Glossary).
   • methotrexate.
   • phenytoin (Dilantin, etc.), and cause phenytoin toxicity.
   Sulfadiazine may *decrease* the effects of
   • birth control pills (oral contraceptives).
   • cyclosporine (Sandimmune), and impair its ability to prevent transplant rejection.
   • penicillin. Avoid concurrent use.
   Sulfadiazine *taken concurrently* with
   • isoniazid, may cause hemolytic anemia (see Glossary).
   • methenamine, may cause crystal formation and kidney damage. Avoid concurrent use.
▷ *Driving, Hazardous Activities:* This drug may cause dizziness and impaired balance. Restrict activities as necessary.
   Aviation Note: The use of this drug *may be a disqualification* for piloting. Consult a designated Aviation Medical Examiner.
   Exposure to Sun: Use caution. This drug may cause photosensitivity (see Glossary).
   Discontinuation: Take the full course prescribed. Your physician should determine when to discontinue this drug.

SULFAMETHOXAZOLE (sul fa meth OX a zohl)

Introduced: 1961 **Prescription:** USA: Yes; Canada: Yes **Available as Generic:** Yes **Class:** Anti-infective, sulfonamides **Controlled Drug:** USA: No; Canada: No

Brand Names: ✦Apo-Sulfamethoxazole, ✦Apo-Sulfatrim [CD], ✦Apo-Sulfatrim DS [CD], Azo Gantanol [CD], Bactrim [CD], Bactrim DS [CD], Bethaprim [CD], Comoxol [CD], Cotrim [CD], Gantanol, ✦Novo-Trimel [CD], ✦Novo-Trimel DS [CD], ✦Nu-Cotrimox, ✦Protrin [CD], ✦Protrin DF [CD], ✦Roubac [CD], Septra [CD], Septra DS [CD], Sulfatrim [CD], ✦Uro Gantanol [CD], Uroplus DS [CD], Uroplus SS [CD]

Sulfamethoxazole

BENEFITS versus RISKS	
Possible Benefits	*Possible Risks*
EFFECTIVE ANTIMICROBIAL ACTION against susceptible bacteria and protozoa	Allergic reactions: mild to severe skin reactions, anaphylaxis, myocarditis
Effective adjunctive prevention and treatment of Pneumocystis carinii pneumonia associated with AIDS	Rare blood cell disorders: aplastic anemia, hemolytic anemia, abnormally low white cell and platelet counts
	Low blood sugar
	Drug-induced liver damage
	Drug-induced kidney damage

▷ **Principal Uses**

 As a Single Drug Product: Uses currently included in FDA approved labeling: (1) Used to treat a variety of bacterial and protozoal infections: chancroid, cystitis and other infections of the urinary tract.

 Other (unlabeled) generally accepted uses: (1) Chlamydia infections; (2) combination therapy of resistant Mycobacterium kansaii infections.

 As a Combination Drug Product [CD]: This drug is available in combination with phenazopyridine, an analgesic that relieves discomfort associated with acute urethral infections. This drug is also available in combination with another antibacterial drug—trimethoprim; in some countries this combination is given the generic name co-trimoxazole. This combination is quite effective in the treatment of certain types of middle ear infection, bronchitis, pneumonia and certain infections of the intestinal tract and urinary tract. It is now used as primary prevention and treatment for Pneumocystis carinii pneumonia associated with AIDS.

How This Drug Works: This drug prevents the growth and multiplication of susceptible bacteria by interfering with their formation of folic acid, an essential nutrient.

Available Dosage Forms and Strengths
 Oral suspension — 500 mg per 5-ml teaspoonful
  Tablets — 500 mg, 1 gram

▷ **Usual Adult Dosage Range:** Initially, 2 grams; then 1 gram every 8 to 12 hours, depending upon the severity of the infection. The total daily dosage should not exceed 3 grams. **Note: Actual dosage and administration schedule must be determined by the physician for each patient individually.**

Conditions Requiring Dosing Adjustments
 Liver function: Patients with compromised livers should be followed closely; however, specific guidelines for decreasing doses are not defined.
 Kidney function: The dose should be decreased in patients with compromised kidneys. In moderate failure, 50% of the usual dose can be given at the normal time.

▷ **Dosing Instructions:** The tablet may be crushed and is preferably taken on an empty stomach, 1 hour before or 2 hours after eating. However, it may be taken with or following food to reduce stomach irritation.

Usual Duration of Use: Use on a regular schedule for 4 to 7 days usually determines effectiveness in controlling responsive infections. Treatment should be continued until the patient is free of symptoms for 48 hours. Limit treatment to no more than 14 days if possible.

Currently a "Drug of Choice"
(when combined with trimethoprim) for preventing pneumonia (due to Pneumocystis carinii) in patients with AIDS.

▷ **This Drug Should Not Be Taken If**
- you are allergic to **any** sulfonamide drug (see Drug Classes).
- you are in the last month of pregnancy.
- you are breast-feeding.

▷ **Inform Your Physician Before Taking This Drug If**
- you are allergic to any sulfonamide derivative: acetazolamide, thiazide diuretics, sulfonylurea antidiabetics (see Drug Classes).
- you are allergic by nature: history of hay fever, asthma, hives, eczema.
- you have impaired liver or kidney function.
- you have a personal or family history of porphyria.
- you have had a drug-induced blood cell or bone marrow disorder.
- you have a G6PG deficiency in your red blood cells (ask your doctor).
- you currently take any oral anticoagulant, antidiabetic drug or phenytoin.
- you plan to have surgery under pentothal anesthesia while taking this drug.

Possible Side-Effects (natural, expected and unavoidable drug actions)
Brownish coloration of the urine, of no significance.
Superinfections, bacterial or fungal (see Glossary).

▷ **Possible Adverse Effects** (unusual, unexpected and infrequent reactions)
If any of the following develop, consult your physician promptly for guidance.

Mild Adverse Effects
Allergic Reactions: Skin rashes, hives, itching, localized swellings, reddened eyes.
Myopia (occasional).
Headache, dizziness, unsteadiness, ringing in the ears.
Loss of appetite, irritation of the mouth and tongue, nausea, vomiting, abdominal pain, diarrhea.

Serious Adverse Effects
Allergic Reactions: Drug fever (see Glossary), swollen glands, painful joints, anaphylaxis (see Glossary). Allergic reaction in the heart muscle (myocarditis), allergic pneumonitis, allergic hepatitis. Severe skin reactions.
Idiosyncratic Reaction: Hemolytic anemia (see Glossary).
Bone marrow depression (see Glossary): fatigue, weakness, fever, sore throat, abnormal bleeding or bruising.
Pancreatitis; kidney damage: bloody or cloudy urine, reduced urine volume.
Psychotic reactions, hallucinations, seizures, hearing loss, peripheral neuropathy (see Glossary).
Severe hypoglycemia (rare).
Methemoglibinemia (rare).
Drug-induced lupus erythematosus (rare).
Problems in blood clotting (hypoprothrombinemia) (rare).

Sulfamethoxazole

▷ **Possible Effects on Sexual Function:** None reported.

▷ **Adverse Effects That May Mimic Natural Diseases or Disorders**
Liver reactions may suggest viral hepatitis.
Lung reactions may suggest an infectious pneumonia.

Natural Diseases or Disorders That May Be Activated by This Drug
Goiter, acute intermittent porphyria, polyarteritis nodosa, systemic lupus erythematosus (questionable).

Possible Effects on Laboratory Tests
Complete blood cell counts: decreased red cells, hemoglobin, white cells and platelets; increased eosinophils (allergic reaction).
Prothrombin time: increased (when taken concurrently with warfarin).
Liver function tests: increased liver enzymes (ALT/GPT, AST/GOT and alkaline phosphatase), increased bilirubin.

CAUTION
1. A large intake of water (up to 2 quarts daily) is necessary to ensure an adequate volume of urine.
2. Shake liquid dosage forms thoroughly before measuring each dose.

Precautions for Use
By Infants and Children: This drug should not be used in infants under 2 months of age.
By Those over 60 Years of Age: Small doses taken at longer intervals often achieve adequate blood and tissue drug levels. Observe for the development of reduced urine volume, fever, sore throat, abnormal bleeding or bruising or skin irritation with itching, particularly in the anal or genital regions.

▷ **Advisability of Use During Pregnancy**
Pregnancy Category: C, however, the drug is contraindicated near the time of the birth of the baby. See Pregnancy Code at the back of this book.
Animal studies: Cleft palate and skeletal birth defects reported in mice and rats.
Human studies: No increase in birth defects reported in 4584 exposures to various sulfonamides during pregnancy.
Avoid use of drug during the last month of pregnancy because of possible adverse effects on the newborn infant.

Advisability of Use if Breast-Feeding
Presence of this drug in breast milk: Yes.
Avoid drug or refrain from nursing.

Habit-Forming Potential: None.

Effects of Overdosage: Headache, dizziness, nausea, vomiting, abdominal cramping, toxic fever, coma, jaundice, kidney failure.

Possible Effects of Long-Term Use: Superinfections, bacterial or fungal. Development of goiter, with or without hypothyroidism. Excessive loss of vitamin C via urine.

Suggested Periodic Examinations While Taking This Drug (at physician's discretion)
Complete blood cell counts, weekly for the first 8 weeks.
Urine analysis weekly.
Liver and kidney function tests.

▷ **While Taking This Drug, Observe the Following**
   Foods: No restrictions.
   Beverages: No restrictions. May be taken with milk.
▷ *Alcohol:* Use caution. Sulfonamide drugs can increase the intoxicating effects of alcohol.
   Tobacco Smoking: No interactions expected.
▷ *Other Drugs*
   Sulfamethoxazole may *increase* the effects of
   - amantadine (Symmetrel) and cause abnormal heart rhythms and CNS stimulation (confusion, disorientation).
   - anticoagulants (Coumadin, etc.), and increase the risk of bleeding.
   - methotrexate (Mexate) and cause severe blood toxicity.
   - sulfonylureas (see Drug Classes), and increase the risk of hypoglycemia.
   - warfarin (Coumadin) and result in bleeding.
   - zidovudine (AZT) and result in zidovudine toxicity.
   Sulfamethoxazole may *decrease* the effects of
   - birth control pills (oral contraceptives).
   - cyclosporine (Sandimmune), and reduce its immunosuppressive effect.
   - penicillins.
▷ *Driving, Hazardous Activities:* This drug may cause dizziness. Restrict activities as necessary.
   Aviation Note: The use of this drug ***may be a disqualification*** for piloting. Consult a designated Aviation Medical Examiner.
   Exposure to Sun: Use caution. Some sulfonamide drugs can cause photosensitivity (see Glossary).

SULFASALAZINE (sul fa SAL a zeen)

Introduced: 1949 **Prescription:** USA: Yes; Canada: Yes **Available as Generic:** USA: Yes; Canada: No **Class:** Bowel anti-inflammatory, sulfonamides **Controlled Drug:** USA: No; Canada: No

Brand Names: Azaline, Azulfidine, Azulfidine EN-tabs, ✦PMS Sulfasalazine, ✦PMS Sulfasalazine E.C., ✦Salazopyrin, ✦Salazopyrin EN, ✦SAS-Enema, ✦SAS Enteric-500, SAS-500

BENEFITS versus RISKS	
Possible Benefits	*Possible Risks*
EFFECTIVE SUPPRESSION OF INFLAMMATORY BOWEL DISEASE SYMPTOMATIC RELIEF IN TREATMENT OF REGIONAL ENTERITIS AND ULCERATIVE COLITIS	Allergic reactions: mild to severe skin reactions Rare blood cell disorders: aplastic anemia, hemolytic anemia, abnormally low white cell and platelet counts Drug-induced liver damage Drug-induced kidney damage Rare seizures

▷ **Principal Uses**
   As a Single Drug Product: Uses currently included in FDA approved labeling:
   (1) Treats inflammatory disease of the lower intestinal tract: regional

Sulfasalazine

enteritis (Crohn's disease) and ulcerative colitis. It is usually taken by mouth, but may also be used in retention enemas.

Other (unlabeled) generally accepted uses: (1) Short-term use in therapy of ankylosing spondylitis; (2) treatment of mild to moderate psoriasis; (3) may help juvenile rheumatoid arthritis.

How This Drug Works: Possible method of this drug's action is an anti-inflammatory action that suppresses the formation of prostaglandins (and related compounds), tissue substances that induce inflammation, tissue destruction and diarrhea.

Available Dosage Forms and Strengths
Oral suspension — 250 mg per 5-ml teaspoonful
Tablets — 500 mg
Tablets, enteric-coated — 500 mg

▷ **Usual Adult Dosage Range:** Initially, 1 to 2 grams every 6 to 8 hours until symptoms are adequately controlled. For maintenance, 500 mg/6 hours. The total daily dosage should not exceed 12 grams. **Note: Actual dosage and administration schedule must be determined by the physician for each patient individually.**

Conditions Requiring Dosing Adjustments
Liver function: It can be a cause of liver damage, and patients should be followed closely.
Kidney function: Empiric decreases in doses should be considered. It should be used with caution in kidney compromise.

▷ **Dosing Instructions:** Preferably taken with 8 ounces of water on an empty stomach, 1 hour before or 2 hours after eating. However, it may be taken with or following food to reduce stomach irritation. Intervals between doses (day and night) should be no longer than 8 hours. The regular tablet may be crushed for administration; the enteric-coated tablet should be swallowed whole without alteration.

Usual Duration of Use: Use on a regular schedule for 1 to 3 weeks usually determines effectiveness in controlling the symptoms of regional enteritis or ulcerative colitis. Long-term use (months to years) requires physician supervision.

▷ **This Drug Should Not Be Taken If**
- you are allergic to *any* sulfonamide drug (see Drug Classes), or to aspirin (or other salicylates).
- you are in the last month of pregnancy.
- you have a urinary or intestinal obstruction or porphyria.
- you are breast-feeding.

▷ **Inform Your Physician Before Taking This Drug If**
- you are allergic to any sulfonamide: acetazolamide, thiazide diuretics or sulfonylurea antidiabetics (see Drug Classes).
- you are allergic by nature: history of hay fever, asthma, hives, eczema.
- you have asthma.
- you have impaired liver or kidney function.
- you have a G6PD deficiency.
- you have a personal or family history of porphyria.
- you have had a drug-induced blood cell or bone marrow disorder.

- you currently take any oral anticoagulant, antidiabetic drug or phenytoin.
- you plan to have surgery under pentothal anesthesia soon.

Possible Side-Effects (natural, expected and unavoidable drug actions)
Brownish coloration of the urine, of no significance.
Superinfections, bacterial or fungal (see Glossary).

▷ **Possible Adverse Effects** (unusual, unexpected and infrequent reactions)
If any of the following develop, consult your physician promptly for guidance.

Mild Adverse Effects
Allergic Reactions: Skin rashes, hives, itching.
Headache, dizziness.
Discoloration of contact lenses.
Ringing in the ears.
Loss of appetite, irritation of the mouth and tongue, nausea, vomiting, abdominal pain, diarrhea.
Skin pigmentation.
Taste disorders.

Serious Adverse Effects
Allergic Reactions: Drug fever (see Glossary), swollen glands, painful joints, anaphylaxis (see Glossary). Allergic pneumonitis, allergic hepatitis. Severe skin reactions.
Idiosyncratic Reaction: Hemolytic anemia (see Glossary).
Bone marrow depression (see Glossary): fatigue, weakness, fever, sore throat, abnormal bleeding or bruising.
Pancreatitis.
Drug-induced lupus erythematosus (rare).
Kidney damage: bloody or cloudy urine, reduced urine volume.
Peripheral neuropathy (see Glossary).
Inflammation of the tissue around the heart (pericarditis).

▷ **Possible Effects on Sexual Function:** Decreased production of sperm, reversible infertility.

▷ **Adverse Effects That May Mimic Natural Diseases or Disorders**
Liver reactions may suggest viral hepatitis.
Lung reactions may suggest an infectious pneumonia.

Natural Diseases or Disorders That May Be Activated by This Drug
Goiter, acute intermittent porphyria.

Possible Effects on Laboratory Tests
Complete blood cell counts: decreased red cells, hemoglobin, white cells and platelets; increased eosinophils (allergic reaction).
Liver function tests: increased liver enzymes (ALT/GPT, AST/GOT and alkaline phosphatase), increased bilirubin.
Sperm count: decreased; abnormal sperm common; effects reversible on discontinuation of drug.

CAUTION
1. A large intake of water (up to 2 quarts daily) is necessary to ensure an adequate volume of urine.
2. Shake liquid dosage forms thoroughly before measuring each dose.

Sulfasalazine

Precautions for Use
   By Infants and Children: Safety and effectiveness for those under 2 years of age are not established.
   By Those over 60 Years of Age: Observe for the development of reduced urine volume, fever, sore throat, abnormal bleeding or bruising or skin irritation with itching, particularly in the anal or genital regions.

▷ **Advisability of Use During Pregnancy**
   Pregnancy Category: B, however, this drug should **not** be used near the time of the birth of the baby. See Pregnancy Code at the back of this book.
   Animal studies: Cleft palate and skeletal birth defects due to sulfonamides reported in mice and rats.
   Human studies: No increase in birth defects reported in 4584 exposures to various sulfonamides during pregnancy.
   Avoid use of drug during the last month of pregnancy because of possible adverse effects on the newborn infant.

Advisability of Use if Breast-Feeding
   Presence of this drug in breast milk: Yes.
   Avoid drug or refrain from nursing.

Habit-Forming Potential: None.

Effects of Overdosage: Headache, dizziness, nausea, vomiting, abdominal cramping, toxic fever, coma, jaundice, kidney failure.

Possible Effects of Long-Term Use: Development of goiter, with or without hypothyroidism. An orange-yellow discoloration of the skin has been reported. This is not jaundice.

Suggested Periodic Examinations While Taking This Drug (at physician's discretion)
   Complete blood cell counts, weekly for the first 8 weeks.
   Urine analysis weekly.
   Liver and kidney function tests.

▷ **While Taking This Drug, Observe the Following**
   Foods: No restrictions. Follow prescribed diet.
   Beverages: No restrictions. May be taken with milk.
▷   *Alcohol:* Use caution. Sulfonamide drugs can increase the intoxicating effects of alcohol.
   Tobacco Smoking: No interactions expected.
▷   *Other Drugs*
     Sulfasalazine may *increase* the effects of
     • anticoagulants (Coumadin, etc.), and increase the risk of bleeding.
     • sulfonylureas (see Drug Classes), and increase the risk of hypoglycemia.
     Sulfasalazine may *decrease* the effects of
     • digoxin (Lanoxin).
     Sulfasalazine **taken concurrently** with
     • Iron salts or calcium may decrease sulfasalazine benefits.
▷   *Driving, Hazardous Activities:* This drug may cause dizziness. Restrict activities as necessary.

Aviation Note: The use of this drug *may be a disqualification* for piloting. Consult a designated Aviation Medical Examiner.

Exposure to Sun: Use caution. Some sulfonamide drugs can cause photosensitivity (see Glossary).

SULFISOXAZOLE (sul fi SOX a zohl)

Introduced: 1949 **Prescription:** USA: Yes; Canada: Yes **Available as Generic:** Yes **Class:** Anti-infective, sulfonamides **Controlled Drug:** USA: No; Canada: No

Brand Names: Azo Gantrisin [CD], Azo-Sulfisoxazole, Eryzole [CD], Gantrisin, Gulfasin, Lipo Gantrisin, ✦Novosoxazole, Pediazole [CD], SK-Soxazole, Sulfalar

BENEFITS versus RISKS	
Possible Benefits	*Possible Risks*
EFFECTIVE ANTIMICROBIAL ACTION against susceptible bacteria and protozoa	Allergic reactions: mild to severe skin reactions, anaphylaxis Rare blood cell disorders: aplastic anemia, hemolytic anemia, abnormally low white cell and platelet counts Drug-induced liver damage Drug-induced kidney damage

▷ **Principal Uses**

As a Single Drug Product: Uses currently included in FDA approved labeling: (1) Used to treat a variety of bacterial and protozoal infections: ear infections, malaria, nocardia, toxoplasmosis and trachoma. It is most commonly used to treat certain infections of the urinary tract.

Other (unlabeled) generelly accepted uses: (1) Treats meningitis caused by Haemophilus influenzae; (2) has a role in chylamydia infections; (3) may help prevent ear infections when used in long-term therapy; (4) can have a role in preventing plague.

As a Combination Drug Product [CD]: This drug is available in combination with phenazopyridine, an analgesic drug that relieves the discomfort associated with acute infections of the urinary bladder and urethra. This combination provides early symptomatic relief while the underlying infection is being eradicated.

How This Drug Works: This drug prevents the growth and multiplication of susceptible bacteria by interfering with their formation of folic acid, an essential nutrient.

Available Dosage Forms and Strengths

Emulsion, prolonged-action — 1 gram per 5-ml teaspoonful
Eye drops — 4%
Eye ointment — 4%
Injection — 400 mg per ml
Pediatric suspension — 500 mg per 5-ml teaspoonful

Sulfisoxazole

Syrup — 500 mg per 5-ml teaspoonful
Tablets — 500 mg

▷ **Usual Adult Dosage Range:** Initially, 2 to 4 grams; then 750 to 1500 mg (1.5 grams) every 4 hours, or 1 to 2 grams every 6 hours, depending upon the severity of the infection. The total daily dosage should not exceed 12 grams. **Note: Actual dosage and administration schedule must be determined by the physician for each patient individually.**

Conditions Requiring Dosing Adjustments
Liver function: This drug can be a rare cause of liver damage, and patients should be followed closely.
Kidney function: In patients with mild to moderate kidney failure, sulfasoxazole can be given every 6 hours in the usual dose. In moderate to severe kidney failure, it can be given every 12 to 24 hours in the usual dose. In severe kidney failure, it can be given once a day. Increased elimination of this drug may be seen in patients with alkaline urine. It should be used with caution in renal compromise.

▷ **Dosing Instructions:** Preferably taken with 8 ounces of water on an empty stomach, 1 hour before or 2 hours after eating. However, it may be taken with or following food to reduce stomach irritation. The tablet may be crushed for administration.

Usual Duration of Use: Use on a regular schedule for 7 to 10 days usually determines effectiveness in controlling responsive infections. Treatment should be continued until the patient is free of symptoms for 48 hours. Limit treatment to no more than 14 days if possible.

▷ **This Drug Should Not Be Taken If**
- you are allergic to *any* sulfonamide drug (see Drug Classes).
- you are in the last month of pregnancy.
- you are breast-feeding.

▷ **Inform Your Physician Before Taking This Drug If**
- you are allergic to any sulfonamide: acetazolamide, thiazide diuretics, sulfonylurea antidiabetic drugs (see Drug Classes).
- you are allergic by nature: history of hay fever, asthma, hives, eczema.
- you have impaired liver or kidney function.
- you have a low glucose-6-phosphate dehydrogenase.
- you have a personal or family history of porphyria.
- you have had a drug-induced blood cell or bone marrow disorder.
- you currently take any oral anticoagulant, antidiabetic drug or phenytoin.
- you plan to have surgery under pentothal anesthesia while taking this drug.

Possible Side-Effects (natural, expected and unavoidable drug actions)
Brownish coloration of the urine, of no significance.
Superinfections, bacterial or fungal (see Glossary).

▷ **Possible Adverse Effects** (unusual, unexpected and infrequent reactions)
If any of the following develop, consult your physician promptly for guidance.
Mild Adverse Effects
Allergic Reactions: Skin rashes, hives, itching, localized swellings, reddened eyes.

Headache, dizziness, unsteadiness, ringing in the ears.
Loss of appetite, irritation of the mouth and tongue, nausea, vomiting, abdominal pain, diarrhea.

Serious Adverse Effects
Allergic Reactions: Drug fever (see Glossary), swollen glands, painful joints, anaphylaxis (see Glossary). Allergic hepatitis. Severe skin reactions.
Idiosyncratic Reaction: Hemolytic anemia (see Glossary).
Bone marrow depression (see Glossary): fatigue, weakness, fever, sore throat, abnormal bleeding or bruising.
Kidney damage: bloody or cloudy urine, reduced urine volume.
Peripheral neuropathy (see Glossary).
Drug-induced parotitis (rare).
Drug-induced systemic lupus erythematosus.
Drug-induced disulfiram reaction.

▷ **Possible Effects on Sexual Function:** None reported.

▷ **Adverse Effects That May Mimic Natural Diseases or Disorders**
Liver reactions may suggest viral hepatitis.

Natural Diseases or Disorders That May Be Activated by This Drug
Goiter, acute intermittent porphyria.

Possible Effects on Laboratory Tests
Complete blood cell counts: decreased red cells, hemoglobin, white cells and platelets; increased eosinophils (allergic reaction).
Blood lupus erythematosus (LE) cells: positive.
Blood amylase and lipase levels: increased (pancreatitis).
Liver function tests: increased liver enzymes (ALT/GPT, AST/GOT and alkaline phosphatase), increased bilirubin.

CAUTION
1. A large intake of water (up to 2 quarts daily) is necessary to ensure an adequate volume of urine.
2. Shake liquid dosage forms thoroughly before measuring each dose.

Precautions for Use
By Infants and Children: This drug should not be used in infants under 2 months of age.
By Those over 60 Years of Age: Small doses taken at longer intervals often achieve adequate blood and tissue drug levels. Watch for development of reduced urine volume, fever, sore throat, abnormal bleeding or bruising or skin irritation with itching, particularly in the anal or genital regions.

▷ **Advisability of Use During Pregnancy**
Pregnancy Category: C. See Pregnancy Code at the back of this book.
Animal studies: Cleft palate and skeletal birth defects due to sulfonamides reported in mice and rats.
Human studies: No increase in birth defects reported in 4287 exposures to this drug during pregnancy.
Avoid use of drug during the last three months of pregnancy because of possible adverse effects on the newborn infant.

Advisability of Use if Breast-Feeding
Presence of this drug in breast milk: Yes.
Avoid drug or refrain from nursing.

Habit-Forming Potential: None.

Effects of Overdosage: Headache, dizziness, nausea, vomiting, abdominal cramping, toxic fever, coma, jaundice, kidney failure.

Possible Effects of Long-Term Use: Superinfections, bacterial or fungal. Development of goiter, with or without hypothyroidism. Excessive loss of vitamin C via urine.

Suggested Periodic Examinations While Taking This Drug (at physician's discretion)
Complete blood cell counts, weekly for the first 8 weeks.
Urine analysis weekly.
Liver and kidney function tests.

▷ **While Taking This Drug, Observe the Following**
Foods: No restrictions.
Beverages: No restrictions. May be taken with milk.
▷ *Alcohol:* Use caution. Sulfonamide drugs can increase the intoxicating effects of alcohol.
Tobacco Smoking: No interactions expected.
▷ *Other Drugs*
Sulfisoxazole may *increase* the effects of
- anticoagulants (Coumadin, etc.), and increase the risk of bleeding.
- methotrexate (Mexate), and cause serious blood toxicity.
- sulfonylureas (see Drug Class Section), or other oral hypoglycemic agents and increase the risk of hypoglycemia.

Sulfisoxazole may *decrease* the effects of
- birth control pills (oral contraceptives).
- penicillins.

▷ *Driving, Hazardous Activities:* This drug may cause dizziness. Restrict activities as necessary.
Aviation Note: The use of this drug ***may be a disqualification*** for piloting. Consult a designated Aviation Medical Examiner.
Exposure to Sun: Use caution. Some sulfonamide drugs cause photosensitivity (see Glossary).

SULINDAC (sul IN dak)

Introduced: 1976 **Prescription:** USA: Yes; Canada: Yes **Available as Generic:** USA: Yes; Canada: Yes **Class:** Mild analgesic, anti-inflammatory **Controlled Drug:** USA: No; Canada: No

Brand Name: +✦Apo-Sulin, Clinoril, Novo-Sundac

BENEFITS versus RISKS	
Possible Benefits	*Possible Risks*
EFFECTIVE RELIEF OF MILD TO MODERATE PAIN AND INFLAMMATION	Gastrointestinal pain, ulceration, bleeding (rare) Rare liver damage Rare kidney damage Rare bone marrow depression (aplastic anemia) Rare auditory and visual hallucinations Rare pancreatitis

Please see the acetic acid nonsteroidal anti-inflammatory drug profile for further information.

SUMATRIPTAN (Soo ma TRIP tan)

Introduced: 1993 **Prescription:** USA: Yes; Canada: Yes **Available as Generic:** USA: No; Canada: No **Class:** Antimigraine drug, serotonin 1 receptor agonist **Controlled Drug:** USA: No; Canada: No
Brand Name: Imitrex

BENEFITS versus RISKS	
Possible Benefits	*Possible Risks*
RAPID AND EFFECTIVE RELIEF OR PREVENTION OF MIGRAINE (NONBASILAR NONHEMIPLEGIC) WELL TOLERATED Relieves photophobia (light sensitivity) Relieves phonophobia (sound sensitivity) Relieves nausea and vomiting	SYNCOPE (fainting) (0.1-1%) Confusion and other mental changes (0.1-1%) Rare myocardial infarction Rare serious atrial and ventricular arrhythmias

▷ **Principal Uses**

As a Single Drug Product: Uses currently included in FDA approved labeling: (1) Acute treatment of migraine with or without aura.

Other (unlabeled) generally accepted uses: (1) Treatment of cluster headache; (2) may have a role in posttraumatic headaches.

How This Drug Works: Sumatriptan acts on blood vessels to cause vasoconstriction (shrinking of the blood vessels). This relieves swelling thought to be the cause of migraine. The drug binds to a receptor arteries such as the basilar artery and in vasculature (blood vessels) associated with the dura mater (part of the lining of the brain).

Available Dosage Forms and Strengths

Sumatriptan succinate (Imitrex) injection
SELFdose system kit which has two syringes with 6 mg in 0.5 ml of liquid

Sumatriptan

in a 1 ml size syringe, a dosing device and instructions. NDC # 0173-0449-03.

Unit-of-use syringes with 6 mg in 0.5 ml of liquid in a 1 ml syringe packaged in a carton containing two syringes. NDC # 0173-0449-01.

6 mg single-dose vials with 0.5 ml of liquid in a 2 ml vial. These vials are packaged in cartons of 5 vials. NDC # 0173-0449-02.

All of the liquid in these products should be a colorless to pale yellow, clear solution. Particles or precipitates should never be present.

Tablets—25 mg

How To Store

Keep out of reach of children. Store at room temperature in a room where the temperature will not exceed 86 degrees. Keep away from heat and light.

▷ Recommended Dosage Ranges (Actual dosage and administration schedule must be determined by the physician for each patient individually.)

Infants and Children: The safety and effectiveness in pediatrics has **not** been determined.

18 to 60 Years of Age: The maximum adult dose of subcutaneous sumatriptan is 6 mg. The dose should be given as soon as possible after the symptoms of acute migraine are recognized. Controlled clinical trials have failed to demonstrate a benefit of repeat injections if the initial injection is unsuccessful. If symptoms return, a second 6 mg injection may be given 12 hours after the first injection was given. If side effects occur, use the lowest dose in the approved dosage range that is effective for you.

Over 65 Years of Age: Safety and effectiveness **not** evaluated in this age group. Since declines in renal and hepatic function and coronary artery disease are more common in those over 65, the possibility of an increase in side effects would be expected.

Conditions Requiring Dosing Adjustments

Liver function: The effect of liver impairment on sumatriptan has not been specifically studied, and dosage or interval adjustments have not been established.

Kidney function: Presently, there are no determined requirements for dosage adjustment in renal compromise.

▷ Dosing Instructions:

This drug must be given subcutaneously, **not intravenously**. Intravenous injection must be avoided because of its potential to cause coronary vasospasm (constriction of the blood vessels which supply the heart). This medicine should be colorless to pale yellow and clear. Be certain to check the medicine before injecting it. Particles should never be present. There is extensive information on self-injection available from your doctor or pharmacist.

Usual Duration of Use:

The maximum dose is two 6 mg doses in 24 hours. This medication relieves existing migraines, and will not change the frequency or number of attacks. Recurring use of this medicine will be needed. If your migraines increase in frequency or severity, consult your doctor. If this medicine is not effective in helping your migraine, consult your doctor.

Possible Advantages of This Drug
Effective subcutaneous treatment of acute nonbasilar nonhemiplegic migraine. Better side-effect profile and treatment of migraine-associated nausea and vomiting and phono and photophobia than other currently available agents.

Currently a "Drug of Choice"
for nonbasilar nonhemiplegic migraine.

▷ **This Drug Should Not Be Taken If**
- you have had an allergic reaction to any dosage form of it previously.
- you are unfamiliar with the subcutaneous route. Particular care must be taken to avoid intravenous use because this may lead to coronary vasospasm (constriction of the blood vessels that supply the heart).
- you have ischemic heart disease with symptoms such as: angina pectoris, silent ischemia or history of MI (myocardial infarction).
- you have Prinzmetal's angina (a specific kind of chest pain).
- you have uncontrolled hypertension (high blood pressure).
- you have basilar or hemiplegic migraine.
- you have (within 24 hours) taken an ergotamine preparation.

▷ **Inform Your Physician Before Taking This Drug If**
- you are pregnant or plan to become pregnant.
- you are breast-feeding.
- you have high blood pressure.
- you have chest pain, heart disease or irregular heartbeats.
- you have had a heart attack.
- you have taken or have prescriptions for other migraine medications.
- you have allergies or trouble taking other medication, whether prescription or over the counter.
- you have liver or kidney disease.
- you are uncertain of how much to take or when to take this medicine.
- you do not understand the subcutaneous injection technique.
- you have Raynaud's syndrome.

Possible Side-Effects (natural, expected and unavoidable drug actions)
Excessive thirst and frequent urination. Transient rises in blood pressure.

▷ **Possible Adverse Effects** (unusual, unexpected and infrequent reactions)
If any of the following develop, consult your physician promptly for guidance.

Mild Adverse Effects
Allergic Reactions: Red itching skin, skin rash and tenderness.
Atypical sensations such as tingling and numbness (0.1–1%). Confusion and other mental changes (0.1–1%), dizziness and vertigo (0.1–1%), flushing (0.1–1%), tightness in the chest or jaw (infrequent), gastroesophageal reflux and diarrhea, pain at the injection site, joint pain, weakness and stiffness (all are 0.1–1%).

Serious Adverse Effects
Syncope (fainting) (0.1–1%), CVA (rare), dysphasia (rare), seizure (rare), subarachnoid hemorrhage (rare), changes in blood pressure and heart rate (0.1–1%), serious changes in heart rate and rhythm (rare), Raynaud's syndrome (less than 0.1%), peptic ulcer (less than 0.1), dyspnea (difficulty

breathing) (0.1–1%), renal calculi (less than 0.1%), Princemetal's angina (rare), myocardial infarction (very rare), acute renal failure (very rare).

▷ **Possible Effects on Sexual Function:** Dysmenorrhea, erection.

Possible Delayed Adverse Effects: None identified.

▷ **Adverse Effects That May Mimic Natural Diseases or Disorders**

Changes in heart rate and rhythmn may mimic a number of cardiac conditions. Drug induced acute renal failure (ARF) may mimic nondrug induced ARF. Drug induced hypertension may mimic hypertension from other causes.

Urological symptoms may mimic benign prostatic hypertrophy. Sumatriptan can mimic Raynaud's syndrome.

Natural Diseases or Disorders That May Be Activated by This Drug
Hypertension.

Possible Effects on Laboratory Tests
Liver function tests: Rare increases in SGOT and SGPT.

CAUTION
1. Do not use sumatriptan if you are pregnant.
2. Call your doctor if you have any pain or tightness in the chest or throat when you use this medicine.
3. Do not use sumatriptan if you have used an ergotamine containing preparation within the last 24 hours.
4. This medication is **not** to be used intravenously.
5. If you are diagnosed as having ischemic heart disease after sumatriptan has been prescribed for you, do not use the medicine again.

Precautions for Use
By Infants and Children:
Safety and effectiveness for those under 18 years of age not established.
By Those over 65 Years of Age: Have not been established.

▷ **Advisability of Use During Pregnancy**
Pregnancy Category: C. See Pregnancy Code at the back of this book.
Animal studies: Sumatriptan has been lethal to rabbit embryos when given in doses that were three fold higher than those produced by a 6 mg dose. Term fetuses from rabbits treated with sumatriptan exhibited an increase in cervicothoracic vascular defects and minor skeletal abnormalities.
Human studies: Adequate studies of pregnant women are not available.
Ask your physician for guidance.

Advisability of Use if Breast-Feeding
Presence of this drug in breast milk: Sumatriptan is excreted in the breast milk of animals, however no human data is available.
Use of this medication in nursing mothers is a benefit to risk decision to be made by a physician.

Habit-Forming Potential: Not clearly defined.

Effects of Overdosage: Patients have received doses of 8 to 12 mg without adverse effects. Healthy volunteers have taken up to 16 mg subcutaneously without serious adverse events. Coronary vasospasm has resulted from intravenous administration of normal doses. Animal data presents: convulsions, tremor, flushing, decreased breathing and activity, cyanosis, ataxia and paralysis.

Possible Effects of Long-Term Use: Not defined.

Suggested Periodic Examinations While Taking This Drug (at physician's discretion)
Liver function tests, electrocardiogram.

▷ **While Taking This Drug, Observe the Following**
Foods: No restrictions.
Beverages: No restrictions.
▷ *Alcohol:* May cause additive sedation.
Tobacco Smoking: No interactions expected.
Marijuana Smoking: May cause additive dizziness, drowsiness and lethargy, may cause additive increases in blood pressure.
▷ *Other Drugs*
Sumatriptan *taken concurrently* with
• ergotamine containing preparations may result in additive vasospasm (prolonged constriction of the blood vessels).
▷ *Driving, Hazardous Activities:* This drug may cause dizziness and drowsiness. Restrict activities as necessary.
Aviation Note: The use of this drug *may be a disqualification* for piloting. Consult a designated Aviation Medical Examiner.
Exposure to Sun: No restrictions.
Exposure to Cold: Use caution until tolerance is determined. Cold may enhance sumatriptan vasoconstriction.
Special Storage Instructions: Keep this medicine out of reach of children.
Observe the Following Expiration Times: There is an expiration date printed on the treatment package. Throw the medication away if it has expired. The autoinjector may be used again.

TACRINE (TA kreen)

Introduced: September 1993 **Prescription:** USA: Yes; Canada: Not available in Canada **Available as Generic:** USA: No **Class:** Cholinesterase inhibitor **Controlled Drug:** USA:No

Brand Names: Cognex

BENEFITS versus RISKS	
Possible Benefits	*Possible Risks*
IMPROVEMENT OF MEMORY IN MILD TO MODERATE ALZHEIMER'S DISEASE	LIVER TOXICITY (20 to 40 %) agitation (4%) hallucinations (2%)

▷ **Principal Uses**
As a Single Drug Product: Uses currently included in FDA approved labeling: (1) Treatment of symptoms of mild to moderate Alzheimer's disease.
Other (unlabeled) generally accepted uses: (1) Significant increases in protective white blood cells (CD4 lymphocytes) occurred when tacrine was used to treat AIDS dementia; (2) some early data indicated a benefit in movement disorders (tardive dyskinesia).

Tacrine

How This Drug Works: Alzheimer's disease is thought to be caused by a loss of nerve cells that make a nerve transmitter (acetylcholine). Tacrine acts to increase levels of neurotransmitter (acetylcholine) in the brain.

Available Dosage Forms and Strengths
Capsules — 10 mg, 20 mg, 30 mg, 40 mg

▷ **Recommended Dosage Ranges (Actual dosage and administration schedule must be determined by the physician for each patient individually.)**
Infants and Children: No data are available on use of this drug in infants and children.
18 to 60 Years of Age: Adult starting dose is 10 mg taken four times a day. The dose can be increased at 6-week intervals if needed. Maximum daily dose is 160 mg.
Over 60 Years of Age: Same as 12 to 60 years of age.

Conditions Requiring Dosing Adjustments
Liver function: Used with great caution in liver compromise.
Kidney function: Dose decreases in kidney compromise are not presently indicated.

▷ **Dosing Instructions:** Tablet may be crushed and is best taken 1 hour before meals.

Usual Duration of Use: Use on a regular schedule for 1 to 4 weeks is usually needed to see clinical improvement in this drug. Dose increases are made at 6-week intervals.
Long-term use (months to years) requires periodic physician evaluation of response and dosage adjustment.

Possible Advantages of This Drug
Improvement of memory and other symptoms of mild to moderate Alzheimer's with fewer side effects of other available agents.

Currently a "Drug of Choice"
for treatment of symptoms of mild to moderate Alzheimer's disease.

▷ **This Drug Should Not Be Taken If**
- you have had an allergic reaction to any dosage form of it previously.
- you have had tacrine-caused hepatoxicity and blood bilirubin levels greater than 3 mg/dl.
- you have bronchial asthma.
- you have a slow heartbeat (bradycardia), an abnormal electrical conduction system in your heart (AV conduction defect) or excessively low blood pressure.
- you have an overly active thyroid (hyperthyroidism).
- you have peptic ulcer disease.
- you have an intestinal or urinary tract obstruction.

▷ **Inform Your Physician Before Taking This Drug If**
- you have a history of seizure disorder.
- you have had liver disease.
- you take a NSAID (see Drug Classes section).
- you take muscle relaxants.
- you have gluacoma (angle closure).

▷ **Possible Adverse Effects** (unusual, unexpected and infrequent reactions)
If any of the following develop, consult your physician promptly for guidance.
Mild Adverse Effects
Allergic Reactions: Skin rash.
Increased sweating.
Muscle aches (5%).
Nausea or vomiting (28%), belching and diarrhea (16%) decreased appetite (9%).
Dizziness (12%), confusion (7%) and insomnia (6%).
Serious Adverse Effects
Allergic Reactions: Anaphylactoid reactions.
Liver toxicity (20 to 40%) starts within 6 to 8 weeks after therapy began.
Agitation (4%), hallucinations (2%).
Purpura (2%).
Excessive urination (3%).
Severe decrease in white blood cells (very rare).
Respiratory compromise (rare).
Slow heart rate or abnormal rhythm (rare).
Low white blood cell count (rare).

▷ **Possible Effects on Sexual Function:** Very rare effect in inducing lactation.

Possible Delayed Adverse Effects: Liver toxicity, rash, low white blood cell count.

▷ **Adverse Effects That May Mimic Natural Diseases or Disorders**
Liver toxicity may mimic acute hepatitis.

Natural Diseases or Disorders That May Be Activated by This Drug
May worsen bronchial asthma and precipitate seizures. May exacerbate peptic ulcer disease.

Possible Effects on Laboratory Tests
Liver function tests: increased SGOT, SGPT and CPK.
Complete blood count: decreased white blood cells.

CAUTION
1. This drug should **not** be stopped abruptly as acute deterioration of cognitive abilities may result.
2. Changes in color of stools (light or very black) should be promptly reported to your doctor.
3. This drug does **not** alter the course of Alzheimer's disease. Over time, the benefit of this drug may be lost.
4. The dose **must** be decreased by 40 mg per day if the liver function levels (transaminases) rise to 3 to 5 times the uper normal value.
5. Blood levels achieved by females are 50% higher than those in men. Dose-related side effects may occur sooner (with lower doses) in women than in men. Therapeutic doses may be lower for women than men.

Precautions for Use
By Infants and Children:
Safety and effectiveness for those under 18 years of age not established.
By Those over 60 Years of Age: No specific changes are presently indicated.

▷ **Advisability of Use During Pregnancy**
Pregnancy Category: C. See Pregnancy Code at the back of this book.
Animal studies: Data not available.
Human studies: Adequate studies of pregnant women are not available.
Consult your doctor.

Advisability of Use if Breast-Feeding
Presence of this drug in breast milk: Unknown.
Monitor nursing infant closely and discontinue drug or nursing if adverse effects develop.

Habit-Forming Potential: None.

Effects of Overdosage: May precipitate a cholinergic crisis—severe nausea and vomiting, slow heartbeat, low blood pressure, extreme muscle weakness, collapse and convulsions.

Suggested Periodic Examinations While Taking This Drug (at physician's discretion)
Assessment of mental status: periodically to check benefit of therapy and potential loss of effectiveness as the underlying disease progresses.
Liver function tests: should be checked every 2 weeks for the first 16 weeks of therapy, then monthly for 2 months and then every 3 months thereafter if the same dose is maintained. If the dose is increased, liver function tests shuld be checked weekly for 7 weeks and then the above schedule should be followed.
Complete blood count: checked periodically or if symptoms of low blood count occur.

▷ **While Taking This Drug, Observe the Following**
Foods: Best **not** taken with food.
Beverages: No restrictions.

▷ *Alcohol:* Occasional small amounts of alcohol acceptable. Frequent use of alcohol may worsen memory impairment and adversely effect liver enzymes.
Tobacco Smoking: No interactions expected.
Marijuana Smoking: Additive dizziness may occur.

▷ *Other Drugs*
Tacrine may *increase* the effects of
• bethanechol (Duvoid, others).
• theophylline (Theo-Dur, others) by doubling the drug level.
• succinlycholine (Anectine, others).
Tacrine may *decrease* the effects of
• anticholinergic medications (see Drug Classes).
The following drugs may *increase* the effects of tacrine
• cimetidine (Tagamet).

▷ *Driving, Hazardous Activities:* This drug may cause confusion. Restrict activities as necessary.
Aviation Note: The use of this drug **may be a disqualification** for piloting. Consult a designated Aviation Medical Examiner.
Exposure to Sun: No restrictions.
Exposure to Heat: Increased sweating may routinely occur with this drug. The combination of increased sweating and hot environments may lead to more rapid dehydration.

Discontinuation: This drug should **not** be abruptly stopped. Some adverse effects are dose related, and may abate if the dose is decreased. Slow withdrawal of the drug is indicated if it is not tolerated and must be stopped.

TAMOXIFEN (ta MOX i fen)

Introduced: 1973 **Prescription:** USA: Yes; Canada: Yes **Available as Generic:** No **Class:** Antiestrogen, anticancer **Controlled Drug:** USA: No; Canada: No

Brand Names: ◆Alpha-Tamoxifen, ◆Apo-Tamox, Nolvadex, ◆Nolvadex-D, ◆Novo-Tamoxifen, ◆Tamofen, ◆Tamone

BENEFITS versus RISKS	
Possible Benefits	*Possible Risks*
EFFECTIVE ADJUNCTIVE TREATMENT IN ADVANCED BREAST CANCER	UTERINE CANCER (increased occurence, percentage not yet defined)
	Severe increase in tumor or bone pain, transient
	Thromophlebitis, pulmonary embolism
	Abnormally high blood calcium levels
	Eye changes: corneal opacities, retinal injury

▷ **Principal Uses**

As a Single Drug Product: Uses currently included in FDA approved labeling: (1) Used as an alternative to estrogens and androgens (male sex hormones) to treat advanced breast cancer in postmenopausal women; (2) treats advanced breast cancer in men that has spread (metastasized) from a prior site; (3) used to delay the reccurance of breast cancer in women.

Other (unlabeled) generally accepted uses: (1) May have a role in treating cancer of the liver or lung; (2) used to stimulate ovulation in premenopausal women with infertility; (3) used to treat rare desmoid tumors; (4) helps prevent osteoporosis in women in whom the drug is being used to prevent the recurrence of cancer; (4) can help retroperitoneal fibrosis.

How This Drug Works: It is thought that by blocking the uptake of estradiol (estrogen), this drug removes or reduces a stimulus to breast cancer cells.

Available Dosage Forms and Strengths

Tablets — 10 mg, 15.2 mg (in Canada), 20 mg (in Canada) and 30.4 mg (in Canada)

▷ **Usual Adult Dosage Range:** 10 to 20 mg twice/day, morning and evening. **Note: Actual dosage and administration schedule must be determined by the physician for each patient individually.**

Conditions Requiring Dosing Adjustments
Liver function: Dose decreases are not defined in patients with compromised livers.

Kidney function: The kidney plays a minor role in the elimination of this drug, however, tamoxifen should be used with caution in renal compromise.

▷ **Dosing Instructions:** The tablet may be crushed and taken either on an empty stomach or with food.

Usual Duration of Use: Use on a regular schedule for 4 to 10 weeks usually determines effectiveness in controlling the growth and spread of advanced breast cancer. In the presence of bone involvement, treatment for several months may be required to evaluate effectiveness. Long-term use (months to years) requires physician supervision and periodic evaluation.

▷ **This Drug Should Not Be Taken If**
- you have had a serious allergic or adverse reaction to it previously.
- you have active phlebitis.
- you have a significant deficiency of white blood cells or blood platelets.
- you are pregnant.

▷ **Inform Your Physician Before Taking This Drug If**
- you have a history of thrombophlebitis or pulmonary embolism.
- you have a history of abnormally high blood calcium levels.
- you have a history of any type of blood cell or bone marrow disorder.
- you have cataracts or other visual impairment.
- you have impaired liver function.
- you plan to have surgery in the near future.

Possible Side-Effects (natural, expected and unavoidable drug actions)
Hot flashes, fluid retention, weight gain.

▷ **Possible Adverse Effects** (unusual, unexpected and infrequent reactions)
If any of the following develop, consult your physician promptly for guidance.

Mild Adverse Effects
Allergic Reaction: Skin rash.
Visual impairment.
Headache, dizziness, drowsiness, depression, fatigue, confusion.
Nausea, vomiting, itching in genital area, loss of hair.

Serious Adverse Effects
Initial "flare" of severe pain in tumor or involved bone.
Development of thrombophlebitis, risk of pulmonary embolism.
Eye changes: corneal opacities, retinal injury.
Development of abnormally high blood calcium levels.
Transient decreases in white blood cells and blood platelets.
Liver toxicity (rare).

▷ **Possible Effects on Sexual Function**
Premenopausal: altered timing and pattern of menstruation.
Postmenopausal: vaginal bleeding.
Priapism.
This drug may be effective in treating the following conditions:
- male infertility due to abnormally low sperm counts.
- male breast enlargement and tenderness.
- chronic female breast pain (mastalgia).

Possible Effects on Laboratory Tests
  Complete blood cell counts: decreased red cells, hemoglobin, white cells and platelets.
  Blood calcium level: increased.
  Blood thyroid hormone levels: T_3, T_4 and free T_4 increased.
  Liver function tests: increased liver enzyme (AST/GOT), increased bilirubin (one case report).
  Sperm count: increased.

CAUTION
  1. If this drug is used prior to your menopause, it may induce ovulation and predispose to pregnancy. Since this drug should not be used during pregnancy, some method of contraception (other than oral contraceptives) is advised.
  2. Do not take any form of estrogen while taking this drug; estrogens can inhibit tamoxifen's effectiveness.
  3. Tamoxifen has recently been shown to cause an increased incidence of uterine cancer. Women who have received or who are receiving this drug should have regular gynecologic examinations. Report menstrual irregularity, abnormal vaginal bleeding or vaginal discharge, pelvic pain or pressure promptly to your doctor.

▷ **Advisability of Use During Pregnancy**
  Pregnancy Category: D. See Pregnancy Code at the back of this book.
  Animal studies: No birth defects due to this drug reported.
  Human studies: Adequate studies of pregnant women are not available.
  This drug can have estrogenic effects. It should not be used during pregnancy.

Advisability of Use if Breast-Feeding
  Presence of this drug in breast milk: Unknown.
  Avoid drug or refrain from nursing.

Habit-Forming Potential: None.

Effects of Overdosage: Severe extension of the pharmacologic effects.

Possible Effects of Long-Term Use: Development of abnormally high blood calcium levels.

Suggested Periodic Examinations While Taking This Drug (at physician's discretion)
  Complete blood cell counts, measurements of blood calcium levels.
  Complete eye examinations if impaired vision occurs.
  Women who have been given or who are now receiving tamoxifen **must** have regular gynecologic examinations.

▷ **While Taking This Drug, Observe the Following**
  Foods: No restrictions.
  Beverages: No restrictions. May be taken with milk.
▷ *Alcohol:* No interactions expected.
  Tobacco Smoking: No interactions expected.
▷ *Other Drugs*
  The following drugs may *decrease* the effects of tamoxifen
  • estrogens.
  • oral contraceptives (those that contain estrogens).

Tamoxifen *taken concurrently* with
- allopurinol may worsen allopurinol toxicity to the liver.
- cyclosporine (Sandimmune) may increase cyclosporine levels and cause toxicity.
- mitomycin will cause increased risk of hemolytic uremic syndrome.
- pneumococcal and perhaps other vaccines will blunt the vaccine's immune response (benefit).
- warfarin (Coumadin) presents an increased risk of bleeding.

▷ *Driving, Hazardous Activities:* This drug may cause dizziness or drowsiness. Restrict activities as necessary.

Aviation Note: The use of this drug **may be a disqualification** for piloting. Consult a designated Aviation Medical Examiner.

Exposure to Sun: No restrictions.

TERAZOSIN (ter AY zoh sin)

Introduced: 1987   **Prescription:** USA: Yes   **Available as Generic:** No   **Class:** Antihypertensive   **Controlled Drug:** USA: No   **Brand Name:** Hytrin

BENEFITS versus RISKS	
Possible Benefits	*Possible Risks*
EFFECTIVE TREATMENT OF MILD TO MODERATE HYPERTENSION when used alone or in combination with other antihypertensive drugs	"First dose" drop in blood pressure with fainting (1%) Fluid retention (5.5%) Rapid heart rate (1.9%)

▷ **Principal Uses**

As a Single Drug Product: Uses currently included in FDA approved labeling: (1) Used to treat mild to moderate hypertension. Also used in combination with other drugs to treat moderate to severe hypertension; (2) treats symptomatic benign prostatic hyperplasia (BPH).

Other (unlabeled) generally accepted uses: (1) Used to help correct symptoms in congestive heart failure; (2) may have a beneficial effect in lowering cholesterol levels.

How This Drug Works: Terazosin blocks some actions of the sympathetic nervous system, causing direct opening of blood vessel walls, lowering blood pressure. In BPH it relaxes the smooth muscle around the bladder neck and prostate allowing opening of the urethra and increased urine flow.

Available Dosage Forms and Strengths
Tablets — 1 mg, 2 mg, 5 mg, 10 mg

▷ **Usual Adult Dosage Range:** Treatment is started with a "test dose" of 1 mg and the patient's response is observed for 2 hours. If terazosin is tolerated, dose can be slowly (as needed and tolerated) increased up to 5 mg/24 hours. Maximum daily dosage should not exceed 20 mg. **Note: Actual dosage and administration schedule must be determined by the physician for each patient individually.**

Conditions Requiring Dosing Adjustments
  Liver function: Dose should be decreased in patients with severe liver problems.
  Kidney function: Dose changes are not needed in patients with severe kidney failure.
▷ **Dosing Instructions:** The tablet may be crushed and taken without regard to food. Best taken at bedtime to avoid orthostatic hypotension (see Glossary).
Usual Duration of Use: Use on a regular schedule for 6 to 8 weeks usually determines effectiveness in controlling hypertension. Two weeks of scheduled use is needed in BPH. See your doctor regularly.
Possible Advantages of This Drug
  May be used to initiate treatment.
  Usually effective with once-a-day dosage.
  Rarely causes depression or impotence.
  Does not alter blood cholesterol, potassium or sugar.
▷ **This Drug Should Not Be Taken If**
  • you have had an allergic reaction to it previously.
  • you are experiencing mental depression.
  • you have angina (active coronary artery disease) and you are not taking a beta-blocking drug. (See your physician.)
▷ **Inform Your Physician Before Taking This Drug If**
  • you have experienced orthostatic hypotension (see Glossary).
  • you have a history of mental depression.
  • you have impaired circulation to the brain, or a history of stroke.
  • you have coronary artery disease.
  • you have impaired liver or kidney function.
  • surgery under general anesthesia is planned soon.
Possible Side-Effects (natural, expected and unavoidable drug actions)
  Orthostatic hypotension (1.3%), drowsiness (5.4%), salt and water retention (5.5%), dry mouth, nasal congestion (5.9%), constipation.
▷ **Possible Adverse Effects** (unusual, unexpected and infrequent reactions)
  If any of the following develop, consult your physician promptly for guidance.
  Mild Adverse Effects
  Allergic Reaction: Skin rash.
  Headache (16.2%), dizziness (19.3%), fatigue (6.9%), weakness (11.3%), nervousness (2.3%), sweating, numbness and tingling (2.9%), blurred vision (1.6%).
  Weight gain.
  Congestion of the nose (5.9%).
  Palpitation (4.3%), rapid heart rate (1.9%), shortness of breath (3.1%).
  Nausea (4.4%), vomiting, diarrhea, abdominal pain.
  Serious Adverse Effects
  Mental depression (0.3%).
▷ **Possible Effects on Sexual Function:** Impotence (1.2%).
Natural Diseases or Disorders That May Be Activated by This Drug
  Latent coronary artery insufficiency.

Terazosin

Possible Effects on Laboratory Tests
Blood total cholesterol, LDL and VLDL cholesterol levels: decreased.
Blood HDL cholesterol level: no effect.
Blood triglyceride levels: no effect.

CAUTION
1. A "first dose" precipitous drop in blood pressue, with or without fainting can happen (usually within 30 to 90 minutes). Limit initial doses to 1 mg taken at bedtime (for first 3 days); stay laying down after taking trial doses.
2. Call your doctor if you plan to use over-the-counter remedies for allergic rhinitis or head colds. Serious drug interactions are possible.

Precautions for Use
By Infants and Children: Safety and effectiveness for those under 12 years of age not established.
By Those over 60 Years of Age: Therapy is started with no more than 1 mg/day for the first 3 days. Any dose increases must be very gradual and closely physician supervised. Orthostatic hypotension can cause falls and injury. Sit or lie down promptly if you feel light-headed or dizzy. Report dizziness or chest pain promptly.

▷ **Advisability of Use During Pregnancy**
Pregnancy Category: C. See Pregnancy Code at the back of this book.
Animal studies: No birth defects found in rat or rabbit studies.
Human studies: Adequate studies of pregnant women are not available.
Use this drug only if clearly needed. Ask your physician for guidance.

Advisability of Use if Breast-Feeding
Presence of this drug in breast milk: Unknown.
Watch infant closely and stop drug or nursing if adverse effects start.

Habit-Forming Potential: None.

Effects of Overdosage: Orthostatic hypotension, headache, flushing, fast heart rate, extreme weakness, irregular heart rhythm, circulatory collapse.

Possible Effects of Long-Term Use: None reported.

Suggested Periodic Examinations While Taking This Drug (at physician's discretion)
Measurements of blood pressure in lying, sitting and standing positions.
Measurements of body weight to detect fluid retention.

▷ **While Taking This Drug, Observe the Following**
Foods: No restrictions. Avoid excessive salt intake.
Beverages: No restrictions. May be taken with milk.
▷ *Alcohol:* Alcohol can exaggerate the blood-pressure-lowering actions of this drug and cause excessive reduction. Use with extreme caution.
Tobacco Smoking: Nicotine can intensify this drug's ability to worsen coronary insufficiency. All forms of tobacco should be avoided.
▷ *Other Drugs*
The following drugs may *increase* the effects of terazosin
- beta-adrenergic-blocking drugs (see Drug Classes Section); severity and duration of the "first dose" response may be increased.
- verapamil and cause excessive lowering of the blood pressure.

The following drugs may *decrease* the effects of terazosin
- estrogens.
- indomethacin (Indocin) and other NSAIDs (see Drug Classes).

▷ *Driving, Hazardous Activities:* This drug may cause dizziness or drowsiness. Restrict activities as necessary.

Aviation Note: The use of this drug *is a disqualification* for piloting. Consult a designated Aviation Medical Examiner.

Exposure to Sun: No restrictions.

Exposure to Cold: Cold environments may increase this drug's ability to cause coronary insufficiency (angina) and hypothermia (see Glossary). Use caution.

Heavy Exercise or Exertion: Excessive exertion can increase likelihood of chest pain. See Angina in Section Two.

Discontinuation: Do not stop this medicine abruptly if it is being used to treat congestive heart failure. Ask your physician for guidance.

TERBUTALINE (ter BYU ta leen)

Introduced: 1974 **Prescription:** USA: Yes; Canada: Yes **Available as Generic:** No **Class:** Antiasthmatic, bronchodilator **Controlled Drug:** USA: No; Canada: No

Brand Names: Brethaire, Brethine, Bricanyl, ◆Bricanyl Spacer

BENEFITS versus RISKS	
Possible Benefits	*Possible Risks*
VERY EFFECTIVE RELIEF OF BRONCHOSPASM	Increased blood pressure Fine hand tremor Irregular heart rhythm (with excessive use)

▷ **Principal Uses**

As a Single Drug Product: Uses currently included in FDA approved labeling: (1) Relieves acute bronchial asthma and reduces frequency and severity of chronic, recurrent asthmatic attacks; (2) also used to relieve reversible bronchospasm associated with chronic bronchitis and emphysema.

Other (unlabeled) generally accepted uses: (1) May have a role in helping ease fetal distress in some patients; (2) used to help stop premature labor; (3) can be an alternative to intravenous isoproterenol in therapy of status asthmaticus; (4) has a role in easing priapism; (5) may be used in combination therapy in patients who have wheals and itching of unknown cause (idiopathic urticaria).

How This Drug Works: By stimulating certain sympathetic nerve terminals, this drug acts to dilate those bronchial tubes that are in sustained constriction, thereby increasing the size of the airway and improving the ability to breathe.

Available Dosage Forms and Strengths
Aerosol — 0.2 mg/actuation and 0.25 mg/actuation (Canada)
Injection — 1 mg per ml
Tablets — 2.5 mg, 5 mg

▷ **Usual Adult Dosage Range:** Aerosol: 0.4 mg taken in 2 separate inhalations 1 minute apart; repeat every 4 to 6 hours as needed. Tablets: 2.5 to 5 mg taken 3 times/day, 6 hours apart. The total daily dosage should not exceed 15 mg. **Note: Actual dosage and administration schedule must be determined by the physician for each patient individually.**

Conditions Requiring Dosing Adjustments
Liver function: This drug is extensively metabolized in the liver, however, guidelines for dosing changes in patients with compromised livers are not available.
Kidney function: In patients with moderate to severe kidney failure, 50% of the usual dose can be given at the usual time. In severe failure, the drug should not be used.

▷ **Dosing Instructions:** Tablets may be crushed and taken on empty stomach or with food or milk. For aerosol, follow the written instructions carefully. Do not overuse.

Usual Duration of Use: According to individual requirements. Do not use beyond the time necessary to terminate episodes of asthma.

Possible Advantages of This Drug
Rapid onset of action.
Long duration of action.
Highly effective relief of asthma.

▷ **This Drug Should Not Be Taken If**
- you have had an allergic reaction to any dosage form of it previously.
- you currently have an irregular heart rhythm.
- you are taking, or have taken within the past 2 weeks, any monoamine oxidase (MAO) type A inhibitor drug (see Drug Classes).

▷ **Inform Your Physician Before Taking This Drug If**
- you are overly sensitive to other drugs that stimulate the sympathetic nervous system.
- you are currently using epinephrine (Adrenalin, Primatene Mist, etc.) to relieve asthmatic breathing.
- you have a seizure disorder.
- you have liver or kidney failure.
- you have any type of heart or circulatory disorder, especially high blood pressure or coronary heart disease.
- you have diabetes or an overactive thyroid gland (hyperthyroidism).
- you are taking any form of digitalis or any stimulant drug.

Possible Side-Effects (natural, expected and unavoidable drug actions)
Aerosol: dryness or irritation of mouth or throat, altered taste. Tablet: nervousness, tremor, palpitation.

▷ **Possible Adverse Effects** (unusual, unexpected and infrequent reactions)
If any of the following develop, consult your physician promptly for guidance.
Mild Adverse Effects
Headache, dizziness, drowsiness, restlessness, insomnia.
Rapid, pounding heartbeat; increased sweating; muscle cramps in arms and legs.
Nausea, heartburn, vomiting.
Increased blood sugar.

Serious Adverse Effects
 Rapid or irregular heart rhythm, intensification of angina, increased blood pressure.
 Lowered blood calcium or potassium (especially with intravenous use).
 Liver toxicity (very rare).

▷ **Possible Effects on Sexual Function:** None reported.

Natural Diseases or Disorders That May Be Activated By This Drug
 Latent coronary artery disease, diabetes or high blood pressure.

Possible Effects on Laboratory Tests
 Blood total cholesterol and LDL cholesterol levels: no effect.
 Blood HDL cholesterol level: increased.
 Blood triglyceride levels: no effect.
 Blood thyroid hormone levels: T_3 increased; T_4 decreased; free T_4 no effect.
 Glucose tolerance test: abnormal test.
 Liver function tests: May be eleveated.

CAUTION
 1. Combination of this drug by aerosol with beclomethasone aerosol (Beclovent, Vanceril) may increase the risk of toxicity due to fluorocarbon propellants. Best to use this aerosol 20 to 30 minutes **before** beclomethasone aerosol. This will reduce the risk of toxicity and will help beclomethasone get into the lungs.
 2. *Avoid excessive use of aerosol inhalation.* The excessive or prolonged use of this drug by inhalation can reduce its effectiveness and cause serious heart rhythm disturbances, including cardiac arrest.
 3. Do not use this drug concurrently with epinephrine. These two drugs may be used alternately if an interval of 4 hours is allowed between doses.
 4. If you do not respond to your usually effective dose, ask your physician for guidance. Do not increase the size or frequency of the dose without your physician's approval.

Precautions for Use
 By Infants and Children: Safety and effectiveness for those under 12 years of age not established.
 By Those over 60 Years of Age: Avoid excessive and continual use. If acute asthma is not relieved promptly, other drugs will be needed. Watch for nervousness, palpitations, irregular heart rhythm and muscle tremors. Use with extreme caution if you have hardening of the arteries, heart disease or high blood pressure.

▷ **Advisability of Use During Pregnancy**
 Pregnancy Category: B. See Pregnancy Code at the back of this book.
 Animal studies: No significant birth defects reported in mouse and rat studies.
 Human studies: Adequate studies of pregnant women are not available.
 Use only if clearly needed. Ask your physician for guidance.

Advisability of Use if Breast-Feeding
 Presence of this drug in breast milk: Yes.
 Monitor nursing infant closely and discontinue drug or nursing if adverse effects develop.

Habit-Forming Potential: None.

Effects of Overdosage: Nervousness, palpitation, rapid heart rate, sweating, headache, tremor, vomiting, chest pain.

Possible Effects of Long-Term Use: Loss of effectiveness. See *CAUTION* category above.

Suggested Periodic Examinations While Taking This Drug (at physician's discretion)
Blood pressure measurements, evaluation of heart status.

▷ **While Taking This Drug, Observe the Following**
Foods: No restrictions.
Beverages: Avoid excessive use of caffeine-containing beverages: coffee, tea, cola, chocolate.

▷ *Alcohol:* No interactions expected.
Tobacco Smoking: No interactions expected.

▷ *Other Drugs*
Terbutaline *taken concurrently* with
- monoamine oxidase (MAO) type A inhibitor drugs may cause excessive increase in blood pressure and undesirable heart stimulation (see Drug Classes).
- theophylline may cause decreased theophylline effectiveness.

The following drugs may *decrease* the effects of terbutaline
- beta blocker drugs may impair its effectiveness (see Drug Classes).

▷ *Driving, Hazardous Activities:* Usually no restrictions. Use caution if excessive nervousness or dizziness occurs.
Aviation Note: The use of this drug *is a disqualification* for piloting. Consult a designated Aviation Medical Examiner.
Exposure to Sun: No restrictions.
Heavy Exercise or Exertion: Use caution. Excessive exercise can induce asthma in some patients.

TERFENADINE (ter FEN a deen)

Introduced: 1977   **Prescription:** USA: Yes; Canada: No   **Available as Generic:** No   **Class:** Antihistamines   **Controlled Drug:** USA: No; Canada: No
Brand Names: ✦Contact Allergy Formula, Seldane, Seldane-D

BENEFITS versus RISKS	
Possible Benefits	*Possible Risks*
EFFECTIVE RELIEF OF ALLERGIC RHINITIS AND ALLERGIC SKIN DISORDERS	RARE HEART RHYTHM DISTURBANCES Infrequent headache Minor digestive disturbances Slight atropinelike effects

▷ **Principal Uses**
As a Single Drug Product: Uses currently included in FDA approved labeling:
(1) Provides symptomatic relief in allergic and related disorders: seasonal and perennial allergic rhinitis (hay fever), allergic conjunctivitis and vasomotor rhinitis.

Terfenadine

Other (unlabeled) generally accepted uses: (1) Helps relieve hives and localized swellings (angioedema) of allergic origin; (2) can decrease or prevent symptoms of grass pollen sensitive asthmatic patients; (3) relieves the symptoms of the common cold; (4) helps prevent exercise induced asthma; (5) can ease the blockage of eustachian tubes seen in otitis media.

How This Drug Works: Antihistamines reduce the intensity of the allergic response by blocking the action of histamine after it has been released from sensitized tissue cells in the eyes, nose and skin.

Available Dosage Forms and Strengths
Suspension — 30 mg per 5-ml teaspoonful (Canada)
Tablets — 60 mg

▷ **Usual Adult Dosage Range:** 60 mg every 12 hours as needed. The total daily dosage should not exceed 120 mg. **Note: Actual dosage and administration schedule must be determined by the physician for each patient individually.**

Conditions Requiring Dosing Adjustments
Liver function: This drug is extensively metabolized in the liver and it is contraindicated in liver compromise.
Kidney function: Changes in dosing do not appear to be needed in renal compromise.

▷ **Dosing Instructions:** The tablet may be crushed and taken with food or milk to prevent stomach irritation.

Usual Duration of Use: Use on a regular schedule for 2 to 3 days usually determines effectiveness in relieving the symptoms of allergic rhinitis and dermatosis. It may be necessary to take this drug throughout the entire pollen season, depending upon individual sensitivity. However, antihistamines should not be taken continually (without interruption) for long-term use. Limit their use to periods that require symptomatic relief. Consult your physician on a regular basis.

Possible Advantages of This Drug
Fast onset of action, relief within 1 hour.
No loss of effectiveness with continual use.
Little drowsiness or impaired mental function.

▷ **This Drug Should Not Be Taken If**
- you have had an allergic reaction to any dosage form of it previously.
- you are currently undergoing allergy skin tests.
- you have severely impaired liver function.
- you are taking erythromycin, clarithromycin, azithromycin, ketoconazole, itraconazole or troleandomycin.

▷ **Inform Your Physician Before Taking This Drug If**
- you have had any allergic reactions or unfavorable responses to antihistamines.
- you have a history of heart rhythm disorders.
- you have a history of liver disease.
- you have bronchial asthma.

Possible Side-Effects (natural, expected and unavoidable drug actions)
Dry nose, mouth or throat.

Terfenadine

▷ **Possible Adverse Effects** (unusual, unexpected and infrequent reactions)
  If any of the following develop, consult your physician promptly for guidance.
  Mild Adverse Effects
   Allergic Reactions: Skin rash, itching.
   Headache, nervousness, fatigue.
   Increased appetite, indigestion, nausea, vomiting.
  Serious Adverse Effects
   Significant heart rhythm disorders (resulting from excessive dosage or interactions with other drugs).
   Liver toxicity (rare).
▷ **Possible Effects on Sexual Function**
   Altered timing and pattern of menstruation.
   Female breast enlargement with milk production.
Possible Effects on Laboratory Tests
   None reported.
CAUTION
  1. Do not exceed recommended doses; high blood levels may cause serious heart rhythm disturbances.
  2. Do not take this drug concurrently with any form of erythromycin, ketoconazole (Nizoral), itraconazole or troleandomycin (TAO).
  3. Report promptly the development of faintness, dizziness, heart palpitation, or chest pain.
  4. Stop this drug 4 days before diagnostic skin testing procedures in order to prevent false negative test results.
  5. Do not use this drug if you have active bronchial asthma, bronchitis or pneumonia. It may thicken bronchial mucus and make it more difficult to remove (by absorption or coughing).
Precautions for Use
  By Infants and Children: Safety and effectiveness for those under 12 years of age are not established.
  By Those over 60 Years of Age: You may be more susceptible to the development of headache and fatigue. Use smaller doses at longer intervals if necessary.
▷ **Advisability of Use During Pregnancy**
  Pregnancy Category: C. See Pregnancy Code at the back of this book.
   Animal studies: No birth defects due to this drug reported.
   Human studies: Adequate studies of pregnant women are not available.
   Use this drug only if clearly needed. Ask your physician for guidance.
Advisability of Use if Breast-Feeding
   Presence of this drug in breast milk: Expected, but not well studied.
   Avoid drug or refrain from nursing.
Habit-Forming Potential: None.
Effects of Overdosage: Possible development of serious heart rhythm disturbances.
Possible Effects of Long-Term Use: None reported.
Suggested Periodic Examinations While Taking This Drug (at physician's discretion)
   Electrocardiograms for those with heart disorders.

▷ **While Taking This Drug, Observe the Following**
   Foods: No restrictions.
   Beverages: No restrictions. May be taken with milk.
▷ *Alcohol:* No interactions expected.
   Tobacco Smoking: No interactions expected.
▷ *Other Drugs:* Terfenadine **taken concurrently** with
   • carbamazepine (Tegretol) may result in carbamazepine toxicity.
   • fluoxetine may result in terfenadine toxicity.
   • ketoconazole (Nizoral) may cause increased blood levels of terfenadine resulting in serious heart rhythm disorders.
   • itraconazole (Sporanox) may cause increased blood levels of terfenadine resulting in serious heart rhythm disorders.
   • macrolide antibiotics (see Drug Classes): erythromycin, azithromycin, clarithromycin, troleandomycin, others, may cause increased blood levels of terfenadine resulting in serious heart rhythm disorders.
   • sotolol may result in abnormal and serious heart rhythm changes.
   Hazardous Activities: No restrictions.
   Aviation Note: The use of this drug *is probably not a disqualification* for piloting. Consult a designated Aviation Medical Examiner.
   Exposure to Sun: Rare cases of photosensitivity have been reported. Use caution.

TETRACYCLINE (te trah SI kleen)

Introduced: 1953   **Prescription:** USA: Yes; Canada: Yes   **Available as Generic:** Yes   **Class:** Antibiotic, tetracyclines   **Controlled Drug:** USA: No; Canada: No
Brand Names: Achromycin, Achromycin V, ✦Acrocidin, ✦Apo-Tetra, Actisite, Aureomycin, Contimycin, Cyclinex, Cyclopar, ✦Medicycline, Mysteclin-F [CD], ✦Neo-Tetrine, ✦Novo-Tetra, ✦Nor-Tet, ✦Novotetra, ✦Nu-Tetra, Panmycin, Retet, Robitet, SK-Tetracycline, Sumycin, Teline, Tetra-C, Tetracap, Tetra-Con, Tetracyn, Tetralan, Tetram, Tropicycline

BENEFITS versus RISKS	
Possible Benefits	*Possible Risks*
EFFECTIVE TREATMENT OF INFECTIONS due to susceptible bacteria and protozoa	ALLERGIC REACTIONS, mild to severe: ANAPHYLAXIS, DRUG-INDUCED HEPATITIS (rare)
	Drug-induced colitis
	Superinfections (bacterial or fungal)
	Rare blood cell disorders: hemolytic anemia, abnormally low white cell and platelet counts

▷ **Principal Uses**
   As a Single Drug Product: Uses currently included in FDA approved labeling: (1) Treats a broad range of infections caused by susceptible bacteria and protozoa (short-term use); and (2) treat severe, resistant pustular acne (long-term use); (3) used in a sustained release form (Actisite) to treat gum disease (periodontitis) in adults.

Tetracycline

Other (unlabeled) generally acepted uses: (1) Combination antibiotic treatment of duodenal ulcers caused by H. pylori; (2) used in vaginal and vulval cysts (gartner) and in vaginal hydrocele; (3) topical tetracycline is useful in chronic eye problems (blepharitis); (4) treats cancer (malignant) fluid (pericardial effusion) build up around the heart; (5) used to treat Stage One Lyme disease; (6) has a role in acne rosacea in decreasing the number of papules or nodules.

As a Combination Drug Product [CD]: This drug is available in combination with amphotericin B, an antifungal antibiotic that is provided to reduce the risk of developing an overgrowth of yeast organisms (superinfection) of the gastrointestinal tract.

How This Drug Works: This drug prevents the growth and multiplication of susceptible bacteria by interfering with their formation of essential proteins.

Available Dosage Forms and Strengths
- Capsules — 100 mg, 250 mg, 500 mg
- Ointment — 3%
- Ointment, ophthalmic — 10 mg per gram
- Solution, topical — 2.2 mg per ml
- Suspension, ophthalmic — 10 mg per ml
- Suspension, oral — 125 mg per 5-ml teaspoonful
- Tablets — 250 mg, 500 mg

▷ **Usual Adult Dosage Range:** 250 to 500 mg/6 hours, or 500 to 1000 mg/12 hours. The total daily dosage should not exceed 4000 mg (4 grams). **Note: Actual dosage and administration schedule must be determined by the physician for each patient individually.**

Conditions Requiring Dosing Adjustments
Liver function: Tetracycline is a cause of hepatoxicity. A benefit to risk decision should be made to use this drug in patients with compromised livers.
Kidney function: Patients with mild to moderate kidney failure can be given the usual dose every 8 to 12 hours. Patients with moderate to severe kidney failure can be given the usual dose every 12 to 24 hours. In severe kidney failure (creatinine clearance less than 10 ml/min), tetracycline should be avoided.

▷ **Dosing Instructions:** The tablet may be crushed and the capsule opened and preferably taken on an empty stomach, 1 hour before or 2 hours after eating. However, to reduce stomach irritation it may be taken with crackers that contain insignificant amounts of iron, calcium, magnesium or zinc. Avoid all dairy products for 2 hours before and after taking this drug. Take at the same time each day, with a full glass of water. Take the full course prescribed.

Usual Duration of Use: The time required to control the acute infection and be free of fever and symptoms for 48 hours. This varies with the nature of the infection. Long-term use (months to years, as for treatment of acne) requires supervision and periodic evaluation. Treatment of Stage One Lyme disease requires longer lengths of therapy (often 3 to 4 weeks). Consult your physician on a regular basis.

Currently a "Drug of Choice"
for the initial treatment of early Lyme disease. (Note: Children under 8 years of age and pregnant/breast-feeding women should use penicillin instead of tetracycline.)

▷ **This Drug Should Not Be Taken If**
- you are allergic to any tetracycline (see Drug Class Section).
- you are pregnant or breast-feeding.
- you have severe liver compromise.

▷ **Inform Your Physician Before Taking This Drug If**
- it is prescribed for a child under 8 years of age.
- you have a history of liver or kidney disease.
- you have systemic lupus erythematosus.
- you are taking any penicillin drug.
- you are taking any anticoagulant drug.
- you plan to have surgery under general anesthesia in the near future.

Possible Side-Effects (natural, expected and unavoidable drug actions)
Superinfections (see Glossary), often due to yeast organisms. These can occur in the mouth, intestinal tract, rectum and/or vagina, resulting in rectal and vaginal itching.
Tooth discoloration (when used in children less than 8 years old).

▷ **Possible Adverse Effects** (unusual, unexpected and infrequent reactions)
If any of the following develop, consult your physician promptly for guidance.
Mild Adverse Effects
Allergic Reactions: Skin rash, hives, itching of hands and feet, swelling of face or extremities.
Loss of appetite, stomach irritation, taste disorders, nausea, vomiting, diarrhea.
Warts (rare).
Irritation of mouth or tongue, "black tongue," sore throat, abdominal cramping or pain.
Serious Adverse Effects
Allergic Reactions: Anaphylactic reaction (see Glossary), asthma, fever, swollen joints and lymph glands.
Serious skin problems (Stenvens-Johnson syndrome, JH).
Drug-induced hepatitis with jaundice.
Permanent discoloration and/or malformation of teeth when taken under 8 years of age, including unborn child and infant.
Impaired vision, increased intracranial pressure.
Drug-induced colitis.
Drug-induced myasthenia gravis.
Worsening of existing systemic lupus erythematosus.
Pancreatitis (rare).
Rare blood cell disorders: hemolytic anemia (see Glossary); abnormally low white blood cell count, causing fever, sore throat and infections; abnormally low blood platelet count, causing abnormal bleeding or bruising.
Impairment of blood clotting.
Increased intracranial pressure (Pseudotumor cerebri).
Kidney problems (rare).

Tetracycline

Drug-induced porphyria.
Drug-induced low blood potassium.
Drug-induced esophageal ulcers.

▷ **Possible Effects on Sexual Function:** Decreased effectiveness of oral contraceptives taken concurrently (several case reports of pregnancy).
Decreased male fertility.

▷ **Adverse Effects That May Mimic Natural Diseases or Disorders**
Drug-induced hepatitis may suggest viral hepatitis.

Natural Diseases or Disorders That May Be Activated by This Drug
Systemic lupus erythematosus.

Possible Effects on Laboratory Tests
Complete blood cell counts: decreased red cells, hemoglobin, white cells and platelets; increased eosinophils (allergic reaction).
Blood lupus erythematosus (LE) cells: positive.
Blood amylase level: increased (toxic effect in pregnant women).
Liver function tests: increased liver enzymes (ALT/GPT, AST/GOT and alkaline phosphatase), increased bilirubin.
Kidney function tests: increased blood creatinine and urea nitrogen (BUN) levels (kidney damage).
Urine sugar tests: false positive results with Benedict's solution and Clinitest.

CAUTION
1. Antacids, dairy products and preparations containing aluminum, bismuth, calcium, iron, magnesium or zinc can prevent adequate absorption of this drug and reduce its effectiveness significantly.
2. Troublesome and persistent diarrhea can develop. If diarrhea persists for more than 24 hours, stop this drug and call your doctor.
3. If general anesthesia is required while taking this drug, the choice of anesthetic agent must be selected carefully to prevent kidney damage.

Precautions for Use
By Infants and Children: If possible, tetracyclines should not be given to children under 8 years of age because of the risk of permanent discoloration and deformity of the teeth. Rarely, infants may develop increased intracranial pressure within the first 4 days of receiving this drug. Tetracyclines may inhibit normal bone growth and development.
By Those over 60 Years of Age: Dosage must be carefully individualized based on kidney function. Natural skin changes may predispose to severe and prolonged itching reactions in the genital and anal regions.

▷ **Advisability of Use During Pregnancy**
Pregnancy Category: D. See Pregnancy Code at the back of this book.
Animal studies: Tetracycline causes limb defects in rats, rabbits and chickens.
Human studies: Information from studies of pregnant women indicates that this drug can cause impaired development and discoloration of teeth and other developmental defects.
It is advisable to avoid this drug completely during entire pregnancy.

Advisability of Use if Breast-Feeding
Presence of this drug in breast milk: Yes.
Avoid drug or refrain from nursing.

Tetracycline

Habit-Forming Potential: None.

Effects of Overdosage: Stomach burning, nausea, vomiting, diarrhea.

Possible Effects of Long-Term Use: Superinfections; rarely, impairment of bone marrow, liver or kidney function.

Suggested Periodic Examinations While Taking This Drug (at physician's discretion)
Complete blood cell counts, liver and kidney function tests.
During extended use, sputum and stool examinations may detect early superinfection due to yeast organisms.

▷ **While Taking This Drug, Observe the Following**
Foods: Avoid cheeses, yogurt, ice cream, iron-fortified cereals and supplements and meats for 2 hours before and after taking this drug. Calcium and iron can combine with this drug and reduce its absorption significantly.
Beverages: Avoid all forms of milk for 2 hours before and after taking this drug.

▷ *Alcohol:* No interactions expected. However, it is best avoided if you have active liver disease.
Tobacco Smoking: No interactions expected.

▷ Other Drugs
Tetracyclines may *increase* the effects of
- oral anticoagulants such as warfarin (Coumadin), and make it necessary to reduce their dosage.
- digoxin (Lanoxin), and cause digitalis toxicity.
- lithium (Eskalith, Lithane, etc.), and increase the risk of lithium toxicity.

Tetracyclines may *decrease* the effects of
- birth control pills (oral contraceptives), and impair their effectiveness in preventing pregnancy.
- penicillins, and impair their effectiveness in treating infections.

Tetracyclines *taken concurrently* with
- isotretinoin may worsen tetracycline induced increased intracranial pressure and cause additive toxicity.
- methoxyflurane anesthesia may impair kidney function.
- warfarin poses an increased risk of bleeding. INR (prothrombin testing) should be checked more frequently, and doses adjusted if needed.

The following drugs may *decrease* the effects of tetracyclines
- antacids (aluminum and magnesium preparations, sodium bicarbonate, etc.) may reduce drug absorption.
- bismuth subsalicylate (Pepto Bismol).
- cholestyramine and other cholesterol lowering resins.
- iron, zinc and mineral preparations may reduce drug absorption.
- sucralfate.

▷ *Driving, Hazardous Activities:* Usually no restrictions. However, this drug may cause nausea or diarrhea. Restrict activities as necessary.
Aviation Note: The use of this drug *may be a disqualification* for piloting. Consult a designated Aviation Medical Examiner.
Exposure to Sun: Use caution. Some tetracyclines can cause photosensitivity (see Glossary).

THEOPHYLLINE (thee OFF i lin)

Introduced: 1900 **Prescription:** USA: Yes; Canada: Yes **Available as Generic:** Yes **Class:** Antiasthmatic, bronchodilator, xanthines **Controlled Drug:** USA: No; Canada: No

Brand Names: Accurbron, ✦Acet-Am, Aerolate, Aminodrox-Forte, ✦Apo-Oxtriphylline, ✦Aquaphyllim, ✦Asbron [CD], Asmalix, Azpan, Brocomar, Bronchial Gelatin Capsule, Broncomar, Bronkotabs, Bronkaid Tablets [CD], Bronkodyl, Bronkolixir [CD], Bronkotabs [CD], Constant-T, Duraphyl, Elixicon, Elixomin, Elixophyllin, For-Az-Ma [CD], Isuprel Compound [CD], Labid, Lanophyllin, Lixolin, Lodrane, Lodrane CR, Marax [CD], Marax DF [CD], Mudrane GG Elixir [CD], Phedral [CD], Physpan, ✦PMS Theophylline, Primatene, ✦Pulmophylline, Quadrinal [CD], Quibron [CD], Quibron-300 [CD], Quibron Plus [CD], Quibron-T Dividose, Quibron-T/SR, Respbid, Slo-bid, Slo-bid Gyrocaps, Slo-Phyllin, Slo-Phyllin GG [CD], Slo-Phyllin Gyrocaps, Somophyllin, Sompphyllin-12, Sustaire, Tedral [CD], Tedral SA [CD], T.E.H. [CD], T.E.P., Thalfed, Theobid Duracaps, ✦Theo-Bronc, Theochron, Theoclear, Theoclear L.A., Theocord, Theo-Dur, Theolair, Theolate [CD], Theolixir, Theomar [CD], Theomax DF, Theon, Theophyl-SR, Theo-24, Theospan-SR, Theo-SR, Theo-Time, Theovent, Theox, Theozine, Therex [CD], ✦Uniphyl, Vitaphen [CD]

BENEFITS versus RISKS	
Possible Benefits	*Possible Risks*
EFFECTIVE PREVENTION AND RELIEF OF ACUTE BRONCHIAL ASTHMA	NARROW TREATMENT RANGE FREQUENT STOMACH DISTRESS Gastrointestinal bleeding
MODERATELY EFFECTIVE CONTROL OF CHRONIC, RECURRENT BRONCHIAL ASTHMA	Central nervous system toxicity, seizures Heart rhythm disturbances
Moderately effective symptomatic relief in chronic bronchitis and emphysema	

▷ **Principal Uses**

As a Single Drug Product: Uses currently included in FDA approved labeling: (1) Used to relieve shortness of breath and wheezing of acute bronchial asthma, and to prevent the recurrence of asthmatic episodes; (2) It is also useful in relieving the asthmaticlike symptoms that are associated with some types of chronic bronchitis, chronic obstructive pulmonary disease and emphysema.

Other (unlabeled) generally accepted uses: (1) May have a role in combination therapy of cystic fibrosis; (2) can help decrease excessive production of red blood cells in kidney transplant patients; (3) may have a role in helping decrease the risk of sudden infant death syndrome; (4) may have a supportive role with steroids and other agents in helping prevent rejection of transplanted kidneys; (5) can help ease essential tremor; (6) decreases risk of breathing cessation in neonatal apnea; (7) helps in treating SIDS children; (8) may have a role in sleep apnea.

As a Combination Drug Product [CD]: Available in combination with several other drugs that help in overall management of bronchial asthma and related conditions. Ephedrine is added to enhance the bronchodilator effects; guaifenesin is added to provide an expectorant effect that thins mucus in the bronchial tubes; mild sedatives such as phenobarbital are added to allay the anxiety that often accompanies acute attacks of asthma.

How This Drug Works: By inhibiting the enzyme phosphodiesterase, this drug produces an increase in the tissue chemical cyclic AMP. This causes relaxation of the muscles in the bronchial tubes and blood vessels of the lung, resulting in relief of bronchospasm, expanded lung capacity and improved lung circulation.

Available Dosage Forms and Strengths
Capsules — 100 mg, 200 mg, 250 mg, 260 mg
Capsules, prolonged-action — 50 mg, 60 mg, 65 mg, 75 mg, 100 mg, 125 mg, 130 mg, 200 mg, 250 mg, 260 mg, 300 mg
Elixir — 27 mg, 50 mg per 5-ml teaspoonful
Oral solution — 27 mg, 53.3 mg per 5-ml teaspoonful
Oral suspension — 100 mg per 5-ml teaspoonful
Syrup — 27 mg, 50 mg per 5-ml teaspoonful
Tablets — 100 mg, 125 mg, 200 mg, 250 mg, 300 mg
Tablets, prolonged-action — 100 mg, 200 mg, 250 mg, 300 mg, 400 mg, 450 mg, 500 mg, 600 mg

▷ **Recommended Dosage Ranges** (Actual dosage and administration schedule must be determined by the physician for each patient individually.)
Infants and Children: For acute attack of asthma (not currently taking theophylline)—loading dose of 5 to 6 mg/kg of body weight.
For acute attack while currently taking theophylline—a single dose of 2.5 mg/kg of body weight, if no indications of theophylline toxicity. Monitor blood levels of theophylline.
For maintenance during acute attack—dosage is based on age:
Up to 6 months of age—0.07 for each week of age + 1.7 = the mg/kg of body weight, given every 8 hours.
6 months to 1 year of age—0.05 for each week of age + 1.25 = the mg/kg of body weight, given every 6 hours.
1 to 9 years of age—5 mg/kg of body weight, every 6 hours.
9 to 12 years of age—4 mg/kg of body weight, every 6 hours.
12 to 16 years of age—3 mg/kg of body weight, every 6 hours.
For chronic treatment to prevent recurrence of asthma—dosage is based on age:
Initially 16 mg/kg of body weight, in 3 or 4 divided doses at 6 to 8 hour intervals, up to a maximum of 400 mg daily. Increase dose as needed and tolerated by increments of 25% every 2 to 3 days. Limit total daily dosage as follows:
Up to 1 year of age—0.3 for each week of age + 8.0 = the mg/kg of body weight, per day.
1 to 9 years of age—22 mg/kg of body weight, per day.
9 to 12 years of age—20 mg/kg of body weight, per day.
12 to 16 years of age—18 mg/kg of body weight, per day.
16 years of age and over—13 mg/kg of body weight or 900 mg per day, whichever is less.

Theophylline

Note: It is advisable to measure blood levels of theophylline periodically during chronic therapy.

16 to 60 Years of Age: For acute attack of asthma (not currently taking theophylline)—loading dose of 5 to 6 mg/kg of body weight.

For acute attack while currently taking theophylline—a single dose of 2.5 mg/kg of body weight, if no indications of theophylline toxicity. Monitor blood levels of theophylline.

For maintenance during acute attack—for nonsmokers: 3 mg/kg of body weight, every 8 hours; for smokers: 4 mg/kg of body weight, every 6 hours.

For chronic treatment to prevent recurrence of asthma—Initially 6 to 8 mg/kg of body weight, in 3 or 4 divided doses at 6 to 8 hour intervals, up to a maximum of 400 mg daily. Increase dose as needed and tolerated by increments of 25% every 2 to 3 days. The total daily dosage should not exceed 13 mg/kg of body weight or 900 mg, whichever is less.

Over 60 Years of Age: For acute attack—same as 16 to 60 years of age.

For maintenance during acute attack—2 mg/kg of body weight, every 8 hours.

Conditions Requiring Dosing Adjustments

Liver function: The dose **must** be lowered, and blood levels obtained frequently.

Kidney function: Levels should be followed closely in severe kidney failure.

▷ **Dosing Instructions:** May be taken with or following food to reduce stomach irritation. The regular capsules may be opened and the regular tablets may be crushed for administration. The prolonged-action dosage forms should be swallowed whole and not altered. Shake the oral suspension well before measuring each dose. Do not refrigerate any liquid dosage forms of this drug.

Usual Duration of Use: Use on a regular schedule for 48 to 72 hours usually determines effectiveness in controlling the breathing impairment associated with bronchial asthma and chronic lung disease. Long-term use (months to years) requires supervision and periodic physician evaluation.

▷ **This Drug Should Not Be Taken If**
- you have had an allergic reaction to it, or to aminophylline, dyphylline or oxtriphylline.
- you have active peptic ulcer disease.
- you have an uncontrolled seizure disorder.

▷ **Inform Your Physician Before Taking This Drug If**
- you have had an unfavorable reaction to any xanthine (see Drug Class Section).
- you have a seizure disorder of any kind.
- you have a history of peptic ulcer disease.
- you have impaired liver or kidney function.
- you take any of the drugs listed in the "Other Drugs" section.
- you have hypertension, heart disease or any type of heart rhythm disorder.

Possible Side-Effects (natural, expected and unavoidable drug actions)

Nervousness, insomnia, rapid heart rate, increased urine volume.

▷ **Possible Adverse Effects** (unusual, unexpected and infrequent reactions)
   If any of the following develop, consult your physician promptly for guidance.
   Mild Adverse Effects
   Allergic Reactions: Skin rash, hives.
   Headache, dizziness, irritability, tremor, fatigue, weakness.
   Loss of appetite, nausea, vomiting, abdominal pain, diarrhea, excessive thirst.
   Flushing of face.
   Serious Adverse Effects
   Idiosyncratic Reactions: Marked anxiety, confusion, behavioral disturbances.
   Central nervous system toxicity: muscle twitching, seizures.
   Heart rhythm abnormalities, rapid breathing, low blood pressure.
   Gastrointestinal bleeding.
   Defects in clotting (coagulation).
   Drug-induced abnormal urine production (SIADH) (rare).
   Drug-induced porphyria (rare).
   Worsening of ulcers.
   Liver toxicity.
   Serious skin disorder (Stevens-Johnson syndrome).
▷ **Possible Effects on Sexual Function:** None reported.
  Natural Diseases or Disorders That May Be Activated by This Drug
   Latent peptic ulcer disease.
  Possible Effects on Laboratory Tests
   Blood uric acid level: increased.
   Fecal occult blood test: positive (large doses may cause stomach bleeding).
  CAUTION
   1. This drug should not be taken at the same time as other antiasthmatic drugs unless your doctor prescribes the combination. Serious overdose could result.
   2. Influenza vaccine may delay the elimination of this drug and cause accumulation to toxic levels.
  Precautions for Use
   By Infants and Children: Do not exceed recommended doses. Watch for toxicity: irritability, agitation, tremors, lethargy, fever, vomiting, rapid heart rate and breathing, seizures. Blood levels needed during long-term use.
   By Those over 60 Years of Age: Small starting doses are indicated. You may be at increased risk for stomach irritation, nausea, vomiting or diarrhea. When used concurrently with coffee (caffeine) or with nasal decongestants, this drug may cause excessive stimulation and a hyperactivity syndrome.
▷ **Advisability of Use During Pregnancy**
   Pregnancy Category: C. See Pregnancy Code at the back of this book.
   Animal studies: Significant birth defects due to this drug reported in mice.
   Human studies: Adequate studies of pregnant women are not available. No increase in birth defects reported in 394 exposures to this drug.
   Avoid this drug during the first 3 months. Use it otherwise only if clearly needed. Ask your physician for guidance.

Theophylline

Advisability of Use if Breast-Feeding
Presence of this drug in breast milk: Yes.
Avoid drug or refrain from nursing.

Habit-Forming Potential: None.

Effects of Overdosage: Nausea, vomiting, restlessness, irritability, confusion, delirium, seizures, high fever, weak pulse, coma.

Possible Effects of Long-Term Use: Gastrointestinal irritation.

Suggested Periodic Examinations While Taking This Drug (at physician's discretion)
Periodic testing of blood theophylline levels, especially with high dosage or long-term use. (See Therapeutic Drug Monitoring Section.)
Time to sample blood for theophylline level: 2 hours after regular (standard) dosage forms; 5 hours after sustained-release dosage forms.
Recommended therapeutic range: 10 to 20 mcg/ml.

▷ **While Taking This Drug, Observe the Following**
Foods: No restrictions.
Beverages: Avoid excessive use of caffeine-containing beverages: coffee, tea, cola; this combination could cause nervousness and insomnia.
▷ *Alcohol:* No interactions expected. May have additive effect on stomach irritation.
Tobacco Smoking: May hasten the elimination of this drug and reduce its effectiveness. Higher doses may be necessary to maintain a therapeutic blood level.

▷ *Other Drugs*
Theophylline may *decrease* the effects of
- lithium (Lithane, Lithobid, etc.), and reduce its effectiveness.

Theophylline *taken concurrently* with
- halothane (anesthesia) may cause heart rhythm abnormalities.
- phenytoin (Dilantin) may cause decreased effects of both drugs. Monitor blood levels and adjust dosages as appropriate.

The following drugs may *increase* the effects of theophylline
- allopurinol (Lopurin, Zyloprim).
- cimetidine (Tagamet).
- ciprofloxacin (Cipro).
- clarithromycin and perhaps azithromycin.
- disulfiram (Antabuse).
- doxycycline and other tetracyclines.
- enoxacin.
- ephedrine.
- erythromycin (E-Mycin, Erythrocin, etc.).
- imipenem-cilastatin (Primaxin).
- influenza vaccine.
- interferon alpha.
- isoniazid.
- mexiletine (Mexitil).
- nicotine (Nicorette, Pro-Step, others).
- norfloxacin (Noroxin).
- oral contraceptives.
- ranitidine (Zantac).

- tacrine (Cognex).
- thiabendazole.
- ticlopidine (Ticlid).
- troleandomycin (TAO).
- verapamil.
- viloxazine.

The following drugs may *decrease* the effects of theophylline
- barbiturates (phenobarbital, etc.).
- beta blocker drugs (see Drug Classes).
- carbamazepine (Tegretol).
- isoproterenol.
- primidone (Mysoline).
- rifampin (Rifadin, Rimactane, etc.).
- sulfinpyrazone.

▷ *Driving, Hazardous Activities:* This drug may cause dizziness. Restrict activities as necessary.

Aviation Note: The use of this drug *may be a disqualification* for piloting. Consult a designated Aviation Medical Examiner.

Exposure to Sun: No restrictions.

Occurrence of Unrelated Illness: Acute viral respiratory infections may decrease drug elimination. Watch for signs of toxicity. Dosing **must** be changed if this occurs.

Discontinuation: Avoid prolonged or unnecessary use of this drug. When your asthma resolves, withdraw this drug gradually over several days.

THIAZIDE DIURETICS

Hydrochlorothiazide (hi droh klor oh THI a zide) **Chlorothiazide** (KLOR oh THI a zide) **Methyclothiazide** (METHI klo THI a zide) **Trichlormethiazide** (TRY klor me THI azide) **Chlorthalidone** (KLOR thal i dohn) **metolazone** (me TOHL a zohn)

Introduced: 1959, 1957, 1959, 1962, 1960, 1974   **Prescription:** USA: Yes; Canada: Yes   **Available as Generic:** USA: Yes; Canada: Yes   **Class:** Antihypertensive, diuretic, thiazides   **Controlled Drug:** USA: No; Canada: No

Brand Names: Hydrochlorothiazide: Aldactazide [CD], Aldoril-15/25 [CD], Aldoril D30/D50 [CD], ♦Apo-Amilzide, ♦Apo-Hydro, ♦Apo-Methazide [CD], ♦Apo-Triazide [CD], Apresazide [CD], Apresoline-Esidrix [CD], Capozide [CD], ♦Co-Betaloc [CD], Diaqua, ♦Diuchlor H, Dyazide [CD], Esidrix, H-H-R, H.H.R., HydroDIURIL, Hydromal, Hydropres [CD], Hydroserpine [CD], Hdroserpine Plus [CD], Hydro-T, Hydro-Z-50, Inderide [CD], Inderide LA [CD], ♦Ismelin-Esidrix [CD], Lopressor HCT [CD], Maxzide [CD], Maxzide-25 [CD], M Dopazide [CD], Mictrin, ♦Moduret [CD], Moduretic [CD], ♦Natrimax, ♦Neo-Codema, Normozide [CD], ♦Novo-Doparil [CD], ♦Novo-Hydrazide, ♦Novo-Spirozine [CD], ♦Novo-Triamzide [CD], Oretic, Oreticyl [CD], ♦PMS Dopazide [CD], Prinzide [CD], Ser-Ap-Es [CD], Serpasil-Esidrix [CD], SK-Hydrochlorothiazide, Thiuretic, Timolide [CD], Trandate HCT [CD], Unipres [CD], ♦Urozide, Vaseretic [CD], ♦Viskazide [CD], Zestoretic [CD], Ziac, Zide, Chlorothiazide: Aldochlor [CD], Diachlor, Diupres [CD], Diurigen, Diuril, SK-Chlorothiazide, ◆Supres [CD], Methyclothiazide: ◆Duretic, Aquatensen, ◆Duretic, Enduron, Trichlormethiazide: Diurese, Marazide II, Metahydrin, Naqua, Naquival [CD], Chlorthalidone: ◆Apo-Chlorthalidone, Combipress [CD], Demi-Regroton [CD], Hygroton, ◆Hygroton-Resperpine [CD], Hylidone, ◆Novothalidone, Regroton [CD], Thalitone, ◆Uridon, Tenoretic, Metolazone: Diulo, Microx, Mykrox, Zaroxolyn

---

BENEFITS versus RISKS

Possible Benefits	*Possible Risks*
EFFECTIVE, WELL-TOLERATED DIURETICS	Loss of body potassium and magnesium
POSSIBLY EFFECTIVE IN MILD HYPERTENSION	(Especialy with higher doses)
ENHANCES EFFECTIVENESS OF OTHER ANTIHYPERTENSIVES	Cardiac arrhythmias caused by decreased electrolytes
Beneficial in treatment of diabetes insipidus	(Recently studied in chlorthalidone and hydrochlorothiazide)
	Increased blood sugar
	Increased blood uric acid
	Increased blood calcium
	Rare blood cell disorders
	Rare liver toxicity (chlorothiazide or hydrochlorothiazide)

▷ **Principal Uses**

As a Single Drug Product: Uses currently included in FDA approved labeling: (1) increase the volume of urine (diuresis) to correct fluid retention (edema) seen in congestive heart failure, corticosteroid or estrogen use and certain types of liver and kidney disease; and (2) starting therapy for high blood pressure (hypertension).

Other (unlabeled) generally accepted uses: (1) Prevention of kidney stones that contain calcium; (2) may help decrease the frequency of hip fractures in the elderly; (3) methyclothiazide has been used to help maintain blood calcium levels in Paget's disease.

As a Combination Drug Product [CD]: Used to treat blood pressure that has not responded to single drug therapy.

How These Drugs Work: By increasing the elimination of salt and water in the urine, these drugs reduce fluid volume and body sodium. They also relax the walls of smaller arteries and the combined effect of these two actions (reduced blood volume in expanded space) results in lowering of the blood pressure.

Available Dosage Forms and Strengths

Hydrochlorothiazide:
 Solution — 50 mg per 5-ml teaspoonful
 Solution, intensol — 100 mg per ml
 Tablets — 25 mg, 50 mg, 100 mg
Chlorothiazide:
 Injection — 500 mg per 20 ml
 Oral suspension — 250 mg per 5 ml teaspoonful
 Tablets — 250 mg, 500 mg

Methyclothiazide:
    Tablets — 2.5 mg, 5 mg
Trichlormethiazide:
    Tablets — 2 mg, 4 mg
Chlorthalidone:
    Tablets — 25 mg, 50 mg, 100 mg
Metolazone:
    Tablets — 0.5 mg, 2.5 mg, 5 mg, 10 mg

▷ **Usual Adult Dosage Range:** Hydrochlorothiazide: As antihypertensive: 50 to 100 mg/day initially; 50 to 200 mg/day for maintenance. As diuretic: 50 to 200 mg/day initially; the smallest effective dose should be determined (see *CAUTIONS*). The total daily dose should not exceed 200 mg, however, this maximum may change in light of recent data.

Chlorothiazide: As antihypertensive: 500 to 1000 mg per day to start and 500 to 2000 mg daily as a maintenance dose. As a diuretic: 500 to 2000 mg per day with use of the smallest effective dose. Daily maximum is 2000 mg.

Methyclothiazide: As antihypertensive or diuretic: 2.5 to 5 mg daily are used. Maximum daily diuretic dose is 10 mg. Pediatric dose: 0.05 to 0.2 mg per kg daily.

Trichlormethiazide: As antihypertensive or diuretic: Therapy may be started with 1 to 4 mg twice daily. Usual maintenance dose is 1 to 4 mg once daily.

Chlorthalidone as antihypertensive: 25 to 50 mg daily to start therapy, then 50 to 100 mg for maintenance. As a diuretic: 50 to 100 mg daily, then maintenance with the smallest effective dose (see *CAUTIONS*). Daily maximum is 200 mg, however, this may change with recently published data.

Note: Actual dosage and administration schedule must be determined by the physician for each patient individually.

Conditions Requiring Dosing Adjustments

Liver function: Electrolyte balance is critical in liver failure, and these drugs may precipitate encephalopathy. Hydrochlorothiazide and chlorothiazide are also a rare cause of cholestatic jaundice and are used with caution in liver failure.

Kidney function: These drugs can be used with caution in patients with mild kidney failure, and are not effective in patients with moderate failure. Contraindicated in patients severe kidney failure, and can be a rare cause of kidney damage.

▷ **Dosing Instructions:** The tablets may be crushed and taken with or following meals to reduce stomach irritation. Best taken in the morning to avoid nighttime urination.

Usual Duration of Use: Use on a regular schedule for 2 to 3 weeks determines effectiveness in lowering high blood pressure. Long-term use (months to years) requires periodic physician evaluation.

▷ **These Drugs Should Not Be Taken If**
- you have had an allergic reaction to any dosage form of it previously.
- your kidneys are not making urine.

▷ **Inform Your Physician Before Taking These Drugs If**
- you are allergic to any form of "sulfa" drug.
- you are pregnant or planning pregnancy.
- you have a history of kidney or liver disease.
- you have a history of pancreatitis.
- you have asthma or allergies to other medicines.
- you have diabetes, gout or lupus erythematosus.
- you take any form of cortisone, digitalis, oral antidiabetic drug or insulin.
- you plan to have surgery under general anesthesia in the near future.

Possible Side-Effects (natural, expected and unavoidable drug actions)
Light-headedness on arising from sitting or lying position (see Orthostatic Hypotension in Glossary).
Increase in blood sugar level, affecting control of diabetes.
Increase in blood uric acid level, affecting control of gout.
Decrease in blood potassium level, causing muscle weakness and cramping.
Decreased blood magnesium, combined with loss of potassium may lead to increased risk of sudden cardiac death, especially if high doses are used for extended periods.

▷ **Possible Adverse Effects** (unusual, unexpected and infrequent reactions)
If any of the following develop, consult your physician promptly for guidance.

Mild Adverse Effects
Allergic Reactions: Skin rashes, hives, drug fever.
Headache, dizziness, blurred or yellow vision.
Reduced appetite, indigestion, nausea, vomiting, diarrhea.

Serious Adverse Effects
Allergic Reactions: Hepatitis with jaundice (see Glossary), anaphylactic reaction (see Glossary), severe skin reactions.
Inflammation of the pancreas—severe abdominal pain.
Bone marrow depression (see Glossary)—fatigue, weakness, fever, sore throat, abnormal bleeding or bruising.
Data from studies of hydrochlorothiazide and chlorthalidone suggest that potassium and magnesium loss associated with higher dose therapy increases the risk of sudden cardiac death.

▷ **Possible Effects on Sexual Function:** Decreased libido (hydrochlorothiazide, chlorthalidone); impotence (chlorothiazide, hydrochlorothiazide).

▷ **Adverse Effects That May Mimic Natural Diseases or Disorders**
Liver reaction may suggest viral hepatitis.

Natural Diseases or Disorders That May Be Activated by These Drugs
Diabetes, gout, systemic lupus erythematosus. People with asthma or other drug allergies may be more likely to have allergic reactions.

Possible Effects on Laboratory Tests
Complete blood counts: decreased red cells, hemoglobin, white cells and platelets.
Blood amylase level: increased (possible pancreatitis).
Blood calcium level: increased.
Blood sodium and chloride levels: decreased.
Blood cholesterol and triglyceride levels: increased, short-term.

Blood glucose level: increased.
Glucose tolerance test (GTT): decreased.
Blood lithium level: increased.
Blood potassium and magnesium level: decreased.
Blood urea nitrogen (BUN) level: increased with long-term use.
Blood uric acid level: increased.
Liver function tests (hydrochlorothiazide and chlorothiazide): increased liver enzymes (ALT/GPT, AST/GOT and alkaline phosphatase), increased bilirubin.

CAUTION
1. A recent study found a strong association between higher doses of hydrochlorothiazide and chlorthalidone and combination drugs containing these diuretics and electrolyte loss and sudden cardiac death. This did appear to be a result of magnesium and potassium loss, and may be circumvented by close following of those electrolytes.
2. Take exactly as prescribed. Excessive loss of sodium and potassium can lead to loss of appetite, nausea, fatigue, weakness, confusion and tingling in the extremities.
3. If you take digitalis (digitoxin, digoxin), adequate potassium is critical. Periodic testing and high-potassium foods may be needed to prevent potassium deficiency—a potential cause of digitalis toxicity. (See Table of High Potassium Foods in Section Six.)

Precautions for Use
By Infants and Children: Overdose could cause serious dehydration. Significant potassium loss can occur within the first 2 weeks of drug use.
By Those over 60 Years of Age: Starting doses may be as low as 12.5 mg. Increased risk of impaired thinking, orthostatic hypotension, potassium loss and blood sugar increase. Overdose or extended use can cause excessive loss of body water, thickening (increased viscosity) of blood and increased tendency for the blood to clot—predisposing to stroke, heart attack or thrombophlebitis (vein inflammation with blood clot).

▷ **Advisability of Use During Pregnancy**
Pregnancy Category: Metolazone: B by manufacturer, D by other independent researchers. All other thiazides in this class are D. See Pregnancy Code at the back of this book.
Animal studies: No birth defects found in rat studies.
Human studies: Reports are conflicting and inconclusive. Use of thiazides can acuse a variety of maternal complications which may cause adverse fetal effects, including death. They should not be used during pregnancy unless a very serious complication occurs for which this drug is significantly beneficial. Ask physician for guidance.

Advisability of Use if Breast-Feeding
Presence of these drugs in breast milk: Yes.
Avoid drug or refrain from nursing.

Habit-Forming Potential: None.

Effects of Overdosage: Dry mouth, thirst, lethargy, weakness, muscle cramping, nausea, vomiting, drowsiness progressing to stupor or coma.

Possible Effects of Long-Term Use: Impaired balance of water, salt, magnesium and potassium in blood and body tissues. Development of diabetes in predisposed individuals. Pathological changes in parathyroid glands with increased blood calcium levels and decreased blood phosphate levels.

Suggested Periodic Examinations While Taking These Drugs (at physician's discretion)
  Complete blood cell counts, measurements of blood levels of sodium, potassium, chloride, sugar and uric acid.
  Kidney and liver function tests.

▷ **While Taking These Drugs, Observe the Following**
  Foods: Ask your doctor if you need to eat foods rich in potassium. See the Table of High Potassium Foods if needed. Follow physician's advice regarding the use of salt. Magnesium should be routinely checked, and supplemented if these medicines have lowered blood levels.
  Beverages: No restrictions. This drug may be taken with milk.
▷ *Alcohol:* Use with caution—alcohol may exaggerate the blood-pressure-lowering effects of this drug and cause orthostatic hypotension.
  Tobacco Smoking: No interactions expected. Follow physician's advice.
▷ *Other Drugs*
  These drugs may *increase* the effects of
  • other antihypertensive drugs; dosage adjustments may be necessary to prevent excessive lowering of blood pressure.
  • lithium, and cause lithium toxicity.
  These drugs may *decrease* the effects of
  • oral antidiabetic drugs (sulfonylureas); dosage adjustments may be necessary for proper control of blood sugar.
  • oral anticoagulants such as warfarin (Coumadin) and require dose adjustments.
  These drugs *taken concurrently* with
  • digitalis preparations (digitoxin, digoxin) requires careful monitoring and dose changes to prevent low potassium levels and serious disturbances of heart rhythm.
  • allopurinol (Zyloprim) may decrease kidney function.
  • calcium may result in the Milk-alkali syndrome: with increased calcium, alkalosis and kidney failure.
  • carbamazepine (Tegretol) may result in low sodium levels and symptomatic hyponatremia.
  • cortisone or other corticosteroid medicines may result in excessive potassium loss with resultant heart rhythm changes and lethargy.
  • nonsteroidal antiinflammatory drugs such as sulindac (Clinoril) and naproxen (Naprosyn, Aleve, Anaprox, others) may result in decreased effectiveness of the thiazide.
  The following drugs may *decrease* the effects of these thiazides
  • cholestyramine (Cuemid, Questran) may interfere with its absorption.
  • colestipol (Colestid) may interfere with its absorption.
  Take cholestyramine and colestipol 1 hour before any oral diuretic.
▷ *Driving, Hazardous Activities:* Use caution until the possible occurrence of orthostatic hypotension, dizziness or impaired vision has been determined.

Aviation Note: The use of this drug **may be a disqualification** for piloting. Consult a designated Aviation Medical Examiner.

Exposure to Sun: Use caution until sensitivity has been determined. This drug can cause photosensitivity (see Glossary).

Exposure to Heat: Caution—excessive perspiring could cause additional loss of salt and water from the body.

Heavy Exercise or Exertion: Avoid exertion that produces light-headedness, excessive fatigue or muscle cramping. Isometric exercises can raise blood pressure significantly. Ask doctor for help regarding participation in this form of exercise.

Occurrence of Unrelated Illness: Vomiting or diarrhea can produce a serious imbalance of important body chemistry. Consult your physician for guidance.

Discontinuation: These drugs should not be stopped abruptly following long-term use; sudden discontinuation can cause serious thiazide-withdrawal fluid retention (edema). The dose should be reduced gradually. It may be advisable to discontinue this drug 5 to 7 days before major surgery. Ask your physician, surgeon and/or anesthesiologist for guidance.

THIORIDAZINE (thi oh RID a zeen)

Introduced: 1959 **Prescription:** USA: Yes; Canada: Yes **Available as Generic:** USA: Yes; Canada: Yes **Class:** Strong tranquilizer, phenothiazines **Controlled Drug:** USA: No; Canada: No

Brand Names: ✦Apo-Thioridazine, Mellaril, Mellaril-S, Millazine, ✦Novoridazine, ✦PMS-Thioridazine, SK-Thioridazine

BENEFITS versus RISKS	
Possible Benefits	*Possible Risks*
EFFECTIVE CONTROL OF ACUTE MENTAL DISORDERS in the majority of patients: beneficial effects on thinking, mood and behavior	SERIOUS TOXIC EFFECTS ON BRAIN with long-term use
	Liver damage with jaundice (infrequent)
Relief of anxiety, agitation and tension	Rare blood cell disorders: abnormally low white blood cell count
Possibly effective in the management of the hyperactivity syndrome in children	

▷ **Principal Uses**

As a Single Drug Product: Uses currently included in FDA approved labeling: (1) Helps manage: moderate to marked depression with significant anxiety and nervous tension; agitation, anxiety, depression and exaggerated fears in the elderly; (2) of use in severe behavioral problems in children characterized by hyperexcitability, combativeness, short attention span and rapid swings in mood (temper tantrums).

Other (unlabeled) generally accepted uses: (1) May have a role in treating alcohol withdrawal in patients who can not tolerate benzodiazepines; (2) can be used to treat unexplained infertility; (3) may help control premature ejaculation and nocturnal emissions in men; (4) can help borderline personality disorder; (5) of use in some chronic pain syndromes; (6) may be of use in hypersexuality.

How This Drug Works: By inhibiting the action of dopamine in certain brain centers, this drug acts to correct an imbalance of nerve impulse transmissions that is thought to be responsible for certain mental disorders. May help control premature ejaculation by inhibiting the muscle (longitudinal) that controls the vas deferens.

Available Dosage Forms and Strengths
  Concentrate — 30 mg, 100 mg per ml
  Oral suspension — 25 mg, 100 mg per 5-ml teaspoonful
    Tablets — 10 mg, 15 mg, 25 mg, 50 mg, 100 mg, 150 mg, 200 mg

▷ **Usual Adult Dosage Range:** Initially, 25 to 100 mg 3 times/day. Dose may be increased by 25 to 50 mg at 3 to 4 day intervals as needed and tolerated. Usual dosage range is 200 to 800 mg daily, divided into 2 to 4 doses. The total daily dosage should not exceed 800 mg. **Note: Actual dosage and administration schedule must be determined by the physician for each patient individually.**

Conditions Requiring Dosing Adjustments
  Liver function: This drug is extensively metabolized in the liver and should be used with caution in liver compromise, and the patient closely monitored.
  Kidney function: Patients with compromised kidneys should be closely followed.

▷ **Dosing Instructions:** The tablets may be crushed and taken with or following meals to reduce stomach irritation.

Usual Duration of Use: Use on a regular schedule for 3 to 4 weeks usually determines effectiveness in controlling psychotic disorders. If not significantly beneficial within 6 weeks, it should be stopped. Long-term use (months to years) requires periodic physician evaluation of response, appropriate dosage adjustment and consideration of continued need.

▷ **This Drug Should Not Be Taken If**
- you are allergic to any of the drugs bearing the brand names listed above.
- you have active liver disease.
- you have cancer of the breast.
- you have a constitutionally low blood pressure.
- you have a current blood cell or bone marrow disorder.

▷ **Inform Your Physician Before Taking This Drug If**
- you are allergic or abnormally sensitive to any phenothiazine (see Drug Classes).
- you have impaired liver or kidney function.
- you have any type of seizure disorder.
- you have diabetes, glaucoma or heart disease.
- you have a history of lupus erythematosus.
- you are taking any drug with sedative effects.
- you plan to have surgery under general or spinal anesthesia in the near future.

Possible Side-Effects (natural, expected and unavoidable drug actions)
> Drowsiness (usually during the first 2 weeks), orthostatic hypotension (see Glossary), blurred vision, dry mouth, nasal congestion, constipation, impaired urination.
>
> Pink or purple coloration of urine, of no significance.

▷ **Possible Adverse Effects** (unusual, unexpected and infrequent reactions)
> **If any of the following develop, consult your physician promptly for guidance.**
>
> *Mild Adverse Effects*
> Allergic Reactions: Skin rash, hives, low-grade fever.
> Lowering of body temperature, especially in the elderly. (See Hypothermia in Glossary.)
> Abnormal body hair growth (hirsutism).
> Urinary incontinence.
> Increased appetite and weight gain.
> Inflammation of the parotid gland.
> Weakness, agitation, insomnia, impaired day and night vision.
> Chronic constipation, fecal impaction.
>
> *Serious Adverse Effects*
> Allergic Reactions: Hepatitis with jaundice (see Glossary), severe skin reactions (Stevens-Johnson syndrome or erythema multiforme).
> Idiosyncratic Reactions: Neuroleptic malignant syndrome (see Glossary).
> Depression, disorientation, seizures, loss of peripheral vision.
> Rapid heart rate, heart rhythm disorders.
> Blood cell disorders: reduced white blood cell count (more common in the elderly).
> Sudden death syndrome (rare).
> Excessive production of urine (SIADH).
> Pituitary tumors (rare).
> Nervous system reactions: Parkinson-like disorders (see Glossary), severe restlessness, muscle spasms involving the face and neck, tardive dyskinesia (see Glossary).
> Retinopathy.
> Liver toxicity (Cholestatic jaundice).
> Abnormally low blood pressure.

▷ **Possible Effects on Sexual Function**
> Decreased male and female libido; inhibited ejaculation (49% to 60%); impotence (54%); impaired female orgasm; priapism (see Glossary).
> Male breast enlargement and tenderness.
> Female breast enlargement with milk production.
> Altered timing and pattern of menstruation.
> False positive pregnancy test results.
> May help control premature ejaculation and nocturnal emissions.

▷ **Adverse Effects That May Mimic Natural Diseases or Disorders**
> Nervous system reactions may suggest true Parkinson's disease.
> Liver reactions may suggest viral hepatitis.
> Reactions resembling systemic lupus erythematosus can occur.

Natural Diseases or Disorders That May Be Activated by This Drug
> Latent epilepsy, glaucoma, diabetes mellitus, prostatism (see Glossary).

Thioridazine

Possible Effects on Laboratory Tests
> Complete blood cell counts: decreased red cells, hemoglobin, white cells and platelets.
> Liver function tests: increased liver enzymes (ALT/GPT, AST/GOT and alkaline phosphatase), increased bilirubin.
> Urine pregnancy tests: falsely positive result with Prognosticon.

CAUTION
> 1. Many over-the-counter medications (see OTC Drugs in Glossary) for allergies, colds and coughs contain drugs that can interact unfavorably with this drug. Ask your doctor or pharmacist for help **before** using any such medications.
> 2. Antacids that contain aluminum and/or magnesium can prevent the absorption of this drug and reduce its effectiveness.
> 3. Obtain prompt evaluation of any change or disturbance of vision.

Precautions for Use
> *By Infants and Children:* **not** recommended in children under 2 years of age. Do not use this drug in the presence of symptoms suggestive of Reye syndrome (see Glossary). Children with acute infectious diseases ("flu-like" infections, chicken pox, measles, etc.) are more prone to develop muscular spasms of the face, back and extremities when this drug is given for any reason.
>
> *By Those over 60 Years of Age:* Small starting doses are advisable. You may be more susceptible to drowsiness, lethargy, constipation, lowering of body temperature (hypothermia) and orthostatic hypotension (see Glossary). This drug can worsen existing prostatism (see Glossary). You may also be more susceptible to Parkinson-like reactions and/or tardive dyskinesia (see discussion of these terms in Glossary). These reactions must be recognized early since they may become unresponsive to treatment and irreversible.

▷ **Advisability of Use During Pregnancy**
> *Pregnancy Category:* C. See Pregnancy Code at the back of this book.
> Animal studies: The results of rodent studies are conflicting.
> Human studies: No increase in birth defects reported in 23 exposures. Adequate studies of pregnant women are not available.
> Avoid drug during the first 3 months. Use it otherwise only if clearly needed. Ask your physician for guidance.

Advisability of Use if Breast-Feeding
> Presence of this drug in breast milk: Yes, in minute amounts.
> Monitor nursing infant closely and discontinue drug or nursing if adverse effects develop.

Habit-Forming Potential: None.

Effects of Overdosage: Marked drowsiness, weakness, tremor, agitation, unsteadiness, deep sleep, coma, convulsions.

Possible Effects of Long-Term Use: Opacities in the cornea or lens of the eye, pigmentation of the retina. Tardive dyskinesia (see Glossary).

Suggested Periodic Examinations While Taking This Drug (at physician's discretion)
Complete blood cell counts, especially between the fourth and tenth weeks of treatment.
Liver function tests, electrocardiograms.
Complete eye examinations—eye structures and vision.
Careful inspection of the tongue for early evidence of fine, involuntary, wavelike movements that could be the beginning of tardive dyskinesia.

▷ **While Taking This Drug, Observe the Following**
Foods: No restrictions.
Nutritional Support: A riboflavin (vitamin B-2) supplement should be taken with long-term use.
Beverages: No restrictions. May be taken with milk.
▷ *Alcohol:* Avoid completely. Alcohol can increase the sedative action of phenothiazines and accentuate their depressant effects on brain function and blood pressure. Phenothiazines can increase the intoxicating effects of alcohol.
Tobacco Smoking: Possible reduction of drowsiness from drug.
Marijuana Smoking: Moderate increase in drowsiness; accentuation of orthostatic hypotension; increased risk of precipitating latent psychoses, confusing the interpretation of mental status and drug responses.

▷ *Other Drugs*
Thioridazine may *increase* the effects of
- all sedative drugs, especially meperidine (Demerol), and cause excessive sedation.
- all atropinelike drugs, and cause nervous system toxicity.

Thioridazine may *decrease* the effects of
- guanethidine (Ismelin, Esimil), and reduce its effectiveness in lowering blood pressure.
- oral hypoglycemic agents (see Drug Classes).

Thioridazine *taken concurrently* with
- lithium (Lithobid, Lithotabs) may impair the effectiveness of lithium and cause nervous system toxicity.
- phenytoin (Dilantin) may increase or decrease blood levels.

The following drugs may *decrease* the effects of thioridazine
- antacids containing aluminum and/or magnesium.
- barbiturates (see Drug Classes).
- benztropine (Cogentin).
- disulfiram (Antabuse).
- trihexyphenidyl (Artane).

▷ *Driving, Hazardous Activities:* This drug can impair mental alertness, judgment and physical coordination. Avoid hazardous activities.
Aviation Note: The use of this drug *is a disqualification* for piloting. Consult a designated Aviation Medical Examiner.
Exposure to Sun: Use caution. Some phenothiazines can cause photosensitivity (see Glossary).
Exposure to Heat: Use caution and avoid excessive heat as much as possible.

This drug may impair the regulation of body temperature and increase the risk of heat stroke.

Exposure to Cold: Use caution and dress warmly. This drug can increase the risk of hypothermia in the elderly.

Discontinuation: After long-term use, do not stop this drug suddenly. Gradual withdrawal over 2 to 3 weeks under physician supervision is recommended. Do not discontinue this drug without your physician's knowledge and approval.

THIOTHIXENE (thi oh THIX een)

Introduced: 1967 **Prescription:** USA: Yes; Canada: Yes **Available as Generic:** USA: Yes; Canada: No **Class:** Strong tranquilizer, thioxanthenes **Controlled Drug:** USA: No; Canada: No **Brand Name:** Navane

BENEFITS versus RISKS	
Possible Benefits	*Possible Risks*
EFFECTIVE CONTROL OF ACUTE MENTAL DISORDERS: beneficial effects on thinking, mood and behavior	SERIOUS TOXIC EFFECTS ON BRAIN with long-term use Liver damage with jaundice (rare) Rare blood cell disorders: abnormally low white blood cell count

▷ **Principal Uses**

As a Single Drug Product: Uses currently included in FDA approved labeling: (1) Used to relieve the psychotic thinking and behavior associated with acute psychoses of unknown nature, episodes of mania and paranoia, and acute schizophrenia.

Other (unlabeled) generally accepted uses: (1) Can be of use in significant borderline personality disorder.

How This Drug Works: Present theory is that, by inhibiting the action of dopamine, this drug acts to correct an imbalance of nerve impulse transmissions (at both D1 and D2 receptors) that is thought to be responsible for certain mental disorders.

Available Dosage Forms and Strengths
Capsules — 1 mg, 2 mg, 5 mg, 10 mg, 20 mg
Concentrate — 5 mg per ml
Injections — 2 mg, 5 mg per ml

▷ **Usual Adult Dosage Range:** Initially, 2 to 5 mg 2 or 3 times daily. Dose may be increased by 2 mg at 3 to 4 day intervals as needed and tolerated. Usual dosage range is 20 to 30 mg daily. The total daily dosage should not exceed 60 mg. **Note: Actual dosage and administration schedule must be determined by the physician for each patient individually.**

Conditions Requiring Dosing Adjustments

Liver function: This drug should be used with caution in liver compromise.
Kidney function: Patients with compromised kidneys should be closely followed.

▷ **Dosing Instructions:** The capsules may be opened and taken with or following meals to reduce stomach irritation. The liquid concentrate must be diluted just before administration by adding it to 8 ounces of water, milk, fruit juice or carbonated beverage.

Usual Duration of Use: Use on a regular schedule for several weeks usually determines effectiveness in controlling psychotic disorders. If not beneficial within 6 weeks, it should be stopped. Long-term use (months to years) requires periodic physician evaluation of response, appropriate dosage adjustment and consideration of continued need.

▷ **This Drug Should Not Be Taken If**
- you have had an allergic reaction to it previously.
- you have active liver disease.
- you have cancer of the breast.
- you have a current blood cell or bone marrow disorder.

▷ **Inform Your Physician Before Taking This Drug If**
- you are allergic or abnormally sensitive to other thioxanthene drugs or any phenothiazine drug (see Drug Classes).
- you have impaired liver or kidney function.
- you have any type of seizure disorder.
- you have diabetes, glaucoma or heart disease.
- you have a history of lupus erythematosus.
- you have Parkinson's disease.
- you have had neuroleptic malignant syndrome.
- you are taking any drug with sedative effects.
- you drink alcohol daily.
- you plan to have surgery under general or spinal anesthesia in the near future.

Possible Side-Effects (natural, expected and unavoidable drug actions)

Mild drowsiness (usually during the first 2 weeks), orthostatic hypotension (see Glossary), blurred vision, dry mouth, nasal congestion, constipation, impaired urination.

▷ **Possible Adverse Effects** (unusual, unexpected and infrequent reactions)

If any of the following develop, consult your physician promptly for guidance.

Mild Adverse Effects

Allergic Reactions: Skin rash, hives, itching.

Lowering of body temperature, especially in the elderly. (See Hypothermia in Glossary.)

Fluid retention, weight gain.

Dizziness, weakness, agitation, insomnia, impaired vision.

Nausea, vomiting.

Serious Adverse Effects

Allergic Reactions: Rare hepatitis with jaundice (see Glossary), anaphylactic reaction (see Glossary).

Idiosyncratic Reactions: Paradoxical worsening of psychotic symptoms. Development of the neuroleptic malignant syndrome (see Glossary).

Abnormal production of urine and loss of blood sodium (SIADH).

Depression, disorientation, seizures.

Deposits in cornea and lens of the eye.

Abnormal fixed eye positioning (Oculogyric crisis).
Drug-induced oculogyric crisis.
Rapid heart rate, heart rhythm disorders.
Blood cell disorders: reduced white blood cell count.
Nervous system reactions: Parkinson-like disorders (see Glossary), severe restlessness, muscle spasms involving the face and neck, tardive dyskinesia (see Glossary).
Severe reduction in blood pressure (rare).

▷ **Possible Effects on Sexual Function**
Altered timing and pattern of menstruation.
Impotence (rare).
Priapism and retrograde ejaculation.
Male breast enlargement and tenderness.
Female breast enlargement with milk production.

▷ **Adverse Effects That May Mimic Natural Diseases or Disorders**
Nervous system reactions may suggest true Parkinson's disease or Reye syndrome (see Glossary).
Liver reactions may suggest viral hepatitis.

Natural Diseases or Disorders That May Be Activated by This Drug
Latent epilepsy, glaucoma, prostatism (see Glossary).

Possible Effects on Laboratory Tests
Complete blood cell counts: decreased red cells, hemoglobin, white cells and platelets; increased eosinophils.
Blood glucose level: increased and decreased (fluctuations).
Liver function tests: increased liver enzymes (ALT/GPT, AST/GOT and alkaline phosphatase), increased bilirubin.
Urine pregnancy tests: falsely positive result with some tests.

CAUTION
1. Many over-the-counter medications (see OTC Drugs in Glossary) for allergies, colds and coughs contain drugs that can interact unfavorably with this drug. Ask your doctor or pharmacist for help **before** using any such medications.
2. Antacids that contain aluminum and/or magnesium may prevent the absorption of this drug and reduce its effectiveness.
3. Obtain prompt evaluation of any change or disturbance of vision.

Precautions for Use
By Infants and Children: Use of this drug is not recommended in children under 12 years of age. Do not use this drug in the presence of symptoms suggestive of Reye syndrome (see Glossary). Children with acute infectious diseases ("flulike" infections, chicken pox, measles, etc.) are more prone to develop muscular spasms of the face, back and extremities when this drug is given.

By Those over 60 Years of Age: Small starting doses are advisable. Increased risk of drowsiness, lethargy, constipation, lowering of body temperature (hypothermia) and orthostatic hypotension (see Glossary). This drug can worsen existing prostatism (see Glossary). You may also be more susceptible to the development of Parkinson-like reactions and/or tardive dyskinesia (see discussion of these terms in Glossary). These reactions must be recognized early since they may become unresponsive to treatment and irreversible.

▷ **Advisability of Use During Pregnancy**
Pregnancy Category: C. See Pregnancy Code at the back of this book.
Animal studies: No birth defects reported in rats, rabbits or monkeys.
Human studies: Adequate studies of pregnant women are not available.
Avoid drug during the first 3 months if possible. Avoid during the last month because of possible effects on the newborn infant.

Advisability of Use if Breast-Feeding
Presence of this drug in breast milk: Expected in small amounts, but no data are available.
Avoid drug or refrain from nursing.

Habit-Forming Potential: None.

Effects of Overdosage: Marked drowsiness, weakness, tremor, agitation, unsteadiness, deep sleep, coma, convulsions.

Possible Effects of Long-Term Use: Opacities in the cornea or lens of the eye, pigmentation of the retina. Tardive dyskinesia (see Glossary).

Suggested Periodic Examinations While Taking This Drug (at physician's discretion)
Complete blood cell counts, especially between the fourth and tenth weeks of treatment.
Liver function tests, electrocardiograms.
Complete eye examinations—eye structures and vision.
Careful inspection of the tongue for early evidence of fine, involuntary, wavelike movements that could indicate the beginning of tardive dyskinesia.

▷ **While Taking This Drug, Observe the Following**
Foods: No restrictions.
Beverages: No restrictions. May be taken with milk.
▷ *Alcohol:* Avoid completely. Alcohol can increase the sedative action of thiothixene and accentuate its depressant effects on brain function and blood pressure. Thiothixene can increase the intoxicating effects of alcohol.
Tobacco Smoking: No interactions expected.
Marijuana Smoking: Moderate increase in drowsiness; accentuation of orthostatic hypotension; increased risk of precipitating latent psychoses, confusing the interpretation of mental status and drug responses.
▷ *Other Drugs*
Thiothixene may *increase* the effects of
- all sedative drugs, especially barbiturates and narcotic analgesics, and cause excessive sedation.
- all atropinelike drugs, and cause nervous system toxicity.

Thiothixene may *decrease* the effects of
- guanethidine (Ismelin, Esimil), and reduce its effectiveness in lowering blood pressure.

Thiothixene *taken concurrently* with
- lithium may result in exaggerated neurotoxicity (rigidity and tremor).

The following drugs may *decrease* the effects of thiothixene
- antacids containing aluminum and/or magnesium.

- barbiturates (see Drug Class Section).
- benztropine (Cogentin).
- trihexyphenidyl (Artane).

▷ *Driving, Hazardous Activities:* This drug can impair mental alertness, judgment and physical coordination.
Avoid hazardous activities.

Aviation Note: The use of this drug *is a disqualification* for piloting. Consult a designated Aviation Medical Examiner.

Exposure to Sun: Use caution until sensitivity has been determined. This drug can cause photosensitivity (see Glossary).

Exposure to Heat: Use caution and avoid excessive heat as much as possible. This drug may impair the regulation of body temperature and increase the risk of heat stroke.

Exposure to Cold: Use caution and dress warmly. This drug can increase the risk of hypothermia in the elderly.

Discontinuation: After a period of long-term use, do not stop this drug suddenly. Gradual withdrawal over 2 to 3 weeks under physician supervision is recommended. Do not discontinue this drug without your physician's knowledge and approval. The relapse rate of schizophrenia after discontinuation is 50% to 60%.

TICLOPIDINE (ti KLOH pi deen)

Introduced: 1985   **Prescription:** USA: Yes   **Available as Generic:** USA: No   **Class:** Platelet inhibitor   **Controlled Drug:** USA: No
Brand Name: Ticlid

BENEFITS versus RISKS
Possible Benefits / *Possible Risks*
SIGNIFICANT REDUCTION IN THE RISK OF STROKE FOR THOSE WITH TRANSIENT ISCHEMIC ATTACK (TIA) OR PREVIOUS STROKE	SIGNIFICANT REDUCTION IN WHITE BLOOD CELL COUNTS (2.4%) Increase (of 8–10%) in total blood cholesterol level Rare drug-induced hepatitis with jaundice

▷ **Principal Uses**

As a Single Drug Product: Uses currently included in FDA approved labeling: Used in selected individuals (who are intolerant to aspirin) to prevent: (1) Recurrent stroke following initial thrombotic stroke.

Other (unlabeled) generally accepted uses: (1) Used in selected individuals with peripheral vascular disease and intermittent claudication to prevent blood clots (thrombosis); (2) used in people who have had bypass surgery to help prevent clot formation and keep the graft working; may have a role in slowing the progression of eye problems (retinopathy) in diabetics; (3) combined with other agents to keep patients with angina from having heart attacks; (4) used in combination therapy to help lessen the symptoms of rheumatoid arthritis; (5) may help prevent strokes in patients who have experienced transient ischemic atacks (TIAs).

How this Drug Works: By inhibiting clumping of blood platelets, this drug prevents the beginning of processes that lead to blood clot formation within atherosclerotic vessels (arterial thrombosis).

Available Dosage Forms and Strengths
Tablets — 250 mg

▷ **Recommended Dosage Ranges (Actual dosage and administration schedule must be determined by the physician for each patient individually.)**
Infants and Children: Dosage not established.
18 to 60 Years of Age: 250 mg twice daily, 12 hours apart, taken with food.
Over 60 Years of Age: Same as 18 to 60 years of age.

Conditions Requiring Dosing Adjustments
Liver function: This drug is contraindicated in patients with severe liver impairment.
Kidney function: Changes in dosing in kidney compromise patients does not appear to be needed.

▷ **Dosing Instructions:** The tablet may be crushed and is best taken with meals to enhance absorption and reduce stomach irritation.

Usual Duration of Use: Use on a regular schedule for 6 to 12 months usually determines effectiveness in preventing stroke. Long-term use (months to years) requires periodic physician evaluation of response and dosage adjustment.

Possible Advantages of This Drug
A 48% reduction in risk of initial stroke during first year following TIA (in contrast to aspirin).
A 33% reduction in risk of recurrent stroke during first year following initial stroke.
Effective in both men and women.

▷ **This Drug Should Not Be Taken If**
- you have had an allergic reaction to it previously.
- you currently have a bone marrow, blood cell or bleeding disorder.
- you have active peptic ulcer disease, Crohn's disease or ulcerative colitis.
- you have severely impaired liver function.
- you are taking aspirin, anticoagulants or cortisonelike drugs.

▷ **Inform Your Physician Before Taking This Drug If**
- you have a history of a drug-induced bone marrow depression or blood cell disorder.
- you have gastric or duodenal ulcers.
- you have impaired liver or kidney function.
- you plan to have surgery in the near future; this drug should be discontinued 10 to 14 days prior to surgery.

Possible Side-Effects (natural, expected and unavoidable drug actions)
Spontaneous bruising (purpura) 2.2%.

▷ **Possible Adverse Effects** (unusual, unexpected and infrequent reactions)
If any of the following develop, consult your physician promptly for guidance.

Ticlopidine

Mild Adverse Effects
Allergic Reactions: Rash (5.1%), itching (1.3%).
Dizziness (1.1%), ringing in the ears.
Loss of appetite (1%), indigestion (7%), nausea (7%), vomiting (1.9%), stomach pain (3.7%), diarrhea (12.5%).

Serious Adverse Effects
Allergic Reactions: Drug-induced hepatitis with jaundice (rare). This usually occurs during the first 4 months of treatment. (See **jaundice** in the Glossary.)
Idiosyncratic Reactions: Decreased production of white blood cells (neutrophils and granulocytes, 2.4%): fever, sore throat, susceptibility to infection.
Very rare aplastic anemia (see Glossary).

▷ **Possible Effects on Sexual Function:** None reported.

▷ **Adverse Effects That May Mimic Natural Diseases or Disorders**
Drug-induced hepatitis may suggest viral hepatitis.

Possible Effects on Laboratory Tests
Complete blood cell counts: decreased red cells, hemoglobin, white cells and platelets.
Bleeding time: increased.
Total cholesterol and triglyceride levels: increased.
Liver function tests: increased liver enzymes (ALT/GPT, AST/GOT and alkaline phosphatase), increased bilirubin.

CAUTION
1. If significantly low white blood cell counts occurs, it usually begins between 3 weeks and 3 months after treatment starts. White blood cell counts **must** be obtained every 2 weeks from the second week to the end of the third month of drug administration.
2. Report promptly any indications of infection: fever, chills, sore throat, cough, etc.
3. Report promptly any abnormal or unusual bleeding or bruising.
4. Do not take any type of aspirin or anticoagulant drug while taking this drug without your physician's approval.
5. Inform all physicians and dentists that you consult that you are taking this drug.

Precautions for Use
By Infants and Children: Safety and effectiveness for those under 18 years of age not established.
By Those over 60 Years of Age: You may be more susceptible to bone marrow depression and blood cell decreases. Observe carefully for any tendency to infections or unusual bleeding or bruising. Report such developments promptly.

▷ **Advisability of Use During Pregnancy**
Pregnancy Category:
B. See Pregnancy Code at the back of this book.
Animal studies: No drug-induced birth defects found in mouse, rat or rabbit studies.
Human studies: Adequate studies of pregnant women are not available. Use this drug only if clearly needed. Ask your physician for guidance.

Advisability of Use if Breast-Feeding
Presence of this drug in breast milk: Unknown.
Avoid drug or refrain from nursing.

Habit-Forming Potential: None.

Effects of Overdosage: Abnormal bleeding or bruising, dizziness, nausea, diarrhea.

Possible Effects of Long-Term Use: None reported.

Suggested Periodic Examinations While Taking This Drug (at physician's discretion)
Complete blood cell counts. See *CAUTION*.
Liver function tests.

▷ **While Taking This Drug, Observe the Following**
Foods: High fat meals may increase absorption by 20%.
Beverages: No restrictions. May be taken with milk.
▷ *Alcohol:* No interactions expected. Avoid if you have active peptic ulcer disease.
Tobacco Smoking: No interactions expected.
▷ *Other Drugs*
Ticlopidine may *increase* the effects of
- aspirin.
- theophylline.
- warfarin (Coumadin) and also increase the risk of hepatitis. The combination is **not** recomended.

Ticlodipine may *decrease* the efects of
- cyclosporine (Sandimmune) and decrease effectiveness.

The following drug may *increase* the effects of ticlopidine
- cimetidine (Tagamet).

The following drugs may *decrease* the effects of ticlopidine
- antacids decrease absorption of ticlopidine.

▷ *Driving, Hazardous Activities:* This drug may cause dizziness. Restrict activities as necessary.
Aviation Note: The use of this drug *may be a disqualification* for piloting. Consult a designated Aviation Medical Examiner.
Exposure to Sun: No restrictions.
Discontinuation: To be determined and guided by your physician.

TIMOLOL (TI moh lohl)

Introduced: 1972   **Prescription:** USA: Yes; Canada: Yes   **Available as Generic:** USA: Yes; Canada: No   **Class:** Antianginal, antiglaucoma, antihypertensive, migraine preventive, beta-adrenergic blocker   **Controlled Drug:** USA: No; Canada: No

Brand Names: ✢Apo-Timolol, ✢Apo-Timop, Blocadren, ✢Timolide [CD], Timoptic, Timoptic Ocudose, Timoptic-XE

Timolol

BENEFITS versus RISKS	
Possible Benefits	*Possible Risks*
EFFECTIVE, WELL-TOLERATED AS: ANTIANGINAL DRUG in effort-induced angina; ANTIGLAUCOMA DRUG in open-angle glaucoma; ANTIHYPERTENSIVE DRUG in mild to moderate hypertension EFFECTIVE PREVENTION OF MIGRAINE HEADACHES Effective adjunct in the prevention of recurrent heart attack (myocardial infarction)	CONGESTIVE HEART FAILURE in advanced heart disease Worsening of angina in coronary heart disease (if drug is abruptly withdrawn) Masking of low blood sugar (hypoglycemia) in drug-treated diabetes Provocation of asthma

▷ **Principal Uses**

As a Single Drug Product: Uses currently included in FDA approved labeling: (1) Treats classical effort-induced angina, certain types of heart rhythm disturbance and high blood pressure; (2) helps lower increased internal eye pressure in chronic open-angle glaucoma; (3) beneficial in preventing the recurrence of heart attacks (myocardial infarction); (4) used to reduce the frequency and severity of migraine headaches.

Other (unlabeled) generally accepted uses: (1) Has been used in people who are afraid to fly on airplanes (air travel phobia); (2) may be helpful in decreasing the incidence of abnormal heart rhythms that arise in the atria of the heart (atrial fibrillation and flutter); (3) helps prevent abnormally increased intraocular pressure following cataract surgery; (4) can be of use in patients with detached retinas which have not torn.

As a Combination Drug Product [CD]: This drug is available in combination with hydrochlorothiazide for the treatment of hypertension. This combination product includes two drugs with different mechanisms of action; it is intended to provide greater effectiveness and convenience for long-term use.

How This Drug Works: By blocking certain actions of the sympathetic nervous system, this drug
- reduces the rate and contraction force of the heart, lowering the ejection pressure of blood and reducing the amount of oxygen the heart needs to work.
- reduces the degree of contraction of blood vessel walls, resulting in their expansion and consequent lowering of blood pressure.
- prolongs the conduction time of nerve impulses through the heart, of benefit in the management of certain heart rhythm disorders.
- slows formation of fluid (aqueous humor) in the anterior chamber of the eye and improves its drainage from the eye, lowering the internal eye pressure.

Available Dosage Forms and Strengths
Eye solutions — 0.25% and 0.5%
Tablets — 5 mg, 10 mg, 20 mg

▷ **Usual Adult Dosage Range:** Varies with indication.
    Antianginal and antihypertensive: Initially, 10 mg 2 times/day; increase dose gradually every 7 days as needed and tolerated. Usual maintenance dose is 10 to 20 mg twice/day. The total daily dosage should not exceed 60 mg.
    Migraine headache prevention: Initially, 10 mg 2 times/day; increase dose as needed to 10 mg in the morning and 20 mg at night.
    Recurrent heart attack prevention: 10 mg twice/day.
    Antiglaucoma: 1 drop in affected eye every 12 to 24 hours.
    Note: Actual dosage and administration schedule must be determined by the physician for each patient individually.

Conditions Requiring Dosing Adjustments
    Liver function: Consideration must be given to empirically decreasing the dose in patients with compromised livers.
    Kidney function: Patients with kidney compromise should be followed closely, and the dose decreased if the medication appears to be accumulating.

▷ **Dosing Instructions:** Preferably taken 1 hour before eating to maximize absorption. The tablet may be crushed for administration. Do not stop this drug abruptly.

Usual Duration of Use: Use on a regular schedule for 10 to 14 days usually determines effectiveness in preventing angina, controlling heart rhythm disorders and lowering blood pressure. Peak benefit may require continual use for 6 to 8 weeks. The long-term use of this drug (months to years) will be determined by the course of your symptoms over time and your response to an overall treatment program (weight reduction, salt restriction, smoking cessation, etc.). Consult your physician on a regular basis.

▷ **This Drug Should Not Be Taken If**
- you have bronchial asthma.
- you have severe obstructive lung disease.
- you have had an allergic reaction to it previously.
- you have Prinzmetal's variant angina (coronary artery spasm).
- you have congestive heart failure.
- you have an abnormally slow heart rate or a serious form of heart block.
- you are taking, or have taken within the past 14 days, any monoamine oxidase (MAO) type A inhibitor drug (see Drug Classes).

▷ **Inform Your Physician Before Taking This Drug If**
- you have had an adverse reaction to any beta blocker (see Drug Class Section).
- you have a history of serious heart disease.
- you have a history of hay fever (allergic rhinitis), asthma, chronic bronchitis or emphysema.
- you have a history of overactive thyroid function (hyperthyroidism).
- you have a history of low blood sugar (hypoglycemia).
- you have impaired liver or kidney function.
- you have Raynaud's phenomenon.
- you have diabetes or myasthenia gravis.
- you currently take any form of digitalis, quinidine or reserpine, or any calcium blocker drug (see Drug Classes).
- you plan to have surgery under general anesthesia in the near future.

Timolol

Possible Side-Effects (natural, expected and unavoidable drug actions)
   Lethargy and fatigability, cold extremities, slow heart rate, light-headedness in upright position (see Orthostatic Hypotension in Glossary).

▷ **Possible Adverse Effects** (unusual, unexpected and infrequent reactions)
   If any of the following develop, consult your physician promptly for guidance.
   Mild Adverse Effects
   Allergic Reactions: Skin rash, itching.
   Loss of hair involving the scalp, eyebrows and/or eyelashes. This effect can occur with use of the oral tablets or the eye drops (used to treat glaucoma). Regrowth occurs with discontinuation of this drug.
   Headache, dizziness, visual disturbances, vivid dreams.
   Indigestion, nausea, vomiting, diarrhea.
   Numbness and tingling in extremities, joint pain.
   Serious Adverse Effects
   Allergic Reactions: Laryngospasm, severe dermatitis.
   Idiosyncratic Reactions: Acute behavioral disturbances: depression, hallucinations.
   Chest pain, shortness of breath, precipitation of congestive heart failure.
   Induction of bronchial asthma (in asthmatic individuals).
   Masking of warning signs of impending low blood sugar (hypoglycemia) in drug-treated diabetes.
   Drug-induced myasthenia gravis.
   Periodic cramping of the leg (intermittent claudication).
   Stopping of breathing (respiratory arrest) (rare).

▷ **Possible Effects on Sexual Function**
   Decreased libido, impaired erection, impotence.
   Note: All of these effects can occur with the use of timolol eye drops at recommended dosage.

▷ **Adverse Effects That May Mimic Natural Diseases or Disorders**
   Reduced blood flow to extremities may resemble Raynaud's phenomenon (see Glossary).

Natural Diseases or Disorders That May Be Activated by This Drug
   Prinzmetal's variant angina, Raynaud's disease, intermittent claudication, myasthenia gravis (questionable).

Possible Effects on Laboratory Tests
   None reported.

CAUTION
   1. **Do not stop this drug suddenly** without the knowledge and guidance of your doctor. Carry a notation on your person that take this drug.
   2. Ask your doctor or pharmacist before using nasal decongestants usually present in over-the-counter cold preparations and nose drops. These can cause sudden increases in blood pressure when taken concurrently with beta blocker drugs.
   3. Report the development of any tendency to emotional depression (rare with this drug).

Precautions for Use
   By Infants and Children: Safety and effectiveness for those under 12 years of age not established. However, if this drug is used, watch for low blood sugar (hypoglycemia) during periods of reduced food intake.

By Those over 60 Years of Age: Unacceptably high blood pressure should be reduced without creating the risks associated with excessively low blood pressure. Small starting doses, and frequent blood pressure checks are needed. Sudden, rapid and excessive reduction of blood pressure can predispose to stroke or heart attack. Observe for dizziness, unsteadiness, tendency to fall, confusion, hallucinations, depression or urinary frequency.

▷ **Advisability of Use During Pregnancy**
Pregnancy Category: C. See Pregnancy Code at the back of this book.
Animal studies: No significant increase in birth defects due to this drug.
Human studies: Adequate studies of pregnant women are not available.
Avoid use of drug during the first 3 months if possible. Use this drug only if clearly needed. Ask your physician for guidance.

Advisability of Use if Breast-Feeding
Presence of this drug in breast milk: Yes.
Monitor nursing infant closely and discontinue drug or nursing if adverse effects develop.

Habit-Forming Potential: None.

Effects of Overdosage: Weakness, slow pulse, low blood pressure, fainting, cold and sweaty skin, congestive heart failure, possible coma and convulsions.

Possible Effects of Long-Term Use: Reduced heart reserve and eventual heart failure in susceptible individuals with advanced heart disease.

Suggested Periodic Examinations While Taking This Drug (at physician's discretion)
Complete blood cell counts (because of adverse effects of other drugs of this class).
Measurements of blood pressure, evaluation of heart function.

▷ **While Taking This Drug, Observe the Following**
Foods: No restrictions. Avoid excessive salt intake.
Beverages: No restrictions. May be taken with milk.
▷ *Alcohol:* Use with caution. Alcohol may exaggerate this drug's ability to lower the blood pressure and may increase its mild sedative effect.
Tobacco Smoking: Nicotine may reduce this drug's effectiveness in treating angina, heart rhythm disorders and high blood pressure. In addition, high doses of this drug may worsen constriction of the bronchial tubes caused by regular smoking.

▷ *Other Drugs*
Timolol may *increase* the effects of
- other antihypertensive drugs, and cause excessive lowering of blood pressure. Dosage adjustments may be necessary.
- amiodarone (Codarone) and cause caridac arrest and bradycardia.
- lidocaine (Xylocaine, etc.).
- reserpine (Ser-Ap-Es, etc.), and cause sedation, depression, slowing of the heart rate and lowering of the blood pressure.
- verapamil (Calan, Isoptin), and cause excessive depression of heart function; monitor this combination closely.

Timolol may *decrease* the effects of
- theophyllines (Aminophyllin, Theo-Dur, etc.), and reduce their antiasthmatic effectiveness.

Timolol *taken concurrently* with
- clonidine (Catapres) requires close monitoring for rebound high blood pressure if clonidine is withdrawn while timolol is still being taken.
- epinephrine (Adrenalin, etc.) may cause marked rise in blood pressure and slowing of the heart rate.
- insulin may hide the symptoms of hypoglycemia (see Glossary).
- oral hypoglycemic agents such as acetohexamide (Dymelor) and glipizide (Glucotrol) may result in prolonged low blood sugar.

The following drugs may *increase* the effects of timolol
- chlorpromazine (Thorazine, etc.)
- cimetidine (Tagamet).
- methimazole (Tapazole).
- propylthiouracil (Propacil).

The following drugs may *decrease* the effects of timolol
- barbiturates (phenobarbital, etc.).
- indomethacin (Indocin), and possibly other "aspirin substitutes" or NSAIDs may impair timolol's antihypertensive effect.
- rifampin (Rifadin, Rimactane).

▷ *Driving, Hazardous Activities:* Use caution until the full extent of dizziness, lethargy and blood pressure change have been determined.

Aviation Note: The use of this drug **may be a disqualification** for piloting. Consult a designated Aviation Medical Examiner.

Exposure to Sun: No restrictions.

Exposure to Heat: Caution advised. Hot environments can exaggerate the effects of this drug.

Exposure to Cold: Caution advised. Cold environments can worsen circulatory deficiency in the extremities that may occur with this drug. The elderly should take precautions to prevent hypothermia (see Glossary).

Heavy Exercise or Exertion: It is advisable to avoid exertion that produces light-headedness, excessive fatigue or muscle cramping. The use of this drug may intensify the hypertensive response to isometric exercise.

Occurrence of Unrelated Illness: Fever can lower blood pressure and require adjustment of dosage. Nausea or vomiting may interrupt the dosing schedule. Ask your doctor for help.

Discontinuation: It is advisable to avoid sudden discontinuation of this drug in all situations; this is especially true in the presence of coronary artery disease. If possible, gradual reduction of dose over a period of 2 to 3 weeks is recommended. Ask your physician for specific guidance.

TOLAZAMIDE (tohl AZ a mide)

Introduced: 1966 **Prescription:** USA: Yes **Available as Generic:** Yes **Class:** Antidiabetic, sulfonylureas **Controlled Drug:** USA: No

Brand Names: Ronase, Tolamide, Tolinase

Tolazamide

BENEFITS versus RISKS	
Possible Benefits	*Possible Risks*
Assistance in regulating blood sugar in noninsulin-dependent diabetes (adjunctive to appropriate diet and weight control)	INCREASED RISK OF CARDIOVASCULAR DEATH HYPOGLYCEMIA, severe and prolonged Drug-induced liver damage Rare bone marrow depression (see Glossary) Hemolytic anemia (see Glossary)

▷ **Principal Uses**
   As a Single Drug Product: Uses currently included in FDA approved labeling: (1) To assist in the control of mild to moderately severe type II diabetes mellitus (adult, maturity-onset) that does not require insulin, but that cannot be adequately controlled by diet alone.
   Other (unlabeled) generally accepted uses: None.

How This Drug Works: This drug (1) stimulates the release of insulin (by a pancreas that is capable of responding to stimulation), and (2) enhances the utilization of insulin by appropriate tissues.

Available Dosage Forms and Strengths
   Tablets — 100 mg, 250 mg, 500 mg

▷ **Usual Adult Dosage Range:** Initially, 100 to 250 mg daily with breakfast. At 4 to 6 day intervals, the dose may be increased by increments of 100 to 250 mg daily as needed and tolerated. The total daily dosage should not exceed 1000 mg (1 gram). A "loading" or priming dose is not necessary and should not be given. **Note: Actual dosage and administration schedule must be determined by the physician for each patient individually.**

Conditions Requiring Dosing Adjustments
   Liver function: May require decreased dosing in severe liver compromise. Can be a rare cause of liver damage, and patients should be followed closely.
   Kidney function: The starting dose should be decreased, and the drug only increased if needed.

▷ **Dosing Instructions:** If the daily maintenance dose is found to be more than 500 mg, the total dose should be divided into 2 equal doses: the first taken with the morning meal, the second with the evening meal. The tablet may be crushed for administration.

Usual Duration of Use: Use on a regular schedule for several weeks usually determines effectiveness in controlling diabetes. Failure to respond to maximal doses within 1 month constitutes a primary failure. Up to 10% of those who respond initially may develop secondary failure of the drug later. The duration of effective use can only be determined by periodic measurement of the blood sugar. Consult your physician on a regular basis.

▷ **This Drug Should Not Be Taken If**
   • you have had an allergic reaction to it previously.
   • you have severe impairment of liver or kidney function.
   • you have type I diabetes.
   • your diabetes is complicated by acidosis (ask your doctor).
   • you are pregnant.

Tolazamide

▷ **Inform Your Physician Before Taking This Drug If**
- you are allergic to other sulfonylurea drugs or to "sulfa" drugs. (See Drug Classes).
- your diabetes has been unstable or "brittle" in the past.
- you do not know how to recognize or treat hypoglycemia (see Glossary).
- you have a history of congestive heart failure, peptic ulcer disease, cirrhosis of the liver, hypothyroidism or porphyria.
- you have G6PD defficiency in your red blood cells (ask your doctor).

Possible Side-Effects (natural, expected and unavoidable drug actions)
If dose is excessive or food intake is delayed or inadequate, abnormally low blood sugar (hypoglycemia) will occur.

▷ **Possible Adverse Effects** (unusual, unexpected and infrequent reactions)
If any of the following develop, consult your physician promptly for guidance.

Mild Adverse Effects
Allergic Reactions: Skin rash, hives, itching, drug fever.
Headache, ringing in the ears.
Indigestion, heartburn, nausea, vomiting, diarrhea.

Serious Adverse Effects
Allergic Reactions: Hepatitis with jaundice (see Glossary).
Idiosyncratic Reactions: Hemolytic anemia (see Glossary); disulfiramlike reaction with concurrent use of alcohol (see Glossary), infrequent with this drug.
Lichenoid skin reactions.
Disulfiram-like reaction with alcohol.
Bone marrow depression (see Glossary): fatigue, weakness, fever, sore throat, abnormal bleeding or bruising.
Increased risk of cardiovascular death versus management by diet or insulin.
Abnormal urine production and lowering of blood sodium (SIADH).
Drug-induced porphyria.
Cholestatic jaundice (rare).

▷ **Possible Effects on Sexual Function**
None reported.

▷ **Adverse Effects That May Mimic Natural Diseases or Disorders**
Liver reactions may suggest viral hepatitis.

Possible Effects on Laboratory Tests
Complete blood cell counts: decreased red cells, hemoglobin, white cells and platelets.
Blood glucose level: decreased.
Liver function tests: increased liver enzymes (ALT/GPT, AST/GOT and alkaline phosphatase), increased bilirubin.

CAUTION
1. This drug must be regarded as only part of a total program of diabetic management. It is not a substitute for a properly prescribed diet and regular exercise.
2. Over a period of time (usually several months), this drug may lose its

effectiveness. Periodic follow-up examinations are necessary to monitor all aspects of response to drug treatment.

Precautions for Use

By Infants and Children: This drug is not effective in type I (juvenile, growth-onset) insulin-dependent diabetes.

By Those over 60 Years of Age: This drug should be used with caution, and with decreased starting doses of 100 mg/day. Dose is slowly increased to prevent hypoglycemic reactions. Repeated episodes of hypoglycemia in the elderly can cause brain damage.

▷ **Advisability of Use During Pregnancy**

Pregnancy Category: C. See Pregnancy Code at the back of this book.
Animal studies: No birth defects due to this drug reported in rats.
Human studies: Adequate studies of pregnant women are not available.
Because uncontrolled blood sugar levels during pregnancy are associated with a higher incidence of birth defects, many experts recommend that insulin (instead of an oral agent) be used as necessary to control diabetes during the entire pregnancy.
Use during pregnancy is not recommended by the manufacturer.

Advisability of Use if Breast-Feeding

Presence of this drug in breast milk: Probably yes.
Avoid drug or refrain from nursing.

Habit-Forming Potential: None.

Effects of Overdosage: Symptoms of mild to severe hypoglycemia: headache, light-headedness, faintness, nervousness, confusion, tremor, sweating, heart palpitation, weakness, hunger, nausea, vomiting, stupor progressing to coma.

Possible Effects of Long-Term Use: Reduced function of the thyroid gland (hypothyroidism). Reports of increased frequency and severity of heart and blood vessel diseases associated with long-term use of this class of drugs are highly controversial and inconclusive. A direct cause-and-effect relationship (see Glossary) is tenuous. Ask your physician for guidance.

Suggested Periodic Examinations While Taking This Drug (at physician's discretion)

Complete blood cell counts, liver function tests, thyroid function tests, periodic evaluation of heart and circulatory system.

▷ **While Taking This Drug, Observe the Following**

Foods: Follow the diabetic diet prescribed by your physician.
Beverages: As directed in the diabetic diet. May be taken with milk.

▷ *Alcohol:* Use with extreme caution. Alcohol can exaggerate this drug's hypoglycemic effect. This drug infrequently causes a marked intolerance of alcohol resulting in a disulfiramlike reaction (see Glossary): facial flushing, sweating, palpitation.

Tobacco Smoking: No interactions expected.

▷ *Other Drugs*

The following drugs may *increase* the effects of tolazamide
- aspirin, and other salicylates.
- birth control pills (oral contraceptives).
- chloramphenicol.

- cimetidine (Tagamet).
- clofibrate (Atromid S).
- colestipol
- fenfluramine (Pondimin).
- fluconazole.
- itraconazole (Sporanox).
- ketoconazole.
- monoamine oxidase (MAO) type A inhibitor drugs (see Drug Classes).
- phenylbutazone (Butazolidin).
- ranitidine (Zantac).
- sulfa antibiotics.

The following drugs may *decrease* the effects of tolazamide
- beta blocker drugs (see Drug Classes).
- bumetanide (Bumex).
- calcium channel blockers (see drug Classes).
- diazoxide (Proglycem).
- ethacrynic acid (Edecrin).
- furosemide (Lasix).
- niacin.
- phenytoin (Dilantin).
- thiazide diuretics (see Drug Class Section).

Tolazamide *taken concurrently* with
- colestipol may result in loss of response to colestipol.

▷ *Driving, Hazardous Activities:* Regulate your dosage schedule, eating schedule and physical activities very carefully to prevent hypoglycemia. Be able to recognize the early symptoms of hypoglycemia so you can avoid hazardous activities and take corrective measures.

Aviation Note: Diabetes *is a disqualification* for piloting. Consult a designated Aviation Medical Examiner.

Exposure to Sun: Use caution until sensitivity has been determined. Some drugs of this class can cause photosensitivity (see Glossary).

Occurrence of Unrelated Illness: Acute infections, illnesses causing vomiting or diarrhea, serious injuries and surgical procedures can interfere with diabetic control and may require insulin. If any of these conditions occur, call your doctor promptly.

Discontinuation: Because of the possibility of secondary failure, it is advisable to evaluate the continued benefit of this drug every 6 months.

TOLBUTAMIDE (tohl BYU ta mide)

Introduced: 1956   **Prescription:** USA: Yes; Canada: Yes   **Available as Generic:** Yes   **Class:** Antidiabetic, sulfonylureas   **Controlled Drug:** USA: No; Canada: No

Brand Names: ✤Apo-Tolbutamide, ✤Mobenol, ✤Novobutamide, Oramide, Orinase, Sk-Tolbutamide

Warning: The brand names Orinase, Ornade and Ornex are similar and can be mistaken for each other; this can lead to serious medication errors. These names represent very different drugs. Orinase is the generic drug tolbutamide; it is used to treat diabetes. Ornade is a combination of chlorpheniramine and phenylpropanolamine; used to treat nasal and sinus congestion. Ornex is a combination of acetaminophen and phenylpropanolamine; used to treat head-colds and sinus pain. Verify that you are taking the correct drug.

BENEFITS versus RISKS	
Possible Benefits	*Possible Risks*
Assistance in regulating blood sugar in noninsulin-dependent diabetes (adjunctive to appropriate diet and weight control)	INCREASED RISK OF CARDIOVASCULAR DEATH HYPOGLYCEMIA, severe and prolonged Drug-induced liver damage Rare bone marrow depression (See Glossary) Hemolytic anemia (See Glossary)

▷ **Principal Uses**
  As a Single Drug Product: Uses currently included in FDA approved labeling: (1) Helps control mild to moderately severe type II diabetes mellitus (adult, maturity-onset) that does not require insulin, but that cannot be adequately controlled by diet alone; (2) has reversed some cases of diabetic coma.
  Other (unlabeled) generally accepted uses: (1) Has been used intravenously to help diagnose tumors which secrete insulin.
How This Drug Works: It is thought that this drug (1) stimulates the release of insulin (by a pancreas that is capable of responding to stimulation), and (2) enhances the utilization of insulin by appropriate tissues.
Available Dosage Forms and Strengths
  Tablets — 250 mg, 500 mg
▷ **Usual Adult Dosage Range:** Initially, 500 mg twice a day. The dose may be increased or decreased every 48 to 72 hours until the minimal amount required for satisfactory control is determined. The usual range is 500 to 2000 mg/24 hours. The total daily dosage should not exceed 3000 mg (3 grams). A "loading" or priming dose is not necessary and should not be given. **Note: Actual dosage and administration schedule must be determined by the physician for each patient individually.**
Conditions Requiring Dosing Adjustments
  Liver function: Consideration should be given to decreasing the dose in patients with compromised livers. Tolbutamide can be a rare cause of liver damage, and patients should be followed closely.
  Kidney function: Dosing decreases are not needed in kidney compromise.
▷ **Dosing Instructions:** May be taken with food (morning and evening meals) to reduce stomach irritation. The tablet may be crushed for administration.
Usual Duration of Use: Use on a regular schedule for 5 to 7 days weeks usually determines effectiveness in controlling diabetes. Failure to respond to maximal doses within 1 month constitutes a primary failure. Up to 15% of those who respond initially may develop secondary failure of the drug within the first year. The duration of effective use can only be determined

by periodic measurement of the blood sugar. See your physician on a regular basis.

▷ **This Drug Should Not Be Taken If**
- you have had an allergic reaction to it previously.
- you have severe impairment of liver or kidney function.
- you are undergoing major surgery.
- you have a severe infection.
- you have diabetes complicated by formation of excess acid (acidosis).
- you are pregnant.

▷ **Inform Your Physician Before Taking This Drug If**
- you are allergic to other sulfonylurea drugs or to "sulfa" drugs. (See Drug Classes).
- your diabetes has been unstable or "brittle" in the past.
- you do not know how to recognize or treat hypoglycemia (see Glossary).
- you have a deficiency of G6PD in your red blood cells (ask your doctor).
- you have a history of congestive heart failure, peptic ulcer disease, cirrhosis of the liver, hypothyroidism or porphyria.

Possible Side-Effects (natural, expected and unavoidable drug actions)
If drug dose is excessive or food intake is delayed or inadequate, abnormally low blood sugar (hypoglycemia) will occur.

▷ **Possible Adverse Effects** (unusual, unexpected and infrequent reactions)
If any of the following develop, consult your physician promptly for guidance.

Mild Adverse Effects
Allergic Reactions: Skin rash, hives, itching, drug fever.
Headache, ringing in the ears, weakness.
Indigestion, heartburn, nausea, vomiting.

Serious Adverse Effects
Allergic Reactions: Hepatitis with jaundice (see Glossary).
Idiosyncratic Reactions: Hemolytic anemia (see Glossary); disulfiramlike reaction with concurrent use of alcohol (see Glossary), infrequent with this drug.
Seizures (rare).
Low blood sodium (SIADH).
Drug-induced porphyria.
Drug-induced urinary tract stones (urolithiasis).
Disulfiram-like reaction.
Bone marrow depression (see Glossary): fatigue, weakness, fever, sore throat, abnormal bleeding or bruising.
Abnormally low thyroid gland function (hypothyroidism).
Increased risk of cardiovascular death versus management by diet or insulin.

▷ **Possible Effects on Sexual Function**
None reported.

▷ **Adverse Effects That May Mimic Natural Diseases or Disorders**
Liver reactions may suggest viral hepatitis.

Natural Diseases or Disorders That May Be Activated by This Drug
Acute intermittent porphyria (see Glossary).

Possible Effects on Laboratory Tests
Complete blood cell counts: decreased red cells, hemoglobin, white cells and platelets.
Blood glucose level: decreased.
Liver function tests: increased liver enzymes (ALT/GPT, AST/GOT and alkaline phosphatase), increased bilirubin.

CAUTION
1. This drug must be regarded as only one part of the total program for the management of your diabetes. It is not a substitute for a properly prescribed diet and regular exercise.
2. Over a period of time (usually several months), this drug may lose its effectiveness in controlling blood sugar levels. Periodic follow-up examinations are necessary to monitor all aspects of response to drug treatment.

Precautions for Use
By Infants and Children: This drug is not effective in type I (juvenile, growth-onset) insulin-dependent diabetes.

By Those over 60 Years of Age: This drug should be used with caution in this age group. Start treatment with 500 mg/day; increase dosage cautiously and monitor closely to prevent hypoglycemic reactions. Repeated episodes of hypoglycemia in the elderly can cause brain damage.

▷ ## Advisability of Use During Pregnancy
Pregnancy Category: C. See Pregnancy Code at the back of this book.
Animal studies: Ocular and bone birth defects reported in rat studies.
Human studies: Adequate studies of pregnant women are not available.
Because uncontrolled blood sugar levels during pregnancy are associated with a higher incidence of birth defects, many experts recommend that insulin (instead of an oral agent) be used as necessary to control diabetes during the entire pregnancy.
Use during pregnancy is not recommended by the manufacturer.

Advisability of Use if Breast-Feeding
Presence of this drug in breast milk: Yes.
Avoid drug or refrain from nursing.

Habit-Forming Potential: None.

Effects of Overdosage:
Symptoms of mild to severe hypoglycemia: headache, light-headedness, faintness, nervousness, confusion, tremor, sweating, heart palpitation, weakness, hunger, nausea, vomiting, stupor progressing to coma.

Possible Effects of Long-Term Use:
Reduced function of the thyroid gland (hypothyroidism). Reports of increased frequency and severity of heart and blood vessel diseases associated with long-term use of this class of drugs are highly controversial and inconclusive. A direct cause-and-effect relationship (see Glossary) is tenuous. Ask your physician for guidance.

Suggested Periodic Examinations While Taking This Drug (at physician's discretion)
Complete blood cell counts, liver function tests, thyroid function tests, periodic evaluation of heart and circulatory system.

Tolbutamide

▷ **While Taking This Drug, Observe the Following**
   Foods: Follow the diabetic diet prescribed by your physician.
   Beverages: As directed in the diabetic diet. May be taken with milk.
▷ *Alcohol:* Use with extreme caution. Alcohol can exaggerate this drug's hypoglycemic effect. This drug infrequently causes a marked intolerance of alcohol resulting in a disulfiramlike reaction (see Glossary): facial flushing, sweating, palpitation.
   Tobacco Smoking: No interactions expected.
▷ *Other Drugs*
   The following drugs may *increase* the effects of tolbutamide
   - aspirin, and other salicylates.
   - chloramphenicol (Chloromycetin).
   - cimetidine (Tagamet).
   - clofibrate (Atromid S).
   - fenfluramine (Pondimin).
   - fluconazole (Diflucan).
   - ketoconazole.
   - itraconazole (Sporanox).
   - monoamine oxidase (MAO) type A inhibitors (see Drug Classes).
   - phenylbutazone (Butazolidin).
   - ranitidine (Zantac).
   - sulfonamide drugs (see Drug Classes).

   The following drugs may *decrease* the effects of tolbutamide
   - beta blocker drugs (see Drug Classes).
   - bumetanide (Bumex).
   - diazoxide (Proglycem).
   - ethacrynic acid (Edecrin).
   - furosemide (Lasix).
   - phenytoin (Dilantin).
   - rifampin (Rifadin, Rimactane).
   - thiazide diuretics (see Drug Classes).

   Tolbutamide *taken concurrently* with
   - digoxin may result in increased risk of digoxin toxicity.
   - insulin will result in additive lowering of the blood sugar.
▷ *Driving, Hazardous Activities:* Regulate your dosage schedule, eating schedule and physical activities very carefully to prevent hypoglycemia. Be able to recognize the early symptoms of hypoglycemia so you can avoid hazardous activities and take corrective measures.
   Aviation Note: Diabetes *is a disqualification* for piloting. Consult a designated Aviation Medical Examiner.
   Exposure to Sun: Use caution. Some drugs of this class can cause photosensitivity (see Glossary).
   Occurrence of Unrelated Illness: Acute infections, illnesses causing vomiting or diarrhea, serious injuries and surgical procedures can interfere with diabetic control and may require insulin. If any of these conditions occur, call your doctor promptly.
   Discontinuation: Because of the possibility of secondary failure, it is advisable to evaluate the continued benefit of this drug every 6 months.

TOLMETIN (TOHL met in)

Introduced: 1976 **Prescription:** USA: Yes; Canada: Yes **Available as Generic:** Yes **Class:** Mild analgesic, anti-inflammatory **Controlled Drug:** USA: No; Canada: No
Brand Names: Tolectin, Tolectin DS, Tolectin 600

BENEFITS versus RISKS	
Possible Benefits	*Possible Risks*
EFFECTIVE RELIEF OF MILD TO MODERATE PAIN AND INFLAMMATION	Increased blood pressure (3-9%) Gastrointestinal pain, ulceration, bleeding (rare) Rare liver damage Rare kidney damage Rare blood cell disorders: hemolytic anemia, abnormally low white blood cell and platelet counts

Please see the new combined acetic acid nonsteroidal anti-inflammatory drug profile for further information.

TRAZODONE (TRAZ oh dohn)

Introduced: 1967 **Prescription:** USA: Yes; Canada: Yes **Available as Generic:** USA: Yes; Canada: No **Class:** Antidepressants **Controlled Drug:** USA: No; Canada: No
Brand Name: Desyrel, ◆Desyrel Dividose, Trialodine

BENEFITS versus RISKS	
Possible Benefits	*Possible Risks*
EFFECTIVE TREATMENT IN ALL TYPES OF DEPRESSIVE ILLNESS, with or without anxiety	Adverse behavioral effects: confusion, disorientation, delusions, hallucinations (all infrequent) Potential for causing heart rhythm disorders (in people with heart disease)

▷ **Principal Uses**
As a Single Drug Product: Uses currently included in FDA approved labeling: (1) Used to provide symptomatic relief in all types of depression, with or without anxiety or agitation.
Other (unlabeled) generally accepted uses: (1) May have a role in reducing the symptoms of agoraphobia; (2) may help drug-induced (such as MAO inhibitors) insomnia; (3) can have a role in cobination therapy of some pain syndromes; (4) may be of help in essential tremor.
How This Drug Works: It is thought that this drug increases the availability of the nerve impulse transmitter serotonin within certain brain centers and thereby relieves the symptoms of emotional depression.

Trazodone

Available Dosage Forms and Strengths
  Tablets — 50 mg, 100 mg, 150 mg, 300 mg

▷ **Usual Adult Dosage Range:** Initially, 50 mg 3 times/day. The dose may be increased by 50 mg daily at intervals of 3 or 4 days as needed and tolerated. The total daily dosage should not exceed 400 mg. **Note: Actual dosage and administration schedule must be determined by the physician for each patient individually.**

Conditions Requiring Dosing Adjustments
  Liver function: Blood levels should be obtained to guide dosing. It can be a rare cause of liver damage, and patients should be followed closely.
  Kidney function: Trazodone metabolites are eliminated by the kidneys, however, dosage adjustment in renal compromise is not defined.

▷ **Dosing Instructions:** Best taken with food to improve absorption. The tablet may be crushed for administration. If excessive drowsiness or dizziness occurs, it is advisable to take a larger portion of the total daily dose at bedtime and to divide the remaining amount into 2 or 3 smaller doses to be taken during the day.

Usual Duration of Use: Use on a regular schedule for 2 to 4 weeks usually determines effectiveness in relieving the symptoms of depression. Long-term use (weeks to months) requires supervision and periodic evaluation by your physician.

▷ **This Drug Should Not Be Taken If**
- you have had an allergic reaction to it previously.
- you are recovering from a recent heart attack (myocardial infarction).
- you have carcinoid syndrome.
- you are taking, or have taken within the past 14 days, any monoamine oxidase (MAO) type A inhibitor (see Drug Classes).

▷ **Inform Your Physician Before Taking This Drug If**
- you have a history of any of the following: alcoholism, epilepsy, heart disease (especially heart rhythm disorders).
- you have impaired liver or kidney function.
- you are pregnant or are breast feeding your infant.
- you are taking any antihypertensive drugs.
- you plan to have surgery under general anesthesia in the near future.

Possible Side-Effects (natural, expected and unavoidable drug actions)
  Drowsiness, light-headedness, blurred vision, dry mouth, constipation.

▷ **Possible Adverse Effects** (unusual, unexpected and infrequent reactions)
  If any of the following develop, consult your physician promptly for guidance.
  Mild Adverse Effects
  Allergic Reaction: Skin rash.
  Headache, dizziness, fatigue, impaired concentration, nervousness, tremors.
  Rapid heart rate, palpitations.
  Peculiar taste, constipation, stomach discomfort, nausea, vomiting, diarrhea.

Weight gain, blurred vision.
Dry mouth (xerostomia).
Urinary retention.
Cavities (dental caries).
Muscular aches and pains.

Serious Adverse Effects
Behavioral effects: Confusion, anger, hostility, disorientation, impaired memory, delusions, hallucinations, nightmares.
Irregular heart rhythms, low blood pressure, fainting.
Erythema multiforme.
Seizures (rare).
Liver toxicity.

▷ **Possible Effects on Sexual Function**
Decreased male libido; increased female libido.
Inhibited ejaculation, impotence, priapism (see Glossary).
Altered timing and pattern of menstruation.

Possible Effects on Laboratory Tests
None reported.

CAUTION
1. If you experience a significant degree of mouth dryness while using this drug, consult your dentist regarding the risk of gum erosion or tooth decay. Ask for his guidance in ways to keep the mouth comfortably moist.
2. It is advisable to withhold this drug if electroconvulsive therapy (ECT) is to be used.

Precautions for Use
By Infants and Children: Safety and effectiveness for use by those under 18 years of age have not been established.
By Those over 60 Years of Age: During the first two weeks of treatment, observe for the development of restlessness, agitation, excitement, forgetfulness, confusion or disorientation. Be aware of possible unsteadiness and incoordination that may predispose to falling. This drug may enhance prostatism (see Glossary).

▷ **Advisability of Use During Pregnancy**
Pregnancy Category: C. See Pregnancy Code at the back of this book.
Animal studies: Fetal deaths and birth defects reported.
Human studies: Adequate studies of pregnant women are not available.
Avoid this drug completely during the first 3 months. Use otherwise only if clearly needed. Ask your physician for guidance.

Advisability of Use if Breast-Feeding
Presence of this drug in breast milk: Yes.
Avoid drug or refrain from nursing.

Habit-Forming Potential: None.

Effects of Overdosage: Marked drowsiness, weakness, confusion, tremors, low blood pressure, rapid heart rate, stupor, coma, possible seizures.

Possible Effects of Long-Term Use: None reported.

Triamcinolone

Suggested Periodic Examinations While Taking This Drug (at physician's discretion)

Complete blood cell counts. (This drug may cause slight reductions in white blood cell counts. This should be monitored closely if infection, sore throat or fever develops.)

Serial blood pressure readings and electrocardiograms.

▷ **While Taking This Drug, Observe the Following**

Foods: No restrictions.

Beverages: No restrictions. May be taken with milk.

▷ *Alcohol:* Avoid completely. This drug can increase markedly the intoxicating effects of alcohol and accentuate its depressant action on brain functions.

Tobacco Smoking: No interactions expected.

▷ *Other Drugs*

Trazodone may *increase* the effects of
- antihypertensive drugs, and cause excessive lowering of blood pressure; dosage adjustments may be necessary.
- drugs with sedative effects, and cause excessive sedation.
- phenytoin (Dilantin), by raising its blood level; observe for phenytoin toxicity.

Trazodone *taken concurrently* with
- clonidine will lessen the therapeutic effect of clonidine.
- fluoxetine (Prozac) may result in an increased trazodone level and toxicity.
- warfarin (Coumadin) may result in a decreased therapeutic benefit of warfarin. Prothrmbin times (INR) should be checked three times a week while combined warfarin and trazodone therapy are undertaken.

▷ *Driving, Hazardous Activities:* This drug may cause dizziness or drowsiness. Restrict activities as necessary.

Aviation Note: The use of this drug *is a disqualification* for piloting. Consult a designated Aviation Medical Examiner.

Exposure to Sun: No restrictions.

Discontinuation: It is advisable to discontinue this drug gradually. Ask your physician for guidance in dosage reduction over an appropriate period of time.

TRIAMCINOLONE (tri am SIN oh lohn)

Introduced: 1985 **Prescription:** USA: Yes; Canada: Yes **Available as**
Generic: No **Class:** Antiasthmatic, cortisonelike drugs **Controlled**
Drug: USA: No; Canada: No

Brand Name: Amcort, Aristocort, Aristocort R, Aristoform D, ✦Aristospan, Articulose LA, ✦Aureocort, Azmacort, Cenocort, Flutex, ✦Kenacomb, Kenacort, Kenaject, Kenalog, Kenalog H, Kenalog IN, Kenalone, Mycogen II, Mycomar, Mytrex [CD], Nasacort, Sk-Triamcinolone, TAC-40, Triacet, ✦Triaderm Mild, ✦Triaderm Regular, Triam-A, Triamolone 40, Triderm, Tri-Kort, Trilog, Tristoject, ✦Viaderm-K.C.

Triamcinolone

BENEFITS versus RISKS	
Possible Benefits	**Possible Risks**
EFFECTIVE CONTROL OF SEVERE, CHRONIC BRONCHIAL ASTHMA	Yeast infections of mouth and throat Suppression of normal cortisone production. Euphoria and psychotic episodes. Cushing's syndrome (moon face, obesity and buffalo hump). Muscle wasting (with long-term use). Osteoporosis (with long-term use).

▷ **Principal Uses**

As a Single Drug Product: Uses currently included in FDA approved labeling: (1) In inhaler form used to treat chronic bronchial asthma in people who require cortisonelike drugs for asthma control. This inhalation dosage form is significantly more advantageous than cortisone taken by mouth (swallowed) or by injection in that it works locally on the tissues of the respiratory tract and does not require absorption and systemic distribution. This prevents the more serious adverse effects that usually result from the long-term use of cortisone taken for systemic effects; (2) the tablet form can be used in a variety of inflammatory disorders; (3) tablet form is used to ease drug reactions.

Other (unlabeled) generally accepted uses: (1) May have a role in postherpetic nerve pain (neuralgia); (2) corticosteroids may be of use in Pneumocystis carinii pneumonia in extreme cases where conventional therapy has not worked; (3) may help Guillain-Barre syndrome; (4) can help myasthenia gravis; (5) short-term therapy of psoriasis.

How This Drug Works: By increasing the amount of cyclic AMP in appropriate tissues, this drug may thereby increase the concentration of epinephrine, which is an effective bronchodilator and antiasthmatic. Additional benefit is due to the drug's ability to reduce local allergic reaction and inflammation in the lining tissues of the respiratory tract.

Available Dosage Forms and Strengths
Inhalation aerosol — 0.1 mg per metered spray
Tablets — 1 mg, 2 mg, 4 mg, 8 mg

▷ **Recommended Dosage Ranges (Actual dosage and administration schedule must be determined by the physician for each patient individually.)**

Infants and Children: Up to 6 years of age—Dosage not established.

6 to 12 years of age—0.1 to 0.2 mg (1 or 2 metered sprays) 3 or 4 times a day. Adjust dosage as needed and tolerated. Limit total daily dosage to 1.2 mg (12 metered sprays).

12 to 60 Years of Age: Initially 0.2 mg (2 metered sprays) 3 or 4 times a day.

For severe asthma—1.2 to 1.6 mg (12 to 16 metered sprays) per day, in divided doses. Adjust dosage as needed and tolerated. Limit total daily dose to 1.6 mg (16 metered sprays).

For tablets: 4 to 48 mg daily for inflammatory conditions.

Over 60 Years of Age: Same as 12 to 60 years of age.

Conditions Requiring Dosing Adjustments
Liver function: This drug is metabolized in the liver. Dosing changes in liver compromise are not defined.
Kidney function: Dosing adjustments do not appear warranted in patients with compromised kidneys.

▷ **Dosing Instructions:** For inhalation form: May be used as needed without regard to eating. Shake the container well before using. Carefully follow the printed patient instructions provided with the unit. Rinse the mouth and throat (gargle) with water thoroughly after each inhalation; do not swallow the rinse water.

For oral tablets: May cause stomach upset, and can be taken with meals or snacks.

Usual Duration of Use: Use on a regular schedule for 1 to 2 weeks usually determines effectiveness in controlling severe, chronic asthma. Long-term use requires the supervision and guidance of the physician.

▷ **This Drug Should Not Be Taken If**
- you have had an allergic reaction to it previously.
- you are experiencing severe acute asthma or status asthmaticus that requires more intense treatment for prompt relief.
- you have a form of nonallergic bronchitis with asthmatic features.
- you have a systemic fungal infection.

▷ **Inform Your Physician Before Taking This Drug If**
- you are now taking or have recently taken any cortisone-related drug (including ACTH by injection) for any reason (see Drug Classes).
- you have a history of tuberculosis of the lungs.
- you have chronic bronchitis or bronchiectasis.
- you have diabetes, glaucoma, myasthenia gravis, or peptic ulcer disease.
- you think you may have an active infection of any kind, especially a respiratory infection.
- you are taking any of the following drugs: warfarin, oral antidiabetic drugs, insulin or digoxin

Possible Side-Effects (natural, expected and unavoidable drug actions)
Yeast infections (thrush) of the mouth and throat.
Irritation of mouth, tongue or throat.

▷ **Possible Adverse Effects** (unusual, unexpected and infrequent reactions)
If any of the following develop, consult your physician promptly for guidance.
Mild Adverse Effects
Allergic Reaction: Skin rash.
Memory loss, weight loss.
Swelling of face, hoarseness, voice change, cough.
Serious Adverse Effects
Allergic reactions: rare.
Bronchospasm, asthmatic wheezing (rare).
Can be a cause of high blood pressure with long-term use.
Edema or swelling, especially with kidney or heart vessel disease.
May cause euphoria, manic depressive illness or paranoid states with long-term oral use.

Can cause a syndrome (Cushing's) characterized by: moon face, obesity, and poorly controlled high blood pressure.
Decrease of circulating T lymphocytes.
Hypertension (rare).
Drug-induced seizures.
Rare electrolyte disturbances.
Excessive thyroid activity (hyperthyroidism).
Long-term use can be associated with osteoporosis.
Long-term oral dosing can result in duodenal ulcer development.
Cataract formation has occurred with long-term use.
Muscle wasting can occur with long-term use.
Pancreatitis (rare).
Toxic megacolon (rare).
Toxic psychosis has occurred with other steroids.

▷ **Possible Effects on Sexual Function:** None reported.

Natural Diseases or Disorders That May Be Activated by This Drug
Latent amebiasis, congestive heart failure, diabetes, glaucoma, hypertension, myasthenia gravis, peptic ulcer.
Cortisone-related drugs (used by inhalation) that produce systemic effects can impair immunity and lead to reactivation of "healed" or quiescent tuberculosis of the lungs. Individuals with a history of tuberculosis should be observed closely during use of cortisonelike drugs by inhalation.

Possible Effects on Laboratory Tests
Blood calcium levels: decreased.
Blood total cholesterol levels: increased.
Blood glucose levels: increased.
Blood potassium levels: decreased.
Blood sodium levels: increased.

CAUTION
1. This drug does not act primarily as a brochodilator and should not be relied upon for the immediate relief of acute asthma.
2. If you were using any cortisone-related drugs for treatment of your asthma *before* transferring to this inhaler drug, it may be necessary to resume the former cortisone-related drug if you experience injury or infection of any kind, or if you require surgery. Be sure to notify your attending physician of your prior use of cortisone-related drugs taken either by mouth or by injection.
3. If you experience a return of severe asthma while using this drug, notify your physician immediately so that additional supportive treatment with cortisone-related drugs by mouth or injection can be provided as needed.
4. It is advisable to carry a card of personal identification with a notation (if applicable) that you have used cortisone-related drugs within the past year. During periods of stress it may be necessary to resume cortisone treatment in adequate dosage.
5. An interval of approximately 5 to 10 minutes should separate the inhalation of bronchodilators such as albuterol, epinephrine, pirbuterol, etc., (which should be used first) and the inhalation of this drug. This sequence will permit greater penetration of triamcinolone into the bron-

chial tubes. The delay between inhalations will also reduce the possibility of adverse effects from the propellants used in the two inhalers.

Precautions for Use
By Infants and Children: Safety and effectiveness for use of the oral inhaler by those under 6 years of age have not been established. To ensure adequate penetration of the drug and to obtain maximal benefit, the use of a spacer device is recommended for inhalation therapy in children.
By Those over 60 Years of Age: Individuals with chronic bronchitis or bronchiectasis should be observed closely for the development of lung infections.

▷ **Advisability of Use During Pregnancy**
Pregnancy Category: D. See Pregnancy Code at the back of this book.
Animal studies: Rat and rabbit studies reveal significant toxic effects on the embryo and fetus and multiple birth defects due to this drug.
Human studies: Adequate studies of pregnant women are not available.
Limit use to very serious illness for which no satisfactory treatment alternatives are available.

Advisability of Use if Breast-Feeding
Presence of this drug in breast milk: Unknown.
Ask your doctor for guidance.

Habit-Forming Potential: With recommended dosage, a state of functional dependence (see Glossary) is not likely to develop.

Effects of Overdosage: Indications of cortisone excess (due to systemic absorption)—fluid retention, flushing of the face, stomach irritation, nervousness.

Possible Effects of Long-Term Use: Significant suppression of normal cortisone production.

Suggested Periodic Examinations While Taking This Drug (at physician's discretion)
Inspection of mouth and throat for evidence of yeast infection.
Assessment of the status of adrenal gland function (cortisone production).
X-ray examination of the lungs of individuals with a prior history of tuberculosis.

▷ **While Taking This Drug, Observe the Following**
Foods: No specific restrictions beyond those advised by your physician.
Beverages: No specific restrictions.
▷ *Alcohol:* No interactions expected.
Tobacco Smoking: No interactions expected. However, smoking can affect the condition under treatment and reduce the effectiveness of this drug. Follow your physician's advice.

▷ *Other Drugs*
The following drugs may *increase* the effects of triamcinolone
• inhalant bronchodilators—albuterol, bitolterol, epinephrine, pirbuterol, etc.
• oral bronchodilators—aminophylline, ephedrine, terbutaline, theophylline, etc.
The following drugs may *decrease* the effects of triamcinolone
• carbamazepine (Tegretol) increases triamcinolone metabolism and may result in decreased effectiveness.

- phenytoin (Dilantin) increases triamcinolone metabolism and may result in decreased effectiveness.
- primidone (Mysoline) increases steroid metabolism and may result in decreased triamcinolone metabolism.
- rifampin.

Triamcinolone *taken concurrrently* with
- oral hypoglycemic agents (see Drug Classes) may result in loss of glucose control.
- thiazide diuretics can result in loss of glucose control.
- vaccines may result in a less than optimal vaccine response.
- warfarin (Coumadin) can result in variation in the degree of anticoagulation. Increased prothrombin time (INR) testing is indicated.

▷ *Driving, Hazardous Activities:* No restrictions.

Aviation Note: The use of this drug and the disorder for which this drug is prescribed *may be disqualifications* for piloting. Consult a designated Aviation Medical Examiner.

Exposure to Sun: No restrictions.

Occurrence of Unrelated Illness: Acute infections, serious injuries, and surgical procedures can create an urgent need for the administration of additional supportive cortisone-related drugs given by mouth and/or injection. Notify your physician immediately in the event of new illness or injury of any kind.

Discontinuation: If the regular use of this drug has made it possible to reduce or discontinue maintenance doses of cortisonelike drugs by mouth, *do not* discontinue this drug abruptly. If you find it necessary to discontinue this drug for any reason, consult your physician promptly. It may be necessary to resume cortisone preparations and to institute other measures for satisfactory management.

Special Storage Instructions: Store at room temperature. Avoid exposure to temperatures above 120 degrees F (49 degrees C). Do not store or use this inhaler near heat or open flame.

TRIAMTERENE (tri AM ter een)

Introduced: 1964 **Prescription:** USA: Yes; Canada: Yes **Available as Generic:** No **Class:** Diuretic **Controlled Drug:** USA: No; Canada: No
Brand Names: ♣Apo-Triazide [CD], Dyazide [CD], Dyrenium, Maxzide [CD], Maxzide-25 [CD], ♣Novo-Triamzide [CD], ♣Nu-Triazide

BENEFITS versus RISKS	
Possible Benefits	*Possible Risks*
EFFECTIVE PREVENTION OF POTASSIUM LOSS when used adjunctively with other diuretics EFFECTIVE DIURETIC IN REFRACTORY CASES OF FLUID RETENTION when used adjunctively with other diuretics	ABNORMALLY HIGH BLOOD POTASSIUM LEVEL with excessive use Rare blood cell disorders: megaloblastic anemia, abnormally low white blood cell and platelet counts Rare kidney stones

Triamterene

▷ **Principal Uses**

As a Single Drug Product: Uses currently included in FDA approved labeling: (1) Used as part of the treatment program for the management of congestive heart failure and disorders of the liver and kidney that are accompanied by excessive fluid retention (edema); (2) Used in conjunction with other measures to treat high blood pressure. It is used primarily in situations where it is advisable to prevent loss of potassium from the body.

Other (unlabeled) generally accepted uses: None.

As a Combination Drug Product [CD]: This drug is available in combination with hydrochlorothiazide, a different kind of diuretic that promotes the loss of potassium from the body. Triamterene is used in this combination to counteract the potassium-wasting effect of the thiazide diuretic.

How This Drug Works: By inhibiting the enzyme system that initiates the sodium-potassium exchange process, this drug prevents the reabsorption of sodium and the excretion of potassium by the kidney. Thus the drug promotes the excretion of sodium (and water with it) and the retention of potassium.

Available Dosage Forms and Strengths

Capsules — 50 mg, 100 mg

▷ **Usual Adult Dosage Range:** Initially, 50 to 100 mg twice daily. The dose is then adjusted according to individual response. The usual maintenance dose is 100 to 200 mg/day, divided into 2 doses. The total daily dosage should not exceed 300 mg. **Note: Actual dosage and administration schedule must be determined by the physician for each patient individually.**

Conditions Requiring Dosing Adjustments

Liver function: The dose should be reduced and used with extreme caution in patients with severe liver disease.

Kidney function: Patients with mild to moderate kidney failure may be given the usual dose every 12 hours. In severe or progressive kidney failure, this medication should **not** be used.

▷ **Dosing Instructions:** May be taken with or following meals to promote absorption of the drug and to reduce stomach irritation. The capsule may be opened for administration. Intermittent or alternate-day use is recommended to minimize the possibility of sodium and potassium imbalance.

Usual Duration of Use: Use on a regular schedule for 3 to 5 days usually determines effectiveness in clearing edema, and for 2 to 3 weeks to determine its effect on hypertension. Long-term use (months to years) requires physician supervision and periodic evaluation.

▷ **This Drug Should Not Be Taken If**
- you have had an allergic reaction to it previously.
- you have severely impaired liver or kidney function.
- your kidney disease is progressive or you have a creatinine greater than 2.5 mg/dl (ask your doctor).
- your blood potassium level is significantly elevated (ask your doctor).

▷ **Inform Your Physician Before Taking This Drug If**
- you have a history of liver or kidney disease.
- you have diabetes or gout.
- you are taking any of the following: antihypertensives, a digitalis preparation, another diuretic, lithium or a potassium preparation.

- you have a history of G6PD deficiency (ask your doctor).
- you have a history of blood cell disorders.
- you plan to have surgery under general anesthesia in the near future.

Possible Side-Effects (natural, expected and unavoidable drug actions)
With excessive use: abnormally high blood potassium levels, abnormally low blood sodium levels, dehydration.
Blue coloration of the urine (of no significance).

▷ **Possible Adverse Effects** (unusual, unexpected and infrequent reactions)
If any of the following develop, consult your physician promptly for guidance.

Mild Adverse Effects
Allergic Reactions: Skin rash, itching.
Headache, dizziness, unsteadiness, weakness, drowsiness, lethargy.
Dry mouth, nausea, vomiting, diarrhea.

Serious Adverse Effects
Allergic Reaction: Anaphylactic reaction (see Glossary).
Symptomatic potassium excess: confusion, numbness and tingling in lips and extremities, fatigue, weakness, shortness of breath, slow heart rate, low blood pressure.
Rare blood cell disorders: megaloblastic anemia, causing weakness and fatigue; abnormally low white blood cell count, causing infection, fever or sore throat; abnormally low blood platelet count, causing abnormal bleeding or bruising.
Abnormal urine production (SIADH).
Hemolytic anemia (in those with deficiency of G6PD in red cells).
Rare formation of kidney stones and kidney toxicity.
Rare liver toxicity.

▷ **Possible Effects on Sexual Function:** None reported.

Possible Effects on Laboratory Tests
Complete blood cell counts: decreased red cells, hemoglobin, white cells and platelets; increased eosinophils (allergic reaction).
Blood glucose level: increased in diabetics.
Blood lithium level: increased.
Blood potassium level: increased.
Blood uric acid level: increased in 17% of users.
Kidney function tests: increased blood creatinine and urea nitrogen (BUN) levels (kidney damage).

CAUTION
1. Do not take potassium supplements or increase your intake of potassium-rich foods while taking this drug.
2. Do not stop this drug abruptly unless abnormally high blood levels of potassium develop.
3. Avoid the liberal use of salt substitutes that contain potassium; these are a potential cause of potassium excess.

Precautions for Use
By Infants and Children: This drug is not recommended for use in children.
By Those over 60 Years of Age: The natural decline in kidney function may predispose to potassium retention in the body. Watch for indications of potassium excess: slow heart rate, irregular heart rhythms, low blood

pressure, confusion, drowsiness. Excessive use of diuretics can cause harmful loss of body water (dehydration), increased viscosity of the blood and an increased tendency of the blood to clot, predisposing to stroke, heart attack or thrombophlebitis.

▷ **Advisability of Use During Pregnancy**
Pregnancy Category: B by the manufacturer, D by one researcher. See Pregnancy Code at the back of this book.
Animal studies: No birth defects due to this drug reported.
Human studies: Adequate studies of pregnant women are not available.
This drug should not be used during pregnancy unless a very serious complication of pregnancy occurs for which this drug is significantly beneficial.

Advisability of Use if Breast-Feeding
Presence of this drug in breast milk: Yes.
Avoid drug or refrain from nursing.

Habit-Forming Potential: None.

Effects of Overdosage: Thirst, drowsiness, fatigue, weakness, nausea, vomiting, confusion, irregular heart rhythm, low blood pressure.

Possible Effects of Long-Term Use: Potassium accumulation to abnormally high blood levels.

Suggested Periodic Examinations While Taking This Drug (at physician's discretion)
Complete blood cell counts.
Measurements of blood sodium, potassium and chloride levels.
Kidney function tests.

▷ **While Taking This Drug, Observe the Following**
Foods: Diets high in high potassium foods (see table) may cause problems. Avoid excessive restriction of salt.
Beverages: No restrictions. May be taken with milk.
▷ *Alcohol:* Use with caution. Alcohol may enhance the drowsiness and the blood-pressure-lowering effect of this drug.
Tobacco Smoking: No interactions expected.

▷ *Other Drugs*
Triamterene may *increase* the effects of
- amantadine (Symmetrel).
- digoxin (Lanoxin).

Triamterene *taken concurrently* with
- captopril (Capoten) or other ACE inhibitors may cause excessively high blood potassium levels.
- H2 blockers (see Drug Classes) may decrease the absorption of triamterione and decrease the therapeutic effect of triamterine.
- indomethacin (Indocin) may increase the risk of kidney damage.
- lithium may cause accumulation of lithium to toxic levels.
- NSAIDs (see Drug Classes) may blunt the blood pressure lowering effect of triamterine.
- potassium preparations may cause excessively high blood potassium levels.

▷ *Driving, Hazardous Activities:* This drug may cause dizziness and drowsiness. Restrict activities as necessary.

Aviation Note: The use of this drug *may be a disqualification* for piloting. Consult a designated Aviation Medical Examiner.

Exposure to Sun: Use caution. This drug may cause photosensitivity (see Glossary).

Discontinuation: With high dosage or prolonged use, it is advisable to withdraw this drug gradually. Sudden discontinuation may cause rebound potassium excretion and resultant potassium deficiency. Ask your physician for guidance.

TRICHLORMETHIAZIDE Try KLOR meth eye a zyde

Introduced: 1961 **Prescription:** USA: Yes; Canada: Yes **Available as Generic:** Yes **Class:** Thiazide diuretics **Controlled Drug:** USA: No; Canada: No
Brand Names: Diurese, Marzide II, Metahydrin, Naqua, Naquival

BENEFITS versus RISKS	
Possible Benefits	*Possible Risks*
Effective, well-tolerated diuretic	Loss of body potassium and magnesium
Helpful in mild hypertension	Cardiac risk caused by electrolyte loss
Increases effectiveness of other antihypertensives	Increased blood sugar
Helps diabetes insipidus	Rare blood cell disorders
	Rare liver toxicity

Please see the combined thiazide diuretic profile for further information.

TRIFLUOPERAZINE (tri floo oh PER a zeen)

Introduced: 1958 **Prescription:** USA: Yes; Canada: Yes **Available as Generic:** USA: Yes; Canada: No **Class:** Strong tranquilizer, phenothiazines **Controlled Drug:** USA: No; Canada: No
Brand Names: ◆Apo-Trifluoperazine, ◆Novo-Flurazine, ◆Solazine, Stelabid [CD], Stelazine, Suprazine, ◆Terfluzine

BENEFITS versus RISKS	
Possible Benefits	*Possible Risks*
EFFECTIVE CONTROL OF ACUTE MENTAL DISORDERS: beneficial effects on thinking, mood and behavior	SERIOUS TOXIC EFFECTS ON BRAIN with long-term use
	Liver damage with jaundice (infrequent)
	Rare blood cell disorders: abnormally low red and white blood cell and platelet counts

▷ **Principal Uses**

As a Single Drug Product: Uses currently included in FDA approved labeling: (1) Treats psychotic thinking and behavior associated with acute psychoses of unknown nature, mania, paranoid states and acute schizophrenia. It is most effective in those who are withdrawn and apathetic and in those with agitation, delusions and hallucinations; (2) approved for treatment of anxiety disorders, but is not a drug of first choice.

Other (unlabeled) generally accepted uses: (1) May have a role in combination therapy of some kinds of chronic pain; (2) may help in combination therapy of chemotherapy induced nausea or vomiting.

How This Drug Works: Present theory is that by inhibiting the action of dopamine, this drug acts to correct an imbalance of nerve impulse transmissions that is thought to be responsible for certain mental disorders.

Available Dosage Forms and Strengths
Concentrate — 10 mg per ml
  Injection — 2 mg per ml
    Tablets — 1 mg, 2 mg, 5 mg, 10 mg

▷ **Usual Adult Dosage Range:** Initially, 1 or 2 mg twice daily. The dose may be increased by 1 or 2 mg at 3 to 4 day intervals as needed and tolerated. Usual dosage range is 10 to 30 mg daily. The total daily dosage should not exceed 40 mg. **Note: Actual dosage and administration schedule must be determined by the physician for each patient individually.**

Conditions Requiring Dosing Adjustments
Liver function: This drug should be used with caution in liver compromise.
Kidney function: Patients with compromised kidneys should be closely followed.

▷ **Dosing Instructions:** The tablets may be crushed and taken with or following meals to reduce stomach irritation.

Usual Duration of Use: Use on a regular schedule for several weeks usually determines effectiveness in controlling psychotic disorders. If not significantly beneficial within 6 weeks, it should be stopped. Long-term use (months to years) requires periodic physician evaluation of response, appropriate dosage adjustment and consideration of continued need.

▷ **This Drug Should Not Be Taken If**
- you are allergic to any of the drugs bearing the brand names listed above.
- you have active liver disease.
- you have cancer of the breast.
- you have a current blood cell or bone marrow disorder.

▷ **Inform Your Physician Before Taking This Drug If**
- you are allergic or abnormally sensitive to any phenothiazine drug (see Drug Classes).
- you have impaired liver or kidney function.
- you have a history of anginal pain (this drug may worsen it).
- you have any type of seizure disorder.
- you have diabetes, glaucoma or heart disease.
- you have a history of lupus erythematosus.
- you are taking any drug with sedative effects.
- you have had neuroleptic malignant syndrome (ask your doctor).
- you plan to have surgery under general or spinal anesthesia in the near future.

Trifluoperazine

Possible Side-Effects (natural, expected and unavoidable drug actions)
- Drowsiness (usually during the first 2 weeks), orthostatic hypotension (see Glossary), blurred vision, dry mouth, nasal congestion, constipation, impaired urination.
- Pink or purple coloration of urine, of no significance.

▷ **Possible Adverse Effects** (unusual, unexpected and infrequent reactions)
If any of the following develop, consult your physician promptly for guidance.

Mild Adverse Effects
- Allergic Reactions: Skin rash, hives, low-grade fever.
- Lowering of body temperature, especially in the elderly. (See Hypothermia in Glossary.)
- Increased appetite and weight gain.
- Dizziness, weakness, agitation, insomnia, impaired day and night vision.
- Chronic constipation, fecal impaction.

Serious Adverse Effects
- Allergic Reactions: Hepatitis with jaundice (see Glossary), severe skin reactions, anaphylactic reaction (see Glossary).
- Idiosyncratic Reactions: Neuroleptic malignant syndrome (see Glossary).
- Depression, disorientation, loss of peripheral vision.
- Serious skin disorders (Stevens-Johnson syndrome).
- Drug-induced glaucoma or abnormal eye positioning (oculogyric crisis).
- Seizures.
- Drug-induced porphyrias.
- Drug-induced pituitary tumors (rare).
- Rapid heart rate, heart rhythm disorders.
- Blood cell disorders: significant reduction in all cellular elements of the blood (reduced counts of red cells, white cells and blood platelets). (See Bone Marrow Depression in the Glossary.)
- Phenothiazine-induced sudden death syndrome (rare).
- Nervous system reactions: Parkinsonlike disorders (see Glossary), severe restlessness, muscle spasms involving the face and neck, tardive dyskinesia (see Glossary) (10% to 20%).

▷ **Possible Effects on Sexual Function**
- Altered timing and pattern of menstruation.
- Male breast enlargement and tenderness.
- Female breast enlargement with milk production.
- Spontaneous male orgasm, paradoxical (1 case reported).
- Inhibited ejaculation, painful ejaculation, priapism (see Glossary).
- Delayed female orgasm.

▷ **Adverse Effects That May Mimic Natural Diseases or Disorders**
- Nervous system reactions may suggest true Parkinson's disease.
- Liver reactions may suggest viral hepatitis.
- Reactions resembling systemic lupus erythematosus may occur.

Natural Diseases or Disorders That May Be Activated by This Drug
- Latent epilepsy, glaucoma, diabetes mellitus, prostatism (see Glossary).

Possible Effects on Laboratory Tests
- Complete blood cell counts: decreased red cells, hemoglobin, white cells and platelets.

Liver function tests: increased liver enzymes (ALT/GPT, AST/GOT and alkaline phosphatase), increased bilirubin.
Urine pregnancy tests: falsely positive result with some.

CAUTION
1. Many over-the-counter medications (see OTC Drugs in Glossary) for allergies, colds and coughs contain drugs that can interact unfavorably with this drug. Ask your doctor or pharmacist for help before using any such medications.
2. Antacids that contain aluminum and/or magnesium may prevent the absorption of this drug and reduce its effectiveness.
3. Obtain prompt evaluation of any change or disturbance of vision.

Precautions for Use

By Infants and Children: Use of this drug is not recommended in children under 6 years of age. Do not use this drug in the presence of symptoms suggestive of Reye syndrome (see Glossary). Children with acute infectious diseases ("flulike" infections, chicken pox, measles, etc.) are more prone to develop muscular spasms of the face, back and extremities when this drug is given.

By Those over 60 Years of Age: Small starting doses are advisable. May be increased risk of: drowsiness, lethargy, constipation, lowering of body temperature (hypothermia) and orthostatic hypotension (see Glossary). This drug may enhance existing prostatism (see Glossary). You may also be more susceptible to the development of Parkinson-like reactions and/or tardive dyskinesia (see discussion of these terms in Glossary). These reactions must be recognized early since they may become unresponsive to treatment and irreversible.

▷ **Advisability of Use During Pregnancy**

Pregnancy Category: C. See Pregnancy Code at the back of this book.
Animal studies: Significant birth defects reported in mouse and rat studies.
Human studies: No increase in birth defects reported in 700 exposures. Adequate studies of pregnant women are not available.
Avoid drug during the first 3 months; avoid during the last month because of possible adverse effects on the newborn infant.

Advisability of Use if Breast-Feeding
Presence of this drug in breast milk: Yes, in minute amounts.
Monitor nursing infant closely and discontinue drug or nursing if adverse effects develop.

Habit-Forming Potential: None.

Effects of Overdosage: Marked drowsiness, weakness, tremor, agitation, unsteadiness, deep sleep, coma, convulsions.

Possible Effects of Long-Term Use: Tardive dyskinesia (see Glossary).

Suggested Periodic Examinations While Taking This Drug (at physician's discretion)
Complete blood cell counts, especially between the fourth and tenth weeks of treatment.
Liver function tests, electrocardiograms.
Complete eye examinations of eye structures and vision.

Careful inspection of the tongue for early evidence of fine, involuntary, wavelike movements that could indicate the beginning of tardive dyskinesia.

▷ **While Taking This Drug, Observe the Following**
Foods: No restrictions.
Nutritional Support: A riboflavin (vitamin B-2) supplement should be taken with long-term use.
Beverages: Caffeine may slightly blunt the calming effect of this medicine. May be taken with milk.

▷ *Alcohol:* Avoid completely. Alcohol can increase the sedative action of phenothiazines and accentuate their depressant effects on brain function and blood pressure. Phenothiazines can increase the intoxicating effects of alcohol.
Tobacco Smoking: Possible reduction of drowsiness from drug.
Marijuana Smoking: Moderate increase in drowsiness; accentuation of orthostatic hypotension; increased risk of precipitating latent psychoses, confusing the interpretation of mental status and drug responses.

▷ *Other Drugs*
Trifluoperazine may *increase* the effects of
- all sedative drugs, especially narcotic analgesics, and cause excessive sedation.
- all atropinelike drugs, and cause nervous system toxicity.

Trifluoperazine may *decrease* the effects of
- guanethidine (Ismelin, Esimil), and reduce its effectiveness in lowering blood pressure.

Trifluoperazine ***taken concurrently*** with
- lithium (Lithobid, Lithotabs) may impair the effectiveness of lithium and cause nervous system toxicity.
- oral hypoglycemic agents (see drug Classes) will blunt the beneficial effects of the oral hypoglycemic agents.

The following drugs may *decrease* the effects of trifluoperazine
- antacids containing aluminum and/or magnesium.
- barbiturates (see Drug Classes).
- benztropine (Cogentin).
- disulfiram (Antabuse).
- trihexyphenidyl (Artane).

▷ *Driving, Hazardous Activities:* This drug can impair mental alertness, judgment and physical coordination. Avoid hazardous activities.
Aviation Note: The use of this drug ***is a disqualification*** for piloting. Consult a designated Aviation Medical Examiner.
Exposure to Sun: Use caution. Some phenothiazines can cause photosensitivity (see Glossary).
Exposure to Heat: Use caution and avoid excessive heat as much as possible. This drug may impair the regulation of body temperature and increase the risk of heat stroke.
Exposure to Cold: Use caution and dress warmly. This drug can increase the risk of hypothermia in the elderly.
Discontinuation: After a period of long-term use, do not stop this drug suddenly. Gradual withdrawal over 2 to 3 weeks under physician supervision

is recommended. Do not discontinue this drug without your physician's knowledge and approval. The relapse rate of schizophrenia after discontinuation is 50–60%.

TRIMETHOPRIM (tri METH oh prim)

Introduced: 1966 **Prescription:** USA: Yes; Canada: Yes **Available as Generic:** USA: Yes; Canada: No **Class:** Anti-infective **Controlled Drug:** USA: No; Canada: No

Brand Names: ◆Apo-Sulfatrim [CD], ◆Apo-Sulfatrim DS [CD], Bactrim [CD], Bactrim DS [CD], Bethaprim [CD], Comoxol [CD], ◆Coptin [CD], Cotrim [CD], ◆Novo-Trimel [CD], ◆NovoTrimel DS [CD], ◆Nu-Cotrimox, Polytrim, Proloprim, ◆Protrin [CD], ◆Protrin DF [CD], ◆Roubac [CD], Septra [CD], Septra DS [CD], Sulfatrim D/S, Trimpex, Uroplus DS [CD], Uroplus SS [CD]

BENEFITS versus RISKS	
Possible Benefits	*Possible Risks*
EFFECTIVE TREATMENT OF INFECTIONS due to susceptible microorganisms Effective adjunctive prevention and treament of Pneumocystis carinii pneumonia associated with AIDS	Rare blood cell disorders: megaloblastic anemia, methemoglobinemia, abnormally low white blood cell and platelet counts

▷ **Principal Uses**

As a Single Drug Product: Uses currently included in FDA approved labeling: (1) Used to treat certain infections of the urinary tract that are not complicated by the presence of kidney stones or obstructions to the normal flow of urine. It is sometimes used to prevent the recurrence of such infections; (2) treats eye infections caused by sensitive organisms.

Other (unlabeled) generally accepted uses: (1) Used in combination with dapsone to treat pneumocystis carinii pneumonia in AIDS patients; (2) may have a role in combination therapy of resistant acne.

As a Combination Drug Product [CD]: This drug is available in combination with sulfamethoxazole; the generic name co-trimoxazole is used in some countries to identify this combination. It is very effective in the treatment of certain urinary tract infections, middle ear infections, chronic bronchitis, acute enteritis and certain types of pneumonia. Now used as primary prevention and treatment of Pneumocystis carinii pneumonia associated with AIDS.

How This Drug Works: This drug prevents the growth and multiplication of susceptible infecting organisms by inactivating the enzyme systems that are necessary for the formation of essential nuclear elements and cell proteins.

Available Dosage Forms and Strengths
    Tablets — 100 mg, 200 mg
    Tablets — 80 mg combined with 400 mg of sulfamethoxazole
    Tablets — 160 mg combined with 800 mg of sulfamethoxazole

Oral suspension — 40 mg combined with 200 mg of sulfamethoxazole per 5-ml teaspoonful

▷ **Usual Adult Dosage Range:** 100 mg every 12 hours for 10 days. For certain pneumonias, the same dose is given every 6 hours. The total daily dosage should not exceed 640 mg. **Note: Actual dosage and administration schedule must be determined by the physician for each patient individually.**

Conditions Requiring Dosing Adjustments
Liver function: This drug should be used with caution in patients with both liver and kidney compromise.
Kidney function: Patients with mild kidney compromise can be given the usual dose every 12 hours. Patients with moderate to severe kidney failure (creatinine clearances of 15 to 50 ml/min) can be given the usual dose every 18 hours. The drug is contraindicated in patients with severe and worsening kidney failure.

▷ **Dosing Instructions:** The tablet may be crushed and taken without regard to meals. However, it may also be taken with or following food if necessary to reduce stomach irritation.

Usual Duration of Use: Use on a regular schedule for 7 to 14 days usually determines effectiveness in controlling responsive infections. The actual duration of use will depend upon the nature of the infection.

Currently a "Drug of Choice"
(when combined with sulfamethoxazole) for preventing pneumonia (due to Pneumocystis carinii) in patients with AIDS.

▷ **This Drug Should Not Be Taken If**
 • you have had an allergic reaction to it previously.
 • you have an anemia due to folic acid deficiency.

▷ **Inform Your Physician Before Taking This Drug If**
 • you have a history of folic acid deficiency.
 • you have impaired liver or kidney function.
 • you are pregnant or breast-feeding.

Possible Side-Effects (natural, expected and unavoidable drug actions)
None with short-term use.

▷ **Possible Adverse Effects** (unusual, unexpected and infrequent reactions)
If any of the following develop, consult your physician promptly for guidance.
Mild Adverse Effects
Allergic Reactions: Skin rash (2.9%), itching, drug fever.
Headache, abnormal taste, sore mouth or tongue, loss of appetite, nausea, vomiting, abdominal cramping, diarrhea.
Serious Adverse Effects
Allergic Reactions: Severe dermatitis with peeling of skin.
Blood cell disorders: megaloblastic anemia, methemoglobinemia, abnormally low white blood cell and platelet counts. (All are rare.)
Worsening of hyperkalemia (increased blood potassium).
Kidney toxicity (rare).
Liver toxicity (rare).
Aspetic meningitis (of questionable causal relationship) (extremely rare).

Trimethoprim

▷ **Possible Effects on Sexual Function:** None reported.

Possible Effects on Laboratory Tests
    Complete blood cell counts: decreased red cells, hemoglobin, white cells and platelets.
    Prothrombin time: increased (when taken concurrently with warfarin).

CAUTION
1. Certain strains of bacteria that cause urinary tract infections can develop resistance to this drug. If you do not show significant improvement within 10 days, consult your physician.
2. Comply with your physician's request for periodic blood counts during long-term therapy.

Precautions for Use
    By Infants and Children: Safety and effectiveness for those under 2 months of age not established.
    By Those over 60 Years of Age: The natural decline in liver and kidney function may require smaller doses. If you develop itching reactions in the genital or anal areas, report this promptly.

▷ **Advisability of Use During Pregnancy**
    Pregnancy Category: C. See Pregnancy Code at the back of this book.
    Animal studies: Birth defects due to this drug reported in rat and rabbit studies.
    Human studies: Adequate studies of pregnant women are not available.
    Avoid use of drug during the first 3 months and during the last 2 weeks of pregnancy. Use this drug otherwise only if clearly needed. Ask your physician for guidance.

Advisability of Use if Breast-Feeding
    Presence of this drug in breast milk: Yes.
    Avoid drug or refrain from nursing.

Habit-Forming Potential: None.

Effects of Overdosage: Headache, dizziness, confusion, depression, nausea, vomiting, bone marrow depression, possible liver toxicity with jaundice.

Possible Effects of Long-Term Use: Impaired production of red and white blood cells and blood platelets.

Suggested Periodic Examinations While Taking This Drug (at physician's discretion)
    Complete blood cell counts.

▷ **While Taking This Drug, Observe the Following**
    Foods: No restrictions.
    Beverages: No restrictions. May be taken with milk.
▷   *Alcohol:* No interactions expected.
    Tobacco Smoking: No interactions expected.
▷   *Other Drugs*
    Trimethoprim may *increase* the effects of
- amantadine (Symmetrel) and also result in increased levels of trimethoprim resulting in toxicity.
- cyclosporine (Sandimmune) and result in increased kidney toxicity.
- dapsone and result in dapsone or trimethoprim toxicity.

- phenytoin (Dilantin), and cause phenytoin toxicity.
- procainamide (Procan SR) and result in procainamide toxicity.

The following drugs may *decrease* the effects of trimethoprim
- cholestyramine and perhaps other cholesterol lowering medicines of the same class will bind trimethoprim and blunt the beneficial effects of trimethoprim by inhibiting absorption.
- rifampin (Rifadin, Rimactane).

▷ *Driving, Hazardous Activities:* No restrictions.

Aviation Note: The use of this drug is probably not a disqualification for piloting. Consult a designated Aviation Medical Examiner.

Exposure to Sun: No restrictions.

VALPROIC ACID (val PROH ik)

Introduced: 1967   **Prescription:** USA: Yes; Canada: Yes   **Available as Generic:** USA: Yes; Canada: No   **Class:** Anticonvulsant   **Controlled Drug:** USA: No; Canada: No

Brand Names: Depa, Depakene, Depakote, Deproic, ◆Epival

BENEFITS versus RISKS	
Possible Benefits	*Possible Risks*
EFFECTIVE CONTROL OF MULTIPLE SEIZURE TYPES: ABSENCE SEIZURES, TONIC-CLONIC SEIZURES, MYOCLONIC SEIZURES, PSYCHOMOTOR SEIZURES when used adjunctively with other antiseizure drugs	LIVER TOXICITY, infrequent but may be severe Rare reduction of blood platelets and impaired platelet function with risk of bleeding Rare pancreatitis Rare liver toxicity

▷ **Principal Uses**

As a Single Drug Product: Uses currently included in FDA approved labeling: (1) Used to manage the following types of epilepsy: simple and complex absence seizures (petit mal); tonic-clonic seizures (grand mal); myoclonic seizures; complex partial seizures (psychomotor, temporal lobe epilepsy). It is sometimes used adjunctively with other anticonvulsants as needed.

Other (unlabeled) generally accepted uses: (1) May help prevent migraine headache attacks; (2) can help relieve the symptoms of trigeminal neuralgia; (3) can have a role in intractable hiccups; (4) has had some use in patients with epilepsy and hepatic porphyria; (4) may be of help in writer's cramp.

How This Drug Works: It is thought that by increasing the availability of the nerve impulse transmitter gamma-aminobutyric acid (GABA), this drug suppresses the spread of abnormal electrical discharges that cause seizures.

Available Dosage Forms and Strengths

Capsules — 250 mg
Capsules, sprinkle — 125 mg
Syrup — 250 mg per 5-ml teaspoonful
Tablets, enteric-coated — 125 mg, 250 mg, 500 mg

Valproic Acid

▷ **Usual Adult Dosage Range:** Initially, 15 mg/kg/24 hours. The dose is increased cautiously by 5 to 10 mg/kg/24 hours every 7 days as needed and tolerated. *The usual daily dose is from 1000 mg to 1600 mg in divided doses.* The total daily dosage should not exceed 60 mg/kg. **Note: Actual dosage and administration schedule must be determined by the physician for each patient individually.**

Conditions Requiring Dosing Adjustments
Liver function: Blood levels should be obtained to guide dosing. It can be a rare cause of fatal liver damage, and patients should be followed closely.
Kidney function: No dosing changes are anticipated in patients with compromised kidneys.

▷ **Dosing Instructions:** Preferably taken 1 hour before meals. However, it may be taken with or following food if necessary to prevent stomach irritation. The regular capsule should not be opened and the tablet should not be crushed for administration. The sprinkle-capsule may be opened and the contents sprinkled on soft food for administration. Do not administer the syrup in carbonated beverages. It may be diluted in water or milk.

Usual Duration of Use: Use on a regular schedule for 2 weeks usually determines effectiveness in reducing the frequency and severity of seizures. Long-term use (months to years) requires physician supervision and periodic evaluation.

▷ **This Drug Should Not Be Taken If**
- you have had an allergic reaction to it previously.
- you have active liver disease.
- you are pregnant.
- you have an active bleeding disorder.

▷ **Inform Your Physician Before Taking This Drug If**
- you have a history of liver disease or impaired liver function.
- you have a history of any type of bleeding disorder.
- you are pregnant or planning pregnancy.
- you have myasthenia gravis.
- you are taking: anticoagulants; other anticonvulsants; antidepressants, either the tricyclic type or monoamine oxidase (MAO) type A inhibitors (see Drug Classes).
- you plan to have surgery or dental extraction in the near future.

Possible Side-Effects (natural, expected and unavoidable drug actions)
Drowsiness and lethargy (5%).

▷ **Possible Adverse Effects** (unusual, unexpected and infrequent reactions)
If any of the following develop, consult your physician promptly for guidance.
Mild Adverse Effects
Allergic Reaction: Skin rash (rare).
Headache, dizziness, confusion, unsteadiness, tremor, slurred speech.
Nausea, indigestion, stomach cramps, diarrhea.
Weight gain.
Bed wetting at night.
Temporary loss of scalp hair.

Serious Adverse Effects
   Idiosyncratic Reactions: Bizarre behavior, psychosis, hallucinations.
   Drug-induced hepatitis with jaundice (see Glossary).
   Drug-induced pancreatitis.
   Possible Reye syndrome (see Glossary).
   Increased blood ammonia level.
   Increased blood glucose.
   Drug-induced porphyria.
   Drug-induced lowered function of the thyroid gland (hypothyroidism).
   Decreased selenium levels.
   Reduced formation of blood platelets and impaired function of platelets, with increased risk of abnormal bleeding.
   Drug-induced pancreatitis (rare)
   Reduced formation of red blood cells (rare).
   Increased pressure in the head (pseudotumor cerebri).
   Can cause a Reye-like syndrome.
▷ **Possible Effects on Sexual Function**
   Altered timing and pattern of menstruation.
   Female breast enlargement with milk production.
   Decreased libido.
   Decreased effectiveness of oral contraceptives taken concurrently (6%).
▷ **Adverse Effects That May Mimic Natural Diseases or Disorders**
   Liver reactions may suggest viral hepatitis.
Possible Effects on Laboratory Tests
   Complete blood cell counts: decreased white cells and platelets.
   Bleeding time: increased.
   Prothrombin time: increased.
   Blood amylase level: increased (possible pancreatitis).
   Liver function tests: increased liver enzymes (ALT/GPT, AST/GOT and alkaline phosphatase), increased bilirubin.
CAUTION
   1. The capsules and tablets should be swallowed whole without alteration to avoid irritation of the mouth and throat.
   2. This drug can impair normal blood clotting mechanisms. In the event of injury, dental extraction, or need for surgery, inform your physician or dentist that you are taking this drug.
   3. Because this drug can impair the normal function of blood platelets, it is advisable to avoid aspirin (which has the same effect).
   4. Over-the-counter drug products that contain antihistamines (allergy and cold remedies, sleep aids) can enhance sedative effects.
Precautions for Use
   By Infants and Children: The concurrent use of aspirin with this drug can cause abnormal bleeding or bruising. Children with mental retardation, organic brain disease or severe seizure disorders may be at increased risk for severe liver toxicity while taking this drug. Observe closely for the development of fever that could indicate the onset of a drug-induced Reye syndrome (see Glossary). Avoid concurrent use of clonazepam (Clonopin); the combined use could result in continuous petit mal episodes.
   By Those over 60 Years of Age: Start treatment with small doses and increase

1026   Valproic Acid

dosage cautiously. Observe closely for excessive sedation, confusion or unsteadiness that could predispose to falling and injury.

▷ **Advisability of Use During Pregnancy**
Pregnancy Category: D. See Pregnancy Code at the back of this book.
Animal studies: Palate and skeletal birth defects reported in mouse, rat and rabbit studies.
Human studies: Adequate studies of pregnant women are not available. There have been several reports of birth defects attributed to the use of this drug during early pregnancy.
Consult your physician regarding the advantages and disadvantages of using this drug. If it is used, it is advisable to keep the dose as low as possible.

Advisability of Use if Breast-Feeding
Presence of this drug in breast milk: Yes, in small amounts.
Monitor nursing infant closely and discontinue drug or nursing if adverse effects develop.

Habit-Forming Potential: None.

Effects of Overdosage: Increased drowsiness, weakness, unsteadiness, confusion, stupor progressing to coma.

Possible Effects of Long-Term Use: None reported.

Suggested Periodic Examinations While Taking This Drug (at physician's discretion)
Complete blood cell counts and baseline liver function tests should be done before treatment is started. During treatment, blood counts should be repeated every month and liver function tests repeated every 2 months.

▷ **While Taking This Drug, Observe the Following**
Foods: No restrictions.
Beverages: Do not administer the syrup in carbonated beverages; this could liberate the valproic acid and irritate the mouth and throat. This drug may be taken with milk.

▷ *Alcohol:* Alcohol can increase the sedative effect of this drug. Also, this drug can increase the depressant effects of alcohol on brain function.
Tobacco Smoking: No interactions expected.

▷ *Other Drugs*
Valproic acid may *increase* the effects of
- anticoagulants (Coumadin, etc.), and increase the risk of bleeding.
- antidepressants, both monoamine oxidase (MAO) type A inhibitors and tricyclics, and cause toxicity.
- nimodipine (Nimotop) and cause nimodipine toxicity.
- phenobarbital, and cause barbiturate intoxication.
- phenytoin (Dilantin), and cause phenytoin toxicity.

Valproic acid *taken concurrently* with
- antacids (Maalox) will decrease absorption and decrease therapeutic benefit.
- antiplatelet drugs: aspirin, dipyridamole (Persantine), sulfinpyrazone (Anturane) may enhance the inhibition of platelet function and increase the risk of bleeding.
- aspirin can lead to valproic acid toxicity.
- cyclosporine (Sandimmune) may increase risk of liver toxicity.

- erythromycin (Ery-Tab, others) may increase the level of valproic acid and result in toxicity. The newer macrolides (azithromycin or clarithromycin) may also cause problems.
- felbamate can lead to increased valproic acid levels.
- isoniazid can cause valproic acid or isoniazid toxicity.

▷ *Driving, Hazardous Activities:* This drug may cause drowsiness, dizziness or confusion. Restrict activities as necessary.

Aviation Note: The use of this drug *is a disqualification* for piloting. Consult a designated Aviation Medical Examiner.

Exposure to Sun: No restrictions.

*Discontinuation: **Do not discontinue this drug suddenly.*** Abrupt withdrawal can cause repetitive seizures that are difficult to control.

VANCOMYCIN (van koh MI sin)

Introduced: 1974 **Prescription:** USA: Yes; Canada: Yes **Available as Generic:** USA: Yes; Canada: No **Class:** Anti-infective **Controlled Drug:** USA: No; Canada: No

Brand Name: Vancocin, Vancoled, Vancor

Note: Vancomycin is used to treat a variety of serious infections. It is given intravenously to treat some infections and orally to treat others. The information provided in this Drug Profile is limited to the use of vancomycin taken by mouth.

BENEFITS versus RISKS	
Possible Benefits	*Possible Risks*
HIGHLY EFFECTIVE IN TREATING ANTIBIOTIC-ASSOCIATED PSEUDOMEMBRANOUS COLITIS	Ringing in ears (tinnitus) Loss of hearing

▷ **Principal Uses**

As a Single Drug Product: Uses currently included in FDA approved labeling: Treatment of (1) antibiotic-associated pseudomembranous colitis caused by *Clostridium difficile*; (2) enterocolitis caused by staphylococcal organisms.

Other (unlabeled) generally accepted uses: None.

How This Drug Works: By inhibiting the formation of bacterial cell walls and the production of RNA, this drug destroys susceptible strains of infecting bacteria.

Available Dosage Forms and Strengths

Capsules — 125 mg, 250 mg

Oral solution — 250 mg per 5-ml teaspoonful and 500 mg per 5-ml teaspoonful

▷ **Recommended Dosage Ranges (Actual dosage and administration schedule must be determined by the physician for each patient individually.)**

Infants and Children: 10 mg/kg of body weight every 6 hours, for 5 to 10 days. The total daily dose should not exceed 2000 mg (2 grams). Repeat course as necessary.

Vancomycin

12 to 60 Years of Age: 125 to 500 mg every 6 hours, for 5 to 10 days. The total daily dose should not exceed 2000 mg (2 grams). Repeat course as necessary.

Over 60 Years of Age: Same as 12 to 60 years of age.

Conditions Requiring Dosing Adjustments
Liver function: The liver is not involved in the elimination of vancomycin.
Kidney function: Oral vancomycin is minimally absorbed.

▷ **Dosing Instructions:** May be taken with or following food to reduce stomach irritation. Because of this drug's unpleasant taste, it is preferable to swallow the capsule whole without alteration. Use a measuring device to ensure accuracy of dose when taking the oral solution. Observe the expiration date.

Usual Duration of Use: Use on a regular schedule for 48 to 72 hours usually determines effectiveness in controlling infection in the colon. If response is prompt, limit treatment to 7 days. If symptoms warrant, continue treatment for 14 to 21 days. Consult your physician on a regular basis.

Currently a "Drug of Choice"
for treating metronidazole treatment failures in antibiotic-associated pseudomembranous colitis caused by *C. difficile*.

▷ **This Drug Should Not Be Taken If**
- you have had an allergic reaction to it previously.

▷ **Inform Your Physician Before Taking This Drug If**
- you have a history of Crohn's disease or ulcerative colitis.
- you have impaired kidney function.
- you have any degree of hearing loss.
- you are taking cholestyramine (Questran) or colestipol (Colestid).

Possible Side-Effects (natural, expected and unavoidable drug actions)
Bitter, unpleasant taste.

▷ **Possible Adverse Effects** (unusual, unexpected and infrequent reactions)
If any of the following develop, consult your physician promptly for guidance.

Mild Adverse Effects
Allergic Reactions: Skin rash (with large doses or prolonged use).
Nausea, vomiting.

Serious Adverse Effects
Ringing or buzzing in ears, sensation of ear fullness, loss of hearing.

▷ **Possible Effects on Sexual Function:** None reported.

Natural Diseases or Disorders That May Be Activated by This Drug
Latent hearing loss.

Possible Effects on Laboratory Tests
None expected.

CAUTION
1. Report promptly the development of fullness, ringing or buzzing in either ear. This may indicate the onset of nerve damage that could lead to hearing loss.
2. Do not take any medication to stop your diarrhea without calling your doctor. The bacterial toxin that causes colitis is eliminated by diarrhea; stopping the elimination could intensify and prolong your illness.

Precautions for Use
By Infants and Children: This drug is usually well tolerated. Some cases may require doses up to 50 mg/kg of body weight daily.
By Those over 60 Years of Age: You may be more susceptible to drug-induced hearing loss. Use the minimum course of treatment required to cure your colitis.

▷ **Advisability of Use During Pregnancy**
Pregnancy Category:
B. See Pregnancy Code at the back of this book.
Animal studies: Rat and rabbit studies reveal no drug-induced birth defects.
Human studies: Adequate studies of pregnant women are not available.
Use this drug only if clearly needed. Ask your physician for guidance.

Advisability of Use if Breast-Feeding
Presence of this drug in breast milk: Yes.
Avoid drug or refrain from nursing.

Habit-Forming Potential: None.

Effects of Overdosage: Possible nausea, vomiting, ringing in ears.

Possible Effects of Long-Term Use: Hearing loss.

Suggested Periodic Examinations While Taking This Drug (at physician's discretion)
Hearing tests.

▷ **While Taking This Drug, Observe the Following**
Foods: No restrictions.
Beverages: No restrictions. May be taken with milk.
▷ *Alcohol:* No interactions expected. Use sparingly; alcohol may aggravate colitis.
Tobacco Smoking: No interactions expected.
▷ *Other Drugs*
The following drugs may *decrease* the effects of vancomycin
  • cholestyramine (Questran).
  • colestipol (Colestid).
Vancomycin *taken concurrently* with
  • aminoglycoside antibiotics such as gentamicin or tobramycin may cause additive toxicity risk to the ears and kidneys.
  • cyclosporine (Sandimmune) may result in increased toxicity risk.
  • warfarin (Coumadin) may cause an increased risk of bleeding.
▷ *Driving, Hazardous Activities:* Usually no restrictions.
Aviation Note: The use of this drug *is probably not a disqualification* for piloting. Consult a designated Aviation Medical Examiner.
Exposure to Sun: No restrictions.
Discontinuation: To be determined by your physician.
Special Storage Instructions: Refrigerate the oral solution.
Observe the Following Expiration Times: Provided on your prescription label by your pharmacist.

VARICELLA VIRUS VACCINE (VAIR a Cella)

Introduced: 1995 **Prescription:** USA: Yes; Canada: Yes **Available as Generic:** USA: No; Canada: No **Class:** Vaccine **Controlled Drug:** USA: No; Canada: No

Brand Names: Varivax

BENEFITS versus RISKS	
Possible Benefits	*Possible Risks*
Prevention of varicella (chicken pox)	Rash (5%)
	Soreness at the injection site
	Anaphylactoid reaction (rare)

▷ **Principal Uses**
  As a Single Drug Product: Uses currently included in FDA approved labeling: (1) Prevention of chicken pox.
  Other (unlabeled) generally accepted uses: None.

How This Drug Works: By stimulating the immune system, the vaccine prepares the body to fight any exposure the the wild type virus.

Available Dosage Forms and Strengths
  Vaccine (multi-dose vial) — a single dose vial of vaccine (1500 PFU per dose)

How To Store
  This product **must** be kept frozen prior to use.
  Author's note: The Center for Disease Control's (CDC) Immunization Practices Committee has recommended that all children 12 to 18 months old should be given varicella vaccine if they have not previously contracted chicken pox. The vaccine is also recomended by the committee for children 19 months to 13 years old. Finally, adults or adolescents who have not had chicken pox and are at risk for exposure should also be given the vaccine.

▷ **Recommended Dosage Ranges (Actual dosage and administration schedule must be determined by the physician for each patient individually.)**
  Infants and Children from one to 12 years old: Not indicated in infants. Children 1 year old or older are given 0.5 ml injected under the skin.
  12 to 55 Years of Age: Same as the children's dose, providing the patient has not had chicken pox.
  Over 55 Years of Age: Not studied.

Conditions Requiring Dosing Adjustments
  Liver function: Not a consideration.
  Kidney function: Not a consideration.

▷ **Dosing Instructions:** This vaccine is to be injected under the skin. It may be given with measles, mumps and rubella vaccine.

Usual Duration of Benefit: Exposure to chicken pox 5 years after vaccination may result in 20% of patients developing mild disease. More experience is needed before the question of repeat vaccination is answered.

Varicella Virus Vaccine 1031

Possible Advantages of This Drug
Prevention of chicken pox.

Currently a "Drug of Choice"
for prevention of chicken pox.

▷ **This Drug Should Not Be Taken If**
- you have had an allergic reaction to any dosage form of it previously.
- you have a history of anaphylactoid reaction to neomycin.
- you have a history of blood diseases, leukemia, or have AIDS.
- you are taking medicines which suppress the immune system.
- you have tuberculosis which has not been treated.
- you are allergic to eggs.
- you are pregnant.
- you have an active infection.

▷ **Inform Your Physician Before Taking This Drug If**
- you are planning pregnancy in the near future.
- you have a condition which may require steroids.

Possible Side-Effects (natural, expected and unavoidable drug actions)
Pain at the injection site.

▷ **Possible Adverse Effects** (unusual, unexpected and infrequent reactions)
If any of the following develop, consult your physician promptly for guidance.
Mild Adverse Effects
Allergic Reactions: Skin rash.
Varicella-like rash (3.4%).
Irritability, fatigue and loss of appetite.
Chills, stiff neck and joint pain.
Serious Adverse Effects
Allergic Reactions: Anaphylactoid reaction.
Idiosyncratic Reactions: None reported.
Febrile seizures (rare).
Pneumonitis (very rare and of questionable causation).

▷ **Possible Effects on Sexual Function:** None reported.

Possible Delayed Adverse Effects: None reported.

▷ **Adverse Effects That May Mimic Natural Diseases or Disorders**
Rash may resemble chicken pox.

Natural Diseases or Disorders That May Be Activated by This Drug
None reported.

Possible Effects on Laboratory Tests
None reported.

CAUTION
1. **Do not** give aspirin or other salicylates to patients who have recently received the vaccine. The risk of Reye's syndrome is associated with such aspirin use.

1032 Venlafaxine

Precautions for Use
By Infants and Children:
Safety and effectiveness for use by those under 12 months of age have not been established.
By Those over 60 Years of Age: Not studied.

▷ **Advisability of Use During Pregnancy**
Pregnancy Category: C. See Pregnancy Code at the back of this book.
Animal studies: Have not been conducted with this vaccine.
Human studies: Information from adequate studies of pregnant women is not available. The manufacturer says that the vaccine should not be given to pregnant women and pregnancy should be avoided for three months following vaccination.

Advisability of Use if Breast-Feeding
Presence of this drug in breast milk: Expected.
Avoid drug or refrain from nursing.

Habit-Forming Potential: None.

Effects of Overdosage: Not defined.

Possible Effects of Long-Term Use: Not intended for long-term use.

Suggested Periodic Examinations While Taking This Drug (at physician's discretion)
None suggested.

▷ **While Taking This Drug, Observe the Following**
Foods: No restrictions.
Beverages: No restrictions.
▷ *Alcohol:* No interactions expected.
Tobacco Smoking: No interactions expected.
▷ *Other Drugs*
Varicella vaccine **taken concurrently** with
- corticosteroids (see Drug Classes) may result in extreme reactions.
- immunosuppressant medicines may result in extreme reactions.

▷ *Driving, Hazardous Activities:* This drug may cause soreness at the injection site. Restrict activities as necessary.
Aviation Note: The use of this drug **is probably not a disqualification** for piloting. Consult a designated Aviation Medical Examiner.
Exposure to Sun: No restrictions.
Occurrence of Unrelated Illness: This vaccination should not be given in the presence of any other active infection.
Special Storage Instructions: This vaccine must be stored frozen.

Author's note: There is now a Vaccine Adverse Event Reporting System (VAERS). The toll free number is 1–800-822-7967.

VENLAFAXINE (Ven la FAX ene)

Introduced: 1993 **Prescription:** USA: Yes **Available as Generic:** USA: No **Class:** Antidepressant **Controlled Drug:** USA: No
Brand Names: Effexor

BENEFITS versus RISKS	
Possible Benefits	**Possible Risks**
EFFECTIVE TREATMENT OF DEPRESSION BETTER SIDE EFFECT PROFILE THAN TRICYCLIC ANTIDEPRESSANTS RAPID ONSET OF EFFECT	INCREASED BLOOD PRESSURE Seizures (rare) Constipation Increased heart rate Increased serum lipids

▷ **Principal Uses**

As a Single Drug Product: Uses currently included in FDA approved labeling: (1) Treatment of depression.

Other (unlabeled) generally accepted uses: (1) May be useful in treatment of obsessive-compulsive disorder.

How This Drug Works: This bicyclic (second generation) antidepressant inhibits the return of (reuptake) of nerve transmitters (serotonin, norepinephrine and dopamine) and helps return normal mood and thinking.

Available Dosage Forms and Strengths

Tablets — 25 mg, 37.5 mg, 50 mg, 75 mg, 100 mg.

▷ **Recommended Dosage Ranges (Actual dosage and administration schedule must be determined by the physician for each patient individually.)**

Infants and Children: Safety and efficacy for those under 18 years of age not established.

18 to 60 Years of Age: Therapy is started with 75 mg per day, given as 25 mg doses 3 times daily.

If needed and tolerated, the dose may be increased at 4 day intervals up to a maximum of 225 mg per day. Some hospitalized patients have been given a maximum of 375 mg per day.

Over 60 Years of Age: Low starting doses and slow increases are indicated. Natural declines in kidney function may lead to drug accumulation at higher doses. This drug may worsen a constipation problem that you already face.

Conditions Requiring Dosing Adjustments

Liver function: The total daily dose must be reduced by 50% in patients with moderate liver compromise. Further dose decreases and individualized dosing is indicated in patients with liver cirrhosis. The drug is changed to an active form in the liver.

Kidney function: In patients with compromised kidneys (creatinine clearance of 10 to 70 ml/min) should be given 75% of the usual daily dose.

▷ **Dosing Instructions:** Food has no clinically significant effect on venlafaxine absorption.

Usual Duration of Use: Use on a regular schedule for 2 weeks usually determines effectiveness in treating depression. Long-term use (months to years) requires periodic physician evaluation of response and dosage adjustment.

Possible Advantages of This Drug

Effective treatment of depression with fewer side effects than other currently available agents. Starts to have a therapeutic effect more rapidly than other available agents.

Venlafaxine

▷ **This Drug Should Not Be Taken If**
  • you have had an allergic reaction to any dosage form of it previously.

▷ **Inform Your Physician Before Taking This Drug If**
  • you have a history of high blood pressure.
  • you have a history of abnormally increased lipids (hyperlipidemia).
  • you are uncertain of how much venlafaxine to take or how often to take it.

Possible Side-Effects (natural, expected and unavoidable drug actions)
Constipation and headache.

▷ **Possible Adverse Effects** (unusual, unexpected and infrequent reactions)
  If any of the following develop, consult your physician promptly for guidance.
Mild Adverse Effects
Allergic Reactions.
Palpitations.
Nausea and vomiting.
Dizziness (may disappear without treatment), fatigue and headache.
Anxiety or insomnia (may stop on its own).
Somnolence (up to 24%).
Blurred vision (6%).
Sweating (25%).
Weight loss (6%), dry mouth (up to 22%).
Small increases in cholesterol (2–3 mg/dl).
Serious Adverse Effects
Allergic Reactions: None reported.
Idiosyncratic Reactions: None reported.
Increased blood pressure.
Seizures (rare).

▷ **Possible Effects on Sexual Function:** Delayed orgasm, abnormal ejaculation, impotence and erectile failure (all infrequent).

Possible Delayed Adverse Effects: None reported.

▷ **Adverse Effects That May Mimic Natural Diseases or Disorders**
None reported.

Natural Diseases or Disorders That May Be Activated by This Drug
None reported.

Possible Effects on Laboratory Tests
Serum cholesterol: Increased slightly.

CAUTION
  1. This drug should **not** be taken with MAO inhibiter (see Glossary) drugs. If you have recently stopped a MAO inhibiter, 14 days should pass before venlafaxine is started.

▷ **Advisability of Use During Pregnancy**
Pregnancy Category: C. See Pregnancy Code at the back of this book.
Animal studies: There was an increase in stillborn rats at 10 times the usual human dose.
Human studies: Adequate studies of pregnant women are not available.
Ask your doctor for guidance.

Advisability of Use if Breast-Feeding
Presence of this drug in breast milk: Unknown.

Monitor nursing infant closely and discontinue drug or nursing if adverse effects develop.

Habit-Forming Potential: None.

Effects of Overdosage: Nausea, vomiting, constipation, seizure potential.

Possible Effects of Long-Term Use: None noted.

Suggested Periodic Examinations While Taking This Drug (at physician's discretion)
Blood pressure checks.

▷ **While Taking This Drug, Observe the Following**
Foods: No restrictions.
Nutritional Support: No special support indicated.
Beverages: No restrictions.
▷ *Alcohol:* May increase somnolence if combined.
Tobacco Smoking: No interactions expected.
Marijuana Smoking: Additive effect on somnolence.
▷ *Other Drugs*
Venlafaxine *taken concurrently* with
- drugs with sedative propertive will increase those effects.
- cimetidine may lead to venlafaxine toxicity.
- MAO inhibitors may lead to undesirable side effects. Do not combine.

▷ *Driving, Hazardous Activities:* This drug may cause somnolence. Restrict activities as necessary.
Aviation Note: The use of this drug *is a disqualification* for piloting. Consult a designated Aviation Medical Examiner.
Exposure to Sun: No restrictions.
Exposure to Heat: No restrictions.
Discontinuation: Talk to your doctor before stopping this medication.

VERAPAMIL (ver AP a mil)

Introduced: 1967 **Prescription:** USA: Yes; Canada: Yes **Available as Generic:** USA: Yes; Canada: No **Class:** Antianginal, antiarrhythmic, antihypertensive, calcium channel blocker **Controlled Drug:** USA: No; Canada: No
Brand Names: ✦Apo-Verap, Calan, Calan SR, Isoptin, Isoptin SR, ✦Novo-Veramil, ✦Nu-Verap, Verelan

BENEFITS versus RISKS	
Possible Benefits	*Possible Risks*
EFFECTIVE PREVENTION OF BOTH MAJOR TYPES OF ANGINA	Congestive heart failure
	Low blood pressure (2.9%)
	Heart rhythm disturbance
EFFECTIVE CONTROL OF HEART RATE IN CHRONIC ATRIAL FIBRILLATION AND FLUTTER	Fluid retention (1.7%)
	Liver damage without jaundice (very rare)
EFFECTIVE PREVENTION OF PAROXYSMAL ATRIAL TACHYCARDIA (PAT)	Swelling of male breast tissue
EFFECTIVE TREATMENT OF HYPERTENSION	

Verapamil

▷ **Principal Uses**

As a Single Drug Product: Uses currently included in FDA approved labeling: Used to treat (1) angina pectoris due to coronary artery spasm (Prinzmetal's variant angina) that occurs spontaneously and is not associated with exertion; (2) classical angina-of-effort (due to atherosclerotic disease of the coronary arteries) in individuals who have not responded to or cannot tolerate the nitrates and beta blocker drugs customarily used to treat this disorder; (3) abnormally rapid heart rate due to chronic atrial fibrillation or flutter; (4) recurrent paroxysmal atrial tachycardia; and (5) primary hypertension.

Other (unlabeled) generally accepted uses: (1) May help prevent abnormal heart rhythms that occur after surgery; (2) can help relieve symptoms and may help reverse hypertrophic cardiomyopathy; (3) may help decrease the severity or occurrence of cluster headaches; (4) used to help control the symptoms of panic attacks; (5) can be of use in postischemic acute kidney failure; (6) may stop the progression of abnormal buildup on the inside of blood vessels (atherosclerosis); (7) may help decrease severity and occurance of nocturnal leg cramps; (8) could have a place in combination therapy of multiple myeloma; (9) can help stuttering; (10) may have a role in Tourette's syndrome.

How This Drug Works: By blocking passage of calcium through certain cell walls (which is necessary for the function of nerve and muscle tissue), this drug slows the spread of electrical activity through the heart and inhibits the contraction of coronary arteries and peripheral arterioles. As a result of these combined effects, this drug
- prevents spontaneous coronary artery spasm (Prinzmetal's type of angina).
- reduces the rate and contraction force of the heart during exertion, thus lowering the oxygen requirement of the heart muscle; this reduces the occurrence of effort-induced angina (classical angina pectoris).
- reduces the degree of contraction of peripheral arterial walls, resulting in their relaxation and consequent lowering of blood pressure. This further reduces the work load of the heart during exertion and contributes to the prevention of angina.
- slows the rate of electrical impulses through the heart and thereby prevents excessively rapid heart action (tachycardia).

Available Dosage Forms and Strengths

Capsules, prolonged-action — 120 mg, 240 mg
Injection — 5 mg per 2 ml
Tablets — 40 mg, 80 mg, 120 mg
Tablets, prolonged-action — 180 mg, 240 mg

▷ **Usual Adult Dosage Range:** Initially, 80 mg 3 or 4 times daily. The dose may be increased gradually at 1 to 7 day intervals as needed and tolerated. The usual maintenance dose is from 240 mg to 480 mg daily in 3 or 4 divided doses. The prolonged-action dosage forms permit once-a-day dosing. The total daily dosage should not exceed 480 mg.

Once-a-day treatment may be initiated with 1 prolonged-action capsule of 120 mg or 1 tablet of 180 mg.

Verapamil

Note: Actual dosage and administration schedule must be determined by the physician for each patient individually.

Conditions Requiring Dosing Adjustments
Liver function: Blood levels should be obtained, and used to guide dosing. In patients with liver compromise, the dose should be decreased to 20–50% of the usual dose and may be given at the usual interval. Verapamil can be a rare cause of liver damage, and patients should be followed closely. Changes in the electrocardiogram may provide an early indication of increasing blood levels.

Kidney function: In severe kidney compromise, the dose should be decreased by 50–75%.

▷ **Dosing Instructions:** Preferably taken with meals and with food at bedtime. The regular tablet may be crushed for administration. The prolonged-action dosage forms (capsules and tablets) should be swallowed whole and not altered. Verelan capsules may be taken without regard to food intake.

Usual Duration of Use: Use on a regular schedule for 2 to 4 weeks usually determines effectiveness in reducing the frequency and severity of angina. Reduction of elevated blood pressure may be apparent within the first 1 to 2 weeks. For long-term use (months to years), the smallest effective dose should be used. Periodic physician evaluation is needed.

Possible Advantages of This Drug
No adverse effects on blood levels of glucose, potassium or uric acid.
Does not increase blood cholesterol or triglyceride levels.
Does not impair capacity for exercise.

Currently a "Drug of Choice"
for (1) initiating treatment of hypertension with a single drug; (2) treating hypertension in African-Americans.

▷ **This Drug Should Not Be Taken If**
- you have had an allergic reaction to it previously.
- you have active liver disease.
- you have a "sick sinus" syndrome (and do not have an artificial pacemaker).
- you have been told that you have a second-degree or third-degree heart block.
- you have low blood pressure systolic pressure below 90.
- you have advanced aortic stenosis (ask your doctor).

▷ **Inform Your Physician Before Taking This Drug If**
- you have had an unfavorable response to any calcium blocker.
- you are currently taking any other drugs, especially digitalis or a beta blocker drug (see Drug Class Section).
- you have had a recent stroke or heart attack.
- you have a history of congestive heart failure or heart rhythm disorders.
- you have impaired liver or kidney function.
- you have a history of drug-induced liver damage.

Possible Side-Effects (natural, expected and unavoidable drug actions)
Low blood pressure (2.9%), fluid retention (1.7%).

Verapamil

▷ **Possible Adverse Effects** (unusual, unexpected and infrequent reactions)
If any of the following develop, consult your physician promptly for guidance.

Mild Adverse Effects
Allergic Reactions: Skin rash, hives, itching, aching joints.
Headache (1.8%), dizziness (3.6%), fatigue (1.1%).
Nausea (1.6%), indigestion, constipation (6.3%).
Sensation of numbness or coldness in the extremities.

Serious Adverse Effects
Serious disturbances of heart rate and/or rhythm, congestive heart failure (0.9%).
Drug-induced liver damage without jaundice (very rare).
Antiplatelet effect and extended time to form blood clots.
Ventricular fibrillation (with intravenous use in patients with atrial fibrillation).
Excessive lowering of blood pressure.
Low blood sugar.

▷ **Possible Effects on Sexual Function**
Altered timing and pattern of menstruation.
Male breast enlargement and tenderness.
Impotence (20%).

Possible Effects on Laboratory Tests
Blood total cholesterol and HDL cholesterol levels: no effect in some; decreased in others.
Blood LDL cholesterol level: no effect.
Blood triglyceride levels: no effect.
Glucose tolerance test (GTT): decreased.
Liver function tests: increased liver enzymes (ALT/GPT and AST/GOT), increased bilirubin (one case report).

CAUTION
1. Be sure to inform all physicians and other health care professionals who provide medical care for you that you take this drug. Note the use of this drug on your card of personal identification.
2. You may use nitroglycerin and other nitrate drugs as needed to relieve acute episodes of angina pain. However, if you detect that your angina attacks are becoming more frequent or intense, notify your physician promptly.
3. If this drug is used concurrently with a beta blocker drug, you may develop excessively low blood pressure.
4. This drug may cause swelling of the feet and ankles. This may not be indicative of either heart or kidney dysfunction.

Precautions for Use
By Infants and Children: Safety and effectiveness for those under 12 years of age not established.
By Those over 60 Years of Age: You may be more susceptible to the development of weakness, dizziness, fainting and falling. Take necessary precautions to prevent injury. Report promptly any changes in your pattern of thirst and urination.

▷ **Advisability of Use During Pregnancy**
Pregnancy Category: C. See Pregnancy Code at the back of this book.
Animal studies: Toxic effects on the embryo and retarded growth of the fetus (but no birth defects) reported in rat studies.
Human studies: Adequate studies of pregnant women are not available.
Avoid this drug during the first 3 months. Use during the last 6 months only if clearly needed. Ask your physician for guidance.

Advisability of Use if Breast-Feeding
Presence of this drug in breast milk: Possibly yes.
Avoid drug or refrain from nursing.

Habit-Forming Potential: None.

Effects of Overdosage: Flushed and warm skin, sweating, light-headedness, irritability, rapid heart rate, low blood pressure, loss of consciousness.

Possible Effects of Long-Term Use: None reported.

Suggested Periodic Examinations While Taking This Drug (at physician's discretion)
Evaluations of heart function, including electrocardiograms; liver and kidney function tests, with long-term use.

▷ **While Taking This Drug, Observe the Following**
Foods: No restrictions. Avoid excessive salt intake.
Beverages: Caffeine levels will be increased if caffeine containing beverages are consumed while you are on verapamil. May be taken with milk.
▷ *Alcohol:* Use with caution until combined effects have been determined. Alcohol may exaggerate the drop in blood pressure, and change the elimination of alcohol experienced by some patients.
Tobacco Smoking: Nicotine can reduce the effectiveness of this drug. Avoid all forms of tobacco.
Marijuana Smoking: Possible reduced effectiveness of this drug; mild to moderate increase in angina; possible changes in electrocardiogram, confusing interpretation.

▷ *Other Drugs*
Verapamil may *increase* the effects of
- carbamazepine (Tegretol), and cause carbamazepine toxicity.
- digitoxin and digoxin, and cause digitalis toxicity.

Verapamil *taken concurrently* with
- aspirin may result in bleeding.
- amiodarone (Codarone) may result in cardiac arrest.
- beta blocker drugs (see Drug Class Section) may affect heart rate and rhythm adversely. Careful monitoring by your physician is necessary if these drugs are taken concurrently.
- cyclosporine (Sandimmune) may result in cyclosporine toxicity and renal compromise.
- dantrolene will cause elevated blood potsssium and depression of the heart.
- disopyramide can cause congestive heart failure.
- lithium (Lithobid, others) may result in lithium toxicity and mania.
- NSAIDs (see Drug Classes) may blunt the therapeutic effect of verapamil on blood pressure.

- oral hypoglycemic agents (see Drug Classes) may lead to excessively low blood sugar.
- phenytoin (Dilantin) may result in decreased effectiveness of verapamil.
- quinidine (Quinaglute, others) can result in quinidine toxicity.
- rifampin will decrease the therapeutic benefit of verapamil.
- sulfinpyrazone increases the removal of verapamil and lessens the therapeutic effect.
- terazocin can lead to excessive decreases in blood pressure.
- theophylline can lead to theophylline toxicity.

The following drugs may *increase* the effects of verapamil
- cimetidine (Tagamet).

▷ *Driving, Hazardous Activities:* Usually no restrictions. This drug may cause dizziness. Restrict activities as necessary.

Aviation Note: Coronary artery disease *is a disqualification* for piloting. Consult a designated Aviation Medical Examiner.

Exposure to Sun: Use caution until sensitivity has been determined. This drug may cause photosensitivity (see Glossary).

Exposure to Heat: Caution advised. Hot environments can exaggerate the blood-pressure-lowering effects of this drug. Observe for light-headedness or weakness.

Heavy Exercise or Exertion: This drug may improve your ability to be more active without resulting angina pain. Use caution and avoid excessive exercise that could impair heart function in the absence of warning pain.

Discontinuation: Do not stop this drug abruptly. Consult your physician regarding gradual withdrawal to prevent the development of rebound angina.

WARFARIN (WAR far in)

Introduced: 1941 **Prescription:** USA: Yes; Canada: Yes **Available as Generic:** USA: No; Canada: No **Class:** Anticoagulant, coumarins
Controlled Drug: USA: No; Canada: No
Brand Names: Coumadin

BENEFITS versus RISKS	
Possible Benefits	*Possible Risks*
EFFECTIVE PREVENTION OF BOTH ARTERIAL AND VENOUS THROMBOSIS	NARROW TREATMENT RANGE Dose-related bleeding (5–7%) Skin and soft tissue hemorrhage with tissue death (rare)
EFFECTIVE PREVENTION OF EMBOLIZATION IN THROMBOEMBOLIC DISORDERS	
HELPS PREVENT RECURRENCE OF HEART ATTACK	

▷ **Principal Uses**

As a Single Drug Product: Uses currently included in FDA approved labeling: Used in: (1) acute thrombosis (clot) or thrombophlebitis of the deep veins; (2) acute pulmonary embolism, resulting from blood clots that originate anywhere in the body; (3) atrial fibrillation, to prevent clotting of blood inside the heart that could result in embolization of small clots to any part of the body; (4) acute myocardial infarction (heart attack), to prevent clotting and embolization and therefore a recurrence of heart attack.

Other (unlabeled) generally accepted uses: (1) Helps prevent embolization from the heart in those individuals with artificial heart valves; (2) may help patients with low blood platelets caused by heparin.

How This Drug Works: The coumarin anticoagulants interfere with the production of four essential blood clotting factors by blocking the action of vitamin K. This leads to a deficiency of these clotting factors in circulating blood and inhibits blood clotting mechanisms.

Available Dosage Forms and Strengths
Injection — 50 mg/vial
Tablets — 1 mg, 2 mg, 2.5 mg, 5 mg, 7.5 mg, 10 mg

▷ **Usual Adult Dosage Range:** Initially, 10 to 15 mg daily for 2 to 3 days. A large loading dose is inappropriate and may be hazardous. For maintenance, 2 to 10 mg/day. The dosage is adjusted according to the prothrombin time. **Note: Actual dosage and administration schedule must be determined by the physician for each patient individually.**

Conditions Requiring Dosing Adjustments
Liver function: Blood testing (prothrombin times) should be obtained to guide dosing. It is contraindicated in patients with liver disease.
Kidney function: This drug should be used with caution in renal compromise, however, as warfarin may cause microscopic kidney stones.

▷ **Dosing Instructions:** The tablet may be crushed and is preferably taken when the stomach is empty, and at the same time each day to ensure uniform results.

Usual Duration of Use: Use on a regular schedule for 3 to 5 days usually determines effectiveness in providing significant anticoagulation. An additional 10 to 14 days is required to determine the optimal maintenance dose for each individual. Long-term use (months to years) requires physician supervision.

▷ **This Drug Should Not Be Taken If**
- you have had an allergic reaction to it previously.
- you have an active peptic ulcer or active ulcerative colitis.
- you are pregnant.
- recent anesthesia (lumbar block) to the spine.
- arterial aneurysm.
- low blood platelets.
- infective pericarditis.
- you have esophageal varices (ask your doctor).
- you have had a recent stroke.

▷ **Inform Your Physician Before Taking This Drug If**
- you are now taking *any other drugs,* either prescription drugs or over-the-counter drug products.
- you are planning pregnancy.
- you have a history of a bleeding disorder.
- you have high blood pressure.
- you have abnormally heavy or prolonged menstrual bleeding.
- you have diabetes.

- you are using an indwelling catheter.
- you have impaired liver or kidney function.
- you plan to have surgery or dental extraction in the near future.

Possible Side-Effects (natural, expected and unavoidable drug actions)
Minor episodes of bleeding may occur even though dosage and prothrombin times are well within the recommended range.

▷ **Possible Adverse Effects** (unusual, unexpected and infrequent reactions)
If any of the following develop, consult your physician promptly for guidance.

Mild Adverse Effects
Allergic Reactions: Skin rash, hives.
Loss of scalp hair.
Loss of appetite, nausea, vomiting, cramping, diarrhea.

Serious Adverse Effects
Allergic Reaction: Drug fever (see Glossary).
Idiosyncratic Reactions: Bleeding into skin and soft tissues causing gangrene of breast, toes and localized areas anywhere (rare).
Hereditary warfarin resistance (rare).
Abnormal bleeding from nose, gastrointestinal tract, lungs urinary tract or uterus.
Pericardial tamponade.
Acute femoral neuropathy (rare)
Kidney problems (tubulointerstitial nephritis) (rare).

▷ **Possible Effects on Sexual Function:** None reported.

▷ **Adverse Effects That May Mimic Natural Diseases or Disorders**
Drug-induced fever may suggest infection.

Natural Diseases or Disorders That May Be Activated by This Drug
Bleeding from "silent" peptic ulcer, intestinal or bladder polyp or tumor.

Possible Effects on Laboratory Tests
Complete blood cell counts: decreased red cells, hemoglobin and white cells.
Bleeding time: increased.
Prothrombin time: increased.
Blood uric acid level: increased (in men).
Liver function tests: increased liver enzymes (ALT/GPT, AST/GOT and alkaline phosphatase).

CAUTION
1. Always carry with you a card of personal identification that includes a statement that *you are taking an anticoagulant drug.*
2. While taking this drug, always consult your physician *before* starting any new drug, changing the dosage schedule of any drug or stopping any drug.

Precautions for Use
By Those over 60 Years of Age: Small starting doses are mandatory. Watch regularly for excessive drug effects: prolonged bleeding from shaving cuts, bleeding gums, bloody urine, rectal bleeding, excessive bruising.

▷ **Advisability of Use During Pregnancy**
Pregnancy Category: D. See Pregnancy Code at the back of this book.
Animal studies: Fetal hemorrhage and death due to this drug reported in mice.

Human studies: Information from studies of pregnant women indicates fetal defects and fetal hemorrhage due to this drug.

The manufacturers state that this drug is contraindicated during entire pregnancy.

Advisability of Use if Breast-Feeding
Presence of this drug in breast milk: Yes.
Avoid drug or refrain from nursing.

Habit-Forming Potential: None.

Effects of Overdosage: Episodes of bleeding from minor surface bleeding (nose, gums, small lacerations) to major internal bleeding: vomiting blood, bloody urine or stool.

Possible Effects of Long-Term Use: None reported.

Suggested Periodic Examinations While Taking This Drug (at physician's discretion)
Regular determinations of prothrombin time are essential to safe dosage and proper control.
Urine analyses for blood.

▷ **While Taking This Drug, Observe the Following**
Foods: A larger intake than usual of foods rich in vitamin K may reduce the effectiveness of this drug and make larger doses necessary. Foods rich in vitamin K include: asparagus, bacon, beef liver, cabbage, cauliflower, fish, green leafy vegetables. Vitamin E may increase risk of bleeding.
Beverages: No restrictions. May be taken with milk.

▷ *Alcohol:* Limit alcohol to one drink daily. Note: Heavy users of alcohol with liver damage may be very sensitive to anticoagulants and require smaller than usual doses.
Tobacco Smoking: Heavy smokers may require relatively larger doses of this drug.

▷ *Other Drugs*
Warfarin may *increase* the effects of
- oral hypoglycemic agents (see Drug Classes).
- phenytoin (Dilantin).

The following drugs may *increase* the effects of warfarin
- acetaminophen (high dose).
- allopurinol.
- amiodarone.
- androgens.
- azithromycin.
- bismuth subsalicylate (Pepto Bismol).
- carbamazepine.
- cephalosporins.
- chloral hydrate.
- chloramphenicol.
- cimetidine.
- ciprofloxacin and other quinolone antibiotics (see drug Classes).
- clarithromycin.
- clofibrate.
- cotrimoxazole.
- dextrothyroxine.

- disulfiram.
- disopyramide.
- erythromycin.
- felbamate.
- gemfibrozil.
- glucagon.
- influenza vaccine.
- isoniazid.
- itraconazole.
- ketoconazole.
- metronidazole.
- miconazole.
- nonsteroidal anti-inflammatory drugs.
- omeprazole.
- phenylbutazone.
- pravastatin.
- propranolol.
- quinidine.
- ranitidine.
- salicylates (aspirin, etc.).
- sertraline.
- simvastatin.
- streptokinase.
- sulfinpyrazone.
- sulfonamides.
- tamoxifen.
- tetracyclines.
- thyroid hormones.
- vancomycin.
- vitamin E.

The following drugs may *decrease* the effects of warfarin
- azathioprine.
- barbiturates.
- birth control pills (oral contraceptives).
- carbamazepine.
- cholestyramine.
- ethchlorvynol.
- glutethimide.
- griseofulvin.
- phytonadione (vitamin K).
- primidone.
- some penicillins.
- spironolactone.
- sucralfate.
- rifampin.
- vitamin K.

▷ *Driving, Hazardous Activities:* No restrictions.

Aviation Note: The use of this drug ***is a disqualification*** for piloting. Consult a designated Aviation Medical Examiner.

Exposure to Sun: No restrictions.

Discontinuation: Do not stop this drug abruptly unless abnormal bleeding occurs. Ask your physician for guidance regarding gradual reduction in dosage over a period of 3 to 4 weeks.

ZALCITABINE (zal SIT a been)

Other Names: Dideoxycytidine, DDC
Introduced: 1987   **Prescription:** USA: Yes   **Available as Generic:** USA: No   **Class:** Antiviral   **Controlled Drug:** USA: No
Brand Name: HIVID

BENEFITS versus RISKS	
Possible Benefits	*Possible Risks*
DELAYED PROGRESSION OF DISEASE IN HIV-INFECTED PATIENTS WITH AIDS OR AIDS-RELATED COMPLEX	DRUG-INDUCED PERIPHERAL NEURITIS Rare drug-induced pancreatitis Rare drug-induced esophageal ulcers Rare drug-induced cardiomyopathy/congestive heart failure Drug-induced arthritis

▷ **Principal Uses**
As a Single Drug Product: Uses currently included in FDA approved labeling: (1) This drug is approved for combination therapy (with zidovudine) of advanced (CD4 cell count less than or equal to 300 cells per cubic millimeter) HIV infection. This drug is not a cure for AIDS, and it does not reduce the risk of transmission of HIV infection to others through sexual contact or contamination of blood.
Other (unlabeled) generally accepted uses: (1) May have a role in pediatric AIDS.

How This Drug Works: By interfering with essential HIV enzyme systems, this drug is thought to prevent the growth and reproduction of HIV particles within infected cells, thus limiting the severity and extent of HIV infection.

Available Dosage Forms and Strengths
Zalcitabine (Hivid) tablets — 0.375 mg
— 0.75 mg

▷ **Recommended Dosage Ranges** (Actual dosage and administration schedule must be determined by the physician for each patient individually.)
Infants and Children: Under investigation.
12 to 60 Years of Age: The recommended combination regimen is: 1 0.75mg tablet orally to be taken with 200 mg of zidovudine every eight hours. The total daily dose for both drugs then becomes: 2.25 mg of zalcitabine and 600 mg of zidovudine. The initial dose does not need to be reduced unless the patient weighs less than 30 kg (66 pounds).

Zalcitabine

Conditions Requiring Dosing Adjustments
Liver function: Liver toxicity may be more likely in people with a prior history of alcohol abuse or liver damage. The patient should be monitored closely, and the dosage reduced or the medication interrupted if toxicity occurs.

Kidney function: Patients with moderate kidney failure can be given zalcitabine 0.75 mg every 12 hours. In severe kidney failure, the patient can be given 0.75 mg every 24 hours.

▷ **Dosing Instructions:** When combination therapy is being given, dose adjustments must be based on the toxicity profiles for each drug. For example: if the patient experiences peripheral neuropathy, or severe oral ulcers, the zalcitibine dose should be decreased or interrupted. Secondly: if the patient experiences anemia or granulocytopenia, the zidovudine dose should be decreased or interrupted. If the zalcitibine is interrupted or stopped, the zidovudine dose should be changed from 200 mg every 8 hours to 100 mg every 4 hours. Zalcitibine is **not** indicated for use as the only therapy. If zalcitibine is stopped, the physician **must** consider alternative antiretroviral therapy.

The largest peak concentration, the time that it takes for the peak to be achieved, and the amount absorbed are all changed if this drug is taken with food. It is better to take this medication on an empty stomach.

Usual Duration of Use: Use on a regular schedule for several months usually determines effectiveness in slowing the progression of AIDS. Long-term use (months to years) requires periodic physician evaluation of response and dosage adjustment.

Possible Advantages of This Drug
Greater potency against HIV.

Does not cause serious depression of bone marrow function (production of blood cells).

Less toxicity than other available drugs.

Less tendency for HIV to develop resistance to this drug.

▷ **This Drug Should Not Be Taken If**
- you have had an allergic reaction to it previously.
- you have had pancreatitis recently.

▷ **Inform Your Physician Before Taking This Drug If**
- you have had allergic reactions to any drugs in the past.
- you are taking any other drugs currently.
- you have a history of pancreatitis or peripheral neuritis.
- you have a history of severe myelosuppression (ask your doctor).
- you have a history of alcoholism.
- you have impaired liver or kidney function.

Possible Side-Effects (natural, expected and unavoidable drug actions)
Mild and infrequent decreases in red blood cell, white blood cell and platelet counts.

▷ **Possible Adverse Effects** (unusual, unexpected and infrequent reactions)
If any of the following develop, consult your physician promptly for guidance.

Mild Adverse Effects
　Allergic Reactions: Skin rash and itching.
　Fever, joint pains.
　Ringing in the ears.
　Mouth sores, nausea, vomiting, diarrhea, stomach pain.
Serious Adverse Effects
　Drug-induced peripheral neuritis (see Glossary), usually occuring after 7 to 18 weeks of treatment. This is more frequent and severe with high doses, and less frequent and mild with low does.
　Drug induced cardiomyopathy/congestive heart failure (rare).
　Drug-induced pancreatitis usually within the first 6 months of treatment (rare).
　Ototoxicity and hearing loss (rare).
　Worsening of preexisting liver disease or hepatoxicity in patients with a history of alcohol abuse.
▷ **Possible Effects on Sexual Function:** None reported.
▷ **Adverse Effects That May Mimic Natural Diseases or Disorders**
　None reported to date.

Possible Effects on Laboratory Tests
　Complete blood cell counts: decreased red cells, white cells and platelets (infrequent and mild).
　Blood amylase level: increased (infrequent).
　Blood glucose level: increased.
　Liver function tests: increased (SGOT, SGPT AND LDH).

CAUTION
1. This drug does not cure HIV infection. Taking it does not reduce the risk of transmitting infection to others through sexual contact or contamination of blood.
2. Report promptly the development of stomach pain with nausea and vomiting; this could indicate the onset of pancreatitis. It may be necessary to discontinue this drug.
3. Report promptly the development of pain, numbness, tingling or burning in the hands or feet; this could indicate the onset of peripheral neuritis. It may be necessary to discontinue this drug.
4. It is advisable to avoid all other drugs that are known to cause pancreatitis or peripheral neuritis; ask your physician for guidance.

Precautions for Use
　By Infants and Children: Safety and effectiveness for use by this age group have not been established. Children may also be at risk for developing drug-induced pancreatitis and peripheral neuritis; monitor closely for significant symptoms.
　By Those over 60 Years of Age: Reduced kidney function may require dosage reduction.
▷ **Advisability of Use During Pregnancy**
　Pregnancy Category: C. See Pregnancy Code at the back of this book.
　Animal studies: This drug has been shown to be teratogenic in mice at doses of 1365 and 2730 times that achieved at the maximum recommended

human dose (MRHD). Increased embryolethality was observed in mice with use of 2730 times the MRHD.

Human studies: Information from adequate studies of pregnant women is not available. The manufacturer recommends that fertile women should not receive zalcitibine unless they are using effective contraception during therapy.

Consult your physician for specific guidance.

Advisability of Use if Breast-Feeding

Presence of this drug in breast milk: Unknown.

Avoid drug or refrain from nursing.

Note: HIV has been found in human breast milk. Breast-feeding may result in transmission of HIV infection to the nursing infant.

Habit-Forming Potential: None.

Effects of Overdosage: Nausea, vomiting, stomach pain, diarrhea, pain in hands and feet.

Possible Effects of Long-Term Use: Peripheral neuritis (see Glossary).

Suggested Periodic Examinations While Taking This Drug (at physician's discretion)

Complete blood cell counts before starting treatment and weekly thereafter until tolerance is established.

Blood amylase levels, fractionated for salivary gland and pancreatic origin.

Triglyceride levels should be tested at baseline (before theray is started) and periodically.

Assessment of CD4 counts.

Measurement of viral load can be the clearest indication of pending failure and reason to change to other agents.

▷ **While Taking This Drug, Observe the Following**

Foods: No restrictions.

Beverages: No restrictions.

▷ *Alcohol:* No interactions expected.

Tobacco Smoking: No interactions expected.

▷ *Other Drugs*

Zalcitabine may *increase* the effects of
- zidovudine (Retrovir), and enhance its antiviral effect against HIV.

Zalcitibine *taken concurrently* with
- didanosine (Videx) may result in additive neurotoxicity.
- other drugs which cause neurotoxicity or pancreatitis are best avoided.

▷ *Driving, Hazardous Activities:* This drug may cause pain and weakness in the extremities. Restrict activities as necessary.

Aviation Note: The use of this drug *is a disqualification* for piloting. Consult a designated Aviation Medical Examiner.

Exposure to Sun: No restrictions.

Discontinuation: Do not stop this drug without your physician's knowledge and guidance.

ZIDOVUDINE (zi DOH vyoo deen)

Other Names: AZT, azidothymidine, Compound S, ZDV
Introduced: 1987 **Prescription:** USA: Yes; Canada: Yes **Available as Generic:** USA: No; Canada: No **Class:** Antiviral **Controlled Drug:** USA: No; Canada: No
Brand Name: Retrovir

BENEFITS versus RISKS	
Possible Benefits	*Possible Risks*
DELAYED PROGRESSION OF DISEASE IN HIV-INFECTED PATIENTS	SERIOUS BONE MARROW DEPRESSION (see Glossary)
REDUCED INCIDENCE OF INFECTIONS IN TREATING ACTIVE AIDS AND AIDS-RELATED COMPLEX	Brain toxicity
	Lip, mouth and tongue sores

▷ **Principal Uses**

As a Single Drug Product: Uses currently included in FDA approved labeling: (1) Used to treat selected patients who have acquired immunodeficiency syndrome (AIDS) or acquired immunodeficiency syndrome-related complex (ARC) caused by human immunodeficiency virus (HIV). This drug is not a cure for AIDS, and it does not reduce the risk of transmission of AIDS infection to others through sexual contact or contamination of blood; (2) recently approved to help prevent transmission of HIV from mother to infant; (3) approved for combination therapy with other agents; (4) approved for children 3 months or older who have laboratory values that indicate HIV infection or HIV immunosuppression; (5) approved for use in HIV positive patients who are as yet asymptomatic.

Other (unlabeled) generally accepted uses: (1) Used to treat Kaposi's sarcoma; (2) helps remove hairy leukoplakia in the mouth; (3) used to treat heart dysfunction in people with HIV; (4) may prevent HIV in health care workers exposed to the AIDS virus; (5) appears to increase AIDs-related low platelet counts.

How This Drug Works: By interfering with essential enzyme systems, this drug is thought to prevent the growth and reproduction of HIV particles within tissue cells, thus limiting the severity and extent of HIV infection.

Available Dosage Forms and Strengths
Capsules — 100 mg
Injection — 10 mg per ml
Syrup — 50 mg per 5-ml teaspoonful

▷ **Usual Adult Dosage Range:** For asymptomatic HIV infection: 100 mg/4 hours while awake (500 mg/day).

For symptomatic HIV infection: Initially 200 mg/4 hours throughout the day and night (no omission for activities or sleep) for 1 month. Smaller and larger doses may be used according to individual patient characteristics. After 1 month, the dose may be reduced to 100 mg/4 hours. Some authors recommend a maximum daily dose of 400 to 600 mg.

For prevention of maternal fetal transmission in pregnancy: 100 mg by mouth five times per day until the start of labor. During labor, AZT is given intravenously (2 mg/kg of total body weight), followed by 1 mg/kg/hour (again based on total body weight). This dose is continues until the unbilical cord is clamped. The infant then receives 1.5 mg/kg every 6 hours.

Note: Actual dosage and administration schedule must be determined by the physician for each patient individually.

Author's note: There is controversy present as to the ideal time to start antiretroviral therapy. Some clinicians wait until the CD4 count has declined to 500 or 400 cells. Since it is now known that HIV does not have a dormant period, many clinicians are starting therapy once the infection is diagnosed.

Conditions Requiring Dosing Adjustments

Liver function: The dose should be decreased by 50% or the dosing interval should be doubled in paients with significant liver compromise. It can be a rare cause of liver damage, and patients should be followed closely.

Kidney function: Specific guidelines for dosage adjustments in patients with compromised kidneys are not available. It should be used with caution in renal compromise.

▷ **Dosing Instructions:** Preferably taken on an empty stomach, but may be taken with or following food. Take exactly as prescribed. The capsule may be opened and the contents mixed with food just prior to administration. It is best to take the caspule with at least 120 ml of water.

Usual Duration of Use: Use on a regular schedule for 10 to 12 weeks usually determines effectiveness in improving the course of symptomatic AIDS infection. Long-term use requires periodic physician evaluation of response and dosage adjustment.

▷ **This Drug Should Not Be Taken If**
- you have had a serious allergic reaction to it previously.
- you have a serious degree of uncorrected bone marrow depression.

▷ **Inform Your Physician Before Taking This Drug If**
- you have a history of either folic acid or vitamin B-12 deficiency.
- you have impaired liver or kidney function.

Possible Side-Effects (natural, expected and unavoidable drug actions)
None reported.

▷ **Possible Adverse Effects** (unusual, unexpected and infrequent reactions)

If any of the following develop, consult your physician promptly for guidance.

Mild Adverse Effects

Allergic Reactions: Skin rash, hives, itching.

Headache (50%), weakness (20%), drowsiness, dizziness, nervousness, insomnia.

Nausea (50%), stomach pain (20%), diarrhea (12%), loss of appetite and vomiting (5% to 11%), altered taste, lip sores, swollen mouth or tongue.

Paresthesias (5%).

Muscle aches (8%), fever, sweating.

Serious Adverse Effects

Confusion, loss of speech, twitching, tremors, seizures (representing brain toxicity).

Eye problems (macular edema).
Muscle toxicity (myopathy).
Bone marrow depression (see Glossary): Fatigue, weakness, fever, sore throat, abnormal bleeding or bruising. Anemia occurs most commonly after 4 to 6 weeks of treatment; abnormally low white blood cell counts occur after 6 to 8 weeks of treatment.
Esophageal ulcers (patients should take this medicine with at least 120 ml of water.
Liver toxicity.

▷ **Possible Effects on Sexual Function**
None reported.

Possible Delayed Adverse Effects: Significant anemia and deficient white blood cell counts may develop after this drug has been discontinued. Myopathy.

▷ **Adverse Effects That May Mimic Natural Diseases or Disorders**
Seizures may suggest the possibility of epilepsy.

Possible Effects on Laboratory Tests
Complete blood cell counts: decreased red cells, hemoglobin, white cells and platelets.

CAUTION
1. This drug is not a cure for AIDS or AIDS-related complex. Nor does it protect completely against other infections or complications. Follow your physician's instructions and take all medications exactly as prescribed.
2. This drug does not reduce the risk of transmitting AIDS to others through sexual contact or contamination of the blood. The use of an effective condom is mandatory. Needles for drug administration should not be shared.

Precautions for Use
By Infants and Children: Zidovudine syrup is used in HIV-infected pediatric patients who are greater than 3 months old. The usual dose is 180 mg/ square meter.
By Those over 60 Years of Age: Impaired kidney function will require dosage reduction.

▷ **Advisability of Use During Pregnancy**
Pregnancy Category: C. See Pregnancy Code at the back of this book.
Animal studies: Rat studies reveal no birth defects.
Human studies: Adequate studies of pregnant women are not available.
Consult your physician for specific guidance.

Advisability of Use if Breast-Feeding
Presence of this drug in breast milk: Unknown.
Avoid drug or refrain from nursing.

Habit-Forming Potential: None.

Effects of Overdosage: Nausea, vomiting, diarrhea, bone marrow depression.

Possible Effects of Long-Term Use: Serious anemia and loss of white blood cells.
Muscle toxicity (myopathy).

Suggested Periodic Examinations While Taking This Drug (at physician's discretion)

Complete blood cell counts before starting treatment and weekly thereafter until tolerance is established. Continual monitoring for bone marrow depression is necessary during entire course of treatment.

Periodic CD4 counts or measurements of viral load are indicators that treatment is failing and demand change of antiretroviral therapy.

▷ **While Taking This Drug, Observe the Following**

Foods: No restrictions.

Beverages: No restrictions. May be taken with milk.

▷ *Alcohol:* No interactions expected.

Tobacco Smoking: No interactions expected.

▷ *Other Drugs*

The following drugs may *increase* the effects of zidovudine and enhance its toxicity
- acetaminophen.
- acyclovir.
- amphotericin B.
- aspirin.
- benzodiazepines (see Drug Class Section).
- cimetidine.
- fluconazole.
- ganciclovir.
- indomethacin.
- interferon beta.
- morphine.
- probenecid.
- sulfonamides (see Drug Class Section).

Zidovudine *taken concurrently* with
- didanosine may result in increased risk of myelosuppression.
- filgrastim (Neupogen) may help maintain the white blood cell count.
- rifampin can lead to decreased zidovudine blood levels.
- trimexate may cause additive hematological toxicity.

▷ *Driving, Hazardous Activities:* This drug may cause dizziness or fainting. Restrict activities as necessary.

Aviation Note: The use of this drug *is a disqualification* for piloting. Consult a designated Aviation Medical Examiner.

Exposure to Sun: No restrictions.

Discontinuation: Do not stop this drug without your physician's knowledge and guidance.

ZOLPIDEM (ZOL pi dem)

Introduced: 1993 **Prescription:** USA: Yes **Available as Generic:** USA: No **Class:** Hypnotic, Imidazopyridine **Controlled Drug:** USA: C-IV*

Brand Names: Ambien

*See Schedules of Controlled Drugs at the back of this book.

BENEFITS versus RISKS	
Possible Benefits	*Possible Risks*
GIVES SHORT-TERM RELIEF OF INSOMNIA WITH MINIMAL SLEEP DISRUPTION (REM)	Habit-forming potential with prolonged use Rebound insomnia upon withdrawal

▷ **Principal Uses**

As a Single Drug Product: Uses currently included in FDA approved labeling: (1) Short-term treatment of insomnia in adults.

Other (unlabeled) generally accepted uses: None at present.

How This Drug Works: This drug attaches (binds) to a specific receptor (omega-1) and: reduces time it takes to fall asleep, increases total sleep time while producing a pattern and benefit of sleep that is similar to normal sleep patterns.

Available Dosage Forms and Strengths
Tablets — 5 mg, 10 mg

▷ **Recommended Dosage Ranges (Actual dosage and administration schedule must be determined by the physician for each patient individually.)**

Infants and Children: Safety and efficacy for those under 18 years of age not established.

18 to 60 Years of Age: Ten mg is given imediately before bedtime. Patients should be reevaluated after taking this drug for ten days.

Over 60 Years of Age: Therapy should be started with 5 mg taken at bedtime. The dose may be cautiously increased to 10 mg at bedtime.

Conditions Requiring Dosing Adjustments

Liver function: The dose should be reduced by 50% in patients with liver compromise.

Kidney function: The half life is doubled in chronic kidney compromise, and the dose must be decreased.

▷ **Dosing Instructions:** The tablet may be crushed and is best taken on an empty stomach. Do **not** stop this drug abruptly if taken for more than 7 days.

Usual Duration of Use: Use on a regular schedule for two nights usually determines effectiveness in treating insomnia. Your physician should be assess the benefit of this drug after 10 days.

Possible Advantages of This Drug
Low occurance of adverse effects.
May produce less of an undesirable effect on normal sleep patterns.

Currently a "Drug of Choice"
for short-term management of insomnia in adults.

▷ **This Drug Should Not Be Taken If**
- you have had an allergic reaction to any dosage form of it previously.

▷ **Inform Your Physician Before Taking This Drug If**
- you have abnormal liver or kidney function.
- you are pregnant or planning pregnancy.
- you have a history of alcoholism or drug abuse.
- you have a history of serious depression or mental disorder.
- you are uncertain of how much zolpidem to take or how often to take it.

Possible Side-Effects (natural, expected and unavoidable drug actions)
Drowsiness, and blurred vision, "hangover" effects following long term use.

▷ **Possible Adverse Effects** (unusual, unexpected and infrequent reactions)
If any of the following develop, consult your physician promptly for guidance.
Mild Adverse Effects
Allergic Reactions: Skin rash.
Drowsiness (2%) and Dizziness (1%).
Nausea and diarrhea (1%).
Muscle tremors (infrequent).
Blurred vision (infrequent).
Serious Adverse Effects
Allergic Reactions: Not defined.
Abnormal thoughts or hallucinations (infrequent).
Rare elevation of liver function tests.
Paradoxical aggression, agitation or suicidal thoughts.

▷ **Possible Effects on Sexual Function:**   None reported.

Possible Effects on Laboratory Tests
Liver function tests: increased SGOT, SGPT and CPK.

CAUTION
1. This drug works quickly. It is best to take it just before bed time.
2. Do **not** drink alcohol while taking this drug.
3. Withdrawal (see Glossary) may occur even if this drug was only taken for a week or two. Ask your doctor for advice before stoping zolpidem.
4. You may experience trouble going to sleep for 1 or 2 nights after stopping this drug (rebound insomnia). This effect is usually short-term.
5. Sleep disturbances may be a symptom of underlying phychological problems. Inform your doctor if unusual behaviors or odd thoughts occur.
6. Drugs which depress the central nervous system may produce additive effects with this drug. Ask your doctor or pharmacist **before** combining other prescription or non-prescription drugs with zolpidem.

Precautions for Use
By Infants and Children:
Safety and effectiveness for those under 18 years of age not established.
By Those over 60 Years of Age: The starting dose should be decreased to 5 mg. Since this drug works quickly, it is best taken immediately before going to bed. You may at increased risk for falls if the drug remains in your system in the morning. Watch for lethargy, unsteadiness, nightmares and paradoxical agitation and anger.

▷ **Advisability of Use During Pregnancy**
Pregnancy Category: B. See Pregnancy Code at the back of this book.
Animal studies: In rats, abnormal skull bone formation was reported. In rabbits, abnormal bone formation was found.
Human studies: Adequate studies of pregnant women are not available.
Use during pregnancy **not** advisable. Ask your doctor for guidance.

Advisability of Use if Breast-Feeding
  Presence of this drug in breast milk: Yes.
  Avoid drug or refrain from nursing.
Habit-Forming Potential: This drug may cause dependence (see Glossary).
Effects of Overdosage: Marked change from letargy to coma. Cardiovascular and respiratory compromise was also reported. The drug flumazenil may help reverse symptoms.
Possible Effects of Long-Term Use: Psychological and/or physical dependence.
Suggested Periodic Examinations While Taking This Drug (at physician's discretion)
  Liver function tests.

▷ **While Taking This Drug, Observe the Following**
  Foods: This drug should **not** be taken with food.
  Beverages: Avoid caffeine-containing beverages: coffee, tea, cola.
▷ *Alcohol:* This drug should **not** be combined with alcohol.
  Tobacco Smoking: Nicotine is a stimulant and should be avoided.
  Marijuana Smoking: May cause additive drowsiness.
▷ *Other Drugs*
  Zolpidem may *increase* the effects of
  • chlorpromazine (Thorazine).
  • narcotics or other CNS depressant drugs.
▷ *Driving, Hazardous Activities:* This drug may cause drowsiness and impair coordination. Restrict activities as necessary.
  Aviation Note: The use of this drug *is a disqualification* for piloting. Consult a designated
  Aviation Medical Examiner.
  Discontinuation: This drug should **not** be stopped abruptly even after a week of use. Ask your doctor for help regarding an appropriate withdrawal schedule.

SECTION THREE

THE LEADING EDGE

This section is designed to help the reader become more fully aware of medications which show promise in novel applications or are FDA approvable. The Leading Edge is also intended to bring information about new concepts in medication delivery which show great promise. Finally, a few interesting medications still in early clinical trials may be included as stars on the horizon.

It is impossible to predict which medicines or delivery systems will achieve final FDA approval or will become used in specific drugs, but many of those successful ones will be covered in subsequent editions. Finally, there will be many potential medicines or delivery systems which could be covered in a given year. The author will choose those which in his opinion offer the most potential to the readers of this book.

MINOCYCLINE (MINNOW si clean)

Novel Application:
This antibiotic has now demonstrated some clear benefits in two studies of patients with rheumatoid arthritis. The way in which this medicine helps this condition has not been clarified, but the results are promising.

ALENDRONATE (a LIN dra nate)

FDA Approvable:
This bisphosphonate medication inhibits specific cells which are responsible for bone resorption. This drug is the first in a new class of medicines which, if approved, appears to be able to actually prevent bone fractures. New data show that this drug decreases the occurrence of new bone fractures by up to 48%. Alendronate may become the biggest weapon against osteoporosis in years.

MANY NAMES PENDING

Medication delivery:
Liposomes, and the encapsulation of medicines in these vehicles or in association with lipids, offers great promise. It appears that much higher doses of some previously toxic drugs can be used with minimal adverse effects. The ability to use higher doses with fewer bad effects may actually translate into clinical cures of a variety of diseases.

LAMIVUDINE (lamb IV you dean)

Star on the horizon:
Protease inhibitors represent a new class of medicines in the war against AIDS. These drugs act at a different point in the life cycle of the virus than the four nucleoside analogs currently available and have shown great promise in decreasing the amount of virus (viral burden or load) challenging a patient.

SECTION FOUR

DRUG CLASSES

Throughout the Drug Profiles, reference is made to various drug classes. The reader may be advised to consult Section Four to become familiar with the drugs which belong to a particular class of drugs that share important characteristics in their chemical composition or in their actions within the body. Often it is important to know that *any* drug (or *all* drugs) within a given class can be expected to behave in a particular way. This may be useful in preventing interactions that could reduce the effectiveness of the drugs in use or result in unanticipated and sometimes hazardous adverse effects.

The presentation of each Drug Class consists of the drug class designation followed by an alphabetic listing of the generic names of the drugs that comprise the class. Following each generic name (and enclosed in parentheses) is the widely recognized brand name(s) of that particular drug. In some instances the number of brand names in use is so large that a complete listing is not possible. In such cases, to be certain that you are consulting the correct drug class, call your pharmacist or physician to determine the generic name of the drug that concerns you and consult the master list to see if it is included there. The generic name listings are sufficiently complete to serve the scope of this book.

The following page lists the names of all the Drug Classes included in this section.

LIST OF DRUG CLASSES

Adrenocortical Steroids
Amebicides
Aminoglycosides
Amphetaminelike Drugs
Analgesics, Mild
Analgesics, Strong (see Opioid Drugs)
Androgens
Angiotensin-Converting Enzyme (ACE) Inhibitors
Angiotensin Two Receptor Antagonists
Anorexiants
Antiacne Drugs
Anti-AIDS Drugs
Antialcholism Drugs
Anti-Alzheimer's Drugs
Antianginal Drugs
Antianxiety Drugs
Antiarrhythmic Drugs
Antiasthmatic Drugs (Bronchodilators)
Antibiotics
Antibiotics, Topical
Anticholinergic Drugs
Anticoagulant Drugs
Anticonvulsant Drugs
Anticystic Fibrosis Agents
Antidepressant Drugs
Antidiabetic Drugs, Oral (see Biguanides or Sulfonylureas)
Antiemetic Drugs
Antiepileptic Drugs (see Anticonvulsants)
Antifungal Drugs
Antiglaucoma Drugs
Antigout Drugs
Antihistamines
Antihypertensive Drugs
Anti-infective Drugs
Antileprosy Drugs
Antimalarial Drugs
Antimigraine Drugs
Antimotion Sickness/Antinausea Drugs (see Antiemetics)
Antiparkinsonism Drugs
Antiplatelet Drugs
Antipsychotic Drugs (Neuroleptics)
Antipyretic Drugs
Antisickle Cell Anemia Drugs
Antispasmodics, Synthetic
Antituberculosis Drugs
Antitussive Drugs
Antiviral Drugs
Appetite Suppressants (see Anorexiants)
Atropinelike Drugs (see Anticholinergic Drugs)
Barbiturates
Benzodiazepines
Beta-Adrenergic Blocking Drugs (Beta Blockers)
Biguanides
Bowel Anti-inflammatory Drugs
Bronchodilators (see Antiasthmatic Drugs)
Calcium Channel Blocking Drugs (Calcium Blockers)
Cephalosporins
Cholesterol-Reducing Drugs
Cortisonelike Drugs (see Adrenocortical Steroids)
Cough Suppressants (see Antitussive Drugs)
Decongestants
Digitalis Preparations
Diuretics
Estrogens
Female Sex Hormones (see Estrogens and Progestins)
Fever-Reducing Drugs (see Antipyretic Drugs)
Fluoroquinolones
Gastrointestinal Drugs
Heart Rhythm Regulators (see Antiarrhythmic Drugs)
Hematopoietic Agents
Histamine (H-2)-Blocking Drugs (H-2 Blockers)
Hypnotic Drugs
Male Sex Hormones (see Androgens)
Macrolide Antibiotics
Mast Cell Stabilizing Agents (see Antiasthmatic Drugs)
Monoamine Oxidase (MAO) Inhibitor Drugs
Muscle Relaxants
Nitrates
Nonsteroidal Anti-inflammatory Drugs (NSAIDs)
Opioid Drugs (Narcotics)
Penicillins
Phenothiazines
Progestins
Proton Pump Inhibitors

Radiopharmaceuticals
Salicylates
Sedatives/Sleep Inducers (see Hypnotic Drugs)
Smoking Deterrents
Sulfonamides ("Sulfa" Drugs)
Sulfonylureas
Tetracyclines
Thiazide Diuretics
Tranquilizers, Minor (see Antianxiety Drugs)
Tranquilizers, Major (see Antipsychotic Drugs)
Vaccines
Vasodilators
Xanthines

ADRENOCORTICAL STEROIDS

(Cortisonelike Drugs)

beclomethasone (Beclovent, Vanceril)
betamethasone (Celestone)
cortisone (Cortone)
dexamethasone (Decadron)
flunisolide (AeroBib)
fluticasone (Flonase)

hydrocortisone (Cortef)
methylprednisolone (Medrol)
prednisolone (Delta-Cortef)
prednisone (Deltasone)
triamcinolone (Aristocort, Azmacort)

AMEBICIDES

(Anti-infectives)

chloroquine (Aralen)
emetine (no brand name)
iodoquinol (Yodoxin)

metronidazole (Flagyl)
paromomycin (Humatin)

AMINOGLYCOSIDES

(Anti-infectives)

kanamycin (Kantrex)
neomycin (Mycifradin, Neobiotic)

paromomycin (Humatin)

AMPHETAMINELIKE DRUGS

amphetamine (no brand name)
benzphetamine (Didrex)
dextroamphetamine (Dexedrine)
diethylpropion (Tenuate, Tepanil)
methamphetamine (Desoxyn)

methylphenidate (Ritalin)
phendimetrazine (Anorex, Plegine)
phenmetrazine (Preludin)
phentermine (Fastin, Ionamin)
phenylpropanolamine (Dexatrim)

ANALGESICS, MILD

acetaminophen (Datril, Tylenol)
aspirin (see Drug Profile, Section Two)
lidocaine/prilocaine cream (Emla)

See Nonsteroidal Anti-inflammatory Drugs (NSAIDs) below

ANDROGENS

(Male Sex Hormones)

fluoxymesterone (Halotestin)
methyltestosterone (Android, Metandren, Oreton)

testosterone (Depotest, Testone)

ANGIOTENSIN-CONVERTING ENZYME (ACE) INHIBITORS

benazepril (Lotensin)
captopril (Capoten)
enalapril (Vasotec)
fosinopril (Monopril)

lisinopril (Prinivil, Zestril)
quinapril (Accupril)
ramipril (Altace)

ANGIOTENSIN TWO RECEPTOR ANTAGONISTS

losartan (Cozaar)

ANOREXIANTS
(Appetite Suppressants)

fenfluramine (Pondimin)
mazindol (Mazanor, Sanorex)

See also Amphetaminelike Drugs

ANTIACNE DRUGS

benzoyl peroxide (Epi-Clear, others)
erythromycin (Eryderm)
isotretinoin (Accutane)

tetracycline (Achromycin V)
tretinoin (Retin-A)

ANTIAIDS DRUGS

didanosine (DDI, Videx)
stavudine (Zerit)
zalcitabine (dideoxycytidine, DDC, Hivid)

zidovudine (AZT, Retrovir)
lamivudine (3TC) (see The Leading Edge)

ANTIALCOHOLISM DRUGS

disulfiram (Antabuse)

naltrexone (Trexan, ReVia)

ANTIALZHEIMER'S DRUGS

tacrine (Cognex)

ANTIANGINAL DRUGS

beta-adrenergic-blocking class (see below)
bepridil (Vascor)
diltiazem (Cardizem)
nicardipine (Cardene)

nifedipine (Adalat, Procardia)
nitrates (see below)
verapamil (Calan, Isoptin)

ANTIANXIETY DRUGS
(Minor Tranqilizers)

See Benzodiazepine class below
buspirone (Buspar)
chlormezanone (Trancopal)

hydroxyzine (Atarax, Vistaril)
lorazepam (Ativan)
meprobamate (Equanil, Miltown)

ANTIARRHYTHMIC DRUGS
(Heart Rhythm Regulators)

acebutolol (Sectral)
amiodarone (Cordarone)
digitoxin (Crystodigin)
digoxin (Lanoxin)
disopyramide (Norpace)
flecainide (Tambocor)
mexiletine (Mexitil)

moricizine (Ethmozine)
procainamide (Procan SR, Pronestyl)
propafenone (Rythmol)
propranolol (Inderal)
quinidine (Quinaglute, Quinidex, Quinora)
tocainide (Tonocard)
verapamil (Calan, Isoptin)

ANTIASTHMATIC DRUGS
(Bronchodilators)

albuterol (Proventil, Ventolin)
aminophylline (Phyllocontin)

bitolterol (Tornalate)
dyphylline (Lufyllin)

ephedrine (Efed II)
epinephrine (Adrenalin, Bronkaid Mist, Primatene Mist)
isoetharine (Bronkosol, Dey-Lute)
isoproterenol (Isuprel)
metaproterenol (Alupent, Metaprel)
oxtriphylline (Choledyl)
pirbuterol (Maxair)
salmeterol (Serevent)
terbutaline (Brethaire, Brethine, Bricanyl)
theophylline (Bronkodyl, Elixophyllin, Slo-Phyllin, others)

Mast Cell Stabilizing Agents

cromolyn sodium (Gastlrocom, Intal)
nedocromil (Tilade)

ANTIBIOTICS

See specific Antibiotic Class (cephalosporins, erythromycins, penicillins, etc.)

ANTIBIOTICS, TOPICAL

(Anti-infectives)

mupirocin (Bactroban)

ANTICHOLINERGIC DRUGS

(Atropinelike Drugs)

atropine
belladonna
hyoscyamine
scopolamine
antidepressants, tricyclic (see Class below)
antihistamines, some (see Class below)
antiparkinsonism drugs, some (see Class below)
antispsmodics, synthetic some (see Class below)
muscle relaxants, some (see Class below)

ANTICOAGULANT DRUGS

anisindione (Miradon)
dicumarol (no brand name)
warfarin (Coumadin)

ANTICONVULSANT DRUGS

(Antiepileptic Drugs)

acetazolamide (Diamox)
carbamazepine (Tegretol)
clonazepam (Klonopin)
clorazepate (Tranxene)
diazepam (Valium)
ethosuximide (Zarontin)
ethotoin (Peganone)
felbamate (Felbatol)
gabapentin (Neurontin)
lamotrigine (Lamictal)
mephenytoin (Mesantoin)
methsuximide (Celontin)
paramethadione (Paradione)
phenacemide (Phenurone)
phenobarbital (Luminal)
phensuximide (Milontin)
phenytoin (Dilantin)
primidone (Mysoline)
trimethadione (Tridione)
valproic acid (Depakene)

ANTICYSTIC FIBROSIS AGENTS

Recombinant DNase

dornase alfa (Pulmozyme)

ANTIDEPRESSANT DRUGS

Bicyclic Antidepressant

fluoxetine (Prozac)
venlafaxine (Effexor)

Tricyclic Antidepressants

amitriptyline (Elavil, Endep)
amoxapine (Asendin)
clomipramine (Anafranil)
desipramine (Norpramin, Pertofrane)
doxepin (Adapin, Sinequan)
imipramine (Janimine, Tofranil)
nortriptyline (Aventyl, Pamelor)
protriptyline (Vivactil)
trimipramine (Surmontil)

Tetracyclic Antidepressant

maprotiline (Ludiomil)

Other Antidepressants

bupropion (Wellbutrin)
fluvoxamine (Luvox)
nefazodone (Serzone)
paroxetine (Paxil)
sertraline (Zoloft)
trazodone (Desyrel)

Monoamine Oxidase (MAO) Inhibitors

See Class below.

ANTIEMETIC DRUGS

(Antimotion Sickness, Antinausea Drugs)

chlorpromazine (Thorazine)
cyclizine (Marezine)
dimenhydrinate (Dramamine)
diphenhydramine (Benadryl)
granisetron (Kytril)
hydroxyzine (Atarax, Vistaril)
meclizine (Antivert, Bonine)
ondansetron (zofran)
prochlorperazine (Compazine)
promethazine (Phenergan)
scopolamine (Transderm Scop)
trimethobenzamide (Tigan)

ANTIFUNGAL DRUGS

(Anti-infectives)

amphotericin B (Fungizone) (a new liposomal form is pending)
fluconazole (Diflucan)
flucytosine (Ancobon)
griseofulvin (Fulvicin, Grifulvin, Grisactin)
itraconazole (Sporanox)
ketoconazole (Nizoral)
miconazole (Monistat)
nystatin (Mycostatin)

ANTIGLAUCOMA DRUGS

acetazolamide (Diamox)
betaxolol (Betoptic)
epinephrine (Glaucon)
pilocarpine (Isopto-carpine)
timolol (Timoptic)

ANTIGOUT DRUGS

allopurinol (Zyloprim)
colchicine (no brand name)
diclofenac (Cataflam, Voltaren)
fenoprofen (Nalfon)
ibuprofen (Advil, Motrin, Nuprin, Rufin)
indomethacin (Indocin)
ketoprofen (Orudis)
Mefenamic acid (Ponstel)
naproxen (Anaprox, Naprosyn)
oxaprozin (Daypro)
piroxicam (Feldene)
probenecid (Benemid)
sulfinpyrazone (Anturane)
sulindac (Clinoril)

ANTIHISTAMINES

astemizole (Hismanal)
azatadine (Optimine)
brompheniramine (Dimetane, others)
carbinoxamine (Clistin, Rondec)
chlorpheniramine (Chlor-Trimeton, Teldrin)
clemastine (Tavist)
cyclizine (Marezine)
cyproheptadine (Periactin)
dimenhydrinate (Dramamine)
diphenhydramine (Benadryl)
doxylamine (Unisom)

loratadine (Claritin, Claritin Extra)
meclizine (Antivert, Bonine)
orphenadrine (Norflex)
pheniramine (component of Triaminic)
promethazine (Phenergan, others)
pyrilamine (component of Triaminic)
terfenadine (Seldane)
tripelennamine (Pyribenzamine, PBZ)
triprolidine (component of Actifed and Sudahist)

ANTIHYPERTENSIVE DRUGS

clonidine (Catapres)
doxazosin (Cardura)
guanabenz (Wytensin)
guanadrel (Hylorel)
guanethidine (Ismelin)
guanfacine (Tenex)

hydralazine (Apresoline)
methyldopa (Aldomet)
minoxidil (Loniten)
prazosin (Minipres)
reserpine (Serpasil)
terazosin (Hytrin)

See also the following Drug Classes

Angiotensin-Converting Enzyme (ACE) Inhibitors (above)
Angiotensin Two Receptor Antagonists (above)

Beta-Adrenergic Blocking Drugs (below)
Calcium Channel Blocking Drugs (below)
Diuretics (below)

ANTI-INFECTIVE DRUGS

See specific Anti-infective Drug Class

Amebicides
Aminoglycosides
Antifungal Drugs
Antileprosy Drugs
Antimalarial Drugs
Antituberculosis Drugs
Antiviral Drugs

Cephalosporins
Fluoroquinolones
Macrolides
Penicillins
Sulfonamides
Tetracyclines

Miscellaneous Anti-infective Drugs

atovaquone (Mepron)
chloramphenicol (Chloromycetin)
clindamycin (Cleocin)
colistin (Coly-Mycin S)
furazolidone (Furoxone)
lincomycin (Lincocin)

nalidixic acid (NegGram)
nitrofurantoin (Furadantin, Macrodantin)
novobiocin (Albamycin)
pentamidine (Pentam-300)
trimethoprim (Proloprim, Trimpex)
vancomycin (Vancocin)

ANTILEPROSY DRUGS

(Anti-infectives)

clofazimine (Lamprene)

dapsone (no brand name)

ANTIMALARIAL DRUGS

(Anti-infectives)

chloroquine (Aralen)
doxycycline (Vibramycin)
hydroxychloraquine (Plaquenil)
mefloquine (Lariam)
primaquine (no brand name)

pyrimethamine (Daraprim)
quinacrine (Atabrine)
quinine (no brand name)
sulfadoxine/pyrimethamine (Fansidar)

ANTIMIGRAINE DRUGS

atenolol (Tenormin)
ergotamine (Ergostat)
methysergide (Sansert)
metoprolol (Lopressor)
nadolol (Corgard)

nifedipine (Procardia)
propranolol (Inderal)
sumatriptan (Imitrex)
timolol (Blocadren)
verapamil (Calan, Isoptin)

ANTIPARKINSONISM DRUGS

amantadine (Symmetrel)
benztropine (Cogentin)
bromocriptine (Parlodel)
diphenhydramine (Benadryl)
levodopa (Dopar, Larodopa)

levodopa/bensarazide (Prolopa)
levodopa/carbidopa (Sinemet, Sinemet CR)
pergolide (Permax)
selegiline (Eldepryl)
trihexyphenidyl (Artane)

ANTIPLATELET DRUGS

(Platelet aggregation inhibitors)

aspirin (Bufferin, Ecotrin, others)
dipyridamole (Persantine)

sulfinpyrazone (Anturane)
ticlopidine (Ticlid)

ANTIPSYCHOTIC DRUGS

(Neuroleptics, Major Tranquilizers)

see Phenothiazine class below
chlorprothixene (Taractan)
clozapine (Clozaril)
haloperidol (Haldol)
loxapine (Loxitane)

molindone (Moban)
pimozide (Orap)
risperidone (Risperdal)
thiothixene (Navane)

ANTIPYRETIC DRUGS

(Fever-Reducing Drugs)

acetaminophen (Panadol, Tylenol, others)
aspirin (Bufferin, Ecotrin, others)

see Nonsteroidal Anti-inflammatory Drugs below

ANTISICKLE CELL ANEMIA DRUGS

hydroxyurea (Hydrea)

ANTISPASMODICS, SYNTHETIC

anisotropine (Valpin)
clidinium (Quarzan)
glycopyrrolate (Robinul)
hexocyclium (Tral)
isopropamide (Darbid)

mepenzolate (Cantil)
methantheline (Banthine)
methscopolamine (Pamine)
propantheline (Pro-Banthine)
tridihexethyl (Pathilon)

ANTITUBERCULOSIS DRUGS

aminosalicylate sodium (Sodium P.A.S.)
capreomycin (Capastat)
cycloserine (Seromycin)
ethambutol (Myambutol)
ethionamide (Trecator-SC)
isoniazid (Laniazid, Nidrazid)
pyrazinamide (no brand name)
rifampin (Rifadin, Rimactane)
rifabutin (Mycobutin)
streptomycin (no brand name)

ANTITUSSIVE DRUGS

(Cough Suppressants)

benzonatate (Tessalon)
codeine (no brand name)
dextromethorphan (Hold DM, Suppress)
diphenhydramine (Benylin)
hydrocodone (Hycodan)
hydromorphone (Dilaudid)
promethazine (Phenergan)

ANTIVIRAL DRUGS

(Anti-infectives)

acyclovir (Zovirax)
amantadine (Symmetrel)
didanosine (Videx)
famciclovir (Famvir)
foscarnet (Foscavir)
ganciclovir (Cytovene)
ribavirin (Virazole)
rimantadine (no brand name)
stavudine (Zerit)
vidarabine (Vira A)
zalcitabine (Hivid)
zidovudine (Retrovir)

BARBITURATES

amobarbital (Amytal)
aprobarbital (Alurate)
butabarbital (Butisol)
mephobarbital (Mebaral)
metharbital (Gemonil)
pentobarbital (Nembutal)
phenobarbital (Luminal, Solfoton)
secobarbital (Seconal)
talbutal (Lotusate)

BENZODIAZEPINES

alprazolam (Xanax)
bromazepam (Lectopam)
chlordiazepoxide (Libritabs, Librium)
clonazepam (Klonopin)
clorazepate (Tranxene)
diazepam (Valium, Vazepam)
flurazepam (Dalmane)
halazepam (Paxipam)
ketazolam (Loftran)
lorazepam (Ativan)
midazolam (Versed)
nitrazepam (Mogadon)
oxazepam (Serax)
prazepam (Centrax)
quazepam (Doral)
temazepam (Restoril)
triazolam (Halcion)

BETA-ADRENERGIC BLOCKING DRUGS

(Beta Blockers)

acebutolol (Sectral)
atenolol (Tenormin)
betaxolol (Kerlone)
bisoprolol (Zebta)
bisoprolol/hydrochlorothiazide (Ziac)
carteolol (Cartrol)
labetalol (Normodyne, Trandate)
metoprolol (Lopressor)
nadolol (Corgard)
penbutolol (Levatol)
pindolol (Visken)
propranolol (Inderal)
timolol (Blocadren)

BIGUANIDES
(Oral Antidiabetic Drugs)

metformin (Glucophage)

BOWEL ANTI-INFLAMMATORY DRUGS
(Inflammatory Bowel Disease Suppressants)

azathioprine (Imuran)
mesalamine (Rowasa, Asacol)
metronidazole (Flagyl)
olsalazine (Dipentum)
sulfasalazine (Azulfidine)

CALCIUM CHANNEL BLOCKING DRUGS
(Calcium Blockers)

bepridil (Vascor)
diltiazem (Cardizem)
felodipine (Plendil)
isradipine (DynaCirc)
nicardipine (Cardene)
nifedipine (Adalat, Procardia)
nimodipine (Nimotop)
verapamil (Calan, Isoptin)

CEPHALOSPORINS
(Anti-infectives)

cefaclor (Ceclor)
cefadroxil (Duricef, Ultracef)
cefamandole (Mandol)
cefazolin (Ancef, Kefzol, Zolicef)
cefixime (Suprax)
cefmetazole (Zefazone)
cefonicid (Monocid)
cefoperazone (Cefobid)
ceforanide (Precef)
cefotaxime (Claforan)
cefotetan (Cefotan)
cefoxitin (Mefoxin)
cefprozil (Cefzil)
ceftazidime (Fortaz, Tazidime, Tazicef)
ceftizoxime (Cefizox)
ceftriaxone (Rocephin)
cefuroxime (Ceftin, Kefurox, Zinacef)
cephalexin (Keflex, Keftab)
cephalothin (Keflin)
cephapirin (Cefadyl)
cephradine (Anspor, Velosef)
moxalactam (Moxam)

CHOLESTEROL-REDUCING DRUGS

cholestyramine (Cholybar, Questran)
clofibrate (Atromid-S)
colestipol (Colestid)
dextrothyroxine (Choloxin)
fenofibrate (Lipidil)
gemfibrozil (Lopid)
lovastatin (Mevacor)
niacin (Nicobid, Slo-Niacin, others)
pravastatin (Pravachol)
probucol (Lorelco)
simvastatin (Zocor)

DECONGESTANTS

ephedrine (Efedron, Ephedsol)
naphazoline (Naphcon, Vasocon)
oxymetazoline (Afrin, Duration, others)
phenylephrine (Neo-Synephrine, others)
phenylpropanolamine (Propadrine, Propagest, others)
pseudoephedrine (Afrinol, Sudafed, others)
tetrahydrozoline (Tyzine, Visine, others)
xylometazoline (Otrivin)

DIGITALIS PREPARATIONS

deslanoside (Cedilanid-D)
digitoxin (Crystodigin)
digoxin (Lanoxicaps, Lanoxin)

DIURETICS

acetazolamide (Diamox)
amiloride (Midamor)
bumetanide (Bumex)
chlorthalidone (Hygroton)
ethacrynic acid (Edecrin)
furosemide (Lasix)
indapamide (Lozol)
metolazone (Diulo, Zaroxolyn)
spironolactone (Aldactone)
thiazide diuretics (see Class below)
triamterene (Dyrenium)

ESTROGENS

(Female Sex Hormones)

chlorotrianisene (Tace)
diethylstilbestrol (DES, Stilphostrol)
estradiol (Estrace, Estraderm, others)
estrogens, conjugated (Premarin)
estrogens, esterified (Estratab, Menest)
estrone (Theelin, others)
estropipate (Ogen)
ethinyl estradiol (Estinyl)
quinestrol (Estrovis)

FLUOROQUINOLONES

(Anti-infectives)

ciprofloxacin (Cipro)
lomefloxacin (Maxaquin)
norfloxacin (Noroxin)
ofloxacin (Floxin)

GASTROINTESTINAL DRUGS

Miscellaneous

metoclopramide (Reglan)
cisapride (Propulsid)

HEMATOPOIETIC AGENTS

filgrastim (Neupogen)

HISTAMINE (H-2)-BLOCKING DRUGS

(H-2 Blockers)

cimetidine (Tagamet)
famotidine (Pepcid)
nizatidine (Axid)
ranitidine (Zantac)

HYPNOTIC DRUGS

(Sedatives/Sleep Inducers)

acetylcarbromal (Paxarel)
chloral hydrate (Aquachloral, Noctec)
estazolam (ProSom)
ethchlorvynol (Placidyl)
ethinamate (Valmid)
flurazepam (Dalmane)
glutethimide (Doriden)
methyprylon (Noludar)
paraldehyde (Paral)
propiomazine (Largon)
quazepam (Doral)
temazepam (Restoril)
triazolam (Halcion)
zolpidem (Ambien)
see also Barbiturate Class (above)

MACROLIDE ANTIBIOTICS
(Anti-infectives)

azithromycin (Zithromax)
clarithromycin (Biaxin)
erythromycin (E-Mycin, Ilosone, Erythrocin, E.E.S.)
troleandomycin (Tao)

MONOAMINE OXIDASE (MAO) INHIBITOR DRUGS
(Type A: Antidepressants)

isocarboxazid (Marplan)
phenelzine (Nardil)
tranylcypromine (Parnate)

MUSCLE RELAXANTS
(Skeletal Muscle Relaxants)

baclofen (Lioresal)
carisoprodol (Rela, Soma, others)
chlorphenesin carbamate (Maolate)
chlorzoxazone (Paraflex, Parafon Forte)
cyclobenzaprine (Flexeril)
dantrolene (Dantrium)
diazepam (Valium)
meprobamate (Equanil, Miltown, others)
metaxalone (Skelaxin)
methocarbamol (Robaxin, others)
orphenadrine (Norflex, others)

NITRATES

amyl nitrate (Amyl Nitrate Vaporole, others)
erythrityl tetranitrate (Cardilate)
isosorbide dinitrate (Isordil, Sorbitrate, others)
isosorbide mononitrate (Ismo, Imdur)
nitroglycerin (Nitrostat, Nitrolingual, Nitrogard, Nitrong, others)
pentaerythritol tetranitrate (Duotrate, Peritrate)

NONSTEROIDAL ANTI-INFLAMMATORY DRUGS (NSAIDS)
(Aspirin Substitutes)
Acetic Acids

diclofenac Potassium (Cataflam)
diclofenac Sodium (Voltaren
etodolac (Lodine)
indomethacin (Indochron E-R, Indocin, Indocin SR)
ketorolac (Toradol)
nabumetone (Relafen)
sulindac (Clinoril)
tolmetin (Tolectin, Tolectin DS)

Fenamates

meclofenamate (Meclomen)
mefenamic acid (Ponstel)

Oxicams

piroxicam (Feldene)

Propionic acids

diflunisal (Dolobid)
fenoprofen (Nalfon)
flurbiprofen (Ansaid)
ibuprofen (Motrin, Nuprin, Rufen, Advil, Medipren, others)
ketoprofen (Orudis, Orvail)
naproxen (Naprosyn)
naproxen sodium (Aleve, Anaprox, Anaprox DS)
oxaprozin (Daypro)
oxyphenbutazone (Oxalid)
suprofen (Profenal)

OPIOID DRUGS

(Narcotics)

alfentanil (Alfenta)
codeine (no brand name)
fentanyl (Sublimaze, Duragesic)
hydrocodone (Hycodan)
hydromorphone (Dilaudid)
levorphanol (Levo-Dromoran)
meperidine (Demerol)
methadone (Dolophine)
morphine (Astramorph, Duramorph, MS Contin, Roxanol)
oxycodone (Roxicodone)
oxymorphone (Numorphan)
propoxyphene (Darvon)
sufentanil (Sufenta)

PENICILLINS

(Anti-infectives)

amoxicillin (Amoxil, Larotid, Polymox, Trimox, others)
amoxicillin/clavulanate (Augmentin)
ampicillin (Omnipen, Polycillin, Principen, Totacillin)
ampicillin/sulbactam (Unasyn)
bacampicillin (Spectrobid)
carbenicillin (Geocillin, Geopen, Pyopen)
cloxacillin (Cloxapen, Tegopen)
dicloxacillin (Dynapen, Pathocil, Veracillin)
methicillin (Staphcillin)
mezlocillin (Mezlin)
nafcillin (Nafcil, Unipen)
oxacillin (Prostaphlin)
penicillin G (Pentids, others)
penicillin V (Pen Vee K, V-Cillin K, Veetids, others)
piperacillin (Pipracil)
ticarcillin (Ticar)
ticarcillin/clavulanate (Timentin)

PHENOTHIAZINES

(Antipsychotic Drugs)

acetophenazine (Tindal)
chlorpromazine (Thorazine)
fluphenazine (Permitil, Prolixin)
mesoridazine (Serentil)
perphenazine (Trilafon)
prochlorperazine (Compazine)
promazine (Sparine)
thioridazine (Mellaril)
trifluoperazine (Stelazine)
triflupromazine (Vesprin)

PROGESTINS

(Female Sex Hormones)

ethynodiol (no brand name)
hydroxyprogesterone (Duralutin, Gesterol L.A., others)
medroxyprogesterone (Amen, Curretab, Provera)
megestrol (Megace)
norethindrone (Micronor, Norlutate, Norlutin)
norgestrel (Ovrette)
progesterone (Gesterol 50, Progestaject)

PROTON PUMP INHIBITORS

(H/K ATPase inhibitors)

lansoprazole (Prevacid)
omeprazole (Prilosec)

RADIOPHARMACEUTICALS

strontium-89 (Metastron)

SALICYLATES

aspirin (ASA, Bufferin, Ecotrin, Empirin, others)
choline salicylate (Arthropan)
magnesium salicylate (Doan's, Magan, Mobidin)
salsalate (Amigesic, Disalcid, Salsitab)
sodium salicylate (no brand name)
sodium thiosalicylate (Rexolate, Tusal)

SMOKING DETERRENTS

nicotine (Habitrol, Nicoderm, Nicotrol, Prostep, Nicorette, others)

SULFONAMIDES

(Anti-infectives)

multiple sulfonamides (Triple Sulfa No. 2)
sulfacytine (Renoquid)
sulfadiazine (no brand name)
sulfamethizole (Thiosulfil)
sulfamethoxazole (Gantanol)
sulfasalazine (Azulfidine)
sulfisoxazole (Gantrisin)

SULFONYLUREAS

(Oral Antidiabetic Drugs)

acetohexamide (Dymelor)
chlorpropamide (Diabinese)
glipizide (Glucotrol)
glyburide (DiaBeta, Micronase)
tolazamide (Ronase, Tolamide, Tolinase)
tolbutamide (Orinase)

TETRACYCLINES

(Anti-infectives)

demeclocycline (Declomycin)
doxycycline (Doryx, Doxychel, Vibramycin)
methacycline (Rondomycin)
minocycline (Minocin)
oxytetracycline (Terramycin)
tetracycline (Achromycin V, Panmycin, Sumycin)

THIAZIDE DIURETICS

bendroflumethiazide (Naturetin)
benzthiazide (Aquatag, Exna, Marazide)
chlorothiazide (Diuril)
cyclothiazide (Anhydron)
hydrochlorothiazide (Esidrix, Hydrodiuril, Oretic)
hydroflumethiazide (Diucardin, Saluron)
methyclothiazide (Enduron, Aquatensen)
polythiazide (Renese)
trichlormethiazide (Metahydrin, Naqua)

VACCINES

(Immune Modulators)

influenza vaccine (Fluogen, Flu-Shield, Fluzone)
varicella virus vaccine (Varivax)

VASODILATORS

(Peripheral Vasodilators)

cyclandelate (Cyclospasmol)
ethaverine (Ethaquin, Isovex)
isoxsuprine (Vasodilan)

nylidrin (Arlidin)
papaverine (Cerespan, Pavabid)

XANTHINES

(Bronchodilators)

aminophylline (Phyllocontin, Truphylline)
dyphylline (Dilor, Lufyllin)
oxtriphylline (Choledyl)

theophylline (Bronkodyl, Slo-Phyllin, Theolair, others)

SECTION FIVE

A GLOSSARY OF DRUG-RELATED TERMS

Glossary

Addiction Although there is disagreement among authorities as to how inclusive this designation should be, addiction is generally recognized to be a state of intense dependence (upon a drug) that is characterized by uncontrollable drug-seeking behavior, *tolerance* for the drug's pleasure-giving effects, and *withdrawal* manifestations when the drug is withheld. These features constitute *physical dependence*—a state of physical incorporation of the drug into the fundamental biochemistry of specific brain activities. (See the terms DEPENDENCE and TOLERANCE for a further account of physical and psychological dependence.)

Adverse Effect or Reaction An abnormal, unexpected, infrequent and usually unpredictable injurious response to a drug. Used in this restrictive sense, the term *adverse reaction* does *not* include effects of a drug which are normally a part of its pharmacological action, even though such effects may be undesirable and unintended. (See SIDE-EFFECT.) Adverse reactions are of three basic types: those due to drug *allergy,* those caused by individual *idiosyncrasy* and those representing *toxic* effects of drugs on tissue structure and function (see ALLERGY, IDIOSYNCRASY and TOXICITY).

Allergy (Drug) An abnormal mechanism of drug response that occurs in individuals who produce injurious antibodies* that react with foreign substances—in this instance, a drug. The person who is allergic by nature and has a history of hay fever, asthma, hives or eczema is more likely to develop drug allergies. Allergic reactions to drugs take many forms: skin eruptions of various kinds, fever, swollen glands, painful joints, jaundice, interference with breathing, acute collapse of circulation, etc. Drug allergies can develop gradually over a long period of time, or they can appear with dramatic suddenness and require life-saving intervention.

Alternative Delivery System (ADS) A term coined to describe a variety of health care forms other than the traditional fee-for-service model such as HMOs, PPOs and others.

---

*Antibodies are special tissue proteins that combine with substances foreign to the body. Protective antibodies destroy bacteria and neutralize toxins. Injurious antibodies, reacting with foreign substances, cause the release of histamine, the principal chemical responsible for allergic reactions.

Analgesic A drug that is used primarily to relieve pain. Analgesics are of three basic types: (1) Simple, nonnarcotic analgesics that relieve pain by suppressing the local production of prostaglandins and related substances—examples are acetaminophen, aspirin and the large group of nonsteroidal anti-inflammatory drugs known as aspirin substitutes (Motrin, Advil, Naprosyn, etc.); (2) Narcotic analgesics or opioids ("like opium" derivatives) that relieve pain by suppressing its perception in the brain—examples are morphine, codeine and hydrocodone (natural derivatives of opium), and meperidine or pentazocine (synthetic drug products); (3) Local anesthetics that prevent or relieve pain by rendering sensory nerve endings insensitive to painful stimulation—an example is the urinary tract analgesic phenazopyridine (Pyridium).

Anaphylactic (Anaphylactoid) Reaction A group of symptoms which represent (or resemble) a sometimes overwhelming and dangerous allergic reaction due to extreme hypersensitivity to a drug. Anaphylactic reactions, whether mild, moderate or severe, often involve several body systems. Mild symptoms consist of itching, hives, nasal congestion, nausea, abdominal cramping and/or diarrhea. Sometimes these precede more severe symptoms such as choking, shortness of breath and sudden loss of consciousness (usually referred to as anaphylactic shock).

Characteristic features of anaphylactic reaction must be kept in mind. It can result from a very small dose of drug; it develops suddenly, usually within a few minutes after taking the drug; it can be rapidly progressive and can lead to fatal collapse in a short time if not reversed by appropriate treatment. A developing anaphylactic reaction is a true medical emergency. Any adverse effect that appears within 20 minutes after taking a drug should be considered the early manifestation of a possible anaphylactic reaction. Obtain medical attention immediately! (See ALLERGY, DRUG and HYPERSENSITIVITY.)

Antihypertensive A drug used to lower excessively high blood pressure. The term *hypertension* denotes blood pressure above the normal range. It does not refer to excessive nervous or emotional tension. The term *antihypertensive* is sometimes used erroneously as if it had the same meaning as *antianxiety* (or tranquilizing) drug action.

Today there are more than 80 drug products in use for treating hypertension. Those most frequently prescribed for long-term use fall into three major groups:

1. drugs that increase urine production (the diuretics)
2. drugs that relax blood vessel walls
3. drugs that reduce the activity of the sympathetic nervous system

Regardless of their mode of action, all these drugs share an ability to lower the blood pressure. It is important to remember that many other drugs can interact with antihypertensive drugs: some add to their effect and cause excessive reduction in blood pressure; others interfere with their action and reduce their effectiveness. Anyone who is taking medications for hypertension should consult with his or her physician whenever drugs are prescribed for the treatment of other conditions as well.

Antipyretic A drug that is used to treat fever because of its ability to lower body temperature that is elevated above the normal. Antipyretics relieve fever through their effects on the temperature regulating center in the hypothalamus of the brain. Their actions cause dilation of the blood vessels (capillary beds) in the skin, bringing overheated blood to the surface for cooling; in addition, the sweat glands are stimulated to provide copious perspiration that cools the body further through evaporation. An antipyretic drug may also be analgesic (acetaminophen), or analgesic and anti-inflammatory (aspirin).

Aplastic Anemia A form of bone marrow failure in which the production of all 3 types of blood cells is seriously impaired (also known as pancytopenia). Aplastic anemia can occur spontaneously from unknown causes, but about one-half of reported cases are induced by certain drugs or chemicals. The offending drug may be difficult to identify; a delay of from one to six months may occur between the use of a causative drug and the detection of anemia. The symptoms reflect the consequences of inadequate supplies of all 3 blood cell types: deficiency of red blood cells (anemia) results in fatigue, weakness and pallor; deficiency of white blood cells (leukopenia) predisposes to infections; deficiency of blood platelets (thrombocytopenia) leads to spontaneous bruising and hemorrhage. Treatment is difficult and the outcome unpredictable. Even with the best of care, approximately 50% of cases end fatally.

Although aplastic anemia is a rare consequence of drug treatment (3 in 100,000 users of quinacrine, for example), anyone taking a drug capable of inducing it should have complete blood cell counts periodically if the drug is to be used over an extended period of time. For a listing of causative drugs, see Section Six, Table 5.

Bioavailability The measurable characteristics of a drug product (usually a tablet or a capsule) that represent how rapidly the active drug ingredient is absorbed into the bloodstream and to what extent it is absorbed. Two types of measurements—(1) blood levels of the drug at certain time intervals after administration, and (2) the duration of the drug's presence in the blood—indicate how much of the drug is available for biological activity and for how long.

Another method of determining a drug product's bioavailability is to measure (1) the cumulative amount of the drug (or any breakdown product after transformation) that is excreted in the urine, and (2) the rate of drug accumulation in the urine.

The two major factors that govern a drug product's bioavailability are the chemical and physical characteristics (the formulation) of the dosage form given, and the functional state of the digestive system of the individual who takes it. A drug product that disintegrates rapidly in a normally functioning stomach and small intestine produces blood levels of the absorbed drug quite promptly. Such a drug product can be demonstrated to possess good bioavailability.

Specially designed laboratory tests are now available to evaluate a drug product's potential bioavailability when taken by the "average" individual.

Bioequivalence It is generally accepted that the ability of a drug product to produce its intended therapeutic effect is directly related to its bioavailability. When a particular drug is marketed by several manufacturers, often in a variety of dosage forms, it is critically important that the drug product selected for use be one that possesses the bioavailability necessary to be effective therapeutically. Substantial variations occur among manufacturers in the formulation of their drug products. Although the principal drug ingredient of products from different firms may be identical chemically, it cannot be assumed that these products possess equal bioavailability and are therefore equal therapeutically.

The bioavailability of any drug product is governed to a large extent by the physical characteristics of its formulation; these in turn determine how rapidly and how completely the drug product disintegrates and releases its active drug component(s) for absorption into the bloodstream. Drug products that contain the same principal drug ingredient but are combined with different inert additives, are coated with different substances or are enclosed in capsules of different composition may or may not possess the same bioavailability. Those that do are said to be bioequivalent, and can be relied upon to be equally effective in achieving therapeutic results.

If you consider having your prescription filled with the generic equivalent of a brand name drug product, ask your physician *and* pharmacist for guidance. This decision requires professional judgment in each case. In many treatment situations, reasonable differences in the bioavailability patterns among drug products are acceptable. In some situations, however, because of the serious nature of the illness, or because it is mandatory that blood levels of the drug be maintained within a narrowly defined range, it is essential to use the drug product that has been demonstrated to possess reliable bioavailability.

Blood Platelets The smallest of the three types of blood cells produced by the bone marrow. Platelets are normally present in very large numbers. Their primary function is to assist the process of normal blood clotting so as to prevent excessive bruising and bleeding in the event of injury. When present in proper numbers and functioning normally, platelets preserve the retaining power of the walls of the smaller blood vessels. By initiating appropriate clotting processes in the blood, platelets seal small points of leakage in the vessel walls, thereby preventing spontaneous bruising or bleeding (that which is unprovoked by trauma).

Certain drugs and chemicals may reduce the number of available blood platelets to abnormally low levels. Some of these drugs act by suppressing platelet formation; other drugs hasten their destruction. When the number of functioning platelets falls below a critical level, blood begins to leak through the thin walls of smaller vessels. The outward evidence of this leakage is the spontaneous appearance of scattered bruises in the skin of the thighs and legs. This is referred to as purpura. Bleeding may occur anywhere in the body, internally as well as superficially into the tissues immediately beneath the skin. See Section Six, Table 5.

Bone Marrow Depression A serious reduction in the ability of the bone marrow to carry on its normal production of blood cells. This can occur as an adverse reaction to the toxic effect of certain drugs and chemicals on bone marrow components. When functioning normally, the bone marrow produces the majority of the body's blood cells. These consist of three types: the red blood cells (erythrocytes), the white blood cells (leukocytes) and the blood platelets (thrombocytes). Each type of cell performs one or more specific functions, all of which are indispensable to the maintenance of life and health.

Drugs that are capable of depressing bone marrow activity can impair the production of all types of blood cells simultaneously or of only one type selectively. Periodic examinations of the blood can reveal significant changes in the structure and number of the blood cells that indicate a possible drug effect on bone marrow activity.

Impairment of the production of red blood cells leads to anemia, a condition of abnormally low red cells and hemoglobin. This causes weakness, loss of energy and stamina, intolerance of cold environments and shortness of breath on physical exertion. A reduction in the formation of white blood cells can impair the body's immunity and lower its resistance to infection. These changes may result in the development of fever, sore throat or pneumonia. When the formation of blood platelets is suppressed to abnormally low levels, the blood loses its ability to quickly seal small points of leakage in blood vessel walls. This may lead to episodes of unusual and abnormal spontaneous bruising or to prolonged bleeding in the event of injury.

Any of these symptoms can occur in the presence of bone marrow depression. These symptoms should alert both patient and physician to the need for prompt studies of blood and bone marrow. See Section Six, Table 5.

Brand Name The registered trade name given to a drug product by its manufacturer. Many drugs are marketed by more than one manufacturer or distributor. Each company adopts a distinctive trade name to distinguish its brand of the generic drug from that of its competitors. Thus a brand name designates a proprietary drug—one that is protected by patent or copyright. Generally, brand names are shorter, easier to pronounce and more readily remembered than their generic counterparts.

Capitation A system where a set amount of money is used to cover the cost of health care for a given person. For instance, a health plan or hospital is paid monthly on a negotiated per person rate where the plan or hospital provides all health services for the people in the plan.

Cause-and-Effect Relationship A possible causative association between a drug and a biologic event—most commonly a side-effect or an adverse effect. Knowledge of a drug's full spectrum of effects (wanted and unwanted) is highly desirable when weighing its benefits and risks. However, it is often impossible to establish that a particular drug is the primary agent responsible for an adverse effect. Meticulous consideration must be given to such factors as the time sequence of drug administration and possible reaction, the use of multiple drugs, possible interactions among these drugs, the effects of the disease under treatment, the physiological and psychological characteristics of the patient and the influence of unrecognized disorders and malfunctions.

The majority of adverse drug reactions occur sporadically, unpredictably and infrequently in the general population. A *definite* cause-and-effect relationship between drug and reaction is established when (1) the adverse effect immediately follows administration of the drug; or (2) the adverse effect disappears after the drug is discontinued (dechallenge) and promptly reappears when the drug is used again (rechallenge); or (3) the adverse effects are clearly the expected and predictable toxic consequences of drug overdosage.

In contrast to the obvious "causative" (definite) relationship, there exists a large gray area of "probable," "possible" and "coincidental" associations associated with varying degrees of uncertainty. These classifications often apply to alleged drug reactions that require a relatively long time to develop, are rare, and for which there are no clear-cut means to show a causal mechanism that links drug and reaction. Clarification of cause-and-effect relationships in these uncertain groups requires carefully designed observation over a long period of time, followed by sophisticated statistical analysis. Occasionally the public is alerted to a newly found "relationship" based upon suggestive but incomplete data. Though early warning is in the public interest, such announcements should make clear whether the presumed relationship is based upon definitive criteria or is simply inferred. It is critical to avoid losing valuable medication use because of poorly designed or reported studies that find their way to the newspaper or television.

The most competent techniques for evaluating cause-and-effect relationships of adverse drug reactions have been devised by the Division of Tissue Reactions to Drugs, a research unit of the Armed Forces Institute of Pathology. Based upon a highly critical examination of all available evidence, the Division's study of 2800 drug-related deaths yielded the following levels of certainty:

No association	5.0%
Coincidental	14.5%
Possible	33.0%
Probable	30.0%
Causative	17.5%

It is significant that expert evaluation of 2800 drug-related cases concluded that only 47.5% could be substantiated as definitely or probably causative.

Contraindication A condition or disease that precludes the use of a particular drug. Some contraindications are *absolute*, meaning that the use of the drug would expose the patient to extreme hazard and therefore cannot be justified. Other contraindications are *relative*, meaning that the condition or disease does not entirely bar the use of the drug but requires that special consideration be given to factors which could aggravate existing disease, interfere with current treatment or produce new injury.

Covered Lives A term used by health maintenance organizations to indicate how many people have enrolled in their plan. From the HMO's point of view, a minimum number of covered lives is necessary to support a certain number of family practice physicians, a certain number of subspecialists and so on. Understanding their logic helps explain why some HMOs have one urologist while others have several.

Critical or clinical pathway An assortment of coordinated measures taken by a hospital or clinic to organize the care of their patients with specific diseases or conditions. All diagnostic tests, treatments, discharge planning and other measures are the result of careful study and practice aimed at providing the maximum benefit to all patients in the most cost-effective manner.

Dependence A term used to identify the drug-dependent states of *psychological dependence* (or *habituation*), and *physical dependence* (or *addiction*). In addition, a third kind of drug-dependence can be included under this term. This might be called *functional dependence*—the need to use a drug continuously in order to sustain a particular body function, the impairment of which causes annoying symptoms of varying degree and significance.

Psychological dependence is a form of neurotic behavior—an "emotional" dependence. It is an obsession to satisfy a particular desire, be it one of self-gratification or one of escape from some real or imagined distress. Psychological dependence is a very human trait seen often in many socially acceptable patterns and practices such as entertainment, gambling, sports and collecting. A common form in today's culture is the increasing reliance upon drugs to help in coping with the everyday problems of living: pills for frustration, disappointment, nervous stomach, tension headache and insomnia. This compulsive drug abuse is characterized by little or no tendency to increase the dose (see TOLERANCE) and no or only minor physical symptoms on withdrawal. Some authorities choose to broaden the definition of addiction to include psychological dependence.

Physical dependence, which is true addiction, includes two elements: *tolerance* and *withdrawal* manifestations. Addicting drugs provide relief from anguish and pain; they also induce a physiological tolerance that requires increasing dose or repeated use to remain effective. These two features foster continued need for the drug and lead to its becoming a functioning component in the biochemistry of the brain. As this occurs, the drug assumes an "essential" role in ongoing chemical processes. (Thus some authorities prefer the term *chemical dependence*.) Sudden removal of the drug from the system causes a major upheaval in body chemistry and provokes a withdrawal syndrome—the intense mental and physical pain experienced by the addict when intake of the drug is stopped abruptly—that is the hallmark of addiction. It must be noted that true addiction is rare, and fear of addiction, even with potent narcotics should never stand in the way of effective pain control.

Functional dependence differs significantly from both psychological and physical dependence. It occurs when a drug relieves an annoying or distressing condition and the body function involved becomes increasingly dependent upon the action of the drug to provide a sense of well-being. Drugs that cause functional dependence are used primarily for the relief of symptoms. They do not act on the brain to produce alteration of mood or consciousness as do those drugs with potential for either psychological or physical dependence. The most familiar example of functional dependence is the "laxative habit." Some types of constipation are made worse by the wrong choice of laxative, and natural bowel function fades as the colon becomes more and more dependent upon the laxative drug.

Disulfiramlike (Antabuselike) Reaction The symptoms that result from the interaction of alcohol and any drug that is capable of provoking the pattern of response typical of the "Antabuse effect." The interacting drug interrupts the decomposition of alcohol by the liver and permits accumulation of a toxic by-product that enters the bloodstream. When sufficient levels of both alcohol and drug are present in the blood, the reaction occurs. It consists of intense flushing and warming of the face, a severe throbbing headache, shortness of breath, chest pains, nausea, repeated vomiting, sweating and weakness. If the amount of alcohol ingested has been large enough, the reaction may progress to blurred vision, vertigo, confusion, marked drop in blood pressure and loss of consciousness. Severe reactions may lead to convulsions and death. The reaction can last from 30 minutes to several hours, depending upon the amount of alcohol in the body. As the symptoms subside, the individual is exhausted and usually sleeps for several hours.

Diuretic A drug that alters kidney function to increase the volume of urine. Diuretics use several different mechanisms to increase urine volume, and these, in turn, have different effects on body chemistry. Diuretics are used primarily to (1) remove excess water from the body (as in congestive heart failure and some types of liver and kidney disease), and (2) treat hypertension by promoting the excretion of sodium from the body.

Disease Management An approach to the prevention and treatment of a specific condition which attempts to identify the frequency of its occurrence in the population, organize available resources, and allocate money to reach the best balance of dollars spent and results achieved.

Divided Doses The total daily dose of a medicine is split into smaller individual doses over the course of a day.

Dosage Forms and Strengths This information category in the individual Drug Profiles (Section Two) uses several abbreviations to designate measurements of weight and volume. These are

```
mcg = microgram = 1,000,000th of a gram (weight)
mg  = milligram = 1000th of a gram (weight)
ml  = milliliter = 1000th of a liter (volume)
gm  = gram      = 1000 milligrams (weight)
```

There are approximately 65 mg in 1 grain.
There are approximately 5 ml in 1 teaspoon.
There are approximately 15 ml in 1 tablespoon.
There are approximately 30 ml in 1 ounce.
1 milliliter of water weighs 1 gram.
There are approximately 454 grams in 1 pound.

Drug, Drug Product Terms often used interchangeably to designate a medicine (in any of its dosage forms) used in medical practice. Strictly speaking, the term *drug*

refers to the single chemical entity that provokes a specific response when placed within a biological system—the "active" ingredient. A *drug product* is the manufactured dosage form—tablet, capsule, elixir, etc.—that contains the active drug intermixed with inactive ingredients to provide for convenient administration.

Drug products which contain only one active ingredient are referred to as single entity drugs. Drug products with two or more active ingredients are called combination drugs (designated [CD] in the lists of brand names in the Drug Profiles, Section Two).

Drug Class A group of drugs that are similar in chemistry, method of action and use in treatment. Because of their common characteristics, many drugs within a class will produce the same side-effects and have similar potential for related adverse reactions and interactions. However, significant variations among members within a drug class can occur. This sometimes allows the physician an important degree of selectivity in choosing a drug if certain beneficial actions are desired or particular side-effects are to be minimized.

Examples: Antihistamines, phentothiazines, tetracyclines (see Section Four).

Drug Fever The elevation of body temperature that occurs as an unwanted manifestation of drug action. Drugs can induce fever by several mechanisms; these include allergic reactions, drug-induced tissue damage, acceleration of tissue metabolism, constriction of blood vessels in the skin with resulting decrease in loss of body heat and direct action on the temperature-regulating center in the brain.

The most common form of drug fever is associated with allergic reactions. It may be the only allergic manifestation apparent, or it may be part of a complex of allergic symptoms that can include skin rash, hives, joint swelling and pain, enlarged lymph glands, hemolytic anemia or hepatitis. The fever usually appears about 7 to 10 days after starting the drug and may vary from low-grade to alarmingly high levels. It may be sustained or intermittent, but it usually persists for as long as the drug is taken. In previously sensitized individuals drug fever may occur within 1 or 2 hours after taking the first dose of medication.

While many drugs are capable of producing fever, the following are more commonly responsible:

allopurinol
antihistamines
atropinelike drugs
barbiturates
coumarin anticoagulants
hydralazine
iodides
isoniazid
methyldopa
nadalol

novobiocin
para-aminosalicylic acid
penicillin
pentazocine
phenytoin
procainamide
propylthiouracil
quinidine
rifampin
sulfonamides

Extension Effect An unwanted but predictable drug response that is a logical consequence of mild to moderate overdosage. An extension effect is an exaggeration of the drug's normal pharmacological action; it can be thought of as a mild form of dose-related toxicity (see OVERDOSAGE and TOXICITY).

Example: The continued "hangover" of drowsiness and mental sluggishness that persists after arising in the morning is a common extension effect of a long-acting sleep-inducing drug (hypnotic) taken the night before.

Example: The persistent intestinal cramping and diarrhea that result from too generous a dose of laxative are extension effects of the drug's anticipated action.

FDA Approvable A stage in the Food and Drug Administration's review and approval process. A medicine is considered FDA approvable once the panel which reviewed the supporting data submitted to the FDA finds that data acceptable. In general, at this point only final details need to be resolved before the drug becomes FDA approved and is made available for general prescription use.

Generic Name The official, common or public name used to designate an active drug entity, whether in pure form or in dosage form. Generic names are coined by committees of officially appointed drug experts and are approved by governmental agencies for national and international use. Thus they are nonproprietary. Many drug products are marketed under the generic name of the principal active ingredient and bear no brand name of the manufacturer.

While the total number of prescriptions written in the United States in 1986 increased by 0.6%, prescriptions specifying the *generic name* of the drug increased by 8.6%. Generically written prescriptions now account for 13.5% of all new prescriptions written in the United States. The drugs most commonly prescribed by generic name are listed below, ranked in descending order of the number of new prescriptions issued.

amoxicillin   erythromycin
penicillin VK   hydrochlorothiazide
ampicillin   acetaminophen/codeine
tetracycline   doxycycline
prednisone   phenobarbital

Genetic Therapy Perhaps the most promising area of therapy in medicine today. Specific healthy genetic material is isolated and inserted into appropriate, but diseased, cells. For example, normal lung genes are given to a person with cystic fibrosis. Still very experimental, it may someday allow people suffering with genetically-based diseases or conditions to receive therapy that changes the effected genes and actually *cure* those conditions.

Habituation A form of drug dependence based upon strong psychological gratification. The habitual use of drugs that alter mood or relieve minor discomforts results from a compulsive need to feel pleasure and satisfaction or to escape emotional distress. The abrupt cessation of habituating drugs does not produce the withdrawal syndrome seen in addiction. Thus habituation is a *psychological dependence.* (See DEPENDENCE for a further account of psychological and physical dependence.)

Hemolytic Anemia A form of anemia (deficient red blood cells and hemoglobin) resulting from the premature destruction (hemolysis) of red blood cells. Several mechanisms can cause hemolytic anemia; among these is the action of certain drugs and chemicals. Some patients are susceptible to hemolytic anemia because of a genetic deficiency in the makeup of their red blood cells. If such people are given certain antimalarial drugs, sulfa drugs or numerous other drugs, some of their red cells will disintegrate on contact with the drug. (About 10% of American blacks have this genetic trait.)

Another type of drug-induced hemolytic anemia is a form of drug allergy. Many drugs in wide use (including quinidine, methyldopa, levodopa and chlorpromazine) are known to cause hemolytic destruction of red cells as a hypersensitivity (allergic) reaction.

Hemolytic anemia can occur abruptly (with evident symptoms) or silently.

The acute form lasts about 7 days and is characterized by fever, pallor, weakness, dark-colored urine and varying degrees of jaundice (yellow coloration of eyes and skin). When drug-induced hemolytic anemia is mild, involving the destruction of only a small number of red blood cells, there may be no symptoms to indicate its presence. Such episodes are detected only by means of laboratory studies (see IDIOSYNCRASY and ALLERGY, DRUG).

For listings of causative drugs, see Section Six, Table 5.

Hepatitislike Reaction Changes in the liver, induced by certain drugs, which resemble those produced by viral hepatitis. The symptoms of drug-induced hepatitis and virus-induced hepatitis are often so similar that the correct cause cannot be established without precise laboratory studies.

Hepatitis due to drugs may be a form of drug allergy (as in reaction to many of the phenothiazines), or it may represent a toxic adverse effect (as in reaction to some of the monoamine oxidase inhibitor drugs). Liver reactions of significance usually result in jaundice and represent serious adverse effects (see JAUNDICE). See Section Six, Table 8.

HMO Abbreviation for Health Maintenance Organization: A health care delivery system that provides a broad spectrum of medical therapies and services by a collective group of practitioners within a common organization.

Hypersensitivity A term subject to varying usages for many years. One common use has been to identify the trait of overresponsiveness to drug action, that is, an intolerance to even small doses. Used in this sense, the term indicates that the nature of the response is appropriate but the degree of response is exaggerated.

The term is more widely used today to identify a state of allergy. To have a *hypersensitivity* to a drug is to be *allergic* to it [see ALLERGY (DRUG)].

Some individuals develop cross-hypersensitivity. This means that once a person has developed an allergy to a certain drug, that person will experience an allergic reaction to other drugs which are closely related in chemical composition.

Example: The patient was known to be *hypersensitive* by nature, having a history of seasonal hay fever and asthma since childhood. His *allergy* to tetracycline developed after his third course of treatment. This drug *hypersensitivity* manifested itself as a diffuse, measleslike rash.

Hypnotic A drug that is used primarily to induce sleep. There are several classes of drugs that have hypnotic effects: antihistamines, barbiturates, benzodiazepines and several unrelated compounds. Within the past 15 years the benzodiazepines, because of their relative safety and lower potential for inducing dependence, have largely replaced the barbiturates as the most commonly used hypnotics. The body usually develops a tolerance to the hypnotic effect after several weeks of continual use. To maintain their effectiveness, hypnotics should be used intermittently for short periods of time.

Hypoglycemia A condition where the amount of glucose (a sugar) in the blood is below the normal range. Since normal brain function depends upon an adequate supply of glucose, reducing the level of glucose in the blood below a critical point will cause serious impairment of brain activity. The resulting symptoms are characteristic of hypoglycemia. Early indications are headache, a sensation resembling mild drunkenness and an inability to think clearly. These may be accompanied by hunger. As the level of blood glucose continues to fall, nervousness and confusion develop. Varying degrees of weakness, numbness, trembling, sweating and rapid heart action follow. If sugar is not provided at this point and the blood glucose level drops further, impaired speech, incoordination and unconsciousness, with or without convulsions, will follow.

Hypoglycemia in any stage requires prompt recognition and treatment. Because of the potential for injury to the brain, the mechanisms and management of hypoglycemia should be understood by all who use drugs capable of producing it.

Hypothermia A state of the body characterized by an unexpected decline of internal body temperature to levels significantly below the norm of 98.6 degrees F or 37 degrees C. By definition, hypothermia means a body temperature of less than 95 degrees F or 35 degrees C. The elderly and debilitated are more prone to develop hypothermia if clothed inadequately and exposed to cool environments. Most episodes are initiated by room temperatures below 65 degrees F or 18.3 degrees C. The condition often develops suddenly, can mimic a stroke and has a mortality rate of 50%. Some drugs, such as phenothiazines, barbiturates and benzodiazepines, are conducive to causing hypothermia.

Idiosyncrasy An abnormal mechanism of drug response that occurs in people who have a peculiar defect in their body chemistry (often hereditary) which produces an effect totally unrelated to the drug's normal pharmacological action. Idiosyncrasy is not a form of allergy. The actual chemical defects responsible for certain idiosyncratic drug reactions are well understood; others are not.

Example: Approximately 100 million people in the world (including 10% of American blacks) have an enzyme deficiency in their red blood cells which causes these cells to disintegrate when exposed to drugs such as sulfonamides (Gantrisin, Kynex), nitrofurantoin (Furadantin, Macrodantin), probenecid (Benemid), quinine and quinidine. As a result of this reaction, these drugs (and others) can cause a significant anemia in susceptible individuals.

Example: Approximately 5% of the population of the United States is susceptible to the development of glaucoma on prolonged use of cortisone-related drugs (see Cortisone Drug Class in Section Four).

Immunosuppressive A drug that significantly impairs (suppresses) the functions of the body's immune system. In some cases, immunosuppression is an intended drug effect (cyclosporine to prevent the immune system from rejecting a transplanted kidney). In other instances, it is an unwanted side-effect as in the long-term use of cortisonelike drugs (to control asthma) suppressing the immune system sufficiently to permit reactivation of a dormant tuberculosis. Immunosuppressant drugs are being used to treat several chronic disorders that are thought to be autoimmune diseases, notably advanced rheumatoid arthritis, ulcerative colitis and systemic lupus erythematosus.

Interaction An unwanted change in the body's response to a drug that results when a second drug that can alter the action of the first is administered at the same time. Some drug interactions can enhance the effect of either drug, producing an overresponse similar to overdosage. Other interactions may reduce drug effectiveness and cause inadequate response. A third type of interaction can produce a seemingly unrelated toxic response with no associated increase or decrease in the pharmacological actions of the interacting drugs.

Theoretically, many drugs can interact with one another, but in reality drug interactions are comparatively infrequent. Many interactions can be anticipated, and the physician can make appropriate adjustments in dosage to prevent or minimize unintended fluctuations in drug response.

Jaundice A yellow coloration of the skin (and the white portion of the eyes) that occurs when excessive bile pigments accumulate in the blood as a result of impaired liver function. Jaundice can be produced by several mechanisms. It may occur as a manifestation of a wide variety of diseases, or it may represent an adverse reaction to a particular drug. At times it is difficult to distinguish between disease-induced jaundice and drug-induced jaundice.

Jaundice due to a drug is always a serious adverse effect. Anyone taking a drug that is capable of causing jaundice should watch closely for any significant change in the color of urine or feces. Dark discoloration of the urine and paleness (lack of color) of the stool may be early indications of a developing jaundice. Should either of these symptoms occur, it is advisable to discontinue the drug and notify the prescribing physician promptly. Diagnostic tests are available to clarify the nature of the jaundice. See Section Six, Table 8.

Lupus Erythematosus (LE) A serious disease of unknown cause that occurs in two forms, one limited to the skin (discoid LE) and the other involving several body systems (systemic LE). Both forms occur predominantly in young women. About 5% of cases of the discoid form convert to the systemic form. Systemic LE is a disorder of the body's immune system which may result in chronic, progressive inflammation and destruction of the connective tissue framework of the skin, blood vessels, joints, brain, heart muscle, lungs and kidneys. Altered proteins in the blood lead to antibody formation which react with certain organ tissues to produce the inflammation and destruction characteristic of the disease. A reduction in the number of white blood cells and blood platelets often occurs. The course of systemic LE is usually quite protracted and unpredictable. While no cure is known, satisfactory management may be achieved in some cases by the judicious use of cortisonelike drugs.

Several drugs are capable of initiating a form of systemic LE quite similar to that which occurs spontaneously. Symptoms may appear as early as 2 weeks or as late as 8 years after starting the responsible drug. The initial symptoms usually consist of low-grade fever, skin rashes of various kinds, aching muscles and multiple joint pains. Chest pains (pleurisy) are fairly common. Enlargement of the lymph glands occurs less frequently. Symptoms usually subside if the drug is stopped, but laboratory evidence of the reaction may persist for many months.

Neuroleptic Malignant Syndrome (NMS) A rare, serious, sometimes fatal idiosyncratic reaction to the use of neuroleptic (antipsychotic) drugs. The principal features of the reaction are hyperthermia (temperatures of 102 to 104 degress F), marked muscle rigidity and coma. Other symptoms include rapid heart rate and breathing, profuse sweating, tremors and seizures. Two thirds of reported cases occurred in men, one third in women. The mortality rate is 15% to 20%.

The following drugs have a potential for inducing this reaction:

amitriptyline + perphenazine (Triavil)
amoxapine (Asendin)
chlorpromazine (Thorazine)
chlorprothixene (Taractan)
clomipramine (Anafranil)
fluphenazine (Permitil, Prolixin)
haloperidol (Haldol)
imipramine (Tofranil, etc.)
levodopa + carbidopa (Sinemet)
loxapine (Loxitane)

metoclopramide (Reglan, Octamide)
molindone (Moban)
perphenazine (Etrafon, Trilafon)
pimozide (Orap)
prochlorperazine (Compazine)
thioridazine (Mellaril)
thiothixene (Navane)
trifluoperazine (Stelazine)
trimeprazine (Temaril)

Orthostatic Hypotension A type of low blood pressure that is related to body position or posture (also called postural hypotension). The individual who is subject to orthostatic hypotension may have a normal blood pressure while lying down, but on sitting upright or standing he or she will experience sudden sensations of lightheadedness, dizziness and a feeling of impending faint that compel him to return quickly to a lying position. These symptoms are manifestations of inadequate blood flow (oxygen supply) to the brain due to a delay in the rise in blood pressure that always occurs as the body adjusts the circulation to the erect position.

Many drugs (especially the stronger antihypertensives) may cause orthostatic hypotension. Individuals who experience this drug effect should report it to their physician so that appropriate dosage adjustment can be made. Failure to correct or to compensate for these sudden drops in blood pressure can lead to severe falls and injury.

The tendency to orthostatic hypotension can be reduced by avoiding sudden standing, prolonged standing, vigorous exercise and exposure to hot environments. Alcoholic beverages should be used cautiously until their combined effect with the drug in use has been determined.

Outcomes Research A current concept in health care evaluation that considers the comparative benefits (gauged by a variety of measures) of using a particular medication over another. This may lead to the cheapest drug **not** being the drug of choice, because the outcomes from the therapy to not stand up over time, or may be subject to significant treatment failure.

Overdosage The meaning of this term should not be limited to the concept of doses that exceed the normal dosage range recommended by the manufacturer. The optimal dose of many drugs (that amount which gives the greatest benefit with least distress) varies greatly from person to person. What may be an average dose for most people will be an overdose for some and an underdose for others. Numerous factors, such as age, body size, nutritional status and liver and kidney function, have significant influence on dosage requirements. Drugs with narrow safety margins often produce indications of overdosage if something delays the elimination of the customary daily dose. In this instance, overdosage results from accumulation of prescribed daily doses. Massive overdosage—as occurs with accidental ingestion of drugs by children or with suicidal intention by adults—is referred to as poisoning.

Over-the-Counter (OTC) Drugs Drug products that can be purchased without prescription. Many are available in food stores, variety stores and newsstands as well as in conventional drug stores. Because of the unrestricted availability, many people do not look upon OTC medicines as drugs. But drugs they are! And like the more potent drug products that are sold only on prescription, they are chemicals that are capable of a wide variety of actions on biological systems. Within the last 30 years, many OTC drugs have assumed greater importance because of their ability to interact unfavorably with widely used prescription drugs. Serious problems in drug management can arise when (1) the patient fails to tell the physician of the OTC drug(s) he or she is taking ("because they really aren't drugs") and (2) the physician fails to specify that his or her question about what medicines are being taken currently *includes all OTC drugs.* During any course of treatment, whether medical or surgical, the patient should consult with the physician regarding any OTC drug that he or she wishes to take.

The major classes of OTC drugs for internal use include:

allergy medicines (antihistamines)
antacids
antiworm medicines
aspirin and aspirin combinations
aspirin substitutes
asthma aids
cold medicines (decongestants)
cough medicines
diarrhea remedies

digestion aids
diuretics
iron preparations
laxatives
menstrual aids
motion sickness remedies
pain relievers
reducing aids
salt substitutes

sedatives and tranquilizers
sleeping pills
stimulants (caffeine)
sugar substitutes (saccharin)
tonics
vitamins

Paradoxical Reaction An unexpected drug response that is not consistent with the known pharmacology of the drug. Such reactions are due to individual sensitivity or variability and can occur in any age group. They are seen more commonly, however, in children and the elderly.

Example: An 80-year-old man was admitted to a nursing home following the death of his wife. He had difficulty adjusting to his new environment and was restless, agitated and irritable. He was given a trial of the tranquilizer diazepam (Valium) to relax him, starting with small doses. On the second day of medication he became confused and erratic in behavior. The dose of diazepam was increased. On the third day he began to wander aimlessly, talked incessantly in a loud voice and displayed anger and hostility when attempts were made to help him. Suspecting the possibility of a paradoxical reaction, the diazepam was discontinued. All behavioral disturbances gradually subsided within 3 days.

Parkinsonlike Disorders (Parkinsonism) A group of symptoms that resembles those caused by Parkinson's disease, a chronic disorder of the nervous system also known as shaking palsy. The characteristic features of parkinsonism include a fixed, emotionless facial expression (masklike in appearance), a prominent trembling of the hands, arms or legs and stiffness of the extremities that limits movement and produces a rigid posture and gait.

Parkinsonism is a fairly common adverse effect that occurs in about 15% of all patients who take large doses of phenothiazines or use them over an extended period of time. If recognized early, the Parkinsonlike features will lessen or disappear with reduced dosage or change in medication. In some instances, however, Parkinsonlike changes may become permanent, requiring appropriate medication.

Peripheral Neuritis (Peripheral Neuropathy) A group of symptoms that results from injury to nerve tissue in the extremities. A variety of drugs and chemicals are capable of inducing changes in nerve structure or function. The characteristic pattern consists of a sensation of numbness and tingling that usually begins in the fingers and toes and is accompanied by an altered sensation to touch and vague discomfort ranging from aching sensations to burning pain. Severe forms of peripheral neuritis may include loss of muscular strength and coordination.

A relatively common form of peripheral neuritis is that seen with the long-term use of isoniazid in the treatment of tuberculosis. If vitamin B-6 (pyridoxine) is not given concurrently with isoniazid, peripheral neuritis may occur in sensitive individuals. Vitamin B-6 can be both preventive and curative in this form of drug-induced peripheral neuritis.

Since peripheral neuritis can also occur as a late complication following many viral infections, care must be taken to avoid assigning a cause-and-effect relationship to a drug which is not responsible for the nerve injury (see CAUSE-AND-EFFECT RELATIONSHIP).

See Section Six, Table 10 for further discussion of drug-induced nerve damage.

Peyronie's Disease A permanent deformity of the penis caused by the formation of dense fibrous (scarlike) tissue within the system of penile vessels that become engorged with blood during the process of erection. During sexual arousal, this inelastic fibrous tissue causes a painful downward bowing of the penis that hampers or precludes satisfactory intercourse. This condition has been associated with the use of phenytoin (Dilantin, etc.) and with most members of the beta blocker class of drugs (see Drug Class, Section Four). See Section Six, Table 11.

Pharmacoeconomics The discipline within Pharmacology that studies specifically the issues of costs versus benefits, utilizing a variety of measures: material and personnel costs, treatment outcomes, quality of patient life, etc. Study results are used in deciding where and how health care resources should be utilized.

Pharmacology The medical science that relates to the development and use of medicinal drugs, their composition and action in animals and man. Used in its broadest sense, pharmacology embraces the related sciences of medicinal chemistry, experimental therapeutics and toxicology.

Example: The widely used sulfonylurea drugs (Diabinese, Dymelor, Orinase, Tolinase) are effective in the treatment of some forms of diabetes because of the accidental discovery that some of their parent "sulfa" drugs produced hypoglycemia (low blood sugar) during their early therapeutic trials as antiinfectives. Subsequent investigation of the mechanisms of action (*pharmacology*) of these drugs revealed that they are capable of stimulating the pancreas to release more insulin.

Pharmacological studies on another group of "sulfa" related drugs—the thiazide diuretics—revealed that they could induce the kidney to excrete more water and salt in the urine. This drug action is of great value in treating high blood pressure and heart failure.

Photosensitivity A drug-induced change in the skin that results in the development of a rash or exaggerated sunburn on exposure to the sun or ultraviolet lamps. The reaction is confined to uncovered areas of skin, providing a clue to the nature of its cause. See Section Six, Table 2.

Porphyria The porphyrias are a group of hereditary disorders characterized by excessive production of prophyrins, essential respiratory pigments of the body. (One porphyrin is a component of hemoglobin, the pigment of red blood cells.) Two forms of porphyria—acute intermittent porphyria and cutaneous porphyria—can be activated by the use of certain drugs. Acute intermittent porphyria involves damage to the nervous system; an acute attack can include fever, rapid heart rate, vomiting, pain in the abdomen and legs, hallucinations, seizures, paralysis and coma. Some examples include barbiturates, "sulfa" drugs, chlordiazepoxide (Librium), chlorpropamide (Diabinese), methyldopa (Aldomet) and phenytoin (Dilantin). Cutaneous porphyria involves damage to the skin and liver. An episode can include reddening and blistering of the skin, followed by crust formation, scarring and excessive hair growth; repeated liver damage can lead to cirrhosis. This form of porphyria can be precipitated by chloroquine, estrogen, oral contraceptives and excessive iron.

Priapism The prolonged, painful erection of the penis usually unassociated with sexual arousal or stimulation. It is caused by obstruction to the outflow (drainage) of blood through the veins at the root of the penis. Erection may persist for 30 minutes to a few hours and then subside spontaneously; or it may persist for up to 30 hours and require surgical drainage of blood from the penis for relief. More than half of the episodes of priapism induced by drugs result in permanent impotence. Sickle cell anemia (or trait) may predispose to priapism; individuals with this disorder should avoid all drugs that may induce priapism.

Drugs reported to induce priapism include the following:

anabolic steroids (male hormonelike drugs: Anadrol, Anavar, Android, Halotestin, Metandren, Oreton, Testred, Winstrol)
chlorpromazine (Thorazine)

cocaine
guanethidine (Ismelin)
haloperidol (Haldol)
heparin
levodopa (Sinemet)
molindone (Moban)
prazosin (Minipress)
prochlorperazine (Compazine)
trazodone (Desyrel)
trifluoperazine (Stelazine)
warfarin (Coumadin)

Prostatism This term refers to the difficulties associated with an enlarged prostate. As the prostate enlarges (a natural development in aging men), it constricts the urethra (outflow passage) where it joins the urinary bladder and impedes urination. This causes a reduction in the size and force of the urinary stream, hesitancy in starting the flow of urine, interruption of urination and incomplete emptying of the bladder. Atropine and drugs with atropinelike effects can impair the bladder's ability to compensate for the obstructing prostate gland, thus intensifying all of the above symptoms.

Raynaud's Phenomenon This term refers to intermittent episodes of reduced blood flow into the fingers or toes, with resulting paleness, discomfort, numbness and tingling. It is due to an exaggerated constriction of the small arteries that supply blood to the digits. Characteristically an attack is precipitated either by emotional stress or exposure to cold. It can occur as part of a systemic disorder (lupus erythematosus, scleroderma), or it can occur without apparent cause (Raynaud's disease). Some widely used drugs, notably beta-adrenergic blockers and products that contain ergotamine, are conducive to the development of Raynaud-like symptoms in predisposed individuals.

Reye (Reye's) Syndrome An acute, often fatal, childhood illness characterized by swelling of the brain and toxic degeneration of the liver. It usually develops during recovery from a flulike infection, measles or chicken pox. Symptoms include fever, headache, delirium, loss of consciousness and seizures. It is one of the 10 major causes of death in children ages 1 to 10 years. Evidence to date suggests that the syndrome may be due to the combined effects of viral infection and chemical toxins (possibly drugs) in a genetically predisposed child. Drugs that have been used just prior to the onset of symptoms include acetaminophen, aspirin, antibiotics and antiemetics (drugs to control nausea and vomiting). Although it has not been definitely established that drugs actually cause Reye syndrome, it is thought that they may contribute to its development or adversely affect its course. Current recommendations are to avoid the use of acetaminophen, aspirin and antiemetic drugs in children with flulike infections, chickenpox or measles.

Secondary Effect A by-product or complication of drug use which does not occur as part of the drug's primary pharmacological activity. Secondary effects are unwanted consequences and may therefore be classified as adverse effects.

Example: The reactivation of dormant tuberculosis can be a *secondary effect* of long-term cortisone administration for arthritis. Cortisone and related drugs (see Drug Class, Section Four) suppress natural immunity and lower resistance to infection.

Example: The cramping of leg muscles can be a *secondary effect* of diuretic (urine-producing) drug treatment for high blood pressure. Excessive loss of potassium through increased urination renders the muscle vulnerable to painful spasm during exercise.

Side-Effect A normal, expected and predictable response to a drug that accompanies the principal (intended) response sought in treatment. Side-effects are part of a drug's pharmacological activity and thus are unavoidable. Most side-effects are undesirable. The majority cause minor annoyance and inconvenience; some may cause serious problems in managing certain diseases; a few can be hazardous.

Example: The drug propantheline (Pro-Banthine) is used to treat peptic ulcer because one of the consequences of its pharmacological action is the reduction of acid formation in the stomach (an intended effect). Other consequences can include blurring of near vision, dryness of the mouth and constipation. These are *side-effects*.

Superinfection (Suprainfection) The development of a second infection that is superimposed upon an initial infection currently under treatment. The superinfection is caused by organisms that are not susceptible to the killing action of the drug(s) used to treat the original (primary) infection. Superinfections usually occur during or immediately following treatment with a broad spectrum antibiotic—one that is capable of altering the customary balance of bacterial populations in various parts of the body. The disturbance of this balance permits the overgrowth of organisms that normally exist in numbers too small to cause disease. The superinfection may also require treatment, using those drugs that are effective against the offending organism.

Example: Recurrent infections of the kidney and bladder often require repeated courses of treatment with a variety of anti-infective drugs. When these are taken by mouth they can suppress the normally dominant types of bacteria present in the colon and rectum, encouraging the overgrowth of yeast organisms which are capable of causing *colitis*. When this occurs, colitis is a *superinfection*.

Tardive Dyskinesia A late-developing, drug-induced disorder of the nervous system characterized by involuntary bizarre movements of the eyelids, jaws, lips, tongue, neck and fingers. It occurs after long-term treatment with the more potent drugs used in the management of serious mental illness. While it may occur in any age group, it is more common in the middle-aged and the elderly. Older, chronically ill women are particularly susceptible to this adverse drug effect. Once developed, the pattern of uncontrollable chewing, lip puckering and repetitive tongue protruding (fly-catching movement) appears to be irreversible. No consistently satisfactory treatment or cure is available. To date, there is no way of identifying beforehand the individual who may develop this distressing reaction to drug treatment, and there is no known prevention. Fortunately, the persistent dyskinesia (abnormal movement) is not accompanied by further impairment of mental function or deterioration of intelligence.

Tolerance An adaptation by the body that lessens responsiveness to a drug on continuous administration. Body tissues become accustomed to the drug's presence and react to it less vigorously. Tolerance can be beneficial or harmful in treatment.

Examples: Beneficial tolerance occurs when the hay fever sufferer finds that the side-effect of drowsiness gradually disappears after 4 or 5 days of continuous use of antihistamines.

Harmful tolerance occurs when the patient with "shingles" (herpes zoster) finds that the usual dose of codeine is no longer sufficient to relieve pain and that the need for increased dosage creates a risk of physical dependence or addiction.

Toxicity The capacity of a drug to dangerously impair body functions or to damage body tissues. Most drug toxicity is related to total dosage: the larger the overdose, the greater the toxic effects. Some drugs, however, can produce toxic reactions when used in normal doses. Such adverse effects are not due to allergy or idiosyncrasy; in many instances their mechanisms are not fully understood. Toxic effects due to overdosage are generally a harmful extension of the drug's normal pharmacological actions and—to some extent—are predictable and preventable. Toxic reactions which occur with normal dosage are unrelated to the drug's known pharmacology and for the most part are unpredictable and unexplainable.

Tyramine A chemical present in many common foods and beverages that causes no difficulties to body functioning under normal circumstances. The main pharmacological action of tyramine is to raise the blood pressure. Normally, enzymes present in many body tissues neutralize this action of tyramine in the quantities in which it is consumed in the average diet. The principal enzyme responsible for neutralizing the blood-pressure-elevating action of tyramine (and chemicals related to it) is monoamine oxidase (MAO) type A. Monoamine oxidase type A serves an important regulatory function that helps to balance several of the chemical processes in the body that control certain activities of the nervous system. Stabilization of the blood pressure is one of these activities. If the action of monoamine oxidase type A is blocked, chemical substances like tyramine function unopposed, and relatively small amounts can cause alarming and dangerous elevations of blood pressure.

Several drugs in use today are capable of blocking the action of monoamine oxidase type A. These drugs are commonly referred to as monoamine oxidase (MAO) type A inhibitors (see Drug Class, Section Four). If an individual is taking one of these drugs and his diet includes foods or beverages that contain a significant amount of tyramine, he may experience a sudden increase in blood pressure. Before this interaction of food and drug was understood, several deaths due to brain hemorrhage occurred in persons taking MAO type A inhibitor drugs as a result of an extreme elevation of blood pressure following a meal of tyramine-rich foods.

It should be noted also that MAO inhibitor drugs can interact with many other drugs and cause serious adverse effects. Consult your physician before taking *any* drug concurrently with one that can inhibit the action of monoamine oxidase, type A or B.

Any protein-containing food that has undergone partial decomposition may present a hazard because of its increased tyramine content. The following foods and beverages have been reported to contain varying amounts of tyramine. Unless their tyramine content is known to be insignificant, they should be avoided altogether while taking a MAO type A inhibitor drug. Consult your physician about the advisability of using any of the foods or beverages on these lists if you are taking such drugs.

FOODS	BEVERAGES
Aged cheeses of all kinds*	Beer (unpasteurized)
Avocado	Chianti wine
Banana skins	Sherry wine
Bean curd	Vermouth
Bologna	
"Bovril" extract	
Broad bean pods	
Chicken liver (unless fresh and used at once)	

*Cottage cheese, cream cheese and processed cheese are safe to eat.

Chocolate
Figs, canned
Fish, canned
Fish, dried and salted
Herring, pickled
Liver, if not very fresh
"Marmite" extract
Meat extracts
Meat tenderizers
Pepperoni
Raisins
Raspberries
Salami
Shrimp paste
Sour cream
Soy sauce
Yeast extracts

NOTE: *Any* high-protein food that is aged or has undergone breakdown by putrefaction probably contains tyramine and could produce a hypertensive crisis in anyone taking MAO type A inhibiting drugs.

Viral load or viral burden A term used in reference to AIDS patients to describe the amount of HIV virus present in the body at any given time. The amount of virus relates to the effectiveness of the drug therapy which is being used, and can be a reason to change medication if the load increases.

WHO Pain Ladder A therapeutic scheme of utilizing increasing strengths of pain medications (analgesics) which include NSAIDs, opiates, and adjuvant drugs to control pain as specified by the World Health Organization. It is *not* an absolute treatment scheme, but should be used to organize the approach to effective analgesia.

SECTION SIX

TABLES OF DRUG INFORMATION

TABLE 1
Drugs That May Adversely Affect the Fetus and Newborn Infant

Following the confirmation in 1961 that the hypnotic drug thalidomide, taken during early pregnancy, could cause major birth defects, interest and concern regarding medicinal drugs as possible teratogens have greatly intensified. Numerous studies have increased our understanding of how drugs can adversely affect the developing fetus and newborn infant; they have also helped to identify those drugs that appear to have potential for causing significant harm to the unborn and newborn child. It is now recognized that some drugs can cause (or contribute to) malformations, retarded growth, functional disorders and death of the fetus or newborn infant. However, in many instances, it is not possible to clearly separate adverse effects due to the mother's disease or disorder from those that may be induced by the drugs used as therapy. Based upon our current knowledge, it is strongly recommended that only those drugs that confer clear and essential benefits should be used during pregnancy.

Drugs that *probably* cause adverse effects when taken during the *first trimester*

aminopterin	fluorouracil	opioid analgesics*
anticonvulsants*	iodides	progestins*
antithyroid drugs	isotretinoin	quinine
cytarabine	kanamycin	streptomycin
danazol	mercaptopurine	testosterone
diethylstilbestrol	methotrexate	warfarin
etretinate	misoprostol	

Drugs that *possibly* cause adverse effects when taken during the *first trimester*

angiotensin converting enzyme inhibitors*	lithium	piperazine
busulfan	mebendazole	rifampin
chlorambucil	monoamine oxidase inhibitors*	tetracyclines*
estrogens*	oral contraceptives	

Drugs that *probably* cause adverse effects when taken during the second and third trimesters

amiodarone	iodides	rifampin
androgens*	kanamycin	streptomycin
angiotensin converting enzyme inhibitors*	lithium	sulfonamides*
antithyroid drugs	nonsteroidal anti-inflammatory drugs*	sulfonylureas*
aspirin		tetracyclines*
benzodiazepines*	opioid analgesics*	thiazide diuretics*
chloramphenicol	phenothiazines*	tricyclic antidepressants*
estrogens*	progestins*	warfarin

Drugs that *possibly* cause adverse effects when taken during the second and third trimesters

acetazolamide	ethacrynic acid	hydroxyzine
clemastine	fluoroquinolones*	promethazine
diphenhydramine	haloperidol	

*See Drug Class, Section Four.

TABLE 2

Drugs That May Cause Photosensitivity on Exposure to Sun

Some drugs are capable of sensitizing the skin to the action of ultraviolet light. This can cause uncovered areas of the skin to react with a rash or exaggerated burn on exposure to sun or ultraviolet lamps. If you are taking any of the following drugs, ask your physician for guidance and use caution with regard to sun exposure.

acetazolamide	doxepin	nortriptyline
acetohexamide	doxycycline	ofloxacin
alprazolam	enoxacin	oral contraceptives
amantadine	estrogen	oxyphenbutazone
amiloride	etretinate	oxytetracycline
aminobenzoic acid	flucytosine	para amino benzoic acid
amiodarone	fluorescein	perphenazine
amitriptyline	fluorouracil	phenobarbital
amoxapine	fluphenazine	phenylbutazone
barbiturates	furosemide	phenylzine
bendroflumethiazide	flutamide	phenytoin
benzocaine	glipizide	piroxicam
benzoyl peroxide	glyburide	polythiazide
benzophenones	gold preparations	prochlorperazine
benzthiazide	griseofulvin	promazine
captopril	haloperidol	promethazine
carbamazepine	hexachlorophene	protriptyline
chlordiazepoxide	hydrochlorothiazide	pyrazinamide
chloroquine	hydroflumethiazide	quinidine
chlorothiazide	ibuprofen	quinine
chlorpromazine	imipramine	sulfonamides
chlorpropamide	indomethacin	sulindac
chlortetracycline	isotretinoin	tetracycline
chlorthalidone	ketoprofen	thiabendazole
ciprofloxacin	lincomycin	thioridazine
clindamycin	lomefloxacin	thiothixene
clofazimine	maprotiline	tolazamide
clofibrate	mesoridazine	tolbutamide
clomipramine	methacycline	tranylcypromine
cyproheptadine	methotrexate	trazodone
dacarbazine	methyclothiazide	tretinoin
dapsone	methyldopa	triamterene
demeclocycline	metolazone	trichlormethiazide
desipramine	minocycline	trifluoperazine
desoximetasone	minoxidil	trifluopromazine
diethylstilbestrol	nabumetone	trimeprazine
diflunisal	nalidixic acid	trimethoprim
diltiazem	naproxen	trimipramine
diphenhydramine	nifedipine	triprolidine
disopyramide	norfloxacin	vinblastine

TABLE 3

Drugs That May Adversely Affect Behavior

In addition to producing side-effects that can alter mood and disturb emotional stability, some drugs are capable of causing unexpected and unpredictable patterns

*See Drug Class, Section Four.

of abnormal thinking and behavior. Such responses are relatively infrequent, but the nature and degree of mental disturbance can, at times, be quite alarming and potentially dangerous for both patient and family. It is now well recognized that such paradoxical responses are often of an idiosyncratic nature, and that someone with a history of a serious mental or emotional disorder is more likely to experience bizarre reactions involving disturbed behavior.

It is often difficult to judge whether a particular aberration of thought or behavior is primarily a feature of the disorder under treatment or an effect of one (or more) drugs the patient may be taking at the time. If in doubt, it is advisable to discontinue any drug with potential for such side-effects and observe for changes during a drug-free period.

Drugs reported to impair *concentration* and/or *memory*

antihistamines*	isoniazid	primidone
antiparkinsonism drugs*	monoamine oxidase	scopolamine
barbiturates*	inhibitor drugs*	
benzodiazepines*	phenytoin	

Drugs reported to cause *confusion, delirium* or *disorientation*

acetazolamide	cortisonelike drugs*	levodopa
aminophylline	cycloserine	meprobamate
antidepressants*	digitalis	para-aminosalicylic acid
antihistamines*	digitoxin	phenelzine
atropinelike drugs*	digoxin	phenothiazines*
barbiturates*	disulfiram	phenytoin
benzodiazepines*	ethchlorvynol	piperazine
bromides	ethinamate	primidone
carbamazepine	fenfluramine	propranolol
chloroquine	glutethimide	reserpine
cimetidine	isoniazid	scopolamine

Drugs reported to cause *paranoid thinking*

bromides	diphenhydramine	isoniazid
cortisonelike drugs*	disulfiram	levodopa

Drugs reported to cause *schizophreniclike behavior*

amphetamines*	fenfluramine	phenylpropanolamine
ephedrine	phenmetrazine	

Drugs reported to cause *maniclike behavior*

antidepressants*	levodopa	inhibitor drugs*
cortisonelike drugs*	monoamine oxidase	

Less apparent—but no less important—are the mood-altering *side-effects* of some drugs which are prescribed primarily for altogether unrelated conditions, with no intention of modifying emotional status. In keeping with the wide variation of individual response to the primary and intended effects of drugs, it is to be expected that emotional and behavioral secondary effects will also be quite unpredictable and will

*See Drug Class, Section Four.

vary enormously from person to person. However, the following experiences have been seen with sufficient frequency to establish recognizable patterns.

Drugs reported to cause *nervousness* (anxiety and irritability)

amantadine
amphetaminelike drugs*
  (appetite suppressants)
antihistamines*
caffeine
chlorphenesin
cortisonelike drugs*
ephedrine
epinephrine
isoproterenol
levodopa
liothyronine (in excessive
  dosage)
methylphenidate
methysergide
monoamine oxidase
  inhibitor drugs*
nylidrin
oral contraceptives
theophylline
thyroid (in excessive
  dosage)
thyroxine (in excessive
  dosage)

Drugs reported to cause *emotional depression*

amantadine
amphetamine* (on
  withdrawal)
benzodiazepines*
carbamazepine
chloramphenicol
cortisonelike drugs*
cycloserine
digitalis
digitoxin
digoxin
diphenoxylate
estrogens
ethionamide
fenfluramine (on
  withdrawal)
fluphenazine
guanethidine
haloperidol
indomethacin
isoniazid
levodopa
methsuximide
methyldopa
methysergide
metoprolol
oral contraceptives
phenylbutazone
procainamide
progesterones
propranolol
reserpine
sulfonamides*
vitamin D (in excessive
  dosage)

Drugs reported to cause *euphoria*

amantadine
aminophylline
amphetamines
antihistamines* (some)
antispasmodics,
  synthetic*
aspirin
barbiturates*
benzphetamine
chloral hydrate
clorazepate
codeine
cortisonelike drugs*
diethylpropion
diphenoxylate
ethosuximide
flurazepam
haloperidol
levodopa
meprobamate
methysergide
monoamine oxidase
  inhibitor drugs*
morphine
pargyline
pentazocine
phenmetrazine
propoxyphene
scopalamine
tybamate

Drugs reported to cause *excitement*

acetazolamide
amantadine
amphetaminelike drugs*
antidepressants*
antihistamines*
atropinelike drugs*
barbiturates* (paradoxical
  response)
benzodiazepines*
  (paradoxical response)
cortisonelike drugs
cycloserine
diethylpropion
digitalis
ephedrine
epinephrine
ethinamate (paradoxical
  response)
ethionamide
glutethimide (paradoxical
  response)
isoniazid
isoproterenol
levodopa
meperidine and MAO
  inhibitor drugs*
methyldopa and MAO
  inhibitor drugs*
methyprylon (paradoxical
  response)
nalidixic acid
orphenadrine
quinine
scopalamine

*See Drug Class, Section Four.

TABLE 4
Drugs That May Adversely Affect Vision

Approximately 3.5% of all adverse drug effects involve impairment of vision or eye damage. Some effects, such as blurring of vision or double vision, may occur shortly after starting a drug. These quickly disappear with adjustment of dosage. More subtle and serious effects, such as cataract development or damage to the retina or optic nerve, may not occur until a drug has been in continuous use for an extended period of time. Some of these changes are irreversible. If you are taking a drug that can affect the eye in any way, promptly report any eye discomfort or change in vision so that appropriate evaluation can be made and corrective action taken as soon as possible.

Drugs reported to cause *blurring of vision*

acetazolamide	chlorthalidone	norfloxacin
antiarthritic/anti-inflam-	ciprofloxacin	oral contraceptives
matory drugs	cortisonelike drugs*	phenytoin
antidepressants*	diethylstilbestrol	sulfonamides*
antihistamines*	etretinate	tetracyclines*
atropinelike drugs*	fenfluramine	thiazide diuretics*

Drugs reported to cause *double vision*

antidepressants*	digitalis	nitrofurantoin
antidiabetic drugs*	digitoxin	norfloxacin
antihistamines*	digoxin	oral contraceptives
aspirin	ethionamide	orphenadrine
barbiturates*	ethosuximide	oxyphenbutazone
benzodiazepines*	etretinate	pentazocine
bromides	guanethidine	phenothiazines*
carbamazepine	hydroxychloroquine	phensuximide
carisoprodol	indomethacin	phenylbutazone
chloroquine	isoniazid	phenytoin
chlorprothixene	levodopa	primidone
ciprofloxacin	mephenesin	propranolol
clomiphene	methocarbamol	quinidine
colchicine	methsuximide	sedatives/sleep inducers*
colistin	morphine	thiothixene
cortisonelike drugs*	nalidixic acid	tranquilizers*

Drugs reported to cause *farsightedness*

ergot	sulfonamides* (possibly)
penicillamine	tolbutamide (possibly)

Drugs reported to cause *nearsightedness*

acetazolamide	ethosuximide	phensuximide
aspirin	methsuximide	spironolactone
carbachol	morphine	sulfonamides*
chlorthalidone	oral contraceptives	tetracyclines*
codeine	penicillamine	thiazide diuretics*
cortisonelike drugs*	phenothiazines*	

Drugs reported to *alter color vision*

acetaminophen	amyl nitrite	atropine
amodiaquine	aspirin	barbiturates*

*See Drug Class, Section Four.

Drugs reported to *alter color vision* (cont.)

belladonna	hydroxychloroquine	primidone
chloramphenicol	indomethacin	prochlorperazine
chloroquine	isocarboxazid	promazine
chlorpromazine	isoniazid	promethazine
chlortetracycline	mephenamic acid	quinacrine
ciprofloxacin	mesoridazine	quinidine
cortisonelike drugs*	methysergide	quinine
digitalis	nalidixic acid	reserpine
digitoxin	norfloxacin	sodium salicylate
digoxin	oral contraceptives	streptomycin
disulfiram	oxyphenbutazone	sulfonamides*
epinephrine	paramethadione	thioridazine
ergotamine	pargyline	tranylcypromine
erythromycin	penicillamine	trifluoperazine
ethchlorvynol	pentylenetetrazol	triflupromazine
ethionamide	perphenazine	trimeprazine
fluphenazine	phenacetin	trimethadione
furosemide	phenylbutazone	

Drugs reported to cause *sensitivity to light* (photophobia)

antidiabetic drugs*	ethionamide	norfloxacin
atropinelike drugs*	ethosuximide	oral contraceptives
bromides	etretinate	paramethadione
chloraquine	hydroxychloroquine	phenothiazines*
ciprofloxacin	mephenytoin	quinidine
clomiphene	methsuximide	quinine
digitoxin	monoamine oxidase	tetracyclines*
doxepin	inhibitor drugs*	trimethadione
ethambutol	nalidixic acid	

Drugs reported to cause *halos around lights*

amyl nitrite	digoxin	paramethadione
chloroquine	hydrochloroquine	phenothiazines*
cortisonelike drugs*	nitroglycerin	quinacrine
digitalis	norfloxacin	trimethadione
digitoxin	oral contraceptives	

Drugs reported to cause *visual hallucinations*

amantadine	digitalis	pentazocine
amphetaminelike drugs*	digoxin	phenothiazines*
amyl nitrite	disulfiram	phenylbutazone
antihistamines*	ephedrine	phenytoin
aspirin	furosemide	primidone
atropinelike drugs*	griseofulvin	propranolol
barbiturates*	haloperidol	quinine
benzodiazepines*	hydroxychloroquine	sedatives/sleep inducers*
bromides	indomethacin	sulfonamides*
carbamazepine	isosorbide	tetracyclines*
cephalexin	levodopa	tricyclic antidepressants*
cephaloglycin	nialamide	tripelennamine
chloroquine	oxyphenbutazone	
cycloserine	pargyline	

*See Drug Class, Section Four.

Drugs reported to impair the use of *contact lenses*

brompheniramine
carbinoxamine
chlorpheniramine
cyclizine
cyproheptadine
dexbrompheniramine
dexchlorpheniramine
dimethindene
diphenhydramine
diphenpyraline
furosemide
oral contraceptives
terfenadine
tripelennamine

Drugs reported to cause *cataracts* or *lens deposits*

allopurinol
busulfan
chlorpromazine
chlorprothixene
cortisonelike drugs*
fluphenazine
mesoridazine
methotrimeprazine
perphenazine
phenmetrazine
pilocarpine
prochlorperazine
promazine
promethazine
thioridazine
thiothixene
trifluoperazine
triflupromazine
trimeprazine

TABLE 5
Drugs That May Cause Blood Cell Dysfunction or Damage

All blood cells originate and mature in the bone marrow. They arise from "stem" cells that have the ability to differentiate into specific cell lines that produce fully developed, distinctive blood cell forms: erythrocytes (red blood cells), leukocytes (white blood cells), thrombocytes (blood platelets); the leukocytes include three varieties: granulocytes, monocytes (macrophages), and lymphocytes. Drugs that adversely affect the formation and development of blood cells can (1) act on any stage of cell production; (2) impair the production of one cell line; (3) influence the production of all cell lines.

Through a variety of mechanisms, some medicinal drugs can adversely affect mature cells circulating in the blood stream. Examples can be found in the tables that follow.

Drugs that cause inevitable (dose-dependent) *aplastic anemia* (see Glossary)

actinomycin D
azathioprine
busulphan
carboplatin
carmustine
chlorambucil
cisplatin
cyclophosphamide
cytarabine
doxorubicin
epirubicin
etoposide
fluorouracil
hydroxyurea
lomustine
melphalan
mercaptopurine
methotrexate
mitomycin
mitozantrone
plicamycin
procarbazine
thioguanine
thiotepa

Drugs that may cause idiosyncratic (dose-independent) *aplastic anemia*

amodiaquine
benoxaprofen
carbimazole
chloramphenicol
chlorpromazine
gold
indomethacin
mepacrine
oxyphenbutazone
penicillamine
phenylbutazone
phenytoin
piroxicam
prothiaden
pyrimethamine
sulfonamides*
sulindac
thiouracils
trimethoprim/sulfamethoxazole

*See Drug Class, Section Four.

Drugs that may *impair red blood cell production* (only)

azathioprine	isoniazid	sulfasalazine
carbamazepine	methyldopa	sulfathiazide
chloramphenicol	penicillin	sulfonamides*
chlorpropamide	pentachlorophenol	sulfonylureas*
dapsone	phenobarbital	thiamphenicol
fenoprofen	phenylbutazone	tolbutamide
gold	phenytoin	trimethoprim/sulfamethoxazole
halothane	pyrimethamine	

Drugs that may significantly *reduce granulocyte cell counts* (various mechanisms)

acetaminophen	disopyramide	phenylbutazone
acetazolamide	ethacrynic acid	phenytoin
allopurinol	fansidar	procainamide
amitriptyline	gentamicin	propranolol
amodiaquine	gold	propylthiouracil
benzodiazepines*	hydralazine	pyrimethamine
captopril	hydrochlorothiazide	quinidine
carbamazepine	imipramine	quinine
carbimazole	indomethacin	ranitidine
cephalosporins*	isoniazid	rifampin
chloramphenicol	levamisole	sodium aminosalicylate
chloroquine	meprobamate	streptomycin
chlorothiazide	methimazole	sulfadoxime
chlorpromazine	methyldopa	sulfonamides*
chlorpropamide	oxyphenbutazone	tetracyclines*
chlorthalidone	penicillamine	tocainide
cimetidine	penicillins*	tolbutamide
clindamycin	pentazocine	trimethoprim/sulfamethoxazole
dapsone	phenacetin	
desipramine	phenothiazines*	vancomycin

Drugs that may significantly *reduce blood platelet counts*

acetazolamide	diazepam	oxyphenbutazone
actinomycin	diazoxide	penicillamine
allopurinol	diclofenac	penicillin
alpha-interferon	digoxin	phenylbutazone
amiodarone	diltiazem	phenytoin
ampicillin	furosemide	piroxicam
aspirin	gentamicin	procainamide
carbamazepine	gold	quinidine
carbenicillin	hydrochlorothiazide	quinine
cephalosporins*	imipramine	ranitidine
chenodeoxycholic acid	isoniazid	rifampin
chloroquine	isotretinoin	sodium aminosalicylate
chlorothiazide	levamisole	sulfasalazine
chlorpheniramine	meprobamate	sulfonamides*
chlorpropamide	methyldopa	thioguanine
chlorthalidone	mianserin	trimethoprim/sulfamethoxazole
cimetidine	minoxidil	
cyclophosphamide	morphine	valproate
danazol	nitrofurantoin	vancomycin
desferrioxamine	oxprenolol	

*See Drug Class, Section Four.

Drugs that cause significant *hemolytic anemia* due to glucose-6-phosphate dehydrogenase (G6PD) deficiency of red blood cells

acetanilid	pamaquine	sulfanilamide
methylene blue	phenazopyridine	sulfapyridine
nalidixic acid	phenylhydrazine	thiazosulfone
naphthalene	primaquine	toluidine blue
niridazole	sulfacetamide	
nitrofurantoin	sulfamethoxazole	

Drugs that may cause *hemolytic anemia* by other mechanisms

antimony	methotrexate	quinidine
chlorpropamide	para-aminosalicylic acid	quinine
cisplatin	penicillamine	rifampin
mephenesin	phenazopyridine	sulfasalazine

Drugs that may cause *megaloblastic anemia*

acyclovir	metformin	primidone
alcohol	methotrexate	pyrimethamine
aminopterin	neomycin	sulfasalazine
azathioprine	nitrofurantoin	tetracycline
colchicine	nitrous oxide	thioguanine
cycloserine	oral contraceptives	triamterene
cytarabine	para-aminosalicylic acid	trimethoprim
floxuridine	pentamidine	vinblastine
fluorouracil	phenformin	vitamin A
hydroxyurea	phenobarbital	vitamin C (large doses)
mercaptopurine	phenytoin	zidovudine

Drugs that may cause *sideroblastic anemia*

alcohol	isoniazid	pyrazinamide
chloramphenicol	penicillamine	
cycloserine	phenacetin	

TABLE 6
Drugs That May Cause Heart Dysfunction or Damage

Drugs of very diverse classes can adversely affect both the function and structure of the heart. Disorders of the heart (that require drug therapy) often determine the nature of adverse effects induced by drugs. Some adverse effects are due to direct pharmacological actions of a drug on heart tissues (as with antiarrhythmic drugs); while other reactions are caused indirectly by altering biochemical balances that influence heart function (as with excessive loss of potassium due to diuretics resulting in abnormal heart rhythms and digitalis toxicity).

Drugs that may cause or contribute to *abnormal heart rhythms* (arrythmias)

aminophylline	beta-adrenergic blocking drugs*	chlorpromazine
amiodarone		cimetidine
amitriptyline	beta-adrenergic bronchodilators*	digitoxin
antiarrythmic drugs*		digoxin
bepridil	carbamazepine	diltiazem

*See Drug Class, Section Four.

Drugs that may cause or contribute to *abnormal heart rhythms* (arrythmias) (cont.)

disopyramide	maprotiline	sotalol
diuretics*	methyldopa	terbutaline
doxepin	mexiletine	theophylline
encainide	milrinone	thiazide diuretics*
fentolterol	phenothiazines*	thioridazine
flecainide	prenylamine	trazodone
isoproterenol	procainamide	tricyclic antidepressants*
ketanserin	quinidine	verapamil
lidocaine	ranitidine	

Drugs that may *depress heart function* (reduce pumping efficiency)

beta-adrenergic blocking drugs*	disopyramide	isoproterenol
cocaine	doxorubicin	nifedipine
daunorubicin	epinephrine	verapamil
diltiazem	flecainide	
	fluorouracil	

Drugs that may *reduce coronary artery blood flow* (reduce oxygen supply to heart muscle)

amphetamines*	ergotamine	vasopressin
beta-adrenergic blocking drugs* (abrupt withdrawal)	fluorouracil	vinblastine
	nifedipine	vincristine
	oral contraceptives	
cocaine	ritodrine	

Drugs that may *impair healing of heart muscle* following heart attack (myocardial infarction)

adrenocortical steroids*   nonsteroidal anti-inflammatory drugs (NSAIDs)*

Drugs that may cause *heart valve damage*

ergotamine   minocycline (blue-black pigmentation)
methysergide

Drugs that may cause *pericardial disease*

actinomycin D	cytarabine	phenylbutazone
anthracyclines	fluorouracil	practolol
bleomycin	hydralazine	procainamide
cisplatin	methysergide	sulfasalazine
cyclophosphamide	minoxidil	

TABLE 7
Drugs That May Cause Lung Dysfunction or Damage

Adverse drug reactions that directly affect the lung are often difficult to distinguish from natural diseases or disorders that involve lung function or structure. As with other organ systems, the lung is subject to both principal types of drug reactions: Type

*See Drug Class, Section Four.

A—those due to known and expected pharmacological drug actions; Type B—those due to unexpected and unpredictable allergic or idiosyncratic reactions on the part of the drug user.

Drugs that may adversely affect *blood vessels of the lung*

Drugs that may cause thrombo-embolism

estrogens*
oral contraceptives (high estrogen type)

Drugs that may cause pulmonary hypertension

amphetamines*
fenfluramine
oral contraceptives
tryptophan

Drugs that may cause vasculitis (blood vessel damage) with or without hemorrhage

aminoglutethimide
amphotericin
cocaine
febarbamate
nitrofurantoin
penicillamine
phenytoin

Drugs that may cause adult respiratory distress syndrome (ARDS)

bleomycin
codeine
cyclophosphamide
dextropropoxyphene
heroin
hydrochlorothiazide
methadone
mitomycin
naloxone
ritodrine
terbutaline
vinblastine

Drugs that may adversely affect the *bronchial tubes*

Drugs that may cause bronchoconstriction (asthma)

acetaminophen
aspirin
beta-adrenergic blocking drugs*
carbachol
cephalosporins*
chloramphenicol
deanol
demeclocycline
erythromycin
griseofulvin
maprotiline
methacholine
methoxypsoralen
metoclopramide
morphine
neomycin
neostigmine
nitrofurantoin
nonsteroidal anti-inflammatory drugs*
penicillins*
pilocarpine
propafenone
pyridostigmine
streptomycin
tartrazine (coloring agent)

Drugs that may cause bronchiolitis (with permanent obstruction of small bronchioles)

penicillamine
sulfasalazine

Drugs that may *damage lung tissues*

Drugs that may cause acute allergic-type pneumonitis

ampicillin
bleomycin
cephalexin
chlorpropamide
gold
imipramine

*See Drug Class, Section Four.

Drugs that may cause acute allergic-type pneumonitis (cont.)

mephenesin	nitrofurantoin	penicillin
mercaptopurine	nomifensine	phenylbutazone
metformin	nonsteroidal	phenytoin
methotrexate	anti-inflammatory	procarbazine
metronidazole	drugs*	sulfonamides*
mitomycin	para-aminosalicylic acid	tetracycline
nalidixic acid	penicillamine	vinblastine

Drugs that may cause chronic pneumonitis and fibrosis (scarring)

amiodarone	ergotamine	pentolinium
bleomycin	gold	practolol
bromocriptine	hexamethonium	sulfasalazine
busulfan	mecamylamine	tocainide
carmustine	melphalan	tolfenamic acid
chlorambucil	methysergide	
cyclophosphamide	nitrofurantoin	

Drugs that may damage the pleura

bromocriptine	methysergide	practolol

TABLE 8
Drugs That May Cause Liver Dysfunction or Damage

The liver is the principal organ that converts drugs into forms that can be readily eliminated from the body. Given the diversity of drugs in use today and the complex burdens they impose upon the liver, it is not surprising that a broad spectrum of adverse drug effects on liver functions and structures has been documented. The reactions range from mild and transient changes in the results of liver function tests to complete liver failure and death. Many drugs may affect the liver adversely in more than one way, as cited below in several listings. The use of the following drugs requires careful monitoring of their effects on the liver during the entire course of treatment.

Drugs that may cause *acute dose-dependent liver damage* (resembling acute viral hepatitis)

acetaminophen (overdose)
salicylates (doses over 2 grams daily)

Drugs that may cause *acute dose-independent liver damage* (resembling acute viral hepatitis)

acebutolol	enflurane	maprotiline
allopurinol	ethambutol	metoprolol
atenolol	ethionamide	mianserin
carbamazepine	halothane	naproxen
cimetidine	ibuprofen	nifedipine
dantrolene	indomethacin	para-aminosalicylic acid
diclofenac	isoniazid	penicillins*
diltiazem	ketoconazole	phenelzine
disulfiram	labetalol	phenindione

*See Drug Class, Section Four.

Drugs that may cause *acute dose-independent liver damage* (resembling acute viral hepatitis) (cont.)

phenobarbital	pyrazinamide	sulfonamides*
phenylbutazone	quinidine	sulindac
phenytoin	quinine	tricyclic antidepressants*
piroxicam	ranitidine	valproic acid
probenecid	rifampin	verapamil

Drugs that may cause *acute fatty infiltration of the liver*

adrenocortical steroids*	phenothiazines*	tetracyclines*
antithyroid drugs	phenytoin	valproic acid
isoniazid	salicylates*	
methotrexate	sulfonamides*	

Drugs that may cause *cholestatic jaundice*

actinomycin D	erythromycin	norethandrolone
amoxicillin/clavulanate	flecainide	oral contraceptives
azathioprine	flurazepam	oxacillin
captopril	flutamide	penicillamine
carbamazepine	glyburide	phenothiazines*
carbimazole	gold	phenytoin
cephalosporins*	griseofulvin	propoxyphene
chlordiazepoxide	haloperidol	propylthiouracil
chlorpropamide	ketoconazole	sulfonamides*
cloxacillin	mercaptopurine	tamoxifen
cyclophosphamide	methyltestosterone	thiabendazole
cyclosporine	nifedipine	tolbutamide
danazol	nitrofurantoin	tricyclic antidepressants*
diazepam	nonsteroidal	troleandomycin
disopyramide	anti-inflammatory	verapamil
enalapril	drugs*	

Drugs that may cause *liver granulomas* (chronic inflammatory nodules)

allopurinol	gold	phenytoin
aspirin	hydralazine	procainamide
carbamazepine	isoniazid	quinidine
chlorpromazine	methyldopa	ranitidine
chlorpropamide	nitrofurantoin	sulfonamides*
diltiazem	penicillin	tolbutamide
disopyramide	phenylbutazone	

Drugs that may cause *chronic liver disease*

Drugs that may cause active chronic hepatitis

acetaminophen (chronic use, large doses)	dantrolene	methyldopa
	isoniazid	nitrofurantoin

Drugs that may cause liver cirrhosis or fibrosis (scarring)

methotrexate	nicotinic acid

*See Drug Class, Section Four.

Drugs that may cause chronic cholestasis (resembling primary biliary cirrhosis)

chlorpromazine/valproic acid (combination)	imipramine	tolbutamide
chlorpropamide/erythromycin (combination)	phenothiazines*	
	phenytoin	
	thiabendazole	

Drugs that may cause *liver tumors* (benign and malignant)

anabolic steroids	oral contraceptives	thorotrast
danazol	testosterone	

Drugs that may cause *damage to liver blood vessels*

adriamycin	dacarbazine	vincristine
anabolic steroids	mercaptopurine	vitamin A (excessive doses)
azathioprine	methotrexate	
carmustine	mitomycin	
cyclophosphamide/cyclosporine (combination)	oral contraceptives	
	thioguanine	

TABLE 9
Drugs That May Cause Kidney Dysfunction or Damage

With regard to medicinal drugs, the kidneys perform two major functions: (1) the alteration (biotransformation) of the drug to facilitate its processing; (2) the elimination of the drug from the body via the excretion of urine. As with drug effects on the liver, many drugs may adversely affect the kidneys in several ways. This is illustrated in the following tables by the appearance of some drug names in more than one listing. The kidneys are quite sensitive to the toxic effects of medicinal drugs. Vigilance and careful monitoring are always advisable during the course of treatment with any of the drugs cited below.

Drugs that may primarily *impair kidney function* (without damage)

amphotericin	demeclocycline	nifedipine
angiotensin converting enzyme inhibitors* (with renal artery stenosis; with congestive heart failure)	diuretics/NSAIDs* (avoid this combination)	nitroprusside
	glyburide	nonsteroidal anti-inflammatory drugs*
	isofosfamide	
	lithium/tricyclic antidepressants* (avoid this combination)	rifampin
beta-adrenergic blocking drugs*		vinblastine
colchicine	methoxyflurane	

Drugs that may cause *acute kidney failure* (due to kidney damage)

Drugs that may damage the kidney filtration unit (the nephron)

acetaminophen (excessive dosage)	bismuth thiosulfate	hydralazine
	carbamazepine	metronidazole
allopurinol	cisplatin	mitomycin
aminoglycoside antibiotics*	cyclosporine	oral contraceptives
	enalapril	penicillamine
amphotericin	ergometrine	phenytoin

*See Drug Class, Section Four.

Drugs that may damage the kidney filtration unit (the nephron) (cont.)

quinidine	streptokinase	thiazide diuretics*
rifampin	sulfonamides*	

Drugs that may cause acute interstitial nephritis

allopurinol	diclofenac	phenindione
amoxicillin	diflunisal	phenobarbital
ampicillin	fenoprofen	phenylbutazone
aspirin	foscarnet	phenytoin
azathioprine	furosemide	piroxicam
aztreonam	gentamicin	pirprofen
captopril	glafenine	pyrazinamide
carbamazepine	ibuprofen	rifampin
carbenicillin	indomethacin	sodium valproate
cefaclor	ketoprofen	sulfamethoxazole
cefoxitin	mefenamate	sulfinpyrazone
cephalexin	methicillin	sulfonamides*
cephalothin	methyldopa	sulindac
cephapirin	mezlocillin	thiazide diuretics*
cephradine	minocycline	tolmetin
cimetidine	nafcillin	trimethoprim
ciprofloxacin	naproxen	vancomycin
clofibrate	oxacillin	warfarin
cloxacillin	penicillamine	
diazepam	penicillin	

Drugs that may cause muscle destruction and associated acute kidney failure

adrenocortical steroids*	cocaine	opioid analgesics*
alcohol	cytarabine	pentamidine
amphetamines*	fenofibrate	phenothiazines*
amphotericin	haloperidol	streptokinase
carbenoxolone	halothane	suxamethonium
chlorthalidone	heroin	
clofibrate	lovastatin	

Drugs that may cause *kidney damage resembling glomerulonephritis or nephrosis*

captopril	lithium	practolol
fenoprofen	mesalamine	probenecid
gold	penicillamine	quinidine
ketoprofen	phenytoin	

Drugs that may cause *chronic interstitial nephritis and papillary necrosis* (analgesic kidney damage)

acetaminophen	phenacetin
aspirin	(all with long-term use)

Drugs that may cause or contribute to *urinary tract crystal or stone formation*

acetazolamide	cytotoxic drugs	magnesium trisilicate
acyclovir	dihydroxyadenine	mercaptopurine

*See Drug Class, Section Four.

Drugs that may cause or contribute to *urinary tract crystal or stone formation* (cont.)

methotrexate
methoxyflurane
phenylbutazone
probenecid
salicylates*
sulfonamides*
thiazide diuretics*
triamterene
uricosuric drugs
vitamin A
vitamin C
vitamin D
warfarin
zoxazolamine

TABLE 10
Drugs That May Cause Nerve Dysfunction or Damage

Medicinal drugs may adversely affect any segment of the nervous system from the brain to peripheral nerves. There is wide variability in the patterns of response to drugs among people—in both therapeutic effects and unwanted adverse effects. Individual variability is determined largely by genetic programming of drug metabolism and responsiveness. The following scheme of classification groups drugs according to the familiar clinical syndromes that represent drug-induced neurological disorders.

Drugs that may cause *significant headache*

amyl nitrate
bromocriptine
clonidine
ergotamine (prolonged use)
etretinate
hydralazine
ibuprofen
indomethacin
labetalol
naproxen
nifedipine
nitrofurantoin
nitroglycerin
perhexilene
propranolol
sulindac
terbutaline
tetracyclines*
theophylline
tolmetin
trimethoprim/sulfamethoxazole

Drugs that may cause *seizures* (convulsions)

ampicillin
atenolol
carbenicillin
cephalosporins*
chloroquine
cimetidine
ciprofloxacin
cycloserine
disopyramide
ether
halothane
indomethacin
isoniazid
lidocaine
lithium
mefenamic acid
nalidixic acid
oxacillin
penicillins* (synthetic)
phenothiazines*
pyrimethamine
terbutaline
theophylline
ticarcillin
tricyclic antidepressants*
vincristine

Drugs that may cause *stroke*

anabolic steroids
cocaine
oral contraceptives
phenylpropanolamine

Drugs that may cause features of *parkinsonism*

amitriptyline
amodiaquine
chloroquine
chlorprothixene
desipramine
diazoxide
diphenhydramine
droperidol
haloperidol
imipramine
levodopa
lithium
methyldopa
metoclopramide
phenothiazines*
reserpine
thiothixene
trifluoperidol

*See Drug Class, Section Four.

Drugs that may cause *acute dystonias* (acute involuntary movement syndromes—AIMS)

carbamazepine
chlorzoxazone
haloperidol
metoclopramide
phenothiazines*
phenytoin
propranolol
tricyclic antidepressants*

Drugs that may cause *tardive dyskinesia* (see Glossary)

haloperidol
phenothiazines*
thiothixene

**Drugs that may cause *neuroleptic malignant syndrome (NMS)*
See this term in the Glossary for a list of causative drugs.**

Drugs that may cause *peripheral neuropathy* (see Glossary)

amiodarone
amitriptyline
amphetamines*
amphotericin
anticoagulants*
carbutamide
chlorambucil
chloramphenicol
chloroquine
chlorpropamide
cimetidine
clioquinol
clofibrate
colchicine
colistin
cytarabine
dapsone
disopyramide
disulfiram
ergotamine
ethambutol
glutethimide
gold
hydralazine
imipramine
indomethacin
isoniazid
methaqualone
methimazole
methysergide
metronidazole
nalidixic acid
nitrofurantoin
nitrofurazone
penicillamine
penicillin
perhexiline
phenelzine
phenylbutazone
phenytoin
podophyllin
procarbazine
propranolol
propylthiouracil
stavudine
streptomycin
sulfonamides*
sulfoxone
thalidomide
tolbutamide
vinblastine
vincristine

Drugs that may cause a *myasthenia gravis* syndrome

aminoglycoside
  antibiotics*
beta-adrenergic blocking
  drugs*
penicillamine
phenytoin
polymixin B
trihexyphenidyl

TABLE 11
Drugs That May Adversely Affect Sexuality

It is well established that certain drugs have the potential for affecting sexual functions in a variety of unintended ways. Many commonly prescribed drugs can cause both obvious and subtle effects on one or more aspects of sexual expression. Patients are usually unaware that changes in sexual performance or response may be related to medications they are taking. If they suspect it, they are often reluctant to discuss the possible association with their physician. In some situations, the sexual dysfunction may be a natural consequence of the disorder under treatment or of a concurrent and undetected disorder, possibilities often overlooked by both practitioner and patient. It is well known that disorders such as diabetes, kidney failure, hypertension, depression and alcoholism may reduce libido and cause failure of erection. In addi-

*See Drug Class, Section Four.

tion, many of the drugs used to treat these conditions may have the ability to augment a subclinical sexual dysfunction through unavoidable pharmacological activity. Such situations require the closest cooperation between therapist and patient in order to correctly assess the possible cause-and-effect relationships and to change therapy appropriately.

Possible Drug Effects on Male Sexuality

1. Increased libido
    androgens (replacement therapy in deficiency states)
    baclofen (Lioresal)
    chlordiazepoxide (Librium) (antianxiety effect)
    diazepam (Valium) (antianxiety effect)
    haloperidol (Haldol)
    levodopa (Larodopa, Sinemet) (may be an indirect effect due to improved sense of well-being)

2. Decreased libido
    antihistamines
    barbiturates
    chlordiazepoxide (Librium) (sedative effect)
    chlorpromazine (Thorazine) 10% to 20% of users
    cimetidine (Tagamet)
    clofibrate (Atromid-S)
    clonidine (Catapres), 10% to 20% of users
    danazol (Danocrine)
    diazepam (Valium) (sedative effect)
    disulfiram (Antabuse)
    estrogens (therapy for prostatic cancer)
    fenfluramine (Pondimin)
    heroin
    licorice
    medroxyprogesterone (Provera)
    methyldopa (Aldomet), 10% to 15% of users
    metoclopramide (Reglan), 80% of users
    perhexilene (Pexid)
    prazosin (Minipress), 15% of users
    propranolol (Inderal) rarely
    reserpine (Serpasil, Ser-Ap-Es)
    spironolactone (Aldactone)
    tricyclic antidepressants (TAD's)

3. Impaired erection (impotence)
    anticholinergics
    antihistamines
    baclofen (Lioresal)
    barbiturates (when abused)
    beta blockers (see Drug Class, Section Four)
    chlordiazepoxide (Librium) (in high dosage)
    chlorpromazine (Thorazine)
    cimetidine (Tagamet)
    clofibrate (Atromid-S)
    clonidine (Catapres), 10% to 20% of users
    cocaine
    diazepam (Valium) (in high dosage)
    digitalis and its glycosides
    disopyramide (Norpace)
    disulfiram (Antabuse) (uncertain)
    estrogens (therapy for prostatic cancer)

ethacrynic acid (Edecrin), 5% of users
ethionamide (Trecator-SC)
fenfluramine (Pondimin)
furosemide (Lasix), 5% of users
guanethidine (Ismelin)
haloperidol (Haldol), 10% to 20% of users
heroin
hydroxyprogesterone (therapy for prostatic cancer)
licorice
lithium (Lithonate)
marijuana
mesoridazine (Serentil)
methantheline (Banthine)
methyldopa (Aldomet), 10% to 15% of users
metoclopramide (Reglan), 60% of users
monoamine oxidase (MAO) type A inhibitors, 10% to 15% of users
perhexilene (Pexid)
prazosin (Minipres) infrequently
reserpine (Serpasil, Ser-Ap-Es)
spironolactone (Aldactone)
thiazide diuretics, 5% of users
thioridazine (Mellaril)
tricyclic antidepressants (TAD's)

4. Impaired ejaculation
    anticholinergics
    barbiturates (when abused)
    chlorpromazine (Thorazine)
    clonidine (Catapres)
    estrogens (therapy for prostatic cancer)
    guanethidine (Ismelin)
    heroin
    mesoridazine (Serentil)
    methyldopa (Aldomet)
    monoamine oxidase (MAO) type A inhibitors
    phenoxybenzamine (Dibenzyline)
    phentolamine (Regitine)
    reserpine (Serpasil, Ser-Ap-Es)
    thiazide diuretics
    thioridazine (Mellaril)
    tricyclic antidepressants (TAD's)

5. Decreased testosterone
    adrenocorticotropic hormone (ACTH)
    barbiturates
    digoxin (Lanoxin)
    haloperidol (Haldol)
    —increased testosterone with low dosage
    —decreased testosterone with high dosage
    lithium (Lithonate)
    marijuana
    medroxyprogesterone (Provera)
    monoamine oxidase (MAO) type A inhibitors
    spironolactone (Aldactone)

6. Impaired spermatogenesis (reduced fertility)
    adrenocorticosteroids (prednisone, etc.)
    androgens (moderate to high dosage, extended use)
    antimalarials

aspirin (abusive, chronic use)
chlorambucil (Leukeran)
cimetidine (Tagamet)
colchicine
co-trimoxazole (Bactrim, Septra)
cyclophosphamide (Cytoxan)
estrogens (therapy for prostatic cancer)
marijuana
medroxyprogesterone (Provera)
methotrexate
metoclopramide (Reglan)
monoamine oxidase (MAO) type A inhibitors
niridazole (Ambilhar)
nitrofurantoin (Furadantin)
spironolactone (Aldactone)
sulfasalazine (Azulfidine)
testosterone (moderate to high dosage, extended use)
vitamin C (in doses of 1 gram or more)

7. Testicular disorders
    Swelling
    —tricyclic antidepressants (TAD's)
    Inflammation
    —oxyphenbutazone (Tandearil)
    Atrophy
    —androgens (moderate to high dosage, extended use)
    —chlorpromazine (Thorazine)
    —cyclophosphamide (Cytoxan) (in prepubescent boys)
    —spironolactone (Aldactone)

8. Penile disorders
    Priapism (see Glossary)
    —anabolic steroids (male hormonelike drugs)
    —chlorpromazine (Thorazine)
    —cocaine
    —guanethidine (Ismelin)
    —haloperidol (Haldol)
    —heparin
    —levodopa (Sinemet)
    —molindone (Moban)
    —prazosin (Minipress)
    —prochlorperazine (Compazine)
    —trazodone (Desyrel)
    —trifluoperazine (Stelazine)
    —warfarin (Coumadin)
    Peyronie's disease (see Glossary)
    —beta blocker drugs (see Drug Class, Section Four)
    —phenytoin (Dilantin, etc.)

9. Gynecomastia (excessive development of the male breast)
    androgens (partial conversion to estrogen)
    BCNU
    busulfan (Myleran)
    chlormadinone
    chlorpromazine (Thorazine)
    chlortetracycline (Aureomycin)
    cimetidine (Tagamet)
    clonidine (Catapres) (infrequently)
    diethylstilbestrol (DES)

digitalis and its glycosides
estrogens (therapy for prostatic cancer)
ethionamide (Trecator-SC)
griseofulvin (Fulvicin, etc.)
haloperidol (Haldol)
heroin
human chorionic gonadotropin
isoniazid (INH, Nydrazid)
marijuana
mestranol
methyldopa (Aldomet)
metoclopramide (Reglan)
phenelzine (Nardil)
reserpine (Serpasil, Ser-Ap-Es)
spironolactone (Aldactone)
thioridazine (Mellaril)
tricyclic antidepressants (TAD's)
vincristine (Oncovin)

10. Feminization (loss of libido, impotence, gynecomastia, testicular atrophy)
conjugated estrogens (Premarin, etc.)

11. Precocious puberty
anabolic steroids
androgens
isoniazid (INH)

Possible Drug Effects on Female Sexuality

1. Increased libido
androgens
chlordiazepoxide (Librium) (antianxiety effect)
diazepam (Valium) (antianxiety effect)
mazindol (Sanorex)
oral contraceptives (freedom from fear of pregnancy)

2. Decreased libido
See list of drug effects on male sexuality. Some of these *may* have potential for reducing libido in the female. The literature is sparse on this subject.

3. Impaired arousal and orgasm
anticholinergics
clonidine (Catapres)
methyldopa (Aldomet)
monoamine oxidase inhibitors (MAOI's)
tricyclic antidepressants (TAD's)

4. Breast enlargement
penicillamine
tricyclic antidepressants (TAD's)

5. Galactorrhea (spontaneous flow of milk)
amphetamine
chlorpromazine (Thorazine)
cimetidine (Tagamet)
haloperidol (Haldol)
heroin
methyldopa (Aldomet)
metoclopramide (Reglan)
oral contraceptives

phenothiazines
reserpine (Serpasil, Ser-Ap-Es)
sulpiride (Equilid)
tricyclic antidepressants (TAD's)

6. Ovarian failure (reduced fertility)
    anesthetic gases (operating room staff)
    cyclophosphamide (Cytoxan)
    cytostatic drugs
    danazol (Danacrine)
    medroxyprogesterone (Provera)

7. Altered menstruation (menstrual disorders)
    adrenocorticosteroids (prednisone, etc.)
    androgens
    barbiturates (when abused)
    chlorambucil (Leukeran)
    chlorpromazine (Thorazine)
    cyclophosphamide (Cytoxan)
    danazol (Danocrine)
    estrogens
    ethionamide (Trecator-SC)
    haloperidol (Haldol)
    heroin
    isoniazid (INH, Nydrazid)
    marijuana
    medroxprogesterone (Provera)
    metoclopramide (Reglan)
    oral contraceptives
    phenothiazines
    progestins
    radioisotopes
    rifampin (Rifadin, Rifamate, Rimactane)
    spironolactone (Aldactone)
    testosterone
    thioridazine (Mellaril)
    vitamin A (in excessive dosage)

8. Virilization (acne, hirsutism, lowering of voice, enlargement of clitoris)
    anabolic drugs
    androgens
    haloperidol (Haldol)
    oral contraceptives (lowering of voice)

9. Precocious puberty
    estrogens (in hair lotions)
    isoniazid (INH, Nydrazid)

TABLE 12
Drugs That May Interact With Alcohol

Beverages containing alcohol may interact unfavorably with a wide variety of drugs. The most important (and most familiar) interaction occurs when the depressant action on the brain of sedatives, sleep-inducing drugs, tranquilizers and narcotic drugs is intensified by alcohol. Alcohol may also reduce the effectiveness of some drugs, and it can interact with certain other drugs to produce toxic effects. Some drugs may increase the intoxicating effects of alcohol, producing further impairment of mental alertness, judgment, physical coordination and reaction time.

While drug interactions with alcohol are generally predictable, the intensity and significance of these interactions can vary greatly from one person to another and from one occasion to another. This is because many factors influence what happens when drugs and alcohol interact. These factors include individual variations in sensitivity to drugs (including alcohol), the chemistry and quantity of the drug, the type and amount of alcohol consumed and the sequence in which drug and alcohol are taken. If you need to use any of the drugs listed in the following tables, you should ask your physician for help concerning the use of alcohol.

Drugs with which it is advisable to avoid alcohol completely

Drug name or class	Possible interaction with alcohol
amphetamines	excessive rise in blood pressure with alcoholic beverages containing tyramine**
antidepressants*	excessive sedation, increased intoxication
barbiturates*	excessive sedation
bromides	confusion, delirium, increased intoxication
calcium carbamide	disulfiramlike reaction**
carbamazepine	excessive sedation
chlorprothixene	excessive sedation
chlorzoxazone	excessive sedation
disulfiram	disulfiram reaction**
ergotamine	reduced effectiveness of ergotamine
fenfluramine	excessive stimulation of nervous system with some beers and wines
furazolidone	disulfiramlike reaction**
haloperidol	excessive sedation
MAO inhibitor drugs*	excessive rise in blood pressure with alcoholic beverages containing tyramine**
meperidine	excessive sedation
meprobamate	excessive sedation
methotrexate	increased liver toxicity and excessive sedation
metronidazole	disulfiramlike reaction**
narcotic drugs	excessive sedation
oxyphenbutazone	increased stomach irritation and/or bleeding
pentazocine	excessive sedation
pethidine	excessive sedation
phenothiazines*	excessive sedation
phenylbutazone	increased stomach irritation and/or bleeding
procarbazine	disulfiramlike reaction**
propoxyphene	excessive sedation
reserpine	excessive sedation, orthostatic hypotension**

*See Drug Class, Section Four.
**See Glossary.

Drug name or class	Possible interaction with alcohol
sleep-inducing drugs (hypnotics)	excessive sedation
—carbromal	
—chloral hydrate	
—ethchlorvynol	
—ethinamate	
—glutethimide	
—flurazepam	
—methaqualone	
—methyprylon	
—temazepam	
—triazolam	
thiothixene	excessive sedation
tricyclic antidepressants*	excessive sedation, increased intoxication
trimethobenzamide	excessive sedation

Drugs with which alcohol should be used only in small amounts (use cautiously until combined effects have been determined)

Drug name or class	Possible interaction with alcohol
acetaminophen (Tylenol, etc.)	increased liver toxicity
amantadine	excessive lowering of blood pressure
antiarthritic/anti-inflammatory drugs	increased stomach irritation and/or bleeding
anticoagulants (coumarins)*	increased anticoagulant effect
antidiabetic drugs (sulfonylureas)*	increased antidiabetic effect, excessive hypoglycemia**
antihistamines*	excessive sedation
antihypertensives*	excessive orthostatic hypotension**
aspirin (large doses or continuous use)	increased stomach irritation and/or bleeding
benzodiazepines*	excessive sedation
carisoprodol	increased alcoholic intoxication
diethylpropion	excessive nervous system stimulation with alcoholic beverages containing tyramine**
dihydroergotoxine	excessive lowering of blood pressure
diphenoxylate	excessive sedation
dipyridamole	excessive lowering of blood pressure
diuretics*	excessive orthostatic hypotension**
ethionamide	confusion, delirium, psychotic behavior
fenoprofen	increased stomach irritation and/or bleeding
griseofulvin	flushing and rapid heart action
ibuprofen	increased stomach irritation and/or bleeding
indomethacin	increased stomach irritation and/or bleeding
insulin	excessive hypoglycemia**
iron	excessive absorption of iron

*See Drug Class, Section Four.
**See Glossary.

Drug name or class	Possible interaction with alcohol
isoniazid	decreased effectiveness of isoniazid, increased incidence of hepatitis
lithium	increased confusion and delirium (avoid all alcohol if any indication of lithium overdosage)
methocarbamol	excessive sedation
methotrimeprazine	excessive sedation
methylphenidate	excessive nervous system stimulation with alcoholic beverages containing tyramine**
metoprolol	excessive orthostatic hypotension**
nalidixic acid	increased alcoholic intoxication
naproxen	increased stomach irritation and/or bleeding
nicotinic acid	possible orthostatic hypotension**
nitrates* (vasodilators)	possible orthostatic hypotension**
nylidrin	increased stomach irritation
orphenadrine	excessive sedation
phenelzine	increased alcoholic intoxication
phenoxybenzamine	possible orthostatic hypotension**
phentermine	excessive nervous system stimulation with alcoholic beverages containing tyramine**
phenytoin	decreased effect of phenytoin
pilocarpine	prolongation of alcohol effect
prazosin	excessive lowering of blood pressure
primidone	excessive sedation
propranolol	excessive orthostatic hypotension**
sulfonamides*	increased alcoholic intoxication
sulindac	increased stomach irritation and/or bleeding
tolmetin	increased stomach irritation and/or bleeding
tranquilizers (mild) —chlordiazepoxide —clorazepate —diazepam —hydroxyzine —meprobamate —oxazepam —phenaglycodol —tybamate	excessive sedation
tranylcypromine	increased alcoholic intoxication

Drugs capable of producing a disulfiramlike reaction** when used concurrently with alcohol

antidiabetic drugs (sulfonylureas)*	disulfiram	procarbazine
calcium carbamide	furazolidone	quinacrine
chloral hydrate	metronidazole	sulfonamides*
chloramphenicol	nifuroxine	tinidazole
	nitrofurantoin	tolazoline

*See Drug Class, Section Four.
**See Glossary.

TABLE 13
High-Potassium Foods

Diuretic drugs that cause loss of potassium from the body are often used to treat conditions that also require a reduced intake of sodium. The high-potassium foods listed below have been selected for their compatibility with a sodium restricted diet (500 to 1000 mg of sodium daily).

Beverages

orange juice	skim milk	tomato juice
prune juice	tea	whole milk

Breads and Cereals

brown rice	muffins	waffles
cornbread	oatmeal	
griddle cakes	shredded wheat	

Fruits

apricot	fig	orange
avocado	honeydew melon	papaya
banana	mango	prune

Meats

beef	haddock	rockfish
chicken	halibut	salmon
codfish	liver	turkey
flounder	pork	veal

Vegetables

baked beans	parsnips	tomato
lima beans	radishes	white potato
mushrooms	squash	
navy beans	sweet potato	

TABLE 14
Your Personal Drug Profile

Knowing as much as possible about your body and your medicines can save your life. Please take the time to fill out this profile with the latest infromation.

Name:

Age:

Weight in kilograms: (pounds divided by 2.2)

Height in inches:

Prescription drug allergies:

Non-prescription drug allergies:

Food allergies:

My kidneys* are: normal_____

mildly_____ moderately_____ severely_____ compromised.

My liver* is: normal_____

mildly_____ moderately_____ severely_____ compromised.

Conditions or diseases that I have or have had:

Prescription and non-prescription medications I take regularly:

*Make certain your dose is decreased if the drug is eliminated by an organ (such as the liver or kidneys) with which you have a problem. To determine which organs are involved, refer to the drug profile and "Conditions Requiring Dosing Adjustments" section for each medication you are taking.

Tables of Drug Information

Prescription and non-prescription medications I take periodically:

I find it very difficult_____
                                             to remember to take medicines.
I find it very easy_____

I become constipated rarely_____   occasionally_____   never_____.

Urination is usually easy_____   rather difficult_____   difficult_____.

The phone number of the nearest Poison Control Center is _____.

I sleep well_____   OK_____   poorly_____   little_____   on most nights.

I have_____   have never_____   had blood problems in the past.

I am considering becoming_____   might be_____   am_____   pregnant.

I want the medications which offer the best balance of **price** and **outcomes** for my specific medical history and present conditions.

Sources

The following sources were consulted in the compilation and revision of this book:

Adverse Drug Reaction Bulletin. Edited by D. M. Davies. Meditext, Weybridge, Surrey, United Kingdom, 1992.
AMA Department of Drugs, *AMA Drug Evaluations,* Chicago: American Medical Association, 1992.
Andreoli, T. E., Carpenter, C. C. J., Plum, F., Smith, L. H., eds., *Cecil Essentials of Medicine.* Philadelphia: W. B. Saunders Co., 1986.
Arndt, K. A., *Manual of Dermatologic Therapeutics,* 4th ed. Boston: Little, Brown and Co., 1989.
Atkinson, A. J., Ambre, J. J., *Kalman and Clark's Drug Assay, The Strategy of Therapeutic Drug Monitoring,* 2nd ed. New York: Masson Publishing USA, 1985.
Avery, G. S., ed., *Drug Treatment,* 2nd ed. Sydney, Australia: ADIS Press, 1980.
Bartlett, John, *Medical Management of HIV,* 1994
Berkow, R., ed., *The Merck Manual,* 15th ed. Rahway, New Jersey: Merck Sharp & Dohme Research Laboratories, 1987.
Billups, N. F., ed., *American Drug Index 1992,* 36th ed. St. Louis: Facts and Comparisons, 1992.
Branch, W. T., *Office Practice of Medicine,* 2nd ed. Philadelphia: W. B. Saunders Co., 1987.
Briggs, G. G., Bodendorfer, T. W., Freeman, R. K., Yaffee, S. J., *Drugs in Pregnancy and Lactation.* Baltimore: Williams & Wilkins, 1983.
Brooke, M. H., *A Clinician's View of Neuromuscular Diseases,* 2nd ed. Baltimore: Williams & Wilkins, 1986.
Canadian Pharmaceutical Association, St. Paul's Hospital British Columbia Center of Excellence for HIV—AIDS, 1995.
Canadian Pharmaceutical Association, *Compendium of Pharmaceuticals and Specialties,* 26th ed. Ottawa: Canadian Pharmaceutical Association, 1991.
Cape, Ronald, *Aging: Its Complex Management.* Hagerstown, Maryland: Harper & Row, 1978.
Clin-Alert. Medford, New Jersey: Clin-Alert, Inc., 1989–1992.
Davies, D. M., ed., *Textbook of Adverse Drug Reactions,* 4th ed. New York: Oxford University Press, 1991.

Diamond, S., Dalessio, D. J., eds., *The Practicing Physician's Approach to Headache*, 4th ed. Baltimore: Williams & Wilkins, 1986.
DrugDex, CD-ROM 1995 edition.
Drug Interaction Facts. Edited by D. S. Tatro. St. Louis: Facts and Comparisons Division, J. B. Lippincott Co., 1995.
Drug Interactions Newsletter. Edited by P. D. Hansten, J. R. Horn. Spokane, Washington: Applied Therapeutics, Inc., 1995.
Drug Newsletter. Edited by B. R. Olin. St. Louis: Facts and Comparisons Division, J. B. Lippincott Co., 1995.
Drug Therapy, Physicians Prescribing Update. Lawrenceville, NJ: Excerpta Medica, 1992.
Dukes, M. N. G., ed., *Meyler's Side Effects of Drugs*, 11th ed. Amsterdam: Excerpta Medica, 1988.
Encyclopedia of Associations, 26th ed., Vol. 1, Part 2, Section 8. Detroit: Gale Research, Inc., 1992.
Facts and Comparisons. Edited by B. R. Olin. St. Louis: Facts and Comparisons Division, J. B. Lippincott Co., 1995.
F.D.A. Drug Bulletin. Rockville, Maryland: Department of Health and Human Services, Food and Drug Administration.
Fraunfelder, F. T., *Drug-Induced Ocular Side Effects and Drug Interactions*, 3rd ed. Philadelphia: Lea & Febiger, 1989.
Goodman, L. S., Gilman, A., eds., *The Pharmacological Basis of Therapeutics*, 8th ed. New York: Macmillan, 1990.
Greenberger, N. J., Arvanitakis, C., Hurwitz, A., *Drug Treatment of Gastrointestinal Disorders*. New York: Churchill Livingstone, 1978.
Handbook of Clinical Pharmacy, 1994.
Hansten, P. D., *Drug Interactions*, 6th ed. Philadelphia: Lea & Febiger, 1992.
Heinonen, O. P., Slone, D., Shapiro, S., *Birth Defects and Drugs in Pregnancy*. Littleton, Massachusetts: PSG Publishing Co., 1977.
Hollister, L. E., *Clinical Pharmacology of Psychotherapeutic Drugs*, 2nd ed. New York: Churchill Livingstone, 1983.
Huff, B. B., ed., *The Physicians' Desk Reference*, 46th ed. Oradell, New Jersey: Medical Economics Company, 1995.
International Drug Therapy Newsletter. Edited by F. J. Ayd. Baltimore: Ayd Medical Communications, 1995.
Jefferson, J. W., Greist, J. H., *Primer of Lithium Therapy*. Baltimore: Williams & Wilkens, 1977.
Journal of the American Medical Association. Edited by G. D. Lundberg. Chicago: American Medical Association, 1995.
Klippel, J. H., ed., Systemic Lupus Erythematosus. *Rheumatic Disease Clinics of North America*, Vol. 14, No. 1, April, 1988. Philadelphia: W. B. Saunders Co.
Koda-Kimbal, *Rational Therapeutics* 1994
Koller, W. C., ed., *Handbook of Parkinson's Disease*. New York: Marcel Dekker, 1987.
Kolodny, R. C., Masters, W. H., Johnson, V. E., *Textbook of Sexual Medicine*. Boston: Little, Brown and Co., 1979.
Lawrence, R. A., *Breast-Feeding*. St. Louis: Mosby, 1980.
Lieberman, M. L., *The Sexual Pharmacy*. New York: New American Library, 1988.
Long, J. W., *Clinical Management of Prescription Drugs*. Philadelphia: Harper & Row, 1984.
McEvoy, G. K., ed., *American Hospital Formulary Service, Drug Information 1995*. Bethesda, Maryland: American Society of Hospital Pharmacists, 1995.
Maddin, S., ed., *Current Dermatologic Therapy*. Philadelphia: W. B. Saunders Co., 1982.
The Medical Letter on Drugs and Therapeutics. Edited by H. Aaron. New Rochelle, New York: The Medical Letter, Inc., 1995.
Melmon, K. L., Morrelli, H. F., *Clinical Pharmacology*, 2nd ed. New York: Macmillan, 1978.

Messerli, F. H., ed., *Current Clinical Practice.* Philadelphia: W. B. Saunders Co., 1987.
Mohler, S. R., *Medication and Flying: A Pilot's Guide.* Boston: Boston Publishing Co., 1982.
The New England Journal of Medicine. Edited by J. P. Kassirer. Boston: The Massachusetts Medical Society, 1995.
Patient Drug Facts. Edited by B. R. Olin. St. Louis: Facts and Comparisons Division, J. B. Lippincott Co., 1992.
Postgraduate Medicine, The Journal of Applied Medicine for the Primary Care Physician. Minneapolis: McGraw-Hill, Inc., 1992.
Raj, P. P., *Practical Management of Pain.* Chicago: Year Book Medical Publishers, Inc., 1986.
Rakel, R. E., ed., *Conn's Current Therapy 1992.* Philadelphia: W. B. Saunders Co., 1992.
Rational Drug Therapy, Pharmacology for Physicians. Bethesda, Maryland: American Society for Pharmacology and Experimental Therapeutics, 1990.
Reynolds, J. E. F., ed. *Martindale, The Extra Pharmacopoeia,* 29th ed. London: The Pharmaceutical Press, 1995.
Rodman, M. J., Smith, D. W., *Clinical Pharmacology in Nursing.* Philadelphia: J. B. Lippincott Co., 1984.
Rogers, C. S., McCue, J. D., eds., *Managing Chronic Disease.* Oradell, New Jersey: Medical Economics Books, 1987.
Sauer, G. C., *Manual of Skin Diseases,* 5th ed. Philadelphia: J. B. Lippincott Co., 1985.
Schardein, J. L., *Drugs As Teratogens.* Cleveland: CRC Press, 1976.
Scientific American Medicine, CD-ROM edition 1995.
Shepard, T. H., *Catalog of Teratogenic Agents,* 6th ed. Baltimore: Johns Hopkins University Press, 1989.
Smith, L. H., Thier, S. O., *Pathophysiology, The Biological Principles of Disease,* 2nd ed. Philadelphia: W. B. Saunders Co., 1985.
Speight, T. M., ed., *Avery's Drug Treatment,* 3rd ed. Auckland: ADIS Press, 1987.
Swash, M., Schwartz, M. S., *Neuromuscular Diseases,* 2nd ed. Berlin: Springer-Verlag, 1988.
Tuchmann-Duplessis, H., *Drug Effects on the Fetus.* Sydney, Australia: ADIS Press, 1975.
USAN 1989 and the USP Dictionary of Drug Names. Edited by M. C. Griffiths. Rockville, Maryland: United States Pharmacopeial Convention, Inc., 1988.
USP Dispensing Information 1995, 12th ed., Vol. 1, *Drug Information for the Health Care Provider.* Rockville, Maryland: United States Pharmacopeial Convention, 1995.
Utian, W. H., *Menopause in Modern Perspective.* New York: Appleton-Century-Crofts, 1980.
Wallach, J., *Interpretation of Diagnostic Tests,* 5th ed. Boston: Little, Brown & Co., 1992.
Wartak, J., *Drug Dosage and Administration.* Baltimore: University Park Press, 1983.
Worley, R. J., ed., *Clinical Obstetrics and Gynecology,* Vol. 24, No. 1: *Menopause.* Hagerstown, Maryland: Harper & Row, 1981.
Young, D. S., *Effects of Drugs on Clinical Laboratory Tests, 1991 Supplement*. Washington: AACC Press, 1991. A therapeutic scheme of utilizing increasing strengths of pain medications (analgesics) which include NSAIDs, opiates, and adjuvant drugs to control pain as specified by the World Health Organization. It is *not* an absolute treatment scheme, but should be used to organize the approach to effective analgesia.

Index

This index contains all the brand and generic drug names included in Section Three and the names and alternative names of the disorders and conditions for which drug management is described in Section Two.

Brand names of drugs appear in italic type and are capitalized.

Each brand name is followed by the generic name of its Drug Profile in Section Three.

The symbol [CD] indicates that the brand name represents a combination drug that contains the generic drug components listed below it. To be fully familiar with any combination drug [CD], it is necessary to read the Drug Profile of each of the components listed. The brand name of a combination drug *may* or *may not* appear in the brand name list of each Drug Profile that is cited in the index as a component of a particular combination drug. The index listing of component drugs for any combination drug product represents the manufacturer's formulation of that brand at the time this information was compiled for publication.

The symbol ✦ before the brand name of a combination drug indicates that the brand name is used in both the United States and Canada, but that the ingredients in the combination product in each country differ. The Canadian drug is marked with the symbol ✦ to distinguish it from the American drug which has the same name.

A generic name with no page designation indicates an active component of a combination drug for which there is no Profile in Section Three. It is included to alert you to its presence, should you wish to consult your physician regarding its significance.

Abitrexate, methotrexate, 615
Accupril, quinapril, 876
Accurbron, theophylline, 966
Accutane, isotretinoin, 523
acebutolol, 31
Acet-Am, theophylline, 966
Acetazolam, acetazolamide, 34
acetazolamide, 34
acetic acids, 38
acetylsalicylic acid. See aspirin, 91
Aches-N-Pain, ibuprofen, 488, 843
Achromycin, tetracycline, 961
Achromycin V, tetracycline, 961
Acrocidin, tetracycline, 961
Acroseb-Dex, dexamethasone, 279
Actifed w/ Codeine (CD)
CONTAINS
  codeine, 247
  pseudoephedrine*
  triprolidine*
Actiprofen, ibuprofen, 488, 843
Actisite, tetracycline, 961
Acular, ketorolac, 38, 534
acyclovir, 44
Adalat, nifedipine, 698
Adalat FT, nifedipine, 698
Adalat PA, nifedipine, 698
Adapin, doxepin, 323
Adrenalin, epinephrine, 334

Adrenomist, epinephrine, 334
Adsorbocarpine, pilocarpine, 798
Advil, ibuprofen, 488, 843
AeroBid, flunisolide, 402
Aerolate, theophylline, 966
Akarpine, pilocarpine, 798
Ak-Chlor, chloramphenicol, 189
Ak-Cide (CD)
CONTAINS
  prednisolone, 815
  sulfacetamide*
Ak-Dex, dexamethasone, 279
AK-Mycin Opththalmic, erythromycin, 342
Akne-Mycin, erythromycin, 342
Ak-Pred, prednisolone, 815
Ak-Tate, prednisolone, 815
Ak-Zol, acetazolamide, 34
Alatone, spironolactone, 913
Alazine, hydralazine, 472
Albert Furosemide, furosemide, 436
albuterol, 47
alcohol. See ethanol, 354
Aldactazide (CD)
CONTAINS
  hydrochlorothiazide, 476, 971
  spironolactone, 913
Aldactone, spironolactone, 913
Aldoclor (CD)
CONTAINS

chlorothiazide, 197, 971
methyldopa*
Aldoril-15/25 (CD)
CONTAINS
  hydrochlorothiazide, 476, 971
  methyldopa*
Aldoril D30/D50 (CD)
CONTAINS
  hydrochlorothiazide, 476, 971
  methyldopa*
alendronate, 1057
Aleve, naproxen, 676, 843
Alka-Seltzer Effervescent Pain Reliever & Antacid (CD)
CONTAINS
  aspirin, 91
  citric acid*
  sodium bicarbonate*
Alka-Seltzer Plus (CD)
CONTAINS
  aspirin, 91
  chlorpheniramine*
  phenylpropanolamine*
Allerdryl, diphenhydramine, 301
Alloprin, allopurinol, 50
allopurinol, 50
Almocarpine, pilocarpine, 798
Alpha-Tamoxifen, tamoxifen, 949
alprazolam, 54
Alprazolam Intensol, alprazolam, 54
Altace, ramipril, 884
Alupent, metaproterenol, 604

---

*The symbol [CD] indicates that the brand name given is a combination drug consisting of generic drug components listed below it. If there is no page numbering following the name of the generic drug component, there is no Drug Profile for that ingredient in this book.

Alvosulfon, dapsone, 271
amantadine, 57
Ambenyl Expectorant (CD)
CONTAINS
codeine, 247
diphenhydramine, 301
Ambenyl Syrup (CD)
CONTAINS
codeine, 247
diphenhydramine, 301
Ambien, zolpidem, 1052
Amcill, ampicillin, 88
Amcort, triamcinolone, 1006
Amen, medroxyprogesterone, 591
Amersol, ibuprofen, 488, 843
Amesec (CD)
CONTAINS
amobarbital*
ephedrine*
aminophylline, 65
amethopterin. *See* methotrexate, 615
amfebutamone. *See* bupropion, 140
amiloride, 61
Aminodrox-Forte, phenobarbital, 787
Aminophyllin, aminophylline, 65
aminophylline, 65
5-aminosalicylic acid. *See* mesalamine, 602
Amitril, amitriptyline, 70
amitriptyline, 70
amlodipine, 74
amoxapine, 78
amoxicillin, 81
amoxicillin/clavulanate, 84
Amoxil, amoxicillin, 81
ampicillin, 88
Ampicin, ampicillin, 88
Ampicin PRB (CD)
CONTAINS
ampicillin, 88
probenecid, 828
Ampilean, ampicillin, 88
Anacin (CD)
CONTAINS
aspirin, 91
caffeine*
Anacin Maximum Strength (CD)
CONTAINS
aspirin, 91
caffeine*
Anacin 3 w/ Codeine #2-4, codeine, 247

Anacin w/ Codeine (CD)
CONTAINS
aspirin, 91
caffeine*
codeine, 247
Anafranil, clomipramine, 225
Ana-Kit, epinephrine, 334
Anaplex, hydrocodone, 477
Anaplex SR, pyridostigmine, 861
Anaprox, naproxen, 676, 843
Anaprox DS, naproxen, 676, 843
Ancasal, aspirin, 91
Ancobon, flucytosine, 399
Ancotil, flucytosine, 399
Anexsia (CD)
CONTAINS
acetaminophen*
hydrocodone, 477
Anexsia 7.5 (CD)
CONTAINS
acetaminophen*
hydrocodone, 477
angiotensin-converting enzyme (ACE) inhibitors,
Ansaid, flurbiprofen, 417, 843
Antabuse, disulfiram, 313
Anti-Diarrheal, loperamide, 572
Antispasmodic (CD)
CONTAINS
atropine*
hyoscyamine*
phenobarbital, 787
scopolamine*
Antivert (CD)
CONTAINS
meclizine*
niacin, 685
Apo-Acetazolamide, acetazolamide, 34
Apo-Allopurinol, allopurinol, 50
Apo-Alpraz, alprazolam, 54
Apo-Amilzide, amiloride, 61
Apo-Amitriptyline, amitriptyline, 70
Apo-Amoxi, amoxicillin, 81
Apo-Ampi, ampicillin, 88
Apo-Atenolol, atenolol, 99
Apo-Benztropine, benztropine, 122
Apo-Capto, captopril, 150

Apo-Carbamazepine, carbamazepine, 154
Apo-Cephalex, cephalexin, 182
Apo-Chlorpropamide, chlorpropamide, 202
Apo-Chlorthalidone, chlorthalidone, 205, 971
Apo-Cimetidine, cimetidine, 467
Apo-Clonidine, clonidine, 234
Apo-Cloxi, cloxacillin, 240
Apo-Diazepam, diazepam, 284
Apo-Diclo, diclofenac, 38
Apo-Diltiaz, diltiazem, 298
Apo-Dipyridamole, dipyridamole, 305
Apo-Doxy, 327
Apo-Doxy-Tabs, 327
Apo-Erythro Base, erythromycin, 342
Apo-Erythro-EC, erythromycin, 342
Apo-Erythro-ES, erythromycin, 342
Apo-Erythro-S, erythromycin, 342
Apo-Fluphenazine, fluphenazine, 409
Apo-Flurazepam, flurazepam, 414
Apo-Furosemide, furosemide, 436
Apo-Haloperidol, haloperidol, 462
Apo-Hydralazine, hydralazine, 472
Apo-Hydro, hydrochlorothiazide, 476, 971
Apo-Ibuprofen, ibuprofen, 488, 843
Apo-Imipramine, imipramine, 489
Apo-Indomethacin, indomethacin, 38, 498
Apo-ISDN, isosorbide dinitrate, 516
Apo-Keto, ketoprofen, 534, 843
Apo-Keto-E, ketoprofen, 534, 843
Apo-Lorazepam, lorazepam, 577
Apo-Methazide (CD)
CONTAINS
hydrochlorothiazide, 476, 971
methyldopa*

Apo-Metoclop,
  metoclopramide, 631
Apo-Metoprolol,
  metoprolol, 634
Apo-Metronidazole,
  metronidazole, 639
Apo-Nadol, nadolol, 664
Apo-Naproxen, naproxen,
  676, 843
Apo-Nifed, nifedipine, 698
Apo-Nitrofurantoin,
  nitrofurantoin, 703
Apo-Oxtriphylline,
  oxtriphylline, 742
Apo-Pen-VK, penicillin V,
  762
Apo-Perphenazine,
  perphenazine, 778
Apo-Pindol, pindolol, 801
Apo-Piroxicam, piroxicam,
  738, 808
Apo-Prazo, prazosin, 811
Apo-Prednisone,
  prednisone, 817
Apo-Primidone, primidone,
  824
Apo-Procainamide,
  procainamide, 835
Apo-Propranolol,
  propranolol, 848
Apo-Quinidine, quinidine,
  880
Apo-Ranitidine, ranitidine,
  467, 888
Apo-Salvent, albuterol, 47
Apo-Spriozide,
  spironolactone, 913
Apo-Sulfamethoxazole,
  sulfamethoxazole, 929
Apo-Sulfatrim (CD)
  CONTAINS
  sulfamethoxazole, 929
  trimethoprim, 1020
Apo-Sulfatrim DS (CD)
  CONTAINS
  sulfamethoxazole, 929
  trimethoprim, 1020
Apo-Sulin, sulindac, 38,
  940
Apo-Tamox, tamoxifen,
  949
Apo-Tetra, tetracycline,
  961
Apo-Thioridazine,
  thioridazine, 977

Apo-Timolol, timolol, 989
Apo-Timop, timolol, 989
Apo-Tolbutamide,
  tolbutamide, 998
Apo-Triazide (CD)
  CONTAINS
  hydrochlorothiazide,
    476, 971
  triamterene, 1011
Apo-Trifluoperazine,
  trifluoperazine, 1015
Apo-Verap, verapamil,
  1035
Apresazide (CD)
  CONTAINS
  hydralazine, 472
  hydrochlorothiazide,
    476, 971
Apresoline, hydralazine,
  472
Apresoline-Esidrix (CD)
  CONTAINS
  hydralazine, 472
  hydrochlorothiazide,
    476, 971
Aquaphyllim, theophylline,
  966
Aquatensen,
  methyclothiazide, 619,
    971
Aralen, chloroquine, 192
Aristocort, triamcinolone,
  1006
Aristoform D,
  triamcinolone, 1006
Aristospan, triamcinolone,
  1006
Arm-a-Med,
  metaproterenol, 604
Arthrotec, misoprostol,
  650
Articulose LA,
  triamcinolone, 1006
ASA. *See* aspirin, 91
5-ASA. *See* mesalamine,
  602
Asacol, mesalamine, 602
A.S.A. Enseals, aspirin, 91
Asasantine (CD)
  CONTAINS
  aspirin, 91
  dipyridamole, 305
Ascriptin (CD)
  CONTAINS
  aluminum hydroxide*

aspirin, 91
calcium carbonate*
magnesium hydroxide*
Ascriptin A/D (CD)
  CONTAINS
  aluminum hydroxide*
  aspirin, 91
  calcium carbonate*
  magnesium hydroxide*
Asendin, amoxapine, 78
Aspergum, aspirin, 91
aspirin, 91
astemizole, 97
Asthmahaler, epinephrine,
  334
Asthmanephrine,
  epinephrine, 334
Astramorph, morphine,
  656
Astramorph PF, morphine,
  656
Astrin, aspirin, 91
Atabrine, quinacrine, 872
Atasol-8, -15, -30 (CD)
  CONTAINS
  acetaminophen*
  codeine, 247
atenolol, 99
Ativan, lorazepam, 577
Atrovent, ipratropium, 509
A/T/S, 342
Augmentin, amoxicillin/
  clavulanate, 84
auranofin, 104
Aureocort, triamcinolone,
  1006
Aventyl, nortriptyline, 715
Axid, nizatidine, 467, 711
Axotal (CD)
  CONTAINS
  aspirin, 91
  butalbital*
Azaline, sulfasalazine, 933
azathioprine, 107
Azdone (CD)
  CONTAINS
  aspirin, 91
  hydrocodone, 477
azidothymidine. *See*
  zidovudine, 1049
azithromycin, 110
Azmacort, triamcinolone,
  1006
Azo Gantanol (CD)
  CONTAINS

---

*The symbol [CD] indicates that the brand name given is a combination drug consisting of generic drug components listed below it. If there is no page numbering following the name of the generic drug component, there is no Drug Profile for that ingredient in this book.

phenazopyridine*
sulfamethoxazole, 929
Azo Gantrisin (CD)
CONTAINS
phenazopyridine*
sulfisoxazole, 937
Azo-Sulfisoxazole,
sulfisoxazole, 937
Azpan, phenobarbital, 787
AZT. *See* zidovudine, 1049
Azulfidine, sulfasalazine, 933
Azulfidine EN-tabs,
sulfasalazine, 933

bacampicillin, 114
Bactopen, cloxacillin, 240
Bactrim (CD)
CONTAINS
sulfamethoxazole, 929
trimethoprim, 1020
Bactrim DS (CD)
CONTAINS
sulfamethoxazole, 929
trimethoprim, 1020
Bactroban, mupirocin, 661
Barbidonna (CD)
CONTAINS
atropine*
phenobarbital, 787
Barbidonna Elixir (CD)
CONTAINS
atropine*
phenobarbital, 787
Barbita, phenobarbital, 787
Bayer Aspirin, aspirin, 91
Bayer Children's Chewable Aspirin, aspirin, 91
Bayer Enteric Aspirin,
aspirin, 91
Bayer Select, ibuprofen, 488, 843
Beclodisk,
beclomethasone, 115
Becloforte,
beclomethasone, 115
beclomethasone, 115
Beclovent,
beclomethasone, 115
Beclovent Rotacaps,
beclomethasone, 115
Beclovent Rotahaler,
beclomethasone, 115
Beconase Nasal Inhaler,
beclomethasone, 115
Beepen VK, penicillin V, 762
beer. *See* ethanol, 354
Belap, phenobarbital, 787
Belladenal (CD)

CONTAINS
atropine*
phenobarbital, 787
Belladenal-S (CD)
CONTAINS
atropine*
phenobarbital, 787
Belladenal Spacetabs (CD)
CONTAINS
atropine*
phenobarbital, 787
Bellergal (CD)
CONTAINS
atropine*
ergotamine, 338
phenobarbital, 787
Bellergal-S (CD)
CONTAINS
atropine*
ergotamine, 338
phenobarbital, 787
Bellergal Spacetabs (CD)
CONTAINS
atropine*
ergotamine, 338
phenobarbital, 787
Benadryl,
diphenhydramine, 301
Benadryl 25,
diphenhydramine, 301
benazepril, 118
Bendopa, levodopa, 545
Benemid, probenecid, 828
Bensylate, benztropine, 122
Benuryl, probenecid, 828
Benylin, diphenhydramine, 301
Benylin Decongestant (CD)
CONTAINS
diphenhydramine, 301
pseudoephedrine*
Benylin Pediatric Syrup,
diphenhydramine, 301
Benylin Syrup w/ Codeine (CD)
CONTAINS
codeine, 247
diphenhydramine, 301
benztropine, 122
Betaloc, metoprolol, 634
Betapen-VK, penicillin V, 762
betaxolol, 126
Bethaprim (CD)
CONTAINS
sulfamethoxazole, 929
trimethoprim, 1020
Betoptic, betaxolol, 126

Betoptic-S, betaxolol, 126
Biaxin, clarithromycin, 216
Biohisdex DHC (CD)
CONTAINS
diphenylpyraline*
hydrocodone, 477
phenylephrine*
Biohisdine DHC (CD)
CONTAINS
diphenylpyraline*
hydrocodone, 477
phenylephrine*
Biquin Durules, quinidine, 880
birth control. *See* oral contraceptives, 732
bitolterol, 130
Blephamide, prednisolone, 815
Blocadren, timolol, 989
Brethaire, terbutaline, 955
Brethine, terbutaline, 955
Brevicon, oral contraceptives, 732
Bricanyl, terbutaline, 955
Bricanyl Spacer,
terbutaline, 955
bromocriptine, 132
Bronalide, flunisolide, 402
Bronchotabs (CD)
CONTAINS
ephedrine*
guaifenesin*
phenobarbital, 787
theophylline, 966
Brondecon (CD)
CONTAINS
guaifenesin*
oxtriphylline, 742
Bronkaid Mist,
epinephrine, 334
Bronkaid Mistometer,
epinephrine, 334
Bronkaid Tablets (CD)
CONTAINS
ephedrine*
guaifenesin*
theophylline, 966
Bronkodyl, theophylline, 966
Bronkolixir (CD)
CONTAINS
ephedrine*
guaifenesin*
phenobarbital, 787
theophylline, 966
Bufferin (CD)
CONTAINS
aspirin, 91
magnesium carbonate*

Bufferin Arthritis Strength
(CD)
CONTAINS
aspirin, 91
magnesium carbonate*
Bufferin Extra Strength
(CD)
CONTAINS
aspirin, 91
magnesium carbonate*
Bufferin w/ Codeine (CD)
CONTAINS
aspirin, 91
codeine, 248
magnesium carbonate*
bumetanide, 137
Bumex, bumetanide, 137
bupropion, 140
Buspar, buspirone, 144
buspirone, 144

Cafergot (CD)
CONTAINS
caffeine*
ergotamine, 338
Cafergot P-B (CD)
CONTAINS
atropine*
caffeine*
ergotamine, 338
phenobarbital, 787
Caladryl (CD)
CONTAINS
calamine*
diphenhydramine, 301
Calan, verapamil, 1035
Calan SR, verapamil, 1035
Calcimar, calcitonin, 147
calcitonin, 147
calcium channel blocking
drugs (calcium
blockers), 1069
*Cama Arthritis Pain
Reliever* (CD)
CONTAINS
aluminum hydroxide*
aspirin, 91
Canesten, clotrimazole, 238
Capoten, captopril, 150
Capozide (CD)
CONTAINS
captopril, 150
hydrochlorothiazide,
476, 971
captopril, 150

Carafate, sucralfate, 923
carbamazepine, 154
carbidopa. *See* levodopa,
545
Carbolith, lithium, 563
Cardene, nicardipine, 689
Cardene SR, nicardipine,
689
Cardioquin, quinidine, 880
Cardizem, diltiazem, 298
Cardizem CD, diltiazem,
298
Cardizem SR, diltiazem,
298
Cardura, doxazosin, 319
carteolol, 159
Cartrol, carteolol, 159
Cataflam, diclofenac, 38
Catapres, clonidine, 234
Catapres-TTS, clonidine,
234
Ceclor, cefaclor, 163
Cedocard-SR, isosorbide
dinitrate, 516
cefaclor, 163
cefadroxil, 166
Cefanex, cephalexin, 182
cefixime, 169
cefprozil, 171
Ceftin, cefuroxime, 179
ceftriaxone, 174
cefuroxime, 179
Cefzil, cefprozil, 171
Cenocort, triamcinolone,
1006
cephalexin, 182
Ceporex, cephalexin, 182
C.E.S., estrogens, 346
Chardonna-2 (CD)
CONTAINS
atropine*
phenobarbital, 787
Chibroxin, nizatidine, 711
Children's Advil,
ibuprofen, 488, 843
Children's Motrin,
ibuprofen, 488, 843
chlorambucil, 185
chloramphenicol, 189
Chloromycetin,
chloramphenicol, 189
Chloronase,
chlorpropamide, 202
Chloroptic,
chloramphenicol, 189

chloroquine, 192
chlorothiazide, 197, 971
chlorotrianisene. *See*
estrogens, 346
Chlorpromanyl,
chlorpromazine, 197
chlorpromazine, 197
chlorpropamide, 202
chlorthalidone, 205, 971
Choledyl, oxtriphylline,
742
Choledyl Delayed-release,
oxtriphylline, 742
Choledyl SA, oxtriphylline,
742
cholestyramine, 206
Cholybar, cholestyramine,
206
Cibacalcin, calcitonin, 147
Cibalith-S, lithium, 563
ciclosporin. *See*
cyclosporine, 265
Ciloxan, ciprofloxacin, 210
cimetidine, 467
Cin-Quin, quinidine, 880
Cipro, ciprofloxacin, 210
ciprofloxacin, 210
cisapride, 213
Citanest Forte,
epinephrine, 334
clarithromycin, 216
Claritin, loratadine, 574
clavulanate. *See*
amoxicillin/
clavulanate, 84
Clavulin, amoxicillin/
clavulanate, 84
Cleocin, clindamycin, 219
Cleocin T, clindamycin,
219
Climestrone, estrogens,
346
clindamycin, 219
Clinoril, sulindac, 38, 940
clofazimine, 223
clomipramine, 225
clonazepam, 230
clonidine, 234
Clopra, metoclopramide,
631
clotrimazole, 238
cloxacillin, 240
Cloxapen, cloxacillin, 240
clozapine, 243
Clozaril, clozapine, 243

*The symbol [CD] indicates that the brand name given is a combination drug consisting of generic drug components listed below it. If there is no page numbering following the name of the generic drug component, there is no Drug Profile for that ingredient in this book.

CoAdvil (CD)
CONTAINS
ibuprofen, 488, 843
pseudoephedrine*
Co-Betaloc (CD)
CONTAINS
hydrochlorothiazide, 476, 971
metoprolol, 634
codeine, 247
Cogentin, benztropine, 122
Cognex, tacrine, 945
Colabid (CD)
CONTAINS
colchicine, 251
probenecid, 828
ColBenemid (CD)
CONTAINS
colchicine, 251
probenecid, 828
colchicine, 251
Colestid, colestipol, 255
colestipol, 255
Combid (CD)
CONTAINS
isopropamide*
prochlorperazine, 839
Combipres (CD)
CONTAINS
chlorthalidone, 205, 971
clonidine, 234
Comoxol (CD)
CONTAINS
sulfamethoxazole, 929
trimethoprim, 1020
Compazine, prochlorperazine, 839
compound S. *See* zidovudine, 1049
Compoz, diphenhydramine, 301
Congest, estrogens, 346
conjugated estrogens. *See* estrogens, 346
Constant-T, theophylline, 966
Contact allergy formula, terfenadine, 958
Contimycin, tetracycline, 961
contraceptives. *See* oral contraceptives, 732
Cope (CD)
CONTAINS
aluminum hydroxide*
aspirin, 91
caffeine*
magnesium hydroxide*
Coptin (CD)
CONTAINS
sulfadiazine, 925
trimethoprim, 1020
Coradur, isosorbide dinitrate, 516
Corgard, nadolol, 664
Coronex, isosorbide dinitrate, 516
Cortalone, prednisolone, 815
Coryphen, aspirin, 91
Coryphen-Codeine (CD)
CONTAINS
aspirin, 91
codeine, 248
Corzide (CD)
CONTAINS
bendroflumethiazide*
nadolol, 664
Cosalide, colchicine, 251
Cotrim (CD)
CONTAINS
sulfamethoxazole, 929
trimethoprim, 1020
Coumadin, warfarin, 1040
Cozaar, losartan, 581
cromolyn, 258
cromolyn sodium. *See* cromolyn, 258
Crystodigin, digitoxin, 293
C-Solve 2, erythromycin, 342
Cuprimine, penicillamine, 757
Curretab, medroxyprogesterone, 591
Cutivate, fluticasone, 421
Cyclinex, tetracycline, 961
Cyclopar, tetracycline, 961
cyclophosphamide, 261
cyclosporin A. *See* cyclosporine, 265
cyclosporine, 265
Cycrin, medroxyprogesterone, 591
Cyronine, liothyronine, 556
Cytomel, liothyronine, 556
Cytotec, misoprostol, 650
Cytovene, ganciclovir, 441
Cytoxan, cyclophosphamide, 261

Dalacin C, clindamycin, 219
Dalacin T, clindamycin, 219
Dalalone, dexamethasone, 279
Dalalone DP, dexamethasone, 279
Dalalone LA, dexamethasone, 279
Dalmane, flurazepam, 414
D-Amp, ampicillin, 88
dapsone, 271
Daraprim, pyrimethamine, 865
Daricon PB, phenobarbital, 787
Daypro, oxaprozin, 738, 843
Dazamide, acetazolamide, 34
DDC. *See* zalcitabine, 1045
DDI. *See* didanosine, 288
Decaderm, dexamethasone, 279
Decadron, dexamethasone, 279
Decadron-LA, dexamethasone, 279
Decadron Nasal Spray, dexamethasone, 279
Decadron Phosphate Ophthalmic, dexamethasone, 279
Decadron Phosphate Respihaler, dexamethasone, 279
Decadron Phosphate Turbinaire, dexamethasone, 279
Decadron w/ Xylocaine (CD)
CONTAINS
dexamethasone, 279
lidocaine*
Decaject, dexamethasone, 279
Decaject LA, dexamethasone, 270
Decaspray, dexamethasone, 279
Delestrogen, estrogens, 346
Delta-Cortef, prednisolone, 815
Deltasone, prednisone, 817
Demerol, meperidine, 595
Demerol APAP (CD)
CONTAINS
acetaminophen*
meperidine, 595
Demi-Regroton (CD)
CONTAINS
chlorthalidone, 205, 971
reserpine*
Demulen, oral contraceptives, 732
Depa, valproic acid, 1023

Depakene, valproic acid, 1023
Depakote, valproic acid, 1023
Depen, penicillamine, 757
Depo-Provera, medroxyprogesterone, 591
Deponit, nitroglycerin, 706
deprenyl. See selegiline, 903
Deproic, valproic acid, 1023
Dermoplast, hydroxychloroquine, 480
Deronil, dexamethasone, 279
desipramine, 275
Desogen, oral contraceptives, 732
Desyrel, trazodone, 1003
Detensol, propranolol, 848
Dex-4, dexamethasone, 279
Dexacen-4, dexamethasone, 279
Dexacen LA-8, dexamethasone, 279
Dexameth, dexamethasone, 279
Dexasone, dexamethasone, 279
Dexasone-LA, dexamethasone, 279
dexamethasone, 279
Dexasone, dexamethasone, 279
Dexo-LA, dexamethasone, 279
Dexone, dexamethasone, 279
Dexone-E, dexamethasone, 279
Dexone-LA, dexamethasone, 279
Dey-Dose, metaproterenol, 604
Dey-Lute, metaproterenol, 604
d4T. See stavudine, 917
DHC Plus, hydrocodone, 477
DiaBeta, glyburide, 452
Diabinese, chlorpropamide, 202

Diachlor, chlorothiazide, 197, 971
Diamox, acetazolamide, 34
Diamox Sequles, acetazolamide, 34
Diamox Sustained release, 34
Diazemuls, diazepam, 284
diazepam, 284
diclofenac, 38
Diclophen (CD)
  CONTAINS
  dicyclomine*
  phenobarbital, 787
didanosine, 288
Di-Delamine, diphenhydramine, 302
dideoxycytidine. See zalcitabine, 1045
dideoxyinosine. See didanosine, 288
Didronel, etidronate, 363
Diflucan, fluconazole, 395
diflunisal, 293
Digitaline, digitoxin, 293
digitoxin, 293
digoxin, 293
Dihydrex, diphenhydramine, 302
dihydrocodeinone. See hydrocodone, 477
di-iodohydroxyquin. See iodoquinol, 507
Dilacor XR, diltiazem, 298
Dilantin, phenytoin, 792
Dilantin w/ Phenobarbital (CD)
  CONTAINS
  phenobarbital, 787
  phenytoin, 792
Dilatrate-SR, isosorbide dinitrate, 516
diltiazem, 298
Dilusol, ethanol, 354
Dimetane Cough Syrup-DC (CD)
  CONTAINS
  brompheniramine*
  codeine, 248
  phenylpropanolamine*
Dimetane Expectorant-C (CD)
  CONTAINS
  brompheniramine*

codeine, 248
phenylpropanolamine*
Dimetane Expectorant-DC (CD)
  CONTAINS
  brompheniramine*
  hydrocodone, 477
  phenylpropanolamine*
Dimetapp-C (CD)
  CONTAINS
  brompheniramine*
  codeine, 248
Dimetapp w/ Codeine (CD)
  CONTAINS
  brompheniramine*
  codeine, 248
Diodoquin, iodoquinol, 507
Dipentum, olsalazine, 723
Di-Phen, phenytoin, 792
Diphendryl, diphenhydramine, 302
Diphenhist, diphenhydramine, 302
diphenhydramine, 301
Diphenylan, phenytoin, 792
diphenylhydantoin. See phenytoin, 792
dipyridamole, 305
Diquinol, iodoquinol, 507
disopyramide, 309
disulfiram, 313
Diuchlor H, hydrochlorothiazide, 476, 971
Diulo, metolazone, 634, 971
Diupres (CD)
  CONTAINS
  chlorothiazide, 197, 971
  reserpine*
Diurese, trichlormethiazide, 971, 1015
Diurigen, chlorothiazide, 197, 971
Diuril, chlorothiazide, 197, 971
Dixarit, clonidine, 234
Dolobid, diflunisal, 293
Dologesic, ibuprofen, 488, 843

---

*The symbol [CD] indicates that the brand name given is a combination drug consisting of generic drug components listed below it. If there is no page numbering following the name of the generic drug component, there is no Drug Profile for that ingredient in this book.

Dolophine, methadone, 611
Donn-Sed, phenobarbital, 787
Donnatal (CD)
CONTAINS
atropine*
phenobarbital, 787
Donphen, phenobarbital, 787
Dopar, levodopa, 545
Doral, quazepam, 869
Dormalin, quazepam, 869
Dormarex 2, diphenhydramine, 302
dornase alpha, 317
Doryx, doxycycline, 327
doxazosin, 319
doxepin, 323
Doxy 100, 200, doxycycline, 327
Doxy Caps, doxycycline, 327
Doxychel, doxycycline, 327
Doxycin, doxycycline, 327
doxycycline, 327
Doxy-Lemmon, doxycycline, 327
Dralzine, hydralazine, 472
Duapred, prednisolone, 815
Duocet (CD)
CONTAINS
acetaminophen*
hydrocodone, 477
Duragesic, fentanyl transdermal, 385
Duralith, lithium, 563
Duramorph, morphine, 656
Durapam, flurazepam, 414
Duraphyl, theophylline, 966
Duraquin, quinidine, 880
Duretic, methylclothiazide, 619, 971
Duricef, cefadroxil, 166
DV, estrogens, 346
Dyazide (CD)
CONTAINS
hydrochlorothiazide, 476, 971
triamterene, 1011
DynaCirc, isradipine, 526
Dyrenium, triamterene, 1011
Dysne-Inhal, epinephrine, 334

Easprin, aspirin, 91
Econopredophthalmic, prednisolone, 815

Ecotrin Preparations, aspirin, 91
EES, erythromycin, 342
Effexor, venlafaxine, 1032
8-Hour Bayer, aspirin, 91
Elavil, amitriptyline, 70
Elavil Plus (CD)
CONTAINS
amitriptyline, 70
perphenazine, 778
Eldepryl, selegiline, 903
Elixicon, theophylline, 966
Elixomin, theophylline, 966
Elixophyllin, theophylline, 966
Eltroxin, levothyroxine, 549
Emex, metoclopramide, 631
Emgel, erythromycin, 342
Emitrip, amitriptyline, 70
Emla cream, lidocaine and prilocaine cream, 553
Empirin, aspirin, 91
Empirin w/ Codeine No. 2, 4 (CD)
CONTAINS
aspirin, 91
codeine, 248
Empracet-30, -60 (CD)
CONTAINS
acetaminophen*
codeine, 248
Empracet w/ Codeine No. 3, 4 (CD)
CONTAINS
acetaminophen*
codeine, 248
Emtec-30 (CD)
CONTAINS
acetaminophen*
codeine, 248
E-Mycin, erythromycin, 342
E-Mycin E, erythromycin, 342
E-Mycin 333, erythromycin, 342
enalapril, 330
Endal-HD, hydrocodone, 377
Endep, amitriptyline, 70
Endocet (CD)
CONTAINS
acetaminophen*
oxycodone, 747
Endodan (CD)
CONTAINS

aspirin, 91
oxycodone, 747
Enduron, methyclothiazide, 619, 971
Enlon, histamine blocking drugs, 467
Enovid, oral contraceptives, 732
Enovil, amitriptyline, 70
Entrophen, aspirin, 91
Epifrin, epinephrine, 334
E-Pilo Preparations (CD)
CONTAINS
epinephrine, 334
pilocarpine, 798
Epimorph, morphine, 656
Epinal Ophthalmic, epinephrine, 334
epinephrine, 334
EpiPen, epinephrine, 334
Epitol, carbamazepine, 154
Epitrate, epinephrine, 334
Epival, valproic acid, 1023
Eramycin, erythromycin, 342
Ercaf (CD)
CONTAINS
caffeine*
ergotamine, 338
Ergodryl (CD)
CONTAINS
caffeine*
diphenhydramine, 302
ergotamine, 338
Ergomar, ergotamine, 338
Ergostat, ergotamine, 338
ergotamine, 338
Erybid, erythromycin, 342
Eryc, erythromycin, 342
Erycette, erythromycin, 342
Eryderm, erythromycin, 342
Erygel, erythromycin, 342
Erymax, erythromycin, 342
Erypar, erythromycin, 342
EryPed, erythromycin, 342
Ery-Tab, erythromycin, 342
Erythrocin, erythromycin, 342
Erythromid, erythromycin, 342
erythromycin, 342
Eryzole (CD)
CONTAINS
erythromycin, 342
sulfisoxazole, 937

Esidrix, hydrochlorothiazide, 476, 971
Eskalith, lithium, 563
Eskalith CR, lithium, 563
Eskaphen B (CD)
  CONTAINS
  ethanol, 354
  phenobarbital, 787
  thiamine*
E-Solve 2, erythromycin, 342
esterified estrogens. *See* estrogens, 346
Estinyl, estrogens, 346
Estrace, estrogens, 346
Estraderm, estrogens, 346
estradiol. *See* estrogens, 346
Estraguard, estrogens, 346
Estratab, estrogens, 346
estriol. *See* estrogens, 346
estrogens, 346
estrogens/progestins. *See* oral contraceptives, 732
estrone. *See* estrogens, 346
estropipate. *See* estrogens, 346
Estrovis, estrogens, 346
ethambutol, 351
ethanol, 354
ethosuximide, 360
Etibi, ethambutol, 351
etidronate, 363
etodolac, 38, 366
Etrafon (CD)
  CONTAINS
  amitriptyline, 70
  perphenazine, 778
Etrafon-A (CD)
  CONTAINS
  amitriptyline, 70
  perphenazine, 778
Etrafon-Forte (CD)
  CONTAINS
  amitriptyline, 70
  perphenazine, 778
etretinate, 366
Euflex, flutamide, 418
Euglucon, glyburide, 452
Eulexin, flutamide, 418
Euthroid (CD)
  CONTAINS
  levothyroxine, 549
  liothyronine, 556

Excedrin (CD)
  CONTAINS
  acetaminophen*
  aspirin, 91
  caffeine*
Excedrin P.M. (CD)
  CONTAINS
  acetaminophen*
  diphenhydramine, 302
Exdol-8, -15, -30 (CD)
  CONTAINS
  acetaminophen*
  caffeine*
  codeine, 247

famciclovir, 371
famotidine, 373, 467
Famvir, famciclovir, 371
Fansidar (CD)
  CONTAINS
  pyrimethamine, 865
  sulfadoxine*
felbamate, 373
Felbatol, felbamate, 373
Feldene, piroxicam, 808
felodipine, 377
Femazole, metronidazole, 639
Feminone, estrogens, 346
Femogen, estrogens, 346
Femogex, estrogens, 346
fenamates (NSAIDs), 380
Fenicol, chloramphenicol, 189
fenoprofen, 384, 843
fentanyl transdermal, 385
Fernisolone-P, prednisolone, 815
filgrastim, 388
finasteride, 393
Fiorinal (CD)
  CONTAINS
  aspirin, 91
  butalbital*
  caffeine*
Fiorinal-C 1/4, -C 1/2 (CD)
  CONTAINS
  aspirin, 91
  caffeine*
  codeine, 248
Fiorinal w/ Codeine (CD)
  CONTAINS
  aspirin, 91
  caffeine*
  codeine, 248

Fiorinal w/ Codeine No. 1, 2, 3 (CD)
  CONTAINS
  aspirin, 91
  butalbital*
  caffeine*
  codeine, 248
500 Kit, Pro-Biosan (CD)
  CONTAINS
  ampicillin, 88
  probenecid, 828
Fivent, cromolyn, 258
Flagyl, metronidazole, 639
Flagystatin, metronidazole, 639
Flonase, fluticasone, 421
Floxin, ofloxacin, 719
fluconazole, 395
flucytosine, 399
flunisolide, 402
Fluogen, influenza vaccine, 499
fluoxetine, 405
fluphenazine, 409
flurazepam, 414
flurbiprofen, 417, 843
Flu-Shield, influenza vaccine, 499
flutamide, 418
Flutex, triamcinolone, 1006
fluticasone, 421
fluvoxamine, 423
Fluzone, influenza vaccine, 499
Folex, methotrexate, 615
foscarnet, 427
Foscavir, foscarnet, 427
fosinopril, 433
Froben, flurbiprofen, 417, 843
Froben-SR, flurbiprofen, 417, 843
Fulvicin P/G, griseofulvin, 455
Fulvicin U/F, griseofulvin, 455
Fumide MD, furosemide, 436
Furadantin, nitrofurantoin, 703
Furalan, nitrofurantoin, 703
Furan, nitrofurantoin, 703

*The symbol [CD] indicates that the brand name given is a combination drug consisting of generic drug components listed below it. If there is no page numbering following the name of the generic drug component, there is no Drug Profile for that ingredient in this book.

Furanite, nitrofurantoin, 703
Furatoin, nitrofurantoin, 703
Furocot, furosemide, 436
furosemide, 436
Furoside, furosemide, 436

ganciclovir, 441
Gantanol, sulfamethoxazole, 929
Gantrisin, sulfisoxazole, 937
Gardenal, phenobarbital, 787
Gastrocrom, cromolyn, 258
Gecil, diphenhydramine, 302
gemfibrozil, 445
Genahist, diphenhydramine, 302
Gen-D-Phen, 302
Genergen, ergotamine, 338
Gen-Nifedipine, nifedipine, 698
Genora, oral contraceptives, 732
Genpril, ibuprofen, 488, 843
Genprin, aspirin, 91
Glaucon, epinephrine, 334
glibenclamide. See glyburide, 452
glipizide, 448
Glucamide, chlorpropamide, 202
Glucophage, metformin, 607
Glucotrol, glipizide, 448
glyburide, 452
Grifulvin V, griseofulvin, 455
Grisactin, griseofulvin, 455
Grisactin Ultra, griseofulvin, 455
griseofulvin, 455
Grisovin-FP, griseofulvin, 455
Gris-PEG, griseofulvin, 455
guanfacine, 459
Guildprofen, ibuprofen, 488, 843
Gulfasin, sulisoxazole, 937
Gynergen, ergotamine, 338
Gynetone, estrogens, 346
Gynogen LA, estrogens, 346

Habitrol, nicotine, 693
Haldol, haloperidol, 462

Haldol LA, haloperidol, 462
Halfprin, aspirin, 91
haloperidol, 462
Halperon, haloperidol, 462
Haltran, ibuprofen, 488, 843
Hexadrol, dexamethasone, 279
Hismanal, astemizole, 97
histamine blocking drugs, 467
HIVID, zalcitabine, 1045
Humulin BR, insulin, 502
Humulin L, insulin, 502
Humulin N, insulin, 502
Humulin R, insulin, 502
Humulin U, insulin, 502
Humulin U Ultralente, insulin, 502
Humulin 70/30, insulin, 502
Hycodan (CD)
CONTAINS
homatropine*
hydrocodone, 477
Hycomine (CD)
CONTAINS
ammonium chloride*
hydrocodone, 477
pyrilamine*
Hycomine Compound (CD)
CONTAINS
acetaminophen*
caffeine*
chlorpheniramine*
hydrocodone, 477
phenylephrine*
Hycomine Pediatric Syrup (CD)
CONTAINS
hydrocodone, 477
phenylpropanolamine*
Hycomine-S (CD)
CONTAINS
ammonium chloride*
hydrocodone, 477
phenylephrine*
pyrilamine*
Hycomine Syrup (CD)
CONTAINS
hydrocodone, 477
phenylpropanolamine*
Hycotuss Expectorant (CD)
CONTAINS
guaifenesin*
hydrocodone, 477
Hydelta-TBA, prednisolone, 815
Hydeltrasol, prednisolone, 815

hydralazine, 472
Hydramine, diphenhydramine, 302
Hydrea, hydroxyurea, 485
Hydro-Chlor, hydrochlorothiazide, 476, 971
hydrochlorothiazide, 476, 971
hydrocodone, 477
HydroDIURIL, hydrochlorothiazide, 476, 971
Hydromal, hydrochlorothiazide, 476, 971
Hydropres (CD)
CONTAINS
hydrochlorothiazide, 476, 971
reserpine*
Hydro-T, hydrochlorothiazide, 476, 971
hydroxychloroquine, 480
hydroxyurea, 485
Hydro-Z-50, hydrochlorothiazide, 476, 971
Hygroton, chlorthalidone, 205, 971
Hygroton-Reserpine (CD)
CONTAINS
chlorthalidone, 205, 971
reserpine*
Hylidone, chlorthalidone, 205, 971
Hytrin, terazosin, 952

ibuprofen, 488, 843
Ibuprofin, ibuprofen, 488, 843
Ibuprohm, ibuprofen, 488, 843
Ibu-Tab, ibuprofen, 488, 843
Iletin I NPH, insulin, 502
Iletin II Pork, insulin, 502
Ilosone, erythromycin, 342
Ilotycin, erythromycin, 342
Imdur, isosorbide mononitrate, 520
imipramine, 489
Imitrex, sumatriptan, 941
Imodium, loperamide, 572
Imodium AD, loperamide, 572
Impril, imipramine, 489
Imuran, azathioprine, 107
Indameth, indomethacin, 38, 498
indapamide, 494

Index

Inderal, propranolol, 848
Inderal-LA, propranolol, 848
Inderide (CD)
  CONTAINS
  hydrochlorothiazide, 476, 971
  propranolol, 848
Inderide LA (CD)
  CONTAINS
  hydrochlorothiazide, 476, 971
  propranolol, 848
Indocid, indomethacin, 38, 498
Indocid PDA, indomethacin, 38, 498
Indocid-SR, indomethacin, 38
Indocin, indomethacin, 38, 498
Indocin SR, indomethacin, 38, 498
Indo-Lemmon, indomethacin, 498
indomethacin, 38, 498
Inflamase, prednisolone, 815
Inflamase Forte, prednisolone, 815
influenza vaccine, 499
INH. *See* isoniazid, 512
Initard, insulin, 502
Insomnal, diphenhydramine, 302
Insulatard NPH, insulin, 502
insulin, 502
Insulin-Toronto, insulin, 502
Intal, cromolyn, 258
Intal Spincaps, cromolyn, 258
Intal Syncroner, cromolyn, 258
iodoquinol, 507
I-Pilopine, pilocarpine, 798
Ipran, propranolol, 848
ipratropium, 509
Ismelin-Esidrix (CD)
  CONTAINS
  guanethidine*
  hydrochlorothiazide, 476, 971

Ismo, isosorbide mononitrate, 520
Iso-BID, isosorbide dinitrate, 516
Isoclor Expectorant (CD)
  CONTAINS
  codeine, 248
  guaifenesin*
  pseudoephedrine*
Isonate, isosorbide dinitrate, 516
isoniazid, 512
isonicotinic acid hydrazide. *See* isoniazid, 512
Isoptin, verapamil, 1035
Isoptin SR, verapamil, 1035
Isopto Carpine, pilocarpine, 798
Isopto Fenicol, chloramphenicol, 189
Isordil, isosorbide dinitrate, 516
Isordil Tembids, isosorbide dinitrate, 516
Isordil Titradose, isosorbide dinitrate, 516
isosorbide dinitrate, 516
isosorbide mononitrate, 520
Isotamine, isoniazid, 512
isotretinoin, 523
isradipine, 526

jack. *See* ethanol, 354
Janimine, imipramine, 489
Jenest 28, oral contraceptives, 732

Keflet, cephalexin, 182
Keflex, cephalexin, 182
Keftab, cephalexin, 182
Kefurox, cefuroxime, 179
Kenacomb, triamcinolone, 1006
Kenacort, triamcinolone, 1006
Kenaject, triamcinolone, 1006
Kenalog, triamcinolone, 1006
Kenalone, triamcinolone, 1006

Kerlone, betaxolol, 126
ketoconazole, 530
ketoprofen, 534, 843
ketorolac, 38, 534
Key-Pred, prednisolone, 815
Kinesed (CD)
  CONTAINS
  atropine*
  phenobarbital, 787
Klonopin, clonazepam, 230
Kolex, 302

labetalol, 539
Labid, theophylline, 966
Lagyl, metronidazole, 639
Lamprene, clofazimine, 223
Lamictal, lamotrigine, 544
lamivudine, 1058
lamotrigine, 544
Laniazid, isoniazid, 512
Lanophyllin, theophylline, 966
Lanoxicaps, digoxin, 293
Lanoxin, digoxin, 293
lansoprazole, 544
Largactil, chlorpromazine, 197
Larodopa, levodopa, 545
Larotid, amoxicillin, 81
Lasaject, furosemide, 436
Lasimide, furosemide, 436
Lasix, furosemide, 436
Ledercillin VK, penicillin V, 762
Lenoltec w/ Codeine No. 1, 2, 3, 4 (CD)
  CONTAINS
  acetaminophen*
  caffeine*
  codeine, 248
Lente Iletin I, insulin, 502
Lente Iletin II Beef, insulin, 502
Lente Iletin II Pork, insulin, 502
Lente Insulin, insulin, 502
Lente Purified Pork, insulin, 502
Leukeran, chlorambucil, 185
Levate, amitriptyline, 70
Levatol, penbutolol, 753

---

*The symbol [CD] indicates that the brand name given is a combination drug consisting of generic drug components listed below it. If there is no page numbering following the name of the generic drug component, there is no Drug Profile for that ingredient in this book.

Levlen, oral contraceptives, 732
levodopa, 545
Levothroid, levothyroxine, 549
levothyroxine, 549
Levoxine, levothyroxine, 549
lidocaine, 553
Limbitrol (CD)
  CONTAINS
  amitriptyline, 70
  chlordiazepoxide*
liothyronine, 556
Lipo Gantrisin, sulfisoxazole, 937
liposome encapsulation, 1058
Liquid Pred, prednisone, 817
lisinopril, 560
Lithane, lithium, 563
lithium, 563
Lithizine, lithium, 563
Lithobid, lithium, 563
Lithonate, lithium, 563
Lithotabs, lithium, 563
Lixolin, theophylline, 966
Lo-Aqua, furosemide, 436
Lodine, etodolac, 38, 366
Lodrane, theophylline, 966
Lodrane CR, theophylline, 966
Loestrin, oral contraceptives, 732
lomefloxacin, 569
Loniten, minoxidil, 646
Lo/Ovral, oral contraceptives, 732
loperamide, 572
Lopid, gemfibrozil, 445
Lopressor, metoprolol, 634
Lopressor HCT (CD)
  CONTAINS
  hydrochlorothiazide, 476, 971
  metoprolol, 634
Lopressor OROS, metoprolol, 634
Lopressor Slow-release, metoprolol, 634
Lopurin, allopurinol, 50
loratadine, 574
lorazepam, 577
Lorazepam Intensol, lorazepam, 577
Lorcet-HD (CD)
  CONTAINS
  acetaminophen*
  hydrocodone, 477
Lorcet Plus (CD)
  CONTAINS
  acetaminophen*
  hydrocodone, 477
Lorelco, probucol, 832
Lortab (CD)
  CONTAINS
  acetaminophen*
  hydrocodone, 477
Lortab ASA (CD)
  CONTAINS
  aspirin, 91
  hydrocodone, 477
losartan, 581
Losec, omeprazole, 725
Lotensin, benazepril, 118
Lotrimin, clotrimazole, 238
Lotrimin AF, clotrimazole, 238
Lotrisone, clotrimazole, 238
lovastatin, 584
Lozide, indapamide, 494
Lozol, indapamide, 494
Ludiomil, maprotiline, 587
Luminal, phenobarbital, 787
Luramide, furosemide, 436
Luvox, fluvoxamine, 423

Macrodantin, nitrofurantoin, 703
Macrodantin MACPAC, nitrofurantoin, 703
Mandrax (CD)
  CONTAINS
  diphenhydramine, 302
  methaqualone*
maprotiline, 587
Marax (CD)
  CONTAINS
  ephedrine*
  hydroxyzine*
  theophylline, 966
Marax DF (CD)
  CONTAINS
  ephedrine*
  hydroxyzine*
  theophylline, 966
Marcaine, epinephrine, 334
Marzide II, trichlormethiazide, 1015
Maxair, pirbuterol, 805
Maxaquin, lomefloxacin, 569
Maxeran, metoclopramide, 631
Maxidex, dexamethasone, 279

Maximum Bayer Aspirin, aspirin, 91
Maxolon, metoclopramide, 631
Maxzide (CD)
  CONTAINS
  hydrochlorothiazide, 476, 971
  triamterene, 1011
*Maxzide-*25 (CD)
  CONTAINS
  hydrochlorothiazide, 476, 971
  triamterene, 1011
Mazepine, carbamazepine, 154
M Dopazide, hydrochlorothiazide, 476, 971
Measurin, aspirin, 91
Mebroin (CD)
  CONTAINS
  mephobarbital*
  phenytoin, 792
Meclodium, meclofenamate, 380, 591
meclofenamate, 380, 591
Meclomen, meclofenamate, 380, 591
Medicycline, tetracycline, 961
Medihaler-Epi Preparations, epinephrine, 334
Medihaler Ergotamine, ergotamine, 338
Medipain 5, hydrocodone, 477
Medi-Phedryl, diphenhydramine, 302
Medipren, ibuprofen, 488, 843
Medi-Profen, ibuprofen, 488, 843
Medrol Acne Lotion, methylprednisolone, 622
Medrol Enpak, methylprednisolone, 622
Medrol Veriderm Cream, methylprednisolone, 622
medroxyprogesterone, 591
mefenamic acid, 380, 594
Mellaril, thioridazine, 977
Mellaril-S, thioridazine, 977
Menest, estrogens, 346

Menrium (CD)
CONTAINS
chlordiazepoxide*
estrogens, 346
Menti-Derm, prednisolone, 815
mepacrine. *See* quinacrine, 872
meperidine, 595
Meprolone, methylprednisolone, 622
mercaptopurine, 598
mesalamine, 602
mesalazine. *See* mesalamine, 602
Mestinon, pyridostigmine, 861
Mestinon-SR, pyridostigmine, 861
Mestinon Timespan, pyridostigmine, 861
Metahydrin, trichlormethiazide, 971, 1015
Metaprel, metaproterenol, 604
metaproterenol, 604
Metastron, strontium, 920
metformin, 607
methadone, 611
methotrexate, 615
methyclothiazide, 619, 971
methylphenidate, 619
methylprednisolone, 622
methysergide, 627
Meticortelone, prednisolone, 815
Meticorten, prednisone, 817
Metizol, metronidazole, 639
metoclopramide, 631
metolazone, 634, 971
metoprolol, 634
Metreton, prednisolone, 815
Metro IV, metronidazole, 639
MetroGel, metronidazole, 639
metronidazole, 639
Metryl, metronidazole, 639
Mevacor, lovastatin, 584
Meval, diazepam, 284

Mexate, methotrexate, 615
mexiletine, 643
Mexitil, mexiletine, 643
Miacalcin, calcitonin, *147*
Micronase, glyburide, 452
Micronephrine, epinephrine, 334
Micronor, oral contraceptives, 732
Microsulfon, sulfadiazine, 925
Microx, metolazone, 634, 971
Mictrin, hydrochlorothiazide, 476, 971
Midamor, amiloride, 61
Midol Caplets (CD)
CONTAINS
aspirin, 91
caffeine*
Midol-IB, ibuprofen, 488, 843
Millazine, thioridazine, 977
Milprem (CD)
CONTAINS
estrogens, 346
meprobamate*
Minestrin, estrogens, 346
Minestrin 1/20, oral contraceptives, 732
Minims, chloramphenicol, 189
Minims Prednisolone, prednisolone, 815
Minipress, prazosin, 811
Minitran Transdermal Delivery System, nitroglycerin, 706
Minizide (CD)
CONTAINS
polythiazide*
prazosin, 811
Minodyl, minoxidil, 646
Mini-Ovral, oral contraceptives, 732
minocycline, 1057
minoxidil, 646
Miocarpine, pilocarpine, 798
misoprostol, 650
Mixtard, insulin, 502
Mixtard Human 70/30, insulin, 502
Moban, molindone, 653

Mobenol, tolbutamide, 998
Modecate, fluphenazine, 409
Modicon, oral contraceptives, 732
Moditen, fluphenazine, 409
Moduret (CD)
CONTAINS
amiloride, 61
hydrochlorothiazide, 476, 971
Moduretic (CD)
CONTAINS
amiloride, 61
hydrochlorothiazide, 476, 971
molindone, 653
Monitan, acebutolol, 31
Monoket, isosorbide mononitrate, 520
Monopril, fosinopril, 433
moonshine. *See* ethanol, 354
morphine, 656
Morphine H.P., morphine, 656
Morphitec, morphine, 656
MOS, morphine, 656
MOS-SR, morphine, 656
Motrin, ibuprofen, 488, 843
Motrin IB, ibuprofen, 488, 843
MS. *See* morphine, 656
MS Contin, morphine, 656
MTX. *See* methotrexate, 615
Mudrane GG Elixir (CD)
CONTAINS
ephedrine*
guaifenesin*
phenobarbital, 787
theophylline, 966
Mudrane GG Tablets, (CD)
CONTAINS
aminophylline, 65
ephedrine*
guaifenesin*
phenobarbital, 787
Mudrane Tablets (CD)
CONTAINS
aminophylline, 65
ephedrine*
phenobarbital, 787
potassium iodide*

---

*The symbol [CD] indicates that the brand name given is a combination drug consisting of generic drug components listed below it. If there is no page numbering following the name of the generic drug component, there is no Drug Profile for that ingredient in this book.

mupirocin, 661
Myambutol, ethambutol, 351
Mycelex, clotrimazole, 238
Mycelex-G, clotrimazole, 238
Mycelex-7, clotrimazole, 238
Myclo, clotrimazole, 238
Mycobutin, rifabutin, 889
Mycogen II, triamcinolone, 1006
Mycomar, triamcinolone, 1006
Myidone, primidone, 824
Mykrox, metolazone, 634, 971
Mymethasone, dexamethasone, 279
Myrosemide, furosemide, 436
Mysoline, primidone, 824
Mysteclin-F (CD)
  CONTAINS
  amphotericin B*
  tetracycline, 961

nabumetone, 38, 663
nadolol, 664
Nadopen-V, penicillin V, 762
nafarelin, 669
Nalcrom, cromolyn, 258
Nalfon, fenoprofen, 384, 843
naltrexone, 673
Napamide, disopyramide, 309
Naprosyn, naproxen, 676, 843
naproxen, 676, 843
Naqua, trichlormethiazide, 971, 1015
Naquival, trichlormethiazide, 971, 1015
Nardil, phenelzine, 782
Nasacort, triamcinolone, 1006
Nasalcrom, cromolyn, 258
Nasatab-LA, griseofulvin, 455
Natisedine, quinidine, 880
Natrimax, hydrochlorothiazide, 476, 971
Natulan, epinephrine, 334
Navane, thiothixene, 982
Naxen, naproxen, 676, 843
NebuPent, pentamidine, 765

nedocromil, 676
NEE, oral contraceptives, 732
nefazodone, 679
Nelova, oral contraceptives, 732
Nelova 1/50 M, oral contraceptives, 732
Nelova 10/11, oral contraceptives, 732
Neo-Codema, hydrochlorothiazide, 476, 971
Neodecadron Eye-Ear, dexamethasone, 279
Neo-Medrol Acne Lotion, methylprednisolone, 622
Neo-Medrol Veriderm, methylprednisolone, 622
Neomycin-Dex, dexamethasone, 279
Neo-Pause, estrogens, 346
Neosar, cyclophosphamide, 261
neostigmine, 682
Neo-Tetrine, tetracycline, 961
Neo-Tric, metronidazole, 639
Neo-Zol, clotrimazole, 238
Nephronex, nitrofurantoin, 703
Neupogen, filgrastim, 388
Neuro-Spasex (CD)
  CONTAINS
  homatropine*
  phenobarbital, 787
Neuro-Trasentin (CD)
  CONTAINS
  adiphenine*
  phenobarbital, 787
Neuro-Trasentin Forte (CD)
  CONTAINS
  adiphenine*
  phenobarbital, 787
Nia-bid, niacin, 685
Niac, niacin, 685
niacin, 685
nicardipine, 689
Nicobid, niacin, 685
Nicoderm, nicotine, 693
Nico-400, niacin, 685
Nicolar, niacin, 685
Nicorette, nicotine, 685
Nicorette DS, nicotine, 685
nicotine, 693
nicotine transdermal system. See nicotine, 693
Nicotinex, niacin, 685
nicotinic acid. See niacin, 685
Nicotrol, nicotine, 685
nifedipine, 698
Niscort, prednisolone, 815
Nitro-Bid, nitroglycerin, 706
Nitrocap TD, nitroglycerin, 706
Nitrocine, nitroglycerin, 706
Nitrodisc, nitroglycerin, 706
Nitro-Dur, nitroglycerin, 706
Nitro-Dur II, nitroglycerin, 706
nitrofurantoin, 703
Nitrogard, nitroglycerin, 706
Nitrogard-SR, nitroglycerin, 706
nitroglycerin, 706
Nitroglyn, nitroglycerin, 706
Nitrol, nitroglycerin, 706
Nitrolin, nitroglycerin, 706
Nitrolingual Spray, nitroglycerin, 706
Nitrong, nitroglycerin, 706
Nitrong SR, nitroglycerin, 706
Nitrospan, nitroglycerin, 706
Nitrostabilin, nitroglycerin, 706
Nitrostat, nitroglycerin, 706
Nitro Transdermal System, nitroglycerin, 706
nizatidine, 467, 711
Nizoral, ketoconazole, 530
Nolvadex-D, tamoxifen, 949
Nonsteroidal Anti-inflammatory Drugs, 843
Norcept-E 1/35, oral contraceptives, 732
Norcet 7 (CD)
  CONTAINS
  acetaminophen*
  hydrocodone, 477
Nordette, oral contraceptives, 732
Norethin 1/35E, 1/50M, oral contraceptives, 732

norfloxacin, 711
Norgesic (CD)
  CONTAINS
  aspirin, 91
  caffeine*
Norgesic Forte (CD)
  CONTAINS
  aspirin, 91
  caffeine*
Norinyl, oral contraceptives, 732
Norlestrin, oral contraceptives, 732
Normatine, bromocriptine, 132
Normodyne, labetalol, 539
Normozide (CD)
  CONTAINS
  hydrochlorothiazide, 476, 971
  labetalol, 539
Norocaine, epinephrine, 334
Noroxin, norfloxacin, 711
Norpace, disopyramide, 309
Norpace CR, disopyramide, 309
Norpramin, desipramine, 275
Nor-Pred, prednisolone, 815
Nor-Q.D., oral contraceptives, 732
Nor-Tet, tetracycline, 761
nortriptyline, 715
Norvasc, amlodipine, 74
Novahistex C (CD)
  CONTAINS
  codeine, 248
  phenylephrine*
Novahistex DH (CD)
  CONTAINS
  diphenylpyraline*
  hydrocodone, 477
  phenylephrine*
Novahistine DH (CD)
  CONTAINS
  hydrocodone, 477
  phenylephrine*
Novahistine DMX Liquid, ethanol, 354
Novamoxin, amoxicillin, 81

Nova-Phenicol, chloramphenicol, 189
Nova-Pred, prednisolone, 815
Novasen, aspirin, 91
Novo-Ampicillin, ampicillin, 88
Novo-Anaprox, naproxen, 676, 843
Novo-Atenolol, atenolol, 99
Novobutamide, tolbutamide, 998
Novo-Captopril, captopril, 150
Novo-Carbamaz, carbamazepine, 154
Novochlorocap, chloramphenicol, 189
Novo-Chlorpromazine, chlorpromazine, 197
Novo-Cimetine, cimetidine, 467
Novo-Cloxin, cloxacillin, 240
Novo-Difenac, diclofenac, 38
Novodigoxin, digoxin, 293
Novodipam, diazepam, 284
Novo-Diradol, dipyridamole, 305
Novodoparil (CD)
  CONTAINS
  hydrochlorothiazide, 476, 971
  methyldopa*
Novoflupam, flurazepam, 414
Novo-Flurazine, trifluoperazine, 1015
Novofuran, nitrofurantoin, 703
Novohydrazide, hydrochlorothiazide, 476, 971
Novo-Hylazin, hydralazine, 472
Novo-Lexin, cephalexin, 182
Novolin L, insulin, 502
Novolin-Lente, insulin, 503
Novolin N, insulin, 502
Novolin-NPH, insulin, 503
NovolinPen, insulin, 502
Novolin R, insulin, 502

Novolin-30/70, insulin, 503
Novolin-Toronto, insulin, 503
Novolin-Ultralente, insulin, 503
Novolinset, insulin, 503
Novo-Lorazepam, lorazepam, 577
Novomethacin, indomethacin, 38, 498
Novo-Metoprol, metoprolol, 634
Novoniacin, niacin, 685
Novo-Nidazole, metronidazole, 639
Novo-Nifedin, nifedipine, 698
Novopen-VK, penicillin V, 762
Novo-Peridol, haloperidol, 462
Novo-Pindol, pindolol, 801
Novopirocam, piroxicam, 808
Novopramine, imipramine, 489
Novo-Pranol, propranolol, 848
Novo-Prazin, prazosin, 811
Novoprednisolone, prednisolone, 815
Novoprednisone, prednisone, 817
Novo-Profen, ibuprofen, 488, 843
Novo-Propamide, chlorpropamide, 202
Novopurol, allopurinol, 50
Novoquinidine, quinidine, 880
Novo-Ranidine, ranitidine, 467, 888
Novoridazine, thioridazine, 977
Novorythro, erythromycin, 342
Novo-Salmol, albuterol, 47
Novosemide, furosemide, 436
Novosorbide, isosorbide dinitrate, 516
Novosoxazole, sulfisoxazole, 937

*The symbol [CD] indicates that the brand name given is a combination drug consisting of generic drug components listed below it. If there is no page numbering following the name of the generic drug component, there is no Drug Profile for that ingredient in this book.

Novospiroton,
    spironolactone, 913
Novospirozine (CD)
    CONTAINS
    hydrochlorothiazide,
        476, 971
    spironolactone, 913
Novo-Sundac, sulindac, 38,
    940
Novo-Tamoxifen,
    tamoxifen, 949
Novo-Tetra, tetracycline,
    961
Novo-Thalidone,
    chlorthalidone, 205,
    971
Novo-Triamzide (CD)
    CONTAINS
    hydrochlorothiazide,
        476, 971
    triamterene, 1011
Novo-Trimel (CD)
    CONTAINS
    sulfamethoxasole, 929
    trimethoprim, 1020
Novo-Trimel DS (CD)
    CONTAINS
    sulfamethoxasole, 929
    trimethoprim, 1020
Novotriphyl, oxtriphylline,
    742
Novotriptyn, amitriptyline,
    70
Novo-Veramil, verapamil,
    1035
    CONTAINS
    sulfamethoxazole, 929
    trimethoprim, 1020
NPH Iletin I, insulin, 503
NPH Iletin II Beef, insulin,
    503
NPH Iletin II Pork, insulin,
    503
NPH Insulin, insulin, 503
NPH Purified Pork, insulin,
    503
NSAIDs, 843
Nu-Alpraz, alprazolam, 54
Nu-Amilzide, amiloride,
    61
Nu-Amoxi, amoxicillin, 81
Nu-Ampi, ampicillin, 88
Nu-Atenolol, atenolol, 99
Nu-Capto, captopril, 150
Nu-Cephalex, cephalexin,
    182
Nu-Cimet, histamine
    blocking drugs, 467
Nu-Clonidine, clonidine,
    234
Nu-Cloxi, cloxacillin, 240

Nu-Cotrimox,
    sulfamethoxazole, 929
Nu-Diclo, diclofenac, 38
Nu-Diltiaz, diltiazem, 298
Nu-Hydral, hydralazine,
    472
Nu-Indo, indomethacin,
    38, 498
Nu-Loraz, lorazepam, 577
Nu-Metop, metoprolol, 634
Nu-Naprox, naproxen, 676,
    843
Nu-Nifed, nifedipine, 698
Nu-Pen-VK penicillin V,
    762
Nu-Pindol, pindolol, 801
Nu-Pirox, piroxicam, 808
Nu-Prazo, prazosin, 811
Nu-Ranit, ranitidine, 467,
    888
Nuprin, ibuprofen, 488,
    843
Nu-Tetra, tetracycline, 961
Nu-Triazide,
    hydrochlorothia-
    zide, 476, 971
Nu-Verap, verapamil,
    1035
Nydrazid, isoniazid, 512
*Nyquil Nightime Cold
    Medicine,* ethanol, 354
Nytol, diphenhydramine,
    302

OCs. See oral
    contraceptives, 732
Octamide,
    metoclopramide, 631
Octocaine, epinephrine,
    334
Ocuflox, ofloxacin, 719
Ocupress, carteolol, 159
Ocusert Pilo-20, -40,
    pilocarpine, 798
Ocu-Chlor,
    chloramphenicol, 189
Ocufen, flurbiprofen, 417,
    843
Oestrilin, estrogens, 346
ofloxacin, 719
Ogen, estrogens, 346
olsalazine, 723
omeprazole, 725
Omnipen, ampicillin, 88
Omnipen Pediatric Drops,
    ampicillin, 88
OMS Concentrate,
    morphine, 656
ondansetron, 729
Ophthochlor,
    chloramphenicol, 189

Ophtho-Chloram,
    chloramphenicol, 189
Ophthocort,
    chloramphenicol, 189
Ophtho-Tate,
    prednisolone, 815
Opticrom, cromolyn, 258
Optipress, carteolol, 159
oral contraceptives, 732
Oradexon, dexamethasone,
    279
Oramide, tolbutamide,
    998
Oramorph SR, morphine,
    656
Orasone, prednisone, 817
Orbenin, cloxacillin, 240
orciprenaline. *See*
    metaproterenol, 604
Oretic, hydrochlorothia-
    zide, 476, 971
Oreticyl (CD)
    CONTAINS
    hydrochlorothiazide,
        476, 971
    reserpine*
Orinase, tolbutamide, 998
Ormazine,
    chlorpromazine, 197
Ortho Cyclen, oral
    contraceptives, 832
Ortho Tri-Cyclen, oral
    contraceptives, 832
Ortho-Novum, oral
    contraceptives, 832
Orudis, ketoprofen, 534,
    843
Orudis E-50, E-100,
    ketoprofen, 534, 843
Orudis SR, ketoprofen,
    534, 843
Oruvail ER, SR,
    ketoprofen, 534, 843
Ovcon, oral
    contraceptives, 732
Ovoquinol, sulfadiazine,
    925
Ovral, oral contraceptives,
    732
Ovrette, oral
    contraceptives, 732
oxaprozin, 738, 843
oxicams, 738
oxpentifylline. *See*
    pentoxifylline, 771
oxtriphylline, 742
Oxycocet (CD)
    CONTAINS
    acetaminophen*
    oxycodone, 747
oxycodone, 747

Palaron, aminophylline, 65
Pamelor, nortriptyline, 715
Panasol-S, prednisone, 817
Panmycin, tetracycline, 961
Paracort, prednisone, 817
Paregoric, morphine, 656
Parfuran, nitrofurantoin, 703
Parlodel, bromocriptine, 132
paroxetine, 750
Pathadryl, diphenhydramine, 302
Paveral, codeine, 248
Paxil, paroxetine, 750
PCE Dispertab, erythromycin, 342
Pediaject, prednisolone, 815
Pediamycin, erythromycin, 342
Pediapred, prednisolone, 815
PediaProfen, ibuprofen, 488, 843
Pediazole (CD)
 CONTAINS
 erythromycin, 342
 sulfisoxazole, 937
Penapar VK, penicillin V, 762
Penbritin, ampicillin, 88
penbutolol, 753
Penglobe, bacampicillin, 114
penicillamine, 757
penicillin V, 762
Penntuss (CD)
 CONTAINS
 chlorpheniramine*
 codeine, 248
Pentacarinat, pentamidine, 765
pentamidine, 765
Pentamycetin, chloramphenicol, 189
Pentasa, mesalamine, 602
pentazocine, 768
pentoxifylline, 771
Pen-V, penicillin V, 762
Pen-Vee, penicillin V, 762
Pen-Vee K, penicillin V, 762

Pepcid, famotidine, 373, 467
Pepcid AC, famotidine, 373, 467
PE Preparations (CD)
 CONTAINS
 epinephrine, 334
 pilocarpine, 798
Pepto Diarrhea Control, loperamide, 572
Peptol, cimetidine, 467
Percocet (CD)
 CONTAINS
 acetaminophen*
 oxycodone, 747
Percocet-Demi (CD)
 CONTAINS
 acetaminophen*
 oxycodone, 747
Percodan (CD)
 CONTAINS
 aspirin, 91
 oxycodone, 747
Percodan-Demi (CD)
 CONTAINS
 aspirin, 91
 oxycodone, 747
pergolide, 774
Peridol, haloperidol, 462
Permax, pergolide, 774
Permitil, fluphenazine, 409
perphenazine, 778
Persantine, dipyridamole, 305
Pertofrane, desipramine, 275
Pethadol, meperidine, 595
pethidine. *See* meperidine, 595
Phenaphen (CD)
 CONTAINS
 aspirin, 91
 phenobarbital, 787
Phenaphen No. 2, 3, 4 (CD)
 CONTAINS
 aspirin, 91
 codeine, 248
 phenobarbital, 787
Phenaphen w/ Codeine No. 2, 3, 4 (CD)
 CONTAINS
 acetaminophen*
 codeine, 248

Phenazine, perphenazine, 778
phenelzine, 782
Phenergan w/ Codeine (CD)
 CONTAINS
 codeine, 248
 promethazine*
phenobarbital, 787
phenobarbitone. *See* phenobarbital, 787
phenytoin, 792
Phyllocontin, aminophylline, 65
Physpan, theophylline, 966
Pilagan, pilocarpine, 798
Pilocar, pilocarpine, 798
pilocarpine, 798
Pilopine HS, pilocarpine, 798
Piloptic 1, 2, pilocarpine, 798
Pilosyst 20/40, pilocarpine, 798
pindolol, 801
P-I-N Forte (CD)
 CONTAINS
 isoniazid, 512
 pyridoxine*
pirbuterol, 805
piroxicam, 808
Pisopyramide, disopyramide, 309
Plaquenil, hydroxychloroquine, 480
Plendil, felodipine, 377
PMB (CD)
 CONTAINS
 estrogens, 346
 meprobamate*
PMS Benztropine, benztropine, 122
PMS Carbamazepine, carbamazepine, 154
PMS Chloramphenicol, chloramphenicol, 189
PMS Dexamethasone, dexamethasone, 279
PMS Diphenhydramine, diphenhydramine, 302
PMS Dopazide (CD)
 CONTAINS
 hydrochlorothiazide, 476, 971
 methyldopa*

---

*The symbol [CD] indicates that the brand name given is a combination drug consisting of generic drug components listed below it. If there is no page numbering following the name of the generic drug component, there is no Drug Profile for that ingredient in this book.

PMS Erythromycin,
    erythromycin, 342
PMS Estradiol, estrogens,
    346
PMS Fluphenazine,
    fluphenazine, 409
PMS Imipramine,
    imipramine, 489
PMS Isoniazid, isoniazid,
    512
PMS Levazine (CD)
    CONTAINS
    amitriptyline, 70
    perphenazine, 778
PMS Methylphenidate,
    methylphenidate, 619
PMS Neostigmine,
    neostigmine, 682
PMS Perphenazine,
    perphenazine, 778
PMS Primidone,
    primidone, 824
PMS Prochlorperazine,
    prochlorperazine, 839
PMS Propranolol,
    propranolol, 848
PMS Pyrazinamide,
    pyrazinamide, 858
PMS Sulfasalazine,
    sulfasalazine, 933
PMS Sulfasalazine E.C.,
    sulfasalazine, 933
PMS Theophylline,
    theophylline, 966
PMS Thioridazine,
    thioridazine, 977
Pneumopent, pentamidine,
    765
Polycillin, ampicillin, 88
Polycillin Pediatric Drops,
    ampicillin, 88
Polycillin-PRB (CD)
    CONTAINS
    ampicillin, 88
    probenecid, 828
Polymox, amoxicillin, 81
Polytrim, trimethoprim,
    1020
Pondocillin, ampicillin, 88
Ponstan, mefenamic acid,
    380, 594
Ponstel, mefenamic acid,
    380, 594
Pravachol, pravastatin,
    808
pravastatin, 808
prazosin, 811
Predcor, prednisolone, 815
Pred Forte, prednisolone,
    815
Pred-G (CD)
    CONTAINS
    gentamicin*
    prednisolone, 815
Pred Mild, prednisolone,
    815
Prednicen-M, prednisone,
    817
prednisolone, 815
prednisone, 817
Prelone, prednisolone, 815
Premarin, estrogens, 346
Prepulsid, cisapride, 213
Prevacid, lansoprazole, 544
prilocaine, 553
Prilosec, omeprazole, 725
primaquine, 822
Primatene, theophylline,
    966
Primatene Mist,
    epinephrine, 334
primidone, 824
Principen, ampicillin, 88
Prinivil, lisinopril, 560
Prinzide (CD)
    CONTAINS
    hydrochlorothiazide,
        476, 971
    lisinopril, 560
Probalan, probenecid, 828
Probampacin (CD)
    CONTAINS
    ampicillin, 88
    probenecid, 828
Proben-C (CD)
    CONTAINS
    colchicine, 251
    probenecid, 828
probenecid, 828
Pro-Biosan, ampicillin, 88
Pro-Biosan 500 Kit (CD)
    CONTAINS
    ampicillin, 88
    probenecid, 828
probucol, 832
procainamide, 835
Procamide SR,
    procainamide, 835
Procan SR, procainamide,
    835
Procardia, nifedipine, 698
Procardia XL, nifedipine,
    698
prochlorperazine, 835
Procytox,
    cyclophosphamide,
    261
Progynon Pellet, estrogens,
    346
Pro-Iso, prochlorperazine,
    839
Prolixin, fluphenazine, 409
Prolopa (CD)
    CONTAINS
    benserazide*
    levodopa, 545
Proloprim, trimethoprim,
    1020
Promapar,
    chlorpromazine, 197
Prometa, metaproterenol,
    604
Promine, procainamide,
    835
Pronestyl, procainamide,
    835
Pronestyl-SR,
    procainamide, 835
Propaderm,
    beclomethasone, 115
Propaderm-C,
    beclomethasone, 115
Propine Ophthalmic,
    epinephrine, 334
propionic acids, 843
propranolol, 848
Propulsid, cisapride, 213
Proscar, finasteride, 393
ProStep, nicotine, 693
Prostigmin, neostigmine,
    682
Protamine, Zinc & Iletin I,
    insulin, 503
*Protamine, Zinc & Iletin II
    Beef,* insulin, 503
*Protamine, Zinc & Iletin II
    Pork,* insulin, 503
Protostat, metronidazole,
    639
Protrin (CD)
    CONTAINS
    sulfamethoxazole, 929
    trimethoprim, 1020
Protrin DF (CD)
    CONTAINS
    sulfamethoxazole, 929
    trimethoprim, 1020
protriptyline, 854
Proventil Inhaler,
    albuterol, 47
Proventil Repetabs,
    albuterol, 47
Proventil Tablets,
    albuterol, 47
Provera,
    medroxyprogester-
    one, 591
Prozac, fluoxetine, 405
PSP-IV, prednisolone, 815
Pulmophylline,
    theophylline, 966
Pulmozyme, dornase
    alpha, 317

Purinethol,
mercaptopurine, 598
Purinol, allopurinol, 50
PVF, penicillin V, 762
PVF K, penicillin V, 762
pyrazinamide, 858
Pyridamole, dipyridamole, 305
pyridostigmine, 861
pyrimethamine, 865

Quadrinal (CD)
  CONTAINS
  ephedrine*
  phenobarbital, 787
  potassium iodide*
  theophylline, 966
quazepam, 869
Questran, cholestyramine, 206
Questran Light, cholestyramine, 206
Quibron (CD)
  CONTAINS
  guaifenesin*
  theophylline, 966
Quibron Plus (CD)
  CONTAINS
  butabarbital*
  ephedrine*
  guaifenesin*
  theophylline, 966
Quibron-T Dividose, theophylline, 966
Quibron-T/SR, theophylline, 966
quinacrine, 872
Quinaglute Dura-Tabs, quinidine, 880
quinapril, 876
Quinate, quinidine, 880
quinestrol. *See* estrogens, 346
Quinidex Extentabs, quinidine, 880
quinidine, 880
Quinobarb (CD)
  CONTAINS
  phenylethylbarbiturate*
  quinidine, 880
Quinora, quinidine, 880
Quin-Release, quinidine, 880

ramipril, 884
ranitidine, 467, 888
Reclomide, metoclopramide, 631
Reglan, metoclopramide, 631
Regonol, pyridostigmine, 861
Regroton (CD)
  CONTAINS
  chlorthalidone, 205, 971
  reserpine*
Regular Iletin I, insulin, 503
Regular Iletin II Beef, insulin, 503
Regular Iletin II Pork, insulin, 503
Regular Iletin II U-500, insulin, 503
Regular Insulin, insulin, 503
Regular Purified Pork Insulin, insulin, 503
Relafen, nabumetone, 38, 663
Respbid, theophylline, 966
Retet, tetracycline, 961
Retrovir, zidovudine, 1049
ReVia, naltrexone, 673
Rheumatrex Dose Pack, methotrexate, 615
Rhodis, ketoprofen, 534, 843
Rhotral, acebutolol, 31
Rhythmim, procainamide, 835
Ridaura, auranofin, 104
rifabutin, 889
Rifadin, rifampin, 892
Rifamate (CD)
  CONTAINS
  isoniazid, 512
  rifampin, 892
rifampicin. *See* rifampin, 892
rifampin, 892
Rimactane, rifampin, 892
Rimactane/INH Dual Pack (CD)
  CONTAINS
  isoniazid, 512
  rifampin, 892
Riphen-10, aspirin, 91
Risperdal, risperidone, 896

risperidone, 896
Ritalin, methylphenidate, 619
Ritalin-SR, methylphenidate, 619
Rival, diazepam, 284
Rivotril, clonazepam, 230
RMS Uniserts, morphine, 656
Robaxisal (CD)
  CONTAINS
  aspirin, 91
  methocarbamol*
Robaxisal-C (CD)
  CONTAINS
  aspirin, 91
  codeine, 248
  methocarbamol*
Robicillin VK, penicillin V, 762
Robidone, hydrocodone, 477
Robimycin, erythromycin, 342
Robitet, tetracycline, 961
Rocephin, ceftriaxone, 174
Rofact, rifampin, 892
Rogaine, minoxidil, 646
Ronase, tolazamide, 994
Ro-Semide, furosemide, 436
Roubac (CD)
  CONTAINS
  sulfamethoxazole, 929
  trimethoprim, 1020
Rounox w/ Codeine (CD)
  CONTAINS
  acetaminophen*
  codeine, 248
Rowasa, mesalamine, 602
Roxanol, morphine, 656
Roxanol 100, morphine, 656
Roxanol SR, morphine, 656
Roxicodone, oxycodone, 747
Roxiprin (CD)
  CONTAINS
  aspirin, 91
  oxycodone, 747
Rufen, ibuprofen, 488, 843
Rynacrom, cromolyn, 258
Rythmodan, disopyramide, 309

---

*The symbol [CD] indicates that the brand name given is a combination drug consisting of generic drug components listed below it. If there is no page numbering following the name of the generic drug component, there is no Drug Profile for that ingredient in this book.

Rythmodan-LA,
  disopyramide, 309

St. Joseph Children's
  Aspirin, aspirin, 91
Sal-Adult, aspirin, 91
Salagen, pilocarpine, 798
Salazopyrin, sulfasalazine,
  933
Salbutamol. *See* albuterol,
  47
salcatonin. *See* calcitonin,
  147
Sal-Infant, aspirin, 91
salmeterol, 900
Salofalk, mesalamine, 602
Sandimmune,
  cyclosporine, 265
Sans-Acne, erythromycin,
  342
Sansert, methysergide, 627
SAS-Enema, sulfasalazine,
  933
SAS Enteric-500,
  sulfasalazine, 933
SAS-500, sulfasalazine, 933
Savacort, prednisolone,
  815
Sectral, acebutolol, 31
Seldane, terfenadine, 958
Seldane-D, terfenadine,
  958
selegiline, 903
Semilente Iletin I, insulin,
  503
Semilente Insulin, insulin,
  503
Semilente Purified Pork,
  insulin, 503
Sensoricaine, epinephrine,
  334
Septra (CD)
  CONTAINS
  sulfamethoxazole, 929
  trimethoprim, 1020
Septra DS (CD)
  CONTAINS
  sulfamethoxazole, 929
  trimethoprim, 1020
Ser-Ap-Es (CD)
  CONTAINS
  hydralazine, 472
  hydrochlorothiazide,
    476, 971
  reserpine*
Serevent, salmeterol,
  900
Serpasil-Apresoline (CD)
  CONTAINS
  hydralazine, 472
  reserpine*

Serpasil-Esidrix (CD)
  CONTAINS
  hydrochlorothiazide,
    476, 971
  reserpine*
sertraline, 907
Serzone, nefazodone, 679
simvastatin, 910
Sincomen, spironolactone,
  913
Sinemet (CD)
  CONTAINS
  carbidopa*
  levodopa, 545
Sinemet CR (CD)
  CONTAINS
  carbidopa*
  levodopa, 545
Sinequan, doxepin, 323
SK-Amitriptyline,
  amitriptyline, 70
SK-Ampicillin, ampicillin,
  88
SK-Chlorothiazide,
  chlorothiazide, 197,
  971
SK-Dexamethasone,
  dexamethasone, 279
SK-Digoxin, digoxin, 293
SK-Dipyridamole,
  dipyridamole, 305
SK-Erythromycin,
  erythromycin, 342
SK-Furosemide,
  furosemide, 436
SK-Hydrochlorothia-
  zide, hydrochlorothiazide, 476, 971
SK-Metronidazole,
  metronidazole, 639
SK-Niacin, niacin, 685
SK-Oxycodone, oxycodone,
  747
SK-Penicillin VK,
  penicillin V, 762
SK-Phenobarbital,
  phenobarbital, 787
SK-Pramine, imipramine,
  489
SK-Prednisone,
  prednisone, 817
SK-Probenecid,
  probenecid, 828
SK-Quinidine sulfate,
  quinidine, 880
SK-Soxazole, sulfisoxazole,
  937
SK-Tetracycline,
  tetracycline, 961
SK-Thioridazine,
  thioridazine, 977

SK-Tolbutamide,
  tolbutamide, 998
SK-Triamcinolone,
  triamcinolone, 1006
Sleep, diphenhydramine,
  302
Sleep-Eze D,
  diphenhydramine, 302
Sleep-Eze 3,
  diphenhydramine, 302
Slo-bid, theophylline, 966
Slo-bid Gyrocaps,
  theophylline, 966
Slo-Niacin, niacin, 685
Slo-Phyllin, theophylline,
  966
Slo-Phyllin GG (CD)
  CONTAINS
  guaifenesin*
  theophylline, 966
Slo-Phyllin Gyrocaps,
  theophylline, 966
smoking cessation adjunct.
  See nicotine, 693
sodium cromoglycate. *See*
  cromolyn, 258
Sofracort, dexamethasone,
  279
Solazine, trifluoperazine,
  1015
Solfoton, phenobarbital,
  787
Solu-Medrol,
  methylprednisol-
  one, 622
Solurex, dexamethasone,
  279
Solurex-LA,
  dexamethasone, 279
Sominex,
  diphenhydramine, 302
Sominex 2,
  diphenhydramine, 302
Somnol, flurazepam, 414
Somophyllin,
  aminophylline, 65
Somophyllin-12,
  aminophylline, 65
Som-Pam, flurazepam,
  414
Sonazine, chlorpromazine,
  197
Sopamycetin,
  chloramphenicol, 189
Sopamycetin/HC,
  chloramphenicol, 189
sorbide nitrate. *See*
  isosorbide dinitrate,
  516
Sorbitrate, isosorbide
  dinitrate, 516

Sorbitrate-SA, isosorbide dinitrate, 516
Span-Niacin-150, niacin, 685
Spectrobid, bacampicillin, 114
Spersacarpine, pilocarpine, 798
Spersadex, dexamethasone, 279
spironolactone, 913
Spironazide, spironolactone, 913
SSD, sulfadiazine, 925
Statex, morphine, 656
Staticin, erythromycin, 342
stavudine, 917
Stelazine, trifluoperazine, 1015
Stemetil, prochlorperazine, 835
Sterane, prednisolone, 815
Sterapred, prednisone, 817
Stievamycin, erythromycin, 342
Storzolamide, acetazolamide, 34
strontium, 920
sucralfate, 923
Sulcrate, sucralfate, 923
sulfadiazine, 925
Sulfalar, sulfisoxazole, 937
sulfamethoxazole, 929
sulfasalazine, 933
Sulfatrim (CD)
 CONTAINS
 sulfamethoxazole, 929
 trimethoprim, 1020
sulfisoxazole, 937
sulindac, 38, 940
sumatriptan, 941
Sumycin, tetracycline, 961
Supasa, aspirin, 91
Superior Pain Medicine, ibuprofen, 488, 843
Supeudol, oxycodone, 747
Suprax, cefixime, 169
Suprazine, trifluoperazine, 1015
Supreme Pain Medicine, ibuprofen, 488, 843
Sus-Phrine, epinephrine, 334
Sustaire, theophylline, 966

Symadine, amantadine, 57
Symmetrel, amantadine, 57
Synalgos (CD)
 CONTAINS
 aspirin, 91
 caffeine*
Synalgos-DC (CD)
 CONTAINS
 aspirin, 91
 caffeine*
 drocode*
Synarel, nafarelin, 669
Syn-Captopril, captopril, 150
Syn-Diltiazem, diltiazem, 298
Synflex, naproxen, 676, 843
Syn-Nadol, nadolol, 664
Synphasic, oral contraceptives, 732
Syn-Pindolol, pindolol, 801
Synthroid, levothyroxine, 549
Syroxine, levothyroxine, 549

TACE, estrogens, 346
tacrine, 945
Tagamet, cimetidine, 467
Talacen (CD)
 CONTAINS
 acetaminophen*
 pentazocine, 768
Talwin, pentazocine, 768
Talwin Compound (CD)
 CONTAINS
 aspirin, 91
 pentazocine, 768
Talwin Compound-50 (CD)
 CONTAINS
 aspirin, 91
 caffeine*
 pentazocine, 768
Talwin Nx (CD)
 CONTAINS
 naloxone*
 pentazocine, 768
Tamofen, tamoxifen, 949
Tamone, tamoxifen, 949
tamoxifen, 949
TBA Pred, prednisolone, 815

Tebrazid, pyrazinamide, 858
Tedral Preparations (CD)
 CONTAINS
 ephedrine*
 phenobarbital, 787
 theophylline, 966
Teebaconin, isoniazid, 512
Teebaconin and Vitamin B6 (CD)
 CONTAINS
 isoniazid, 512
 pyridoxine*
Tegison, etretinate, 366
Tegopen, cloxacillin, 240
Tegretol, carbamazepine, 154
Tegretol Chewable Tablets, carbamazepine, 154
Teline, tetracycline, 961
Temaril, ethanol, 354
Tenex, guanfacine, 459
Tenoretic (CD)
 CONTAINS
 atenolol, 99
 chlorthalidone, 205, 971
Tenormin, atenolol, 99
T.E.P., theophylline, 966
terazosin, 952
terbutaline, 955
terfenadine, 958
Terfluzine, trifluoperazine, 1015
Tetra-C, tetracycline, 961
Tetracap, tetracycline, 961
Tetra-Con, tetracycline, 961
tetracycline, 961
Tetracyn, tetracycline, 961
Tetralan, tetracycline, 961
Tetram, tetracycline, 961
T-4. *See* levothyroxine, 549
T-Gesic (CD)
 CONTAINS
 acetaminophen*
 hydrocodone, 477
THA, tacrine, 945
Thalfed, theophylline, 966
Thalitone, chlorthalidone, 205, 971
Theobid Duracaps, theophylline, 966
Theo-Bronc, theophylline, 966

---

*The symbol [CD] indicates that the brand name given is a combination drug consisting of generic drug components listed below it. If there is no page numbering following the name of the generic drug component, there is no Drug Profile for that ingredient in this book.

1154 Index

Theochron, theophylline, 966
Theoclear, theophylline, 966
Theocord, theophylline, 966
Theo-Dur, theophylline, 966
Theolair, theophylline, 966
Theolixer, phenobarbital, 787
Theomax DF, theophylline, 966
Theon, theophylline, 966
theophylline, 966
theophylline ethylenediamine. *See* aminophylline, 65
Theophyl-SR, theophylline, 966
Theo-24, theophylline, 966
Theospan-SR, theophylline, 966
Theovent, theophylline, 966
Theox, theophylline, 966
Theozine, theophylline, 966
thiazide diuretics, 971
thioridazine, 977
thiothixene, 982
Thiuretic, hydrochlorothiazide, 476, 971
Thorazine, chlorpromazine, 197
Thorazine SR, chlorpromazine, 197
thyrocalcitonin. *See* calcitonin, 147
Thyroid USP, levothyroxine, 549
Thyrolar (CD)
  CONTAINS
  levothyroxine, 549
  liothyronine, 556
thyroxine. *See* levothyroxine, 549
Ticlid, ticlopidine, 986
ticlopidine, 986
Tilade, nedocromil, 676
Timolide (CD)
  CONTAINS
  hydrochlorothiazide, 476, 971
  timolol, 989
timolol, 989
Timoptic, timolol, 989
Tipramine, imipramine, 489
Tobradex, dexamethasone, 279

Tofranil, imipramine, 489
Tolamide, tolazamide, 994
tolazamide, 994
tolbutamide, 998
Tolectin, tolmetin, 38, 1003
Tolectin DS, tolmetin, 38, 1003
Tolectin 600, tolmetin, 38, 1003
Tolinase, tolazamide, 994
tolmetin, 38, 1003
Toprol, metoprolol, 634
Toprol XL, metoprolol, 634
Toradol, ketorolac, 38, 534
Tornalate, bitolterol, 130
Totacillin, ampicillin, 88
Trandate, labetalol, 539
Trandate HCT (CD)
  CONTAINS
  hydrochlorothiazide, 476, 971
  labetalol, 539
Transderm-Nitro, nitroglycerin, 706
trazodone, 1003
Trental, pentoxifylline, 771
Trexan, naltrexone, 673
Triacet, triamcinolone, 1006
Triadapin, doxepin, 323
Triaderm, triamcinolone, 1006
Trialodine, trazodone, 1003
Triam-A, triamcinolone, 1006
triamcinolone, 1006
Triaminic Expectorant w/ Codeine (CD)
  CONTAINS
  codeine, 248
  guaifenesin*
  phenylpropanolamine*
Triaminic Expectorant DH (CD)
  CONTAINS
  guaifenesin*
  hydrocodone, 477
  pheniramine*
  phenylpropanolamine*
  pyrilamine*
Triamolone 40, triamcinolone, 1006
Triaderm, triamcinolone, 1006
triamterene, 1011
Triaphen-10, aspirin, 91
Triavil (CD)
  CONTAINS

  amitriptyline, 70
  perphenazine, 778
trichlormethiazide, 971, 1015
Tridil, nitroglycerin, 706
trifluoperazine, 1015
triiodothyronine. *See* liothyronine, 556
Trikacide, metronidazole, 639
Tri-Kort, triamcinolone, 1006
Trilafon, perphenazine, 778
Tri-Levlen, oral contraceptives, 732
Trilog, triamcinolone, 1006
trimethoprim, 1020
Trimox, amoxicillin, 81
Trimpex, trimethoprim, 1020
Tri-Norinyl, oral contraceptives, 732
Triostat, liothyronine, 556
Triphasil, oral contraceptives, 732
Triptil, protriptyline, 854
Triquilar, oral contraceptives, 732
Trisem (CD)
  CONTAINS
  sulfadiazine, 925
  pheniramine*
  phenylpropanolamine*
  pyrilamine*
Trisoralen (CD)
  CONTAINS
  sulfadiazine, 925
  sulfamerazine*
  sulfamethazine*
  pheniramine*
  phenylpropanolamine*
  pyrilamine*
Tristoject, triamcinolone, 1006
Tropicycline, tetracycline, 961
Truphylline, aminophylline, 65
T-Stat, erythromycin, 342
T-3. *See* liothyronine, 556
Tussend (CD)
  CONTAINS
  hydrocodone, 477
  pseudoephedrine*
Tussend Expectorant (CD)
  CONTAINS
  guaifenesin*
  hydrocodone, 477
  pseudoephedrine*

Tussionex (CD)
　CONTAINS
　hydrocodone, 477
　phenyltoloxamine*
Tuss-Ornade, ethanol, 354
Twilite, diphenhydramine, 302
Tycolet (CD)
　CONTAINS
　acetaminophen*
　hydrocodone, 477
Tylenol w/ Codeine (CD)
　CONTAINS
　acetaminophen*
　codeine, 248
Tylenol w/ Codeine Elixir (CD)
　CONTAINS
　acetaminophen*
　codeine, 248
Tylenol w/ Codeine No. 1, 2, 3, 4 (CD)
　CONTAINS
　acetaminophen*
　codeine, 248
Tylox (CD)
　CONTAINS
　acetaminophen*
　oxycodone, 747

Ultracaine, epinephrine, 334
Ultracef, cefadroxil, 166
Ultralente Iletin I, insulin, 503
Ultralente Insulin, insulin, 503
Ultralente Purified Beef, insulin, 503
Ultramiclosine Griseofulvin, griseofulvin, 455
Unipres (CD)
　CONTAINS
　hydralazine, 472
　hydrochlorothiazide, 476, 971
　reserpine*
Uridon, chlorthalidone, 205, 971
Uniphyl, theophylline, 966
Unisom Sleepgels, diphenhydramine, 302
Uritol, furosemide, 436
Uro Gantanol (CD)
　CONTAINS
　phenazopyridine*
　sulfamethoxazole, 929
Uroplus DS (CD)
　CONTAINS
　sulfamethoxazole, 929
　trimethoprim, 1020
Uroplus SS (CD)
　CONTAINS
　sulfamethoxazole, 929
　trimethoprim, 1020
Urozide, hydrochlorothiazide, 476, 971
Uticillin VK, penicillin V, 762
Utimox, amoxicillin, 81

Valdrene, diphenhydramine, 302
Valergen-10, estrogens, 346
Valium, diazepam, 284
valproic acid, 1023
Valrelease, diazepam, 284
Vancenase AQ Nasal Spray, beclomethasone, 115
Vancenase Nasal Inhaler, beclomethasone, 115
Vanceril, beclomethasone, 115
Vancocin, vancomycin, 1027
Vancoled, vancomycin, 1027
vancomycin, 1027
Vancor, vancomycin, 1027
Vaponefrin, epinephrine, 334
varicella virus vaccine, 1030
Varivax, varicella virus vaccine, 1030
Vaseretic (CD)
　CONTAINS
　enalapril, 330
　hydrochlorothiazide, 476, 971
Vasocidin, prednisolone, 815
Vasotec, enalapril, 330
Vazepam, diazepam, 284
V-Cillin K, penicillin V, 762

VC-K 500, penicillin V, 762
Veetids, penicillin V, 762
Velosulin, insulin, 503
Velosulin Cartridge, insulin, 503
Velosulin Human, insulin, 503
venlafaxine, 1032
Ventodisk, albuterol, 47
Ventolin Inhaler, albuterol, 47
Ventolin Rotacaps, albuterol, 47
Ventolin syrup, albuterol, 47
Ventolin Tablets, albuterol, 47
verapamil, 1035
Verban (CD)
　CONTAINS
　colchicine, 251
　podophyllin*
Verelan, verapamil, 1035
Verin, aspirin, 91
Viaderm-KC, neostigmine, 682
Vibramycin, doxycycline, 327
Vibra-Tabs, doxycycline, 327
Vibra-Tabs C-Pak, doxycycline, 327
Vick's Formula 44D, ethanol, 354
Vicodin (CD)
　CONTAINS
　acetaminophen*
　hydrocodone, 477
Vicodin ES (CD)
　CONTAINS
　acetaminophen*
　hydrocodone, 477
Videx, didanosine, 288
Viskazide (CD)
　CONTAINS
　hydrochlorothiazide, 476, 971
　pindolol, 801
Visken, pindolol, 801
Vistacrom, cromolyn, 258
vitamin B-3. *See* niacin, 685
Vitaphen, phenobarbital, 787

*The symbol [CD] indicates that the brand name given is a combination drug consisting of generic drug components listed below it. If there is no page numbering following the name of the generic drug component, there is no Drug Profile for that ingredient in this book.

1156 Index

Vivactil, protriptyline, 854
Vivol, diazepam, 284
vodka. *See* ethanol, 354
Volmax controlled release tablets, albuterol, 47
Voltaren, diclofenac, 38
Voltaren Ophthalmic, diclofenac, 38
Voltaren SR, diclofenac, 38
Vytone, iodoquinol, 507

Wal-ben, diphenhydramine, 302
Wal-dryl, diphenhydramine, 302
warfarin, 1040
Wehydryl, diphenhydramine, 302
Wellbutrin, bupropion, 140
Wesprin, aspirin, 91
whiskey. *See* ethanol, 354
white lightning. *See* ethanol, 354
White Premarin, estrogens, 346
Wigraine (CD)
  CONTAINS
    atropine*
    caffeine*
    ergotamine, 338
Wigrettes, ergotamine, 338
wine. *See* ethanol, 354
Winpred, prednisone, 817
Wyamycin E, erythromycin, 342
Wyamycin S, erythromycin, 342
Wymox, amoxicillin, 81

Xanax, alprazolam, 54

Yodoxin, iodoquinol, 507

zalcitabine, 1045
Zantac, ranitidine, 467, 888
Zantac-C, ranitidine, 467, 888
Zarontin, ethosuximide, 360
Zaroxolyn, metolazone, 634, 971
ZDV. *See* zidovudine, 1049
Zenole, indomethacin, 38, 498
Zerit, stavudine, 917
Zestoretic (CD)
  CONTAINS
    hydrochlorothiazide, 476, 971
    lisinopril, 560
Zestril, lisinopril, 560
Zetran, diazepam, 284
Ziac (CD)
  CONTAINS
    bisoprolol*
    hydrochlorothiazide, 476, 971
Zide, hydrochlorothiazide, 476, 971
zidovudine, 1049
Zinacef, cefuroxime, 179
Zithromax, azithromycin, 110
Zocor, simvastatin, 910
Zofran, ondansetron, 729
Zoloft, sertraline, 907
zolpidem, 1052
Zonalon, doxepin, 323
Zorprin, aspirin, 91
Zovia, oral contraceptives, 732
Zovirax, acyclovir, 44
Zurinol, allopurinol, 50
Zydone (CD)
  CONTAINS
    acetaminophen*
    hydrocodone, 477
Zyloprim, allopurinol, 50

About the Authors:

JAMES J. RYBACKI, Pharm. D., was born in Oneonta, New York. He received his prepharmacy education at Creighton University, and his Doctor of Pharmacy degree from The University of Nebraska Medical Center, College of Pharmacy in Omaha. Over twenty-three years of hospital experience have included early efforts in gas-liquid chromatography research characterizing human drug metabolites, and data collection for the College of American Pathologists helping to establish normal values for laboratory studies. He is a member of the clinical faculty at the University of Maryland School of Pharmacy and has provided clinical rounding and hospital experience for Pharm. D. and Bachelor students at Dorchester General Hospital. He is Board Certified in Pain Management at the Diplomat level by the American Academy of Pain Management, and provides ongoing pain management consulting. Dr. Rybacki is actively involved in the postmarketing monitoring of medicines via The Drug Surveillance Network, a nationwide association of clinical pharmacists, and he is an approved External New Drug Application reviewer for the Canadian Drug Ministry. He lives in Easton, Maryland.

Dr. Rybacki's efforts in drug information and clinical pharmacy include eight years of active practice which were provided at Dorchester General Hospital in Cambridge, Maryland including infectious disease, pharmacokinetic, nutrition support, pain management and pharmacologic consultations at Dorchester General Hospital. Through the Occupational Health Unit, he has offered independent pain management and pharmacologic consultations nationwide. He has advised the World Health Organization's Expert Committee regarding revisions as well as selection of drugs to be listed in the next edition of *The Use of Essential Drugs* and is an assistant editor for the Drugdex drug information system. His past role as Vice President Clinical Services has bought him added expertise in overseeing Occupational Health, Physical Medicines, Laboratory Services, Imaging, Cardiology, Respiratory Therapy, Cancer Programs and Continuing Medical Education. He has served as conference coordinator for the first and second annual Dorchester General Hospital Pain conferences, and served as seminar coordinator for the Eastern Shore of Maryland for the "Take Control" physician and public pain education programs with Johns Hopkins.

Dr. Rybacki is president of The Clearwater Group, and provides seminars on medical cost containment, infectious disease, pain management and therapeutics, drug information support to employers, insurance companies, HMOs, the legal profession, educational tapes on medicines and independent pharmacological evaluations. He was recently selected for full membership in the American College of Clinical Pharmacy, is a member of the steering committee of the Society For Clinical Densitometry and is a board certified Forensic Examiner. He is a lifetime member of Who's Who in Global Business.

Dr. Rybacki has been a guest and guest host on numerous radio and television shows, and participates in numerous medical speakers bureaus including Miles, Dupont Pharma, and Glaxo. He has been selected for the Lederle and Bristol Myers Distinguished Speakers in Medicine faculty. He has published numerous articles in professional journals on use of medicines in critical care, therapeutics and cost containment. The 1994 and 1995 editions of *The Essential Guide to Prescription Drugs* were co-authored by Dr. Rybacki. He produces and hosts "The Medicine Man", a nationally syndicated live radio show as well as provides updates and news in medicine via The Medicine Man Minute on the Health Radio Network. Dr. Rybacki believes that the new art of prescribing medicines lies in cost containment without sacrifice of clinical outcomes.

JAMES W. LONG, M.D., was born in Allentown, Pennsylvania. He received his premedical education from the University of Maryland and his medical degree from the George Washington University School of Medicine in Washington, D.C. For twenty years he was in the private practice of internal medicine in the Washington metropolitan area, and for over thirty-five years he was a member of the faculty of the George Washington University School of Medicine. He has served with the Food and Drug Administration, the National Library of Medicine, and the Bureau of Health Manpower of the National Institutes of Health. Prior to his retirement, Dr. Long was director of Health Services for the National Science Foundation in Washington. He lives in Oxford, Maryland.

Controlled Drug Schedules

Schedule I: These medicines are those with a high abuse and dependence potential. Typically, the only use for these substances are for research purposes. Examples include LSD and heroin. A prescription cannot be legally written for these drugs for medicinal use.

Schedule II: These medicines have therapeutic uses and have the highest abuse and dependence potential for drugs with medicinal purposes. Examples include analgesics such as morphine (MS Contin) and meperidine (Demerol). A written prescription is required and refills are **not** allowed.

Schedule III: Medicines in this schedule have an abuse and dependence potential that is less than those in schedule II, but greater than those in schedule IV. These medicines have clear medicinal uses and include such medicines as hydrocodone, codeine and paregoric in combination. Common names include: Tylenol number three with codeine and Tenuate. A telephone prescription is permitted for medications in this class, however, it must be converted to a written form by a pharmacist. Prescriptions for these medicines may be refilled, but only five times in six months.

Schedule IV: This schedule contains medicines with less abuse and dependence potential than those in schedule III. Examples of medicines in this schedule include propoxyphene (Darvon), diazepam (Valium) and chlordiazepoxide or (Librium). Prescriptions for these medicines may be refilled, but only five times in six months.

Schedule V: These medicines have the lowest abuse and dependence potential. Medicines in this class include diphenoxylate (Lomotil) and loperamide (Imodium). Drugs in this class which require a prescription are handled the same as any nonscheduled prescription medicine. Some drugs in this class do not require a prescription, and can be sold only with the approval of a pharmacist. The buyer is required to sign a log book when the drug is dispensed. Examples include codeine and hydrocodone in combination with other active, nonnarcotic drugs sold in preparations that have limited quantities of codeine or hydrocodone for control of diarrhea or cough.

Pregnancy Risk Categories

Definitions of FDA Pregnancy Categories

Category A: Adequate and well-controlled studies in pregnant women are **negative** for fetal abnormalities. Risk to the fetus is remote.

Category B: Animal reproduction studies are **negative** for fetal abnormalities. Data from adequate and well-controlled studies in pregnant women are not available.

OR

Animal reproduction studies are **positive** for fetal abnormalities. Adequate and well-controlled studies in pregnant women are **negative** for fetal abnormalities. Risk to the fetus is relatively unlikely.

Category C: Animal reproduction studies are **positive** for fetal abnormalities. Information from adequate and well-controlled studies in pregnant women is not available.

OR

Information from animal reproduction studies **and** from adequate and well-controlled studies in pregnant women is not available. Benefits of the drug may justify potential risks to the fetus.

Category D: Studies in pregnant women and/or premarketing (investigational) or postmarketing uses show **positive** evidence of human fetal risk. The drug is only used in serious disease or in life-threatening situations where safer medicines will not work or cannot be used.

Category X: Animal reproduction studies and/or human pregnancy studies are **positive** for fetal abnormalities.

OR

Studies in pregnant women and/or premarketing (investigational) or postmarketing (phase four) experience shows **positive** evidence of human fetal risk.

AND

Potential fetal risks outweigh possible benefits of the drug. These medicines **should never** be used in pregnancy.

The FDA is currently evaluating these pregnancy categories, and may opt to modify them.